Merenstein & Gardner's *Handbook of*

Neonatal Intensive Care

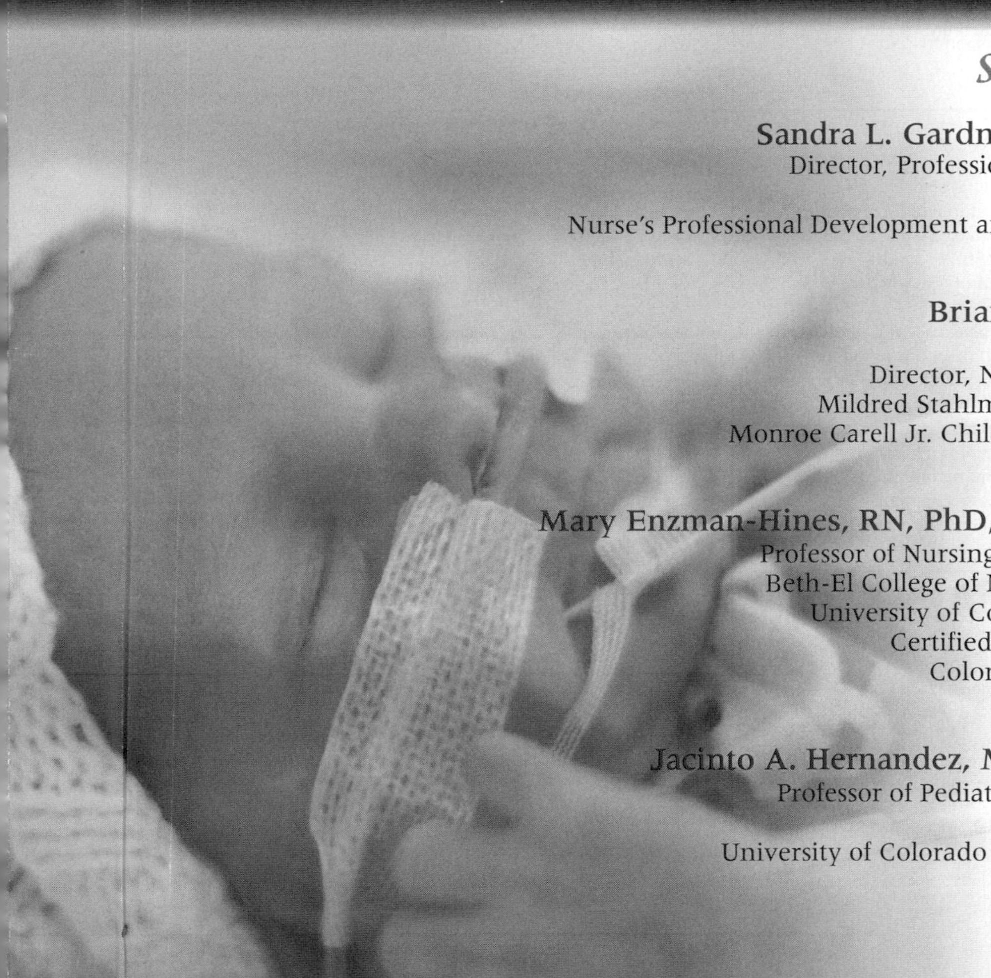

seventh edition

Sandra L. Gardner, RN, MS, CNS, PNP
Director, Professional Outreach Consultation;
Co-Director,
Nurse's Professional Development and Practice Association, LLC
Aurora, Colorado

Brian S. Carter, MD, FAAP
Professor of Pediatrics
Director, Neonatal Follow-up Program
Mildred Stahlman Division of Neonatology
Monroe Carell Jr. Children's Hospital at Vanderbilt
Nashville, Tennessee

Mary Enzman-Hines, RN, PhD, CNS, CPNP, AHN-BC
Professor of Nursing, DNP Program Coordinator
Beth-El College of Nursing and Health Sciences
University of Colorado at Colorado Springs;
Certified Pediatric Nurse Practitioner
Colorado Springs Health Partners
Colorado Springs, Colorado

Jacinto A. Hernandez, MD, PhD, MHA, FAAP
Professor of Pediatrics, Section of Neonatology
Department of Pediatrics
University of Colorado Denver School of Medicine;
Chairman Emeritus
Department of Neonatology
The Children's Hospital
Aurora, Colorado

MOSBY
ELSEVIER

MOSBY
ELSEVIER

3251 Riverport Lane
St. Louis, Missouri 63043

MERENSTEIN & GARDNER'S HANDBOOK OF NEONATAL CARE ISBN: 978-0-323-06715-7

Notices

Knowledge and best practice in this field are constantly changing. As new research and experience broaden our understanding, changes in research methods, professional practices, or medical treatment may become necessary.

Practitioners and researchers must always rely on their own experience and knowledge in evaluating and using any information, methods, compounds, or experiments described herein. In using such information or methods they should be mindful of their own safety and the safety of others, including parties for whom they have a professional responsibility.

With respect to any drug or pharmaceutical products identified, readers are advised to check the most current information provided (i) on procedures featured or (ii) by the manufacturer of each product to be administered, to verify the recommended dose or formula, the method and duration of administration, and contraindications. It is the responsibility of practitioners, relying on their own experience and knowledge of their patients, to make diagnoses, to determine dosages and the best treatment for each individual patient, and to take all appropriate safety precautions.

To the fullest extent of the law, neither the Publisher nor the authors, contributors, or editors assume any liability for any injury and/or damage to persons or property as a matter of products liability, negligence or otherwise, or from any use or operation of any methods, products, instructions, or ideas contained in the material herein.

Library of Congress Cataloging-in-Publication Data

Merenstein & Gardner's handbook of neonatal intensive care / [edited by] Sandra L. Gardner ... [et al.].—7th ed.
p. ; cm.
Rev. ed. of: Handbook of neonatal intensive care / [edited by] Gerald B. Merenstein, Sandra L. Gardner. 6th ed. c2006.
Includes bibliographical references and index.
ISBN 978-0-323-06715-7 (pbk. : alk. paper) 1. Neonatal intensive care—Handbooks, manuals, etc. 2. Pediatric nursing—Handbooks, manuals, etc. I. Merenstein, Gerald B. II. Gardner, Sandra L. III. Handbook of neonatal intensive care. IV. Title: Merenstein and Gardner's handbook of neonatal intensive care.
[DNLM: 1. Intensive Care, Neonatal. 2. Infant, Newborn, Diseases—therapy. WS 421 M559 2011]
RJ253.5.H36 2011
618.92′01—dc22

2009053732

Managing Editor: Maureen Iannuzzi
Developmental Editor: Laurie Sparks
Publishing Services Manager: Deborah L. Vogel
Senior Project Manager: Jodi M. Willard
Design Direction: Jessica Williams

Printed in the United States of America

Last digit is the print number: 9 8 7 6 5 4 3

We dedicate this edition to the memory of Gerald B. Merenstein, MD—our friend, colleague, and mentor who was also a wonderful husband, father, and grandfather. As the inspiration for this text, Gerry contributed to the fields of neonatal and pediatric care through his dedication to nurses, nurse practitioners, child health associates, interns, residents, fellows, neonates, and their families. We miss him every day and know that his empathy, knowledge, teaching, and compassion influences all of us, as well as the newborns, children, and families that he and we serve.

SLG BSC MEH JAH

In memory of Stephanie Marie Gardner, whose three days of life did have a purpose.

SLG

To my family: Angel, Sean, Yvonne, Rebecca, and Jacquelyn; colleagues; and all the children and families who have allowed me to journey with them through both joyous and difficult times in their lives.

BSC

To my husband, Jim Hines, and to my children, Jennifer and Steve Hagedorn, for their enduring source of love, confidence, and encouragement; and to all the families who have informed my practice and knowledge about caring for fragile infants.

MEH

To the Newborn Infant; my wife, Pam; and beloved sons, Gabriel and Jacinto.

JAH

In Memoriam

Jimmie Lynne Scholl Avery

L. Joseph Butterfield, MD

Lula O. Lubchenco, MD

William A. Silverman, MD

CONTRIBUTORS

Karen M. Adams, RN, BSN
School Nurse
Houston Independent School District
Houston, Texas

Marianne Sollosy Anderson, MD
Assistant Clinical Professor, Department of Pediatrics
Division of Neonatology and Developmental Biology
David Geffen School of Medicine at University of California–Los Angeles
Los Angeles, California

Jaime Arruda, MD
Assistant Professor
University of Colorado Denver School of Medicine
Denver, Colorado

Wanda Todd Bradshaw, RN, MSN, NNP-BC, PNP, CCRN
Assistant Clinical Professor
NNP Specialty Director
Duke University School of Nursing;
Neonatal Nurse Practitioner
Duke Health System
Durham, North Carolina

Vivian D. Brown, RNC
Staff Nurse
Seton Medical Center—Williamson
Round Rock, Texas;
Co-Director, Nurse's Professional Development and Practice Association, LLC
Round Rock, Texas

Deanne Buschbach, RN, MSN, NNP, PNP
NNP Coordinator and Lactation Consultant Team Leader
Duke University Medical Center;
Clinical Associate
Duke University School of Nursing
Durham, North Carolina

Angel Carter, RN, MSN, NNP-BC
Coordinator, Neonatal Follow-Up Clinic
Monroe Carell Jr. Children's Hospital at Vanderbilt
Nashville, Tennessee

Brian S. Carter, MD, FAAP
Professor of Pediatrics
Director, Neonatal Follow-up Program
Mildred Stahlman Division of Neonatology
Monroe Carell Jr. Children's Hospital at Vanderbilt
Nashville, Tennessee

Susan B. Clarke, MS, RNC-NIC, CPN
Clinical Nurse Specialist
Outreach & Continuing Education
The Children's Hospital;
Clinical Senior Instructor
University of Colorado Denver College of Nursing
Aurora, Colorado

C. Michael Cotten, MD, MHS
Associate Professor of Pediatrics
Department of Neonatology
Duke University Medical Center
Durham, North Carolina

Donna K. Daily, MD, MA
Associate Professor of Pediatrics
Director, NICU Developmental Follow-Up Clinic
Monroe Carell Jr. Children's Hospital at Vanderbilt
Nashville, Tennessee

Lorraine A. Dickey, MD, MBA, FAAP
Chief, Division of Neonatology
Medical Director, Forrest C. Moyer NICU
Lehigh Valley Health Network
Allentown, Pennsylvania

David J. Durand, MD
Director, Department of Neonatology
Children's Hospital & Research Center
Oakland, California

Nancy English, PhD, RN
Fetal Concerns, Director and Coordinator
Colorado High-Risk Maternity and Newborn Program
University of Colorado Health Sciences Center
The Children's Hospital
Aurora, Colorado

Mary Enzman-Hines, RN, PhD, CNS, CPNP, AHN-BC
Professor of Nursing, DNP Program Coordinator
Beth-El College of Nursing and Health Sciences
University of Colorado at Colorado Springs;
Certified Pediatric Nurse Practitioner
Colorado Springs Health Partners
Colorado Springs, Colorado

Lucy Fashaw, RNC, BSN
Professional Research Assistant
Pediatric Clinical Translational Research Center
University of Colorado Denver Health Sciences Center
The Children's Hospital
Aurora, Colorado

Loretta P. Finnegan, MD
President, Finnegan Consulting, LLC
Perinatal Addiction and Women's Health
Avalon, New Jersey;
Founder and Former Director of Family Center
Jefferson Medical College of Thomas Jefferson University
Philadelphia, Pennsylvania

Mackenzie S. Frost, MD
Assistant Professor of Pediatrics
Saint Christopher's Hospital for Children
Philadelphia, Pennsylvania

Sandra L. Gardner, RN, MS, CNS, PNP
Director, Professional Outreach Consultation;
Co-Director, Nurse's Professional Development and Practice Association, LLC
Aurora, Colorado

Joshua Brian Glenn, MD
Chief Pediatric Surgical Resident
Monroe Carell Jr. Children's Hospital at Vanderbilt
Nashville, Tennessee

Anita Duhl Glicken, MSW
Professor and Section Head, Pediatrics,
Director, Child Health Associate/Physician Assistant Program
University of Colorado Denver School of Medicine
Denver, Colorado

Edward Goldson, MD
Professor, Department of Pediatrics
University of Colorado Denver School of Medicine
The Children's Hospital
Aurora, Colorado

Marie Hastings-Tolsma, PhD, CNM
Associate Professor, Nurse Midwifery
University of Colorado Denver College of Nursing
Aurora, Colorado

William W. Hay, Jr., MD
Professor of Pediatrics
Co-Director (Child and Maternal Health Program) Colorado Clinical Translational Science Institute;
Scientific Director, Perinatal Research Center
University of Colorado Health Sciences Center
Perinatal Research Center
Aurora, Colorado

Ray D. Hayes, DO
Neonatal-Perinatal Medicine Fellow
Wake Forest University Baptist Medical Center
Winston-Salem, North Carolina

Taru Hays, MD
Professor of Pediatrics
Director of Clinical Hematology
University of Colorado at Denver Health Sciences Center
The Children's Hospital
Aurora, Colorado

Jacinto A. Hernandez, MD, PhD, MHA, FAAP
Professor of Pediatrics, Section of Neonatology
Department of Pediatrics
University of Colorado Denver School of Medicine;
Chairman Emeritus
Department of Neonatology
The Children's Hospital
Aurora, Colorado

Deandra Hoover, APRN, MSN, PNP-BC, NNP-BC
Certified Pediatric Nurse Practitioner
Certified Neonatal Nurse Practitioner
Neonatal Intensive Care Unit
Palmetto Health Richland
Columbia, South Carolina

Victor Iskersky, MD, FAAP
Associate Professor of Pediatrics
Assistant Professor of Obstetrics and Gynecology
University of South Carolina School of Medicine;
Chief of Neonatology and Medical Director of the NICU
Palmetto Health Richland
Columbia, South Carolina

Juley C. Jenkins, BA, BS
Clinical Coordinator, Radiology
University of Colorado Denver Health Sciences Center
The Children's Hospital
Aurora, Colorado

James E. Jones, DO
Neonatology Fellow
Wake Forest University Baptist Medical Center
Brenner Children's Hospital, Neonatal Intensive Care Nursery
Forsyth Medical Center, Neonatal Intensive Care Nursery
Winston-Salem, North Carolina

M. Douglas Jones, Jr., MD
Professor
Department of Pediatrics, Section of Neonatology
University of Colorado Denver School of Medicine
Aurora, Colorado

Beena D. Kamath, MD, MPH
Assistant Professor of Pediatrics
Cincinnati Children's Hospital Medical Center
Cincinnati, Ohio

Jacqueline A. Keller, MS, RD, CSP
NICU Clinical Dietitian Specialist
The Children's Hospital
Aurora, Colorado

Patricia M. Kenney, MN, APRN, FNP-BC
Level III Neonatal Intensive Care Unit
Palmetto Health Richland
Columbia, South Carolina

Howard W. Kilbride, MD
Professor of Pediatrics
University of Missouri—Kansas City;
Chief, Section of Neonatal Medicine
Children's Mercy Hospitals and Clinics
Kansas City, Missouri

Susan Landers, MD, FAAP, FABM
Neonatologist, Pediatrix Medical Group
Seton Medical Center and Dell Children's Medical Center of Central Texas
Austin, Texas

Ruth A. Lawrence, MD, DD, FABM
Professor of Pediatrics and Obstetrics/Gynecology
Director of Breastfeeding and Human Lactation Study Center
University of Rochester Medical Center
Galisano Children's Hospital
Rochester, New York

Mary Kay Leick-Rude, RNC, MSN, PCNS
Clinical Nurse Specialist
Children's Mercy Hospitals and Clinics
Kansas City, Missouri

Suzanne M. Lopez, MD, FAAP
Associate Professor of Pediatrics
Medical Director, UT NNP/PA
Director, Neonatal-Perinatal Medicine Fellowship Program
University of Texas Health Sciences Center–Houston
Houston, Texas

Harold N. Lovvorn III, MD, FACS, FAAP
Assistant Professor of Pediatric Surgery
Monroe Carell Jr. Children's Hospital at Vanderbilt
Nashville, Tennessee

Carolyn Houska Lund, RN, MS, FAAN
Neonatal Clinical Nurse Specialist
ECMO Coordinator
Intensive Care Nursery
Children's Hospital & Research Center Oakland
Oakland, CA;
Associate Clinical Professor
Department of Family Health Care Nursing
University of California
San Francisco, California

Marilyn Manco-Johnson, MD
Professor of Pediatrics
Hemophilia and Thrombosis Center
University of Colorado Denver School of Medicine and The Children's Hospital
Aurora, Colorado

Anne Matthews, RN, PhD, FACMG
Associate Professor of Genetics
Director, Genetic Counseling Training Program
Department of Genetics
Case Western Reserve University
Cleveland, Ohio

Jane E. McGowan, MD
Professor of Pediatrics
Drexel University College of Medicine;
Medical Director, NICU
St. Christopher's Hospital for Children
Philadelphia, Pennsylvania

Mary Miller-Bell, Pharm D
Clinical Pharmacist
Duke University Hospital;
Clinical Associate Professor
Duke University School of Nursing
Duke University Medical Center
Durham, North Carolina

Susan Niermeyer, MD, MPH, FAAP
Professor of Pediatrics
University of Colorado Denver School of Medicine
The Children's Hospital
Aurora, Colorado

Priscilla M. Nodine, RN, CNM, PhD(c)
Instructor, OB/GYN Department
University of Colorado Denver School of Medicine
Aurora, Colorado

Steven L. Olsen, MD
Neonatologist
Section of Neonatology
Children's Mercy Hospital
Kansas City, Missouri

Annette S. Pacetti, RNC, MSN, NNP-BC
Neonatal Nurse Practitioner
Monroe Carell Jr. Children's Hospital at Vanderbilt
Nashville, Tennessee

Peter J. Porcelli, MD
Associate Professor of Pediatrics (Neonatology)
Department of Pediatrics
Wake Forest University Baptist Medical Center
Winston-Salem, North Carolina

Webra Price-Douglas, RN, PhD, CRNP, IBCLC
Coordinator, Maryland Regional Neonatal Transport Program
Johns Hopkins Hospital and University of Maryland Medical Center
Baltimore, Maryland

Nathaniel H. Robin, MD, FACMG
Professor of Genetics and Pediatrics
University of Alabama at Birmingham
Birmingham, Alabama

Donna J. Rodden, RN, BSN
Nurse Manager, Perinatal Clinical Translational Research Center
The Children's Hospital/University of Colorado Denver Health Sciences Center
Aurora, Colorado

Mario A. Rojas, MD, MPH
Associate Professor of Pediatrics
Director, Patient-Oriented Research
Mildred Stahlman Division of Neonatology
Monroe Carell Jr. Children's Hospital at Vanderbilt
Nashville, Tennessee

Paul J. Rozance, MD
Assistant Professor of Pediatrics, Neonatal Medicine
University of Colorado Health Sciences Center
Aurora, Colorado

Margaret G. Rush, MD, FAAP
Chief of Staff
Program Director, Neonatal-Perinatal Medicine
Medical Director, Neonatal Transport
Monroe Carell Jr. Children's Hospital at Vanderbilt
Vanderbilt Medical Center
Nashville, Tennessee

Kelly Shirley, RN, APRN, MSN
Neonatal Nurse Practitioner Coordinator
Monroe Carell Jr. Children's Hospital at Vanderbilt
Vanderbilt Medical Center
Nashville, Tennessee

Roberta Siegel, MSW
Assistant to the Chair
Department of Pediatrics
University of Colorado Denver School of Medicine
The Children's Hospital
Aurora, Colorado

Alisa L. Starbuck, MSN, RN, NNP-BC
Director, Pediatric Critical Care
Brenner Children's Hospital
Winston-Salem, North Carolina

Jill Stiens, MS, RD, LD, CNSC
Clinical Nutrition Specialist, Neonatology
Children's Mercy Hospital and Clinics
Kansas City, Missouri

John D. Strain, MD, FACR, CAQ
Clinical Professor in Radiology
Chairman, Department of Radiology
University of Colorado Denver Health Sciences Center
The Children's Hospital
Aurora, Colorado

Julie R. Swaney, MDiv
Manager, Spiritual Care Services
Associate Clinical Professor
University of Colorado Denver School of Medicine
Aurora, Colorado

David T. Tanaka, MD
Professor of Pediatrics
Duke University;
Neonatologist
Duke University Medical Center
Durham, North Carolina

Elizabeth H. Thilo, MD
Associate Professor of Pediatrics, Section of Neonatology
University of Colorado Denver School of Medicine;
Neonatologist, University of Colorado Hospital and The Children's Hospital
Aurora, Colorado

Mohan P. Venkatesh, MD
Assistant Professor Department of Pediatrics, Section of Neonatology
Baylor College of Medicine and Texas Children's Hospital
Houston, Texas

M. Terese Verklan, PhD, CCNS, RNC
Associate Professor/Neonatal Clinical Nurse Specialist
The University of Texas Health Science Center at Houston
School of Nursing, Department of Systems and Technology
Houston, Texas

Susan M. Weiner, PhD(c), MSN, RNC-OB, CNS
Research Nurse Coordinator II
Adjunct Faculty, School of Nursing
Thomas Jefferson University
Philadelphia, Pennsylvania

Leonard E. Weisman, MD
Professor of Pediatrics
Baylor College of Medicine;
Director, Perinatal Center
Texas Children's Hospital
Houston, Texas

Luther C. Williams, MD
Professor of Clinical Pediatrics
Division of Pediatric Cardiology
University of South Carolina School of Medicine
Columbia, South Carolina

Linda Lee Wood, RN, BSN, CCRN, IBCLC
Clinical Nurse IV, Newborn Intensive Care Unit
The Children's Hospital/University of Colorado Denver
Aurora, Colorado

Amy M. Wood, MD
Instructor, Department of Pediatrics, Division of Neonatology
University of Colorado Denver School of Medicine
Aurora, Colorado

REVIEWERS

Debbie Fraser Askin, MN, RNC-NIC
St. Boniface General Hospital and Centre for Nursing and Health Studies
Athabasca University
Winnipeg, Manitoba, Canada

Bobby Bellflower, DNSc, NNP-BC
Assistant Professor/Option Coordinator, NNP Program
University of Tennessee Health Science Center;
Neonatal Nurse Practitioner
LeBonheur Children's Medical Center
Memphis, Tennessee

Catherine M. Bendel, MD, FAAP
Perinatal Section, Associate Professor of Pediatrics
University of Minnesota Medical School
Minneapolis, Minnesota

Carol Turnage Carrier, MSN, RN, CNS
Clinical Nurse Specialist
Texas Children's Hospital;
Newborn Center and Clinical Instructor
University of Texas Health Science Center, School of Nursing
Houston, Texas

Robert Castro, MD
Clinical Professor of Pediatrics
Stanford University School of Medicine
Palo Alto, California

Diane Dale, RNC, MN
NICU/PICU Clinical Nurse Specialist
Providence Tarzana Medical Center
Tarzana, California;
Instructor
University of Phoenix
Southern California Campus
Woodland Hills, California

Karen C. D'Apolito, RN, PhD, APRN, NNP
Program Director
Neonatal Nurse Practitioner Program
Vanderbilt University School of Nursing
Nashville, Tennessee

Melissa Marie Dunham, RN, NNP-BC
Neonatal Nurse Practitioner
The Medical University of South Carolina
Charleston, South Carolina

Manuel Durand, MD
Professor of Pediatrics
University of Southern California
Keck School of Medicine of USC
Los Angeles County–USC Medical Center
Los Angeles, California

Veronica M. Guilfoy, MD
Assistant Professor of Pediatrics
Indiana University School of Medicine
Department of Pediatrics, Section of Neonatology
Indianapolis, Indiana

Noah Hillman, MD
Assistant Professor
Division of Pulmonary Biology/Neonatology
Cincinnati Children's Hospital
Cincinnati, Ohio

Nadine A. Kassity-Krich, RN, MBA
NRP Regional Trainer
Public Health Certificate
Health Care Consultant
San Diego, California

Andrea M. Kline, RN, MS, CPNP-AC/PC, CCRN, FCCM
Pediatric Nurse Practitioner
Children's Memorial Hospital
Chicago, Illinois

Jane S. Lee, MD, MPH
Assistant Professor of Pediatrics
Columbia University College of Physicians & Surgeons;
Attending Neonatologist
Children's Hospital of New York-Presbyterian
New York, New York

Carie Linder, RNC, BSN, ARNP
Advanced Registered Nurse Practitioner
Wesley Medical Center
Wichita, Kansas;
Registered Nurse, Certified
Integris Baptist Medical Center
Oklahoma City, Oklahoma

Mindy Morris
Neonatal Nurse Practitioner
Children's Hospital of Orange County
Orange, California

Suhas Madhukar Nafday, MD, MRCP (IRE), FAAP
Director of Newborn Services
Director, Neonatal Hypothermia Program
Children's Hospital at Montefiore Medical Center
Albert Einstein College of Medicine
Bronx, New York

Steven L. Olsen, MD
Neonatologist
Section of Neonatology
Children's Mercy Hospital
Kansas City, Missouri

Melissa Otoya, RNC, BSN
RN, Clinician III, Neonatal Intensive Care Unit
University of Virginia Health System
Charlottesville, Virginia

Leslie A. Parker, PhD(c), NNP-BC
Neonatal Nurse Practitioner
Clinical Assistant Professor
University of Florida—College of Nursing and College of Medicine
Gainesville, Florida

Sharyl L. Sadowski, MS, APN, NNP-BC
Certified Neonatal Nurse Practitioner
Neonatal Outreach Educator
University of Illinois at Chicago
Chicago, Illinois

Patricia Scheans, MS, NNP-BC
Clinical Support for Neonatal Care
Legacy Health
Portland, Oregon

Elizabeth Sharpe, ARNP, MSN, NNP-BC
Pediatric Medical Group
West Palm Beach, Florida

Caroline L. Steele, MS, RD, CSP, IBCLC
Clinical Nutrition Manager
Children's Hospital of Orange County
Orange, California

Bonnie E. Stephens, MD
Neonatologist
Developmental and Behavioral Pediatrician
Assistant Professor of Pediatrics
Warren Alpert Medical School
Brown University
Providence, Rhode Island

Mollie Frances Tripp, RN, MSN, NNP-BC
Clinical Instructor
East Carolina University College of Nursing;
Neonatal Nurse Practitioner Program
Children's Hospital of Eastern Carolina;
Clinical Instructor
Neonatal Nurse Practitioner Program
Children's Hospital of Eastern Carolina
East Carolina University College of Nursing
Greenville, North Carolina

M. Terese Verklan, PhD, CCNS, RNC
Associate Professor/Neonatal Clinical Nurse Specialist
The University of Texas Health Science Center at Houston
Houston, Texas

Robin L. Watson, MN, CCRN
Clinical Nurse Specialist
Harbor-UCLA Medical Center
Torrance, California

PREFACE

The concept of the team approach is important in neonatal intensive care. Each health care professional must not only perform the duties of his or her own role but must also understand the roles of other involved professionals. Nurses, physicians, other health care providers, and parents must work together in a coordinated and efficient manner to achieve optimal results for patients in the neonatal intensive care unit (NICU).

Because this team approach is so important in the field of neonatal intensive care, we believe it is necessary that this book contain input from major fields of health care—nursing and medicine. Both nurses and physicians have edited and co-authored every chapter.

The book is divided into six units, all of which have been reviewed, revised, and updated for the seventh edition. Unit One presents evidence-based practice and the need to scientifically evaluate neonatal therapies, emphasizing randomized controlled trials as the ideal approach. Units Two through Five are the clinical sections, which have been fully updated for this edition. The chapters within these sections include highlighted clinical directions for quick reference, Parent Teaching boxes to aid in discharge instructions, and Critical Findings boxes to prioritize assessment data.

The combination of physiology and pathophysiology and separate emphasis on clinical application in this text is designed for neonatal intensive care nurses, nursing students, medical students, and pediatric, surgical and family practice housestaff. This text is comprehensive enough for nurses and physicians, yet basic enough to be useful to families and all ancillary personnel.

Unit Six presents the psychosocial aspects of neonatal care. The medical, psychological and social aspects of providing care for the ill neonate and family are discussed in this section. This section in particular will benefit social workers and clergy, who often deal with family members of neonates in the NICU.

In this handbook we present physiologic principles and practical applications and point out areas as yet unresolved. **Material that is clinically applicable is set in purple type so that it can be easily identified.**

INTRODUCTION

In 1974 as the Perinatal Outreach Educator at The Children's Hospital in Denver, Colorado, I took a folder to Gerry Merenstein, MD, at Fitzsimmons Army Medical Center to discuss his lectures for the first outreach education program in La Junta, Colorado. When we finished, he removed from his desk drawer a 1-inch thick compilation of the neonatal data, graphs, nomograms, and diagrams he had created for the medical housestaff during his fellowship. Giving the document to me, he asked that I review it and let him know what I thought. Several weeks later, I told him it was good *except* there was no nursing care or input, which is essential in every NICU. So Gerry asked, "Want to write a book?"—and the idea for the *Handbook* was born!

With this seventh edition in 2010, we celebrate 25 years of publication of the *Handbook of Neonatal Intensive Care*. Gerry and I co-edited this book for 21 years until his death in December 2007. To fulfill my promise that Gerry's name would always be on the book, this seventh edition and all subsequent editions will be known as *Merenstein & Gardner's Handbook of Neonatal Intensive Care.* Instead of editing this edition alone or with another physician, I decided to convene an editorial team consisting of myself, a nurse colleague, and two neonatologists. Together we bring 150 years of clinical practice, research, teaching, writing, and consulting in neonatal, pediatric, and family care to this seventh edition. This is my opportunity to introduce you to the new co-editors.

Mary Enzman-Hines, RN, PhD, CNS, CPNP, AHN-BC, is currently Professor and Graduate Department Chair of Nursing and Program Coordinator of the Doctorate in Nursing Practice at Beth-El College of Nursing and Health Sciences at the University of Colorado in Colorado Springs. Early in her nursing career, Mary worked in the NICU and PICU as a staff nurse, charge nurse, and head nurse. After completing her PNP program and her master's degree, Mary became the Neonatal and Pediatric Clinical Nurse Specialist at Denver Health and Hospital where she created a beginning, intermediate, and advanced orientation for nurses in the NICU and PICU. At the University of Colorado, Mary accepted the practitioner/teacher role in maternal-child services, overseeing clinical practice in the NICU and pediatric units where nursing students were placed from the nursing program. When University Hospital and The Children's Hospital combined their pediatric services, Mary became the Clinical Nurse Specialist in Research and Education, where she consulted in the NICU, PICU, and pediatric medical-surgical areas. In this role she was a founding member of the interdisciplinary Pain Management Team and provided consultation throughout The Children's Hospital for pain management issues. In 1996 Mary became a nursing faculty member at Beth-El College of Nursing and Health Sciences, where she created a student health center and a school-based clinic for schoolchildren in the community and where she maintains a pediatric practice at Colorado Springs Health Partners. Mary is well published in the areas of pediatric, neonatal, and family health care, as well as in legal issues in maternal-child nursing. Mary is also a nurse researcher in the areas of pain, chronic illness, holistic nursing, and technology in health care.

Brian S. Carter, MD, FAAP, is a graduate of David Lipscomb College in Nashville, Tennessee, and of the University of Tennessee's College of Medicine in Memphis, Tennessee. Brian completed his residency in pediatrics at Fitzsimmons Army Medical Center in Aurora, Colorado. He completed his fellowship in neonatal-perinatal medicine at the University of Colorado Health Sciences Center in Denver. During the "Baby Doe" era, Brain trained in bioethics and, in addition to clinical neonatology and neonatal follow-up, he has dedicated most of his academic career to the advancement of clinical ethics in neonatology and pediatric palliative care. Brian has been recognized nationally for his efforts in both of these fields. Currently he is Professor of Pediatrics in the Mildred Stahlman Division of Neonatology at Vanderbilt University Medical Center, where he serves on the Ethics Committee and mentors students, residents, and fellows in the areas of clinical ethics, neonatology, pain management, and palliative care. Brian, Marcia Levetown, MD, and Sarah Friebert, MD, co-edit the book *Palliative Care for Infants, Children, and Adolescents: A Practical Handbook,* whose second edition will be published in 2010 by Johns Hopkins University Press.

Jacinto A. Hernandez, MD, PhD, MHA, FAAP, is a graduate of the School of Medicine of the University of San Marcos in Lima, Peru. Jacinto's postgraduate education includes a specialty in pediatrics and a subspecialty in neonatology at the Children's Hospital National Medical Center and George Washington University in Washington, DC, and at the University of Colorado Denver School of Medicine; a PhD at the University of San Marcos; and a Master's in Health Administration at the University of Colorado Denver School of Business. Jacinto has spent all of his professional life in academic medicine, first at the University of San Marcos as Associate Professor of Pediatrics, and subsequently at the University of Colorado Denver School of Medicine as Professor of Pediatrics. As a physician and professor, Jacinto's activities have been carried out at The Children's Hospital of Denver in Aurora, Colorado, where he has been Director of the Newborn Intensive Care Unit, Chairman of the Department of Neonatology, an active staff neonatologist, and president of the medical staff. Jacinto has distinguished himself both clinically and academically, has written numerous publications in the field of neonatal medicine, and has participated as an invited professor at innumerable international events. Jacinto has been recognized with numerous awards for his scientific achievements, professional qualities, and fruitful work as a superb clinical physician.

Borrowing from the words of Brian Carter in the introduction to the sixth edition of the *Handbook:*

> *The goals of care should be patient- and family-centered. It is the patient we treat, but it is the family, of whatever construct, with whom the baby will go home. Indeed, it is the family who must live with the long-term consequences of our daily decisions in caring for their baby.*

These goals include the provision of skilled professional care. An effective neonatal intensive care team consists of educated professionals of many disciplines—none of us can do it alone.

It has been my honor and privilege to work with these co-editors, who are all patient- and family-centered, and with the amazing editing team of Laurie Sparks and Jodi Willard for this seventh edition.

Sandra L. Gardner, RN, MS, CNS, PNP
Senior Editor

CONTENTS

1 EVIDENCE-BASED CLINICAL PRACTICE

ANITA DUHL GLICKEN, M. DOUGLAS JONES, JR., AND MARY ENZMAN-HINES

Spectacular therapeutic disasters have made it clear that informal let's-try-it-and-see methods of testing new proposals are risky, now more than ever. Because there are no certainties in medicine and nursing, every clinical test of a new treatment is, by definition, a step into the unknown. Silverman described how painfully slow health care providers were to embrace a culture of skepticism. The use of experimentation and the scientific method has ultimately led to our present views of how to ask and answer clinical questions.[41] Mistakes have also occurred at the other extreme, as well, resulting in a failure to adopt therapies that are of proven benefit or an assumption that the risks associated with changing practice justify complacency about current treatments. It is wrong to assume that traditional clinical practices have been studied in appropriately selected populations of sufficient size to accurately predict their efficacy, benefit, safety, side effects, and cost.

Evidence-based practice (EBP) is a systematic way to improve patient and organization outcomes. EBP stresses that clinical decision making involves the consideration of evidence from multiple sources: systematic research, the clinician's clinical experience, and the patients being served.[4] Furthermore, EBP presents an opportunity to enhance patient health and illness outcomes, increase staff satisfaction, and reduce health care expenses. Unfortunately, EBP is not easily integrated into existing clinical settings and changes in routine practice are even more difficult to implement.[18] Integrating EBP requires decisions about health care based on the best available, current, valid, and relevant evidence.[18] The current state of science has provided limited rigorous clinical trials to direct change within clinical practice.

QUALITY OF EVIDENCE

As new therapies are integrated into practice, health care providers must continue to increase existing knowledge of the health and health problems of newborns. Providers must learn to overcome impatience with asking specific questions about the quality of evidence regarding risks and benefits of new practices. Clinical questions arise through practice and careful reading of research literature. **Evidence-based practice begins with questions that can best be answered by the careful design and conduct of clinical trials.**

It is not the purpose of this chapter to provide a detailed review of the various research designs that permit reliable scientific inference. Rather, our purpose is to promote the propositions that (1) challenge clinical observations and wisdom by subjecting them to systematic study and (2) encourage careful assessment and critique of research that supports or challenges the use of new and established clinical practices.

Clinical observations, although valuable in shaping research questions, are limited by selective perception—a desire to see a strategy work or fail to work. At times, a single case or case study may prompt us to question whether we should consider changing current practice. In some situations, much can be learned from carefully maintained databases. However, such knowledge is gained only when we

Please note that the **PURPLE** type in each chapter is intended to make it easier to identify clinically applicable material.

have formed databases with clear intentions and have collected the necessary data.

Sinclair and Bracken[43] described four levels of clinical research used to evaluate safety and efficacy, based on their ability to provide an unbiased answer. In ascending order, these are (1) single case or case series reports without controls, (2) nonrandomized studies with historical controls, (3) nonrandomized studies with concurrent controls, and (4) randomized controlled trials (RCTs). For a variety of reasons, case-controlled and prospective studies with historic controls are sometimes the only feasible way to approach clinical questions.[21,25] **RCTs have been identified as the strongest design for evaluating the effects of therapy.** RCTs test hypotheses by using randomly assigned treatment and control groups of adequate size to examine the efficacy and safety of a new therapy. In theory, random assignment of the treatment balances unknown or unmeasured factors that might otherwise bias the outcome of the trial. A ***meta-analysis*** combines and reports the results of several trials. Tyson[47] has suggested criteria for identifying proven therapies in current literature (Box 1-1). Although conclusions drawn from systematic reviews of RCTs have been regarded as the strongest level of evidence, evidence from descriptive and qualitative studies should be factored into clinical decisions when either randomized trials are not available or additional information is sought related to personal experiences or perspectives on care. Evidence-based practice, using knowledge gained from qualitative studies, recognizes the expertise of individual clinicians and parents in evaluating health care provision. **Price,[36] using a qualitative methodology, explored the experience of parents with a child in the neonatal intensive care unit (NICU) and revealed how non-technical aspects of care, such as comforting infants after painful procedures, were as important to parents as the "technical aspects."**

BOX 1-1 PROVEN THERAPIES

Reported to be beneficial in a well-performed meta-analysis of all trials

or

Beneficial in at least one multicenter trial or two single-center trials

Modified from Tyson JE: Use of unproven therapies in clinical practice and research: how can we better serve our patients and their families? *Semin Perinatol* 19:98, 1995.

Wigert[51] used a phenomenological hermeneutic design to elicit the experiences of having an infant in the NICU. Parents experienced a tension between exclusion and participation in their infant's care with an emphasis on exclusion. In a qualitative study, Charchuk and Simpson[12] described a similar situation of parents experiencing a lack of disclosure of their infant's condition and a lack of control. Raines[37] used a qualitative design to describe nurses' expertise in the NICU. Through analysis, Raines described how neonatal nurses, after learning technical skills, could focus on parental needs.

PRESSURES TO INTERVENE

Although RCTs are cited as providing the best evidence for guiding clinical decisions, they take time, and it is difficult to delay introduction of promising therapies. The pressure to intervene and change practice before studies are conducted or completed has many sources. Ian Chalmers,[9] in considering the struggle to gather scientific evidence in a climate of firmly held beliefs, has illustrated some of the pressures facing the scientific investigator (Figure 1-1). Bryce and Enkin[8] discussed myths about RCTs that lead to reasons to not conduct them. One myth is that randomization is unethical. This might be true in the rare instance that an intervention is dramatically effective and lifesaving. The more common situation is one in which there is relatively poor evidence for both the current and the alternative strategy. To compare an established strategy whose benefit is not scientifically supported (even though widely acclaimed) with one that is openly "experimental" is not unethical; in fact, both are "experimental." It is continued use of an unstudied practice that might more readily be labeled "unethical."

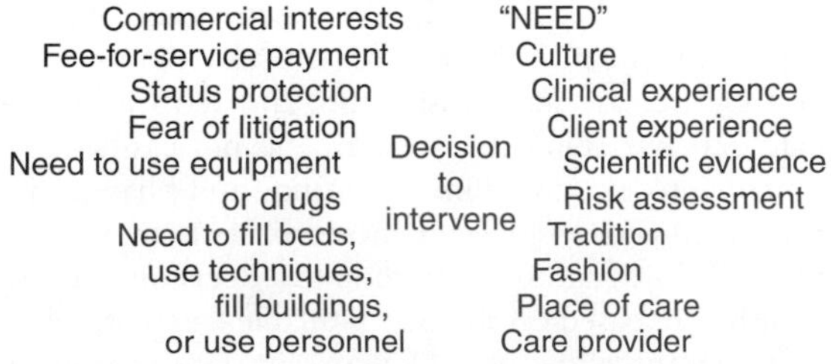
Commercial interests
Fee-for-service payment
Status protection
Fear of litigation
Need to use equipment
or drugs
Need to fill beds,
use techniques,
fill buildings,
or use personnel
Decision
to
intervene
"NEED"
Culture
Clinical experience
Client experience
Scientific evidence
Risk assessment
Tradition
Fashion
Place of care
Care provider

FIGURE 1-1 Pressures to intervene. (From Chalmers I: Scientific inquiry and authoritarianism in perinatal care and education, *Birth* 10:3, 1983.)

Pressure to intervene is, however, often overpowering. Believing that an infant is in trouble, interventions occur through a cascade of interventions,[32] one leading to the next and each carrying risk. One of the most frequently cited examples is the epidemic of blindness associated with use of oxygen in newborns.[40,41] Oxygen, used since the early 1900s for resuscitation and treatment of cyanotic episodes, was noted in the 1940s to "correct" periodic breathing in premature infants. After World War II and introduction of new gas-tight incubators, an epidemic of blindness occurred, resulting from retrolental fibroplasia (RLF). Silverman pointed out that although many causes were suspected, it was not until 1954 that a multicenter, controlled trial confirmed the association between high oxygen concentrations and RLF.[40] Frequently forgotten, however, is that in subsequent years, mortality was increased in infants cared for with an equally experimental regimen of strict restriction of oxygen administration and many survivors had spastic diplegia. In the 1960s, introduction of microtechniques for measuring arterial oxygen tension permitted better monitoring of oxygen therapy, with a reduction in mortality, spastic diplegia, and RLF, now called *retinopathy of prematurity* (ROP). ROP is currently limited to extremely low-birth-weight (ELBW) infants;[40] research continues to explore causes, preventive measures, and treatments (see Chapter 23).

The desire to see an intervention "work" encourages practitioners and investigators to seek early signs of benefit. Long-term effects are frequently overlooked. One reason is that they may not be foreseen. Consider the example of diethylstilbestrol (DES). DES administration to pregnant women was introduced in 1947 without clinical trials to prevent miscarriage, fetal death, and preterm delivery.[8,22] It was thought to be effective after uncontrolled studies despite controlled trials summarized in an overview (meta-analysis) by Goldstein et al[23] (Table 1-1) that showed the opposite. Clearly, DES was not effective, but it continued to be used until the 1970s, when the Food and Drug Administration (FDA) finally disapproved its use. The unforeseen result was that female children born to mothers who were given DES had structural abnormalities of the genital tract, pregnancy complications, decreased fertility, and an increased risk for vaginal adenocarcinoma in young women. Male children had epididymal cysts. The Centers for Disease Control and Prevention (CDC) has even considered the possibility of effects in grandchildren of exposed women.[17] This is not the only example of physicians continuing to use therapies that have been shown in RCTs to be of no benefit.[11]

TABLE 1-1 EFFECTS OF DIETHYLSTILBESTROL (DES) ON PREGNANCY OUTCOMES

	TYPICAL ODDS RATIO*	95% CONFIDENCE LIMITS
Miscarriage	1.20	0.89–1.62
Stillbirth	0.95	0.50–1.83
Neonatal death	1.31	0.74–2.34
All three	1.38	0.99–1.92
Prematurity	1.47	1.08–2.00

Data from Goldstein PA, Sacks HS, Chalmers TC: Hormone administration for the maintenance of pregnancy. In Chalmers I, Enkin M, Keirse M, editors: *Effective care in pregnancy and childbirth,* New York, 1989, Oxford University Press.

*An odds ratio is an estimate of the likelihood (or odds) of being affected by an exposure (e.g., a drug or treatment), compared with the odds of having that outcome without having been exposed. Women receiving DES did not have fewer stillbirths, premature births, or miscarriages than women who were untreated.

The costs of long-term studies and follow-up surveillance are numerous. However, when effects are measurable later in life (e.g., psychological problems, ability to function in school), cost should not determine study design. Even when randomized trials are conclusive, unanswered questions remain: Will a technology or treatment have the same effect in all settings? Has an "appropriate" target population been selected? Are there long-term unforeseeable consequences?

EVALUATION OF THERAPIES

The major cause of death in premature infants is respiratory failure from respiratory distress syndrome (RDS) (see Chapter 23). Previously called *hyaline membrane disease* (HMD), this syndrome of expiratory grunting, nasal flaring, chest wall retractions, and cyanosis unresponsive to high oxygen concentrations was a mystery until the 1950s.[41]

The evaluation of various therapies for RDS contrasts the value of controlled and uncontrolled trials. Sinclair[42] noted that uncontrolled studies were more likely to show benefit than controlled trials. In 19 uncontrolled studies, 17 popular therapies showed "benefit." In 18 controlled studies, only 9 demonstrated benefit. An untrained reviewer of the research might base clinical practice on faulty conclusions of uncontrolled trials

Surfactant Therapy

In contrast to many proposed treatments, surfactant therapy in premature infants has been well studied in RCTs.[20a,25] Studies have evaluated the use of surfactant in treatment of RDS, including the optimal source and composition of surfactant and prophylactic versus rescue treatment. Morbidity (including pneumothorax, periventricular or intraventricular hemorrhage, bronchopulmonary dysplasia [BPD], and patent ductus arteriosus) and mortality rates in treatment and control groups have been compared. A recent summary of these RCTs shows increased survival rates, improved oxygenation and ventilation, and a decrease in the incidence of pneumothorax.[20a] Effects on BPD are less consistent. Although RCTs involving thousands of newborns have clearly demonstrated the benefits of surfactant therapy, unanswered questions remain. Research is needed to define the optimal dose, optimal number of treatments, and most efficacious formulation.[20a]

Corticosteroid Therapy

Misuse of corticosteroids in perinatal medicine illustrates the consequences of failure to practice evidence-based medicine. Many practitioners initially declined to use single doses of antenatal steroids to promote maturation of the immature fetal lung and prevent RDS despite strong supportive evidence, demonstrating a failure to use a proven therapy. At the same time, other practitioners administered repeated doses despite lack of evidence of additional benefit and questions about safety, representing unproven use of a proven therapy. Postnatal glucocorticoids, administered to the infant after birth, were widely used despite weak evidence of long-term benefit and suggestions of possible harm, illustrating use of an uncertain therapy.[27,28]

ANTENATAL CORTICOSTEROID THERAPY: SINGLE COURSE

Antenatal administration of corticosteroids to pregnant women who threatened to deliver prematurely was first shown in 1972 to decrease neonatal mortality rate and the incidence of RDS and intraventricular hemorrhage (IVH) in premature infants.[29] In 1990, Crowley et al[15] used meta-analysis to evaluate 12 RCTs of maternal corticosteroid administration involving more than 3000 women. The data showed that maternal corticosteroid treatment significantly reduced the risk for neonatal mortality, RDS, and IVH. After two decades of published clinical trials[10,13,14,26] and the consensus development conference statement on "Effects of Corticosteroids for Fetal Maturation on Perinatal Outcomes,"[33] antenatal corticosteroid treatment of women at risk for preterm delivery between 24 and 34 weeks of gestation has been shown to be effective and safe in enhancing fetal lung maturity and reducing neonatal mortality. Yet adoption by caretakers was inexplicably slow.[26]

ANTENATAL CORTICOSTEROID THERAPY: REPEATED COURSES

Repeated courses of antenatal corticosteroids have been shown in humans and animals to improve lung function and the quantity of pulmonary surfactant.[16,24] They may also have adverse effects on lung structure, fetal somatic growth, and neonatal adrenocortical function, as well as poorly understood effects on blood pressure, carbohydrate homeostasis, and psychomotor development.[16,31] A 2000 NIH Consensus Development Conference found limited high-quality studies on the use of repeated courses of antenatal steroids.[34] The consensus statement discouraged routine use of repeated courses of antenatal corticosteroids. Results since 2000 are conflicting, with studies finding variously that repeated doses of antenatal corticosteroids are beneficial,[15] of no benefit,[17] or possibly harmful.[34] The paucity of school-age follow-up assessment of infants who received multiple courses has recently been re-emphasized.[2] The American College of Obstetricians and Gynecologists continues to advise that repeated courses of antenatal corticosteroids should be limited to patients enrolled in RCTs.[14]

POSTNATAL STEROID THERAPY

Despite early calls for caution in the use of postnatal corticosteroids to decrease the risk for chronic lung disease and limit ventilator time,[29] they were used liberally in the 1990s.[45,46] A number of years passed before RCTs of postnatal corticosteroid administration included long-term follow-up. Taken together, these studies showed positive short-term effects on the lungs. They also showed increased blood pressure and blood glucose concentrations in the short term; increased incidence of septicemia and gastrointestinal perforation in the intermediate term; and with dexamethasone administered soon after birth, abnormal neurodevelopmental outcome, including cerebral palsy, in the long term.[19,26,42,46,49] An increased risk for septicemia should have been anticipated, because it was first identified in an RCT by Reese et al[38] over 50 years earlier.

In 2002, the American Academy of Pediatrics (Committee on Fetus and Newborn) and the Canadian Paediatric Society (Fetus and Newborn Committee) advised against the use of systemic dexamethasone. They suggested that aside from "exceptional clinical circumstances," use of corticosteroids should be limited to patients enrolled in RCTs that include assessment of long-term developmental outcomes.[1] A 2005 re-analysis of many of the same data by Doyle et al[19] suggests that relative risks and benefits of postnatal corticosteroids vary with level of risk for BPD. When the risk for BPD or death is high, the risk for developmental impairment from postnatal corticosteroids might be outweighed by benefit.[20] Watterberg et al have suggested that hydrocortisone might have the benefits of dexamethasone on the lungs without adverse neurologic effects.[50] Much remains to be learned about postnatal use of corticosteroids to determine dose, timing, duration, type of steroid, benefits, and risks.

SYSTEMATIC REVIEW IN PERINATAL CARE AND THE BIRTH OF EVIDENCE-BASED MEDICINE

Evidence-based medicine (EBM) has been defined as the "conscientious, explicit, and judicious use of current best evidence in making decisions about the care of individual patients"[35] Examples from the literature, such as those cited in the preceding sections, illustrate how the application of the principles of evidence-based medicine offers a strong argument countering those who assert that EBM is nothing more than "typical practice using good clinical judgment." Proponents of EBM argue that the principal four steps of evidence-based practice—formulating a clinical question, retrieving relevant information, critically appraising the relevant information, and applying the evidence to patient care—provide a foundation for practice that leads to improved newborn outcomes and avoidance of repeating medical disasters. It is interesting to note that the roots of the EBM movement can be found in perinatal medicine.

Believing that the results of perinatal controlled trials had to be summarized in a manner useful to practitioners, Chalmers et al[11] and other perinatal professionals from various countries developed a registry of RCTs. They reviewed a vast amount of literature from published trials, sought out unpublished trials, and encouraged those who had begun, but not completed, studies to make them known to the registry. Once gathered, the studies' findings were summarized in "overviews."

A systematic review (or meta-analysis) pools the results of independently conducted RCTs whose study methods are reasonably similar, both in the selection and characteristics of participants and in the treatments that are offered. The results produce unbiased estimates of the effect of an intervention on clinical outcomes and are distinguished from nonsystematic reviews in which author opinions often are reported along with the evidence. Tables 1-1 and 1-2 were developed after pooling the results of different studies.

From these systematic reviews, practitioners can learn the strengths or weakness of clinical trials and evaluate the claims of benefit for implementing a strategy. The result of the efforts of Chalmers et al was the 1989 publication of a remarkably useful book, *Effective Care in Pregnancy and Childbirth*.[11] At the end of their book, they reported their own views of the reviewed treatments based on conclusions formed in the preceding articles. They found that although some strategies and forms of care were useful, others were questionable. Some interventions believed to be useful were not useful, of little benefit, or in fact, even harmful. In 1991, a companion publication, *Effective Care of the Newborn Infant*,[43] compiled and reviewed neonatal RCTs.

Multiple networks have been developed to perform multicenter RCTs. This is particularly useful, providing an opportunity to see whether treatments have similar effects in different practice settings. It is also useful in that practitioners in individual settings may not always see enough cases to reach robust conclusions. Rare conditions and rare outcomes are better understood when trials are replicated or their findings are pooled. Systematic

TABLE 1-2 MORTALITY AFTER PROPHYLACTIC SURFACTANT COMPARED WITH SURFACTANT TREATMENTS*

AUTHOR	PROPHYLACTIC	TREATMENT	RELATIVE RISK†	95% CONFIDENCE INTERVAL
Dunn	09/62	08/60	1.09	0.45, 2.65
Kendig	29/235	49/244	0.62	0.62, 0.94
Merritt	29/102	23/101	1.25	0.78, 2.00
Typical effect			0.85	0.63, 1.14

Data from Soll RF, McQueen MC: Respiratory distress syndrome. In Sinclair JC, Bracken MB, editors: *Effective care of the newborn infant,* Oxford, England, 1992, Oxford University Press.
*In this table it can be seen that mortality was not different when the results of the two treatments were compared.
†None of the relative risk estimates were statistically significant.

reviews provide the opportunity to understand these findings in the context of clinical practice. About the same time the Chalmers et al book was published, the **Cochrane Collaboration was established, again largely through the efforts of Ian Chalmers** *(www.cochrane.org/index0.htm).* The Cochrane Collaboration is a worldwide group with over 50 Collaborative Review Groups whose members prepare, maintain, and disseminate systematic reviews based primarily on the results of RCTs. These reviews are published electronically in the Cochrane Library, which contains the Cochrane Database of Systematic Reviews (CDSR: *www.cochrane.org/reviews/index.htm*), along with editorial comments on these reviews. Comments come from an international group of individuals and institutions dedicated to summarizing randomized controlled trials relevant to health care. In addition to the Collaborative Review Groups, there are now 12 Cochrane Centers in the world. These centers provide support for the review groups. The Neonatal Group is based at McMaster University in Hamilton, Ontario, Canada; and the Pregnancy and Childbirth Group is based at the University of Liverpool, Liverpool, England. Cochrane Neonatal Reviews are available at the National Institute of Child Health and Human Development (NICHD) Cochrane Neonatal Internet home page; approximately 250 overviews are listed.[32]

Additional sources of high-grade integrative literature are also available to the practicing clinician. Critical appraisal of published research takes considerable time, and several groups assemble high-grade literature using a uniform methodology that is typically described to readers as a supplementary article. Reading this article once can inform the practitioner if the method used to assemble a review or guideline is sufficiently rigorous. Also, a number of sites do not produce integrative literature but collect it from a number of sources. Some of these sites discuss the quality of the information presented. If we cannot appraise the method used to collect this information, we should always proceed with caution. Additional reliable sites include the following:

- The Database of Abstracts of Reviews of Effectiveness (DARE) *(www.crd.york.ac.uk/crdweb/),* a collection of international reviews including those from the Cochrane Collaboration. Reviewers at the National Health Service Center for Reviews and Dissemination at the University of York, England, provide quality oversight including detailed structured abstracts that describe the methodology, results, and conclusions of the reviews. The quality of the reviews is discussed along with implications for health care.
- National Guidelines Clearinghouse *(www.guidelines.gov/browse/guideline_index.arpx),* maintained by the U.S. Department of Health and Human Services, Agency for Health Care Research and Quality (AHRQ), in partnership with the American Medical Association (AMA) and the American Association of Health Plans (AAHP). This site provides a wide range of clinical practice guidelines from institutions and organizations. Structured abstracts facilitate critical appraisal, and abstracts on the same topic can be compared on a side-by-side table, allowing comparisons of relevance, generalizability, and rigor of research findings. Links also are provided to the full text of each guideline, when available.

Admittedly, there are problems with EBM. Conducting systematic reviews is time-consuming; thus not many are available. Often, the power of randomized controlled trials, especially in neonatology, is low. The evidence in published studies does not always apply to our specific patient. In addition, locating relevant evidence is time-consuming and may require access to online resources and a higher level of information-seeking skills than is available. Finally, although recognizing that medical expertise and scientific knowledge are crucial components of neonatal care, these rigorous, objective, scientific evaluations create the potential to overlook valuable experiential knowledge of the NICU provided by practitioners and parents.

Reasons to use an evidence-based approach have been well documented. According to Asztalos,[2] there are basically **two reasons to try to keep up with the literature: (1) to maintain clinical competence; and (2) to solve specific clinical problems.** Phillips and Glasziou[35] suggest that clinicians seek information "just in time" (as a clinician seeing patients) and "just in case" (to keep up with a clinical specialty). The former can be achieved by actively searching for information in filtered, summarized clinical point-of-care resources. *FirstConsult*, *DynaMed*, *Clinical Medicine*, and *UpToDate* fall into this category. The latter, "just in case" learning, also called *surveillance of the literature,* is best achieved by using technology tools to survey the current original literature. These tools include auto-alerts and RSS feeds in PubMed or online databases and journals. Learning about these ever-changing resources is a challenge. Many hospitals and clinics are beginning to include a clinical librarian or informationist as part of the health care team.[4–7,30,36,44,48] **At the end of this chapter is a list of additional evidence-based medicine resources.** To use these resources effectively, individuals must become familiar with the principles and value of evidence-based patient care. **EBM can be practiced successfully at the individual level; in addition, an individual clinician can act as a change agent and advocate for evidence-based institutional practice.**

As stated by Silverman[40]:

> Since ours is the only species on the planet that has achieved rates of newborn survival which exceed 90 percent, it seems to me we must demand the highest order of evidence possible before undertaking widespread actions that may affect the full lifetimes of individuals in the present, as well as in future generations. Here a strong case can be made for a slow and measured pace of medical innovation.

REFERENCES

1. American Academy of Pediatrics, Committee on Fetus and Newborn: Postnatal corticosteroids to treat or prevent chronic lung disease in preterm infants, *Pediatrics* 109:330, 2002.
2. Asztalos E: The need to go beyond: evaluating antenatal corticosteroid trials with long-term outcomes, *J Obstet Gynaecol Can* 29:429, 2007.
3. Reference deleted in proofs.
4. Brackenbury T, Burroughs E, Hewitt L: A qualitative examination of current guidelines for evidence-based practice in child language intervention, *Lang Speech Hear Serv Sch* 39:78, 2008.
5. Brandes S: Experience and outcomes of medical librarian rounding, *Med Ref Serv Q* 26:85, 2007.
6. Brettle A, Hulme C, Ormandy P: The costs and effectiveness of information skills training and mediated searching: qualitative results from the empiric project, *Health Info Libr J* 23:239, 2006.
7. Brettle A, Hulme C, Ormandy P: Effectiveness and information skills training and mediated searching: qualitative result from the empiric project, *Health Info Libr J* 24:24, 2007.
8. Bryce RL, Enkin MW: Six myths about controlled trials in perinatal medicine, *Am J Obstet Gynecol* 151:707, 1985.
9. Chalmers I: Scientific inquiry and authoritarianism in perinatal care and education, *Birth* 10:151, 1983.
10. Chalmers I, editor: *Oxford database of perinatal trials*, Oxford, England, 1988, Oxford University Press.
11. Chalmers I, Enkin M, Keirse M: *Effective care in pregnancy and childbirth*, New York, 1989, Oxford University Press.
12. Charchuk M, Simpson C: Hope, disclosure, and control in the neonatal intensive care unit, *Health Commun* 17(2):191, 2005.
13. Collaborative Santiago Surfactant Group: Collaborative trial of prenatal thyrotropin-releasing hormone and corticosteroids for prevention of respiratory distress syndrome, *Am J Obstet Gynecol* 178(1 Pt 1):33, 1998.
14. Committee on Obstetric Practice: Antenatal corticosteroid therapy for fetal maturation, *Obstet Gynecol* 111:805, 2008.
15. Crowley P, Chambers I, Keirse MJ: The effects of corticosteroid administration before preterm delivery: an overview of the evidence from controlled trials, *Br J Obstet Gynaecol* 97:11, 1990.
16. Crowther CA, Haslam RR, Hiller JE, et al: Neonatal respiratory distress syndrome after repeat exposure

to antenatal corticosteroids: a randomized controlled trial, *Lancet* 367:1913, 2006.
17. Crowther CA, Harding JE: Repeat doses of prenatal corticosteroids for women at risk of preterm birth for preventing neonatal respiratory disease, *Cochrane Database Syst Rev* (3): CD003935' 2007. DOI, 10.1002/14651858.CD003935.pub2.
18. Dawes M, Davies P, Gray A: *Evidence based practice: a primer for health care professionals*, New York, 2004, Churchill Livingstone.
19. Doyle L, Halliday HL, Ehrenkranz RA, et al: Impact of postnatal systemic corticosteroids on mortality and cerebral palsy in preterm infants: effect modification by risk for chronic lung disease, *Pediatrics* 115:655, 2005.
20. Eichenwald EC, Stark AR: Are postnatal steroids ever justified to treat severe bronchopulmonary dysplasia? *Arch Dis Child Fetal Neonatal Ed* 92:334, 2007.
20a. Engle WA: and the Committee on Fetus and Newborn: Surfactant-replacement therapy for respiratory distress in the preterm and term neonate, *Pediatrics* 121:419, 2008.
21. Finer NN, Craft A, Vaucher YE, et al: Postnatal steroids: short-term gain, long-term pain? *J Pediatr* 137:9, 2000.
22. Fletcher RH, Fletcher SW, Wagner EH: *Clinical epidemiology*, ed 2, Baltimore, 1988, Williams & Wilkins.
23. Goldstein PA, Sacks HS, Chalmers TC: Hormone administration for the maintenance of pregnancy. In Chalmers I, Enkin M, Keirse M, editors: *Effective care in pregnancy and childbirth*, New York, 1989, Oxford University Press.
24. Guinn DA, Atkinson MW, Sullivan L, et al: Single vs weekly courses of antenatal corticosteroids for women at risk of preterm delivery: a randomized controlled trial, *JAMA* 286:1581, 2001.
25. Halliday HL: Surfactants: past, present and future, *J Perinatol* 28(Suppl 1):S47, 2008.
26. Jobe AH: Glucocorticoids in perinatal medicine: misguided rockets?, *J Pediatr* 137:1, 2000.
27. Jobe AH, Mitchel BR, Gunkel JH: Beneficial effects of the combined use of prenatal corticosteroids and postnatal surfactant on preterm infants, *Am J Obstet Gynecol* 168:508, 1993.
28. LeFlore JL, Salhab WA, Broyles RS, et al: Association of antenatal and postnatal dexamethasone exposure with outcomes in extremely low birth weight neonates, *Pediatrics* 110:275, 2002.
29. Liggins GC, Howie RN: A controlled trial of antepartum glucocorticoid treatment for prevention of the respiratory distress syndrome in premature infants, *Pediatrics* 50:515, 1972.
30. Mann M, Sander L, Weightman A: Signposting best evidence: a role for information professionals, *Health Info Libr J* 23(Suppl 1):S61, 2006.
31. Mildenhall LJF, Battin MR, Morton SMB, et al: Exposure to repeat doses of antenatal corticoids is associated with altered cardiovascular status after birth, *Arch Dis Child* 91:F56, 2006.
32. National Institute of Child Health and Human Development: Cochrane Neonatal Home Page: www.nichd.nih.gov/cochrane.
33. National Institutes of Health Consensus Development Conference Statement: Effects of corticosteroids for fetal maturation on perinatal outcomes, *JAMA* 273:413, 1995.
34. National Institutes of Health: Antenatal corticosteroids revisited: repeat courses, *NIH Consensus Statement 2000* 17:1, 2000.
35. Phillips R, Glasziou P: Evidence based practice: the practicalities of keeping abreast of clinical evidence while in training, *Postgrad Med J* 84:450, 2008.
36. Price PJ: Parents' perceptions of the meaning of quality nursing care, *ANS Adv Nurs Sci* 16(1):33, 1993.
37. Raines D: Parents' values: a missing link in the neonatal intensive care equation, *Neonatal Netw* 15(3):7, 1996.
38. Reese AB, Blodi FC, Locke JC, et al: Results of use of corticotropin (ACTH) in treatment of retrolental fibroplasia, *AMA Arch Ophthalmol* 47:551, 1952.
39. Reference deleted in proofs.
40. Silverman WA: *RLF: a modern parable*, New York, 1980, Grune & Stratton.
41. Silverman WA: *Human experimentation: a guided step into the unknown*, New York, 1985, Oxford University Press.
42. Sinclair JC: Prevention and treatment of respiratory distress syndrome, *Pediatr Clin North Am* 13:711, 1966.
43. Sinclair JC, Bracken MB: *Effective care of the newborn infant*, New York, 1992, Oxford University Press.
44. Spak JM, Glovver JG: The personal librarian program: an evaluation of a Cushing/Whitney Medical Library outreach initiative, *Med Ref Serv Q* 26:15, 2007.
45. Stark AR, Carlo WA, Tyson JE, et al: Adverse effects of early dexamethasone treatment on extremely low-birth-weight infants, *N Engl J Med* 344:95, 2001.
46. Stoll BJ, Temprosa M, Tyson JE, et al: Dexamethasone therapy increases infection in very low birth weight infants, *Pediatrics* 104:63, 1999.
47. Tyson JE: Use of unproven therapies in clinical practice and research: how can we better serve our patients and their families?, *Semin Perinatol* 19:98, 1995.
48. Urquhart C, Turner J, Durbin J, et al: Changes in information behavior in clinical teams after introduction of a clinical librarian service, *J Med Lib Assoc* 95:14, 2007.

49. Watterberg KL: Postnatal steroids for bronchopulmonary dysplasia: where are we now?, *J Pediatr* 150:327, 2007.
50. Watterberg KL, Gerdes JS, Cole CH, et al: Prophylaxis of early adrenal insufficiency to prevent bronchopulmonary dysplasia: a multicenter trial, *Pediatrics* 114:1649, 2004.
51. Wigert H: Mothers' experiences of having their newborn child in a neonatal intensive care unit, *Scand J Caring Sci* 20:35, 2006.

EVIDENCE-BASED MEDICINE RESOURCES

Databases of Evidence and Search Engines

ACP Journal Club (www.acponline.org/journals/acpjc/jcmenu.htm): Evidence-based evaluative summaries of articles taken from 100 clinical journals, written by MDs and others, with comments from MDs.

Campbell Collaboration (www.campbellcollaboration.org/): An independent, international, non-profit organization that aims to help people make well-informed decisions about the effects of interventions in the social, behavioral, and educational arenas. The vision of the Campbell Collaboration is to bring about positive social change and to improve the quality of public and private services across the world by preparing, maintaining, and disseminating systematic reviews of existing social science evidence. The Campbell Collaboration's substantive priorities include, though are not confined to, education, social welfare, and crime and justice.

Cochrane Library (www.thecochranelibrary.com): Premier evidence-based medicine resource composed of the following:

- **Database of Systematic Reviews** containing systematic reviews and meta-analyses conducted by Cochrane Study Groups.
- **Database of Reviews of Effects** including systematic reviews and meta-analyses from non-Cochrane sources, many with structured abstracts with comments on the reviews.
- **Center Register of Controlled Trials:** Indexes many trials not included in MEDLINE.

HTA and NHS EED Include evidence-based reviews of technology and economic issues.

ClinicalTrials.gov (http://clinicaltrials.gov/ct/gui): Provides regularly updated information about federally and privately supported clinical research in human volunteers. Gives information about a trial's purpose, who may participate, locations, and phone numbers for more details.

Current Controlled Trials (www.controlled-trials.com/): Allows users to search, register, and share information about randomized controlled trials.

Google Coop Netting the Evidence: (http://decenturl.com/google/nettingtheevidence): Andrew Booth, a pioneer in evidence-based information practice at the University of Sheffield, created one of the first lists of evidence-based health care resources on the Internet. He has taken this one step further with a Google Coop site that limits your Google search to over 100 authoritative, evidence-based websites. Type a condition and diagnostic method or treatment into the search box to quickly find resources with an evidence-based approach.

HSTAT (http://hstat.nlm.nih.gov/): A free, web-based resource of full-text documents that provide health information and support health care decision making. HSTAT's audience includes health care providers, health service researchers, policy makers, payers, consumers, and the information professionals who serve these groups.

NHS Centre for Reviews and Dissemination (www.york.ac.uk/inst/crd/) Resource for systematic reviews of health economics and technology assessment. Also maintains the DARE, Health Technology Assessment, and NHS Economic Evaluation databases included in Cochrane.

National Institutes of Child Health and Human Development (NICHD) Cochrane Neonatal (www.nichd.nih.gov/cochrane/): Resource for systematic reviews of child health topics.

SUMSearch: (http://sumsearch.uthscsa.edu/) Identifies sources of evidence-based information using this metasearch engine.

TRIP Database: (www.tripdatabase.com/) Locates high-quality, evidence-based medical literature using this metasearch engine. Some resources in the results list may require subscription.

WHO Clinical Trial Search Portal (www.who.int/trialsearch/): Enables researchers, health practitioners, consumers, journal editors, and reporters to search more easily and quickly for information on clinical trials.

Databases of Guidelines

CMA Infobase, Clinical Practice Guidelines (www.cma.ca/): Click on Clinical Resources tab; requires membership. Excellent access to guidelines and other point-of-care resources.

Guidelines International Network (G-I-N) (www.g-i-n.net/): Guidelines organized by health topic. Links to worldwide sources of guidelines.

National Guideline Clearinghouse (www.guideline.gov/): Use "Detailed Search" link on left for more specific searches. A U.S. resource for evidence-based clinical practice guidelines. A display tool allows side-by-side comparison of guidelines.

NHS National Institute for Clinical Excellence (NICE) (www.nice.org.uk/): Evidence-based guidance on technology use, clinical care, and interventional procedures.

Scottish Intercollegiate Guidelines Network (SIGN) (www.sign.ac.uk/): Use link on left to view guidelines by topic. Distribution point for Scottish national clinical guidelines.

U.S. Preventive Services Task Force (USPSTF) (www.ahrq.gov/clinic/uspstfix.htm): A collection of materials related to the work of an independent panel of experts in primary care and prevention that systematically reviews the evidence of effectiveness and develops recommendations for clinical preventive services.

Evidence-Based Medicine Resources

Canadian Centres for Health Evidence (www.cche.net/): Based in Alberta, this centre provides resources and support for evidence-based practice.

Centre for Evidence-Based Medicine(Oxford) (www.cebm.net/): Major website for learning about, practicing, and teaching EBM. The Toolbox provides valuable resources for learning and practice.

Centre for Evidence-Based Medicine(Toronto) (www.cebm.utoronto.ca/): In addition to learning resources, this site provides focused syllabi for specialties and a glossary.

Cochrane Collaboration (www.cochrane.org/): This international non-profit and independent organization is dedicated to making up-to-date, accurate information about the effects of health care readily available worldwide through systematic review of medical research.

Core Library for Evidence-Based Practice (www.shef.ac.uk/scharr/ir/netting/): This resource provides a directory of a wide variety of evidence-based learning and practice materials.

Evidence Based Medicine Tool Kit (www.med.ualberta.ca/ebm/): A collection of tools for identifying, assessing, and applying relevant evidence for better health care decision making.

PedsCCM Evidence-Based Medicine Resources (http://pedsccm.org/EBJournal_Club_intro.php): An online collection of resources and training tools for the pediatric professional.

Student's Guide to the Medical Literature (http://140.226.6.124/SG/): A guide suitable for anyone new to evidence-based medicine, written by a former UCD-AMC medical student for other students.

Understanding Evidence-based Healthcare: A Foundation for Action (http://apps1.jhsph.edu/cochrane/CUEwebcourse.htm): A web course created by the U.S. Cochrane Center that is designed to help the user understand the fundamentals of evidence-based health care concepts and skills. The 6-module course can be done in 15-minute segments and takes a minimum of 5 to 6 hours. Course registration is free and open to all. The hosts request that participants commit to completing the evaluations.

Users' Guides to the Medical Literature, first edition: (http://pubs.ama-assn.org/misc/usersguides.dtl; secondedition:www.JAMAevidence.com): Excellent self-paced learning modules based on the *JAMA Users' Guide* series, featuring interactive activities designed to reinforce learning.

History of Evidence-Based Medicine

Chronology of the Cochrane Collaboration (www.cochrane.org/cochrane/cchronol.htm): A source of information about the development of the Cochrane Collaboration and its significance to evidence-based health care.

Controlled Trials from History at the James Lind Library (www.jameslindlibrary.org/) Excellent source of historical examples of RCTs; perfect for presentations on evidence-based health care.

Teaching Evidence-Based Medicine

Centre for Evidence-Based Medicine (Oxford) (www.cebm.net/?o=1021): Major website for learning about, practicing, and teaching EBM. The Toolbox provides valuable resources for learning and practice.

Evidence Based Medicine Teaching Materials (www.ebmny.org/teach.html): Resource list that includes courses, teaching tools, presentation materials, and a link to a systematic review of the effectiveness of teaching critical appraisal skills.

Fresno Test of Evidence Based Medicine (http://grinch.uchsc.edu/education/ebhc/fresno-test.pdf): This validated test measures competence in searching for and evaluating medical literature.

Richardson WS: Teaching evidence-based practice on foot, *ACP J Club* 143(2):A10, 2005. This article describes methods for teaching evidence-based medicine during rounds.

Syllabi For Practicing EBM (www.cebm.utoronto.ca/syllabi/): These syllabi, taken from the book *Evidence-Based Medicine: How to practice and teach EBM* include scenarios and teaching materials for 14 different fields, including general practice, geriatrics, physiotherapy, nursing, child health, complementary medicine, gastroenterology, and purchasing.

Tips for learners [and teachers] of evidence-based medicine, *CMAJ* 2004-2005 (www.cmaj.ca/cgi/collection/evidence_based_medicine_series/): This series is devoted to helping clinicians understand and apply the basic principles of EBM. The series also targets teachers of EBM principles and offers tips for teaching key concepts. Be sure to advance to page 2 to see all of the articles in the series. Teachers should click on the "Online Appendix" links for teaching advice.

Websites

Centers for Health Evidence
www.cche.net/usersguides/main.asp

Directory of EBM sites and resources
www.herts.ac.uk/lis/subjects/health/ebm.htm.

EBM Toolbox
www.cebm.net/toolbox.asp.

Evidence-Based Medicine: What It Is and What It Isn't
www.cods.edu/cebd-i/articles/article01.htm

Health Information Research Unit (HIRU)
http://hiru.mcmaster.ca/

Health Care Information Resources: Evidence-Based Health Care Practitioners Links
www-hsl.mcmaster.ca/resources/ebpractice.htm.

Users Guide to the Medical Literature
www.shef.ac.uk/scharr/ir/userg.html

Texts

Craig J, Snyth R: *The evidence-based practice manual for nurses*, New York, 2007, Churchill Livingstone.

Dawes M, Davies P, Gray A: *Evidence based practice: a primer for health care professionals*, New York, 2004, Churchill Livingstone.

Dicenso A, Guyat G, Ciliska D: *Evidence based nursing: a guide to clinical practice*, St Louis, 2005, Mosby.

Friedland DJ, Go AS, Davoren JB, et al: *Evidence-based medicine: a framework for clinical practice*, Stamford, Conn, 1998, Appleton-Lange.

Greenhalgh T: *How to read a paper: the basics of evidence-based medicine*, ed 2, London, 2001, BMJ Publishing Group.

Malloch K, Porter-Grady T: *Introduction to evidence-based practice in nursing and health care*, Boston, 2006, Jones & Bartlett Publishers.

Melnyk B, Fineout-Overholt E: *Evidence based practice in nursing and healthcare*, Philadelphia, 2005, Lippincott Williams & Wilkins.

Riegelman RK: *Studying a study and testing a test: how to read the medical evidence*, ed 4, Boston, 2000, Little, Brown.

Sackett DL, Richardson WS, Rosenberg W, et al: *Evidence-based medicine: how to practice and teach EBM*, Edinburgh, 2000, Churchill Livingstone.

Articles

Ambalavanan N, Whyte RK: The mismatch between evidence and practice: common therapies in search of evidence [Review], *Clin Perinatol* 30:305, 2003.

Gonzalez de Dios J: Bibliometric analysis of systematic reviews in the Neonatal Cochrane Collaboration: its role in evidence-based decision making in neonatology [Spanish], *An Pediatr (Barc)* 60:417, 2004.

Kramer MS: Randomized trials and public health interventions: time to end the scientific double standard [Review], *Clin Perinatol* 30:351, 2003.

The Learning and Information Services: University of Hertfordshire, maintains an updated and selective, but substantial list of references on the theory and methodology of evidence-based medicine/healthcare. Retrospective references are available as well from 1993 to 2002. Retrieved from www.herts.ac.uk/lis/subjects/health/ebm.htm#refs.

Shulman ST: Neonatology, then and now, *Pediatr Ann* 32:562, 2003.

Sinclair JC: Evidence-based therapy in neonatology: distilling the evidence and applying it in practice [Review], *Acta Paediatr* 93:1146, 2004.

Sinclair JC, Haughton DE, Bracken MB, et al: Cochrane neonatal systematic reviews: a survey of the evidence for neonatal therapies, *Clin Perinatol* 30:285, 2003.

Strand M, Phelan KJ, Donovan EF: Promoting the uptake and use of evidence: an overview of the problem [Review], *Clin Perinatol* 30:389, 2003.

2 PRENATAL ENVIRONMENT: EFFECT ON NEONATAL OUTCOME

PRISCILLA M. NODINE, JAIME ARRUDA, AND MARIE HASTINGS-TOLSMA

The human fetus develops within a complex maternal environment. Structurally defined by the intrauterine/intraamniotic compartment, the character of the prenatal environment is determined largely by maternal variables. The fetus depends totally on the maternal host for respiratory and nutritive support and is significantly influenced by maternal metabolic, cardiovascular, and environmental factors. In addition, the fetus is limited in its ability to adapt to stress or modify its surroundings. This creates a situation in which the prenatal environment exerts a tremendous influence on fetal development and well-being. This influence lasts well beyond the period of gestation, often affecting the newborn in ways that have profound significance for both immediate and long-term outcome.

There is great utility in identifying maternal factors that adversely affect the condition of the fetus. Providers of obstetric care have long used this information to identify the "at-risk" population and design interventions that prevent or reduce the occurrence of fetal and neonatal complications. **It is equally important that neonatal care providers obtain a clear picture of the prenatal environment and use this information before birth to anticipate the newborn's immediate needs and make appropriate preparations for resuscitation and initial nursery care.** After birth, an awareness of the likely sequelae of environmental compromise helps focus ongoing assessment and aids in clinical problem solving.

The purpose of this chapter is to help neonatal care providers evaluate maternal influences on the prenatal environment, identify significant environmental risk factors, and anticipate the associated neonatal problems. Information on the assessment and treatment of specific neonatal problems is provided throughout this text and is not repeated here. For a more extensive discussion of perinatal physiology and complicated pregnancies, refer to the references cited at the end of this chapter.

PHYSIOLOGY

Two variables have a critical influence on fetal well-being throughout gestation: utero-placental functioning and inherent maternal resources. The interplay of these factors is a major determinant of fetal oxygenation, metabolism, and growth. Alterations in the development and function of the placenta also influence fetal growth and development. The fetus may be affected to the point that survival is threatened. Likewise, extrauterine well-being may be compromised.

The placenta has a dual role in providing nutrients and metabolic fuels to the fetus. First, placental secretion of endocrine hormones, chiefly human chorionic somatomammotropin (HCS), increases throughout pregnancy, causing progressive changes in maternal metabolism. The net effect of these changes is an increase in maternal glucose and amino acids available to the fetus, especially in the second half of pregnancy. Second, the placenta is instrumental in the transfer of these (and other) essential nutrients

Please note that the **PURPLE** type in each chapter is intended to make it easier to identify clinically applicable material.

from the maternal to the fetal circulation and, conversely, of metabolic wastes from the fetal to the maternal system. Adequate maternal and fetal blood flow through the placenta is essential throughout the entire pregnancy.

Fetal respiration also depends on adequate placental function. Respiratory gases (oxygen and carbon dioxide) readily cross the placental membrane by simple diffusion, with the rate of diffusion determined by the PO_2 (or PCO_2) differential between maternal and fetal blood.

Although the placenta mediates the transport of respiratory gases, carbohydrates, lipids, vitamins, minerals, and amino acids, the maternal reservoir is their source. Maternal-fetal transfer depends on the characteristics and absolute content of substances within the maternal circulation, the relative efficiency of the maternal cardiovascular system in perfusing the placenta, and the function of the placenta itself.[155] The fetal environment can be disrupted by inappropriate types or amounts of substances (e.g., ethanol) in the maternal circulation, decreases or interruptions in placental blood flow (e.g., placental abruption), or abnormalities in placental function (e.g., small placenta). Maternal nutrition, exercise, and disease can impair placental uptake and transfer of substances across the placenta to the fetus.

COMPROMISED FETAL ENVIRONMENT

Maternal Disease

DIABETES

The prevalence of diabetes mellitus and gestational diabetes mellitus (GDM) is increasing worldwide. Diabetes is the most common endocrine disorder affecting pregnancy, and approximately 2% to 7% of pregnant women in the United States are diagnosed with GDM annually.[32] Despite major reductions in mortality over the past several decades, the infant of a diabetic mother (IDM) continues to have a considerable perinatal disadvantage. The physiologic changes in maternal glucose use that accompany pregnancy, coupled with either a preexisting hyperglycemia (as found in types 1 and 2 diabetes) or an inability to mount an appropriate insulin response (as seen in patients with gestational diabetes) result in a significantly abnormal fetal environment. This is because of the increased level of maternal glucose, often in concert with episodic hypoglycemia and ketone exposure. Early in pregnancy, this environment may have a teratogenic effect on the embryo, accounting for the dramatic increase in spontaneous abortions and congenital malformations in the offspring of diabetic women with poor metabolic control.[8] During the second and third trimesters, the mechanics of placental transport dictate that fetal glucose levels depend on, but are slightly less than, maternal levels.[126] Assuming adequate placental function and perfusion, elevations in maternal glucose lead to fetal hyperglycemia and increased fetal insulin production. Repeated or continued elevations in blood glucose result in fetal hyperinsulinism, alterations in the use of glucose and other nutrients, and altered patterns of growth and development.[8,126]

Fetal macrosomia (greater than the 90th percentile for weight) occurs in 25% to 42% of diabetic pregnancies because of hyperinsulinemia. These macrosomic infants suffer increased morbidity and mortality from unexplained death in utero, birth trauma, hypertrophic cardiomyopathy, vascular thrombosis, neonatal hypoglycemia, hyperbilirubinemia, erythrocytosis, and respiratory distress.[93] Macrosomic infants have double the risk for shoulder dystocia during vaginal birth and are at greater risk for death during the last 4 to 6 weeks of gestation.[170] Brachial plexus injury and facial nerve palsy also can result from shoulder dystocia.[72] Finally, macrosomic infants are at higher risk for dysfunctional labor patterns and operative vaginal deliveries, which can also contribute to their higher rate of birth trauma.

In addition to the basic metabolic disturbances, diabetes predisposes the pregnant woman to several other complications, including gestational hypertension, preeclampsia, renal disease, and vascular disease.[8] As a consequence, the fetus may be compromised further by chronic hypoxia and other insults, which can lead to intrauterine demise, prematurity, growth restriction, cardiovascular problems, respiratory distress syndrome (RDS), and long-term neurologic problems.[37] In terms of predicting perinatal morbidity and mortality, the "prognostically bad signs of pregnancy," first identified by Pedersen in the 1960s, are especially significant. **The occurrence of any of these signs, which include diabetic ketoacidosis, hypertension, pyelonephritis, and maternal noncompliance, continue to be useful predictors of increased fetal and neonatal risk.**[46]

In preparing for the delivery of an IDM, the neonatal team should consider the classification of maternal diabetes (type 1 or 2, or gestational). In addition, the quality of metabolic control throughout the pregnancy and labor, maternal complications, and the duration of the pregnancy should be considered, along with indicators of fetal growth and well-being. In cases in which the newer generation sulfonylurea (i.e., glyburide) has been used, an increased incidence of neonatal jaundice may be anticipated.[77]

THYROID DISEASE

Thyroid disorders are the second most common endocrine disorder seen in pregnancy.[9] The thyroid hormones *triiodothyronine* (T_3) and *thyroxine* (T_4) cross the placenta in small amounts, though the significance of the transfer has not been well elucidated. The fetus depends on maternal T_4 in the first trimester of pregnancy. At 8 to 10 weeks' gestation, the fetal thyroid begins to concentrate iodine and produce T_4. During the second and third trimester, the fetus is independent of maternal status. At approximately 24 weeks, thyroid-stimulating immunoglobulins (TSIs) or thyroid-stimulating hormone (TSH) receptor *Abs,* which are classes of immunoglobulin G (IgG), cross the placenta and stimulate fetal thyroid. Iodine is readily transferred from mother to fetus. The fetal thyroid gland concentrates iodine and synthesizes its own hormones as early as 10 to 12 weeks' gestation; this is independent of maternal thyroid function. Maternal thyroid hormones are believed to be important for fetal neurologic development in the first trimester.[3] Significant decreases in intelligence quotient (IQ) of offspring of mothers with untreated hypothyroidism in early gestation have been shown in some studies.[70,96] Whereas subclinical hypothyroidism does not need to be treated,[26] severe maternal hypothyroidism may result in increased neurodevelopmental delay in offspring, pregnancy loss, prematurity, preeclampsia, low birth weight, and abruptio placenta.[25] Treatment with replacement hormone during pregnancy is well tolerated by the fetus and reduces these risks.[3]

Maternal hyperthyroidism presents a different situation. Thyroid-stimulating antibodies, commonly found in patients with Graves' disease, as well as many of the drugs used to treat hyperthyroidism, cross the placenta and can have a significant effect on the fetus. Antibodies, including long-acting thyroid stimulant (LATS) and TSI, can increase fetal thyroid hormone production. High levels are associated with fetal and neonatal hyperthyroidism. Untreated maternal thyrotoxicosis has been linked to preterm delivery, intrauterine growth restriction (IUGR), low birth weight, and stillbirth. In rare cases, the offspring of women with Graves' disease may themselves have this condition. In fetuses and newborns, this is evidenced by elevations in heart rate, growth restriction, prematurity, goiter, and congestive heart failure. The perinatal mortality rate is high.[26] Administration of antithyroid medication to the mother can decrease thyroid hormone production in both the mother and the fetus but may result in fetal hypothyroidism and goiter.[1]

Another maternal antibody, TSH-binding inhibitor immunoglobulin, also crosses the placenta and can prevent the expected fetal thyroid response to TSH. The result is a transient fetal and neonatal hypothyroidism. Iodine deficiency in the mother is another cause of fetal and neonatal hypothyroidism and, in its severe form, leads to cretinism because of the fetus's dependence on maternal iodine reserves.[1]

PHENYLKETONURIA

Phenylketonuria (PKU) is an inherited disorder in which an enzymatic defect precludes conversion of the essential amino acid *phenylalanine* to *tyrosine.* This metabolic derangement is evidenced by an accumulation of excessive amounts of phenylalanine and alternative pathway by-products in the blood, and these are toxic to the central nervous system. Historically, PKU resulted in virtually certain mental retardation; affected individuals often were institutionalized and rarely reproduced. With the advent of universal neonatal screening in the United States since the 1960s and effective dietary treatment to prevent hyperphenylalaninemia during infancy and early childhood, genetically affected persons may avoid the devastating effects of this disease, have relatively normal development, and become pregnant. For women who do conceive, PKU poses a significant environmental risk for their developing fetus. The care of these women and their infants presents a unique perinatal challenge.

An estimated 3000 healthy young women of childbearing age with successfully treated PKU are in the United States.[104] However, most discontinued their special diet in childhood because, at the time, most doctors believed it was safe to do so. Unfortunately, their blood phenylalanine levels are very high when they become pregnant if they are eating a normal diet. In up to 90% of such cases, the offspring will be microcephalic and/or have mental retardation. These babies also have an increased incidence of low birth weight, cardiac defects, and characteristic facial features regardless of whether they are themselves affected with PKU.[97,98] They cannot be helped by the PKU diet, or they suffer from brain damage caused entirely by their mothers' high phenylalanine levels during pregnancy. To prevent such damage, these women should resume their special PKU diets during preconception. Studies have identified improved long-term outcomes when desirable phenylalanine levels (2 to 8 mg/dL) are achieved at least 3 months before pregnancy and maintained throughout gestation.[102] Phenylalanine levels drop quickly once dietary restrictions are instituted, and there is a strong correlation between maternal blood levels and neonatal outcome.[102]

About 1 baby in 14,000 inherits PKU when both parents have the PKU gene and both pass it on to their baby. Neonatal blood screening will identify these PKU babies. If this screening is performed within the first 24 hours of life, the American Academy of Pediatrics recommends re-screening at 1 to 2 weeks of age to avoid missed cases of PKU. Once identified, PKU babies should be fed a special formula that contains protein but no phenylalanine, started within the first 7 to 10 days of life, and they must remain on an individualized, restricted diet throughout childhood/adolescence, and generally for life. In some instances, breastfeeding may be possible.[88] When treatment is discontinued too soon, risks include blindness, learning disabilities, behavioral disturbances, and a decrease in IQ. When no treatment is instituted at all, phenylalanine accumulates in the bloodstream and causes brain damage and mental retardation.

RENAL DISEASE

Maternal adaptation to pregnancy involves major changes in renal function and structure. Renal hemodynamic changes begin early in pregnancy and before significant expansion of plasma volume. Renal blood flow increases in the first trimester by 35% to 60% and then decreases from the second trimester to term. Additional changes include an increase in the glomerular filtration rate (GFR) and effective renal plasma flow, a decrease in renal vascular resistance, an activation of the renin-angiotensin-aldosterone system, and increased retention of sodium and water. These changes place unique demands on the renal system. Women with preexisting renal disease may have a successful pregnancy outcome with proper prenatal care; however, some women do experience fetal loss and deterioration in renal function. Furthermore, moderate or severe renal dysfunction complicates pregnancy and increases maternal and fetal risks and adverse outcomes.[16]

Renal disease in pregnancy may occur as a result of urinary tract infections, glomerular disease, or severe hypertension or as a complication of systemic diseases including diabetes and systemic lupus erythematosus.[84] Regardless of the underlying etiologic factors, pregnancy outcome relates most closely to these factors: the presence of hypertension and the degree of renal insufficiency before and during pregnancy.[84] Many women with renal disorders are hypertensive before pregnancy, and they often develop a superimposed pregnancy-induced hypertension leading to preeclampsia.[83] Even those with previously normal blood pressures run an increased risk for developing hypertension during pregnancy. The presence of hypertension in these pregnancies represents a significant risk to the fetus and is strongly associated with IUGR, preterm delivery, and perinatal loss.

Drug therapy to control chronic hypertension has been shown to have a beneficial effect on fetal outcome and generally is continued throughout pregnancy. Renal insufficiency, as measured by creatinine clearance or serum creatinine level, also has implications for fetal outcome. Mild to moderate renal insufficiency (serum creatinine less than 1.5 mg/dL) is associated with a generally favorable outcome, whereas severe insufficiency (serum creatinine greater than 1.6 mg/dL) often carries an increased risk for perinatal death. Persistent proteinuria also may increase fetal loss, and a urinary protein excretion rate higher than 0.5 g/24 hr may be an independent predictor of fetal outcome.[112] As a rule, the number of preterm deliveries and growth-restricted infants increases with increasing blood pressure and decreasing renal function.

Bacteriuria occurs in 2% to 7% of pregnancies. If untreated, asymptomatic bacteriuria may lead to pyelonephritis or acute cystitis. Risks for the fetus are preterm birth and IUGR. Fetal death is an additional risk with pyelonephritis. Prophylactic antibiotics (suppressive therapy) should be given to women with persistent or frequent recurrence of bacteriuria or a history of pyelonephritis in pregnancy.[147]

Two special circumstances are dialysis during pregnancy and pregnancy after renal transplant. Women undergoing dialysis rarely become pregnant. When pregnancy does occur, it is associated with significant perinatal morbidity and mortality, with spontaneous abortions reaching 50%. Hemodialysis also is associated with numerous complications, including placental abruption, polyhydramnios, IUGR, preterm labor, and pregnancy loss.[56,106] The risk may be lower with ambulatory peritoneal dialysis.[56] Pregnancy after transplantation is more common and has a better prognosis than pregnancy managed by dialysis.[84] A long interval from transplantation to conception and use of a low dose of prednisone are predictive of successful outcome.[16] **Infants born after maternal transplantation are commonly preterm. A wide range of perinatal problems have been noted, thus requiring specialized care at a tertiary center. Other complications may include growth restriction, RDS, congenital anomalies, adrenocortical insufficiency, hyperviscosity, seizures, and neonatal sepsis.**[66] Concerns persist about neonatal complications if exposure to immunosuppressive therapy occurred while in utero. The criteria used to predict fetal outcome with other renal patients (i.e., hypertension, renal insufficiency) also have predictive value in post-transplantation pregnancies. Acute renal failure in pregnancy is associated with a maternal mortality rate of 20% and an increased fetal mortality rate.[80]

NEUROLOGIC DISORDERS

The risks that accompany pregnancies complicated by maternal neurologic disorders vary according to the individual disease entity and pertain to both the course of the mother's disease and pregnancy outcome. The physiologic and hormonal changes of pregnancy can influence the course of chronic neuromuscular disorders, such as epilepsy, multiple sclerosis, and myasthenia gravis. The medications used to control these disorders can be particularly problematic for the fetus.

The prevalence of *maternal seizure disorders* is about 4 in every 1000 pregnancies, and most are treated with antiepileptic drugs (AEDs). The disorders and/or the AEDs have been associated with increased fetal and neonatal risks, including spontaneous abortion, prematurity, small for gestational age, congenital defects, intrauterine demise, neonatal depression, and hemorrhage. Significant numbers of epileptic women experience an increase in seizure activity during pregnancy. This is probably because of decreased compliance with medication regimens, physiologic changes associated with pregnancy, and gestational changes in plasma levels of anticonvulsant drugs.[91,108] There is evidence that maternal seizures may compromise fetal oxygenation, possibly because of diminished placental blood flow or maternal hypoxemia resulting from post-seizure apnea. For these reasons, control of maternal seizure activity with anticonvulsants is one of the primary goals of prenatal care.

Placental transport of anticonvulsants does occur, resulting in fetal levels that approximate or, in some cases, exceed maternal levels.[21] Although the majority of infants born to women with epilepsy are normal, these infants are at increased risk for poor outcomes.[153] **Many studies have demonstrated an increased incidence of congenital defects in the offspring of epileptic women treated with anticonvulsants. Estimates of risks vary, but studies report a 2½-fold increased risk over the general population when AED monotherapy is used and a 5-fold increased risk when multiple AEDs are used during pregnancy.**[108,110] The teratogenic potential of most individual AEDs remains unclear, but valproate seems to be consistently associated with the highest rates of congenital malformations and the use of other AEDs is recommended if possible during pregnancy.[20,160] Although many newer AEDs are listed as class B medications in pregnancy, reports of teratogenicity are just now surfacing, so caution should be used with all anticonvulsants.[53,75] **The most common major congenital malformations associated with AEDs are neural tube defects (e.g., spina bifida), orofacial defects (e.g., cleft lip, cleft palate), heart malformations (e.g., ventricular septal defect), urogenital defects (e.g., hypospadias), and skeletal abnormalities (e.g., radial ray defects, phalangeal hypoplasias).**[107] The influence of the seizure disorder itself, as well as genetic makeup, cannot be ignored. Maternal folic acid supplementation has been shown to improve pregnancy outcomes for women taking AEDs.[130,160]

Infants born to mothers treated with anticonvulsants, especially barbiturates, may exhibit signs of generalized depression, including decreased respiratory effort, poor muscle tone, and feeding difficulties. They also may have symptoms indicative of drug withdrawal (see Chapter 11). These symptoms are usually present in the first week of life and include tremors, restlessness,

hypertonia, and hyperventilation.[21] In addition, abnormal clotting and hemorrhage in the offspring of women treated with phenytoin, phenobarbital, and primidone have been reported. This appears to be caused by a decrease in vitamin K–dependent clotting factors. Hemorrhage usually starts within the first 24 hours, is often severe, and may result in death. Infants born to these mothers should have cord blood clotting studies done, vitamin K prophylaxis on admission to the nursery, and close observation. Reports of long-term sequelae for the infants of epileptic mothers with AED use during pregnancy, especially the third trimester, include possible cognitive and behavioral deficiencies.[107]

Multiple sclerosis (MS) frequently strikes women during their reproductive years. The onset of MS usually is insidious; the course is marked by a seemingly capricious cycle of exacerbation and remission. A wide range of sensory, motor, and functional changes is associated with this disease; the type and severity of symptoms vary dramatically from one individual to another and in any one patient over time. The disease is a T-cell–mediated autoimmune disease of the central nervous system triggered by unknown exogenous agents in individuals with specific genetics.[73] Pregnancy usually is well tolerated and may be associated with MS stability or improvement. The reported effects of the disease on pregnancy outcomes, including risk for malformations, cesarean section rates, newborn birth weight, and rate of preterm delivery, are inconsistent. Some report no increase in adverse pregnancy outcomes,[114,169] whereas other groups report a higher cesarean rate as well as a greater number of low-birth-weight infants in mothers with MS.[45] Alterations in neural function, fatigue, and general weakness may play a role in pregnancy outcomes. During the postpartum period, a higher-than-expected relapse rate has been identified and is associated with hormonal changes.[52,163] However, in women with MS, the disease process itself is not a threat to fetal or neonatal well-being. **The priority for neonatal care providers is to determine the extent of the mother's disability, including her level of fatigue and her ability to care for her infant. The availability of appropriate support systems, both personal and professional, should be assessed, and needed follow-up and referrals should be made.**

Even though the prognosis for these infants is excellent, some factors associated with MS are potentially problematic. Bladder dysfunction, common in women with MS, often results in urinary tract infections during pregnancy. Associated fetal and neonatal problems include preterm delivery and sepsis. Early identification and prompt treatment with appropriate antibiotics should minimize these risks. An additional area of concern is the variety of drugs administered to MS patients. Immunosuppressants are frequently used during severe exacerbations. The placental transport and fetal risk vary with the individual agent used. Prednisone and intravenous steroids generally are considered safe for use in pregnancy.[73] Azathioprine also is generally considered safe because the fetal liver lacks the enzyme that converts azathioprine to its active metabolites, thus protecting the fetus from any teratogenic effects from this drug. However, neonatal hematologic and immune impairment have been reported in some exposed infants.[60] Cyclophosphamide has been associated with skeletal defects, growth retardation, and preterm labor[19] and is best avoided during pregnancy. Cyclosporine is not teratogenic; however, it may be associated with prematurity and growth restriction. Early in-utero exposure to interferon beta is controversial.[124] Other drug therapies should be evaluated carefully before use because definitive knowledge about safety in pregnancy may be lacking.[60] A final consideration is a long-term one: the incidence of MS in the offspring of a parent with the disease is 4%, compared with 0.1% in the general population.[73]

Myasthenia gravis (MG) is a chronic autoimmune disease that causes neuromuscular dysfunction and is encountered rarely in pregnancy; only 1 in 20,000 pregnancies is complicated by MG.[81] Cells of the immune system make proteins called *antibodies* that block nerve impulses to the muscles. Antibodies to acetylcholine receptor (AchR) have been found in most affected persons. Distinguishing features include generalized weakness and muscle fatigue with activity. Persons with MG also may experience respiratory compromise and difficulty swallowing.[81] The course of MG during pregnancy is unpredictable and may vary in different pregnancies in the same woman.[59] Exacerbations occur in approximately 40% of pregnancies and remission in 30%, with the remaining 30% experiencing no change. During the first trimester and the first month postpartum, exacerbations are more likely.[81] Corticosteroids can be used to maintain the remissions of MG and should be continued on the lowest possible doses throughout the pregnancy and postpartum period. Immunosuppressive agents like methotrexate, cyclophosphamide, and mycophenolate mofetil are contraindicated in pregnancy, but azathioprine and cyclosporine A are sometimes used and plasmapheresis and intravenous immunoglobulins can be effective in the treatment of myasthenic crises during pregnancy. Instrumental delivery may be needed in the second stage as MG mothers are more likely to become exhausted.[81]

Infants born to myasthenic mothers may be affected by the drug therapy and the underlying immunologic dysfunction. Increased rates of premature rupture of membranes (PROM), preterm delivery, and cesarean birth have been reported.[59] **An additional risk stems from transplacentally acquired antiacetylcholine receptor antibodies, which cause approximately 12% of these newborns to experience a transient, self-limited course of MG.** It is difficult to predict which pregnancies will result in an affected infant, although infants born to women with very high AChR antibody titers may be at highest risk.[81] **Affected infants usually present at birth or within the first 24 hours of life with generalized weakness, a feeble cry, diminished suck and swallow, and a decreased respiratory effort that may require mechanical support.[59] Therefore plans should be made in advance for delivery of the mother with MG, and intensive care facilities for the newborn should be available immediately. Symptoms from neonatal MG generally subside within a few weeks after birth and do not recur.**

MG is not a contraindication to pregnancy and can usually be managed well with relatively safe and effective therapies, including maternal rest. Standard therapies for some obstetric complications, such as preeclampsia and preterm labor, may need to be altered in women with MG.[81] Vaginal delivery is recommended if possible. Breast feeding is not contraindicated but depends on maternal medications and infant and maternal health postpartum.

SYSTEMIC LUPUS ERYTHEMATOSUS

Systemic lupus erythematosus (SLE) is an autoimmune disease that presents primarily in women of childbearing age. The pathogenesis involves the production of autoantibodies and immune complexes. The clinical effects of lupus range from mild or subclinical disease to serious illness affecting multiple organ systems. The leading causes of death are infections and renal failure. In pregnancy, SLE is associated with an increased incidence of preeclampsia, thrombotic events, spontaneous abortion, preterm delivery, IUGR, and stillbirths.[113,152] Outcome is best when infections, renal disease, and hypertension do not complicate pregnancy and when pregnancy occurs with prolonged disease remission.[49,137] Reported frequency of SLE flares in pregnancy is 15% to 60%.[2] When necessary, treatments used with pregnancies complicated by SLE include anti-inflammatory, antimalarial, immunosuppressive, and biological drugs and/or anticoagulants.[49]

The neonatal manifestations of SLE are rare and are attributed to the placental transfer of maternal antibodies to the fetus. Usual findings of neonatal lupus include a transient lupus-like rash (erythematous lesions of the face, scalp, and upper thorax), thrombocytopenia, and hemolysis.[2] These findings generally are transient and clear within a few months. **A strong association has been established between maternal antibodies to the anti-Ro/SS-A and anti-La/SS-B antigens and congenital heart block, a rare manifestation of neonatal lupus syndrome.**[2] The fetal heart block may be detected with antenatal testing; some authors believe that antenatal fetal surveillance with nonstress tests should begin at 28 weeks' gestation. **Infants are treated with cardiac pacemakers after delivery; however, about one third of affected infants die within 3 years.**[164]

HEART DISEASE

Significant changes in cardiovascular function accompany normal pregnancy. Plasma and red blood cell volumes rise, heart rate and cardiac output increase, and peripheral vascular resistance falls. These changes facilitate increased uterine blood flow, placental perfusion, and fetal oxygenation and growth. They also increase maternal oxygen consumption and cardiovascular workload and can further compromise the cardiovascular status of women with preexisting serious heart disease. Approximately 2% to 4% of childbearing-age women have concomitant heart disease.[86] Pregnancy creates a risk for maternal cardiovascular complications, but especially for those with underlying heart disease, and includes an increased incidence of thromboembolism and sudden death.[85,146] In some cases, such as Eisenmenger's syndrome and primary pulmonary hypertension, the risk to maternal survival is so great that pregnancy is contraindicated. In general, how well the woman with heart disease tolerates pregnancy depends on the specific disease process and the degree to which her cardiac status is compromised.[123]

Maternal heart disease also affects the fetus. Fetal risks are the result of genetic factors, alterations in placental perfusion and exchange, and the effect of maternally administered drugs. **The genetic risk is demonstrated by the increased incidence of congenital heart defects that occur in the offspring of parents who have such a defect.** The exact risk depends on the specific parental lesion, mode of inheritance, and exposure to environmental triggers.[23]

Alterations in placental perfusion and gas exchange occur when the mother's condition involves chronic hypoxemia or a significant decrease in cardiac output. These factors increase the threat to the fetus, with fetal risk increasing as maternal cardiac status declines. Chronic maternal hypoxemia results in a decrease in oxygen available to the fetus and is associated with fetal loss, prematurity, and IUGR.[168] Significant reductions in maternal cardiac output create decreased uterine blood flow and diminished placental perfusion with a resulting impairment in the exchange of nutrients, oxygen, and metabolic wastes. **Possible fetal and neonatal consequences include spontaneous abortion, IUGR, neonatal asphyxia, central nervous system (CNS) damage, and intrauterine, intrapartum, or neonatal death.**[85]

A wide variety of drugs are used in the management of maternal cardiovascular disease. Although sometimes it is difficult to differentiate drug effects from the effects of the underlying disease, some associations between drug administration and fetal outcomes can be made. Anticoagulants are used to decrease the risk for thromboembolism, especially in women with artificial valves, a history of thrombophlebitis, or rheumatic heart disease. **Oral anticoagulants, specifically warfarin sodium (Coumadin), have been associated with fetal malformations, including nasal hypoplasia and epiphyseal stippling, when administered during the first trimester. They also have been associated with eye and CNS abnormalities when administered later in pregnancy. The incidence of warfarin embryopathy is estimated to be 15% to 25%.** Warfarin also is associated with maternal and fetal hemorrhage. Because of these risks, warfarin is contraindicated in pregnancy except in special circumstances such as pregnancy in women with prosthetic heart valves.[38] Heparin is considered the preferred agent for anticoagulation therapy during pregnancy. **Heparin does not cross the placenta; therefore it does not result in fetal anticoagulation or neonatal hemorrhage (although maternal hemorrhage still may occur), nor has it been associated with congenital defects. Low-molecular-weight heparin is another alternative for anticoagulation during pregnancy.**[51] In general, patients being treated with low-molecular-weight heparin during pregnancy are converted to unfractionated heparin during the final weeks of pregnancy because of the ease of rapid reversal of anticoagulation for labor and delivery. Some studies, however, did not demonstrate any difference in bleeding complications for gravidas continued on low-molecular-weight heparin versus those who were converted to unfractionated heparin.[89]

Antiarrhythmic medications and cardiac glycosides used during pregnancy cross the placenta to varying degrees. They have not been implicated in fetal malformations and, although several have been associated with minor complications, generally are considered safe for use in pregnancy.[136] Reported complications include uterine contractions (quinidine, disopyramide), decreased birth weight (digoxin, disopyramide), and maternal hypotension with a sudden decrease in placental perfusion (verapamil).

Antihypertensives and diuretics also have been used in the treatment of cardiovascular disease during pregnancy. Labetalol and methyldopa are commonly used in pregnant women with chronic hypertension. These medications have been studied in prospective trials that revealed no adverse fetal or maternal outcomes.[58,157] Their use in the first trimester has also demonstrated safety. Atenolol has been associated with fetal growth restriction and abnormal placental growth.[24,54] Calcium channel blockers, such as nifedipine, are also safely used during pregnancy without an increase in major birth defects or adverse neonatal outcomes.[143] Diuretic use in pregnancy remains an area of some controversy. Fetal and neonatal compromise can result from diuretic-induced electrolyte and glucose imbalance and decreased placental perfusion caused by maternal hypovolemia. The use of thiazide diuretics has been linked to neonatal liver damage and thrombocytopenia. In general, diuretic use is restricted to women with pulmonary edema or acute cardiac or renal failure. Antihypertensive medications are not clearly shown to reduce the risk for preeclampsia in the hypertensive patient.[143]

Although a great number of complications are possible, remember that, with few exceptions, most of the drugs used in the treatment of maternal heart disease can be used in pregnancy if the maternal condition warrants it. **Angiotensin-converting enzyme inhibitors are contraindicated in pregnancy because of an association with fetal injury (renal dysfunction, fetal oliguria, oligohydramnios, fetal skull hypoplasia) and fetal death.**

RESPIRATORY DISEASE

Respiratory function is altered even in normal pregnancy. Changes include a decrease in lung volume and increases in oxygen consumption, tidal volume, and minute ventilation. Significant decreases in maternal respiratory function and oxygenation can result in fetal growth restriction and fetal hypoxia with negative outcomes, but careful management of respiratory disease during pregnancy generally results in a favorable outcome.

Asthma is the most common respiratory disease in pregnancy, occurring in 3% to 12% of women, and the prevalence among pregnant women is rising.[115] For about two thirds of pregnant women, the course of asthma changes.[140] Infants born to women whose asthma is well controlled usually do well; unstable or worsening disease, especially status asthmaticus, increases fetal risk.[14] Commonly used asthma medications (e.g., long-acting beta agonists, inhaled corticosteroids, oral corticosteroids, other bronchodilators, and cromones) are generally considered safe for use in pregnancy. **However, limited studies have associated maternal bronchodilator use and cromone exposure with an elevated risk for fetal gastroschisis**[99] **and a slight increase in fetal musculoskeletal malformation,**[150] **respectively.** Additional research is needed to help determine whether a real risk exists and to guide asthma treatment during pregnancy. Presently, clinical evidence supports pharmacologic asthma control because the fetus is at greater risk from inadequate control of asthma than from asthma medications.[14]

Fetal risks related to maternal asthma depend on the severity of the condition. Controlled asthma carries few risks for the fetus. However, severe or uncontrolled asthma increases the risk for infant death and the incidence of low birth weight, IUGR, preterm birth (possibly influenced by steroid use), and the need for cesarean delivery.[82] Risks are higher in poorly controlled asthma patients.[15] Noncompliance with treatment, respiratory tract infections, allergens and irritants, smoking, gastroesophageal reflux, and exercise can lead to asthma exacerbations.[115]

Cystic fibrosis (CF) was once considered a lethal childhood disease, but the life expectancy of a person with CF has increased, and is currently at about 35 years.[127] With careful planning and appropriate medical care, women with CF of childbearing age may conceive and have successful pregnancies with good neonatal outcomes, especially if their nutritional state and lung function remain good.[67] Women with severe disease may be cautioned to avoid conception because there is a risk for significant deterioration during gestation. Women who are positive for *Burkholderia cepacia* in sputum also have a worse prognosis.[67] Pregnancy in women with CF is likely to be associated with increased health care utilization and more antibiotic use compared with that of non-pregnant women with CF; high rate of gestational diabetes (12%) compared with non-CF pregnancies; and aggressive interventions to ensure weight gain, including the use of total parenteral nutrition for some.[33,119,154] Women with CF may experience pulmonary infections, which should be treated promptly and vigorously with antibiotics, fluids, and respiratory therapy. **Fetal risks related to CF include prematurity, IUGR, and perinatal death, caused primarily by maternal hypoxemia and infection. Because all infants born to mothers with CF will be heterozygous carriers for CF (at least), genetic counseling and carrier testing of the father are important components of preconceptual care and early prenatal care.**[154]

Maternal Behavior

Maternal health behavior is an important component of neonatal and childhood health and may even be the single most important factor for the overall health of a child.[120] Health behaviors evaluated here are smoking, substance abuse, and nutrition, but other maternal behaviors also influence pregnancy outcomes, such as sleep patterns and exercise. Appropriate preconceptual and prenatal counseling regarding maternal health behaviors can help optimize neonatal health.[71,128]

SMOKING

From 16% to 25% of women in the United States smoke during pregnancy,[125,158] with approximately 60% of smokers continuing to smoke through pregnancy. Of those who quit during pregnancy, half resume smoking by 6 months postpartum,[101] putting children at risk for second-hand smoke. It is well established that maternal smoking is a risk factor for stillbirths, IUGR, placental abruption, placental previa, PROM, and preterm labor.[158] Long-term effects include childhood obstructive airway disease, sudden infant death syndrome (SIDS), neurodevelopmental abnormalities, and childhood cancer,[158] and concerns about exposure to second-hand smoke continue to escalate. The exact mechanism by which fetal growth is restricted or fetal health is compromised is not entirely clear; reduced uterine artery blood flow, reduced placental blood flow resulting from vasoconstriction or smaller fetal capillaries in the placental capillary bed, elevated nicotine and carbon monoxide levels, and chronic fetal hypoxia all may play a role.[71,94] Fetal risk increases with the number of cigarettes smoked, maternal anemia, and poor nutrition.[69] **The babies of smokers may undergo withdrawal-like symptoms manifested by jittery movements and may be more difficult to soothe.**[95]

Eliminating or reducing smoking, especially by the end of the first trimester, can improve fetal growth and health. Smoking cessation programs consistently implemented during prenatal visits have been shown to significantly improve smoking cessation rates.[109] The use of nicotine patches to facilitate smoking cessation during pregnancy is controversial.[125] Smoking cessation during pregnancy must be a major priority in counseling women preconceptually and prenatally because these are times when women may be most receptive to quitting because of a strong desire for a healthy pregnancy and baby.[109]

SUBSTANCE ABUSE

Prenatal substance abuse rates vary greatly; however, it is estimated that about 11% of childbearing women have used illegal substances.[17] Use of drugs and alcohol by the mother places the fetus and newborn at risk for a plethora of structural, functional, and developmental problems. Perinatal morbidity is related to the direct effects of the abused substance on the developing fetus, its sudden withdrawal, the interactions of multiple abused substances, the nutritional effects of addiction on the mother, and the social and health care implications of substance abuse.[13,44,159]

Alcohol is one of the most commonly abused substances during pregnancy. Although known to be a teratogen since the 1970s, about 40% of women in the United States drink some alcohol during pregnancy and about 3% to 5% drink heavily throughout pregnancy.[62] Alcohol in the maternal circulation crosses the placenta, resulting in direct fetal exposure to alcohol and its metabolites.[22] **There may be a wide range of effects on the exposed fetus; these include developmental and behavioral abnormalities, spontaneous abortion, stillbirth, craniofacial malformations, growth restriction, preterm birth, CNS dysfunction, and organ or joint abnormalities.**[13,22,55] The mechanism of fetal injury is not entirely clear but is likely related to three main factors: a teratogenic effect, hypoxia as a result of increased oxygen consumption, and a diminished ability to use amino acids in protein synthesis.[22] The expression of fetal alcohol effects ranges from subtle to extreme and depends on the timing of exposure, the dose, and the genetic response of the mother and fetus to the effects of alcohol. Secondary factors such as maternal age, nutritional status, general health, and the effects of other abused substances also may influence outcome.[141,166] When the more severe effects are exhibited, the condition is known as ***fetal alcohol syndrome (FAS)***. **FAS is characterized by growth restriction, physical dysmorphic features including facial anomalies (small palpebral fissures, low nasal bridge, indistinct philtrum, thin upper lip, shortened lower jaw), and neurologic dysfunction, including mental retardation and neurodevelopmental deficits.**[134] **Other physical abnormalities involve the heart, skeletal system, and ears. "Fetal alcohol spectrum disorders (FASD)" is an umbrella term for FAS and other less physically noticeable yet long-term effects of alcohol exposure on the fetus.**[22] **Infants with FASD also may exhibit problems with suck, tremors, irritability, and hypertonus related to alcohol withdrawal.** Continued abnormalities in motor, behavioral, and intellectual development often persist into childhood. Safe levels of alcohol intake have not been established; therefore women should be advised to avoid alcohol intake during pregnancy.

Chemical dependency in pregnancy is a complex problem and creates a high-risk patient. The mother's reporting of drug use often is unreliable; frequently, more than one substance is involved, and there may be a cycle of drug use and periodic abstinence during pregnancy. In addition, a host of medical and social problems are associated with maternal drug abuse. Substance abusers generally have poor health; infectious diseases such as pneumonia, sexually transmitted disease (including human immunodeficiency virus [HIV] infection and acquired immunodeficiency syndrome [AIDS]), urinary tract infections, and hepatitis are common.[13,34] Nutrition and prenatal care often are inadequate; anemia frequently is seen. These factors contribute to a poor pregnancy outcome and make it difficult to isolate the effects of any one drug on the fetus. However, several generalizations can be made. The majority of drugs used by the mother, including opiates (e.g., methadone, heroin), barbiturates, and sedative-hypnotic drugs, cross the placenta and affect the fetus. **Fetal risks include growth restriction, malformations, intrauterine demise, prematurity, asphyxia, CNS dysfunction, and neurobehavioral abnormalities. Fetal drug dependence does occur and is associated with neonatal abstinence syndrome (NAS), which is manifested by CNS irritability and gastrointestinal dysfunction**[17,34] (see Chapter 11).

Cocaine use by the mother merits special attention. Cocaine is a CNS stimulant that produces vasoconstriction, tachycardia, and hypertension in both the mother and the fetus. **Its use during pregnancy has been linked to growth restriction, smaller head circumference, genitourinary tract anomalies, placental abruption, stillbirths, RDS, congenital infection, NAS, and cerebral infarcts, as well as impaired performance as measured with the Brazelton behavioral assessment tool.**[13,121]

All prenatal care providers should thoroughly assess pregnant women for alcohol and substance abuse at each prenatal visit, and treatment interventions should be initiated when abuse is identified. Toxicology screening of maternal blood or urine can verify suspicions of abuse; however, universal screening is not currently recommended. **Neonatal urine or meconium screening can provide an accurate indication of exposure when there are clinical indications of drug effect.** Laws in some states consider prenatal drug exposure to be a form of child abuse; thus the practitioner may be required to report positive drug tests in pregnant women or their newborns. (See Chapter 11 for a more complete discussion of complications in drug-exposed neonates.)

MATERNAL NUTRITION, MALNUTRITION, AND OBESITY

Maternal nutritional status and placental function during pregnancy can significantly influence the growth, development, and health of the fetus and newborn. Nutritional problems that interfere with fetal cell division (increases in cell number) can have permanent consequences. If the fetus is at a stage in which cells are only enlarging (increases in cell size), then nutritional deficits may be reversed if a healthy maternal dietary intake is resumed soon enough in the pregnancy. All women presenting for prenatal care should be questioned about their usual dietary intake and should have their weight and height assessed so that body mass index (BMI) can be determined and appropriate nutrition counseling initiated. BMI can be calculated by dividing a woman's prepregnancy weight in kilograms by her height in meters squared; it is the most frequently used single tool in determining obesity. If a woman's prepregnancy weight is unknown, the value obtained at the first prenatal visit should be used. Although the BMI values for classification vary, the Institute of Medicine (IOM) employs the relative weight classification and prepregnancy BMI values as follows[117]:

- Underweight: less than 19.8
- Healthy weight: 19.8 to 26
- Overweight: 26.1 to 29
- Obese: greater than 29

Optimal ranges for weight gain in singleton pregnancies are also based on the IOM recommendations. As a general rule, weight gain should be as follows: underweight women should gain 28 to 40 lb; normal-weight women, 25 to 35 lb; overweight women, 15 to 25 lb; obese women, up to 15 lb. The optimal weight gain for women carrying twins is 35 to 45 lb.[117] The IOM guidelines are continually being evaluated, but at least one study confirms that following these guidelines can improve pregnancy outcomes.[78] However, fewer than half of women gain the recommended weight during pregnancy,[165] with 43.3% of women gaining above the IOM guidelines.[149]

Prenatal nutrition involves more than appropriate weight gain; a variety of healthy foods should be consumed, providing essential nutrients. The dietary reference intakes (DRIs) increase for most nutrients during pregnancy. Protein, iron, vitamin A, and iodine requirements nearly double, yet some nutrient requirements do not change much.[156] Other maternal factors that should be considered when counseling women on nutrition include age, parity, preconceptual nutritional status, preexisting medical conditions, current medical conditions complicating the pregnancy, food likes and dislikes, and cultural influences. Each woman's counseling should be individualized, and referral to a nutrition specialist and other medical specialists may be indicated.[39]

Malnourished and underweight mothers have more perinatal losses and preterm births, and their newborns have lower Apgar scores and more frequently are of low birth weight (less than 2500 g). This is especially true of significantly underweight women (low BMI) and women with eating disorders, such as anorexia and bulimia, who fail to gain adequate weight during pregnancy.[165] Small-for-gestational-age (SGA) newborns, defined as below the tenth percentile birth weight for gestational age, have higher mortality rates in the perinatal period and are at risk for later problems such as insulin resistance and poor school performance.[165] However, it may be difficult to draw direct correlations between inadequate maternal diet and fetal growth unless the nutritional disturbances are severe. Many fetuses grow well despite suboptimal maternal nutrition, in part because of the complexities of placental transport and the ability of the fetus to be preferentially supplied with some nutrients.

Although reduced birth weight is associated with inadequate carbohydrate, protein, and total caloric intake, inappropriate amounts of other nutrients may also affect the fetus. Vitamin and mineral deficiencies have been linked to miscarriage and stillbirth, congestive heart failure (thiamine), megaloblastic anemia (folic acid, B_{12}), congenital anomalies including neural tube defects (folic acid, zinc, copper), and skeletal abnormalities (vitamin D, calcium).[90,161] Vitamin overdosage, especially of the fat-soluble vitamins, also has been implicated in fetal abnormalities. Vitamin A overdose has been associated with kidney malformations, neural or cranial defects, and hydrocephalus; vitamin D overdose has been linked with cardiac, neurologic, and renal defects.[39]

Obesity has become an epidemic in the United States and other developed countries. Obstetricians and gynecologists now cite obesity as the leading health problem confronting women today. It is a complex problem resulting from a combination of genetic, cultural, behavioral, socioeconomic, and environmental influences. Obesity affects all organ systems and contributes to a multitude of physiologic complications such as cardiovascular disease, gestational diabetes, infections, preeclampsia, and other adverse perinatal outcomes.[27,29]

Overweight, obese, and morbidly obese women (BMI greater than 40) are at risk for chorioamnionitis, preeclampsia, stillbirth, cesarean delivery, instrumental delivery, postpartum hemorrhage, perineal lacerations, and prolonged hospital stay. **Their offspring may suffer macrosomia, shoulder dystocia, meconium aspiration, fetal distress, early neonatal death, complications from cesarean birth, and birth defects.**[47] A 1% decrease in the number of obese pregnant women in the United States would result in 16,000 fewer cesarean births per year.[35]

In addition, obese women may be struggling with associated psychosocial problems such as poor self-esteem, guilt about weight, depression, and ridicule from family and others. Some may not seek prenatal care until pregnancy is well into the second or third trimester. Thus obese women should be considered at high risk for childbearing complications, and these women and their fetus/newborn should be monitored closely throughout gestation and the perinatal period. When problems are identified, individualized intervention strategies should be implemented in an attempt to promote normal birth weight (appropriate for gestational age [AGA]) and improve perinatal outcomes. In conclusion, maternal health behavior, including smoking, nutrition, and drug use, before and during pregnancy is associated with adverse outcomes for the newborn and also long-term health risks of the newborn well into adulthood. Supportive, informed prenatal care for pregnant women at risk is essential to improved newborn health.[28]

Obstetric Complications

ANTEPARTUM BLEEDING

Maternal cardiovascular support is crucial to fetal well-being. Chronic blood loss can lead to maternal anemia and a related decrease in oxygen-carrying capacity. Uncompensated acute bleeding results in diminished blood volume, decreased systolic pressure, decreased cardiac output, and ultimately decreased placental perfusion. The net effect on the fetus is decreased oxygenation and impaired nutrient delivery.

Gestational bleeding in the first or second trimester of pregnancy has been linked to increased risks of preterm labor, preterm birth, PROM, and low birth weight.[36] The most common causes of hemorrhage late in pregnancy include placental abruption and placenta previa. In an abruption, a normally implanted placenta separates from the uterine wall before the time of delivery, resulting in maternal bleeding and a functional decrease in uteroplacental size. A relationship between hypertensive disorders, cocaine use, and cigarette smoking and an increased incidence of abruptions has been reported.[12,61] The risk for abruption was four times higher in women with preterm PROM. In the presence of an intrauterine infection, the relative risk increased ninefold.[11] The separation may be partial or complete, involving peripheral and/or central portions of the placenta. Fetal compromise relates to the extent of the separation and to the frequent need for preterm delivery. When the abruption is small and bleeding is minimal, the pregnancy may continue without significant fetal compromise; however, remember that the decrease in uteroplacental surface area is irreversible and reduces the absolute placental capability. As the fetus grows or experiences additional stressors, its ability to tolerate the abruption may change. Extensive abruptions are poorly tolerated by both fetus and mother; the resulting maternal hemorrhage and decreased placental function lead to fetal asphyxia and, without immediate intervention, to intrauterine demise.[36,41]

A ***placenta previa*** exists when the placenta lies abnormally low in the uterus and to some extent covers or encroaches on the internal cervical os. In the latter part of pregnancy, the normal elongation of the lower uterine segment and changes in the cervix disrupt the attachment of the overlying placenta.[116] This generally presents as episodic, painless maternal bleeding, often accompanied by preterm labor. To avoid active labor with resulting maternal hemorrhage, fetal lung maturity is assessed at 35 to 37 weeks. If the lungs are sufficiently mature, a cesarean section is scheduled before the onset of labor. **Fetal compromise relates to the extent of the previa, severity of maternal hemorrhage, degree of the resulting fetal hypoxia, and gestational age at delivery.**[145]

Other placental abnormalities leading to antepartum bleeding include velamentous insertion and vasa previa. A ***vasa previa*** occurs when naked fetal vessels traverse the cervical os below the level of the fetal presenting part; it is associated with a high perinatal mortality rate. A ***velamentous insertion*** is defined as the insertion of the umbilical cord into the chorioamnionic membranes rather than the mass of the placenta.[131]

HYPERTENSIVE DISORDERS OF PREGNANCY

Chronic hypertension in pregnancy, defined as hypertension diagnosed before pregnancy or before 20 weeks' gestation, complicates 1% to 6% of births in the United States each year. **Chronic hypertension is associated with IUGR, preterm birth, placental abruption, and stillbirth.**[58] The degree of fetal compromise is related to the degree and control of maternal hypertension. Women with chronic hypertension have a 25% risk for developing superimposed preeclampsia.[133]

Gestational hypertension was defined by the Working Group on Research on Hypertension in Pregnancy as hypertension arising after 20 weeks in the absence of proteinuria.[133]

Preeclampsia, a type of pregnancy-induced hypertension, is a condition in which hypertension, accompanied by proteinuria and edema, develops during the second half of pregnancy in women with or without preexisting hypertensive disease. It is most common in primigravidae in obese women, in women with multiple gestations and molar pregnancies, in women with a family history of this disorder, and those with a history of pregestational diabetes mellitus.[144] As a perinatal complication, preeclampsia is significant because of its high toll in terms of both maternal and fetal well-being.

Pregnancy is normally associated with vasodilation and decreased peripheral vascular resistance. The net effect is that, even though there is a significant increase in blood volume, maternal blood pressure does not increase during pregnancy. In contrast, pregnancy-induced hypertension is associated with vasoconstriction and an increase in peripheral vascular resistance and arterial pressure. The result is a reduction in blood flow to the vital organs, including the kidney, liver, brain, and uterus; reduced maternal blood volume; and a host of maternal hepatic, CNS, and coagulation abnormalities. The major effect on the intrauterine environment is placental insufficiency caused by significant reductions in uteroplacental blood flow and the development of placental vascular abnormalities. **Associated fetal and neonatal risks include IUGR, prematurity with all of its attendant problems, perinatal asphyxia, and perinatal death.** The risk to the infant increases with earlier onset and increasingly severe maternal disease, such as chronic hypertension with superimposed preeclampsia.[144] **Maternal seizures (eclampsia) further compromise the fetus by promoting hypoxemia and acidosis, which can result in intrauterine demise.**

HELLP syndrome, a severe form of pregnancy-induced hypertension manifested by **h**emolysis, **e**levated **l**iver **e**nzymes, **l**ow **p**latelets, and renal function abnormalities, carries a high risk for fetal and maternal death. In mild cases of HELLP syndrome, conservative management may facilitate improvement in the condition before delivery, but the risk for IUGR remains. In many cases of HELLP syndrome, immediate delivery is indicated regardless of the gestational age of the fetus.[142] The use of steroids in HELLP has been shown to improve maternal oliguria, mean arterial pressure, mean increase in platelet count, mean increase in urinary output, and liver enzyme elevations. However, no evidence suggests an improvement in maternal and perinatal mortality or morbidity with the use of maternal steroids except with regard to improvement in fetal lung maturity.[105]

Drugs commonly used to treat pregnancy-induced hypertension include magnesium sulfate, hydralazine, labetalol, nifedipine, and other antihypertensive agents. Magnesium sulfate is the most commonly used agent in the United States for the prevention of maternal seizures and has been shown to be more effective than phenytoin (Dilantin).[57]

Hypotonia and CNS depression have been reported as neonatal side effects, yet no correlation has been found between neonatal magnesium level and Apgar score.[132] These effects are more likely the result of coexisting complications, such as prematurity and asphyxia.[139] Hydralazine and other antihypertensives are used in the treatment of severe maternal hypertension; actions include relaxation of the arterial bed, decreased vascular resistance, and decreased blood pressure. Maternal response to antihypertensives must be monitored carefully, because precipitous decreases in blood pressure reduce placental perfusion and further compromise the fetus.

INFECTION

Group B streptococcus (GBS) is a major cause of sepsis, meningitis, and death among newborn infants. It is estimated that 10% to 30% of all pregnant women are colonized with GBS in the vagina or rectum. The American College of Obstetricians and Gynecologists (ACOG) Committee on Obstetric Practice now recommends "vaginal or rectal group B streptococci screening cultures at 35 to 37 weeks of gestation for all pregnant women." Treatment for women with a positive culture, GBS bacteriuria in the current pregnancy, or a previously GBS-infected infant is usually penicillin.[30]

PRETERM LABOR

Preterm birth, defined as any birth before 37 weeks' gestation, poses an unparalleled threat to neonatal survival and well-being. Its cost, both human and economic, is staggering, and its prevention is a primary focus of modern obstetric care. Prevention is best accomplished through an aggressive effort to identify women at risk and close follow-up to achieve early recognition and appropriate intervention should preterm labor occur.[10] Unfortunately, many women continue to receive inadequate prenatal care or no care at all. Even women who obtain early and ongoing care often fail to recognize the signs of preterm labor and delay reporting symptoms until intervention becomes difficult if not impossible.[42]

Risk assessment markers in clinical use today include measurements of cervical length and the biochemical marker fetal fibronectin. ***Fetal fibronectin*** is a glycoprotein secreted by fetal membranes. Its presence in cervical-vaginal secretions between 22 and 35 weeks' gestation has been associated with an increased risk for preterm labor and delivery. Its absence (high negative predictive value) can be used to identify patients who are at low risk for preterm delivery.[10] ***Cervical length*** is assessed by three consecutive measurements using transvaginal ultrasound. The average length of the cervix varies with gestational change but is approximately 4 cm in length from 26 weeks. The length of the cervix has been inversely correlated to the risk for preterm birth.[76] Thus a combination of fetal fibronectin and cervical length may be used to assess the risk for preterm delivery for a given patient.[118]

Although in many specific instances, a definitive cause cannot be identified, it is possible to identify several factors that generally are associated with preterm labor and delivery.[10] **When preterm labor cannot be halted, it culminates in the delivery of a physiologically immature infant. The result is a host of neonatal problems that relate largely to the degree of immaturity** and also to compounding problems such as infant anomalies or maternal disease and to the events that led to the preterm delivery (e.g., asphyxia resulting from a bleeding placenta previa). **Problems commonly encountered in preterm infants include respiratory distress, asphyxia, hyperbilirubinemia, metabolic disturbances, fluid and electrolyte imbalance, neurologic and behavioral problems, infection, nutritional deficits and feeding problems,**

ineffective thermoregulation, cardiovascular disturbances, chronic respiratory disease, and hematologic disturbances.

Although hydration often is used as a first-line measure for preterm uterine activity, the data do not support the efficacy of hydration as a treatment for preterm labor.[148]

Beta-sympathomimetic agents, such as ritodrine hydrochloride and terbutaline sulfate, are commonly used as a means of interrupting preterm labor. They achieve their tocolytic action by maximizing the $beta_2$-adrenergic effects on the uterus, with a resulting decrease in uterine smooth muscle contractility.[42] Although these drugs are effective in prolonging gestation, they are associated also with maternal, fetal, and neonatal complications.[10] Mothers may experience tachycardia and dysrhythmias, hyperglycemia, hypokalemia, anxiety, nausea, and vomiting. Myocardial ischemia and pulmonary edema are rare but serious maternal side effects. The fetus also may develop tachycardia and hyperglycemia. **Neonates born after beta-sympathomimetic therapy may develop a rebound hypoglycemia in response to in utero hyperglycemia and overproduction of insulin. Beta-sympathomimetic tocolytic agents increase fetal aortic blood flow and fetal cardiac output that might increase fetal systolic pressure and cerebral blood flow, which can lead to an increased incidence of intracranial bleeding in immature fetal brains.**[122]

Magnesium sulfate has also been employed as a tocolytic. Magnesium sulfate decreases muscle contractility, thereby inhibiting uterine activity and effectively interrupting preterm labor. **Neonatal consequences of maternal magnesium administration include decreased muscle tone and drowsiness, as well as decreases in serum calcium level.**[42] A recent double-blind randomized control trial has suggested that magnesium sulfate given to preterm babies may decrease rates of gross motor dysfunction.[43]

Prostaglandins play an important role in the onset of labor. ***Prostaglandin synthetase inhibitors,*** such as indomethacin, are a class of pharmacologic agents that interfere with the body's synthesis of prostaglandin, thereby inhibiting prostaglandin-mediated uterine contractions. These drugs have been used to treat preterm labor. They can cause in utero constriction, or closure, of the ductus arteriosus with resulting development of fetal pulmonary hypertension and congestive heart failure. They also may lead to oligohydramnios and must be used with caution, especially late in the third trimester. **Other neonatal risks include decreased platelet activity and gastrointestinal irritation.**[18] The use of selective cyclooxygenase (COX-2) inhibitors in preterm labor treatment is being investigated.[100]

Calcium channel blockers, such as nifedipine, also have a demonstrated ability to interfere with the labor process. Uterine contractility is directly related to the presence of free calcium. Increased calcium concentration enhances muscle contractility, whereas decreased calcium levels inhibit contractility.[42] Calcium antagonists block the entry of calcium into cells and inhibit uterine muscle contraction. In animal studies, these drugs have been associated with fetal acidosis.[50] However, lower umbilical artery pH values or lower Apgar scores have not been associated with nifedipine.[87]

The use of ***progesterone*** suppositories in preterm labor prevention was recently investigated by daFonseca et al.[44a] The study involved 142 women with high-risk singleton pregnancies treated with either 100 mg progesterone or placebo vaginal suppository. The study found statistically significant differences in the frequency of uterine activity and rate of preterm delivery in women treated with progesterone.[10] Intramuscular progesterone injection has also been studied in the prevention of recurrent preterm birth. In women with a history of preterm birth, there appears to be a beneficial effect of intramuscular progesterone to prevent recurrent preterm birth. No evidence supports the use of progesterone as a prophylactic agent in other women at risk for preterm birth such as women with short cervix or twin gestation.[48]

Corticosteroid treatment of pregnant women who deliver prematurely was first introduced in 1972 to enhance fetal lung maturity. In 1994, the National Institutes of Health (NIH) sponsored a Consensus Development Conference on the Effect of Corticosteroids for Fetal Maturation on Perinatal Outcomes. **The consensus panel concluded that giving a single course of corticosteroids to pregnant women at risk for preterm birth reduced the risk for death, RDS, and intraventricular hemorrhage in preterm infants.** The 1994 panel noted that the optimal benefit of antenatal corticosteroid therapy lasts 7 days. Since then, the use of repeated courses of antenatal corticosteroids became widespread in the United States, England, and Australia. In 2000, the NIH reconvened to present research of repeated courses of antenatal corticosteroid therapy. In studies in preterm animals, multiple doses of antenatal corticosteroids improved lung function when compared with a single dose. Human studies suggested possible benefits in reduction of the incidence and severity of RDS and the incidence of patent ductus arteriosus. **Little or no evidence supported a reduction in mortality rate or reductions in the incidence of intraventricular hemorrhage, chronic lung disease, sepsis, necrotizing enterocolitis, or retinopathy of prematurity with repeated antenatal corticosteroid therapy. Some of the suggested fetal risks of repeated antenatal corticosteroid therapy include decreased somatic and brain growth, adrenal suppression, neonatal sepsis, chronic lung disease, and death.** The current clinical recommendations based on the 2000 NIH Consensus Statement are as follows[6]:

- All pregnant women between 24 and 34 weeks' gestation who are at risk for preterm delivery within 7 days should be considered candidates for antenatal treatment with a single course of corticosteroids.
- Treatment consists of two doses of 12 mg of betamethasone given intramuscularly 24 hours apart or four doses of 6 mg of dexamethasone given intramuscularly 12 hours apart.
- Repeated courses of corticosteroids should not be used routinely. In general, it should be reserved for patients enrolled in randomized controlled trials.

ENVIRONMENTAL EFFECTS OF LABOR ON THE FETUS

Effects of Contractions

During labor, the dynamics of uterine contractions alter the intrauterine environment and influence the fetus. A "healthy" fetus is equipped to withstand the challenge of labor, but when the fetus is compromised or the labor is dysfunctional, the fetus can be taxed beyond its capacity, placing it at risk for further compromise, asphyxia, or intrauterine death.

Strong uterine contractions are characterized by decreased blood flow through the intervillous spaces in the placenta. As blood flow decreases, a corresponding decline in placental gas exchange occurs and the fetus must depend on its existing reserves to maintain oxygenation until placental blood flow is reestablished. The net effect is that fetal Pao_2 decreases as the consequence of uterine contraction. In the fetus with adequate reserves, the fall in Pao_2 is not drastic; the fetus remains adequately oxygenated and so can tolerate the stress of labor.

Fetal Reserve

The factors that influence fetal reserve fall into two general categories: those that diminish reserves and those that exhaust reserves. When fetal oxygen reserves are diminished, the fetus has less-than-optimal oxygenation at the onset of a contraction. This may occur as a consequence of any condition that decreases placental exchange, including reduced placental surface area caused by abruption, placenta previa, an abnormally small placenta, decreased placental perfusion caused by maternal hypotension or hypertension, or maternal hypoxemia. Oxygen reserves can be diminished also as a result of a reduction in fetal oxygen-carrying capacity, as in severe anemia or acute fetal hemorrhage.[79]

A fetal reserve that is adequate at the onset of labor can be exhausted by factors that place unusual demands on the fetus. Exhaustion of reserves occurs with contractions that last for a prolonged period, are of extremely high intensity, or occur with increased frequency and without an adequate recovery period between individual contractions.[79] This is often a consequence of the use of oxytocic agents to induce or augment labor.

Determination of cord gases at delivery can be used to determine the timing of a hypoxic or neurologic event. A base excess of equal to or less than 12 mmol/L generally is defined as the threshold that may be associated with hypoxic injury.[135] Fetal pulse oximetry may also be used. Decreased fetal pulse oximetry values, especially prolonged and recurrent recordings less than 30%, are correlated with abnormal fetal heart rate patterns, indicating an association with fetal compromise and metabolic acidosis.[151]

Fetal Response to Contraction-Induced Hypoxia

When the fetal oxygen reserve is diminished or exhausted, uterine contractions can precipitate a significant fall in Pao_2. The fetus is quite limited in its ability to compensate for this hypoxemia. The adult mechanism, which involves increasing total cardiac output by increasing heart rate, does not play a major role in the fetal response. Instead, the fetus responds with a redistribution of cardiac output as a means of maintaining critical function; blood flow to the brain and heart increases, whereas perfusion of less critical organs is reduced.[7] This mechanism enables the fetus to survive brief episodes of hypoxia, but severe and prolonged hypoxic episodes are poorly tolerated.

Acute hypoxemia leads to the development of acidosis and also produces a reflex bradycardia as a result of vagal stimulation, both of which further compromise fetal oxygenation. In addition, myocardial hypoxia has a direct bradycardic effect.[7] These mechanisms give rise to one of the classic signs of fetal distress, the late deceleration, in which the peak of uterine pressure, which also represents the nadir of intervillous blood flow and the onset of fetal hypoxemia, is followed by a decline in fetal heart rate. Late decelerations are significant in that they help identify the fetus that cannot tolerate labor because of inadequate oxygen reserves and they allow for the implementation of measures to enhance fetal reserve, improve placental perfusion, or interrupt labor.[167]

Late decelerations are particularly ominous when accompanied by loss of fetal heart rate variability and/or fetal baseline tachycardia, because these findings are indicative of fetal acidosis. In the preterm infant, the findings of decreased variability and tachycardia, with or without late decelerations, correlate highly with acidosis, depression, and low Apgar scores.[167]

Other Factors That Evoke a Fetal Response During Labor

HEAD COMPRESSION

Pressure on the fetal head during labor, especially with pushing efforts in the second stage, also produces a vagal response and a reflex slowing of the fetal heart rate. In general, this does not indicate hypoxia or fetal compromise and often is seen in a healthy fetus. The deceleration that accompanies head compression, also called an ***early deceleration,*** is differentiated from the late deceleration of fetal asphyxia by its timing in relation to a contraction. In early deceleration, the heart rate begins to fall as a contraction builds, reaching its lowest point as the contraction peaks. As the contraction subsides, the heart rate returns to baseline. The result is a uniformly shaped dip that mirrors the shape of the contraction. In comparison, a late deceleration also has a uniform shape but lags behind the contraction, with the fall in heart rate beginning at or slightly after the contraction peak and continuing to fall as the contraction subsides. With a late deceleration, the heart rate does not return to baseline until well after the contraction has ended.

CORD COMPRESSION

Compression of the umbilical cord occurs when the cord is looped around fetal body parts, when it is knotted or prolapses, or when amniotic fluid is scant (oligohydramnios). During labor, cord compression may be exacerbated by contractions and descent of the fetus, resulting in varying degrees of occlusion of the umbilical vessels and diminution of blood flow. Partial venous occlusion may be manifested by fetal heart rate acceleration, whereas significant occlusion precipitates a rapid fall in heart rate, caused at least in part by vagal reflex. ***Variable decelerations*** can be spontaneous, occurring at any time, or periodic, occurring with contractions. They typically have an abrupt descent in heart rate and may be V, U, or W shaped—hence the term *variable deceleration.* Periodic variable decelerations are identified by a decline in heart rate that generally begins before the contraction peaks but, unlike early decelerations, falls rapidly and does not mirror the shape of the contraction. Typically, recovery of the heart rate also is rapid. However, when the occlusion is severe or of long duration or if the fetus has diminished oxygen reserves, recovery may be slow, indicating fetal hypoxia and, in essence, incorporating a component of late deceleration within the variable deceleration.[167]

When variable decelerations are persistent and worsening during labor in the presence of oligohydramnios, intrapartum amnioinfusions have significantly decreased fetal heart rate abnormalities, acidemia at birth, and rates of cesarean birth.[129] An ***amnioinfusion*** involves infusion of fluid into the uterine cavity via an intrauterine pressure catheter (IUPC). This fluid provides cushioning of the umbilical cord, which may reduce the frequency and severity of the cord compression. Amnioinfusions have also been used when thick meconium is present in amniotic fluid to provide a diluting effect that can reduce the amount of meconium present in the infant's trachea. However, a recent study showed no benefit of amnioinfusion on moderate to severe meconium aspiration syndrome or perinatal death.[64]

MATERNAL PAIN MEDICATION

Maternal anesthesia and/or analgesia has the potential to affect the infant, either during labor and delivery or in the newborn period. The risk is increased if the fetus is preterm or is otherwise compromised. This is not to say that there is no place for these drugs in obstetric care—only that they must be used judiciously and with a clear understanding of the risks and benefits involved. Table 2-1 summarizes the effects of commonly used analgesic and anesthetic agents on the fetus and newborn.[4,68]

TABLE 2-1 **FETAL AND NEONATAL EFFECTS OF MATERNAL ANALGESIA AND ANESTHESIA DURING LABOR**

DRUG	POSSIBLE FETAL AND NEONATAL SIDE EFFECTS
Narcotics	Fetal and neonatal effects are related to the dose, route, and timing of maternal administration and may be reversed by the administration of a narcotic antagonist (naloxone): CNS depression Fetal bradycardia Depressed respiratory effort Decreased muscle tone and reflexes Decreased responsiveness
Paracervical block	Fetal bradycardia and asphyxia related to decreased uterine blood flow and direct fetal myocardial depression
Epidural and spinal block	Fetal bradycardia and asphyxia related to maternal hypotension Fetal/neonatal toxicity Neonatal respiratory depression after epidural containing fentanyl
General (inhalation) anesthesia	Fetal and newborn effects related to the duration and depth of maternal anesthesia include the following: CNS depression Respiratory depression Decreased responsiveness

CNS, Central nervous system.

ASSESSMENT OF FETAL WELL-BEING

Over the past 20 to 30 years, the capability to assess fetal well-being has advanced from simple auscultation of the fetal heart to direct physiologic and biochemical measurement of fetal status. With these advances, an appreciation of the similarities between the fetus and newborn, as well as a more complete understanding of the unique features of fetal life, has been gained. This knowledge reinforces the importance of viewing fetal physiology as a precursor of neonatal function and especially as a significant influence on the success with which the fetus will complete the adaptations required by the birth process.

The goal of antepartum fetal surveillance is to answer the following questions: What is the safest environment for a fetus at the gestational age at which the testing is taking place? Is the fetus more likely to survive in utero for the week after testing, or does the fetus have a significant risk for in utero death based on the degree of environmental or intrinsic intolerance demonstrated through testing? In the case of preterm infants, this may mean delivery at a gestational age at which there is a high likelihood for respiratory, neurologic, cardiac, gastrointestinal, and immunologic immaturity that will require neonatal intensive care.

The obstetric practitioner has several tools available to help answer the preceding questions. First and foremost is the identification of maternal conditions that may predispose the fetus to in utero compromise. Examples of such conditions include type 1 diabetes mellitus, chronic hypertension, collagen vascular disease, antiphospholipid antibody disease, maternal cardiac or pulmonary disease, preeclampsia, blood group isoimmunization, in utero infection, PROM, and maternal substance abuse. This list is not all-inclusive but demonstrates several commonly encountered conditions for which antepartum fetal surveillance is warranted.

Once the decision is made to assess fetal well-being, four modalities are available in general practice to help the practitioner and patient answer questions about the optimal environment for the fetus at any given time—fetal movement counts, the contraction stress test, the nonstress test, and the fetal biophysical profile. Two additional tools often used by maternal-fetal medicine specialists in certain clinical situations are Doppler flow studies and percutaneous umbilical cord blood sampling (PUBS). None of these tools is used as the sole determinant for delivery; rather, each is used in conjunction with the entire clinical picture. The choice of testing method also is clinically driven; each method is useful in certain clinical settings, but no one method is the correct choice in all situations.

Although most of the procedures used to monitor fetal well-being are decidedly high-tech, the simple "kick count," or *fetal movement survey*, is a low-tech, low-cost screening tool. Many women with an intrauterine fetal demise have no identifiable risk factors that would place them in a fetal testing protocol. Fetal motor activity reflects the fetal condition in utero, and a decrease in or absence of fetal movements often presages fetal death. This is one reason that many institutions ask their patients to begin a fetal movement counting protocol at 26 to 32 weeks of gestation. Although there are continuing study results, some centers have demonstrated a significant decrease in the incidence of fetal mortality after the institution of a fetal movement counting protocol.

There are several different approaches to fetal movement counting. None has been shown to be superior.[7] One approach is to have the patient choose a certain time every day to rest in the lateral position and count fetal movements. The perception of 10 distinct fetal movements within 2 hours constitutes a reassuring session. The most important aspect of this type of testing is to emphasize to the patient the importance of notifying her practitioner immediately if the fetal movement counting has not met the established criteria. A system must be in place in which patients have immediate access to health care personnel 24 hours per day.

The ***contraction stress test (CST)*** is used in an attempt to evaluate fetal response to uterine contractions.[74] The principle behind the CST is that uterine contractions cause a transient interruption in uteroplacental perfusion. With normal fetal reserve, this intermittent interruption is well tolerated. With inadequate or exhausted reserve, late fetal heart rate decelerations appear. Because late decelerations during labor had been associated with fetal hypoxia and acidosis, it was reasoned that similar interpretations could be applied to contractions induced in the antepartum patient. Thus the CST is considered a test of uteroplacental reserve.

During a CST, uterine contraction activity is evoked with either the use of maternal nipple stimulation or an intravenous infusion of oxytocin. The fetal heart rate is charted using graph paper attached to a monitor that uses a continuous wave ultrasound transducer placed on the maternal abdomen over the uterus. The minimum number of spontaneous or evoked contractions necessary for adequate testing is three contractions of 40 seconds' duration in a 10-minute period. The results are interpreted as follows:

- A negative CST result is one in which no late fetal heart rate decelerations occur during the examination.
- In a positive CST result, late decelerations occur after 50% or more of the contractions, even if contraction frequency is fewer than three in 10 minutes.
- A suspicious or equivocal finding is one in which intermittent late or significant variable decelerations occur.
- A CST result is considered unsatisfactory if fewer than three contractions occur per 10 minutes or a poor-quality tracing is obtained.

In many clinical situations, a positive CST warrants delivery of the fetus because of suspected in utero hypoxemia during periods of uterine contraction. However, there are numerous exceptions to this rule. For example, if a positive CST is noted in the presence of maternal diabetic ketoacidosis, a correction of the underlying metabolic process may reverse the fetal acidosis and a negative CST may be obtained subsequently. Thus the delivery of a neonate who has metabolic acidosis and is preterm can be avoided.

The ***nonstress test (NST)*** is a tool used to indirectly assess the integrity of the fetal autonomic nervous system. The fetal heart is under the dual influences of the sympathetic and parasympathetic nervous systems. By approximately 28 weeks' gestation, 85% of fetuses demonstrate fetal heart rate accelerations in response to fetal movement. Lack of these intermittent fetal heart rate accelerations usually indicates a fetal sleep cycle. However, many other intrinsic and extrinsic factors, including fetal acidosis, may lead to an absence of these intermittent accelerations in heart rate. Examples include but are not limited to medication exposure, maternal smoking, uteroplacental insufficiency, and fetal structural or chromosomal anomaly. Factors leading to maternal acidosis (severe anemia, congenital heart disease, and sepsis) also can result in fetal acidosis and nonreactive NST.

The NST is performed with the patient in a semi-Fowler's or lateral tilt position. As in the CST, the fetal heart rate is monitored with an external transducer. NSTs are interpreted as either reactive or nonreactive. An accepted definition of a reactive NST is an increase in fetal heart rate of 15 beats/min for 15 seconds above the baseline heart rate occurring twice in a 20-minute period.[7] Some centers may require that the fetal heart rate accelerations be associated with fetal movements, as well as perceived by the maternal patient. A nonreactive test is defined as lacking the necessary fetal heart rate accelerations during a 40-minute period. The following may be candidates for nonstress testing:

- Women who have diabetes that must be controlled with insulin
- Women who have pregnancy-induced hypertension or intrinsic renal disease
- Women in whom fetal IUGR or postdate pregnancy has been determined
- Women who have reported decreased fetal movement

The NST has certain advantages over the CST. It does not entail the production of uterine contractions, and so there are fewer potential problems or contraindications to the NST. Because the NST is quicker and easier to conduct, it is often the first-line screening test of fetal well-being. Its disadvantages are that it does not evaluate uteroplacental reserve and that it has a higher false-positive rate than the CST.

When the NST is nonreactive, an option that is often used in lieu of the CST or delivery of the fetus is the ***biophysical profile*** (Table 2-2). This test combines the NST with real-time ultrasound evaluation of the fetus. Although there are several different biophysical profile (BPP) scoring systems, the one most generally accepted assigns a numerical score of 0 or 2 for the absence or presence, respectively, of five different parameters. These include fetal movement, tone, "breathing" movements, amniotic fluid volume, and the NST. One advantage to evaluation of several different fetal biophysical variables is enhanced specificity of testing with a diminished incidence of delivery for false-positive results. The presence or absence of acute markers (movement, tone, breathing, and NST) helps reflect fetal status at the time of testing. Evaluation of amniotic fluid volume as a marker is indirect evidence that the portions of the fetal CNS that control that activity are intact and functioning and therefore not acidotic. However, the absence of a given marker may be difficult to interpret, because it may simply reflect normal periodicity.

The biophysical activities that mature first in fetal development disappear last as acidosis worsens. Fetal tone (flexion and extension) is present at 7½ to 8½ weeks after the last menstrual period. This activity, as well as gross body movement, is mediated in the cortex and nuclei of the CNS. Fetal movement is present by 9 weeks. Fetal breathing movements (i.e., rhythmic breathing movements of 35 seconds or more) are generally seen by 20 weeks' gestation. The CNS center responsible for control of this activity is the ventral surface of the fourth ventricle. The final acute marker to mature is fetal heart rate acceleration in response to movement (reactive NST) seen in the later second trimester. The posterior hypothalamus and medulla control this activity. Given that the first marker to appear in development is the last to disappear with worsening fetal acidosis, the absence of fetal tone has been found to be associated with high perinatal morbidity and mortality.[162]

TABLE 2-2 BIOPHYSICAL PROFILE SCORING

BIOPHYSICAL VARIABLE	NORMAL (2)	ABNORMAL (0)
Fetal breathing—At least one episode of at least 30 seconds during a 30-minute observation	Present	Absent
Gross body movement—At least three body or limb movements during a 30-minute observation	≥3	≤2
Fetal tone—One episode of extension or flexion of limbs or trunk during a 30-minute observation	Present	Absent
Reactive nonstress test—At least two episodes of 15 beats/min fetal heart rate accelerations during 30-minute observation	Yes	No
Amniotic fluid volume—At least one pocket of at least 1 cm × 1 cm in two directions	Present	Absent
Normal Score: 8-10		

Chronic sustained fetal hypoxia or acidosis may produce a protective redistribution of cardiac output away from less vital fetal organs (e.g., kidney, lung) toward the essential organs (e.g., brain, heart, adrenal glands). Redistribution of fetal blood flow may be so profound that renal perfusion decreases to the point that oligohydramnios is established. When the largest vertical amniotic fluid pocket within the uterus is less than 1 cm, the perinatal mortality rate is as high as 110/1000.[31]

A BPP score of 8 or 10 is normal; a score of 6 is equivocal, and the profile should be repeated in 12 to 24 hours. A score of 4 or less is abnormal. Management in the presence of an abnormal BPP depends on the gestational age and the maternal and/or fetal factors contributing to the altered state.

The BPP employs the advantages of real-time ultrasonography to observe fetal behavior.[103] One of its major advantages is as an intermediate step in the evaluation of a fetus with a nonreactive NST before a time-consuming CST is performed. It is also a useful tool for patients with contraindications to the CST, such as premature labor, premature rupture of membranes, unexplained vaginal bleeding, or multiple gestations. The modified BPP, which combines an acute marker (NST) with the chronic marker of fetal well-being (amniotic fluid index [AFI]), has been shown by some centers to be as predictive of fetal well-being as the full BPP. Because evaluation of the AFI is less time consuming and requires less technical skill, this may be an acceptable alternative for many centers. Finally, it should be noted that though widely used, there is insufficient evidence from randomized trials to support the use of BPP as a test of fetal well-being in high-risk pregnancies.[92]

No matter which of these testing modalities is used, the patient should be counseled as to the predictive value of a "normal" test. The incidence of stillbirth within 1 week of a reactive NST is 1.9/1000; for a negative CST, it is 0.3/1000; and for a normal BPP, it is 0.8/1000.[7] Although some investigators have reported a decreased incidence of fetal mortality after initiation of a fetal movement counting program for "low-risk" patients, enough data are not yet available to apply these numbers to the general population.[111]

The role of ***Doppler flow assessment*** of the fetal arterial and venous systems in the prediction of in utero well-being is increasingly accepted. Measurement of umbilical artery velocity is used as a method of fetal surveillance for growth-restricted fetuses. Specifically, decreased or absent end-diastolic flow may appear days before conventional antenatal tests become abnormal. In cases such as these, at a minimum, intensive fetal surveillance is advised.[63] Reversal of diastolic flow is highly predictive of in utero fetal demise within 24 hours and warrants immediate intense investigation or delivery. No role for Doppler velocimetry in conditions other than in growth restriction has been demonstrated.[7]

The dramatic improvement in ultrasound image quality over the past 15 years also has made it possible to directly sample fetal blood and tissue. The technique of ***percutaneous umbilical blood sampling (PUBS)*** has given the obstetrician access to the fetal circulation with relative safety for both the fetus and mother. In this procedure, real-time ultrasonography is used to guide the insertion of a needle into the umbilical vein or artery. Samples of fetal blood can be obtained, or, as in the case of red cell isoimmunization, transfusions can be carried out. The fetal loss rate is generally quoted as 1% to 2%.[5,138]

REFERENCES

1. Abalovich M, Amino N, Barbour LA, et al: Management of thyroid dysfunction during pregnancy and postpartum: an Endocrine Society Clinical Practice Guideline, *J Clin Endocrinol Metab* 92(Suppl 8):S1, 2007.
2. Adams-Waldorf KM, Nelson JL: Autoimmune disease during pregnancy and the microchimerism legacy of pregnancy, *Immunol Invest* 37:631, 2008.
3. Alexander EK: Timing and magnitude of increases in levothyroxine requirements during pregnancy in women with hypothyroidism, *N Engl J Med* 351:241, 2004.
4. American Academy of Pediatrics, American College of Obstetricians and Gynecologists, and March of Dimes Birth Defects Foundation: *Guidelines for perinatal care*, ed 6, Elk Grove Village, Ill, 2007, The Academy.
5. American College of Obstetricians and Gynecologists (ACOG) Committee Opinion: Fetal pulse oximetry, *Obstet Gynecol* 98:523, 2001.
6. American College of Obstetricians and Gynecologists (ACOG) Committee Opinion: Antenatal corticosteroid therapy for fetal maturation, *Int J Gynaecol Obstet* 78:95, 2002.
7. American College of Obstetricians and Gynecologists (ACOG) Practice Bulletin: Antepartum fetal surveillance, *Int J Gynaecol Obstet* 68:175, 2000.
8. American College of Obstetricians and Gynecologists (ACOG) Practice Bulletin: Gestational diabetes, *Obstet Gynecol* 98(3):525, 2001.

9. American College of Obstetricians and Gynecologists (ACOG) Practice Bulletin: Thyroid disease in pregnancy, *Obstet Gynecol* 100(2):387, 2002.
10. American College of Obstetricians and Gynecologists (ACOG) Practice Bulletin: Management of preterm labor, *Obstet Gynecol* 101:1039, 2003.
11. Ananth CV, Oyelese Y, Srinivas N, et al: Preterm premature rupture of membranes, intrauterine infection, and oligohydramnios: risk factors for placental abruption, *Obstet Gynecol* 104:71, 2004.
12. Ananth CV, Smulian JC, Vintzileos AM: Incidence of placental abruption in relation to cigarette smoking and hypertensive disorder during pregnancy: a meta-analysis of observational studies, *Obstet Gynecol* 93:622, 1999.
13. Araojo R, McCure S, Feibus K: Substance abuse in pregnant women: making improved detection and good clinical outcome, *Clin Pharmacol Ther* 83:521, 2008.
14. Asthma and Pregnancy—update 2004, National Asthma Education Prevention Program Working Group on Managing Asthma During Pregnancy: Recommendations for pharmacologic treatment—update 2004. In *NIH U.S. Department of Health and Human Services, National Heart, Lung and Blood Institute,* NIH Publication No. 05-3279 2004.
15. Bakhireva LN, Schatz M, Jones KL, et al: Organization of Teratology Information Specialists Collaborative Research Group: Asthma control during pregnancy and the risk of preterm delivery or impaired fetal growth, *Ann Allergy Asthma Immunol* 101:137, 2008.
16. Bar J, Ben-Rafael Z, Padoa A, et al: Prediction of pregnancy outcome in subgroups of women with renal disease, *Clin Nephrol* 53:437, 2000.
17. Bell J, Harvey-Dodds L: Pregnancy and injecting drug use, *Br Med J* 336:1303, 2008.
18. Besinger R, Niebyl JR, Keyes WG, et al: Randomized comparative trial of indomethacin for the long term treatment of preterm labor, *Am J Obstet Gynecol* 164:981, 1991.
19. Briggs G, Freeman RK, Yaffe SJ: *Drugs in pregnancy and lactation: a reference guide to fetal and neonatal risk*, ed 7, Baltimore, 2005, Lippincott Williams & Wilkins.
20. Bromfield EB, Dworetzky BA, Wyszynski DF, et al: Valproate teratogenicity and epilepsy syndrome, *Epilepsia*, Epub ahead of print, *PMID:*18557775, 2008.
21. Buehler BA, Stempel LE: Anticonvulsant therapy during pregnancy. In Rayburn WF, Zuspan FP, editors: *Drug therapy in obstetrics and gynecology*, ed 3 St Louis, 1992, Mosby.
22. Burd L, Roberts D, Olson M, et al: Ethanol and the placenta: a review, *J Matern Fetal Neonatal Med* 20:361, 2007.
23. Burns J: Congenital heart disease: risk to offspring, *Arch Dis Child* 58:947, 1983.
24. Butters L, Kennedy S, Rubin PC: Atenolol in essential hypertension during pregnancy, *Br Med J* 301:1103, 1990.
25. Casey BM, Dashe JS, Wells CE, et al: Subclinical hypothyroidism and pregnancy outcomes, *Obstet Gynecol* 105:239, 2005.
26. Casey BM, Dashe JS, Wells CE, et al: Subclinical hyperthyroidism and pregnancy outcomes, *Obstet Gynecol* 107:337, 2006.
27. Castro LC, Avina RL: Maternal obesity and pregnancy outcomes, *Curr Opin Obstet Gynecol* 14:601, 2002.
28. Catalano PM: Management of obesity in pregnancy, *Obstet Gynecol* 109:419, 2007.
29. Catalano PM, Ehrenberg HM: The short- and long-term implications of maternal obesity on the mother and her offspring, *Br J Obstet Gynaecol* 113:1126, 2006.
30. Centers for Disease Control and Prevention: Perinatal group B streptococcal disease after universal screening recommendations—United States, 2003-2005, *MMWR* 56:701, 2007.
31. Chamberlain PFD, Manning FA, Morrison I, et al: Ultrasound evaluation of amniotic fluid volumes. I. The relationship of marginal and decreased amniotic fluid volumes to perinatal outcome, *Am J Obstet Gynecol* 150:250, 1984.
32. Cheng YW, Caughey AB: Gestational diabetes: diagnosis and management, *J Perinatol* Epub ahead of print, *PMID:*18633419, 2008.
33. Cheng EY, Goss CH, McKone EF, et al: Aggressive prenatal care results in successful fetal outcomes in CF women, *J Cyst Fibros* 5:85, 2006.
34. Christensen C: Management of chemical dependence in pregnancy, *Clin Obstet Gynecol* 51:445, 2008.
35. Chu SY, Kim SY, Schmid CH, et al: Maternal obesity and risk of cesarean delivery: a meta-analysis, *Obes Rev* 8:385, 2007.
36. Clark SL: Placenta previa and abruptio placentae. In Creasy RK, Resnik R, editors: *Maternal-fetal medicine*, ed 4, Philadelphia, 1999, Saunders.
37. Coetzee EJ, Levitt NS: Maternal diabetes and neonatal outcome, *Semin Neonatal* 5:221, 2000.
38. Cotrufo M, De Feo M, De Santo LS, et al: Risk of warfarin during pregnancy with mechanical valve prostheses, *Obstet Gynecol* 100(5 Pt 1):1040, 2002.
39. Cox JT, Phelan ST: Nutrition during pregnancy, *Obstet Gynecol Clin North Am* 35:369, 2008.
40. Reference deleted in proofs.
41. Crane JM, van der Hof MC, Dodds L, et al: Neonatal outcomes with placenta previa, *Obstet Gynecol* 93:541, 1999.
42. Creasy RK, Iams JD: Preterm labor and delivery. In Creasy RK, Resnik R, editors: *Maternal-fetal medicine*, ed 4, Philadelphia, 1999, Saunders.

43. Crowther CA, Hiller JE, Doyle LW, et al: Effect of magnesium sulfate given for neuroprotection before preterm birth: a randomized controlled trial, *JAMA* 290:2669, 2003.
44. Curet LB, Hsi AC: Drug abuse during pregnancy, *Clin Obstet Gynecol* 45:73, 2002.
44a. daFonseca EB, Bittar RE, Carvalho MH, Zugaib M: Prophylactic administration of progesterone by vaginal suppository to reduce the incidence of spontaneous preterm birth in women at increased risk: A randomized placebo-controlled double-blind study, *Am J Obstet Gynecol* 188:419, 2003.
45. Dahl J, Myhr KM, Daltveit AK, et al: Pregnancy, delivery, and birth outcome in women with multiple sclerosis, *Neurology* 65:1961, 2005.
46. Diamond MP, Salyer SL, Vaughn WK, et al: Reassessment of White's classification and Pedersen's prognostically bad signs of diabetic pregnancies in insulin-dependent diabetic pregnancies, *Am J Obstet Gynecol* 156:599, 1987.
47. Dietl J: Maternal obesity and complications during pregnancy, *J Perinat Med* 33:100, 2005.
48. Dodd A, Flenady VJ, Cincotta R, et al: Progesterone for the prevention of preterm birth: a systematic review, *Obstet Gynecol* 112:127, 2008.
49. Doria A, Tincani A, Lockshin M: Challenges of lupus pregnancies, *Rheumatology* 47:iii9, 2008.
50. Ducsay CA, Thompson JS, Wu AT, et al: Effects of calcium entry blocker (nicardipine) tocolysis in rhesus macaques: fetal plasma concentrations and cardiorespiratory changes, *Am J Obstet Gynecol* 157:1482, 1987.
51. Dulitzki M, Pauzner R, Langevitz P, et al: Low-molecular-weight heparin during pregnancy and delivery: preliminary experience with 41 pregnancies, *Obstet Gynecol* 87:380, 1996.
52. Dwosh E, Guimond C, Duquette P, et al: The interaction of MS and pregnancy: a critical review, *Int MS J* 10:38, 2003.
53. Eadie MJ: Antiepileptic drugs as human teratogens, *Expert Opin Drug Saf* 7:195, 2008.
54. Easterling TR, Brateng D, Schmucker B, et al: Prevention of preeclampsia: a randomized trial of atenolol in hyperdynamic patients before onset of hypertension, *Obstet Gynecol* 93:725, 1999.
55. Elloit EJ, Bower C: Alcohol and pregnancy: the pivotal role of the obstetrician, *Aust NZ J Obstet Gynaecol* 48:227, 2008.
56. Elliott JP, O'Keefe DF, Schon DA, et al: Dialysis in pregnancy: a critical review, *Obstet Gynecol Surv* 46:319, 1991.
57. Evidence from the Collaborative Eclampsia Trial: Which anticonvulsant for women with eclampsia? *Lancet* 345:1455, 1995.
58. Ferrer RL, Sibai BM, Mulrow CD, et al: Management of mild chronic hypertension during pregnancy: a review, *Obstet Gynecol* 96:849, 2000.
59. Ferrero S, Pretta S, Nicolette A, et al: Myasthenia gravis: management issues during pregnancy, *Eur J Obstet Gynecol Reprod Biol* 121:128, 2005.
60. Ferrero S, Pretta S, Ragni N: Multiple sclerosis: management issues during pregnancy, *Eur J Obstet Gynecol Reprod Biol* 115:3, 2004.
61. Fleming AD: Abruptio placentae, *Crit Care Clin* 7:865, 1991.
62. Floyd RL, Sidhu JS: Monitoring prenatal alcohol exposure, *Am J Med Genet C Semin Med Genet* 127C(1):3, 2004.
63. Forouzan I: Absence of end-diastolic flow velocity in the umbilical artery: a review, *Obstet Gynecol Surv* 50:219, 1995.
64. Fraser W, Hotmeyr J, Lede R, et al: Amnioinfusion for the prevention of the meconium aspiration syndrome, *N Engl J Med* 353:946, 2005.
65. Reference deleted in proofs.
66. Ghafari A, Sanadgol H: Pregnancy after renal transplantation: ten-year-center experience, *Transplant Proc* 40:251, 2008.
67. Gilljam M, Antoniou M, Shin J, et al: Pregnancy in cystic fibrosis: fetal and maternal outcomes, *Chest* 118:85, 2000.
68. Goetzl LM: ACOG Practice Bulletin. Clinical management guidelines for obstetrician-gynecologists: obstetric analgesia and anesthesia, *Obstet Gynecol* 100:177, 2002.
69. Gruslin A, Perkins SL, Manchanda R, et al: Maternal smoking and fetal erythropoietin levels, *Obstet Gynecol* 95:561, 2003.
70. Haddow JE, Palomaki G, Allan W, et al: Maternal thyroid deficiency during pregnancy and subsequent neurophysiological development of the child, *N Engl J Med* 341:549, 1999.
71. Haslam C, Lawrence W: Health-related behavior and beliefs of pregnant smokers, *Health Psychol* 23:486, 2004.
72. Henriksen T: The macrosomic infant: a challenge in current obstetrics, *Acta Obstet Gynecol Scand* 87:134, 2008.
73. Houtchens MK: Pregnancy and multiple sclerosis, *Semin Neurol* 27:434, 2007.
74. Huddleston J: Continued utility of the contraction stress test? *Clin Obstet Gynecol* 45:1005, 2002.
75. Hunt S, Russell A, Smithson WH, et al: Topiramate in pregnancy: preliminary experience from the UK Epilepsy and Pregnancy Register, *Neurology* 71:272, 2008.
76. Iams JD, Goldenberg RL, Meis PJ, et al: The length of the cervix and the risk of spontaneous premature delivery, *N Engl J Med* 334:567, 1996.

77. Jacobson GF, Ramos GA, Ching JY, et al: Comparison of glyburide and insulin for the management of gestational diabetes in a large managed care organization, *Am J Obstet Gynecol* 93:118, 2005.
78. Jain NJ, Denk CE, Kruse LK, et al: Maternal obesity: can pregnancy weight gain modify risk of selected pregnancy outcomes? *Am J Perinatol* 24:291, 2007.
79. James DK, Steer PJ, Weiner CP, et al: *High risk pregnancy: management options*, ed 3, Philadelphia, 2006, Saunders.
80. Jones DC, Hayslett JP: Outcome of pregnancy in women with moderate or severe renal insufficiency, *N Engl J Med* 335:226, 1996.
81. Kalidindi M, Ganpot S, Tahmesebi T, et al: Myasthenia gravis and pregnancy, *J Obstet Gynecol* 27:30, 2007.
82. Karima M, Davar R, Mirzaei M, et al: Pregnancy outcomes in asthmatic women, *Iran J Allergy Asthma Immunol* 7:105, 2008.
83. Karmon A, Sheiner E: The relationship between urinary tract infection during pregnancy and preeclampsia: causal, confounded or spurious?, *Arch Gynecol Obstet* 277:479, 2008.
84. Kashanizadeh N, Nemati E, Sharifi-Bonab M, et al: Impact of pregnancy on the outcome of kidney transplantation, *Transplant Proc* 39:1136, 2007.
85. Khairy P, Ouyang DW, Fernandes SM, et al: Pregnancy outcomes in women with congenital heart disease, *Circulation* 113:517, 2006.
86. Khandelwal M, Rasanen J, Ludormirski A, et al: Evaluation of fetal and uterine hemodynamics during maternal cardiopulmonary bypass, *Obstet Gynecol* 88:667, 1996.
87. King JF, Flenady V, Papatsonis D, et al: Calcium channel blockers for inhibiting preterm labour: a systematic review of the evidence and a protocol for administration of nifedipine, *Aust NZ J Obstet Gynaecol* 43:192, 2003.
88. Kirby R: Maternal phenylketonuria: a new cause for concern, *J Obstet Gynecol Neonatal Nurs* 28:227, 1999.
89. Kominiarek MA, Angelopoulos SM, Shapiro NL, et al: Low-molecular-weight heparin in pregnancy: peripartum bleeding complications, *J Perinatol* 27:329, 2007.
90. Kovacs C: Vitamin D in pregnancy and lactation: maternal, fetal, and neonatal outcomes from human and animal studies, *Am J Clin Nutr* 520S:88, 2008.
91. Krishnamurthy KB: Pregnancy and epilepsy: update on pregnancy registries, *Curr Treat Options Neurol* 10:246, 2008.
92. Lalor JG, Fawole B, Alfirevic Z, et al: Biophysical profile for fetal assessment in high risk pregnancies, *Cochrane Database Syst Rev* 23(1):CD000038, 2008.
93. Langer O, Yogev Y, Most O, et al: Gestational diabetes: the consequences of not treating, *Am J Obstet Gynecol* 192:989, 2005.
94. Larsen LG, Clausen HV, Jansson L: Stereologic examination of placentas from mothers who smoke during pregnancy, *Am J Obstet Gynecol* 186:531, 2002.
95. Law KL, Stroud L, LaGasse L, et al: Smoking during pregnancy and newborn neurobehavior, *Pediatrics* 111:1318, 2003.
96. Lazarus JH, Kokandi A: Thyroid disease in relation to pregnancy: a decade of change, *Clin Endocrinol* 46:381, 2000.
97. Lenke RR, Levy HL: Maternal phenylketonuria and hyperphenylalaninemia: an international survey of the outcome of untreated and treated pregnancies, *N Engl J Med* 303:1202, 1980.
98. Lenke RR, Levy HL: Maternal phenylketonuria: results of dietary therapy, *Am J Obstet Gynecol* 142:548, 1982.
99. Lin S, Munsie JP, Herdt-Losavio ML, et al: Maternal asthma medication use and the risk of gastrochisis, *Am J Epidemiol* 168:73, 2008.
100. Loudon JA, Groom KM, Bennett PR: Prostaglandin inhibitors in preterm labour, *Best Pract Res Clin Obstet Gynaecol* 17:731, 2003.
101. Ma Y, Goins KV, Pbert L, et al: Predictors of smoking cessation in pregnancy and maintenance postpartum in low-income women, *Matern Child Health J* 9:393, 2005.
102. Maillot F, Lilburn M, Baudin J, et al: Factors influencing outcomes in the offspring of mothers with phenylketonuria during pregnancy: the importance of variation in maternal blood phenylalanine, *Am J Clin Nutr* 88:700, 2008.
103. Manning FA, Morrison I, Lange IR, et al: Fetal assessment based on fetal biophysical profile scoring: experience in 12,620 referred high risk pregnancies. I. Perinatal mortality by frequency and etiology, *Am J Obstet Gynecol* 151:343, 1985.
104. March of Dimes Birth Defects Foundation, 2004: www.marchofdimes.com.
105. Matchaba P, Moodley J: Corticosteroids for HELLP syndrome in pregnancy, *Cochrane Database Syst Rev* 1: CD002076, 2004.
106. Maurer G, Ambriola D: Pregnancy following renal transplant, *J Perinat Neonat Nurs* 8:28, 1994.
107. Meador KJ, Pennell PB, Harden CL, et al: Hope Work Group: Pregnancy registries in epilepsy: a consensus statement on health outcomes, *Neurology* 71:1109, 2008.
108. Meador KJ, Reynolds MW, Crean S, et al: Pregnancy outcomes in women with epilepsy: a systematic review and meta-analysis of the published pregnancy registries and cohorts, *Epilepsy Res* 81:1, 2008.
109. Melvin C, Dolan MP, Windsor RA, et al: Recommended cessation counseling for pregnant women who smoke: a review of evidence, *Tob Control* 9:1, 2000.

110. Montouris G: Importance of monotherapy in women across the reproductive cycle, *Neurology* 69:S10, 2007.
111. Moore TR, Piacquadio K: A prospective evaluation of fetal movement screening to reduce the incidences of antepartum fetal death, *Am J Obstet Gynecol* 160:1075, 1989.
112. Moroni G, Pontincelli C: The risk of pregnancy in patients with lupus nephritis, *J Nephrol* 16:161, 2003.
113. Motta M, Tincani A, Meroni P, et al: Follow-up of children exposed antenatally to immunosuppressive drugs, *Rheumatology* 47:iii32, 2008.
114. Mueller BA, Zhang J, Critchlow CW: Birth outcomes and need for hospitalization after delivery among women with multiple sclerosis, *Am J Obstet Gynecol* 186:446, 2002.
115. Murphy VE, Clifton VL, Gibson PG: Asthma exacerbations during pregnancy: incidence and association with adverse pregnancy outcomes, *Thorax* 61:169, 2006.
116. Mustafa SA, Brizot ML, Carvalho MH, et al: Transvaginal ultrasonography in predicting placenta previa at delivery: a longitudinal study, *Ultrasound Obstet Gynecol* 20:356, 2002.
117. National Academy of Science: Nutrition during Pregnancy. I. Weight Gain. II. Nutritional Supplements. In *I.O.M. National Academy of Science, Food and Nutrition Board, Committee on Nutrition Status During Pregnancy*, Washington DC, 1990, National Academy Press.
118. Ness A, Visintine J, Ricci E, et al: Use of fetal fibronectin and transvaginal ultrasound cervical length to triage women with suspected preterm labor: a randomized trial, *Am J Obstet Gynecol* 195:567, 2006.
119. Odegaard I, Stray-Pederson B, Hallberg K, et al: Maternal and fetal morbidity in pregnancies of Norwegian and Swedish women with cystic fibrosis, *Acta Obstet Gynecol Scand* 81:698, 2002.
120. Odent M: The rise of preconceptual counseling vs the decline of medicalized care in pregnancy, *Birth Psychology* 2002. Accessed September 13, 2006, from http://birthpsychology.com/primalhealth/primal10.html.
121. Ogunyemi D, Hernandez-Loera GE: The impact of antenatal cocaine use on maternal characteristics and neonatal outcomes, *J Matern Fetal Neonatal Med* 15:253, 2004.
122. Papatsonis DNM, Kok JH, van Geijn HP, et al: Neonatal effects of nifedipine and ritodrine for preterm labor, *Obstet Gynecol* 95:477, 2000.
123. Patel A, Asopa S, Tang AT, et al: Cardiac surgery during pregnancy, *Tex Heart Inst J* 35:307, 2008.
124. Patti F, Cavallaro T, Lo Fermo S, et al: Is in utero early-exposure to interferon beta a risk factor for pregnancy outcomes in multiple sclerosis?, *J Neurol* Epub ahead of print, *PMID:* 18677640, 2008.
125. Pauly JR, Slokin TA: Maternal tobacco smoking, nicotine replacement and neurobehavioral development, *Acta Paediatr* 97:1331, 2008.
126. Pedersen J: *The pregnant diabetic and her newborn*, ed 2, Baltimore, 1977, Williams & Wilkins.
127. Pinkerton K: *Cystic fibrosis life expectancy: 2006*, Accessed September 14, 2008, from http://ezinearticles.com/?Cystic-Fibrosis-Life-Expectancy&id=353570.
128. Pirie PL, Lando H, Curry SJ, et al: Tobacco, alcohol, and caffeine use and cessation in early pregnancy, *Am J Prev Med* 18:54, 2000.
129. Pitt C, Sanchez-Ramos L, Kaunitz AM, et al: Prophylactic amnioinfusion for intrapartum oligohydramnios: a meta-analysis of randomized controlled trials, *Obstet Gynecol* 96:861, 2000.
130. Pittschieler S, Brezinka C, Jahn B, et al: Spontaneous abortion and the prophylactic effect of folic acid supplementation in epileptic women undergoing antiepileptic therapy, *J Neurol* Epub ahead of print, *PMID:*18677647 2008.
131. Quintero R, Sepulveda W, Romero R, et al: Cord: Velamentous insertion. In *Fetal echocardiography 2009: An intense review course*, Accessed July 11, 2009, from www.thefetus.net/1999.
132. Roberts J: Pregnancy-related hypertension. In Creasy RK, Resnick R, editors: *Maternal fetal medicine*, ed 4 Philadelphia, 1999, Saunders.
133. Roberts JM, Pearson GD, Cutler JA, et al: Summary of the NHLBI Working Group on Research on Hypertension During Pregnancy, *Hypertens Pregnancy* 22:109, 2003.
134. Rosen TS, Bateman DA: Infants of addicted mothers. In Fanoroff AA, Martin RL, editors: *Neonatal-perinatal medicine*, ed 7 St Louis, 2001, Mosby.
135. Ross MG, Gala R: Use of umbilical artery base excess: algorithm for the timing of hypoxic injury, *Am J Obstet Gynecol* 187:1, 2002.
136. Rotmensch HH, Elkayam U, Frishman W: Antiarrhythmic drug therapy during pregnancy, *Ann Intern Med* 98:487, 1993.
137. Ruiz-Irastorza G, Khamashta MA: Lupus and pregnancy: ten questions and some answers, *Lupus* 17:416, 2008.
138. Sarno AP, Wilson RD: Fetal cardiocentesis: a review of indications, risks, applications and technique, *Fetal Diagn Ther* 23:237, 2008.
139. Scardo JA, Hogg BB, Newman RB, et al: Favorable hemodynamic effects of magnesium sulfate in preeclampsia, *Am J Obstet Gynecol* 174:1249, 1995.
140. Schatz M, Dombrowski MP, Wise R, et al: Asthma morbidity during pregnancy can be predicted by severity classification, *J Allergy Clin Immunol* 112:283, 2003.

141. Shankar K, Ronis MJ, Badger TM: Effects of pregnancy and nutritional status on alcohol metabolism, *Alcohol Res Health* 30:55, 2007.
142. Sibai BM: The HELLP syndrome (hemolysis, elevated liver enzymes, and low platelets): much ado about nothing? *Am J Obstet Gynecol* 162:311, 1990.
143. Sibai BM: Chronic hypertension in pregnancy, *Obstet Gynecol* 100:1358, 2002.
144. Sibai BM: Diagnosis and management of gestational hypertension and preeclampsia, *Obstet Gynecol* 102:181, 2003.
145. Sinha P, Kuruba N: Ante-partum haemorrhage: an update, *J Obstet Gynaecology* 28:377, 2008.
146. Siu SC, Sermer M, Colman JM, et al: Prospective multicenter study of pregnancy outcomes in women with heart disease, *Circulation* 104:515, 2001.
147. Smaill F, Vasuez JC: Treatment of asymptomatic bacteriuria in pregnancy, *Cochrane Database Syst Rev* 18(2): CD00490, 2007.
148. Stan C, Boulvain M, Hirsbrunner-Amagbaly P, et al: Hydration for treatment of preterm labour, *Cochrane Database Syst Rev* 2: CD003096, 2002.
149. Stotand NE, Cheng YW, Hopkins LM, et al: Gestational weight gain and adverse neonatal outcomes among term infants, *Obstet Gynecol* 108:635, 2006.
150. Tata LJ, Lewis SA, McKeever TM, et al: Effect of maternal asthma, exacerbations and asthma medication use on congenital malformations in offspring: a UK population-based study, *Thorax* 63:981, 2008.
151. Tekin A, Ozkan S, Caliskan E, et al: Fetal pulse oximetry: correlation with intrapartum fetal heart rate patterns and neonatal outcome, *J Obstet Gynaecol Res* 34:824, 2008.
152. Tincani A, Bazzani C, Zingarelli S, et al: Lupus and the antiphospholipid syndrome in pregnancy and obstetrics: clinical characteristics, diagnosis, pathogenesis, and treatment, *Semin Thromb Hemost* 34:267, 2008.
153. Tomson T, Perucca E, Battino D: Navigating toward fetal and maternal health: the challenge of treating epilepsy in pregnancy, *Epilepsia* 45:1171, 2004.
154. Tonelli MR, Aitken ML: Pregnancy in cystic fibrosis, *Curr Opin Pulm Med* 13:537, 2007.
155. Tropper PJ, Petrie RH: Placental exchange. In Lavery JP, editor: *The human placenta: clinical perspectives*, Rockville, Md, 1987, Aspen Publications.
156. Trumbo P, Schlicker S, Yates AA, et al: Dietary reference intakes for energy, carbohydrates, fiber, fat, fatty acids, cholesterol, protein and amino acids, *J Am Diet Assoc* 102:1621, 2002.
157. Umans JG, Lindheimer MD: Antihypertensive treatment. In Lindheimer MD, Roberts JM, Cunningham FG, editors: *Chesley's hypertensive disorders in pregnancy*, ed 2 Norwalk, Conn, 1998, Appleton & Lange.
158. U.S. Department of Health and Human Services: The health consequences of smoking: a report of the Surgeon General: 2004. In Centers for Disease Control and Prevention Office on Smoking and Health editor: Accessed, November 13, 2008. from www.cdc.gov/tobacco/data_statistics/sgr/sgr_2004/index.htm#full.
159. U.S. Department of Health and Human Services: *National survey on drug use and health: 2006*, Accessed, November 12, 2008. from www.oas.samhsa.gov/NSDUH/2k6NSDUH/2k6Results.pdf.
160. Vajda FJ: Treatment options for pregnant women with epilepsy, *Expert Opin Pharmacother* 9:1859, 2008.
161. Van Mieghem T, Van Schoubroeck D, Depiere M, et al: Fetal cerebral hemorrhage caused by vitamin K deficiency after complicated bariatric surgery, *Obstet Gynecol* 112:434, 2008.
162. Vintzileos AM, Campbell WA, Rodes JF: Fetal biophysical profile scoring: current status, *Clin Perinatol* 16:661, 1989.
163. Vukusic S, Hutchinson M, Hours M, et al: Pregnancy and multiple sclerosis (the PRIMS study): clinical predictors of post-partum relapse, *Brain* 127:1353, 2004.
164. Waltuck J, Buyon JP: Autoantibody associated congenital heart block: outcome in mothers and children, *Ann Intern Med* 120:544, 1994.
165. Wells CS, Schwalberg R, Noonan G, et al: Factors influencing inadequate and excessive weight gain in pregnancy: Colorado 2000-2002, *Matern Child Health J* 10:55, 2006.
166. West JR, Blake CA: Fetal alcohol syndrome: an assessment of the field, *Exp Biol Med* 230:354, 2005.
167. Westgate JA, Wibbens B, Bennet L, et al: The intrapartum deceleration in center stage: a physiologic approach to the interpretation of fetal heart rate changes in labor, *Am J Obstet Gynecol* 197:236, 2007.
168. Whittemore R: Congenital heart disease: its impact on pregnancy, *Hosp Pract* 18:65, 1983.
169. Worthington J, Jones R, Crawford M, et al: Pregnancy and multiple sclerosis: a three-year prospective study, *J Neurol* 241:228, 1994.
170. Zhang X, Decker A, Platt RW, et al: How big is too big? The perinatal consequence of fetal macrosomia, *Am J Obstet Gynecol* 198:517.e1, 2008.

3 PERINATAL TRANSPORT AND LEVELS OF CARE

MARIO A. ROJAS, KELLY SHIRLEY, AND MARGARET G. RUSH

Perinatal transport is the timely and appropriate transfer of high-risk pregnant mothers to health care facilities in which expertise and resources for optimal care are available to improve mortality and morbidity of both the mother and her fetus. If transfer of the mother is not possible because of risk outweighing potential benefit, the objective then shifts to optimizing delivery and birth of the high-risk infant. In the latter situation, it is necessary to have adequately trained professionals to resuscitate and stabilize the infant before his or her transfer to a medical center that has the appropriate expertise and resources.

For perinatal transport to effectively support high-risk mothers and their fetuses, as well as sick newborn infants, each country, state, or region must identify its perinatal resources with respect to physical and human capabilities. This review should include classification of levels of care and expertise, as well as mapping of resources as they exist within specific geographic areas. Classification of perinatal resources according to the different levels of care as recommended by the American Academy of Pediatrics and the American College of Obstetricians and Gynecologists in their *Guidelines for Perinatal Care*[4] will direct organization, identification of resources and roles of patient referral and retrieval centers, as well as reveal the natural elevation of care within the geographic area of question (Table 3-1). Historically, regionalization has been recommended as the most effective and cost-efficient use of perinatal resources.[8,11,12,36,45] The implementation of this important strategy is subject to qualitative variance depending on the characteristics of the health care system and resources where it is applied. In countries in which universal health care is the norm, regionalization is more easily implemented, whereas in market-driven health care systems in which deregionalization is predominant, these provisions for care become more challenging.* Whatever the circumstances, perinatal providers must use innovative strategies to maintain high-quality perinatal transport systems.[19,22]

Because all hospitals cannot provide all levels of perinatal care, interhospital transport of pregnant women and neonates is an essential component of any regional perinatal effort. Women who are at risk for complications and pose significant risk for adverse outcomes or whose neonates are likely to require intensive care support should be considered candidates for referral during the antepartum period.[25] Similarly, it is accepted medical practice to transfer a neonate to a hospital that can provide the services needed or anticipated to be needed if the birth hospital cannot provide that level of service.†

Once resources are identified and classified, a model for integration of perinatal services may be constructed. Strategic planning at this level will direct the design of the organizational structure of the perinatal transport system, including identification of leadership functions, the different member nurseries/units and their roles, and the definition and process for perinatal elevation of care. This integration will then allow for the creation of a system for continuous data collection and analysis, facilitating a systems approach to problem solving and the implementation of quality improvement strategies within the system.[27]

Please note that the **PURPLE** type in each chapter is intended to make it easier to identify clinically applicable material.

*References 19, 22, 25, 36, 41, 57.

†References 8, 11, 12, 19, 25, 36, 41, 45, 57.

TABLE 3-1 RECOGNIZED LEVELS OF PERINATAL AND NEONATAL CARE AND THEIR EXPECTED CAPABILITIES

	MATERNAL	NEONATAL		
	RISK-ORIENTED PRENATAL CARE	BASIC NEONATAL CARE	PATIENT CHARACTERISTICS	PERSONNEL
Level 1	Medical screening examination/Patient triage Initial treatment and stabilization Maternal-fetal monitoring/prenatal ultrasound/BPP Non-stress test/stress test 30-minute response time for cesarean section 24-hour clinical laboratory services 24-hour radiology services 24-hour blood bank services	Resuscitation and stabilization (NRP; S.T.A.B.L.E.): Initiation of respiratory support (nasal cannula, oxygen hood, NCPAP, and Neopuff™) Surfactant administration Peripheral IV access/IV fluids Initiation of antibiotics Initiation of PGE_1 when a congenital heart defect is suspected	Uncomplicated maternity and neonatal care Emergency management of unexpected complications Healthy term infants Stable late-preterm infants 35-37 weeks' gestation	Obstetrician Pediatrician Family physicians Certified nurse midwife Pediatric nurse practitioner 24-hour anesthesia availability
Level 2 A	15-minute response time for cesarean section Complicated cases not requiring intensive care	Level 1 care AND Special care nursery	Complete maternity and neonatal care for uncomplicated and most high-risk patients (infants >32 weeks and >1500 g)	Neonatologist Pediatric neonatal hospitalist 24-hour in-house anesthesia for obstetrics
Level 2 B		Capability to provide mechanical ventilation for up to 24 hours or continuous positive airway pressure		Neonatologist
Level 3	Provision of comprehensive perinatal health care services for women and neonates of all risk categories Complicated cases requiring intensive care Labor <34 weeks' gestation	Provision of comprehensive perinatal health care services for women and neonates of all risk categories	Intensive care patients Anticipated need for neonatal surgery	Maternal-fetal specialist Neonatologist Obstetrician
Level 3 A		Provide comprehensive care for infants >28 weeks' gestation and weighing >1000 g Sustained mechanical ventilation		Pediatric surgeon for minor surgical procedures
Level 3 B		Provide comprehensive care for infants ≤28 weeks' gestation and weighing <1000 g Sustained mechanical ventilation High-frequency ventilation Inhaled nitric oxide		Full range of pediatric medical and surgical subspecialties
Level 3 C	Provision of comprehensive perinatal health care services at and above those of subspecialty care facilities Responsibility for regional perinatal health care service organization and coordination	Extracorporeal life support Open heart surgery for congenital cardiac malformations		Pediatric cardiothoracic surgeon

BPP, Biophysical profile; *NCPAP*, nasal continuous positive airway pressure; *NRP*, Neonatal Resuscitation Program; *PGE_1*, prostaglandin E_1; *S.T.A.B.L.E.*, S.T.A.B.L.E. program.

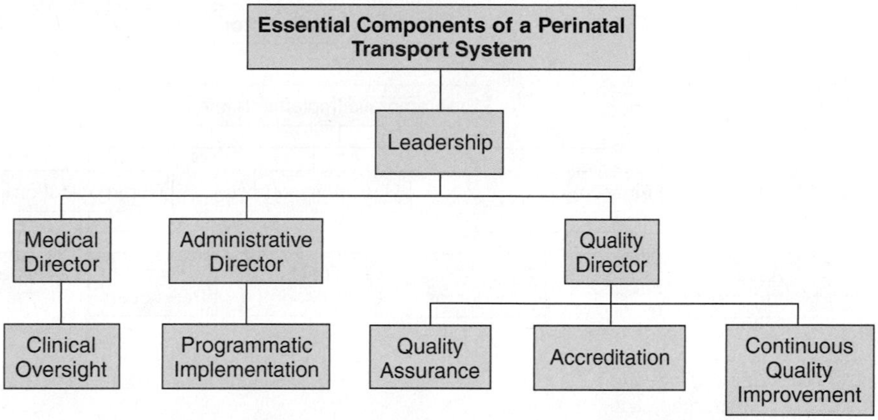

FIGURE 3-1 Organizational structure of perinatal transport system.

REGIONAL PERINATAL REFERRAL AND TRANSPORT SYSTEM

Independent of the health care system with which one identifies (universal versus market driven), the referral system must identify a subspecialty care regional perinatal center, for which the responsibility of coordinating interfacility perinatal transfer lies. Although many different models provide clinical care in transport, the transport system should include the minimal components of (1) leadership (both medical and administrative), (2) communication, and (3) quality assurance (Figure 3-1).

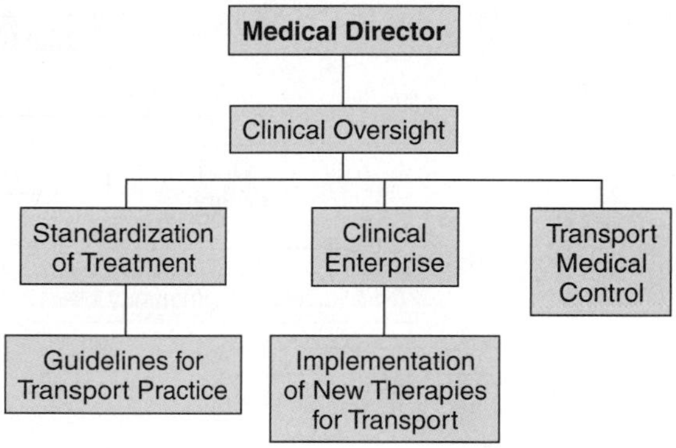

FIGURE 3-2 Role of medical director.

Leadership

One proposed model is the implementation of a leadership team that comprises a medical director, administrative director, and quality director. This team approach enables collaborative and timely oversight of the transport system with potential for growth and quality improvement. The medical director should be a physician with expertise in transport medicine. The medical director's role includes overseeing the following[37] (Figure 3-2):

- Development, implementation, and monitoring of patient care and transport standards
- Scope of practice of team members
- Team selection
- Training and continuing education
- Support of perinatal partnerships and advocacy

The administrative director working in conjunction with the medical director oversees the budget and day-to-day management of the transport process, including maintenance of equipment. The administrative director should possess clinical transport knowledge paired with strong administrative qualities, because this role includes oversight of finance, human resources, and communication operations (Figure 3-3).[37] The quality director should be a health care provider with a professional background in continuous quality improvement, process analysis, and management. In association with the medical director and administrator, the quality director is responsible for the development and maintenance of a transport database for operational management, quality assurance, and analysis. This administrator should also be able to apply the basic concepts of quality improvement and management to implement novel interventions aimed at improving the perinatal transport system (Figure 3-4).[27]

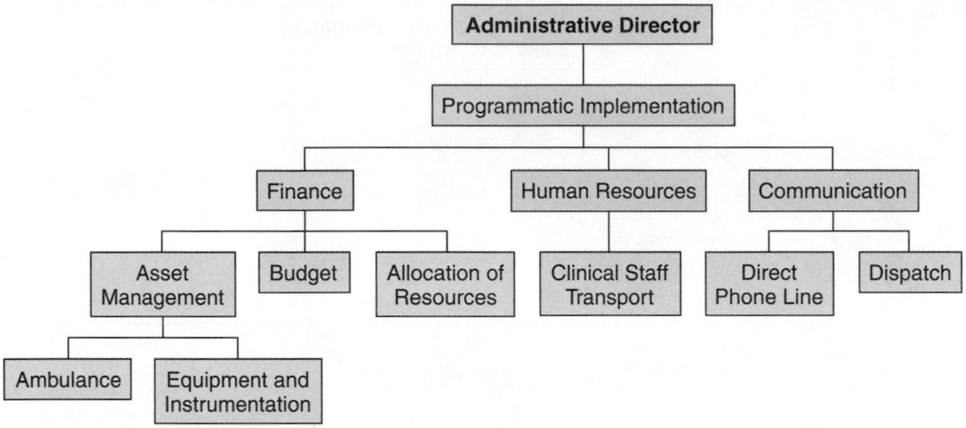

FIGURE 3-3 Role of administrative director.

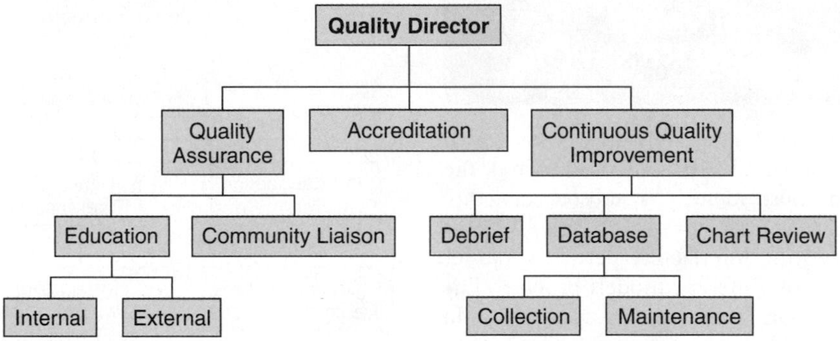

FIGURE 3-4 Role of quality director.

Communication

As indicated in Table 3-1, a regional subspecialty perinatal care center should be responsible for coordination of perinatal transport (level 3C). Integral to the regional transport system is the creation of a centralized communication center with a perinatal regional hotline.[20] The communication center is responsible for coordinating maternal and neonatal transports within the different levels of care. Roles within this center include referring physician, dispatcher, bed locator, and transport medical control officer (obstetrician and neonatologist). The inclusion of specialized personnel in the initial communication process may support rendering institutions appropriate treatment strategies while decreasing diagnostic discordance.[46]

For purposes of basic communication, a central dedicated telephone line is recommended to provide direct, easy, and immediate access to the regional system. This access should be staffed 24 hours per day, 7 days per week and should be unencumbered. This model also includes the transfer of the referral call to the transport medical control officer, thereby greatly simplifying the process for the referral-consultation. The ability to support communication among the referring physician, the dispatcher, and the medical control officer simultaneously can speed up decision making and the initiation of transport. Once in transport, communication among the transport team, the referring physician, and the medical control officer becomes integral to the care provided (Figure 3-5). Changes in patient status, bed status, equipment needs, and weather need to be communicated in a timely manner. This information may demand a review of the transport plan and is best facilitated through a central communication center.[20,37] The organization of a perinatal regional hotline has been shown

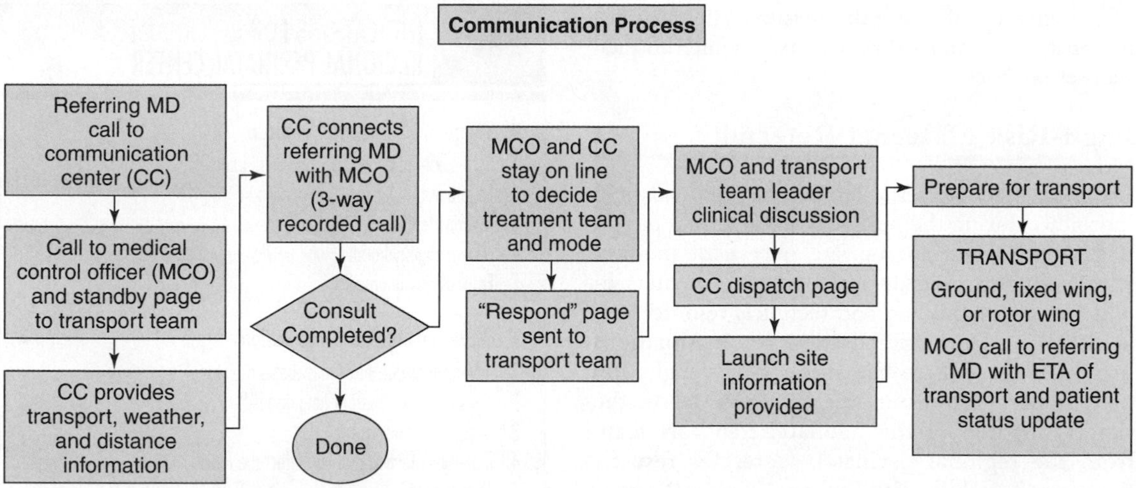

FIGURE 3-5 Working model of Vanderbilt Transport Communication Tool (unpublished), version September 2008. (Contributed by S. Brodtrick, D. Quinn, and M. Cortez.)

to increase significantly both in utero and neonatal transports, allowing for safe, 24-hour, on-call management of perinatal transports and the collection of epidemiologic indicators relative to perinatal transfers.[20]

The rapidly advancing field of telecommunications offers a wide variety of opportunities for transmitting medical information, subject to proper consideration of privacy and confidentiality requirements. This medium permits the use of satellite technology and video-conferencing equipment to conduct a real-time consultation between medical specialists in two geographically different areas. Store-and-forward telemedicine involves acquiring medical data (e.g., medical images, biosignals) and then transmitting this data to a medical specialist for assessment offline. It does not require the presence of both parties at the same time. These technologies may facilitate appropriate referral of patients according to complexity and may decrease incidence of inappropriate transfer or diagnostic discordance, allowing for optimal use of resources.[45,52] Furthermore, these innovative strategies have the potential to overcome de-regionalization of services by creating virtual regional networks for perinatal transport.

Quality

The regional subspecialty perinatal care center, as noted in Table 3-1, is responsible for regional outreach support, education, and continuous quality oversight. Traditionally, quality improvement was assigned to the medical director. However, in light of current health care complexities and regulatory specifications surrounding the quality and safety of patient care, it is recommended that this role be assigned to an individual with the expertise to effectively evaluate programmatic performance at all levels of the organizational structure. This continuous evaluation of the process will facilitate modification of the transport system when potential problems are identified.[27]

The leadership team should oversee overall transport performance. The systematic collection and analysis of carefully selected performance indicators such as patient demographics, management and outcome, safety, logistics, equipment malfunction, and cost will drive quality initiatives. A quality review of individual transports, incidence reports, and occurrence debriefs will enhance this process.[37,55] Using a transport validated physiologic score (e.g., the **t**ransport **r**isk **i**ndex of **p**hysiologic **s**tability [TRIPS]) to evaluate patient status before, during, and after transport can assist team and transport performance.[34,37]

In addition, quality assurance may be implemented through continuing education both internally and externally. Transport programs must create individualized internal training programs that effectively provide current and continuous education to ensure maintenance of appropriate skills for high-quality perinatal transport. A similar program must be adapted to provide educational resources to the referring hospital where training in pretransport resuscitation and stabilization is imperative. Ensuring competence in these areas has the potential to improve short-term and long-term morbidity of sick infants, offsetting the negative effects of de-regionalization and distance between interhospital transfer facilities.[7,37]

High-Risk Maternal Referral

The most effective method to decrease mortality and morbidity during the perinatal and neonatal period is the timely and appropriate referral of mothers with high-risk pregnancies to medical centers in which both the human and technical resources are available to address complications.[14,20] **In situations in which the risk to the mother outweighs the benefit of her transfer during active labor, the timely dispatch of the neonatal transport team from the regional perinatal center for resuscitation and stabilization of the high-risk neonate may be considered the optimal approach to delivery of care.**

Adequate referral of high-risk perinatal patients begins with high-quality antepartum surveillance.[48] Indications for referral to a regional center are shown in Box 3-1. Early identification of factors that can affect pregnancy outcome is important in developing appropriate diagnostic and treatment plans. Optimal perinatal care implies having well-trained and up-to-date obstetricians at all levels of care during both the antepartum and intrapartum period. These physicians should be experts in identifying maternal-fetal risk factors and complications through their knowledge, clinical skills, and expertise in prenatal ultrasound and fetal monitoring.[1,17,40,42] In situations in which this level of expertise is not available, medical and nursing personnel should be specifically trained to identify high-risk pregnancies with the objective of pursuing early referral. Consultation and referral decisions for the high-risk mother should be based on the results of a thorough evaluation of each patient and specific guidelines. Communication between the referral center and the regional perinatal center may be facilitated through the use of video-medicine technology.[18]

BOX 3-1 INDICATIONS FOR REFERRAL TO A REGIONAL PERINATAL CENTER

A. Prenatal Ultrasound Diagnosis

1. Complex fetal genetic or congenital anomalies
2. Severe intrauterine growth restriction[44]
3. Hydrops fetalis
4. Severe oligohydramnios and polyhydramnios
5. Fetal airway anomalies

B. Maternal Medical Complications

1. Advanced or uncontrolled diabetes mellitus
2. Severe organic heart or lung disease
3. Severe renal disease
4. Maternal infection that can affect the fetus
5. Thyrotoxicosis

C. Maternal Surgical Complications

1. Acute abdominal emergency
2. Trauma requiring intensive care
3. Thoracic emergency requiring intensive care

D. Obstetric Complications

1. Premature onset of labor
2. Premature rupture of membranes
3. Third trimester bleeding
4. Severe preeclampsia or hypertension
5. Multiple gestations
6. Rh isoimmunization

Neonatal Referral

Despite efforts to identify high-risk perinatal patients during the antepartum period, as many as 30% to 50% of infants who ultimately require additional neonatal care may not be recognized until the late intrapartum or early neonatal period.[33] For this reason, **all hospitals that provide obstetric services must be prepared for the birth, resuscitation, stabilization, and treatment of premature or term sick infants.** The Neonatal Resuscitation Program (NRP)[3,6,42] sponsored by the American Heart Association and the American Academy of Pediatrics is an excellent resource for training individuals and maintaining resuscitation skills in both a regional program and an individual hospital setting. **Certification (and renewal) of NRP training should be a universal standard for all delivery room and nursery staff.** Beyond the immediate delivery room setting, supportive care should be offered and maintained until the transport team has arrived and assumed care (Box 3-2). This continuance of care is well standardized within the S.T.A.B.L.E. program.[28,51] This program is the only neonatal continuing education program to focus exclusively on the post-resuscitation and/or pre-transport stabilization care of neonates.

BOX 3-2 S.T.A.B.L.E. PRE-TRANSPORT STABILIZATION OF THE NEWBORN

Sugar and safe care
Temperature
Airway
Blood pressure
Lab work
Emotional support for the family

Modified from Karlsen K: *The S.T.A.B.L.E Program: post-resuscitation/pre-transport stabilization care of sick infants—guidelines for neonatal healthcare providers,* ed 5, Park City Utah, 2006, S.T.A.B.L.E., Inc.

NEONATAL TRANSPORT

Stabilization of patients and preparation for transport should begin before the transport team arrives. In consultation, the referring center (physician) and transport medical control officer (MCO) may address additional areas of attention based on specific patient clinical assessment and presumptive diagnosis. Although the reasons for neonatal referral may be quite diverse and based on needs of infants relative to the capabilities of the referring center, the most common indications include respiratory distress, prematurity, congenital anomalies (surgical and nonsurgical), and suspected congenital heart disease. Stabilization and support of these infants may require frequent interhospital communication (referring physician and transport medical control officer) to identify specific medical interventions. The importance of this form of continuing dialogue with respect to accuracy in diagnosis, management, and changes in patient status cannot be stressed enough. Again, the use of video-telemedicine may facilitate the accuracy of these interactions.[7,18]

When the transport team arrives, the receiving hospital generally assumes control of the infant's care, although a certain degree of flexibility and cooperation with the referring staff are maintained. In the event that a community EMS service is used for transport, the referring physician retains medical control until the patient reaches the regional referral center.

Team Configuration

Transport teams may be composed of a variety of medical personnel, including neonatologists, neonatal nurse practitioners, registered nurses, respiratory therapists, paramedics, and emergency medical technicians.[34,35] **The two general categories of transport teams are *dedicated* and *non-dedicated,* with a third hybrid model now emerging in many institutions.** Dedicated teams are those whose members perform neonatal transport on a full-time basis. They generally are not assigned to any other major clinical responsibilities. Non-dedicated teams are composed of members who, although available for transport, are primarily involved with other clinical duties. The hybrid model takes advantage of the well-trained pool of neonatal intensive care unit (NICU) staff, as in the case of the non-dedicated team, but allows for a timely response to transport, as in the dedicated team model. The decision about which type of team to use depends largely on institutional factors. These factors often include the acuity of care level managed in the unit, annual volume of transports, financial support, and national, state, or local laws regulating the expanded role of nurses and respiratory therapists in health care.[23] Regardless of the team composition, the team must have the cumulative expertise to resuscitate, stabilize, and provide critical care throughout the transport.

Dedicated transport teams originated in the 1980s when large metropolitan hospitals began to experience an increase in the demand for neonatal transports. These teams often are composed of a nurse designated as team leader and a second nurse or a respiratory therapist as a partner, with a physician or nurse practitioner added to the team when a neonate is critically ill and more advanced procedures may be anticipated.[16,17,30,35] Nurse-led teams have been shown (1) to provide better continuity of care, improved documentation, better maintenance of transport equipment, improved team availability, and stronger liaisons with referring hospitals and (2) to reduce overall operating costs.[37] The principal advantage to dedicated teams includes their immediate around-the-clock availability and their advanced training in neonatal resuscitation and stabilization procedures. However, the additional personnel necessary for dedicated teams may make these teams expensive to maintain.

Non-dedicated teams usually are made up of staff nurses and respiratory therapists within the NICU.[16,35] The advantage to having a unit-based, non-dedicated transport team is the large pool of trained personnel available around the clock. Qualifications of team members can be based on their daily bedside critical care experience and supplemental education, such as certification as a neonatal resuscitation provider. The primary disadvantage to this team design is that the transport nurse's patient assignments must be absorbed by the unit nursing staff until he or she returns. However, unit-based teams usually are very cost effective because critical care skills are maintained during regular patient care, advanced skill training may be more focused, and administrative oversight duties are diminished.[35]

The ***hybrid model*** recognizes the advantage of pulling the transport team from bedside providers while ensuring immediate, around-the-clock availability. Using this model, transport team members are identified through an interview process and receive additional training for transport care. The personnel then rotate service between bedside care and transport service based on schedule, allowing for a dedicated transport team 24 hours per day, 7 days per week. This model allows for timely dispatch, with no change in patient assignments at the bedside. In addition, this model takes advantage of ongoing bedside critical care training and provides for appropriate skill maintenance. These teams may be nurse-led or may integrate respiratory therapy, physician, or nurse practitioner leadership, based on patient acuity.

Transport Education

A minimum of 2 years of level III neonatal critical care staff experience is a basic requirement for the nursing and respiratory therapy components of most neonatal transport services. **Nurses and respiratory therapists who specialize in neonatal transport should have a basic understanding of neonatal pathophysiology, resuscitation and stabilization techniques, ventilatory management, and radiographic interpretation.** In the event of a critically ill patient, a nurse practitioner or physician may serve as team leader with respect to high-level procedures and patient management.[29,30]

Most transport programs will develop training programs individualized to local needs, with the level of training dependant on whether the providers are nurse-led or physician-led. The scope of practice and curriculum is overseen by the medical director. Although no standard curriculum for transport providers exists, guidelines have been published by the American Academy of Pediatric Taskforce on Interhospital Transport.[2,37] Programs using air transport should ensure that all providers, including physicians who may be involved occasionally, have education on air safety, survival methods, and flight physiology (including air transport effects of barometric pressure, g-force, humidity change, potential temperature loss, noise, and vibration). In addition, the program must ensure continuing education for all aspects of transport to include updates on care management, maintenance of skills, reviewing of practice standards, and new management strategies.[37,49]

Mode of Transport

When initiating a neonatal transport program, the first step should be to identify the geographic catchment area, total number and location of perinatal resources, distance in miles/kilometers, and duration of transport time (ground versus air) between the different levels of care. An important factor is the particular characteristics of the topography of the catchment area, which will help determine the ratio of ground-to-air transport resources required. In areas with good roads and low traffic volume, ground transport may be the only transport system required.[14,26,37,50] Selecting the proper mode of transport (ambulance, helicopter, or fixed-wing aircraft) depends on many variables including environmental conditions. Severity of disease and clinical status of the patient should guide the overall plan for mode of transport. In general, when transport time exceeds 2 hours, air transport is more appropriate.[37] However, local ground transport capabilities to-from a referring hospital and airport must be known when fixed-wing air transport is used.

Equipment and Medications

The equipment and medications necessary for neonatal transport are similar to those used in the NICU. Equipment must be light, compact, durable, and motion and g-force tolerant. All electronic equipment should have its own independent power supply (AC/DC capability), adequate visual and audio alarms, and lack of electromagnetic interference.[14,37] Table 3-2 provides a list of common transport equipment and medications.

Novel Interventions

Because the objective of the perinatal transport team is to bring the intensive care environment to the newborn infant, it is **fundamental that initial resuscitation and stabilization be performed by skilled practitioners in order for the team to**

TABLE 3-2 **EQUIPMENT AND MEDICATIONS FOR NEONATAL TRANSPORT***

PHYSIOLOGIC MONITORING AND SAFETY	AIRWAY AND SUCTION EQUIPMENT	RESPIRATORY EQUIPMENT	PROCEDURE EQUIPMENT	IV FLUID AND ACCESS	MEDICATIONS	REFRIGERATED MEDICATION
BP cuffs, #2-#4 (2 each) Electrodes (2 of each available size) Pulse oximeter probes (2) Dispensable thermometers (2) Skin temperature probes (8) Rectal probe (1) Warming pad portable: chemical (2) 4×4 gauze pads (2) Nonstick gauze pads (2) Bowel bag (1) Sterile rolled gauze (2) Ear protectors (2) Hats (2) Flashlight (2) Tape measures (2)	Laryngoscope (2) Laryngoscope blades (2 of each size) Laryngoscope light bulbs (3) AA batteries (4) Endotracheal tubes (3 of each size) Stylettes (4) CO_2 detector (2 self-contained, sterile) Closed suction catheter (2 of each size) Meconium aspiration device (2) Bulb suction (2) Suction catheters (2 of each size) Saline bullets (4) Replogle (2 of each size) Orogastric tubes (2 of each size)	Anesthesia bags (2 per T-PICU infant resuscitator) Self-inflating bag (2) Oxygen mask (2) Facemasks (2 of each size) Infant nasal cannula (2) CPAP prongs (2 of each size) Neonatal flow sensor (2) CPAP circuit (1) Ventilator circuit (1) Point-of-care blood gas equipment (1-2)	Sterile towels (1) UAC tray (1) Single-lumen umbilical catheters (2 of each size) Double-lumen umbilical catheters (2 of each size) Umbilical tape (2) Povidone iodine (3) Scalpels #11 and #15 (1 each) 4.0 silk suture (4) Dressing for umbilical line (2) Needle aspiration/chest tube kit (2) Transducer (2) Chest tubes, 10 Fr/12 Fr (2 of each size) Heimlich valve (2) Sterile gloves (5 of each size)	D_5W 50 mL (2) NS 250 mL (1) $D_{10}W$ 500 mL (1) $D_{50}W$ 50 mL (1) Heparin sodium 1000 mcg/mL vial (3) Syringes, 3 mL/1 mL (6 each) IV catheter, #22 and #24 gauge (5 each) Access kit, including dressing, tourniquet (2) Butterfly needle (3 of each size) Arm board (2) Heel warmers (2) Lancets (2 of infant and preemie size) Syringes (5 of each size)	Epinephrine 1:10,000 (2) Naloxone 1 mg/1 mL (2) 4.2% sodium bicarbonate (2) Dopamine (2) Dobutamine (2) Acyclovir (1) Ampicillin (2) Gentamicin (2) Vitamin K for injection (1) Eye ointment (2) Lidocaine HCl (1) Adenosine (1) Vecuronium (1) Sterile saline for injection (2) Abboject needle (2) Fentanyl (2) Midazolam (2) Phenobarbital (2)	Exogenous surfactant (1) PGE (2)

*( ) designates numbers of pieces of equipment to be carried in transport kit.
CPAP, Continuous positive airway pressure; *NS,* normal saline; *PGE,* prostaglandin E; *UAC,* umbilical artery catheter; *T-PICU,* T-piece infant care unit.

successfully continue to offer appropriate high-quality intensive care during the transport of the baby. Level I and level II centers should be equipped with surfactant, nasal continuous positive airway pressure (NCPAP) systems, and oxygen-air blenders to give prompt and effective respiratory support while maintaining blood saturation levels within acceptable limits awaiting the arrival of the transport team. Adequate management of the premature infant with surfactant deficiency will include supporting adequate recruitment of the lung and minimizing barotrauma. **Acquiring the requisite skills to intubate and administer surfactant appropriately and to administer early NCPAP has the potential to improve patient survival, decrease the need for mechanical ventilation,[15,47,48,53,54] and decrease morbidity in situations in which duration of transport may be prolonged for**

hours because of unforeseen delays. Although the use of NCPAP in the delivery room is not a novel intervention,[56] its use as an early intervention in the delivery room for infants with respiratory failure is accepted as a common approach for the management of premature infants with respiratory distress syndrome (RDS) and term infants with mild to moderate respiratory failure. Because surfactant is an expensive medication, level I and level II centers can maintain 1 or 2 ampules in their pharmacy to be restocked by the perinatal transport team before transport. The use of NCPAP during transport has also been evaluated recently and has been shown to be a safe and efficacious intervention for respiratory support.[39]

The use of a resuscitation device such as the T-piece infant resuscitator (Neopuff™ Infant Resuscitator, Fisher & Paykel Healthcare) may help decrease the variability of pressures administered to the neonate during resuscitation, stabilization, or administration of surfactant. This device also has the potential to minimize lung damage while supporting lung recruitment with the use of positive end-expiratory pressure (PEEP).[9,43] This system can also temporarily replace the need for mechanical ventilation if NCPAP is unsuccessful in maintaining respiratory stability.

Another important intervention for perinatal transport is the **administration of prostaglandin E_1 (PGE_1) in patients in whom a suspicion of congenital heart diseases is supported with a positive hyperoxia test.** Adequate knowledge of dosing and preparation is fundamental to the successful use of this medication that can prevent patients with ductal dependent lesions from becoming clinically unstable and developing severe hypoxemia and metabolic acidosis before the arrival of the transport team. The need for intubation and ventilator support to prevent apnea varies depending on the anticipated length of transfer and the dose of PGE_1 necessary to maintain the infant asymptomatic.[10,21] Knowledge by the referring physician of the performance and interpretation of the hyperoxia test will facilitate the decision to start PGE_1 and should be part of the maintenance-of-skills program. We recommend that both level I and level II nurseries maintain in stock a vial of PGE_1.

In recent years, **inhaled nitric oxide (iNO) has been used on transport to support term and near-term infants with hypoxemic respiratory failure** that does not respond to conventional mechanical ventilation.[31] The use of this therapeutic gas can be lifesaving and may decrease associated morbidities. Its use during transport will require certain adaptations for both ground and air transport in order to use this gas safely and effectively. Another novel intervention is the **use of whole-body cooling or head cooling during transport to minimize brain damage from severe hypoxic ischemic encephalopathy.** The use of passive and active cooling before and during transport as a therapy for neonatal encephalopathy has been reported in the literature, but more studies are required to determine the safety and efficacy of this intervention.[5]

Patients managed during transport with other more-complex interventions such as high-frequency jet ventilation (HFJV) and extracorporeal membrane oxygenation (ECMO) have been reported in the literature. Their use for routine transport cannot be recommended because of the complexity of training, equipment, and logistics required to administer these interventions.[13,38] Every country and regional perinatal center must determine its priorities for transport based on epidemiologic studies conducted in its catchment area to support the demand with appropriate resources for adequate perinatal transport.

FAMILY-CENTERED CARE FOR TRANSPORT

Separation of the infant and mother (parents) is often the consequence of neonatal transport. **This physical separation affects both bonding and attachment, increasing the stress surrounding the delivery of an ill infant.**[28,32,51] Creative ways to minimize the negative impacts of this separation must be incorporated into the transport process.

Before departure from the referring facility, the transport team should meet with the parents of the infant, communicating the plan for transport, providing information with regard to the receiving hospital (to include phone numbers, directions, and unit-specific guidelines), and answering any questions the parents may have. The transport team should identify a phone number that may be used to communicate with the parents once the infant is transported. In addition, **the transport team should enable the parents to see and touch the infant before departure and should provide the parents with a photograph of their infant.**[37]

Upon arrival at the receiving medical center, a transport team member should call the parents to update them on the condition and the safe arrival of their baby in the receiving facility. At this time, the transport team should give the parents the names of those who will be responsible for the care of the infant. Once the infant is admitted into the receiving unit, the receiving physician should communicate directly with the parents and referring physician. **Engaging the parents in the caregiving process as soon as possible empowers parents** and assists the health care team in devising a care plan that will be mutually acceptable and in the best interest of the infant.

Facilitation of communication with parents may be improved with the use of video-telemedicine.[24] This technology would enable the parents to see their infant in the receiving center and speak directly with the nurses or physicians caring for their infant.

FUTURE OF NEONATAL TRANSPORT

Research, innovation, and maintenance of regionalization represent the future for perinatal transport. The mandate for highly motivated leadership able to apply epidemiologic, research, and quality-improvement methodology to the area of perinatal transport is essential for progress. The development and evaluation of new interventions, as well as the evaluation of what we consider "standard therapies," are imperative to better outcomes. The inclusion of continuous quality improvement at the top leadership level of the organizational structure of the perinatal transport system and the systematic collection of relevant data within an identified perinatal region represents the backbone for research in standing and new technologies. **Special attention must be centered toward the community in order to improve resuscitation and stabilization efforts.** In addition, benchmarking with regard to morbidity and mortality outcomes for transported patients will provide clarity for evaluation of the transport experience. The ultimate focus of this effort is to improve maternal and neonatal outcomes. Ultimate success will depend on the level of multidisciplinary participation of government, community, and private industry stakeholders.

REFERENCES

1. Abbrescia K, Sheridan B: Complications of second and third trimester pregnancies, *Emerg Med Clin N Am* 21:695, 2003.
2. American Academy of Pediatrics, Task Force on Interhospital Transport, MacDonald MG, Ginzburg HM, editors: *Guidelines for air and ground transport of neonatal and pediatric patients*, ed 2, Elk Grove Village, Ill, 1999, The Academy.
3. American Academy of Pediatrics, American Heart Association, Kattwinkel J, editor: *Textbook of neonatal resuscitation*, ed 5, Elk Grove Village, Ill, 2006, The Academy.
4. American Academy of Pediatrics, American College of Obstetricians and Gynecologists: Interhospital care of the perinatal patient. In *Guidelines for perinatal care*, ed 6, Elk Grove Village, Ill, 2007, The Academy.
5. Anderson ME, Longhofer TA, Phillips W, et al: Passive cooling to initiate hypothermia for transported encephalopathic newborns, *J Perinatol* 27:592, 2007.
6. Annibale DJ, Cahill JB, Tuttle DS, et al: Preparation of the critically ill neonate for transport, *J South Carolina Med Assoc* 98:129, 2002.
7. Arad I, Gofin R, Baras M, et al: Neonatal outcome of inborn and transported very-low-birth-weight infants: relevance of perinatal factors, *Eur J Obstet Gynecol Reprod Biol* 83:151, 1999.
8. Bartels DB, Wypij D, Wenzlaff P, et al: Hospital volume and neonatal mortality among very low birth weight infants, *Pediatrics* 117:2206, 2006.
9. Bennett S, Finer NN, Rich W, et al: A comparison of three neonatal resuscitation devices, *Resuscitation* 67:113, 2005.
10. Browing-Carmo KA, Barr P, West M, et al: Transporting newborn infants with suspected duct dependent congenital heart disease on low-dose prostaglandin E_1 without routine *mechanical* ventilation, *Arch Dis Child Fetal Neonatal Ed* 92:F117, 2007.
11. Chien LY, Whyte R, Aziz K, et al: Improved outcome of preterm infants when delivered in tertiary care centers, *Obstet Gynecol* 98:247, 2001.
12. Cifuentes J, Bronstein J, Phibbs CS, et al: Mortality in low birth weight infants according to level of neonatal care at hospital of birth, *Pediatrics* 109:745, 2002.
13. Coppola CP, Tyree M, Larry K, et al: A 22-year experience in global transport extracorporeal membrane oxygenation, *J Pediatr Surg* 43:46, 2007.
14. Cornette L: Contemporary neonatal transport: problems and solutions, *Arch Dis Child Fetal Neonatal Ed* 89:F212, 2004.
15. Dani C, Bertini G, Pezzati M, et al: Early extubation and nasal continuous positive airway pressure after surfactant treatment for respiratory distress syndrome among preterm infants < 30 weeks gestation, *Pediatrics* 113:e560, 2004.
16. Danzig D: Neonatal transport teams: a survey of functions and roles, *Neonatal Netw* 3:41, 1984.
17. Devoe LD: Antenatal fetal assessment: contraction stress test, nonstress test, vibroacoustic stimulation, amniotic fluid volume, biophysical profile, and modified biophysical profile—an overview, *Semin Perinatol* 32:247, 2008.
18. Di Lieto A, De Falco M, Campanile M, et al: Regional and international prenatal telemedicine network for computerized antepartum cardiotocography, *Telemed J E Health* 14:49, 2008.

19. Dobrez D, Gerber S, Budetti P: Trends in perinatal regionalization and the role of managed care, *Obstet Gynecol* 108:839, 2006.
20. Dupuis O, Gaucherand P, Mellier G: et le Comité de pilotage de la cellule des transferts périnatals: Perinatal regional hotline organisation and rate of perinatal transfer: results from 2003 and 2004 in the French Rhône-alps area—a two year study of 4079 transfers, *J Gynecol Obstet Biol Reprod* 35:702, 2006.
21. Ferrarese P, Marra A, Doglioni N, et al: Routine mechanical ventilation for transferred neonates with duct-dependent congenital heart disease, *Arch Dis Child Fetal Neonatal Ed* 92:F422, 2007.
22. Gerber SE, Dobrez DG, Budetti P: Managed care and perinatal regionalization in Washington State, *Obstet Gynecol* 98:139, 2001.
23. Gomez M: Hiring, staffing, and team composition. In McClosky K, Orr R, editors: *Pediatric transport medicine*, St Louis, 1995, Mosby.
24. Gray JE, Safran C, Davis RB, et al: Baby CareLink: using the Internet and telemedicine to improve care for high-risk infants, *Pediatrics* 106:1318, 2000.
25. Heller G, Richardson DK, Schnell R, et al: Are we regionalized enough? Early-neonatal deaths in low-risk births by the size of delivery units in Hesse, Germany 1990–1999, *Int J Epidemiol* 31:1061, 2002.
26. Hon K-LE, Olsen H, Leung T-F: Air versus ground transportation of artificially ventilated neonates: comparative differences in selected cardiopulmonary parameters, *Pediatr Emerg Care* 22:107, 2006.
27. Kaluzny AD, McLaughlin CP: *Continuous quality improvement in health care: theory, implementation, and applications*, Gaithersburg, Md, 1994, Aspen Publishers.
28. Karlsen K: The S.T.A.B.L.E. Program: post-resuscitation/pre-transport stabilization care of sick infants—guidelines for neonatal healthcare providers, ed 5, Park City Utah, 2006, S.T.A.B.L.E., Inc.
29. King BR, Foster RL, Woodward GA, et al: Procedures performed by pediatric nurses: how "advanced" is the practice? *Pediatr Emerg Care* 17:410, 2001.
30. King BR, King TM, Foster RL, et al: Pediatric and neonatal transport teams with and without a physician, *Pediatr Emerg Care* 23:77, 2007.
31. Kinsella JP, Schmidt JM, Griebel J, et al: Inhaled nitric oxide treatment for stabilization and emergency medical transport of critically ill newborns and infants, *Pediatrics* 95:773, 1995.
32. Klaus MH, Kennell JH: *Maternal-infant bonding: the impact of early separation or loss on family development*, St Louis, 1976, Mosby.
33. Ledger WJ: Identification of the high risk mother and fetus: does it work? *Clin Perinatol* 6:125, 1980.
34. Lee SK, Zupanic JAF, Pendray MR, et al: Transport risk index of physiologic stability: a practical system for assessing infant transport care, *J Pediatr* 139:220, 2001.
35. Lee SK, Zupancic JAF, Sale J, et al: Cost-effectiveness and choice of infant transport systems, *Med Care* 40:705, 2002.
36. Lui K, Abdel-Latif ME, Allgood CL, et al: The New South Wales and Australian Capital Territory Neonatal Intensive Care Unit Study Group: Improved outcomes of extremely premature outborn infants: effects of strategic changes in perinatal and retrieval services, *Pediatrics* 118:2076, 2006.
37. Lupton BA, Pendray MR: Regionalized neonatal emergency transport, *Semin Neonatol* 9:125, 2004.
38. Mainali ES, Greene C, Rozycki HJ, et al: Safety and efficacy of high-frequency jet ventilation in neonatal transport, *J Perinatol* 27:609, 2007.
39. Murray PG, Stewart MJ: Use of nasal continuous positive airway pressure during retrieval of neonates with acute respiratory distress, *Pediatrics* e754:121, 2008.
40. Nabhan AF, Abdelmoula YA: Amniotic fluid index versus single deepest vertical pocket as a screening test for preventing adverse pregnancy outcome, *Cochrane Database Syst Rev* 3: CD006593, 2008 DOI:10.1002/14651858.CD006593.pub2.
41. Neto MT: Perinatal care in Portugal: effects of 15 years of a regionalized system, *Acta Paediatr* 95:1349, 2006.
42. Niermeyer S, the contributors and reviewers for the Neonatal Resuscitation Guidelines: International guidelines for neonatal resuscitation: and excerpt from the guidelines 2000 for cardiopulmonary resuscitation and emergency cardiovascular care—international consensus on science, *Pediatrics* 106:e29, 2000. Accessed July 11, 2009, from www.pediatrics.org/cgi/content/full/106/3/e29.
43. Oddie S, Wyllie J, Scally A: Use of self-inflating bags for neonatal resuscitation, *Resuscitation* 67:109, 2005.
44. Pedersen NG, Figueras F, Wojdemann KR, et al: Early fetal size and growth as predictors of adverse outcome, *Obstet Gynecol* 112:765, 2008.
45. Phibbs CS, Baker LC, Caughey AB, et al: Level and volume of neonatal intensive care and mortality in very-low-birth-weight infants, *N Engl J Med* 356:2165, 2007.
46. Philpot C, Day S, Marcdante K, et al: Pediatric interhospital transport: diagnostic discordance and hospital mortality, *Pediatr Crit Care Med* 9:15, 2008.
47. Reininger A, Khalak R, Kendig JW, et al: Surfactant administration by transient intubation in infants 29 to 35 weeks' gestation with respiratory distress syndrome decreases the likelihood of later mechanical ventilation: a randomized control trial, *J Perinatol* 25:703, 2005.
48. Rojas MA, Lozano JM, Rojas MX, et al: For the Colombian Neonatal Research Network: Very early surfactant without mandatory ventilation in premature infants treated with early continuous positive airway pressure: a randomized control trial, *Pediatrics* 123:137, 2009.

49. Skeoch CH, Jackson L, Wilson AM, et al: Fit to fly: practical challenges in neonatal transfers by air, *Arch Dis Child Fetal Neonatal Ed* 90:F456, 2005.
50. Svenson JE, O'Connor JE, Lindsay B: Is air transport faster? A comparison of air versus ground transport times for interfacility transfers in a regional referral system, *Air Med J* 24:170, 2003.
51. Taylor RM, Price-Douglas W: The S.T.A.B.L.E. Program post-resuscitation/pretransport stabilization care of sick infants, *J Perinat Neonat Nurs* 22:159, 2008.
52. Tsai SH, Kraus J, Wu H-R, et al: The effectiveness of video-telemedicine for screening of patients requesting emergency air medical transport (EAMT), *J Trauma* 62:504, 2007.
53. Verder H, Albertsen P, Ebbeson F, et al: Nasal continuous positive airway pressure and early surfactant therapy for respiratory distress syndrome in newborns of less than 30 weeks' gestation, *Pediatrics* 103:e24, 1999.
54. Verder H, Robertson B, Greisen G, et al: Surfactant therapy and nasal continuous positive airway pressure for newborns with respiratory distress syndrome, *N Engl J Med* 331:1051, 1994.
55. Woodward WGA, Insoft RM, Pearson-Shaver AL, et al: The state of pediatric interfacility transport: consensus of the second national pediatric and neonatal interfacility transport medicine leadership conference, *Pediatr Emerg Care* 18:38, 2002.
56. Wung JT, Driscol JM Jr, Epstein RA, et al: A new device for CPAP by nasal route, *Crit Care Med* 3:76, 1975.
57. Yu VY, Doyle LW: Regionalized long-term follow-up, *Semin Neonatol* 9:135, 2004.

4 DELIVERY ROOM CARE

SUSAN NIERMEYER AND SUSAN B. CLARKE

The purpose of immediate delivery room care is to support the newborn's respiratory and circulatory systems during the transition from fetal to neonatal life. Normal physiologic changes at birth include expansion of the lungs with air, initiation of gas exchange across the alveolar membrane, and closure of circulatory shunts that were necessary during intrauterine life. **When delivery is complicated by perinatal conditions leading to asphyxia, the aim of resuscitation is to reverse hypoxia, hypercarbia, and acidosis.** The survival and outcome of distressed newborns depend on timely and effective intervention in the first few minutes after birth.

Information in this chapter provides the reader with a clearer understanding of the physiologic events that take place in a distressed neonate and the current evidence and controversies behind the techniques used in delivery room resuscitation.

All resuscitation efforts begin with the basic techniques of thermal control, clearing of the airway, and stimulation of breathing.[2,38] Advanced resuscitation includes assessment of oxygenation, supplemental oxygen administration (if needed), bag-and-mask ventilation, endotracheal intubation, chest compressions, and use of medications and volume expansion. Delivery room emergencies may require the basic elements of resuscitation, as well as more advanced procedures that may be called for during stabilization in the delivery room and transitional nursery. Finally, the essential elements of successful resuscitation are care of the family, perinatal decision making, and teamwork among health care professionals.

PHYSIOLOGY

At birth, rapid physiologic transition from the intrauterine to extrauterine environment must be made. **Effective, regular respirations should be initiated within 30 to 45 seconds of delivery.** Environmental factors, such as a relatively cool ambient temperature and tactile stimulation, assist in initiating respiration. The changes in $Pa{O_2}$ and $Pa{CO_2}$ resulting from clamping the umbilical cord affect chemoreceptors and aid in the reflexive initiation of respiration. The initial breath may generate from 20 to 70 cm H_2O of negative intrathoracic pressure to replace lung liquid with air inside the alveoli.[55] A rapid decrease in pulmonary vascular resistance and an increase in pulmonary blood flow occur after expansion of the lungs with air. This results in increased pulmonary perfusion and oxygenation.[54] Removal and absorption of fetal lung fluid is also necessary. Resorption of fetal lung liquid across the respiratory epithelium accelerates during labor, resulting in net clearance of liquid from the potential airspaces.[8] Colloid osmotic pressure and the relatively lower postnatal hydrostatic pressure of blood within the pulmonary circuit assist in absorbing alveolar fluid after delivery. During this process, fetal right-to-left shunts through the ductus arteriosus and foramen ovale gradually close (Figure 4-1; Table 4-1).[21]

ASPHYXIA AND APNEA

Asphyxia is defined as inadequate tissue perfusion that fails to meet the metabolic demands of the tissues for

Please note that the **PURPLE** type in each chapter is intended to make it easier to identify clinically applicable material.

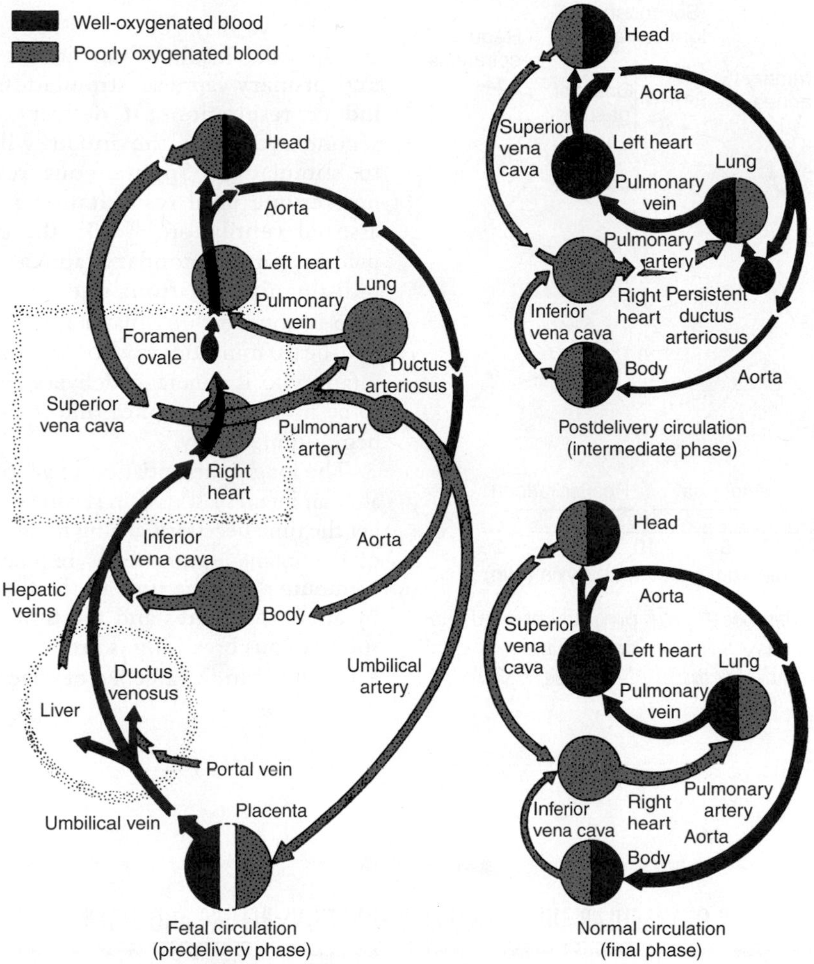

FIGURE 4-1 Blood circulation before and after birth. (From Babson SG, Pernoll ML, Brenda GL: *Diagnosis and management of the fetus and neonate at risk: a guide for team care*, ed 4, St Louis, 1980, Mosby.)

oxygen and waste removal. **Asphyxia is characterized by progressive hypoxemia (↓Po_2), hypercarbia (↑Pco_2), and acidosis (↓pH).**[15] Hypoxic tissues convert from aerobic metabolism to anaerobic glycolysis, producing lactate and metabolic acidosis that is initially buffered by bicarbonate.[18] When the buffering capacity is exhausted, acidosis occurs. Acidosis and hypoxemia initially result in reflexive, compensatory cardiovascular changes. After early tachycardia, cardiac output decreases and generalized peripheral vasoconstriction occurs to maintain a blood pressure adequate for perfusion of vital organs. Prolonged asphyxia results in eventual bradycardia and hypotension as severe acidosis and cardiac failure occur.

Asphyxia may occur in utero or postnatally. In either circumstance, a well-defined series of respiratory events follow (Figure 4-2).[18] During ***primary apnea,*** respiratory movements cease after a brief period of rapid breathing. At the same time, heart rate falls and neuromuscular tone diminishes. Intrauterine asphyxia may result in the passage of meconium before birth. If the asphyxial insult continues, the heart rate falls further, blood pressure falls, hypotonia worsens, and a series of spontaneous deep gasps occur. Gasping continues but becomes weaker and more irregular and then finally ceases. After the last gasp, a period of ***secondary apnea*** begins.[18,38]

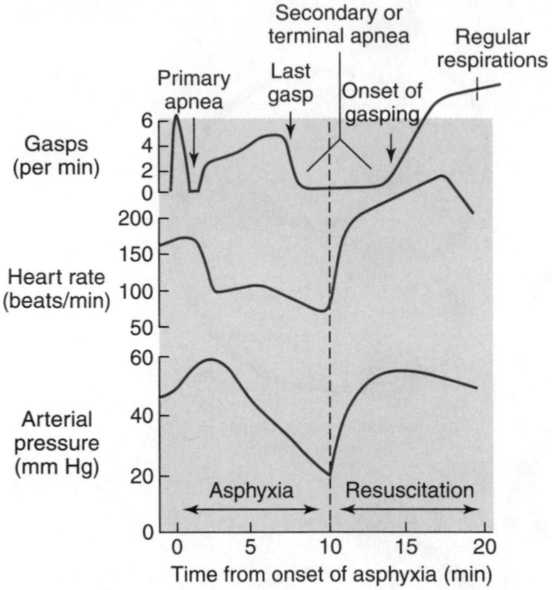

FIGURE 4-2 Changes in physiologic parameters during asphyxiation and resuscitation of rhesus monkey fetus at birth. (From Dawes GS: *Foetal and neonatal physiology: a comparative study of the changes at birth*, St Louis, 1968, Mosby.)

Delivery may occur at any point during an asphyxial insult. **If an infant is born during primary apnea, stimulation will usually induce respirations. If delivery occurs during secondary apnea, the infant will not respond to stimulation. Spontaneous respirations will not resume until resuscitation is initiated with assisted ventilation.**[1,18,38] **In the clinical setting, primary and secondary apnea are essentially indistinguishable from one another.** The infant who is not breathing may have a heart rate below 100 beats/min and may be hypotonic. Thus any infant who is apneic at delivery must be assumed to be in secondary apnea, and resuscitation should begin immediately.

The longer the initiation of ventilation is delayed after an infant's last gasp in secondary apnea, the longer the time necessary during resuscitation for return of the infant's spontaneous respiration. **For every 1-minute delay, the time to the first gasp increases by about 2 minutes and the time to the onset of spontaneous breathing is prolonged by more than 4 minutes.**[1] In the absence of effective resuscitation

TABLE 4-1

COMPARISON OF VASCULAR AND PULMONARY FUNCTIONS BEFORE AND AFTER BIRTH

BODY STRUCTURE	FETAL FUNCTION	EXTRAUTERINE FUNCTION
Aorta	Carries oxygenated blood from left ventricle and deoxygenated blood from pulmonary arteries to fetal organs and placenta	Carries oxygenated blood from left ventricle into systemic circulation
Ductus venosus	Shunts most of the oxygenated blood from placenta to inferior vena cava	Disappears within 2 weeks after birth; becomes ligamentum venosum
Foramen ovale	Connects right and left atria; permits oxygenated blood from right atrium to bypass right ventricle and pulmonary circuit and go directly into left atrium	Functionally closes soon after birth; anatomically seals during childhood
Ductus arteriosus	Shunts blood from pulmonary artery directly into aorta	Functionally closes soon after birth; eventually becomes ligamentum arteriosum
Umbilical arteries and vein	Carry blood to and from placenta, the organ of respiration before birth	Clamped at birth, obliterating placental connections; become ligaments
Lungs	Distended with fluid; minimal pulmonary circulation; fetal respiratory movements	Expanded and aerated; pulmonary circulation allows CO_2 and O_2 exchange; organ of respiration

after delivery, apnea and decreased cardiac output result in progressive biochemical deterioration.[1,18]

Severe fetal and neonatal asphyxia impair the physiologic transitions to extrauterine life. The normally high fetal pulmonary vascular resistance may not decrease in the presence of pulmonary hypoexpansion, persistent acidosis, and hypoxemia. Consequently, the pulmonary circuit continues to carry low volumes of blood. Oxygen transfer is impeded, perpetuating hypoxemia (Figure 4-3).[54] As part of persistent pulmonary hypertension of the newborn, normal closure of fetal shunts is delayed by high pulmonary vascular resistance and pulmonary hypoperfusion, hypoexpansion, and hypoxemia. This results in persistent right-to-left shunting through the ductus arteriosus and foramen ovale. Lung fluid clearance also may be delayed because of poor lung inflation or pulmonary hypoperfusion and hypoxemia. In addition, intraalveolar fluid may accumulate as a result of leakage from damaged pulmonary capillaries, resulting in pulmonary edema. With worsening hypoxemia and acidosis, myocardial function begins to fail, cardiac output falls, and perfusion decreases to vital body organs, including the brain, kidney, and intestine, setting the stage for postasphyxial injury of these organs.[15]

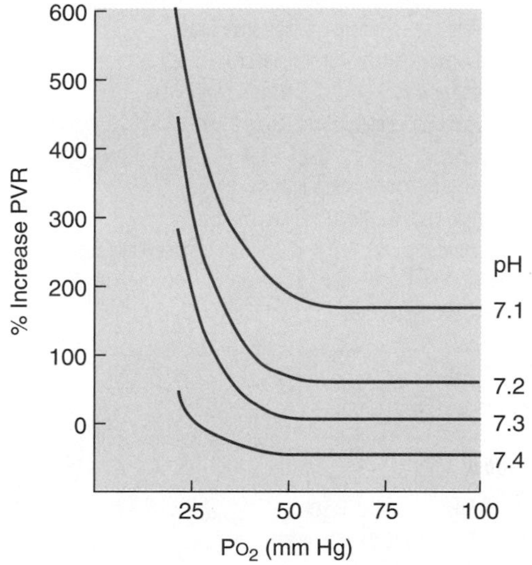

FIGURE 4-3 Pulmonary vascular resistance in calf. *PVR,* Pulmonary vascular resistance. (From Rudolph AM, Yuan S: Response of the pulmonary vasculature to hypoxia and H ion concentration changes, *J Clin Invest* 45:399, 1966.)

RESUSCITATION OF THE NEWBORN

Preparation for Resuscitation

Immediate, effective resuscitation of the newborn infant can reduce or prevent morbidity and mortality. **Much of neonatal resuscitation focuses on accurate assessment and initiation of ventilation. Application of basic procedures often is all that is necessary to successfully resuscitate a depressed infant.[49] However, effective resuscitation requires anticipation, adequate preparation of equipment and personnel, and teamwork.[6,50,74]**

Elements of the antepartum and intrapartum histories may identify the infant at risk for perinatal asphyxia (Box 4-1). However, any normal pregnancy may become high-risk at the onset of previously

BOX 4-1 CONDITIONS THAT MAY REQUIRE AVAILABILITY OF SKILLED RESUSCITATION AT DELIVERY

Intrapartum Problems

- Fetal distress
  - Persistent late decelerations
  - Severe variable decelerations without baseline variability
  - Bradycardia
  - Meconium-stained amniotic fluid
  - Cord prolapse
- Prolonged, unusual, or difficult labor
- Emergency operative or assisted delivery
- Breech presentation with vaginal delivery
- Narcotic administration to mother within 4 hours of delivery

Medical/Obstetric/Genetic Problems

- Diabetes mellitus
- Suspected or confirmed maternal infection
- Substance abuse
- Third trimester bleeding
- Pregnancy-induced hypertension
- Abnormal amniotic fluid volume
- Prolonged rupture of membranes
- Multiple gestation
- Low-birth-weight infant
- Prematurity
- Isoimmunization
- Fetal congenital anomalies

unexpected or undetected intrapartum complications, including maternal hemorrhage, cord prolapse, and meconium staining of the amniotic fluid. Although prevention, detection, and treatment of fetal asphyxia are the responsibilities of the obstetric team, therapeutic intervention should be coordinated between obstetric and neonatal services to ensure a timely delivery and effective, coordinated resuscitation.

In the mid-1980s, the American Heart Association (AHA) and the American Academy of Pediatrics (AAP) addressed the need for a national training program for neonatal resuscitation in the United States by developing the **Neonatal Resuscitation Program (NRP). The NRP provides the materials and training necessary for health care professionals to put into practice the scientific consensus established and updated periodically by the International Liaison Committee on Resuscitation (ILCOR).** In 2000 and 2005, the guidelines were revised based on a rigorous process of evidence evaluation.[33,45] These changes have been incorporated into the fifth edition of the *Textbook of Neonatal Resuscitation*.[38] Evidence review is ongoing, and revised guidelines will be published in the Fall of 2010. **The program's widespread acceptance ensures consistent awareness of current scientific consensus, use of proper equipment, and preparation of personnel to work as a team using shared knowledge and performance skills.**

The NRP recommends the following[38]

> At every delivery, there should be at least one person whose only responsibility is the baby and who is capable of initiating resuscitation. Either that person or another who is immediately available should have the skills necessary to perform a complete resuscitation, including endotracheal intubation and administration of medications.

When a high-risk delivery is anticipated, *two* persons whose sole responsibility is resuscitation of the infant should be present and their roles designated in advance. Multiple births require a full team of personnel with complete equipment for each newborn.

The pediatric staff must be familiar with the prenatal and intrapartum history of the mother and fetus (see Box 4-1), because this information affects the initial level of resuscitation preparation.

Resuscitation equipment (Box 4-2) and drugs (Table 4-2) should always be readily available,

BOX 4-2 EQUIPMENT USED DURING NEONATAL RESUSCITATION

Thermal Management

- Radiant warmer
- Warmed blankets or towels
- Infant stocking cap
- Food-grade plastic wrap or polyethylene bags
- Chemically activated warming pad

Airway

- Bulb syringe
- Mechanical suction
- Suction catheters—5-6, 8, 10, 14 Fr
- 8 Fr feeding tube and 20-mL syringe
- Meconium aspirator/suction device
- Shoulder roll

Breathing

- Bag-and-mask ventilation
  - Oxygen source with flowmeter and tubing
  - Neonatal resuscitation bag with 100% oxygen capability and manometer or pressure release valve and/or T-piece device
  - Facemasks—newborn and premature sizes
  - Oral airways—newborn and premature sizes
  - Pulse oximeter
  - Oxygen blender and compressed air source
- Intubation
  - Laryngoscope with extra batteries
  - Straight blades—No. 0 and No. 1 with extra bulbs
  - Endotracheal tubes—2.5, 3.0, 3.5, 4.0 mm internal diameter
  - Stylet
  - Tape, skin preparation
  - Scissors
  - CO_2 detector
  - Laryngeal mask airway

Circulation

- Stethoscope
- Wall clock or stopwatch
- Cord clamp
- Medications (see Table 4-2)
- Sterile gloves

BOX 4-2 EQUIPMENT USED DURING NEONATAL RESUSCITATION—cont'd

- Alcohol sponges, povidone-iodine solution
- Umbilical vessel catheterization tray
- Umbilical catheters—3.5 and 5 Fr
- Three-way stopcocks
- Umbilical tape
- Suture material
- Intravenous catheters, tubing, fluid
- Needles—25, 23, 22, 20, 18 gauge
- Syringes—1, 3, 5, 10, 20, 50 mL
- Cardiorespiratory monitor
- Procedure light

TABLE 4-2 MEDICATIONS FOR NEONATAL RESUSCITATION

MEDICATION	CONCENTRATION TO ADMINISTER	DOSAGE/ROUTE	TOTAL DOSE/INFANT			RATE/ PRECAUTIONS	INDICATIONS FOR USE
			WEIGHT (kg)	*TOTAL mL*			
Epinephrine	1:10,000	0.1-0.3 mL/kg IV (0.01-0.03 mg/kg) (preferred)	1	0.1-0.3		Give rapidly	Heart rate <60 beats/min after 30 sec of adequate ventilation and chest compressions
			2	0.2-0.6		Use 2 different size syringes—one size for IV dosage and another size for ETT dosage	
			3	0.3-0.9			
			4	0.4-1.2			
		or					
		0.3-1 mL/kg ET (0.03-0.1 mg/kg)	1	0.3-1			
			2	0.6-2			
			3	0.9-3			
			4	1.2-4			
			WEIGHT (kg)	*TOTAL mL*			
Volume expanders	Normal saline solution Lactated Ringer's solution Whole blood	10 mL/kg IV	1	10		Give over 5-10 min	Evidence of acute bleeding with signs of hypovolemia; poor response to resuscitation
			2	20			
			3	30			
			4	40			
			WEIGHT (kg)	*TOTAL mg*	*TOTAL mL*		
Naloxone hydrochloride	1 mg/mL	0.1 mL/kg (0.1 mg/kg) IV, IM	1	0.1	0.1		Severe respiratory depression and history of maternal narcotic administration within past 4 hr Give only after adequate ventilation and heart rate have been established
			2	0.2	0.2		
			3	0.3	0.3		
			4	0.4	0.4		

ETT, Endotracheal tube; *IM*, intramuscular; *IV*, intravenous.

functional, and assembled for immediate use in a designated location—ideally in a specific area of the delivery/birthing room. Consumable supplies and small equipment can be stored on specially constructed wall shelves or on a radiant warmer/intensive-care bed equipped with easily accessible storage (Figures 4-4 and 4-5).

Prepare for neonatal resuscitation by performing the following:

- Preheat the radiant warmer.
- Assemble consumable supplies: warm linens, bulb syringe, suction catheter, cord clamp, and appropriate personal protection.
- Check suction equipment for function, and set the vacuum regulator control not to exceed 100 mm Hg.

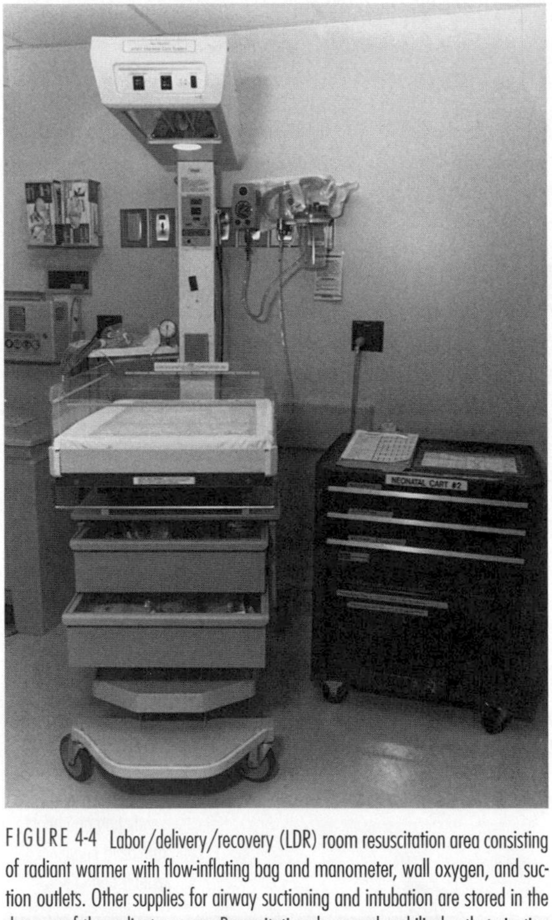

FIGURE 4-4 Labor/delivery/recovery (LDR) room resuscitation area consisting of radiant warmer with flow-inflating bag and manometer, wall oxygen, and suction outlets. Other supplies for airway suctioning and intubation are stored in the drawers of the radiant warmer. Resuscitation drugs and umbilical catheterization trays are kept in a separate resuscitation cart accessible from all LDR rooms.

- Turn on the air/oxygen flow to the ventilation bag, and check all connections, flow-control valves, pressure-release valve, and manometer function to enable the ventilation bag to deliver up to 30 to 40 cm H_2O pressure. Ensure that an appropriate-size facemask is available.
- Check the laryngoscope for a bright light source and appropriate blades (size 0 for premature infants and size 1 for term infants); tighten the bulb.
- Check the availability of appropriate-size endotracheal tubes (2.5 to 4 mm internal diameter [ID]).
- Locate a stethoscope of appropriate size and confirm that it is functioning properly.
- Check the ancillary equipment (i.e., umbilical catheter supplies, intravenous [IV] solutions, unexpired resuscitation drugs).
- If the clinical situation warrants, draw up and label emergency medications for ready administration, using the estimated fetal weight, and obtain O-negative packed red blood cells for emergency transfusion.

The steps of neonatal resuscitation follow the standard ABCs of resuscitation:

A—Airway
B—Breathing
C—Circulation

With the ABCs as an overall framework for neonatal resuscitation, the components of the procedure can be examined sequentially:

A—Establish an airway
Position the infant
Clear secretions from the mouth, nose, and trachea (in some cases)
Perform endotracheal intubation, if necessary
B—Initiate breathing
Provide tactile stimulation
Provide free-flow oxygen, if indicated
Provide positive-pressure ventilation
C—Maintain circulation
Provide chest compressions
Administer epinephrine, volume expander

At each step of the resuscitation procedure, whether uncomplicated or extended, the cycle of evaluation/decision/action repeats. Evaluation includes simultaneous assessment of respirations,

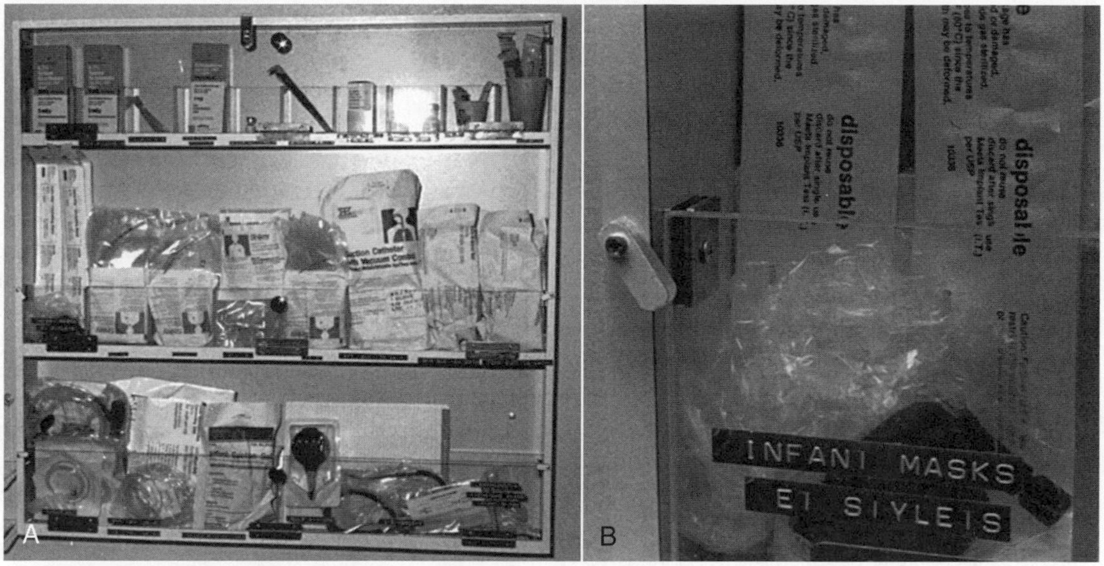

FIGURE 4-5 A, Wall-mounted storage bin. Unit consists of three Plexiglas shelves; each shelf is divided by Plexiglas into smaller compartments. Each compartment is labeled. Shelves can be opened for cleaning. Each shelf is held in place by hinge and magnet. B, Hinge and magnet device used to ensure closure of Plexiglas shelves.

heart rate, and color (Figure 4-6).[33] The importance of establishing an airway and initiating breathing cannot be overemphasized in neonatal resuscitation. **Expansion of the lungs with air and adequate ventilation are the keys to successful resuscitation.** Successful performance of these steps often obviates the need for further intervention, but inadequate lung expansion and ventilation cannot be overcome by performing chest compressions or administering medications.

Apgar Score

The Apgar score provides a comprehensive, objective measure of the infant's condition in the first minutes after birth (Figure 4-7). **The Apgar score does not serve as an indicator of the need for resuscitation; rather, it quantifies an infant's response to the extrauterine environment and resuscitative measures.** In term and preterm infants, the Apgar score remains a valuable predictor of infants who will need ongoing support in the immediate perinatal period and those who are at higher mortality risk in the neonatal period.[17]

Although perinatal asphyxia may be associated with low Apgar scores, it is possible for an infant to have a low Apgar score without having asphyxia.[35] For example, an infant born to a mother who received general anesthesia may be flaccid and have depressed reflexes and poor respiratory efforts. Such infants usually respond rapidly to bag-and-mask ventilation, and no further intervention is necessary. However, an infant may have an equally low Apgar score as a result of intrauterine asphyxia and may require prolonged resuscitative efforts. An infant with a mid-range Apgar score between 6 and 7 may be using homeostatic mechanisms to maintain an adequate central blood pressure and cardiac output. **Apgar scores should be assigned at 1 and 5 minutes, and every 5 minutes thereafter until the score is 7 or greater.** A complete description of the timing and nature of resuscitative steps is vital to interpreting a low Apgar score.[3]

Although the Apgar score is not used to guide resuscitation, the experienced clinician performs a rapid visual assessment of an infant at the moment of birth. This rapid assessment incorporates two elements from the Apgar score, as well as two key questions that influence the overall conduct of the resuscitation.

Rapid Assessment After Birth

In the first few seconds after birth, a rapid visual assessment of the baby should be performed to

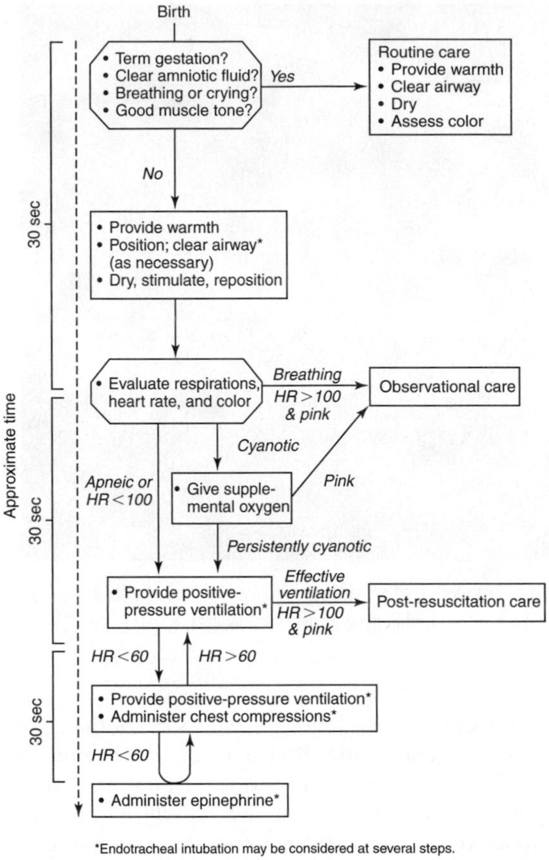

FIGURE 4-6 Throughout resuscitation, the infant's respirations, heart rate, and color are evaluated as a basis for decisions and actions. (From Kattwinkel J, editor: *Textbook of neonatal resuscitation*, ed 5, Elk Grove Village, Ill, 2006, American Academy of Pediatrics and American Heart Association.)

answer the following questions,[33] which can be summarized by the acronym TART:

- Is the baby term?
- Is the amniotic fluid clear?
- Is the baby breathing or crying? (respiratory effort)
- Is there good muscle tone?

If the answer to all of these questions is "yes," the baby can remain with the mother to receive routine care as described in the Routine Care and Initial Steps of Resuscitation section that follows.

If the answer to any of the questions is "no," the infant should be evaluated under a radiant heat source during the initial steps of resuscitation. If meconium is present, the vigor of the infant may alter the initial steps.

If meconium is present, evaluate the vigor of the infant:

- Does the baby have strong respiratory efforts?
- Is there good muscle tone?
- Is the heart rate greater than 100 beats/min?

If the answer to all of the questions is "yes," the airway may be cleared as described in the Position and Clear the Airway section. If the answer to any of the questions is "no," the infant requires endotracheal intubation for suctioning.[38,74] In this circumstance, return to the initial steps of resuscitation and complete them after intubation for suctioning of meconium.

Routine Care and Initial Steps of Resuscitation

The care of every infant at birth includes (1) warmth, (2) clearing the airway (positioning

Sign	Score		
	0	1	2
A Appearance (color)	Blue, pale	Body pink Extremities blue	Completely pink
P Pulse (heart rate)	Absent	Below 100	Above 100
G Grimace (reflex, irritability to suctioning)	No response	Grimace	Cough or sneeze
A Activity (muscle tone)	Limp	Some flexion	Well flexed
R Respiration (breathing efforts)	Absent	Weak, irregular	Strong cry

FIGURE 4-7 Practical epigram of Apgar score. (From Butterfield J, Covey M: Practical epigram of the Apgar score, *JAMA* 181:353, 1962.)

and suctioning as necessary), and (3) support of breathing with drying and tactile stimulation.

Whether part of routine care or during the initial steps of resuscitation, many of the actions can be performed simultaneously, especially if more than one person is caring for the infant.

PROVIDE WARMTH

- Dry the infant, and place him or her directly on the mother's chest; cover both with warm linen (routine care).

or

- Place the infant under a radiant heat source, drying him or her thoroughly and removing the wet linen.

or

- Wrap preterm infants less than 28 weeks' gestation in a polyethylene sheet or bag of food-grade plastic from the shoulders to the toes (without drying) and place under a radiant heat source.[67,68]

POSITION AND CLEAR THE AIRWAY (AS NECESSARY)

- Ensure that the infant's neck is slightly extended when positioning him or her on the mother's chest; wipe secretions from the mouth and nose, or suction with a bulb syringe as necessary (routine care).

or

- Position the infant supine and flat with the neck slightly extended. A rolled blanket or towel may be used under the shoulders.
- Turn the head (or the head and body) to the side to allow secretions to pool in the cheek, and then remove with a bulb syringe or suction catheter. Suction the mouth and then the nose to clear the airway. The mouth is suctioned first to clear the largest volume of secretions; when the nasopharynx is suctioned, a reflex cough, sneeze, or cry often results. Deep pharyngeal suction in an infant not requiring positive-pressure ventilation or intubation should not be performed during the first few minutes after birth to avoid vagal stimulation, resultant bradycardia, and delay in rise in Pa_{O_2}.[13,22]

or

- If meconium is present, evaluate the vigor of the infant before drying (as described earlier) to decide if endotracheal intubation is needed.[74]

STIMULATE AND REPOSITION

- Provide tactile stimulation by briefly rubbing the back or gently slapping or flicking the feet.
- Continue gentle rubbing of trunk, extremities, or head to support early respiratory efforts in the newborn.
- Keep the head and neck in a slightly extended position to maintain an open airway.

Evaluate the Infant

Evaluation of the infant is a continuous, ongoing process. Subsequent action is guided by evaluation during each step of resuscitation and decisions about whether the response is adequate.

EVALUATE RESPIRATIONS

- Rate and depth of respirations (chest wall movement, air exchange) must be adequate; **apnea and gasping respirations both require positive-pressure ventilation.**

EVALUATE HEART RATE

- **The heart rate should be greater than 100 beats/min.** Feel the base of the umbilical cord or listen over the left side of the chest with a stethoscope to count the heart rate. Count the heart rate in 6 seconds and multiply by 10 for the beats per minute. Indicate each beat (for other team members) by tapping the forefinger on the bed or tapping the thumb and index finger together.

EVALUATE COLOR

- **The lips and trunk should be pink.** Term, healthy babies may take more than 10 minutes to achieve a preductal oxygen saturation above 95% and nearly an hour to achieve the same level in the postductal circulation.[30,52,60]
- Give free-flow oxygen if the infant is breathing but remains centrally cyanotic. Peripheral cyanosis (acrocyanosis) is not an indication for supplemental oxygen. The goal of oxygen administration should be normoxia, not hyperoxia.[66]

Positive-Pressure Ventilation

Indications for positive-pressure ventilation in the newborn infant include the following:

- **Apnea or gasping respirations despite a brief period of tactile stimulation**

- A heart rate less than 100 beats/min
- Central cyanosis despite free-flow oxygen

Prolonged tactile stimulation or administration of supplemental oxygen to a baby who is not breathing effectively or who has a heart rate less than 100 beats/min only delays appropriate treatment. If supplemental oxygen is unavailable, positive-pressure ventilation should be initiated with room air.[45] **When supplemental oxygen is available, it should be administered with the goal of achieving normoxia and avoiding hyperoxia. Ongoing research in animals and humans has demonstrated that room air is equivalent to 100% oxygen for positive-pressure ventilation in many newly born infants. The exclusive use of 100% oxygen for postnatal resuscitation, as previously recommended, can result in hyperoxia and predisposition to changes induced by generation of oxygen free radicals.**[64,65] The concentration and duration of supplemental oxygen administration should be individualized to patient needs. **Pulse oximetry, initiated as soon as feasible, can help guide oxygen administration.**[19,63] **Ideally, it should be possible to administer oxygen in concentrations from 21% to 100% in the delivery setting. This has special importance for preterm infants who are more vulnerable to oxygen injury yet may need concentrations greater than 21%.**[59,70]

Chest Compressions

- If, after 30 seconds of effective positive-pressure ventilation with supplemental oxygen, the heart rate is less than 60 beats/min, begin chest compressions. Consider intubation, and prepare emergency drugs (see Table 4-2).

Administration of Epinephrine and Volume Expansion

- If the heart rate remains below 60 beats/min despite 30 seconds of effective positive-pressure ventilation with oxygen and another 30 seconds of ventilation, oxygen, and chest compressions, administer epinephrine.
- If the baby is not responding to resuscitation, including administration of epinephrine, and there is evidence of blood loss or hypovolemia, consider administration of a volume expander.

Each of the major steps in neonatal resuscitation should be accomplished in approximately 30 seconds. The initial rapid assessment can be performed in the first few seconds after birth to determine whether routine care can be provided to the infant, who remains with the mother, or whether more extensive evaluation and resuscitation will be necessary during the initial steps. The initial steps of resuscitation can be performed concurrently with evaluation of heart rate, respirations, and color, especially if more than one person is present to care for the infant. **Positive-pressure ventilation and chest compressions should each be performed for 30-second intervals before moving to the next level of intervention. When oxygen concentrations less than 100% are used to initiate positive-pressure ventilation and an adequate response in heart rate does not occur, steps to improve lung inflation should be taken and the oxygen concentration should be increased before initiating chest compressions.**

An infant who has received more than the initial steps of resuscitation will require close monitoring for additional or recurrent problems during the postnatal transition and may need supportive care such as continued oxygen administration. Infants who require more than brief positive-pressure ventilation should be monitored in a nursery setting in which they can receive ongoing care.[38]

Skills Necessary for Neonatal Resuscitation

INITIAL STEPS: SUCTIONING FOR MECONIUM-STAINED AMNIOTIC FLUID

Meconium-stained amniotic fluid is seen most often in infants of more than 34 weeks' gestational age, especially in term and post-term neonates. Passage of meconium may be associated with asphyxia. Severe fetal acidosis can result in fetal gasping, leading to in utero aspiration of meconium.[75] Suctioning the mouth and hypopharynx at delivery of the head and again after delivery is complete *was* advocated to help prevent meconium aspiration.[14,28] Current evidence no longer advises routine intrapartum suctioning for infants with meconium-stained amniotic fluid.[14,28,33]

Infants with meconium-stained amniotic fluid who are not vigorous at birth require tracheal intubation for suctioning. *Vigor* is defined by effective spontaneous respirations, a heart rate

of greater than 100 beats/min, and good muscle tone. A large, multicenter, controlled trial examining management of vigorous infants with meconium-stained fluid found no difference in the incidence of respiratory distress (meconium aspiration or other respiratory distress) between groups who received routine airway management and endotracheal intubation for suctioning.[74] In that trial, infants were suctioned on the perineum, but results from a subsequent study suggest that intrapartum suctioning does not prevent the meconium aspiration syndrome.[62]

Nevertheless, any infant born with meconium-stained amniotic fluid who develops signs of airway obstruction or needs positive-pressure ventilation should first have the trachea suctioned and cleared of any meconium present.

If meconium is present in the amniotic fluid, perform the initial steps in the following manner:

- If the infant is vigorous, suction the mouth, posterior pharynx, and nose as necessary once the infant is under the radiant heat source and proceed with drying, stimulation, and removal of wet linen.
- If the infant is depressed, clear the oropharynx with a large-bore catheter and suction the trachea under direct visualization using an endotracheal tube, adapter, and mechanical suction or a meconium suction device (Figure 4-8). Dry and stimulate the infant, and remove wet linen after the airway has been cleared.[34]
- Suction the stomach when airway management is complete and vital signs are stable (usually after 5 minutes). Clearing meconium from the stomach decreases the risk for postnatal regurgitation and aspiration; however, suctioning too soon after birth can provoke apnea and bradycardia by vagal stimulation and complicate the initial resuscitation.

ADMINISTRATION OF FREE-FLOW OXYGEN

Supplemental oxygen should be administered after the initial steps if the infant remains centrally cyanotic.[33] The administration of oxygen is guided ideally by pulse oximetry.[19,33] Delivered at a flow rate of 5 L/min, oxygen may be administered by mask or by holding the oxygen tubing in a cupped hand over the infant's face. The delivered oxygen concentration decreases rapidly as the tubing or mask is withdrawn from the face.

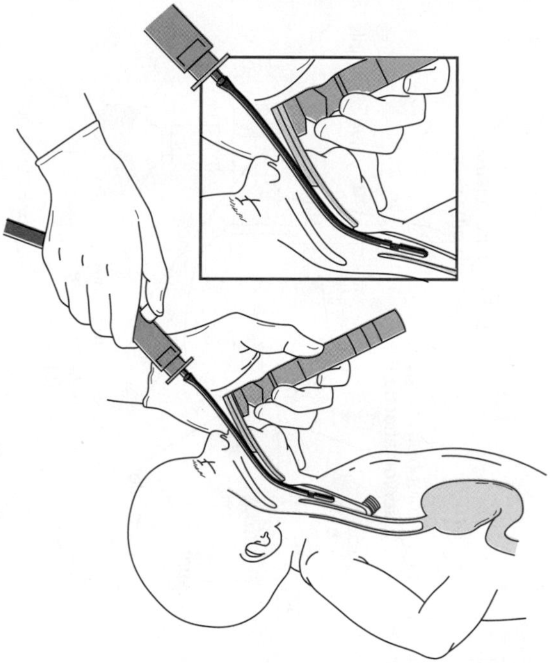

FIGURE 4-8 Equipment for suctioning meconium from the airway. Both meconium aspirator and meconium suction device connect to wall suction. (From Kattwinkel J, editor: *Textbook of neonatal resuscitation*, ed 5, Elk Grove Village, Ill, 2006, American Academy of Pediatrics and American Heart Association.)

Once the infant becomes pink, gradually withdraw the oxygen tubing or the mask from the infant's face. If cyanosis persists, reevaluate the quality of respirations and the heart rate; perform a brief physical examination; and consider bag-and-mask ventilation or intubation if there is evidence of respiratory distress.

BAG-AND-MASK VENTILATION

The indications for bag-and-mask ventilation include (1) apnea unresponsive to brief stimulation or gasping respirations, (2) heart rate of less than 100 beats/min, and (3) persistent cyanosis despite free-flow oxygen. The equipment for bag-and-mask ventilation can be either a self-inflating bag with an oxygen reservoir and pressure-release valve or pressure gauge, a flow-inflating bag (anesthesia bag) with a flow-control valve and pressure gauge, or a T-piece resuscitation device.

Although used widely, ***self-inflating bags*** do not deliver consistent tidal volumes or inflation pressures, even in the hands of providers who resuscitate frequently. Some data suggest, however, that

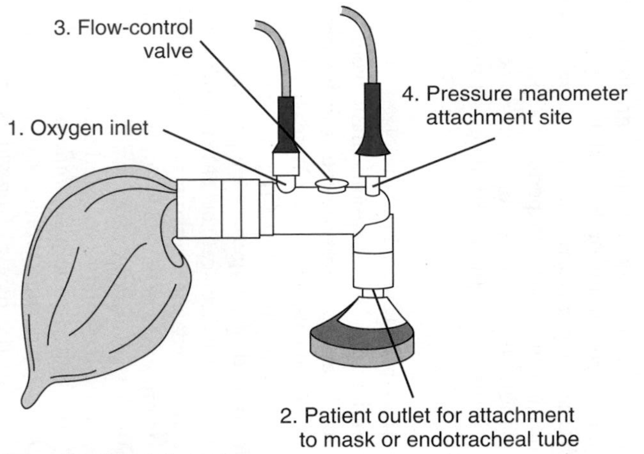

Parts of a flow-inflating bag

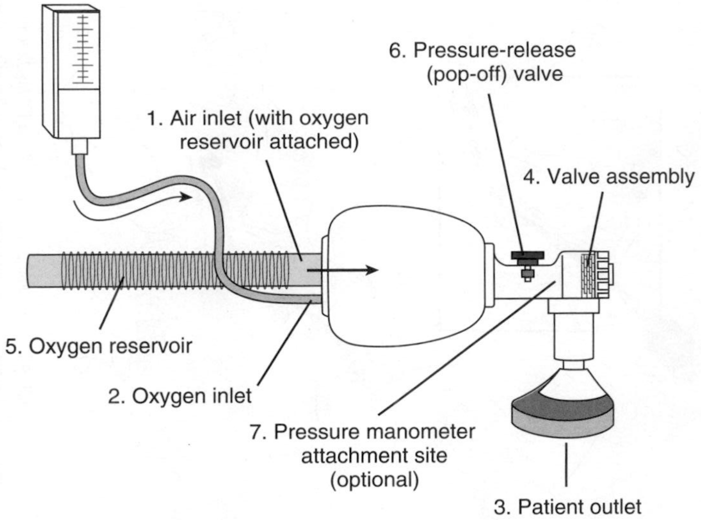

Parts of a self-inflating bag

Flow-inflating bags. Flow-inflating bags contain an inflatable gas reservoir that must be connected to a compressed gas source to refill between breaths.

Advantages:
- Ability to deliver 21% to 100% oxygen and any desired inspiratory pressure
- Ability to maintain a positive end-expiratory pressure
- In-line manometer

Disadvantages:
- The bag must be connected to an external compressed air source to inflate.
- Practice and experience are required to deliver desired tidal volumes and pressures.
- Very high inspiratory pressures may cause overinflation or pneumothorax.

Self-inflating bags. Self-inflating bags fill with ambient air and are independent of an external oxygen or compressed air source.

Advantages:
- Simple to use
- Self-inflation (useful backup system in case compressed gas source fails or is not available)

Disadvantages:
- Maximum pressure-limiting pop-off valve, usually set by the manufacturer at 30 to 35 cm H_2O, may preclude adequate ventilation in a noncompliant lung. (Some models have a manual override device that will allow increased inspiratory pressures.)
- A reservoir must be attached to deliver 90% to 100% oxygen.
- Free-flow oxygen cannot be delivered reliably through the patient outlet.
- The bag does not routinely deliver end-expiratory pressure and difficult to retrofit it with an in-line manometer.

FIGURE 4-9 Flow-inflating bag and self-inflating bag. (From Kattwinkel J, editor: *Textbook of neonatal resuscitation*, ed 5, Elk Grove Village, Ill, 2006, American Academy of Pediatrics and American Heart Association.)

self-inflating bags may offer advantages over flow-inflating bags when in the hands of inexperienced operators.[32,36] Self-inflating bags cannot be used reliably to deliver free-flow oxygen, and they require a special adapter to deliver continuous positive airway pressure (CPAP) (Figure 4-9). Ideally they would be fitted with a CPAP device and a manometer for use with newborns.[32] ***Flow-inflating bags*** require a complete seal between mask and face to deliver a tidal volume. They offer the capability to achieve high peak pressures, deliver CPAP, and administer free-flow oxygen. The volume of the bag should generally be between 200 and 750 mL.[38] Larger bags are more difficult to handle and are predisposed to overly large tidal volumes, especially for preterm infants. A ***T-piece resuscitation device,*** as opposed to a bag, can achieve desired inflation pressures and respiratory times more consistently (at least in mechanical models) but requires setting the inspiratory pressure and PEEP before use and may be more difficult to adjust during resuscitation (Figure 4-10).[25,32]

The facemask should be selected to ensure that it is the appropriate size to cover the chin, mouth, and nose but not the eyes. Masks are commonly available in term and premature sizes and may be obtained to fit even very low-birth-weight infants. Flexible, translucent masks with a cushioned rim generally provide the best seal with minimal trauma and allow monitoring of mouth position and secretions.[76]

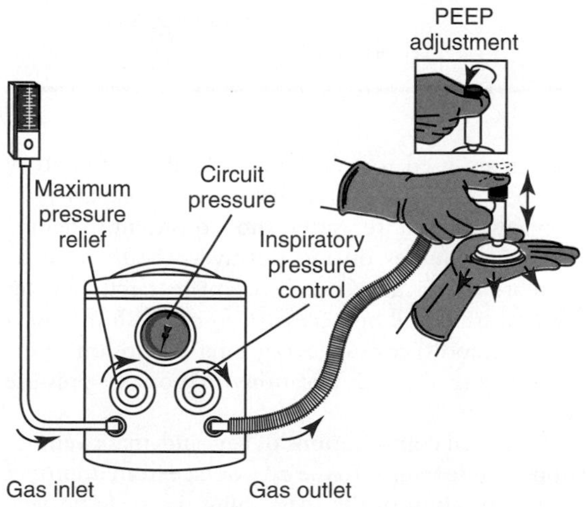

FIGURE 4-10 T-piece resuscitator. (From Kattwinkel J, editor: *Textbook of neonatal resuscitation*, ed 5, Elk Grove Village, Ill, 2006, American Academy of Pediatrics and American Heart Association.)

Perform the following steps:

- Set the flowmeter to deliver 5 to 10 L/min. Flow rates at the higher end of the range are necessary to achieve higher pressures and faster ventilation rates with a flow-inflating bag.
- Test equipment before use. Equipment failure can cause resuscitation failure!
- Position the infant with the neck slightly extended, avoiding compression of soft tissues of the neck by holding the mask to the face with the thumb and index finger and resting the third, fourth, and fifth fingers along the mandible.
- Apply an opening breath with initial pressures of 20 to 30 cm H_2O; pressure as high as 30 to 40 cm H_2O may be necessary in term infants not breathing spontaneously. Most apneic preterm infants respond to initial inflation pressures of 20 to 25 cm H_2O.[33]
- Ventilate at a rate of 40 to 60 breaths/min with pressures of 15 to 20 cm H_2O for normal lungs or up to 20 to 40 cm H_2O for diseased lungs. When surfactant is administered immediately after birth, rapid compliance changes may require equally rapid adjustment of ventilation pressures and oxygen concentration.
- Observe the heart rate. Prompt improvement in heart rate is the best indicator of adequate ventilation. If inadequate, (1) reapply the facemask for a better seal, (2) reposition the head, (3) suction secretions, (4) open the infant's mouth slightly, and (5) increase pressure.[38]
- Reevaluate respirations, heart rate, and color.
- Provide CPAP after spontaneous respirations have returned. End-expiratory pressure decreases lung injury and improves compliance and gas exchange.[46,51] CPAP may have a role in maintaining lung volumes in premature infants and aiding the absorption of lung fluid.[44]
- Insert an orogastric catheter (8 Fr feeding tube) after several minutes of bag-and-mask ventilation or if there is evidence of gastric distention.
- Measure the insertion depth of the catheter by holding the tip at the bridge of the nose and measuring to the earlobe and then midway between the xiphoid and the umbilicus.[38]
- Insert the catheter through the mouth, not the nose, because newborns are obligate nose-breathers.
- Aspirate gastric contents with a 20-mL syringe and leave the catheter open.
- Tape the catheter to the infant's cheek.

TABLE 4-3 COMPLICATIONS DURING RESUSCITATION AND STABILIZATION

PROBLEM	CAUSE	DIAGNOSIS	REMEDIES
Persistent cyanosis	Inadequate oxygenation		
	Inadequate F_{IO_2}	Check flowmeter	Always have available 100% O_2
	Disconnected O_2 line	Check all connections	Reconnect line
	Empty O_2 cylinder	Check O_2 source	Replace O_2 cylinder
	Inadequate ventilation		
	Inadequate facemask seal	Diminished breath sounds; little chest wall movement; air leak around mask	Readjust facemask; seal tightly against skin
	Compression of airway	Diminished breath sounds; little chest wall movement	Apply upward force to mandible to counteract downward force holding facemask in place; extend neck slightly
	Insufficient insufflation pressure	Diminished breath sounds; little chest wall movement	Increase insufflation pressure until breath sounds are audible and chest movement seen
	Compression of lungs by distended stomach	Diminished breath sounds; little chest wall movement; visibly distended stomach	Place orogastric tube
	Malpositioned ET tube	Check tube position with laryngoscope Check breath sounds	Reinsert into trachea Withdraw until breath sounds are bilaterally equal Tape ET tube in place
	Pneumothorax	Check breath sounds Check for chest asymmetry Transillumination Chest x-ray examination	Decompress tension pneumothorax
Bradycardia	Same as for persistent cyanosis	Auscultation of precordium or palpation of umbilical cord base; pulse oximeter or cardiac monitor	Same as for persistent cyanosis External cardiac compression if heart rate less than 60 beats/min after 30 sec of effective ventilation with supplemental oxygen
	Vagal stimulation Perinatal myocardial ischemia	Lack of response to oxygenation, ventilation, and chest compressions	Stop oropharyngeal suctioning Emergency epinephrine/volume expander administration

The adequacy of bag-and-mask ventilation must be continuously assessed by monitoring of heart rate, auscultation of breath sounds, visualization of chest wall movement, and observation of skin color. Peak inspiratory pressure should be limited to that necessary to see an improvement in heart rate and chest wall movement and to hear good air exchange on auscultation of the chest. Infants with collapsed or fluid-filled alveoli may occasionally require inspiratory pressures of 40 to 60 cm H_2O or higher.[62,69] Inspiratory pressures cannot be judged clinically; bags fitted with in-line pressure manometers or T-piece devices are recommended in the delivery room.[38] Data suggest that the neonatal respiratory system responds slowly to mechanical inspiratory pressure[9]; prolonged inspiratory times have been used to achieve an adequate inspiratory volume and establish functional residual capacity.[55,69] Devices that more easily and consistently deliver targeted volumes during positive-pressure ventilation are the focus of much recent research. Further clinical trials will be necessary to establish the optimal method(s) for achieving lung expansion while minimizing the complications of positive-pressure ventilation.

Potential complications of bag-and-mask ventilation include trauma to the eyes or face from improper size or position of the mask, lung injury (especially in preterm infants), air leak (pneumothorax, subcutaneous air), gastric distention elevating the diaphragm, and direct lung compression in the case of a diaphragmatic hernia (Table 4-3). Complications

TABLE 4-3 COMPLICATIONS DURING RESUSCITATION AND STABILIZATION—cont'd

PROBLEM	CAUSE	DIAGNOSIS	REMEDIES
Hypothermia	Evaporative heat loss; conductive heat loss	Specific signs overlap those of asphyxia and shock Low core temperature	Dry infant; remove wet linen Use polyethylene bags Cover wet hair Keep under radiant warmer
Hyperthermia	Excessive warming Maternal fever	Apnea High core temperature	Servocontrol of warming devices
Hypoglycemia	Glucose stores used before birth or during resuscitation	Specific symptoms overlap those of asphyxia and shock Low blood sugar	Bolus 2 mL/kg of $D_{10}W$ Maintenance infusion of $D_{10}W$
Hemorrhage	Inadequately secured umbilical arterial or venous line	Pallor Poor capillary refilling Leakage of blood	Keep all intravascular tubing connection sites in plain view Tape UAC/UVC in place in addition to suturing lines
	Liver laceration		Perform chest compressions with correct position/depth

ET, Endotracheal; *UAC*, umbilical artery catheter; *UVC*, umbilical venous catheter.

can be minimized by using gentle technique and equipment of correct size, careful monitoring of pressures, and insertion of an orogastric tube when indicated.

ENDOTRACHEAL INTUBATION

Endotracheal intubation may be performed at several points during neonatal resuscitation.[38] Intubation is indicated when (1) tracheal suctioning is needed, as with meconium-stained amniotic fluid in a nonvigorous infant, (2) bag-and-mask ventilation is ineffective or prolonged positive-pressure ventilation is needed, (3) chest compressions are necessary, or (4) epinephrine administration is necessary. Additional indications for endotracheal intubation include extreme prematurity, surfactant administration, and suspected diaphragmatic hernia.

Equipment for intubation is listed in the "Airway" and "Breathing" sections in Box 4-2.

Select an uncuffed, uniform-diameter endotracheal tube of the correct size (Table 4-4). A variety of sizes (2.5 to 4 mm internal diameter) should be available, because estimated weights may be inaccurate or airway anomalies may exist. **Orotracheal intubation is preferable to nasotracheal intubation during acute resuscitation because it can be performed rapidly and without additional equipment.**

Perform the following steps:

- Shorten the selected endotracheal tube to 13 cm (or the length appropriate for the fixation method used), and prepare the laryngoscope, tape, suction, oxygen, bag, and mask.
- Position the infant with the neck slightly extended.
- Provide free-flow oxygen.
- Hold the laryngoscope with the left hand; open the mouth with the right index finger and gently insert the blade.
- Lift the laryngoscope upward and outward so that the blade is nearly parallel to the surface beneath the infant.
- Visualize landmarks; identify the epiglottis, vocal cords, and glottis (Figure 4-11). If the esophagus is seen, withdraw the blade until the epiglottis drops down. If only the tongue is visible, advance the blade further until it enters the vallecula or passes under the epiglottis.

- Apply gentle external pressure over the cricoid, which may help visualize the vocal cords. Pressure may be applied with the little finger of the hand holding the laryngoscope or by an assistant.
- Insert the endotracheal tube from the right corner of the mouth to the level of the vocal cord guideline at the tip of the tube.
- Limit each intubation attempt to 20 seconds to avoid hypoxia.
- Confirm endotracheal tube position by exhaled CO_2 detector and by auscultation for bilaterally equal breath sounds in the axillae and absence of breath sounds over the stomach. Observe chest wall movement. Note the centimeter marking at the lip (Table 4-5).
- Secure the endotracheal tube and obtain a chest x-ray.
- Shorten the endotracheal tube to 4 cm beyond the lips, if necessary.

Complications of intubation include hypoxia caused by prolonged intubation attempts or lack of supplemental oxygen; tube malposition; apnea or bradycardia caused by hypoxia or vagal stimulation; and trauma to the oropharynx, trachea, vocal cords, or esophagus (see Table 4-3). Exhaled CO_2 detection devices, commonly used to confirm endotracheal tube position in children, may be helpful even in newborn infants weighing less than 2 kg.[5] To prevent complications, provide free-flow oxygen during intubation, use gentle technique, and limit each intubation attempt to 20 seconds.

TABLE 4-4 ENDOTRACHEAL TUBE SIZE

TUBE SIZE (mm) (INSIDE DIAMETER)	WEIGHT (g)	GESTATIONAL AGE (wk)
2.5	<1000	<28
3.0	1000-2000	28-34
3.5	2000-3000	34-38
3.5-4.0	>3000	>38

From Kattwinkel J, editor: *Textbook of neonatal resuscitation*, ed 5, Elk Grove Village, Ill, 2006, American Academy of Pediatrics and American Heart Association.

TABLE 4-5 DEPTH OF ENDOTRACHEAL INSERTION

WEIGHT (kg)	DEPTH OF INSERTION (cm FROM THE UPPER LIP)
1*	7
2	8
3	9
4	10

From Kattwinkel J, editor: *Textbook of neonatal resuscitation*, ed 5, Elk Grove Village, Ill, 2006, American Academy of Pediatrics and American Heart Association.
*Babies weighing less than 750 g may require only 6 cm insertion.

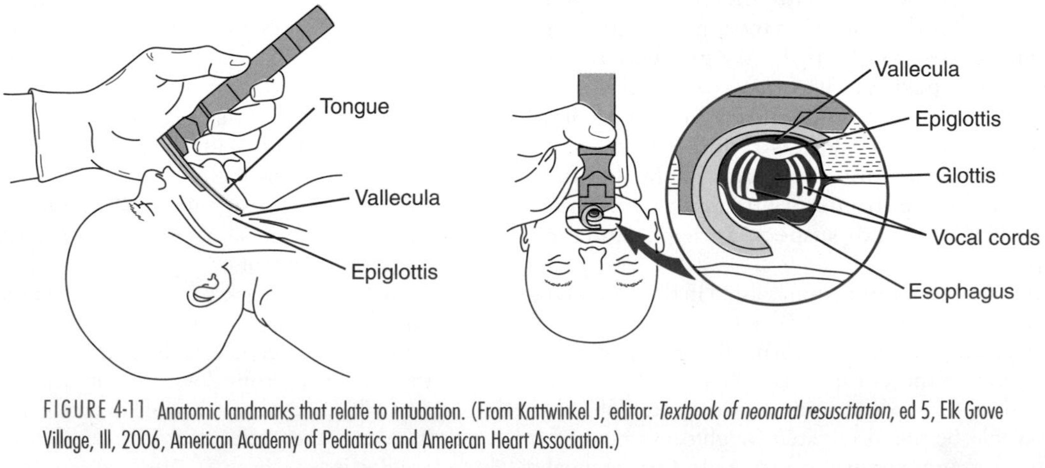

FIGURE 4-11 Anatomic landmarks that relate to intubation. (From Kattwinkel J, editor: *Textbook of neonatal resuscitation*, ed 5, Elk Grove Village, Ill, 2006, American Academy of Pediatrics and American Heart Association.)

CHEST COMPRESSIONS

Indications for chest compressions include a heart rate less than 60 beats/min despite effective positive-pressure ventilation with supplemental oxygen for 30 seconds. Follow the sequence of (A) airway, (B) breathing, and (C) circulation in providing resuscitative support. Even if the heart rate is less than 60 beats/min shortly after delivery, the airway should be cleared and positive-pressure ventilation should be given for 30 seconds before beginning chest compressions. Often, adequate ventilation alone will result in a rapid increase in heart rate.[49] Beginning chest compressions too early may interfere with the effectiveness of positive-pressure ventilation and actually delay an infant's response to resuscitation.

Perform the following steps:

- Position the infant with the neck slightly extended.
- Provide firm support for the back.
- Perform compressions using the two-thumb (preferred) or two-finger technique (Figure 4-12).

Position: Lower third of sternum[26,47]
Rate: 90 times/min
Depth: One third of the anterior-posterior diameter of the chest
Support: Encircling fingers or hand under back

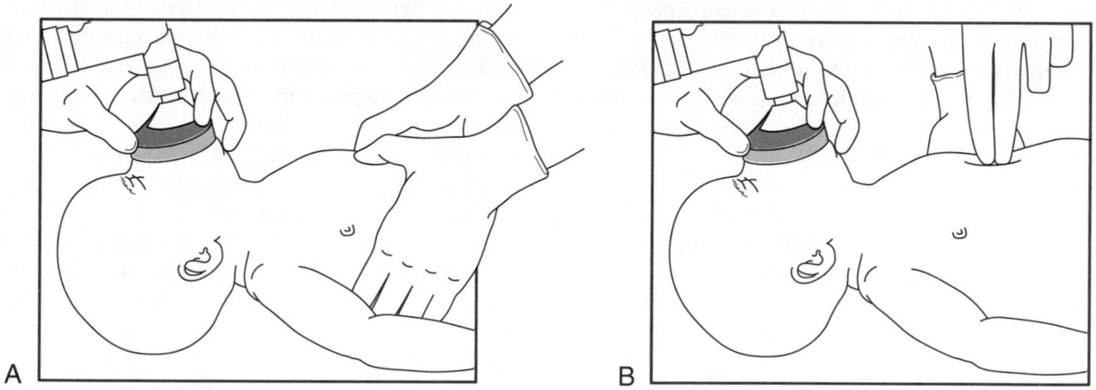

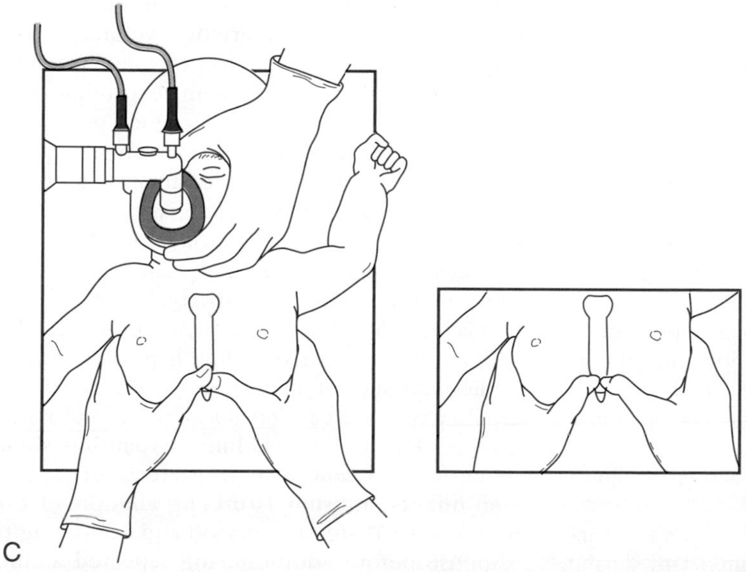

FIGURE 4-12 Two-thumb (***A***, preferred) and two-finger (**B**) methods of chest compression. **C**, The two-thumb method uses two thumbs placed one over the other or side by side (depending on the size of the baby) to compress the sternum; encircle the chest with the hands so that your fingers support the spine. (From Kattwinkel J, editor: *Textbook of neonatal resuscitation*, ed 5, Elk Grove Village, Ill, 2006, American Academy of Pediatrics and American Heart Association.)

- **Provide 90 compressions/min and interpose 30 breaths/min with a 3:1 ratio of compressions to breaths (120 events/min).**[11,33]
- Evaluate the heart rate after 30 seconds.
- Continue chest compressions until the heart rate is greater than 60 beats/min.
- Administer epinephrine if the heart rate remains less than 60 beats/min despite at least 30 seconds of adequate positive-pressure ventilation and another 30 seconds of coordinated ventilations and chest compressions.

When response to positive-pressure ventilation and chest compressions is poor, reevaluate for technical problems and conditions interfering with ventilation. Confirm that oxygen is connected properly and that concentrations are adequate to achieve normoxia (see Table 4-3). To ensure a patent airway, place an endotracheal tube and confirm proper position. Ventilate with pressures to expand the chest and breaths interposed between compressions. Evaluate the infant for pneumothorax, diaphragmatic hernia, or hypovolemia (see "Delivery Room Emergencies" section).

Complications of chest compressions include liver laceration, rib fractures, and pneumothorax. To prevent complications, check the position of compressions, maintain contact with the chest during the release portion of the compression cycle, and avoid excessive force during compressions.

MEDICATIONS

The indications for drug administration during newborn resuscitation include the following:

- **Epinephrine:** Heart rate less than 60 beats/min despite at least 30 seconds of adequate ventilation and another 30 seconds of coordinated ventilation and chest compressions
- **Volume expanders:** Evidence of acute bleeding or signs of hypovolemia; poor response to other resuscitative measures

Perform the following steps (see Table 4-2):

- Calculate the correct dosage of each drug based on the newborn's weight.
- Prepare each drug for administration, draw up the appropriate concentration and volume, and label the syringe.
- Administer each drug by the correct route and at the proper rate.
- Reevaluate for desired effect and take follow-up action.

Epinephrine increases the rate and strength of cardiac contractions. Perhaps more important during resuscitation is its action as a peripheral vasoconstrictor, directing cardiac output to the central circulation and increasing coronary perfusion pressure.[42,45] **Epinephrine is most effective when administered by umbilical venous catheter in a dose of 0.1 to 0.3 mL/kg of 1:10,000 concentration. Endotracheal administration in a one-time dose of 0.3 to 1 mL/kg can be considered while obtaining venous access.** Expansion of plasma and blood volume may also be necessary to maintain cardiac output, blood pressure, and peripheral perfusion.

Volume expansion should be considered when there is evidence of acute blood loss (e.g., abruptio placentae, bleeding from placenta previa, fetal-maternal hemorrhage, umbilical cord tear, acute neonatal hemorrhage) or poor response to resuscitation (e.g., pallor, bradycardia, exaggerated tachycardia). **Normal saline is the preferred solution for volume expansion in a dose of 10 mL/kg by umbilical venous catheter.**

Complications of drug administration include extravasation with intravascular administration, hepatic injury with low umbilical venous catheters, and unpredictable absorption with endotracheal administration. The use of resuscitation drugs also may result in complications from their adverse pharmacologic effects. Epinephrine, administered in high doses, increases the risk for significant hypertension and a hyperadrenergic state, which may result in germinal matrix hemorrhage or myocardial damage.[7] Absorption of epinephrine after endotracheal administration is erratic.[43] Volume overload may result from administration of repeated doses of volume expanders. Rapid volume expansion, resulting in acute elevation of systolic blood pressure, has been associated with intraventricular hemorrhage.[27]

Distressed newborns have impaired autoregulation of cerebral blood flow, with blood flow directly related to the systolic blood pressure. Increased cerebral blood flow and elevated systolic pressures may be responsible for intraventricular hemorrhage in the presence of a capillary bed insulted by acidosis and hypoxia.[42] Autopsy studies also suggest that increased cerebral venous capillary pressure can initiate intraventricular hemorrhage (Figure 4-13). **Volume expansion should be performed cautiously in preterm or asphyxiated infants, infusing 10 mL/kg aliquots of fluid over a 5- to 10-minute period and evaluating the response before administering repeated aliquots**

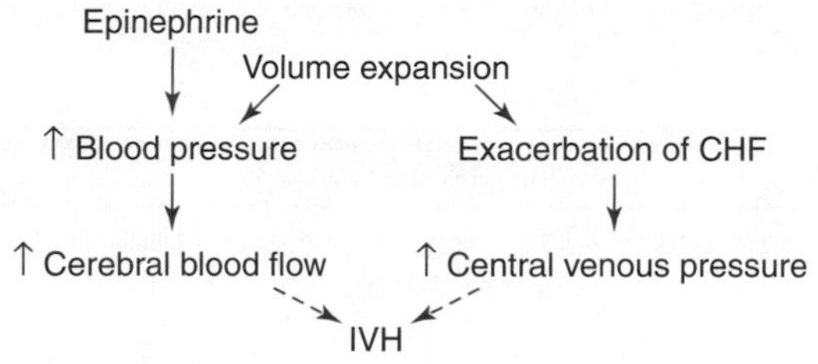

FIGURE 4-13 Potential adverse effects of rapid volume expansion in the setting of asphyxia or prematurity. *CHF*, Congestive heart failure; *IVH*, intraventricular hemorrhage.

of fluid. The exception to this rule is the infant who has experienced acute perinatal hemorrhage with hypovolemia. These infants should have the circulatory fluid volume restored as rapidly as possible. Complications of medication administration can be prevented by choosing the correct dose, rate, and route of administration and positioning umbilical lines carefully. The infant should be evaluated for adverse effects and response to fluid volume after each medication/volume dose.

Sodium bicarbonate is no longer recommended for use during resuscitation immediately after birth. Although acidosis frequently persists after a prolonged resuscitation, many infants correct an acidosis spontaneously once the asphyxiating circumstances are relieved and adequate ventilation is established. Metabolic correction of pH is a slow process that takes several hours, and treatment with sodium bicarbonate is not necessary. Sodium bicarbonate results in worsened acidosis in the setting of impaired ventilation; bicarbonate also may worsen intracellular acidosis. Furthermore, bicarbonate adds a high sodium load, which may directly depress myocardial performance.[4,31]

Naloxone hydrochloride is indicated during acute resuscitation only in the very specific circumstance of severe neonatal respiratory depression and narcotic administration to the mother in the last 4 hours. Naloxone is not part of the routine resuscitation of an apneic infant.[33] Establishment of gas exchange with positive-pressure ventilation is the first priority for any infant who does not have adequate spontaneous respirations after birth. No randomized controlled trials of naloxone for treatment of apnea have been conducted in the delivery room setting. **Furthermore, naloxone hydrochloride is contraindicated in infants of narcotic-addicted mothers, because administration can result in severe abstinence syndrome, including seizures.**

Calcium and atropine have little role in delivery room settings. Calcium is indicated for hypocalcemia or hyperkalemia, both of which are infrequent problems in the delivery room. Atropine may mask hypoxia-related bradycardia.[57]

DELIVERY ROOM EMERGENCIES

Certain conditions can present as emergencies in the delivery room (Table 4-6).[40,53] These conditions may require extensive resuscitation or result in a poor response to resuscitation. Some situations require special intervention immediately; most merit the involvement of a neonatal nurse practitioner, pediatrician, or neonatologist for management. Coordinated teamwork, with techniques and communication skills acquired through simulation training, can help ensure rapid and effective stabilization.[29,71] Surgical intervention is necessary to complete the treatment of diaphragmatic hernia, abdominal wall defects, and neural tube defects. See Box 4-3 for an outline of emergency procedures in the delivery room setting.

CARE DURING THE TRANSITION FROM THE DELIVERY ROOM TO THE NURSERY

After the infant is stabilized and vigorous, perform elective procedures, such as clamping and shortening the umbilical cord, footprinting and identification, applying ophthalmic prophylaxis, and weighing. A vigorous, stable infant may breast feed immediately and be held by the parents. The infant may be placed skin-to-skin with the mother or wrapped in double blankets. A stocking cap prevents heat loss from the large surface area of the head and wet hair. The stable infant may complete the transition period with the mother under appropriate observation.

The infant who has required more extensive resuscitation in the delivery room should be transferred to a special care or intensive care nursery when adequate spontaneous or controlled ventilation has been established, the heart rate is greater than 100 beats/min, and the infant has been dried and protected from excessive heat loss. Note the time of the infant's first respiratory

TABLE 4-6 DELIVERY ROOM EMERGENCIES

CONDITION	SIGNS AND SYMPTOMS	ONGOING PROBLEMS	INITIAL RESPONSES
Pneumothorax	Cyanosis, respiratory distress, unequal breath sounds, bradycardia, displaced heart sounds	Continuing asphyxia, shock (poor venous return)	Transilluminate chest, perform needle thoracentesis, evaluate chest tube placement
Choanal atresia; oral/pharyngeal airway anomalies	Noisy respirations, pink when crying but cyanotic when quiet, cannot pass suction catheter per nares	Respiratory distress, intermittent hypoxemia and bradycardia	Supplemental oxygen, oral airway, and prone positioning; or intubation (lower airway anomalies may require emergency tracheostomy)
Extreme prematurity	Respiratory distress	Continuing hypoxemia, hypothermia, possible sepsis, hypovolemia	Intubate, place umbilical lines, evaluate for artificial surfactant, begin antibiotics, consider transport to neonatal center
Sepsis	Respiratory distress, hypotonia, poor perfusion, foul odor	Continuing hypoxemia, shock	Intubate, place umbilical lines, administer antibiotics
Severe asphyxia	Prolonged apnea, bradycardia, poor perfusion, pallor, hypotonia, seizures	Hypoxemia, shock, multiorgan system injury	Intubate, place umbilical lines, give volume expander and vasopressors for shock, consider transport to neonatal center
Hydrops fetalis	Body wall edema, ascites, pallor, poor perfusion, respiratory distress, possibly unequal breath sounds (pneumothorax), distant heart sounds (pericardial effusion)	Hypoxemia, anemia, shock, potential for multiorgan system injury	Intubate, perform posteriolateral needle thoracentesis bilaterally if unable to ventilate; consider paracentesis if ascites compromises ventilation; place chest tube for pneumothorax, place umbilical lines, evaluate need for partial exchange transfusion, consider transport to neonatal center
Pulmonary hypoplasia and oligohydramnios	Respiratory distress; flattened, deviated nose; infraorbital creases; low-set, crumpled ears; small chin; deformities of the extremities	Hypoxemia, pneumothorax, pulmonary hypoplasia	Intubate, place umbilical lines, monitor closely for pulmonary air leak, consider transport to neonatal center
Congenital diaphragmatic hernia	Respiratory distress with asymmetric breath sounds, barrel chest and scaphoid abdomen, point of maximal cardiac intensity shifted to side opposite hernia	Hypoxemia, pulmonary hypertension, contralateral pneumothorax	Intubate, decompress bowel with orogastric tube to low intermittent suction, place umbilical lines, arrange transport to neonatal center
Abdominal wall defect	Midline abdominal wall defect at base of umbilical cord (omphalocele) or lateral to cord insertion (gastroschisis) with externalization of abdominal contents	Hypovolemia, respiratory distress, hypothermia, ischemic injury to externalized abdominal contents, infection	Protect exposed tissue with evaporative barrier; begin parenteral fluids at 1.5 times maintenance; place an orogastric tube to low intermittent suction, position infant side-lying with support of exposed organs, monitor temperature and urine output, arrange transport to a neonatal center with pediatric surgery
Neural tube defects	Open spinal defect (myelomeningocele), cranial defect with outpouching brain tissue (occipital or frontal encephalocele), failure of formation of skull and brain (anencephaly)	Prolonged apnea, infection, hypothermia	Provide supportive care unless prenatal diagnosis of lethal anomaly has allowed formation of a plan for limited support; protect exposed tissue with gauze soaked in warmed saline and evaporative barrier; arrange transport to a neonatal center with specialists in spinal defects

BOX 4-3 EMERGENCY PROCEDURES IN THE DELIVERY ROOM

A. Umbilical vessel catheterization (see Chapter 7)
B. Thoracentesis and chest tube placement (see Chapter 23)
C. Partial exchange transfusion for anemia (see Chapter 20)
   1. Indications: Profound chronic anemia (hematocrit [Hct] <25%), as in the setting of hydrops. Distinct from situations of acute loss of blood volume, chronic anemia results in normal blood volume per kilogram, necessitating partial exchange transfusion to rapidly raise the hematocrit.
   2. Procedure
      a. Obtain O-negative packed red blood cells (PRBCs) by emergency release if necessary. PRBCs should be as fresh as possible to minimize risk for hyperkalemia.
      b. Insert a low umbilical vein catheter, and attach a four-way stopcock (exchange set).
      c. Perform an isovolumetric exchange by alternating withdrawal and infusion of 5- to 10-mL aliquots of patient blood and PRBCs to a total exchange volume of approximately 20 mL/kg. The formula is as follows:

$$\text{Exchange volume} = \text{Estimated dry wt} \times \text{Blood volume/kg} \\ (\text{desired Hct} - \text{current Hct}) \div \text{Hct of PRBCs}$$

      This equation can be used to estimate the rise in hematocrit for a given exchange volume and a given hematocrit of exchange blood.
      d. Alternatively, place both a low umbilical vein catheter (UVC) and an umbilical artery catheter (UAC). Withdraw from the UAC while infusing PRBCs per the UVC at the same rate to the total exchange volume.
   3. Risks
      a. Thrombotic, embolic events
      b. Infection
      c. Bleeding (from mechanical complications or depletion of clotting factors)
      d. Hyperkalemia (consider use of washed PRBCs for nonemergent partial volume exchanges)
D. Prophylactic administration of exogenous surfactant (see Chapter 23)
   1. Indications
      a. Prematurity
      b. Respiratory distress
      c. Presumed surfactant deficiency
   2. Procedure
      a. Calculate the appropriate dose of surfactant based on birth weight.
      b. Confirm correct endotracheal tube position by centimeter markings at the lip (see Table 4-5) and careful auscultation. Chest x-ray film confirmation is ideal if surfactant is administered during stabilization in the nursery.
      c. Suction the endotracheal tube to clear secretions.
      d. Monitor heart rate and oxygen saturation with pulse oximetry.
      e. Administer surfactant according to manufacturer's directions or experimental protocol. Administration options include rapid bolus and gradual infusion combined with positioning of the infant and hand or mechanical ventilation.
      f. Refrain from suctioning for at least 4 hours after surfactant administration.
      g. Monitor chest wall rise, saturations, and arterial blood gases, and adjust ventilator support accordingly.
   3. Complications
      a. Hypoxemia
      b. Air leak
      c. Pulmonary hemorrhage

effort and when sustained, regular respirations occur. **Transfer the infant in a warmed transport incubator with necessary support measures such as supplemental oxygen or positive-pressure ventilation and pulse oximetry monitoring of heart rate and oxygen saturations.** Delay elective procedures until the infant is physiologically stable.[39] Depending on the level of care required by the infant and the level of care available in the institution, the infant may need to be transported from the birth setting to receive appropriate care after resuscitation (see Chapter 3).

In the intensive care nursery, place the infant on a preheated open warmer with servo control. Avoid overwarming, because hyperthermia may be associated with respiratory depression and worsened neurologic outcome after asphyxial insults.[41,48] Continue adequate cardiopulmonary monitoring, including ECG, respiratory rate and pattern, and monitoring of oxygen saturation with pulse oximetry. Obtain serum glucose by heelstick and blood pressure by a Doppler device and blood pressure cuff. If an umbilical venous catheter was inserted during the initial resuscitation for medication administration, remove this catheter. Begin a peripheral intravenous infusion if blood glucose is low or volume expansion is indicated; alternatively, consider rapid placement of a low umbilical vein catheter (UVC) to administer glucose or volume expander. Evaluate for placement of a central umbilical venous line for maintenance fluid administration and/or an arterial line for blood sampling and continuous arterial pressure monitoring. Confirm endotracheal tube and umbilical line placement with an x-ray examination.

CARE OF THE FAMILY AND PERINATAL DECISION MAKING

Encouraging the presence of the father or another mature support person in the delivery room is common obstetric practice and should not interfere with delivery room care. Ideally, members of the obstetric and neonatal resuscitation team should introduce themselves to the parents/birth companion before the delivery. Parents have a great deal of anxiety concerning procedures performed on their newborn; a few moments spent describing routine procedures will help allay their fears and avoid misinterpretation. When problems are anticipated, a calm, professional explanation of neonatal assessment and life support measures is necessary. Parental awareness that the medical and nursing staff have anticipated and prepared for possible problems can partially relieve their anxieties. Care must be taken, however, to avoid instilling undue alarm. Care providers should understand ethical principles and the impact of their personal moral and ethical beliefs on decisions made about resuscitation.[73]

If an infant requires resuscitation or prolonged assessment and support, the attending staff's primary obligation is to provide this care and communicate with the parents. Parents should be encouraged to have contact with their baby, but the presence of the father or a support person must not be allowed to interfere with or delay the delivery of care. The pediatric staff should tell the parents what is happening at the earliest possible opportunity, because lack of communication prolongs anxiety for the parents. A few brief statements to explain the status of the baby and procedures can relieve the anguish of silence. **Especially when a difficult resuscitation is anticipated, it is ideal to designate, in advance, a team member who can keep parents informed.**[72]

When severe perinatal problems are suspected prenatally and confirmed after birth, such as extreme prematurity (gestational age less than 23 weeks, birth weight less than 400 g), anencephaly, or trisomy 13 or 18, discussions may be held in advance with obstetric care providers and the family about limiting the extent of resuscitative measures.[23,45,56,58,73] Current data suggest that resuscitation of these infants is very unlikely to result in survival or survival without disability.[24,61] When problems are unanticipated, information is uncertain, or there has been no time for decision making before delivery, intervention in the delivery room may be warranted.[10,12] This approach allows time for complete information to be gathered and discussed with the family. If appropriate, support measures can be withdrawn later in the nursery (see Chapter 32).[20,37]

When an infant fails to respond to intensive resuscitative measures in the delivery room, a decision, in consultation with the parents, must be made as to when to stop support. **Survival is unlikely if no heart rate has been obtained after 10 minutes.**[16,17,34,77] **Discontinuation of resuscitation may be appropriate if, after 10 minutes of full resuscitative effort, there is no return of spontaneous circulation.**[34] The data for infants who have an inadequate response to resuscitation remain less clear. The probability of survival diminishes and the probability of cerebral palsy increases with the length of time during which Apgar scores remain below 4. For example, if the Apgar score remains below 4 at 20 minutes, the probability of cerebral palsy in surviving infants is greater than 50%.[37] It is essential to rapidly identify remediable causes of poor response to resuscitation.

SUMMARY

In summary, anticipation and recognition of fetal and neonatal problems indicating delivery room resuscitation depend upon a knowledgeable and prepared staff working as a team to effectively and efficiently communicate and respond in a critical situation. By applying current evidence in performing the skills necessary for neonatal resuscitation, evaluating the infant's response, and taking the time to discuss resuscitation options and outcomes with the parents and resuscitation team, successful delivery room care and stabilization of the newborn is more likely.

REFERENCES

1. Adamson K, Behrman GS, Dawes GS, et al: Resuscitation by positive pressure ventilation and tris-hydroxymethyl aminomethane of rhesus monkeys asphyxiated at birth, *J Pediatr* 65:807, 1964.
2. American Academy of Pediatrics and American College of Obstetricians and Gynecologists: *Guidelines for perinatal care*, ed 6, Elk Grove Village, Ill, 2007, American Academy of Pediatrics and American College of Obstetricians and Gynecologists.
3. American Academy of Pediatrics Committee on Fetus and Newborn and American College of Obstetricians and Gynecologists Committee on Obstetric Practice: The Apgar score, *Pediatrics* 117:1444, 2006.
4. Aschner JL, Poland RL: Sodium bicarbonate: basically useless therapy, *Pediatrics* 122(4):831, 2008.
5. Aziz HF, Martin JB, Moore JJ: The pediatric end-tidal carbon dioxide detector role in endotracheal intubation in newborns, *J Perinatol* 19:110, 1999.
6. Bailey C, Kattwinkel J: Establishing a neonatal resuscitation team in community hospitals, *J Perinatol* 10:294, 1990.
7. Berg RA, Otto CW, Kern KB, et al: A randomized, blinded trial of high-dose epinephrine versus standard-dose epinephrine in a swine model of pediatric asphyxial cardiac arrest, *Crit Care Med* 24:1695, 1996.
8. Bland RD, Nielson DW: Developmental changes in lung epithelial ion transport and liquid movement, *Annu Rev Physiol* 54:373, 1992.
9. Boon AW, Milner AD, Hopkins IE: Lung expansion, tidal exchange and formation of the functional residual capacity during resuscitation of asphyxiated neonates, *J Pediatr* 95:1031, 1979.
10. Boyle RJ, Kattwinkel J: Ethical issues surrounding resuscitation, *Clin Perinatol* 26:779, 1999.
11. Burchfield DJ, Erenberg A, Mullett MD, et al: Why change the compression and ventilation rates during CPR in neonates? Neonatal Resuscitation Steering Committee, American Heart Association and American Academy of Pediatrics, *Pediatrics* 93:1026, (letter) 1994.
12. Byrne PJ, Tyebkhan JM, Laing LM: Ethical decision-making and neonatal resuscitation, *Semin Perinatol* 18:36, 1994.
13. Carrasco M, Martell M, Estol PC: Oronasopharyngeal suction at birth: effects on arterial oxygen saturation, *J Pediatr* 130:832, 1997.
14. Carson BS, Losey RW, Bowes WA, et al: Combined obstetric and pediatric approach to prevent meconium aspiration syndrome, *Am J Obstet Gynecol* 126:712, 1976.
15. Carter BS, Haverkamp AD, Merenstein GB: The definition of acute perinatal asphyxia, *Clin Perinatol* 20:287, 1993.
16. Casalaz DM, Marlow N, Speidel BD: Outcome of resuscitation following unexpected apparent stillbirth, *Arch Dis Child Fetal Neonatal Ed* 78:F112, 1998.
17. Casey BM, McIntire DD, Leveno KJ: The continuing value of the Apgar score for the assessment of newborn infants, *N Engl J Med* 344:467, 2001.
18. Dawes GS: *Foetal and neonatal physiology: a comparative study of the changes at birth*, St Louis, 1968, Mosby.
19. Dawson JA, Davis PG, O'Donnell CP, et al: Pulse oximetry for monitoring infants in the delivery room: a review, *Arch Dis in Child Fetal Neonatal Ed* 92:F4, 2007.
20. Doroshow RW, Hodgman JE, Pomerance JJ, et al: Treatment decisions for newborns at the threshold of viability: an ethical dilemma, *J Perinatol* 20:379, 2000.
21. Emmanouilides GC, Moss AJ, Duffie ER, et al: Pulmonary artery pressure changes in human newborn infants from birth to 3 days of age, *J Pediatr* 65:327, 1964.
22. Estol PC, Piriz H, Basalo S, et al: Oro-naso-pharyngeal suction at birth: effects on respiratory adaptation of normal term vaginally born infants, *J Perinat Med* 20:297, 1992.
23. Finer NN, Barrington KJ: Decision-making in delivery room resuscitation: a team sport, *Pediatrics* 102(3):644, 1998.
24. Finer NN, Horbar JD, Carpenter JH: Cardiopulmonary resuscitation in the very low birth weight infant: the Vermont Oxford Network experience, *Pediatrics* 104:428, 1999.
25. Finer NN, Rich W, Craft A, et al: Comparison of methods of bag and mask ventilation for neonatal resuscitation, *Resuscitation* 49:299, 2001.
26. Finholt DA, Kettrick RG, Wagner HR, et al: The heart is under the lower third of the sternum: implications for external cardiac massage, *Am J Dis Child* 140:646, 1986.
27. Goldberg RN, Chung D, Goldman SL, et al: The association of rapid volume expansion and intraventricular hemorrhage in the preterm infant, *J Pediatr* 96:1060, 1980.
28. Hageman JR, Conley M, Francis K, et al: Delivery room management of meconium staining of the amniotic fluid and the development of meconium aspiration syndrome, *J Perinatol* 8:127, 1988.
29. Halamek LP: The simulated delivery-room environment as the future modality for acquiring and maintaining skills in fetal and neonatal resuscitation, *Semin Fetal Neonatal Med* 13:448, 2008.
30. Harris AP, Sendak MJ, Donham RT: Changes in arterial oxygen saturation immediately after birth in the human neonate, *J Pediatr* 109:117, 1986.
31. Hein HA: The use of sodium bicarbonate in neonatal resuscitation: help or harm? *Pediatrics* 91:496, 1993.
32. Hussey SG, Ryan CA, Murphy BP: Comparison of three manual ventilation devices using an intubated

mannequin, *Arch Dis Child Fetal Neonatal Ed* 89:F490, 2004.
33. International Consensus on Cardiopulmonary Resuscitation (CPR) and Emergency Cardiovascular Care (ECC) Science and Treatment Recommendations: Part 7: Neonatal resuscitation, *Circulation* 112(Suppl 22):III-91–III-99, 2005 and Part 13: Neonatal resuscitation guidelines, *Circulation* 112(Suppl 22): IV-188-IV-195, 2005..
34. Jain L, Ferre C, Vidyasagar D, et al: Cardiopulmonary resuscitation of apparently stillborn infants: survival and long-term outcome, *J Pediatr* 118:778, 1991.
35. Jain L, Vidyasagar D: Controversies in neonatal resuscitation, *Pediatr Ann* 24:540, 1995.
36. Kanter RK: Evaluation of mask-bag ventilation in resuscitation of infants, *Am J Dis Child* 141:761, 1987.
37. Kattwinkel J: Very difficult questions in neonatal resuscitation, *NRP Instructor Update* 5(3 pt, Suppl):1S, 1996.
38. Kattwinkel J, editor: *Textbook of neonatal resuscitation*, ed 5, Elk Grove Village, Ill, 2006, American Academy of Pediatrics and American Heart Association.
39. Kattwinkel J, Cook LJ, Hurt H, et al: Resuscitating the newborn infant. Perinatal Continuing Education Program, Book I. Maternal and fetal evaluation and immediate newborn care, Elk Grove Village, Ill, 2007, American Academy of Pediatrics.
40. Khan NS, Luten RC: Neonatal resuscitation, *Emerg Med Clin North Am* 12:239, 1994.
41. Lieberman E, Lang J, Richardson DK, et al: Intrapartum maternal fever and neonatal outcome, *Pediatrics* 105:8, 2000.
42. Loe HC, Lassen NA, Friis-Hansen B: Impaired autoregulation of cerebral flow in the distressed newborn infant, *J Pediatr* 94:118, 1979.
43. Lucas VW Jr, Preziosi MP, Burchfield DJ: Epinephrine absorption following endotracheal administration: effects of hypoxia-induced low pulmonary blood flow, *Resuscitation* 27:31, 1994.
44. Morley CJ, Davis PG: Continuous positive airway pressure: scientific and clinical rationale, *Curr Opin Pediatr* 20:119, 2008.
45. Niermeyer S, Kattwinkel J, Van Reempts P, et al: International Guidelines for Neonatal Resuscitation: an excerpt from the Guidelines 2000 for Cardiopulmonary Resuscitation and Emergency Cardiovascular Care: International Consensus on Science, *Pediatrics* 106:E29, Accessed, July 18, 2009, from http://pediatrics.aappublications.org/cgi/reprint/106/3/e29 and *Circulation* 102(Suppl 1):1–343, 2000.
46. Nilsson R, Grossmann G, Robertson B: Bronchiolar epithelial lesions induced in the premature rabbit neonate by short periods of artificial ventilation, *Acta Pathol Microbiol Scand (A)* 88:359, 1980.
47. Orlowski JP: Optimum position for external cardiac compression in infants and young children, *Ann Emerg Med* 15:667, 1986.
48. Perlman JM: Maternal fever and neonatal depression: preliminary observations, *Clin Pediatr* 38:287, 1999.
49. Perlman JM, Risser R: Cardiopulmonary resuscitation in the delivery room: associated clinical events, *Arch Pediatr Adolesc Med* 149:20, 1995.
50. Price WR, Eastlack M, Hall DA, et al: Implementing a neonatal resuscitation quality improvement committee, *J Perinat Neonatal Nurs* 7:57, 1993.
51. Probyn ME, Hooper SB, Dargaville PA, et al: Positive end expiratory pressure during resuscitation of premature lambs rapidly improves blood gases without adversely affecting arterial pressure, *Pediatr Res* 56:198, 2004.
52. Reddy VK, Holzman IR, Wedgwood JF: Pulse oximetry saturations in the hours of life in normal term infants, *Clin Pediatr (Phila)* 38:87, 1999.
53. Ringer SA, Stark AR: Management of neonatal emergencies in the delivery room, *Clin Perinatol* 16:23, 1989.
54. Rudolph AM: High pulmonary vascular resistance after birth. I. Pathophysiologic considerations and etiologic classification, *Clin Pediatr* 19:585, 1980.
55. Scarpelli EM: Perinatal lung mechanics and the first breath, *Lung* 162:61, 1984.
56. Seri I, Evans J: Limits of viability: definition of the gray zone, *J Perinatol* 28(Suppl 1):S4, 2008.
57. Sims DG, Heal CA, Bartle SM: Use of adrenaline and atropine in neonatal resuscitation, *Arch Dis Child* 70:F3, 1994.
58. Southgate M, Annibale DJ: Clinical ethics and neonatology: integrating emerging disciplines, *Neonatal Intensive Care* 8:42, 1995.
59. Tin W, Gupta S: Optimum oxygen therapy in preterm babies, *Arch Dis Child Fetal Neonatal Ed* 92:F143, 2007.
60. Toth B, Becker A, Seelbach-Gobel B: Oxygen saturation in healthy newborn infants immediately after birth measured by pulse oximetry, *Arch Gynecol Obstet* 266:105, 2002.
61. Tyson JE, Younes N, Verter J, et al: Viability, morbidity, and resource use among newborns of 501- to 800-g birth weight: National Institute of Child Health and Human Development Neonatal Research Network, *JAMA* 276:1645, 1996.
62. Vain NE, Szyld EG, Prudent LM, et al; for the Meconium Study Network: Oropharyngeal and nasopharyngeal suctioning of meconium-stained neonates before delivery of their shoulders: multicentre, randomized controlled trial, *Lancet* 364:597, 2004.
63. Vento M, Aguar M, Leone TA, et al: Using intensive care technology in the delivery room: a new concept for the resuscitation of extremely preterm neonates, *Pediatrics* 122:1113, 2008.

64. Vento M, Asensi M, Sastre J, et al: Resuscitation with room air instead of 100% oxygen prevents oxidative stress in moderately asphyxiated term neonates, *Pediatrics* 107:642, 2001.
65. Vento M, Sastre J, Asensi M, et al: Oxidative stress in asphyxiated term infants resuscitated with 100% oxygen, *J Pediatr* 142:242, 2003.
66. Verklan MT, Padhye N, Turner C: Oxygen saturations in the first 30 minutes of life, *Adv Neonatal Care* 8:231, 2008.
67. Vohra S, Frent G, Campbell V, et al: Effect of polyethylene occlusive skin wrapping on heat loss in very low birth weight infants at delivery: a randomized trial, *J Pediatr* 134:547, 1999.
68. Vohra S, Roberts RS, Zhang B: Heat loss prevention (HeLP) in the delivery room: a randomized controlled trial of polyethylene occlusive skin wrapping in very preterm infants, *J Pediatr* 145:750, 2004.
69. Vyas H, Field D, Milner AD, et al: Determinants of the first inspiratory volume and functional residual capacity at birth, *Pediatr Pulmonol* 2:189, 1986.
70. Wang CL, Anderson C, Leone TA, et al: Resuscitation of preterm neonates by using room air or 100% oxygen, *Pediatrics* 121:1083, 2008.
71. Weinstock P, Halamek LP: Teamwork during resuscitation, *Ped Clin North Am* 55(4):1011, 2008.
72. Wheeler CA, Tudhope AE: Development of a neonatal intensive care nursery resuscitation and triage team: impact on nursing care and infant outcome, *Neonatal Netw* 13:53, 1994.
73. Wilder MA: Ethical issues in the delivery room: resuscitation of extremely low birth weight infants, *J Perinat Neonatal Nurs* 14:44, 2000.
74. Wiswell TE: Meconium in the Delivery Room Trial Group: delivery room management of the apparently vigorous meconium-stained neonate—results of the multicenter collaborative trial, *Pediatrics* 105:1, 2000.
75. Wiswell TE, Bent RC: Meconium staining and the meconium aspiration syndrome, *Pediatr Clin North Am* 40:955, 1993.
76. Wood FE, Morley CJ, Dawson JA, et al: Improved techniques reduce face mask leak during simulated neonatal resuscitation: Study 2, *Arch Dis Child Fetal Neonatal Ed* 93:F230, 2008.
77. Yeo CL, Tudehope DI: Outcome of resuscitated apparently stillborn infants: a ten year review, *J Paediatr Child Health* 30:129, 1994.

5 INITIAL NURSERY CARE

SANDRA L. GARDNER AND JACINTO A. HERNANDEZ

A neonate must demonstrate a condition of well-being before being considered a normal, low-risk infant. **Neonatal intensive care professionals must understand the normal neonate to care for the sick neonate.** This chapter discusses the initial assessment, transitional period, and gestational age characteristics that are of fundamental clinical importance for the provision of quality initial nursery care by all health care providers.

Physical, biologic, and physiologic changes occur so rapidly after birth that the assessment of the newly born can be divided into four distinctive periods: at delivery, during transition, during the first 24 hours of life, and at discharge. Each of these assessments has a specific purpose. One should consider these evaluations in relation to the age of the newborn infant (minutes, hours, days, and weeks) rather than to the location of the mother and infant in the hospital or to arbitrary nursery routines.

The evaluation at delivery is aimed at determining the condition of the infant at the time of birth (Apgar score)[6] and at detecting life-threatening emergencies. The examination during the next few hours (transition period) is used to evaluate the infant's adjustment to extrauterine life. The complete newborn examination by a qualified health care provider should be performed at about 12 to 24 hours.[3] It is the most important examination, because many findings can be treated or complications can be avoided. Finally, the assessment/evaluation at discharge is of the utmost importance. Although it is not as detailed as the complete examination, it is aimed at establishing the infant's readiness to leave the hospital and to be cared for by the mother. During this examination, the health care professional demonstrates the baby's unique abilities and answers the parents' questions. This is a good time to provide support and encouragement as the parents begin to incorporate the new member into their family.

ASSESSMENT AND CARE AT DELIVERY

Before the delivery, one should obtain pertinent facts about the pregnancy, such as parity, gravidity, fetal losses, estimated birth weight and gestational age of the fetus, and, of course, any problems present in the current pregnancy.[61] Health care providers should note whether the mother was screened for group B streptococcus and whether she received any antibiotic treatment.[3,17]

During labor, one can observe the frequency and duration of contractions and the mother's reaction to contractions. Passage of meconium, rupture of membranes, fetal distress, and other signs will alert the attendants to impending problems.

The initial respiratory effort and heart rate, part of the Apgar evaluation (see Chapter 4, Figure 4-7), are noted even before 60 seconds, because one does not wait for the 1-minute Apgar to begin resuscitative procedures if the infant is limp and not breathing (see Chapter 4). If the baby is vigorous, the care provider may place him or her on the mother's abdomen or in her arms; Apgar assessment can be done there or in a bassinet or warmer. Scoring is repeated at 5 minutes. Under some conditions, such as prolonged resuscitation, it is helpful to have a score at 10 or 15 minutes. Between the 1- and 5-minute Apgar assessments, one systematically evaluates the baby for potential or apparent medical emergencies.

The Apgar score standardizes initial newborn assessment[4] and continues to be a predictor of neonatal survival. A retrospective analysis found that for both preterm and term infants, neonatal survival increases with increasing Apgar scores; low 5-minute scores (e.g., 0 to 3) are associated with the highest risk for neonatal death.[16]

With practice and experience, the professional will be able to identify approximate gestational age

Please note that the **PURPLE** type in each chapter is intended to make it easier to identify clinically applicable material.

from the physical appearance. One quick and effective way to estimate gestational age is by measuring foot length. Foot length of appropriate-for-gestational-age preterm infants has been correlated with gestational age (Table 5-1). In short gestation (i.e., 25th to 34th week), there is a consistent, incremental increase in the mean foot length of 0.5 cm every 2 weeks. Measurement of foot length from the posterior prominence of the heel to the tip of the first (great) toe with a millimeter ruler is a rapid and simple method of assessing maturation of all newborns, even the very ill, very-low-birth-weight (VLBW) infant. With this method, as with other physical measurements of gestational age, one must consider the standard deviation in interpreting the results.

TABLE 5-1 FOOT LENGTH BY GESTATIONAL AGE*

GESTATIONAL AGE (wk)	FOOT LENGTH (cm)				
	NO. OF INFANTS	MEAN	MEDIAN	SD	RANGE
24	6	4.22	4.1	0.17	3.8-4.4
25	12	4.5	4.5	0.08	4.4-4.6
26	16	4.72	4.7	0.07	4.65-4.9
27	19	4.99	5.0	0.14	4.8-5.2
28	18	5.23	5.2	0.13	5.0-5.5
29	22	5.47	5.4	0.129	5.3-5.7
30	27	5.75	5.75	0.23	5.6-6.2
31	24	5.95	6.0	0.19	5.7-6.23
32	21	6.22	6.2	0.13	6.0-6.4
33	25	6.5	6.5	0.26	6.3-6.9
34	24	6.77	6.8	0.20	6.5-7.1
35	20	7.1	7.0	0.15	6.8-7.3
36	22	7.27	7.27	0.21	7.0-7.6
37	24	7.51	7.5	0.24	7.4-8.0
38	40	7.92	8.0	0.23	7.6-8.3
39	42	8.22	8.3	0.32	7.9-8.6
40	56	8.6	8.7	0.37	8.2-8.9
41	22	8.75	8.9	0.30	8.3-9.1
42	12	9.1	9.2	0.33	8.7-9.3
43	8	9.27	9.3	0.25	8.9-9.6

From Hernandez JA, Lazarte R, Pisano D, et al: Foot length and gestational age in the very-low-birth-weight infant, *The Children's Hospital Pediatric Update,* September 1987, p 4.
SD, Standard deviation.
*Applies to both male and female infants.

After turning the infant to a prone position, further inspection will reveal congenital abnormalities such as spina bifida, imperforate anus, skeletal abnormalities, or genital defects. Internal abnormalities should be suspected if an "empty" or scaphoid abdomen (diaphragmatic hernia) or profuse oral or nasopharyngeal mucus (tracheoesophageal [TE] fistula) is present. Choanal atresia may present as apnea after respirations have been established. If closing the infant's mouth results in cyanosis and/or apnea, this is a positive test result for choanal atresia. Examination of the umbilical cord and vessels may give a clue to other abnormalities. The size and amount of Wharton's jelly, especially if the cord is thin, suggest problems in intrauterine nutrition. A single umbilical artery may be a clue to other anomalies (e.g., genitourinary, gastrointestinal, cardiovascular, central nervous system [CNS], twin-to-twin transfusion, and respiratory).

EVALUATION AND CARE DURING THE TRANSITIONAL PERIOD

Physiologic Changes and Clinical Stages

The initial evaluation, assessment, and, management of a newborn must be directed toward promoting and facilitating normal adaptation to extrauterine life and early detection of significant health problems so that they can be evaluated and treated promptly and appropriately.[47]

The obligatory change of environment at birth necessitates adjustment to extrauterine environment so that the newborn experiences a complex series of biologic, physiologic, and metabolic changes. These changes are essential for survival. Every infant must complete this process of transition successfully to survive in the extrauterine environment. For a small percentage of newborns, transition is never achieved; for a slightly larger number, transition is delayed or complicated. For most newborns, transition is so smooth it appears uneventful.

With the first breath of life and the cutting of the umbilical cord, all neonates begin the transition from intrauterine to extrauterine life. Three major changes take place at birth. First, fluid in the alveoli is reabsorbed, allowing diffusion of air into the surrounding blood vessels. Second, because the umbilical arteries and vein are clamped, the low-resistance placental circuit is gone and systemic blood pressure increases. Third, pulmonary vascular resistance is decreased as a result of mechanical distention of the alveoli and increased oxygen content in the alveoli. Oxygen is a potent pulmonary vasodilator.

During the first few hours after birth, the normal newborn progresses through a fairly predictable sequence of events, recovering from the stress of birth and adapting to extrauterine life. Intrapartum and immediate neonatal events result in sympathetic discharges reflected in changes in heart rate, color, respiration, motor activity, gastrointestinal function, and temperature.[47] **Awake and sleep states affect a neonate's behavior and ability to respond to the environment.** A newborn may go from one state to another quite frequently in the nursery and at home (see Critical Findings: Newborn States and Considerations for Caregiving in Chapter 13). Figure 5-1 shows the

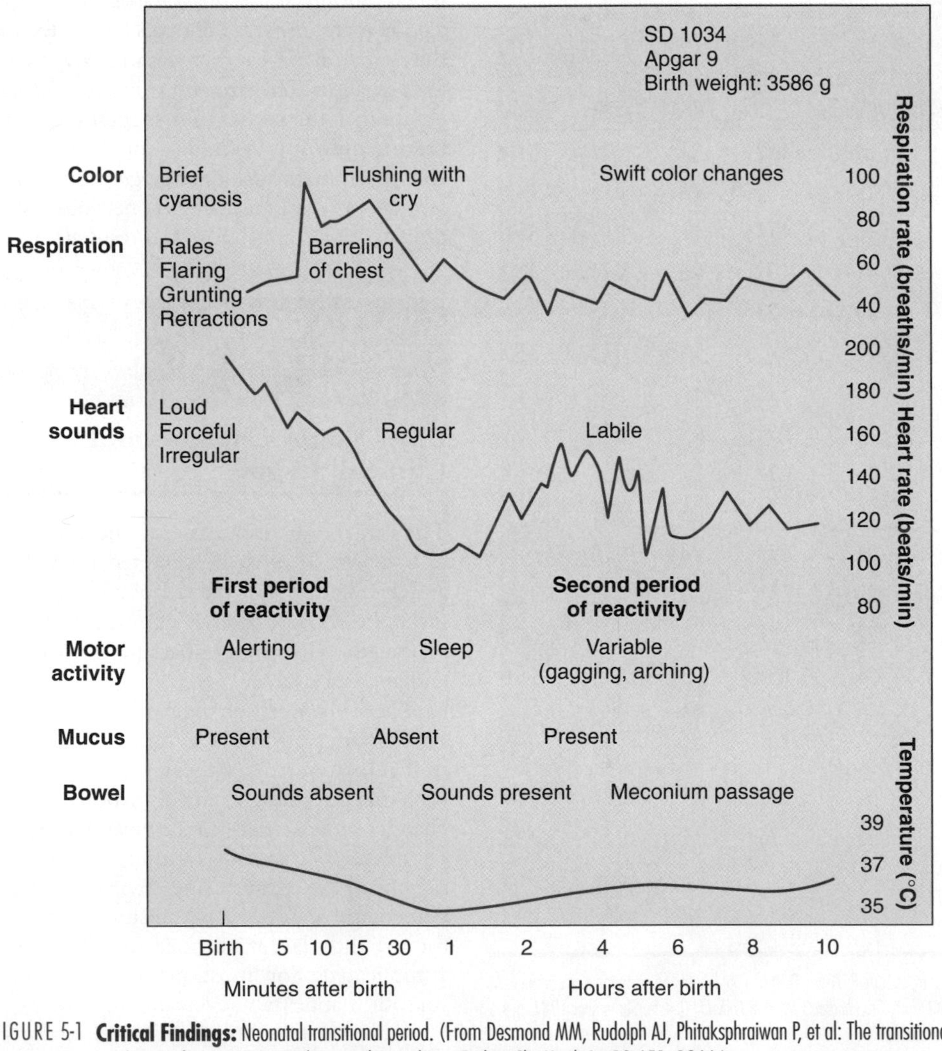

FIGURE 5-1 **Critical Findings:** Neonatal transitional period. (From Desmond MM, Rudolph AJ, Phitaksphraiwan P, et al: The transitional care nursery: a mechanism for preventive medicine in the newborn, *Pediatr Clin North Am* 13:651, 1966.)

classic description by Desmond of the transitional period, which includes the three stages shown in Box 5-1. Failure to establish this pattern of transition requires careful observation and investigation.

Management of the Newborn During Transition

Traditionally, care in "normal newborn" nurseries was based on the optimistic assumption that most newborns have no difficulty with transition after birth and that term infants, in particular, do exceedingly well. With this philosophy, nursery care was geared toward the 85% to 90% of newborns who do well rather than the 10% to 15% with transitional complications.[47] Modern nursery care recognizes the complexity of transitioning to extrauterine life and the reality of serious disease even in term newborns.

NEWBORN SHOULD BE TREATED AS A RECOVERY PATIENT

During the immediate neonatal period, an "intensive care" concept has been introduced into care of the newly born. **All newborns are to be cared for, regarded, and observed as recovering patients until they have successfully completed a smooth transition.**

SKILLED PROVIDERS SHOULD CARE FOR THE NEWBORN

Current standards of care[3] require skilled health care providers (24 hours/day) to care for newborns during the first minutes after birth (e.g., in the delivery room; birth center) and in the follow-up period (e.g., in the birth room; mother-baby area; newborn nursery).[47] All personnel caring for the newborn must be familiar with the transitional changes after birth and deviations from normal transitional

BOX 5-1 TRANSITIONAL PERIOD

First Stage (0-30 min) = First Period of Reactivity

- Rapid increase in heart rate to the range of 160-180 beats/min (0-15 min)
- Gradual decrease in heart rate over 30 min to baseline rate between 100-120 beats/min
- Irregular respirations (first 15 min), peak respiratory rates between 60-80 breaths/min
- Rales present on auscultation
- Grunting, flaring, and retractions may be noted, and brief periods of apnea (<10 sec in duration)
- Plethora
- Alert with spontaneous startle reactions, gustatory movements, tremors, crying, and side-to-side head movements
- Decrease in body temperature
- Generalized increase in motor activity, with increased muscle tone
- Bowel sounds absent, and abdomen distended
- Production of saliva minimal

Second Stage (30 min–2 hr) = Period of Decreased Responsiveness

- Newborn either sleeps or has a marked decrease in motor activity
- Muscle tone returns to normal, but responsiveness is diminished
- Fast, shallow, synchronous breathing (60 breaths/min) without dyspnea occurs
- Newborn's color is pale but pink with excellent perfusion and capillary refill
- Increase in anterior-posterior diameter (barreling) of the chest is usually present
- Heart rate decreases into the range of 100-120 beats/min or lower; the newborn is relatively less responsive to external stimuli
- Abdomen is rounded, and bowel sounds are audible; peristaltic waves may be visible, and meconium may be passed
- Oral mucus is absent
- Spontaneous jerks and twitches are common, but the newborn quickly returns to rest

Third Stage (2-8 hr) = Second Period of Reactivity

- Return of and possible exaggeration of responsiveness
- Labile heart rate: periods of tachycardia
- Brief periods of rapid respirations
- Abrupt changes in tone, color, and bowel sounds
- Possible prominence of oral mucus; gagging and vomiting not unusual
- Possible clearing of meconium from the bowel
- Increased responsiveness to endogenous and exogenous stimuli
- Newborn hunger cues; quiet alert periods when maternal bonding is established

Modified from Hernandez JA, Thilo E: Routine care of the full-term newborn. In Osborn LC, DeWitt TG, First LR, et al, editors: *Pediatrics*, St Louis, 2005, Mosby.

TABLE 5-2 ROUTINE CARE ON ADMISSION TO TRANSITION NURSERY*

ROUTINE CARE	TIME	DRUG/DOSE	COMMENTS
Glucose screening (see Chapter 15)	At 30-60 minutes of age		By POC glucometer device Abnormal screen: glucose <40 mg/dL
Eye prophylaxis	Within 1 hour of age	Erythromycin (0.5%) or tetracycline (1%) eye ointment: apply ribbon in each conjunctival sac	Eye prophylaxis for ophthalmia neonatorum Bacteriocidal effect depends on tissue concentration of drug and microorganisms
Vitamin K_1	Within 1 hour of age	0.5-1 mg IM as a single dose for infants <1.5 kg or >1.5 kg **or**	Prophylaxis for hemorrhagic disease of the newborn. Vitamin K concentrations are physiologically low in breast milk so that exclusively breast-fed infants are at increased risk for vitamin K deficiency as are infants with fat malabsorption (e.g., biliary atresia, cystic fibrosis, alpha$_1$-antitrypsin deficiency) and prolonged treatment with antibiotics. (See Chapter 12 for use of sucrose and topical analgesia to be used for pain relief for injections.)
		2 mg PO	Repeated oral dosing (e.g., first feed, 1 week, 4 weeks, 8 weeks) is necessary; increased risk for late-onset hemorrhagic disease when infant receives only one dose. PO intake contraindicated in preterms, sick infants with diarrhea or cholestasis or receiving antibiotics

Modified from Hernandez JA, Thilo E: Routine care of the full-term newborn. In Osborn LC, DeWitt TG, First LR, et al, editors: *Pediatrics*, St Louis, 2005, Mosby.
IM, Intramuscular; *PO*, orally; *POC*, point-of-care.
*Routine care is required wherever (e.g., labor-delivery-recovery; labor-delivery-recovery-postpartum; birth center; mother-baby unit; nursery) the newly born infant is cared for after birth.

events. After a normal, low-risk pregnancy and birth, primary evaluation and care of the newborn must be provided by educated, professional neonatal nurses who consult advanced practice nurses and/or physician(s) when appropriate.[3,47]

STANDARDS FOR ROUTINE CARE AND PHYSIOLOGIC MONITORING DURING TRANSITION MUST BE MAINTAINED

Both parent-infant bonding and careful neonatal monitoring during the transition period should be addressed in delivery/birth room and nursery routines. After birth, the stable, pink newborn whose Apgar score is greater than 7 at 5 minutes can be rewrapped in warm, dry blankets and given to the parents to hold. Early breast feeding and skin-to-skin contact are acceptable if the neonate is stable and continuous observation is provided. **After birth, at 15-minute intervals, *every* newborn must be assessed for general condition, respiratory effort, color, muscle tone, and temperature; all assessments must be documented.**[47]

When the neonate is admitted to the transition nursery (or recovered with the parents), anthropometric measurements (e.g., weight, length, head circumference) and vital signs are evaluated and recorded. Routine care in Table 5-2 includes glucose screening, eye prophylaxis, and administration of vitamin K_1. **By 30 minutes of age, *every* newborn, regardless of where the baby is being cared for, must be examined by a neonatal nurse.** During the first 6 hours after birth, heart rate, respirations, blood pressure, degree of alertness, and color of skin and mucous membranes should be assessed frequently and the findings recorded. This period is when clinical signs of the most threatening infections, cardiopulmonary diseases, and major congenital abnormalities appear. Table 5-3 presents a useful scoring system for assessing the pattern of respirations for signs of respiratory distress; findings should be documented. For indirectly measured blood pressure, the range of normal is 65 to 95 mm Hg systolic and 30 to 60 mm Hg diastolic, with an average mean blood

TABLE 5-3 CLINICAL RESPIRATORY DISTRESS SCORING SYSTEM*

	0	1	2
Respiratory rate (breaths/min)	60	60-80	>80 or apneic episode
Cyanosis	None	In room air	In 40% FIO_2
Retractions	None	Mild	Moderate to severe
Grunting	None	Audible with stethoscope	Audible without stethoscope
Air entry†	Clear	Delayed or decreased	Barely audible

From Downes JJ, Vidyasager DD, Boggs TR, et al: Respiratory distress syndrome in newborn infants: I. New clinical scoring system (RDS score) with acid-base and blood-gas correlates, *Clin Pediatr* 9:325, 1970.

FIO_2, Fraction of inspired oxygen; *RDS*, respiratory distress syndrome.

*The respiratory distress syndrome score is the sum of the individual scores for each of the five observations.

†Air entry represents the quality of inspiratory breath sounds as heard in the midaxillary line.

pressure of 50 to 55 mm Hg in term infants. The blood pressure value will steadily increase from birth over the transitional period.[47]

Abnormal Transition

Regardless of gestational age or route of delivery, the sequence of clinical behavior just described is common to all well newborns. Preterm infants may exhibit variations in the duration of the transitional phases—shorter phase 1 or longer phase 2—but the patterns are similar. **Knowledge of the normal changes occurring during transition enables early recognition of a newborn who is not making a normal extrauterine adaptation.**[47]

Failure to make a normal transition to extrauterine life may result from obstetric anesthesia or analgesia, neonatal illness, or stress such as perinatal asphyxia and its sequelae. **If the infant's pulse, respirations, color, and activity have not stabilized within the normal ranges *after 1 hour of life,* a problem should be suspected and investigated.**

Observation for risk factors for abnormal transition is essential. A variety of conditions may result in significant deviation from the normal sequence of events during transition. Table 5-4 lists factors that may alter the sequence or pattern of changes expected to occur after birth and that result in either a healthy newborn or a newborn with significant illness. When caring for a newborn with an altered or delayed transition, the factors in Table 5-4 must be considered. **The health care provider's challenge is to discriminate between signs of diseases that produce an ill newborn from the dynamic, rapidly changing features that accompany the physiologic adjustments of normal or altered transition but that still result in a healthy neonate.**[47] Box 5-2 lists clinical manifestations of abnormal transition.

PHYSICAL ASSESSMENT OF THE NEWBORN

Data Collection

HISTORY

Good perinatal care requires the identification of social, demographic, and medical-obstetric risk factors that correlate with fetal outcome. This must be an ongoing process, because high-risk patients may be identified on the first prenatal visit, during follow-up prenatal visits, or not until the intrapartum and postpartum periods. **Review of the perinatal history is important in determining significant factors for neonatal health management.** Identification of an at-risk maternal situation is essential to plan and organize care for an at-risk neonate. Review of the perinatal history includes antepartum and intrapartum events (see Chapter 2) and events of the neonatal course, such as normal or

TABLE 5-4 MATERNAL, OBSTETRIC, NEONATAL CONDITIONS THAT INCREASE THE RISK OF ABNORMAL TRANSITION

Maternal factors	Chronic hypertension Pregnancy-induced hypertension Diabetes mellitus Renal disease Infection Abuse of tobacco, alcohol, or illicit drugs Collagen vascular diseases Hemizygous hemoglobinopathies Certain maternal medications
Obstetric factors	Rh or other isoimmunization Fetal growth restriction Decreased fetal movements Multiple gestation Oligohydramnios or polyhydramnios Premature rupture of membranes Third-trimester bleeding Delivery by cesarean section
Neonatal factors	Prematurity (<37 weeks) Postmaturity (>42 weeks) Small for gestational age Large for gestational age Infection Metabolic abnormalities Birth trauma Major malformations Anemia Apgar 0-4 at 1 minute or need for resuscitation at delivery

From Hernandez JA, Thilo E: Routine care of the full-term newborn. In Osborn LC, DeWitt TG, First LR, et al, editors: *Pediatrics,* St Louis, 2005, Mosby.

abnormal transition, timing and onset of symptoms, and the ability to feed.

SIGNS AND SYMPTOMS

Unlike the verbalizing adult patient, the nonverbal neonate communicates needs primarily by behavior. Through objective observations and evaluations, the neonatal care provider interprets this behavior into information about the individual infant's condition. Assessment of the neonate includes the following:

- Estimation of gestational age
- Physical examination
- Neurologic examination
- Brazelton examination

BOX 5-2 NEONATAL CLINICAL MANIFESTATIONS SIGNALING ABNORMAL TRANSITION

- Persistent tachypnea, flaring, grunting, and retractions (respiratory score >4; duration >first hour of life); fixed bradycardia
- Diffuse and persistent rales, retractions, flaring, and grunting (respiratory score >4; duration >first hour of life)
- Persistent cyanosis (persistent oxygen saturation <90% in room air) and prolonged requirements for supplemental oxygen (after 2-3 hr of age)
- Episodes of prolonged apnea (>20 sec) and bradycardia (<80 beats/min)
- Marked pallor or ruddiness
- Temperature instability, persistently (after 2-3 hr of age) low temperature (<36.5° C)
- Poor capillary filling (>3 sec) and blood pressure instability
- Unusual neurologic behavior (lethargy, decreased activity with marked and persistent hypotonia, irritability, excessive tremors and jitteriness)
- Excessive oral secretions, drooling, and choking/coughing spells, cyanosis

Modified from Hernandez JA, Thilo E: Routine care of the full-term newborn. In Osborn LC, DeWitt TG, First LR, et al, editors: *Pediatrics*, St Louis, 2005, Mosby.

All care providers must not only be familiar with these tools but also be proficient in performing and interpreting them.

Assessment of Growth and Gestational Age. An assessment of gestational age should be done on *all* newborns to assign a newborn classification, determine neonatal mortality risk, generate a problem list of potential morbidities, and quickly initiate appropriate screening procedures and/or interventions for recognized morbidities.[61] Gestational age can be assessed by obstetric methods and by pediatric methods.

The obstetric methods for determining maturity will have already been performed by the time the newborn reaches the nursery. However, the newborn's care providers should be familiar with dating a pregnancy. Dating the last menstrual period (LMP) could be the most accurate method if the mother is sure of the dates of her last menstrual period. Some women will have spotting or even a light period after becoming pregnant, making them unsure of the time of conception. The use of birth control pills may also make the time of ovulation and conception unknown; therefore pregnancy tests are useful in confirming the pregnancy but not the timing of conception.

The most accurate assessment is the ultrasonographic examination during the first trimester. Ultrasonography is preferred because it confirms conception, assesses gestation, and evaluates fetal growth.

Pediatric methods of determining gestational age are based on physical characteristics and neurologic examination. **Within 2 hours of birth,[3] every newborn should have an assessment of gestational age by physical characteristics.** Numerous tables, charts, and graphs are available for determining gestation. Some tables are more subjective than others, but at least one form should be used by all nurseries.

Three of the available charts for determining gestational age by physical characteristics are shown in Figures 5-2, 5-3, and 5-4. Figure 5-2 does not place much emphasis on the neurologic assessment, which may not be valid in the first 24 hours because of birth recovery.[2] To use this chart, an X or ditto marks (″) are placed in each appropriate slot. Then an age is assigned according to a line drawn through the point where most of the marks have been placed. The disadvantage of this system is the subjectivity of the chart; the advantage is that items relate to gestational age, not a score. The examiner must therefore be experienced to offset the possibility of error in the chart.

Figure 5-4 incorporates physical maturity and neuromuscular maturity on an equal basis. An X is placed in the appropriate box for each category. The score for the neuromuscular and physical maturity is added and noted under the maturity rating column. Weeks of gestation are assigned according to the maturity rating score.

Accuracy in estimation of gestational age is important, because for VLBW infants, small differences in gestational age result in large differences in outcome and may be a criterion in decision making by parents and professionals as they decide whether comfort care or intensive care is used.[25,58] Research has shown that estimation of gestational age in very immature preterm infants is inaccurate.[25] For preterm infants of 22 to 28 weeks' gestation, estimates of gestational age (by the scoring system shown in Figure 5-4) exceeded the gestational age (by dates) by 1.3 to 3.3 weeks.[25] These inaccuracies must be considered in decision making, and better scoring systems are needed.[25,58]

To use these charts accurately, the examiner must assess the following physical characteristics.[61,84]

Vernix. At 20 to 24 weeks, vernix is produced by sebaceous glands. **Note the amount and distribution of vernix on the baby's skin (best done in the delivery room).** Vernix is high in fat content and protects the skin from the aqueous amniotic fluid and bacteria. At 36 weeks, the white, cheese-like material begins to decrease and disappears by 41 weeks.

Skin. **In early gestation, the skin of the fetus is very transparent and veins are easily seen. As gestation progresses, the skin becomes tougher, thicker, and less transparent.**

By 37 weeks, very few vessels are visible. From 36 weeks to delivery, fat deposits begin to form and grow. In a postterm infant, desquamation will be prominent at the ankles, wrists, and possibly palms and soles. As gestation progresses, the loss of vernix and subcutaneous tissue causes wrinkling. **Note skin turgor, color, texture, and the prominence of vessels, especially on the abdomen.**

Lanugo. At 20 weeks, fine, downy hair (lanugo) appears over the entire body of the fetus. At 28 weeks, it begins to disappear around the face and anterior trunk. At term, a few patches of lanugo may still be present over the shoulders. **Note the distribution of lanugo, first on the face and anterior trunk and then on the rest of the body.**

Hair on the Head. Hair appears on the head at 20 weeks. At 20 to 23 weeks, the eyelashes and eyebrows develop. From 28 to 36 weeks, the hair is fine and woolly and sticks together. It appears disheveled and sticks out in bunches from the head. At term, the hair lies flat on the head, it feels silky, and single strands are identifiable. **Note the quality and distribution of the hair, and feel its texture.** Scalp hair abnormalities (e.g., growth pattern, hypopigmentation, quantity, distribution, texture) may be external markers of genetic, metabolic, and neurologic disorders.

Sole Creases. Sole creases develop from toe to heel, progressing with gestational age. An infant with intrauterine growth restriction (IUGR) and early loss of vernix may have more sole creases than expected. **By 12 hours after birth, the skin has dried to a point that sole creases are no longer a valid indicator of gestational age.** Note the development of sole creases as they progress from the superior to inferior aspects of the foot (Figure 5-5).

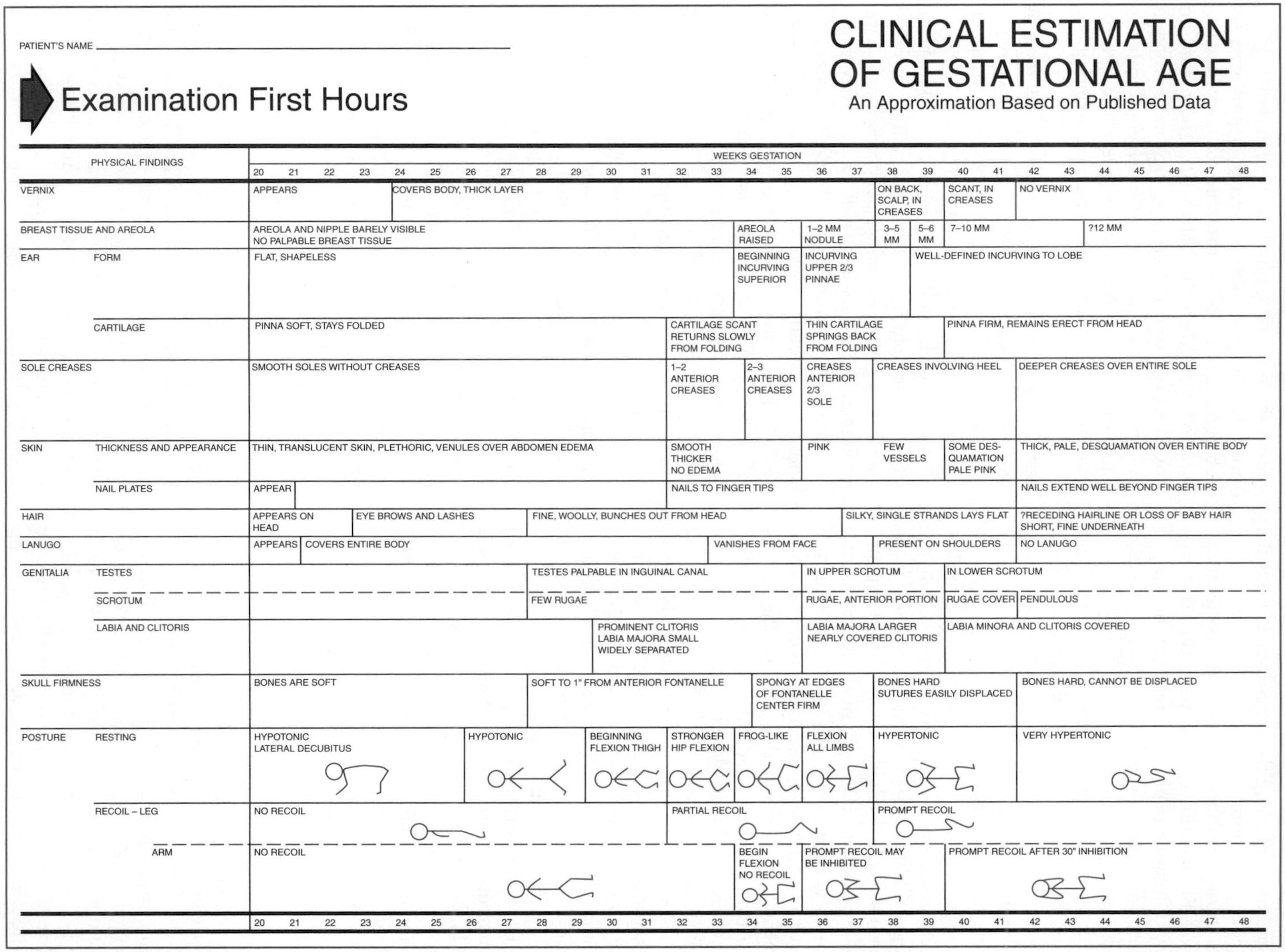

PATIENT'S NAME ____________

Examination First Hours

CLINICAL ESTIMATION OF GESTATIONAL AGE

An Approximation Based on Published Data

WEEKS GESTATION 20 21 22 23 24 25 26 27 28 29 30 31 32 33 34 35 36 37 38 39 40 41 42 43 44 45 46 47 48

PHYSICAL FINDINGS		Findings (20 → 48 weeks)
VERNIX		APPEARS; COVERS BODY, THICK LAYER; ON BACK, SCALP, IN CREASES; SCANT, IN CREASES; NO VERNIX
BREAST TISSUE AND AREOLA		AREOLA AND NIPPLE BARELY VISIBLE NO PALPABLE BREAST TISSUE; AREOLA RAISED; 1–2 MM NODULE; 3–5 MM; 5–6 MM; 7–10 MM; ?12 MM
EAR	FORM	FLAT, SHAPELESS; BEGINNING INCURVING SUPERIOR; INCURVING UPPER 2/3 PINNAE; WELL-DEFINED INCURVING TO LOBE
	CARTILAGE	PINNA SOFT, STAYS FOLDED; CARTILAGE SCANT RETURNS SLOWLY FROM FOLDING; THIN CARTILAGE SPRINGS BACK FROM FOLDING; PINNA FIRM, REMAINS ERECT FROM HEAD
SOLE CREASES		SMOOTH SOLES WITHOUT CREASES; 1–2 ANTERIOR CREASES; 2–3 ANTERIOR CREASES; CREASES ANTERIOR 2/3 SOLE; CREASES INVOLVING HEEL; DEEPER CREASES OVER ENTIRE SOLE
SKIN	THICKNESS AND APPEARANCE	THIN, TRANSLUCENT SKIN, PLETHORIC, VENULES OVER ABDOMEN EDEMA; SMOOTH THICKER NO EDEMA; PINK; FEW VESSELS; SOME DES-QUAMATION PALE PINK; THICK, PALE, DESQUAMATION OVER ENTIRE BODY
	NAIL PLATES	APPEAR; NAILS TO FINGER TIPS; NAILS EXTEND WELL BEYOND FINGER TIPS
HAIR		APPEARS ON HEAD; EYE BROWS AND LASHES; FINE, WOOLLY, BUNCHES OUT FROM HEAD; SILKY, SINGLE STRANDS LAYS FLAT; ?RECEDING HAIRLINE OR LOSS OF BABY HAIR SHORT, FINE UNDERNEATH
LANUGO		APPEARS; COVERS ENTIRE BODY; VANISHES FROM FACE; PRESENT ON SHOULDERS; NO LANUGO
GENITALIA	TESTES	TESTES PALPABLE IN INGUINAL CANAL; IN UPPER SCROTUM; IN LOWER SCROTUM
	SCROTUM	FEW RUGAE; RUGAE, ANTERIOR PORTION; RUGAE COVER; PENDULOUS
	LABIA AND CLITORIS	PROMINENT CLITORIS LABIA MAJORA SMALL WIDELY SEPARATED; LABIA MAJORA LARGER NEARLY COVERED CLITORIS; LABIA MINORA AND CLITORIS COVERED
SKULL FIRMNESS		BONES ARE SOFT; SOFT TO 1" FROM ANTERIOR FONTANELLE; SPONGY AT EDGES OF FONTANELLE CENTER FIRM; BONES HARD SUTURES EASILY DISPLACED; BONES HARD, CANNOT BE DISPLACED
POSTURE	RESTING	HYPOTONIC LATERAL DECUBITUS; HYPOTONIC; BEGINNING FLEXION THIGH; STRONGER HIP FLEXION; FROG-LIKE; FLEXION ALL LIMBS; HYPERTONIC; VERY HYPERTONIC
	RECOIL – LEG	NO RECOIL; PARTIAL RECOIL; PROMPT RECOIL
	ARM	NO RECOIL; BEGIN FLEXION NO RECOIL; PROMPT RECOIL MAY BE INHIBITED; PROMPT RECOIL AFTER 30" INHIBITION

FIGURE 5-2 **Critical Findings:** Clinical estimation of gestational age: examination in the first hour. (From Kempe CH, Silver HK, O'Brien D: *Current pediatric diagnosis and treatment*, ed 3, Los Altos, Calif, 1974, Lange Medical.)

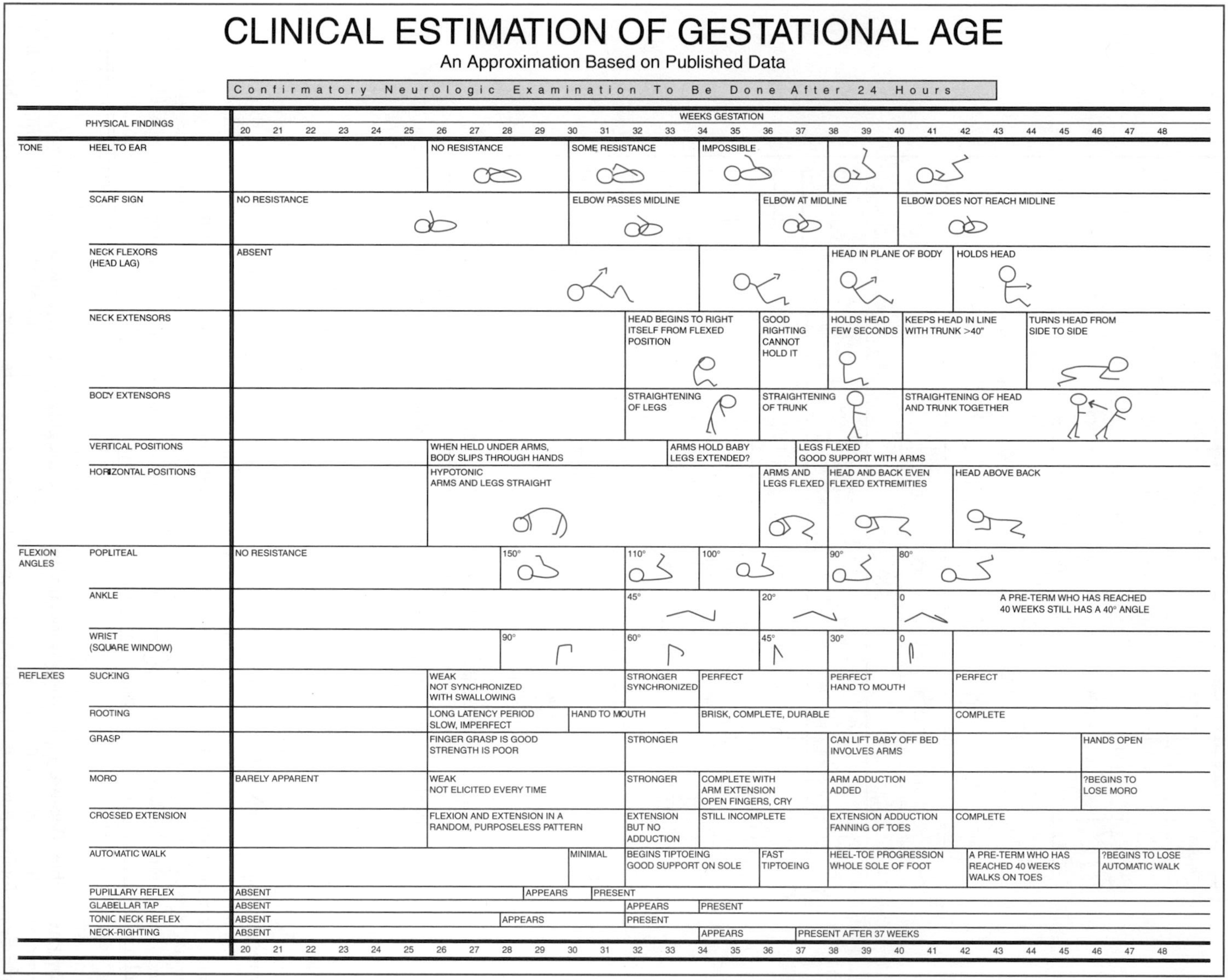
CLINICAL ESTIMATION OF GESTATIONAL AGE
An Approximation Based on Published Data
Confirmatory Neurologic Examination To Be Done After 24 Hours
PHYSICAL FINDINGS
WEEKS GESTATION
20 21 22 23 24 25 26 27 28 29 30 31 32 33 34 35 36 37 38 39 40 41 42 43 44 45 46 47 48
TONE
HEEL TO EAR
NO RESISTANCE
SOME RESISTANCE
IMPOSSIBLE
SCARF SIGN
NO RESISTANCE
ELBOW PASSES MIDLINE
ELBOW AT MIDLINE
ELBOW DOES NOT REACH MIDLINE
NECK FLEXORS (HEAD LAG)
ABSENT
HEAD IN PLANE OF BODY
HOLDS HEAD
NECK EXTENSORS
HEAD BEGINS TO RIGHT ITSELF FROM FLEXED POSITION
GOOD RIGHTING CANNOT HOLD IT
HOLDS HEAD FEW SECONDS
KEEPS HEAD IN LINE WITH TRUNK >40°
TURNS HEAD FROM SIDE TO SIDE
BODY EXTENSORS
STRAIGHTENING OF LEGS
STRAIGHTENING OF TRUNK
STRAIGHTENING OF HEAD AND TRUNK TOGETHER
VERTICAL POSITIONS
WHEN HELD UNDER ARMS, BODY SLIPS THROUGH HANDS
ARMS HOLD BABY LEGS EXTENDED?
LEGS FLEXED GOOD SUPPORT WITH ARMS
HORIZONTAL POSITIONS
HYPOTONIC ARMS AND LEGS STRAIGHT
ARMS AND LEGS FLEXED
HEAD AND BACK EVEN FLEXED EXTREMITIES
HEAD ABOVE BACK
FLEXION ANGLES
POPLITEAL
NO RESISTANCE
150°
110°
100°
90°
80°
ANKLE
45°
20°
0
A PRE-TERM WHO HAS REACHED 40 WEEKS STILL HAS A 40° ANGLE
WRIST (SQUARE WINDOW)
90°
60°
45°
30°
0
REFLEXES
SUCKING
WEAK NOT SYNCHRONIZED WITH SWALLOWING
STRONGER SYNCHRONIZED
PERFECT
PERFECT HAND TO MOUTH
PERFECT
ROOTING
LONG LATENCY PERIOD SLOW, IMPERFECT
HAND TO MOUTH
BRISK, COMPLETE, DURABLE
COMPLETE
GRASP
FINGER GRASP IS GOOD STRENGTH IS POOR
STRONGER
CAN LIFT BABY OFF BED INVOLVES ARMS
HANDS OPEN
MORO
BARELY APPARENT
WEAK NOT ELICITED EVERY TIME
STRONGER
COMPLETE WITH ARM EXTENSION OPEN FINGERS, CRY
ARM ADDUCTION ADDED
?BEGINS TO LOSE MORO
CROSSED EXTENSION
FLEXION AND EXTENSION IN A RANDOM, PURPOSELESS PATTERN
EXTENSION BUT NO ADDUCTION
STILL INCOMPLETE
EXTENSION ADDUCTION FANNING OF TOES
COMPLETE
AUTOMATIC WALK
MINIMAL
BEGINS TIPTOEING GOOD SUPPORT ON SOLE
FAST TIPTOEING
HEEL-TOE PROGRESSION WHOLE SOLE OF FOOT
A PRE-TERM WHO HAS REACHED 40 WEEKS WALKS ON TOES
?BEGINS TO LOSE AUTOMATIC WALK
PUPILLARY REFLEX
ABSENT
APPEARS
PRESENT
GLABELLAR TAP
ABSENT
APPEARS
PRESENT
TONIC NECK REFLEX
ABSENT
APPEARS
PRESENT
NECK-RIGHTING
ABSENT
APPEARS
PRESENT AFTER 37 WEEKS
20 21 22 23 24 25 26 27 28 29 30 31 32 33 34 35 36 37 38 39 40 41 42 43 44 45 46 47 48

FIGURE 5-3 **Critical Findings:** Clinical estimation of gestational age: examination after the first 24 hours. (From Kempe CH, Silver HK, O'Brien D: *Current pediatric diagnosis and treatment*, ed 3, Los Altos, Calif, 1974, Lange Medical.)

Neuromuscular maturity

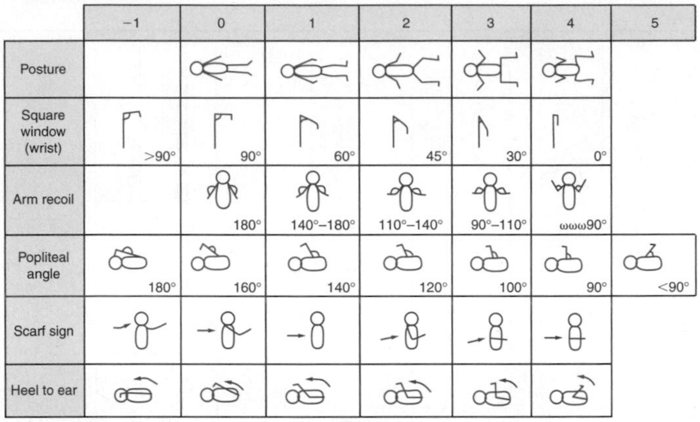

-1
0
1
2
3
4
5
Posture
Square window (wrist)
>90°
90°
60°
45°
30°
0°
Arm recoil
180°
140°–180°
110°–140°
90°–110°
ωωω90°
Popliteal angle
180°
160°
140°
120°
100°
90°
<90°
Scarf sign
Heel to ear

Physical maturity

	-1	0	1	2	3	4	5
Skin	Sticky, friable, transparent	Gelatinous red, translucent	Smooth pink, visible veins	Superficial peeling and/or rash, few veins	Cracking pale areas, rare veins	Parchment deep, cracking, no vessels	Leathery, cracked, wrinkled
Lanugo	None	Sparse	Abundant	Thinning	Bald areas	Mostly bald	
Plantar surface	Heel-toe 40–50 mm: −1 <40 mm: −2	>50 mm no crease	Faint red marks	Anterior transverse crease only	Creases ant. 2/3	Creases over entire sole	
Breast	Imperceptible	Barely perceptible	Flat areola, no bud	Stippled areola 1–2 mm bud	Raised areola, 3–4 mm bud	Full areola, 5–10 mm bud	
Eye/ear	Lids fused loosely: −1 tightly: −2	Lids open; pinna flat, stays folded	Sl. curved pinna; soft, slow recoil	Well-curved pinna; soft but ready recoil	Formed and firm, instant recoil	Thick cartilage, ear stiff	
Genitals male	Scrotum flat, smooth	Scrotum empty, faint rugae	Testes in upper canal, rare rugae	Testes descending, few rugae	Testes down, good rugae	Testes pendulous, deep rugae	
Genitals female	Clitoris prominent, labia flat	Prominent clitoris, small labia minora	Prominent clitoris, enlarging minora	Majora and minora equally prominent	Majora large, minora small	Majora cover clitoris and minora	

Maturity rating

Score	Weeks
−10	20
−5	22
0	24
5	26
10	28
15	30
20	32
25	34
30	36
35	38
40	40
45	42
50	44

FIGURE 5-4 **Critical Findings:** Clinical estimation of gestational age (revised to include extremely premature infants). (From Ballard JL, Khoury JC, Wedig K, et al: New Ballard score, expanded to include extremely premature infants, *J Pediatr* 119:417, 1991.)

Eyes. In the third month of fetal life, the eyelids fuse; they reopen between 26 and 30 weeks. **In neonates of 27 to 34 weeks' gestation, examination of the anterior vascular capsule of the lens is useful in assessing gestational age.** Gestational age is determined by assessing the level of remaining embryonic vessels on the lens (Figure 5-6). Before 27 weeks, the hazy cornea prevents visualization of the vascular system. After 34 weeks, only remnants of the vascular system are visible. Because rapid atrophy occurs in the vascular system, an ophthalmoscopic examination should be performed during the first physical examination or within 24 to 48 hours after birth.

Ears. Before 34 weeks, the pinna of the ear is a slightly formed, cartilage-free double thickness of skin. When it is folded, it remains folded. As **gestation progresses, the pinna develops more cartilage, resulting in better form, so that it recoils when folded (Figure 5-7).** Check ear recoil by folding the ear in half or into a three-corner-hat shape. Consistently folding it the same way helps the care provider develop a baseline for judging maturity. **Note the form and cartilage development of the ear. Examine both ears to be sure they are the same and without defects.**

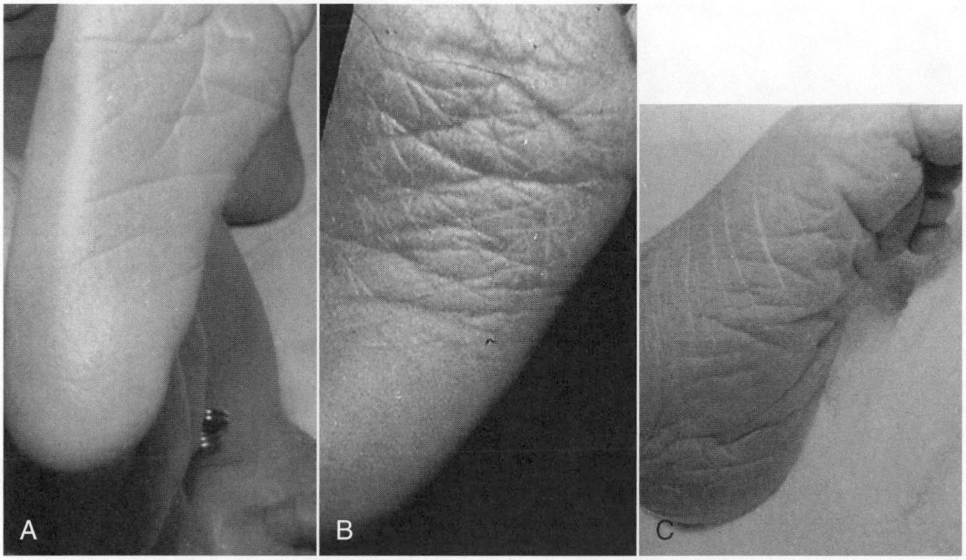

FIGURE 5-5 Sole creases at different gestational ages. **A**, Age 31 to 33 weeks' gestation. **B**, Age 34 to 38 weeks' gestation. **C**, Term.

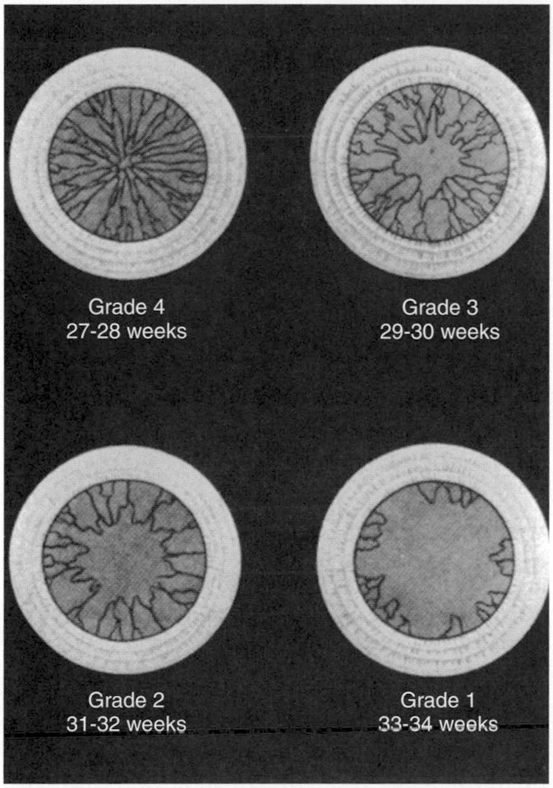

FIGURE 5-6 Anterior vascular capsule and gestational age. (From Hittner H, Hirsch NJ, Rudolph AJ: Assessment of gestational age by examination of the anterior vascular capsule of the lens, *J Pediatr* 91:455, 1977.)

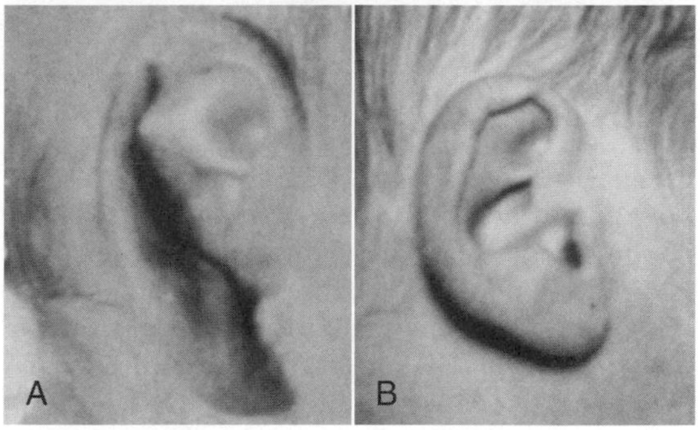

FIGURE 5-7 Ear form and gestational age. **A**, Age 34 to 38 weeks' gestation. **B**, Term.

Breast Development. Breast development is the result of the growth of glandular tissue related to high maternal estrogen levels and fat deposition. The areola is raised in an infant of 34 weeks' gestation. **Note the size, shape, and placement of both breasts.** Palpate the breast nodule and determine its size. If the infant is growth restricted, breast size may be less than expected at term.

Genitalia

Male Genitalia. At 28 weeks, the testes begin to descend from the abdomen. By 37 weeks, they are high in the scrotum. By 40 weeks, the testes are completely descended and the scrotum is covered with rugae. As gestation progresses, the scrotum

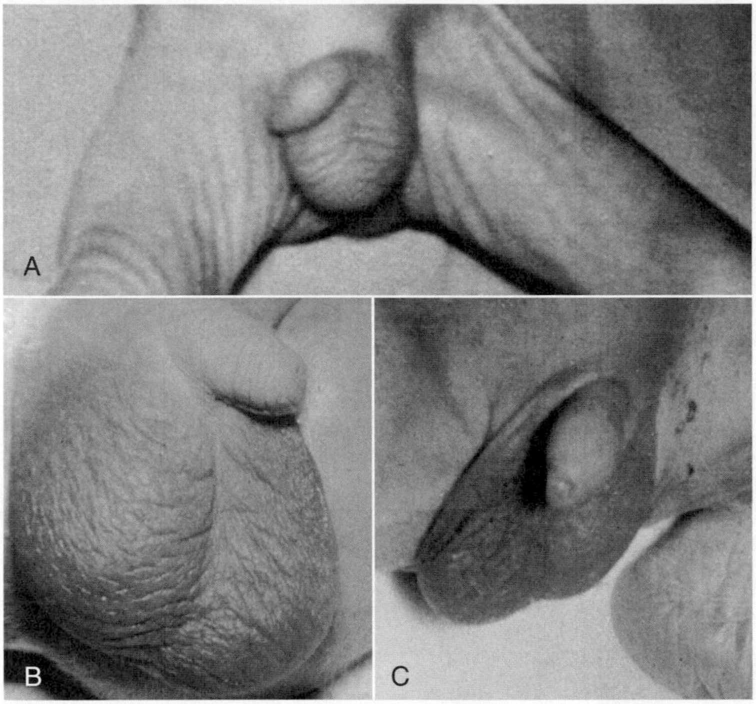

FIGURE 5-8 Male genitalia and gestational age. **A**, Age 28 to 35 weeks' gestation. **B**, Term. **C**, Age 42 or more weeks' gestation.

becomes more pendulous (Figure 5-8). **Note the presence of rugae on the scrotum and its size in relation to the position of the testes.** When examining the baby for descended testes, put the fingers of one hand over the inguinal canal to prevent the testes from ascending into the abdominal cavity and palpate the scrotal sac with the other hand.

Female Genitalia. Early in the female's gestation, the clitoris is prominent with small and widely separated labia. By 40 weeks, the fat deposits have increased in size so that the labia majora completely cover the labia minora (Figure 5-9). **Note the labial development in relation to the prominence of the clitoris.**

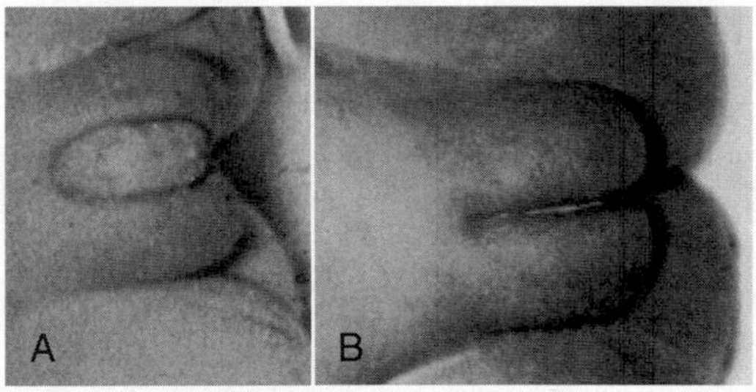

FIGURE 5-9 Female genitalia and gestational age. **A**, Age 30 to 36 weeks' gestation. **B**, Term.

Newborn Classifications. **The clinical estimate of gestation is defined by weeks of gestation into the following categories (Figures 5-10 and 5-11):**

- Preterm (PR)—through 37 completed weeks
  Late Preterm (LP)—34 to 36$\frac{6}{7}$ weeks[27]
- Full-term (F)—38 through 41 completed weeks
- Postterm (PO)—42 weeks or more

Intrauterine growth curves for the 10th and 90th percentiles are represented in Figure 5-10. **Small-for-gestational-age (SGA) infants are those below the 10th percentile.** Appropriate-for-gestational-age **(AGA) infants are those between the 10th and 90th percentiles. Large-for-gestational-age (LGA) infants are above the 90th percentile. Based on birth weight, the infant's intrauterine growth will be SGA, AGA, or LGA.**

Using the clinical estimate of gestational age **(in weeks) and the birth weight (in grams), one determines the newborn's classification. The combined gestational age and weight criteria shown in Figure 5-10 form nine possible newborn classifications: preterm, full-term, and postterm large-for-gestational-age (PRLGA, FLGA,**

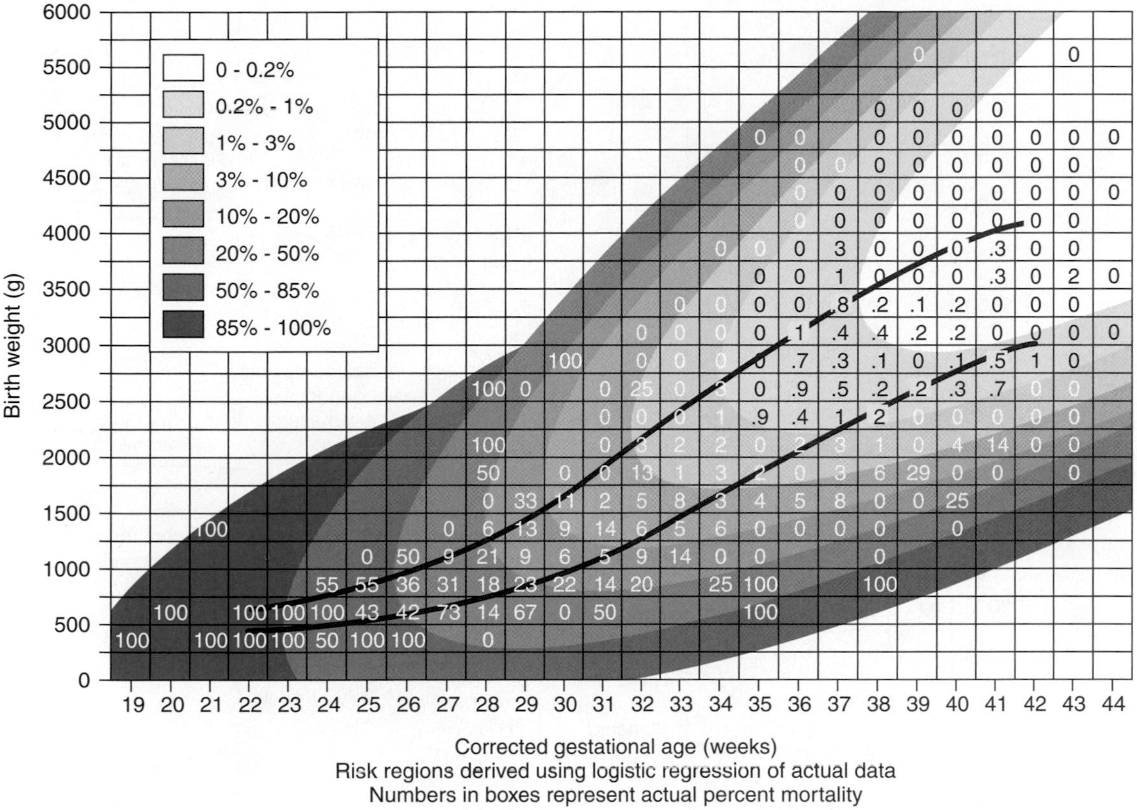

FIGURE 5-10 Neonatal mortality risk by birth weight and gestational age. (From Johnson JL, Merenstein G, Coll J, et al: Colorado intrauterine growth curve 1980-1992: the new Lubchenco growth curve, *Pediatr Res* 35:274A, 1994.)

and POLGA); preterm, full-term, and postterm appropriate-for-gestational-age (PRAGA, FAGA, and POAGA); and preterm, full-term, and postterm small-for-gestational-age (PRSGA, FSGA, and POSGA).

Using Figure 5-10, it is possible to plot the newborn weight in grams against the clinical gestational age (marking an X on the chart) by determining to which of the nine categories the newborn belongs and then classifying and noting his or her classification on the record.

Neonatal Mortality Risk. Neonatal mortality risk (NMR), the chance of dying in the neonatal period, can be determined from graphs such as that shown in Figure 5-10 and is based on birth weight and gestational age. This figure is based on the Lubchenco Perinatal Database, University of Colorado Hospital, 1980 to 1992. On the chart, the area of least risk is the FAGA infant. Deviations from this area of least risk in relation to either weight or gestational age increase the newborn's mortality risk.

Mortality has changed over time because an increasingly physiologic basis of care has been used, coupled with sophisticated professional care, technology, transport systems, and aggressive management to handle increasingly at-risk populations. For example, before recent years, LGA infants were at increased risk for mortality; this is no longer true because of earlier recognition and better obstetric management (see Chapter 2). Babies with greater than 10% risk for neonatal mortality usually require level II or III care. Note the infant's NMR on the chart (see Figure 5-10), and insert an entry in the newborn record. **NOTE:** To determine the appropriate NMR, read to the right of the vertical lines and above the horizontal line.

Examination of NMR in Figure 5-10 also reveals that two infants with the same birth weight but with

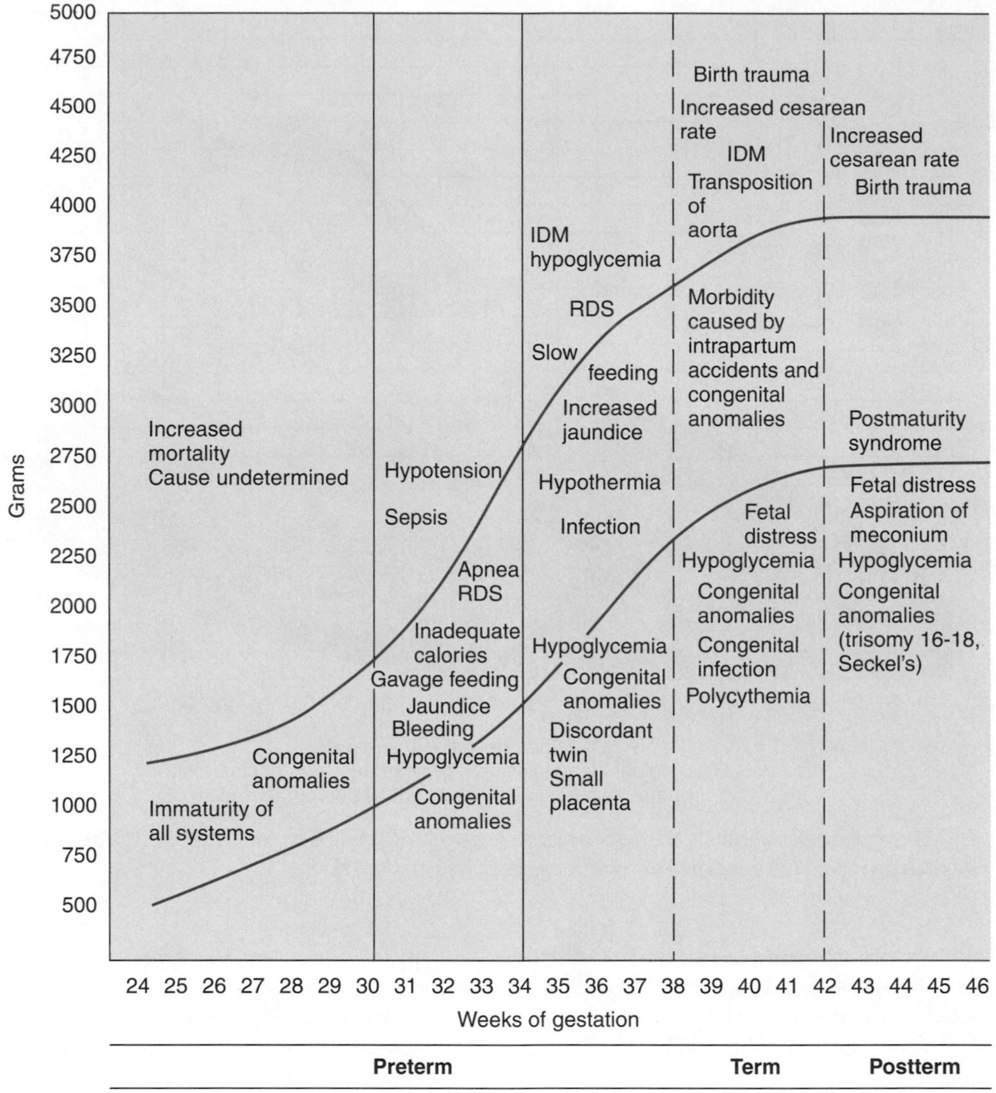

FIGURE 5-11 **Critical Findings:** Specific neonatal morbidity by birth weight and gestational age based on statistics from Newborn and Premature Center at the University of Colorado Medical Center. *IDM,* Infant of diabetic mother; *RDS,* respiratory distress syndrome. (From Lubchenco LO: *The high-risk infant,* Philadelphia, 1976, Saunders.)

different gestational ages may have very different risks for death. For example, infant A may have a birth weight of 2000 g and a gestational age of 33 weeks. Plotting these values on Figure 5-10, one determines the NMR for this infant at 2%. Infant B, on the other hand, may also weigh 2000 g but have a gestational age of 39 weeks. The infant's risk is 0%. Infant A thus has a mortality risk 10 times greater than that of infant B, even though they have the same birth weight.

Within the National Institutes of Child Health and Human Development (NICHD) Neonatal Research Network, mortality for newborns weighing 501 to 1500 grams decreased from 23% (1987-88), to 17% (1993-94), to 14% (1999-2000). However, within each birth weight category, survival free of major morbidity (e.g., chronic lung disease/bronchopulmonary dysplasia [CLD/BPD], necrotizing enterocolitis [NEC], grade 3 or 4 intraventricular hemorrhage [IVH]) did not change significantly. **Because mortality (and morbidity) are highest in infants of the lowest birth weights and gestational ages, VLBW and extremely low birth weight (ELBW) infants have better outcomes when born in a facility that can provide the appropriate subspecialty care.**[11,18,57,88] Infants requiring transfer to another facility have a greater risk for morbidity and mortality when compared with infants born in a tertiary care center; this advantage is inversely related to gestational age.[57] **These research findings have prompted recommendations that high-risk infants (e.g., <32 weeks' gestational age) be born in a facility capable of providing the anticipated appropriate level of neonatal intensive care.**[3]

Neonatal Morbidity Risk. Neonatal morbidity risk (see Figure 5-11) is determined by deviations of intrauterine growth and newborn classification. **Classification of the newborn assists in identification, observation, screening, and treatment of the most commonly occurring problems. For every newborn, formulate a problem list based on the morbidities common to the newborn classification. Observe, screen, intervene, and refer as necessary to prevent complications.**

SGA/IUGR infants are at increased risk for morbidities (e.g., perinatal depression, hypothermia, hypoglycemia, polycythemia, infection) immediately after birth. **There is also an association between size at birth, altered physiologic development, and long-term developmental and health problems (especially heart disease and stroke).**[21]

LATE-PRETERM ("NEAR-TERM") INFANTS

In the United States, 39 weeks has become the most common length of gestation.[24] Since 1981, preterm birth rate has increased by 30%.[48] In 2004, the prematurity rate in the United States was 12.5%. Two thirds of the increase in the rate was due to increasing rates of "near-term" births, so that 8.5% of all U.S. births for 2002 were neonates of 34 to 36⁶⁄₇ weeks of gestation.[48] A 2006 March of Dimes study showed that 75% of all singleton preterm births are 34 to 36 weeks' gestation and that 36 completed weeks of gestation accounts for 40.1% of all singleton preterm births.[24] Because these infants are at increased risk for health and developmental problems when compared with full-term infants, this trend has been called a growing public health problem.[48]

Historically, infants of 34 to 38 weeks' gestational age have been considered "slightly preterm"[59] or "borderline prematures."[77] Use of this terminology reminded heath care providers to have a higher index of suspicion related to morbidities when compared with term infants. In the early 1990s, the terminology "near term" began to be used in the literature. These "near term" infants not only are cared for in special care nurseries but also are found in normal newborn nurseries, mother-baby care, and labor/delivery/recovery/postpartum (LDR/LDRP),[40] because they are "considered functionally full term and management decisions are made accordingly."[87,p.372]

In 2005 at the National Institutes of Health (NIH) meeting,[74] a proposal was made to use the term "late-preterm" rather than "near-term" to reflect the increased morbidity (and mortality) of this group of biologically and physiologically immature neonates.[27] A retrospective chart review of late-preterm infants showed that they have significantly more morbidities. At 34 to 35 weeks, all the common morbidities are more frequent: (1) respiratory distress syndrome (RDS) is twice as common after cesarean section, (2) perinatal depression, (3) hypoglycemia, (4) jaundice, (5) sepsis, (6) feeding problems, and (7) apnea.[8] In this same study, RDS was five times more common at 37 to 38 weeks' gestation after cesarean section.[8] **This is consistent with other studies of elective cesarean section, as follows:**

- Those born at 37 to 38 weeks' gestation were 120 times more likely to receive ventilator support for surfactant deficiency than infants born at 39 to 41 weeks.[64]
- Timing of elective section is a risk factor for RDS.[46,91]
- Risk for respiratory morbidity is increased at any gestation less than 40 weeks (at 39 weeks, risk is doubled but not statistically significant; at 38 weeks, risk is triple; at 37 weeks, risk is fourfold).[46]
- Risks for iatrogenic RDS (i.e., 0.4%) are greatly reduced if delivery occurs at 39 weeks' gestation.[46,69,72,91]

Another study of "late-preterm" infants (i.e., 35-36⁶⁄₇ weeks' gestation) showed that they had more clinical problems, longer lengths of stay, and higher costs when compared with full-term newborns.[87] Table 5-5 shows the difference in occurrence of

TABLE 5-5 MORBIDITIES IN LATE-PRETERM ("NEAR-TERM") VERSUS FULL-TERM NEONATES

	FREQUENCY	
MORBIDITY	LATE PRETERM ("NEAR TERM")	FULL TERM
Temperature instability	10%	0%
Hypoglycemia	15.6%	5.3%
Intravenous infusions	26.7%	5.3%
Respiratory distress	28.9%	4.2%
Jaundice	54.4%	37.9%
Apnea/bradycardia	4.4%	0%
Sepsis evaluation	36.7%	12.6%
Poor feeding	76%	28.6%

Data from Wang M, Dorer D, Fleming M, et al: Clinical outcomes of near-term infants, *Pediatrics* 114:372, 2004.

morbidities between late-preterm infants (with good Apgar scores and appropriate size) and their full-term contemporaries. In addition to more acute respiratory morbidity, research shows late-preterms have more BPD/CLD, neurologic complications, rehospitalizations, and mortality.[10,28,31,82,83]

Late-preterm infants not only have more morbidities but also have been shown to have increased mortalities. While the mortality rates for full-term neonates were stable at 2.5/100,000 live births, the rate for moderately preterm (32-36 weeks' gestation) rose from 8.9 to 9.2/100,000 live births from 2001 to 2002.[48] All causes of infant mortality (i.e., birth defects, sudden infant death syndrome, respiratory distress syndrome) decreased in the United States from 1990 to 2000 except prematurity/LBW, which actually increased. A more recent study shows that late-preterms have higher mortality rates throughout infancy when compared with term infants. Late-preterm infant mortality rates were threefold higher than those of term infants (7.9 versus 2.4 deaths/1000 live births).[83] In the first month of life, deaths in the early and late neonatal period were sixfold and threefold those of term infants. Postneonatal deaths were twice as high as term infants, and during the first year of life, late-preterms were four times as likely to die as were term infants.[83]

Clearly, late-preterm infants are not term infants and need close observation, a high level of suspicion, assessment, and timely intervention by all care providers.[7,29,40] **Regardless of the geographic location of the late-preterm, these immature infants require more nursing time and care than do full-term infants.**[40] **If the level of care cannot be provided in the infant's current geographic area, these infants should be transferred to a higher-care unit (either within or outside the facility)**[40] **as soon as possible.**

Physical Examination

The purpose of the physical examination is (1) to discover common variations of normal or obvious defects, (2) to quickly initiate intervention or referral for deviations from normal, and (3) to establish a database for serial observations and comparisons. The best data are obtained from the neonate when the physical examination is organized to limit stress, maximize interaction with the examiner, and not overwhelm the newborn. **To maximize data and minimize stress, the physical examination should proceed in an orderly fashion from the least stressful to the more stressful aspects of the examination.** (See the Critical Findings box on p. 95.) However, the examination is usually recorded in an orderly manner from head to toe.

When one appreciates how stressful it is to the newborn to be undressed, it becomes obvious that as much as possible should be done without exposing the infant. Warm hands and instruments are essential, and a warm environment helps. Before touching the infant or removing any covers, observe the face, head, and hands as they appear.

OBSERVATION

Observation of the neonate provides pertinent data without touching him or her. General condition, anomalies, resting posture, and respirations should be observed.

General Condition. The general condition of the infant should be assessed by noting the color, activity, and neonatal state.

Color. **The color of the newborn is normally pink. Acrocyanosis, or peripheral cyanosis of the hands and feet, is commonly present in the first 24 hours of life and may be the result of immature circulation or cold stress.** Ecchymotic areas, especially on the presenting part, are common; however, they may be confused with cyanosis. To differentiate

Critical Findings

PHYSICAL EXAMINATION OF THE NEWBORN

I. Observation examination
  A. General condition
    1. Color
    2. Activity and neonatal state
  B. Crying
  C. Anomalies
  D. Resting posture
  E. Respirations
II. Quiet examination
  A. Auscultation
    1. Heart
    2. Lungs
    3. Abdomen
  B. Palpation
    1. Fontanels
    2. Abdomen
  C. Inspection
    1. Eyes
    2. Blood pressure
III. Head-to-Toe examination
  A. Skin
  B. Head
    1. Ears
    2. Nose
    3. Mouth
  C. Thorax
    1. Breast
    2. Clavicles
  D. Genitalia
  E. Rectum
  F. Back
  G. Extremities
    1. Upper
    2. Lower

the two, apply pressure to the area. An ecchymotic area remains blue with pressure, whereas a cyanotic area will blanch.

General cyanosis and central cyanosis of the lips, mouth, and mucous membranes may indicate CNS, heart, or lung disease. Jaundice appearing at birth or within the first 12 hours of life is abnormal. Physiologic jaundice appears after 24 hours, but jaundice may indicate other abnormalities. **Pallor at or directly after birth is a sign of circulatory failure, anoxia, edema, or shock.** Pallor of anoxia is associated with bradycardia and the pallor of anemia with tachycardia. **Plethora, a beef-red color, may indicate polycythemia and is confirmed by hemoglobin and hematocrit determinations.** However, lack of plethora does not rule out polycythemia or hyperviscosity.

Activity and Neonatal State. **Activity and the neonatal state at the beginning of the examination and appropriate changes throughout the examination should be observed.** If the infant is asleep, is it quiet or rapid-eye-movement (REM) sleep? Spontaneous, symmetric movements are normal. Tremors and twitching movements of short duration are normal in relation to states of coldness or startling. Good muscle tone is established with adequate oxygenation soon after birth.

Flaccidity, floppiness, or poor muscle tone should be noted. Spasticity, hyperactivity, opisthotonos, twitching, hypertonicity, tremors, or seizures may be indicative of CNS damage. Asymmetry may result from intrauterine pressure or birth trauma rather than a CNS insult. **A lack of crying or evasive behavior in response to the manipulations of a physical examination is abnormal.**

Crying. **Attempts to calm and console a crying infant during this part of the examination assist in better data collection during the quiet examination.** Crying is beneficial in (1) ductal closure and transition from fetal to neonatal cardiorespiratory status, (2) improving pulmonary capacity, (3) maintaining homeostasis, (4) facilitating vocal tract development, and (5) cueing and care-eliciting behavior. Negative effects include (1) changes in cardiovascular (e.g., tachycardia, hypoxia, changes in cerebral blood flow, increases in the risk for brain injury and cardiac dysfunction)[63] and endocrine systems; (2) stress production and energy drainage[63]; and (3) strong, sometimes negative feelings in care providers.

Although uniquely individual, types of cries that reflect the infant's state and contextual basis have been identified as birth, distress call, hunger, pain, spontaneous, and pleasure.[20] At birth, the term neonate has a loud, lusty cry (a signal of robustness and wellness), whereas the preterm's cry may be weak or absent. Observe the infant's ability to quiet himself or herself when crying. High responsivity of the newborn to sustained handling, undressing, and being put down is associated with more infant crying.

A **high-pitched cry** suggests CNS irritation from increased intracranial pressure, injury, infection, or abnormality. **Weak crying,** no crying, or constant, irritable crying may indicate brain injury, infection, or abnormality. **Hoarse cries or crowing inspirations** result from laryngeal inflammation, injury, vocal cord dysfunction (e.g., paresis/paralysis), or anomalies. A **weak, groaning cry or expiratory grunt** is indicative of respiratory disease.

Anomalies. Obvious bodily malformations such as omphalocele, cleft lip and palate, imperforate anus, syndactyly, polydactyly, spina bifida, or myelomeningocele should be observed and recorded as anomalies. Odd facies or body appearances that are often associated with specific syndromes also should be noted.

Resting Posture. Resting posture should be observed while the infant is quiet and not disturbed. The infant's posture systematically develops according to gestational age: (1) from extension to flexion of the lower extremities, and (2) to flexion of the upper extremities. Asymmetry may result from intrauterine pressure or birth trauma. The infant may take a position of comfort assumed in utero.

Respirations. Respirations should be evaluated while the infant is at rest and before any manipulation. The normal rate is 30 to 60 breaths/min. Count the respiratory rate and rhythm, noticing the infant's use of accessory muscles. Respiration is normally abdominal or diaphragmatic.

After the first hour of life, a respiratory rate of more than 60 breaths/min indicates tachypnea. Tachypnea is the earliest sign of many neonatal respiratory, cardiac, metabolic, and infectious illnesses. Tachypnea, apnea, dyspnea, or cyanosis may indicate cardiorespiratory distress. Labored respirations include retractions, flaring nares, and expiratory grunt. Maternal epidural analgesia with fentanyl has been shown to cause respiratory depression in neonates because fentanyl freely diffuses from the epidural space to maternal blood, equilibrating within 10 to 30 minutes and freely transporting across the placenta with slightly higher concentrations in the fetal compartment.[55] Neonatal respiratory depression secondary to fentanyl epidural analgesia is more common when mothers receive large amounts of fentanyl during labor; naloxone administration reverses the respiratory depression.[55]

If the infant is swaddled, the observation examination will not be as extensive as is possible when the infant is unclothed in an incubator or under a radiant warmer. If the infant is swaddled, unwrap gently so that observations of the thorax, abdomen, genitalia, and extremities may also be done during this phase of the examination.

Without touching the infant, one can rule out a multitude of conditions. In fact, more than 80% of the newborn examination is made through observation.

Quiet Examination. *Quiet examination* is defined as any part of the examination in which data are best collected from the quiet, cooperative newborn. The heart, lungs, head and neck, scalp and skull, abdomen, eyes, and blood pressure are areas that should be checked during the quiet examination. Using pacifiers, warming hands and stethoscopes, and holding and gently manipulating the infant are ways to avoid overwhelming the baby and to prevent crying.

AUSCULTATION

Heart. Auscultation of the heart, lungs, and abdomen is most effective when the infant is quiet. When the infant is quiet and at rest, auscultate the heart rate, rhythm, and regularity at the apex. The normal rate is 120 to 160 beats/min at a regular rhythm. Sinus dysrhythmia is normal and may be heard. The point of maximal intensity (PMI) of the neonatal heart is lateral to the midclavicular line at the third to fourth interspace. Note the PMI.

A rate of less than 80 beats/min is bradycardia. Newborns with persistent bradycardia may have complete heart block caused by maternal systemic lupus erythematosus (see Chapter 2). A rate greater than 160 beats/min is tachycardia, which may be associated with respiratory problems, anemia, or congestive heart failure when accompanied by cardiomegaly, hepatomegaly, and generalized edema.

Murmurs are noted for loudness, quality, location, and timing. They are best auscultated at the base of the third or fourth interspace. Heart murmurs in the newborn period are very common, perhaps as frequent as 10% of the population (see Chapter 24). Note dextrocardia—heart sounds audible on the right side of the chest. Pneumothorax, pneumomediastinum, dextrocardia, and diaphragmatic hernia result in muffled heart sounds or a shift in PMI. To complete the cardiac assessment, careful attention to the femoral pulses is necessary; diminished femoral pulses suggest coarctation of the aorta (see Chapter 24). Often newborns with serious congenital heart disease do not present with clinical signs and symptoms of their anomaly. Recent research has studied the use of pulse oximetry (e.g., postductal [lower extremity] saturations <92%-95%) to screen newborns for congenital heart disease.[65] Use of pulse oximetry to screen for critical congenital heart disease in the first days of life has been successful[65] but may depend on variables such as probe placement, educational level of the nurse, and familiarity with pulse oximetry.[79]

Lungs. **Normally, the lungs and chest are resonant after birth and fine rales may be present for the first few hours. Auscultation reveals bronchial breath sounds bilaterally. Air entry should be good, particularly in the midaxilla. A normal respiratory rate is 30 to 60 breaths/min.**

Hyperresonance suggests pneumomediastinum, pneumothorax, or diaphragmatic hernia. **Decreased resonance** is a result of decreased aeration—atelectasis, pneumonia, or respiratory distress syndrome. **Expiratory grunt** suggests difficulty in aeration and oxygenation. Peristaltic sounds heard in the chest may be caused by a diaphragmatic hernia.

Abdomen. Bowel sounds are normally heard shortly after birth.

PALPATION

Palpation of the fontanels and abdomen is best accomplished before the infant begins crying, because guarded muscles and the normally tense fontanels of the crying infant give little useful data.

Scalp and Skull. **Temporary deformation of the head is caused by pressures during labor and delivery.** The head circumference measurements may be altered so that the occipitofrontal circumference (OFC) on the first day of life may be smaller than on the second or third. **Caput succedaneum** is an edematous area over the presenting part of the scalp that extends across suture lines and resolves in 24 to 48 hours. A **cephalhematoma** is a soft mass of blood in the subperiosteal space on the surface of the skull bone. The blood mass does not extend across suture lines and resolves in 6 to 8 weeks.

Deviating from the normal, **skull fractures may be linear or depressed, palpable or nonpalpable.** Skull fractures are more common with forceps delivery. **Craniotabes,** softening of the skull bones, is caused by maternal vitamin D deficiency.[90]

The **anterior fontanel,** a diamond-shaped space normally measuring from 1 to 4 cm, may be gently palpated at the junction of the sagittal suture and coronal suture and between the two parietal bones. Normally the anterior fontanel softly pulsates with the infant's pulse, becomes slightly depressed when the infant sits upright and is quiet, and may bulge when the infant cries. Within 24 to 48 hours after birth, the initial molding of the head and overlap of the sutures resolve, resulting in a larger fontanel and in suture lines that should be palpated as depressions.

The **posterior fontanel,** formed at the juncture of the sagittal suture and the lambdoidal suture, is palpated between the occipital and parietal bones. Normally it is triangular shaped and barely admits a fingertip.

A **bulging, tense, or full fontanel** may be associated with increased intracranial pressure caused by birth injury, bleeding, infection, or hydrocephalus. A **depressed fontanel,** a very late sign in the newborn, may indicate dehydration. A **third fontanel,** located along the sagittal suture between the anterior and posterior fontanels, may be a sign of congenital infection or Down syndrome or may be a normal variant.

Sutures are palpable ridges between skull bones. The coronal suture is located between the frontal and two parietal bones. The sagittal suture intersects the two parietal bones, and the lambdoidal suture lies between the occipital and the two parietal bones. With increasing gestational age, the suture edges become firmer and with gentle palpation are felt as hard ridges. Sutures may be open to a varying degree or may be overlapped because of molding. Lack of normal expansion may indicate microcephaly or craniosynostosis. Abnormally rapid expansion indicates hydrocephalus or increased intracranial pressure.

Abdomen. **The abdomen will appear slightly scaphoid at birth but will become distended as the bowel fills with air. Gentle palpation of the**

abdomen for organs or masses reveals that the spleen tip can be felt from the infant's left side and is sometimes 2 to 3 cm below the left costal margin. The liver is palpable 1 to 2 cm below the right costal margin. Superficial veins over the abdominal wall may be prominent.

A markedly scaphoid abdomen coupled with respiratory difficulty may indicate a diaphragmatic hernia. **Abdominal distention and lack of bowel sounds** may occur because of intestinal obstruction, paralytic ileus, ascites, imperforate anus, meconium plug, peritonitis, omphalocele, Hirschsprung's disease, or necrotizing enterocolitis. The infant should be observed for **abdominal wall defects**, such as umbilical hernia, omphalocele (a herniation into the base of the umbilical cord), and gastroschisis (a defect of the abdominal wall).

The **umbilical cord** may also be observed and inspected while the abdomen is being palpated. The diameter of the cord varies, depending on the amount of Wharton's jelly present. **Two arteries and one vein are normally present in the umbilical cord.** The umbilical cord begins to dry soon after birth, becomes loose from the skin by 4 to 5 days, and falls off by 7 to 10 days. Redness/umbilical erythema, foul odor, or wetness/oozing of the cord may indicate omphalitis. Persistent drainage may indicate a patent urachus, umbilical fistula, or cysts.

INSPECTION

Head and Neck. **The head and neck of a newborn make up 25% of the total body surface.** The head is usually 2 cm larger than a newborn's chest. Normal head circumference ranges between 32 and 38 cm for a FAGA infant. Note the size, shape, symmetry, and general appearance.

Microcephaly is characterized by a small head size in proportion to body size. **Craniosynostosis** is a small head size caused by early closure of sutures. **Hydrocephalus** is a condition in which an increase in cerebrospinal fluid creates an abnormally large and growing head.

Eyes. **Inspection of an infant's eyes is best accomplished when the infant is found in the quiet alert state or when the infant has been aroused to wakefulness during the examination.** The eyes cannot be observed while the baby is crying. Tipping the baby backward and raising him or her slowly or shading the infant's eyes from bright light often causes the eyes to open.

The newborn's eyes open spontaneously, look toward a light source, fix, focus, and follow. Uncoordinated eye movements are common. Subconjunctival or scleral hemorrhages are a common result of the pressures of labor and birth. The size, shape, and structure of the eye should be noted.

The **pupils** of the normal newborn respond to light by constricting. **Red reflex** is normally present and indicates an intact lens. Tears are not normally produced until 2 months of age. The iris is usually dark blue until 3 to 6 months of age. Doll's eye maneuvers are normally associated with eyes that follow movement of the head, often with a lag and/or nystagmus.

Discharge from the eyes may represent irritation or infection. A lateral upward slope of the eyes with an epicanthal fold may indicate syndromes of mental, physical, or chromosomal aberrations. The **absence of red reflex** may indicate tumors or congenital cataracts accompanying rubella, galactosemia, or disorders of calcium metabolism. **Chorioretinitis** is often found in congenital viral diseases such as cytomegalovirus and toxoplasmosis. White speckles on the iris known as ***Brushfield's spots*** are associated with Down syndrome and developmental delay or are a normal variant. **Scleral blueness** is associated with osteogenesis imperfecta and scleral yellowness with jaundice. Brain injury may be indicated by a constricted pupil, unilaterally dilated fixed pupil, nystagmus, or strabismus.

Blood Pressure. Blood pressure (BP) with non**invasive Doppler devices is best determined (1) by using the appropriate-size cuff for upper and lower extremities (e.g., using the same size cuff for the leg pressure that was used for the arm pressure results in a falsely elevated leg pressure), (2) by obtaining the measurement when the infant is asleep or before the infant is upset, and (3) by using the mean BP to monitor changes.[23] Blood pressure increases in the first 24 hours of life,** is higher in more mature infants (e.g., birth weight and gestational age) and in newborns whose mothers smoke,[44] and increases with increasing postnatal age.[22] Although blood pressure screening is not specifically recommended by the American Academy of Pediatrics (AAP),[3] we recommend it. **The blood pressure should be checked in all four extremities to screen for coarctation of the aorta. Because the blood pressure proximal to the area**

of obstruction is higher than the blood pressure distal to the area of obstruction, blood pressure in the upper extremities is higher (more than 15 mm Hg higher) than in the lower extremities (Figures 5-12 and 5-13).

The only study to evaluate the efficacy of upper and lower extremity blood pressure variations was recently conducted on 40 healthy neonates.[23] This study showed that with the current Doppler devices, normal neonates may have a wide variation in blood pressures between limbs. The researchers concluded that a difference of 20 mm Hg is more likely due to random variability than to coarctation and recommended that if weak/absent pulses are present and coarctation is suspected, an echocardiogram is necessary.[23]

Head-to-Toe Examination. **The infant's crying will not affect the data to be gathered in the head-to-toe examination.**

Skin. **As each body part is examined, the skin is also inspected. Vernix,** a white, cheeselike material that contains quantities of α-tocopherol and surfactant proteins that provide significant protection from infection, normally covers the body of the fetus and decreases with increased gestational age. Discoloration of the vernix occurs with intrauterine distress, postmaturity, hemolytic disease, and breech presentations.

The color of the skin is normally pink. Mongolian spots caused by the presence of pigmented cells may cover the sacral-gluteal areas of infants of color (e.g., black, Hispanic, Asian). The degree of generalized pigmentation varies and is less intense in the newborn period than later in life. **Nevus flammeus** may be present at the nape of the neck or on the eyelids.

Note the size, shape, color, and degree of ecchymosis, erythema, petechiae, or hemangiomas. Meconium staining, which occurs in 10% to 20% of newborns, is indicative of prior fetal distress. Erythema toxicum appears as a generalized red rash in the first 3 days of life. **Milia** caused by retained sebum are pinpoint white spots on the cheeks, chin, and bridge of the nose.

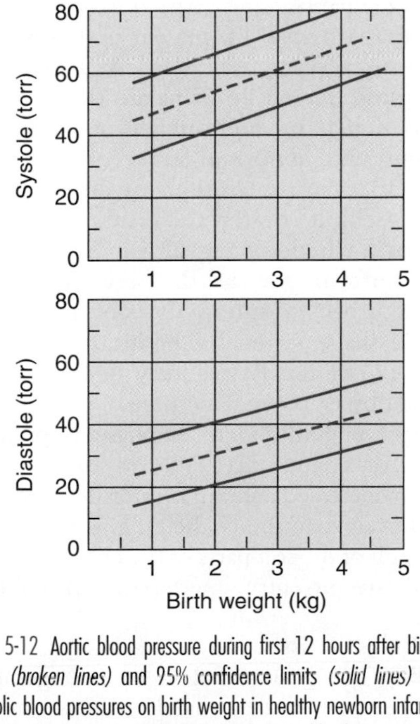

FIGURE 5-12 Aortic blood pressure during first 12 hours after birth. Linear regression *(broken lines)* and 95% confidence limits *(solid lines)* of systolic and diastolic blood pressures on birth weight in healthy newborn infants. (From Versmold HT, Kitterman JA, Phibbs RH, et al: Aortic blood pressure during the first 12 hours of life in infants with birth weight 610 to 4220 grams. *Pediatrics* 67:607, 1981.)

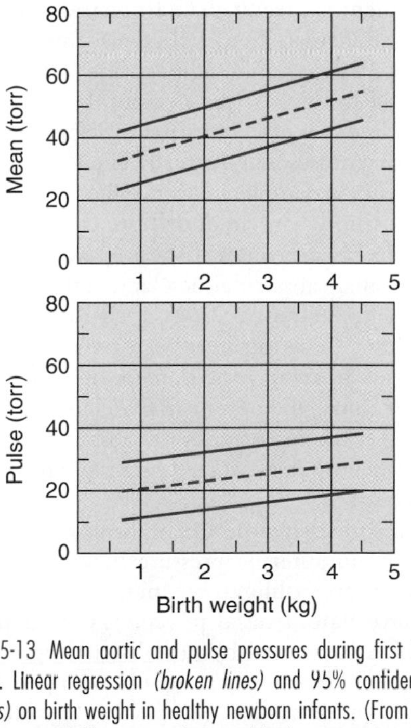

FIGURE 5-13 Mean aortic and pulse pressures during first 12 hours after birth. Linear regression *(broken lines)* and 95% confidence limits *(solid lines)* on birth weight in healthy newborn infants. (From Versmold HT, Kitterman JA, Phibbs RH, et al: Aortic blood pressure during the first 12 hours of life in infants with birth weight 610 to 4220 grams. *Pediatrics* 67:607, 1981.)

The normal texture of a neonate's skin is soft. A preterm infant's skin is more translucent than a term infant's skin. Slight desquamation may occur as skin becomes dry. Moderate to severe desquamation occurs in postterm infants with IUGR. Puffy, shiny skin is symptomatic of edema. Localized edema of a presenting part is caused by trauma and is only temporary. Edema should be distinguished from increased subcutaneous fat. Lanugo coverage decreases with increasing gestational age.

Tissue turgor is the sensation of fullness derived from the presence of hydrated subcutaneous tissue and intrauterine nutrition. Test the elasticity of the skin by grasping a fold of skin between the thumb and forefinger. When released, the skin should promptly spring back to the surface of the body. A loss of normal skin turgor resulting in peaking of the skin is a late sign of dehydration. A generalized hardness of the skin is a sign of sclerema that occurs in debilitated, stressed infants.

Ears. Cartilage development and ear form progress according to gestational age. Observe the external ears for size, shape, and position. The angle of placement of the ears is almost vertical. If the angle of placement is greater than 10 degrees from vertical, it is abnormal. The level of placement is determined by drawing an imaginary line from the outer canthus of the eye to the occiput. If the ear intersects the line, it is placed normally. Slapping hands or other sharp noises will normally elicit a twitching in the eyelid or a complete Moro reflex.

Malformed or malpositioned (low-set or rotated) ears are often associated with renal and chromosomal abnormalities and other congenital anomalies. Abnormalities such as skin tags or sinuses may be associated with renal tract abnormalities or hearing loss. Forceps or difficult deliveries may injure the outer ear. Congenital deafness is suspected if the infant does not respond to noise. It is confirmed by standardized hearing screening tests and follow-up.

Nose. Note the shape and size of the nose. Deformities caused by intrauterine pressure may be temporary. Neonates are obligatory nasal breathers and must have patent nasal passages. Check the patency of the alae nasi by (1) obstructing one nostril, closing the mouth, and observing breathing from the open nostril, (2) placing a stethoscope under the nostrils that will "fog" the diaphragm and auscultate breathing, or (3) passing a soft catheter (if necessary).

Abnormal configuration may be associated with congenital syndromes. Obstructions can be caused by drugs, infections, tumors, nasal discharge, nasal cysts, and mucus. Choanal atresia, a membranous or bony obstruction in the nasal passage, may be unilateral or bilateral. Choanal atresia is characterized by the noisy breathing, cyanosis, and apnea of the quiet infant (mouth closed) as opposed to the pink color of the same crying infant (mouth open).

Mouth. The mouth may be examined here or at the end of the examination when the infant is crying loudly with a wide-open mouth. At birth, a normal infant can suck and swallow (this ability develops at 32 to 34 weeks' gestation) and root and gag (this ability develops at 36 weeks' gestation). Elicit each.

Lips and mucous membranes are normally pink. Observe the lips and mucous membranes for pallor and cyanosis. If the infant is well hydrated, the membranes should be moist. Open the mouth to look for anomalies. Palpate the hard and soft palates for a membranous cleft or submucous cleft. Epithelial pearls are common along the gum margins and the palate.

Natal teeth may be present and may require removal to prevent aspiration. A large tongue (macroglossia), cleft lip or palate (including submucous cleft), or high-arched palate may be associated with abnormal facies or be an isolated finding. If copious secretions or distress in feeding is present, it is often the result of esophageal atresia or tracheoesophageal fistula.

Thorax. Conformation of the newborn chest is cylindric with an anteroposterior ratio of 1:1. Note the shape, symmetry, position, and development of the thorax. Asymmetry of the chest may be caused by diaphragmatic hernia, paralysis of the diaphragm, pneumothorax, emphysema, pulmonary agenesis, or pneumonia. Fullness of the thorax caused by increased anteroposterior diameter occurs with an overexpansion of the lung. Retractions, an inward pull of the soft parts of the chest while inhaling, indicate air-entry interference or pulmonary disease.

Breasts. Breast tissue systematically develops according to gestational age. Enlargement of breasts because of maternal hormones occurs in either sex on the second or third day. Milky secretions may be present. Unilateral redness or firmness indicates infection.

Clavicles. **Observe and palpate the area above each clavicle. A fracture of the clavicle is evidenced by a palpable mass, crepitation, tenderness at the fracture site, and limited arm movements on the affected side.**

Genitalia. Male and female genitalia systematically develop according to gestational age. **Ambiguous genitalia** result from incomplete or altered differentiation and require urology consultation.

Male Genitalia. **Inspect the genitalia for the presence and position of the urethral opening.** Palpate the testes either in the inguinal canal or scrotum. The scrotum appears large and pendulous with the presence of descended testes. A tight prepuce may be found. In dark-skinned races, darker pigmentation of the genitalia is normal. **Hypospadias** exists if the urethral opening is on the ventral surface of the penis. **Epispadias** exists if the opening is on the dorsal surface. Inguinal or scrotal swelling, discoloration, palpable masses, and pain/tenderness with palpation may be an **inguinal hernia, testicular torsion, trauma, tumor,** or **hydrocele**—a collection of fluid in the scrotal sac.

Female Genitalia. **Inspect the genitalia for the presence and position of the urethral opening.** The introitus is posterior to the clitoris. A vaginal skin tag is a visible hymenal ring.

Edema of the genitalia in both sexes is common in breech deliveries. Note the presence of a hydrocele or hernia. Fecal urethral discharge may indicate **rectourethral fistulas.**

Rectum. **Visualize and check the patency of the anal opening by waiting for meconium passage (it is optional to check patency by gently inserting a soft rubber catheter; do not use rigid objects such as glass rectal thermometers).** Observe the anatomy, and feel the muscle tone. Meconium is normally present during the first days of life.

Imperforate anus, irritation, or fissures may be present. Meconium passage before birth suggests fetal intrauterine distress. Failure to pass meconium within 48 hours suggests obstruction. **Meconium ileus** is associated with cystic fibrosis.

Back. Place the infant in a prone position and observe for a flat and straight **vertebral column.** Separate the buttocks to observe the coccygeal area. To check incurving reflex, stroke one side of the vertebral column. The baby will turn the buttocks toward the side stroked. **Deviations from normal include curvature of the vertebral column, pilonidal dimple, pilonidal sinus, spina bifida, or myelomeningocele.** A study of spinal congenital dermal sinuses found an increased incidence (>50%) of neurologic deficit, intradural tumors, or tethered cords; recommendations included a prompt radiologic evaluation and neurosurgical consult so that timely intervention could preserve or improve neurologic function.[1]

Extremities

Upper Extremities. **Note the size, shape, and symmetry of the arms and hands.** Observe and feel for fractures, paralysis, and dislocations. Count and inspect the fingers. The hands are normally clenched into fists. The infant is capable of adduction, flexion, internal rotation, extension, and symmetry of movement. Note the tone of the muscles. Flexion develops with increasing gestational age.

Simian creases may indicate chromosomal abnormalities that are frequent causes of deformity. **Polydactyly and syndactyly** of the fingers may be found. **Osteogenesis imperfecta** is characterized by multiple fractures and deformities. **Palsies** caused by fractures, dislocations, or injury to the brachial plexus are recognized by limited movement of the extremity. **Fractures** may also be present with edema, palpable crepitus, or the "palpable spongy mass sign" over the clavicle.

Lower Extremities. **Note the size, shape, and symmetry of the feet and legs.** Note the normal position of flexion (develops according to gestational age) and abduction. Note symmetry of movement, thigh folds, and gluteal folds. A full range of motion is possible, including the "frog position"—a rotation of the thighs with the knees flexed. Observe and feel for fractures, paralysis, and dislocations. Palpate femoral pulses.

Polydactyly and syndactyly of the toes may exist. **Osteogenesis imperfecta,** a rare genetic defect of collagen production that results in brittle bones, manifests as multiple fractures and deformities. Paralysis of both legs is caused by severe trauma or congenital anomaly of the spinal cord. Unilateral or bilateral **developmental dysplasia of the hip (e.g., congenital dislocated hip),** which is more common in females and breech presentations, causes a hip clunk when the baby's legs are abducted into the frog position. Although soft clicks are common, a sharp click indicates dislocation. Fractures may be present and are characterized by limited movement and edematous, crepitant areas. Chromosomal abnormalities are frequent causes of deformity.

Recoil is a test of flexion development and muscle tone. Recoil systematically develops as flexion develops in the lower extremities first and then in the upper extremities. Extend the legs and then release. Both legs should return promptly to the flexed position in accordance with the gestational age of the infant. Extend the arms alongside the body. On release, prompt flexion should occur at the elbows.

Hypotonia causes the infant to become limp and "floppy," with little control. The extremities fall without resistance when the infant is raised off the bed. Recoil may be partial or absent. Causes of hypotonia include neuromuscular disorders, CNS dysfunction, sepsis, and congenital disorders. **Hypertonia** causes the infant to tremble and startle easily. The fists are tightly clenched, arms flexed, and legs stiffly extended.

NEUROLOGIC EXAMINATION

Clinical, electric, and anatomic studies of the nervous systems of premature and full-term neonates have confirmed the belief that the CNS of the human fetus matures at a fairly constant rate. Neurologic findings, clinical signs, and electroencephalogram (EEG) findings specifically correlating to gestational age have been established.[26,54] However, there are recognized limitations in clinical applications of the neurologic evaluation. **The evaluation is of little value in the first 24 hours of life unless there is an obvious palsy or seizure.** Because a newborn is recovering from the stress of birth, the neurologic examination is not valid until after the infant has successfully completed the transition to extrauterine life. Therefore the neurologic examination should be performed after the first 24 hours of life (see Figure 5-3). If the infant is ill or has obstetric anesthesia or analgesia, the neurologic examination may not be valid even after 24 hours.

BRAZELTON EXAMINATION

The Neonatal Behavioral Assessment Scale[12] assesses the interactive behavior of the newborn. This psychologic scale for the neonate enables assessment of the infant's individual capabilities for social relationships. Clinical application of the Brazelton scale includes neonatal research and evaluation of infant capabilities after illness, prematurity, or maternal medications. **A modified version of the Brazelton examination is useful in teaching parents about their individual infant's patterns of behavior, temperament, and states.**

By understanding the uniqueness of their infant, parents may more intelligently assess and interpret their baby's cues for interaction and distance. If the parents know their infant's individual strengths and weaknesses, they will be more capable of realistically reacting to him or her. It is important for the care provider to elicit the parents' assessment of their infant's behavior and responsiveness. Unrealistic expectations or incorrect parental perceptions may exist. The care provider therefore uses this opportunity for parent teaching, counseling, and possibly referral.

The Brazelton examination is usually performed at 2 to 3 days of life, at discharge, or on the follow-up visit at 1 to 2 weeks. This examination assesses the infant's best performance in response to stimulation and handling by the examiner. For research purposes, the scoring technique by a certified examiner is required. For clinical use, knowledge of the specific techniques and interpretation of results is all that is required. Because the state of consciousness influences a newborn's reactions, the most important variable in the examiner's observation is knowledge of the infant's state (see Chapter 13, Critical Findings: Newborn States and Considerations for Caregiving on p. 276). **Performing the examination with the parents present provides the opportunity for parental participation and observation of their infant's response.**

Maternal use of antidepressants and smoking have recently been shown to alter the newborn's neurobehavioral examination. Neonates exposed to selective serotonin reuptake inhibitors (SSRIs) late in pregnancy exhibit the following mild and spontaneously resolving behaviors[73,76]:

- Tremors/tremulousness
- Restlessness/irritability
- Abnormal crying
- Rigidity
- Fewer state changes
- More active sleep with startles and arousal

A recent retrospective, cohort study of term and preterm infants exposed to SSRIs in the last trimester of pregnancy found behavioral manifestations (in the first 3 days of life; resolving by 3-5 days) of exposure in all preterm and 69.1% of term infants, as well as a 4 times longer length of stay in the exposed preterms.[38]

CARE OF THE WELL NEWBORN INFANT

Mother-Infant Bonding and Interventions

FREQUENCY OF ASSESSMENTS

During the transitional period, vital signs should be recorded frequently enough to monitor the infant's condition and provide appropriate care:

- If the infant is distressed (elevated heart rate or respiratory rate, retracting and/or nasal flaring), vital signs may be required every ½ to 1 hour.
- If the baby's vital signs are normal on admission (heart rate 120 to 160 beats/min, respiratory rate 30 to 60 breaths/min, and temperature 36° to 36.5° C [96.8° to 97.7° F]), he or she should be monitored and the data charted every 30 minutes until the infant's condition has remained stable for 2 hours.
- Vital signs should be recorded at least once every 8 hours.
- Measuring the temperature rectally is ***contraindicated*** in newborn infants because of the risk for rectal perforation (see Chapter 6).

Weight, length, and head circumference should be graphed on the appropriate intrauterine growth chart to show at which percentile the baby falls. The parameters should be set at less than 10%, between 10% and 90%, and greater than 90%. **Determine the weight/length ratio (Figure 5-14), which normally increases with fetal age because the fetus becomes heavier for length as term approaches.** In intrauterine growth retardation, the weight/length ratio decreases because the rate of growth in weight is affected more than length. Severe and prolonged intrauterine malnutrition may affect head, weight, and length ratios.

PREVENTIVE PRACTICES

Determination of the infant's gestational age provides a reference point for individualizing care. Whether the infant is term and admitted to the normal newborn nursery or preterm and admitted to the intensive care nursery, attention to care practices that support development and neurologic integrity is essential in preventing iatrogenic disruptions or injury.

In utero, the fetus depends on the mother's physiologic systems to automatically regulate its own. At birth, the neonate's basic physiologic needs (feeding, elimination, heat balance, communication) are met in new and different ways. Emerging from physiologic dependence into a physiologically independent neonatal state introduces new variables for both mother and baby in the development of their extrauterine relationship. **For both term and preterm newborns, the primary developmental task is to reestablish biorhythmic balance by (1) establishing homeostasis through self-regulation of states (e.g., arousal and sleep/wake cycles), (2) processing, storing, and organizing internal and external stimuli, and (3) establishing a reciprocal relationship with primary care providers and the environment.**

Although biorhythmic balance is internally determined, caregiving interaction between newborn and parent or caregiver either facilitates or disturbs this transition. After birth, balance is facilitated by contact with familiar surroundings (the mother's body).[13,32] The mother's sensorimotor (auditory, tactile, visual), thermal, and nutrient stimuli provide regulatory effects on the infant's behavior (activity level, sucking, sleep and wake cycles, stress management, and circadian rhythms) and physiology (endocrine secretion, oxygen consumption, and cardiovascular status).[13,32] **Full-term newborns placed on the mother's chest immediately -after delivery display the following stereotypic innate sequence of prefeeding behavior[89]:**

- No sucking activity in the first 15 minutes
- Rooting and sucking activity begins and reaches maximum intensity at 45 minutes
- First hand-to-mouth movement at 35 minutes
- Spontaneous and unassisted finding of nipple and initiation of breast feeding at about 55 minutes of age

Within the first 90 minutes after birth, neonates cared for in close body contact with the mother are quiet.[20] However, infants separated from their mothers during this period and cared for in a crib cry and exhibit a "separation distress call" (also seen in several other mammalian species) that ceases at reunion.[20]

Certain care practices (e.g., separation of the mother and infant, gastric suction, noise levels in the newborn nursery) **that have become "routine" in maternal/child care are (1) based on few scientific foundations, (2) disrupt maternal and infant regulation and establishment of innate behaviors,**

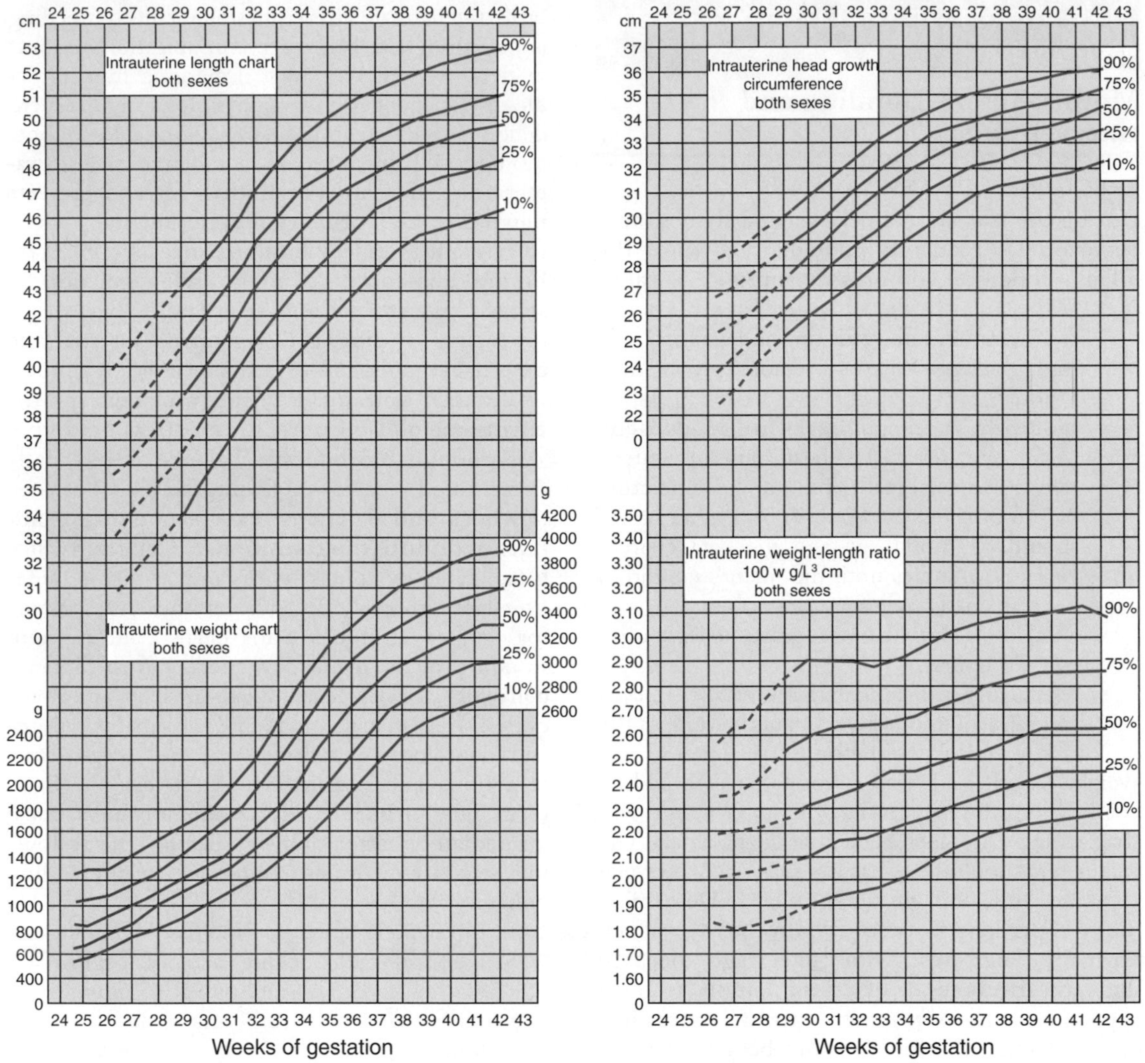

FIGURE 5-14 Colorado intrauterine growth charts. (From Lubchenco LO, Hansman C, Boyd E, et al: Intrauterine growth in length and head circumference as estimated from live births at gestational ages from 26-43 weeks, *Pediatrics* 37:403, 1966.)

(3) may have hidden consequences that surpass human adaptability, and (4) may contribute to behavioral deviations that result from violations of an innate agenda.[53,66,68] For example, gastric suction after birth evokes aversive reflexes (e.g., retching, combative movements, increased mean arterial blood pressure, and varied heart rate, including bradycardia), disrupts development of early feeding behaviors, is unpleasant, and has no advantages in a healthy term infant after normal pregnancy, vaginal delivery, and clear amniotic fluid.[5,89] Use of maternal analgesia may interfere with the newborn's spontaneous breast-seeking and breast-feeding behavior.

During transition of a term neonate, prone position has been shown to improve oxygenation, decrease heart and respiratory rates, and encourage more favorable behavioral states.[80] In the newborn nursery, the lack of diurnal rhythm in noise levels and care-providing activities disrupts reestablishment of biorhythmic balance, sleep and wake cycles, and state lability. **Significant differences in nighttime sleep and wake patterns exist between newborns cared for in the nursery (exposed to more light, noise, crying, and noncontingent care) and newborns rooming with the mother (more quiet sleep and less crying).**[52] In another study, 20 white, term infants exposed to soothing music in the newborn nursery spent less time in high arousal states (i.e., nonalert waking and crying) and had fewer behavioral state changes.[50]

For full-term babies who must have heelstick blood work, heartbeat sounds and white noise (at 85 dB) have been shown to have a calming effect, as measured by less-pronounced behavioral responses and reduced adrenocortical release.[51] **Placing full-term babies skin-to-skin in whole-body contact with their mothers or breast feeding during heelstick procedures reduces heart rate, crying (by 91%), and grimacing (by 84%).**[14,45] **Healthy preterm infants (e.g., 32-36 weeks postmenstrual age) receiving heel sticks experienced diminished pain response when held skin-to-skin by their mothers for 30 minutes before and after the procedure.**[49] **The proximity and caregiving of the mother provide the term and preterm infants with a barrier against outside stimulation and an ability to increase their threshold to noxious stimuli.**[32]

If adaptation to extrauterine life of full-term neonates is influenced either positively or negatively by nursery care practices, **adaptation of preterm or sick neonates may be even more influenced by early care and handling.** Use of stress-reduction techniques to prevent fluctuations in blood pressure, vital signs, and oxygenation often is not initiated until after the preterm infant has been admitted and stabilized in the neonatal intensive care unit (NICU). **Individualized developmental care (e.g., dimmed lights, decreased noise, gentle handling, contingent stimuli) (see Chapter 13) may be delayed in the urgency of expeditious assessment, diagnosis, and life-supporting interventions by care providers in the delivery room and on admission to the nursery.** However, the physiologic, anatomic, and psychologic transition to extrauterine life makes neonates, especially preterm or sick neonates, extremely vulnerable to the stress of resuscitation and initial nursery care.

Minimizing stress and conserving energy should accompany establishing and maintaining an airway, adequate oxygenation and ventilation, and circulatory support. An immature preterm infant (under 32 weeks' gestation) (see Chapter 13) who is physiologically unstable may deteriorate if not handled gently and protected from overstimulation. **Rapid fluctuations in oxygenation and blood pressure, overwhelming stimuli, too-rapid volume expansion, suction, unrelieved pain, and hypothermia contribute to the incidence of intraventricular hemorrhage that occurs most commonly in the first 24 hours after birth (see Chapters 4, 6, 7, 12, 23, and 26). In preterm infants, "routine" procedures such as bathing result in increased heart rate and blood pressure, motor stress behaviors, changes in stability and reorganizational behavior, hypoxia, and increased intracranial pressure (see Chapter 13).** Overwhelmed by external stimuli, a neonate's global response to stress may be apnea and bradycardia.

Based on the infant's ability to tolerate an intervention and the benefits of early assessment and intervention, the admission process should be prioritized to (1) provide life-supportive care, (2) conserve energy, and (3) collect data and complete the health care record. Table 5-6 outlines developmental interventions for neonatal admissions and initial nursery care that decrease stress, reduce energy consumption, improve oxygenation and respiratory and heart rates, and prevent iatrogenic stress and injury. **Developmentally supportive care should begin immediately after birth.**

KANGAROO CARE

Skin-to-skin "kangaroo" care (KC) benefits both parents and neonates (see Box 13-2). For the neonate, KC improves self-regulation, reduces stress and crying, facilitates breast feeding, reduces pain, and facilitates neurodevelopment, maturation, and later mental health outcomes.* For the mother, KC helps reverse the negative effects of preterm birth and separation; it also increases maternal oxytocin levels, which enhances both early and long-term maternal-infant interactions.[32,34,35,75]

A randomized controlled trial of KC in healthy term newborns immediately after birth (i.e., initiated within the first 15-20 minutes of life; duration

*References 13, 32-34, 36, 56, 68, 70.

TABLE 5-6 DEVELOPMENTAL INTERVENTIONS DURING ADMISSION AND INITIAL NURSERY CARE

Oxygenation	Apply noninvasive monitor (see Chapter 7) Titrate F_{IO_2} to maintain saturation at 92% to 94% (see Chapters 7 and 8) Handle gently, minimally (see Chapters 13 and 23) Kangaroo care improves gaseous exchange, especially in preterm infants <1000 g[39] Position prone to maximize oxygenation (see Chapter 13 and below) Delay or defer bathing[78] (see Chapter 19)
Thermoregulation	Maintain temperature axillary (36.5° to 37.5° C in term infants); skin (36° to 36.5° C in preterm infants) (see Chapter 6) Skin-to-skin contact (kangaroo care) provided by mothers or fathers to preterm/term newborns warms better than incubator care[19] Prewarm linen, scales, radiant warmer; incubator (see Chapter 6) Decrease heat loss with position (i.e., prone, flexion) (see Chapters 6 and 13) Use warm water on skin before applying probe, electrodes (see Chapter 19) Delay or defer bathing[78] (see Chapter 19)—healthy term infants with axillary temperature >36.8° C can be bathed after 1 hour of age when appropriate care is taken to support thermal stability.[85] Offer parents opportunity to bathe baby[9,67] (see Chapters 6 and 13)
Nutrition	Screen at-risk and symptomatic infants for hypoglycemia (see Chapter 15) Provide fluids and/or calories (orally or intravenously) (see Chapters 14 through 17) Decrease energy expenditures by decreasing internal (i.e., hypothermia, hypoxia) and external (i.e., noise, light) stressors (see Chapters 13 and 15)
Pain	Minimize painful stimuli (see Chapters 12 and 13) Relieve pain with pharmacologic management (see Chapter 12) Provide comfort measures (e.g., pacifier, containment, grasping) (see Chapters 12 and 13) Use venipuncture rather than heelstick (see Chapter 12) Use kangaroo care or breast feeding during painful procedures[14,45,49]
Environmental stimuli	Tactile: (see Chapter 13) Handle gently and minimally Support and contain in flexion Provide rest periods between procedures, handling Visual: (see Chapter 13) Shield from bright, direct light Dim lights as soon as possible Cover oxygen hood, face with wash cloth Cover incubator with blanket or cover Auditory: (see Chapter 13) Talk quietly Respond quickly to alarms Parents to softly talk to infant Keep ill neonates away from crying babies[52]
Position	Promote flexion in side-lying position with blankets, rolls (see Chapter 13) Prone (oxygenation better; less apnea; quiet, more restful sleep; decreased caloric expenditure; decreased reflux)[80] (see Chapter 13) Swaddle (see Chapter 13) Avoid supine if newborn is hypoxic and has an oxygen requirement; otherwise, always position all well, term newborns supine (see Chapter 13)

TABLE 5-6 DEVELOPMENTAL INTERVENTIONS DURING ADMISSION AND INITIAL NURSERY CARE—cont'd

Assess and interpret newborn cries	Assess avoidance and approach behaviors so that care is individualized (see Chapter 13) Support infant strengths and adaptive and coping behaviors (see Chapter 13) Modulate environmental and caregiver stimuli based on infant cues (contingent on cues rather than noncontingent stimuli and interaction) (see Chapter 13) Teach parents infant cues (see Chapter 13)

for 1 hour) showed a significant difference from the control group (i.e., brought to the nursery in the first 15-20 minutes of life). The newborns in the KC trial demonstrated the following, as compared with the control group[37,86]:

- State organization (e.g., longer sleep period, more quiet sleep)
- Motor system modulation (e.g., more flexor and fewer extensor postures/movements)
- Stable skin temperature and blood glucose level

A randomized controlled trial (RCT) of healthy preterms (33-35 weeks' gestation) found that KC for 3 hours improved breathing patterns and resulted in no apnea, bradycardia, or periodic breathing or temperature instability.[62] A recent meta-analysis of 30 RCTs showed that early skin-to-skin contact between mothers and their infants results in the following significant benefits[71]:

- Better breast feeding
- More affectionate maternal behaviors
- Less infant crying
- Better cardiorespiratory stability

Kangaroo care not only prevents hypothermia but also is effective in treating hypothermia. KC warms healthy, low-risk, hypothermic preterm infants better (90%) than does incubator care (60%).[19] In studies of fathers providing KC after cesarean section (compared with babies in cribs/incubators), outcomes included the following[30]:

- Their full-term newborns had significant increase in the axillary temperature and blood glucose levels.
- The newborns cried less and were calmer.
- The newborns reached a drowsy state earlier.
- The fathers were able to facilitate their infant's prefeeding behavior.
- The fathers should be the primary caregivers during separation of the mother and baby.

Because of this research evidence, both the AAP[5] and the Centers for Disease Control and Prevention (CDC) recommend use of skin-to-skin (kangaroo care) for the term newborn after birth. The AAP recommends that full-term neonates should immediately be placed into kangaroo care after birth and remain there until after the first breast feeding.[5] The CDC[81] recommends that the full-term newborn remain in KC throughout the postpartum period as a strategy to facilitate breast feeding.

SURVEILLANCE FOR POTENTIAL COMPLICATIONS

Complications of common morbidities (see Figure 5-11) are prevented by classification, assessment, and screening of all newborns at birth. Preterm SGA/IUGR infants have more gross motor and neurologic dysfunction but less cerebral palsy (CP) than AGA infants do. SGA infants are at increased risk for mortality and cognitive disorders needing special education when compared with AGA infants. Complications of the morbidities listed in Figure 5-11 are thoroughly discussed in the appropriate chapters.

PARENT TEACHING

Transitional care, neonatal assessment, and initial care need not take place in a nursery in which the newborn and family are isolated from each other. Alternative settings for initial care include birthing rooms, recovery rooms in which family and baby are kept together, the mother's postpartum room, or at a home visit. **In fact, keeping the family together not only facilitates bonding but also provides unique opportunities for teaching parents about the uniqueness and individuality of their newborn.**[67,75] At this time, parents are most

Parent Teaching[3,29,40-42]

- Every encounter with the parents is a teaching opportunity, so that by the time of discharge, parents are totally competent to care for their infant. Assess each individual family's ability to care for their infant and readiness for discharge.
- Teach parents how to care for the newborn's skin, umbilicus, and circumcision site and the appropriate urination/stooling patterns for newborns.
- Teach parents about the nutritional needs of their newborn, how to breast/bottle feed, and burp their baby. Develop a feeding plan with the parents for the late-preterm infant, and teach parents how and why to adhere to the plan for a late-preterm infant.
- Teach parents how to take an axillary temperature on their newborn and maintain the axillary temperature between 36.5° and 37.4° C (97.7° and 99.3° F) with clothes, blankets and an appropriate environmental temperature.
- The presence and clinical significance of jaundice are determined before discharge (see Chapter 21), appropriate follow-up care has been determined, and the importance is stressed to parents. Parents are taught how to assess jaundice at home.
- Teach parents the importance of follow-up care, either at a clinic, physician's office, or home visit, within 24 to 48 hours after discharge for late-preterm infants.
- Give parents the newborn immunization record with documentation of what immunizations their infant has received and the importance of follow-up for childhood immunizations.

receptive to information about the baby, who is the center of attention.

The assessments of gestational age and physical condition are best performed with the mother and father in attendance so that deviations from normal such as caput, cleft lip, cleft palate, or clubfoot can be explained. Eliciting parental cooperation is important. For example, when the major concern is "Will the procedure hurt?" a response such as "It is routine" will not comfort and reassure well-informed, noninterventionist consumers. Rather, a more physiologically oriented explanation about the condition being screened, why their particular infant is at increased risk, and what interventions are available encourages parental cooperation.

Professional care providers are only temporary caregivers. It is the care providers' responsibility to help parents become confident, primary caregivers of their own infants. **Actively involving parents in the care and treatment of their newborn further solidifies their position as primary caregivers.**[67,75] Encouraging active parental involvement enhances the parents' self-esteem and confidence in their abilities[75]; thus the care providers' actions must tell the parents, "You are able to care for this baby." A recent RCT comparing the ability of parents to perform the baby's first bath in the mother's room versus a nurse bathing the baby in the admission nursery found no difference in temperature changes irrespective of who bathed the baby or where the bath was given.[67] The newborn heat loss experienced with bathing was significant and returned to normal in 1 hour. **Parents in the study wanted the opportunity to bathe their infants and gained confidence in their parenting skill/ability.** With the supervision of the nurse, ensuring an environment to reduce heat loss (e.g., warm, draft-free room, temperature assessment, warm water, use of kangaroo care after the bath) and using the bath as a teaching opportunity, parents can bathe their infants.

At discharge, performing the physical examination in the room with the parents offers a final opportunity to teach, counsel, and advise them before they take their new baby home. Information about feeding, cord care, bathing, elimination patterns, safety, signs of illness, medications, and the importance of follow-up care is essential for parents of a full-term, healthy newborn (see the Parent Teaching box above). It is also essential for parents taking home an infant after prolonged hospitalization. In addition, a modified version of the Brazelton examination on all neonates enables parents to become familiar with a newborn's competencies for reacting to and shaping his or her environment and with strategies for parental intervention. Developing written materials for parents about normal newborn care and documenting teaching sessions and return demonstrations ensure that no important information is forgotten. See Chapter 31 for discharge planning and teaching strategies.

Parent Teaching[3,29,40-42]—cont'd

- Teach parents appropriate safety precautions:
  - Verbal and written information about recognizing signs and symptoms of a "sick"/"ill" infant, how the infant acts, and whom to notify.[41]
  - Proper use of car seats including positioning with supports, facing the rear in the backseat, middle of rear seat preferably with an adult seated next to the preterm to enable ongoing observation of the infant during travel.
  - Proper positioning supine for sleep: "Back to Sleep." Model "Back to Sleep" by placing babies who are in cribs only on their backs to sleep. ***All*** care providers (e.g., parents, grandparents, day-care providers, babysitters) should sleep babies supine (see Chapter 13).
  - Importance of a smoke-free environment because second-hand smoke is associated with an increased risk for developing health problems.
  - ***Never*** shake the baby! Babies are shaken by frustrated caregivers when the infant continues to cry.[15] Dangers of shaking infants include blindness, brain damage, developmental delays, seizures, paralysis, and death. (See Resource Materials for Parents, p. 112.)
  - Information, in writing, about all medications for their infant including name, action, dose, route, side effects, schedule (see Chapter 10).
- Teach parents the importance of their own self-care: need for adequate sleep/rest, nutrition/hydration, privacy, stress management, recreation, and sex.

REFERENCES

1. Ackerman L, Menezes A: Spinal congenital dermal sinuses: a 30-year experience, *Pediatrics* 112:641, 2003.
2. Allen MC, Capute A: Tone and reflex development before term, *Pediatrics* 85(suppl):393, 1990.
3. American Academy of Pediatrics, and American College of Obstetricians and Gynecologists: *Guidelines for perinatal care*, ed 6, Washington, DC, 2007, The Academy.
4. American Academy of Pediatrics, Committee on Fetus and Newborn; American College of Obstetricians and Gynecologists, Committee on Obstetric Practice: The APGAR score, *Pediatrics* 117:1444, 2006.
5. American Academy of Pediatrics, Section on Breastfeeding: Breastfeeding and the use of human milk, *Pediatrics* 115:496, 2005.
6. Apgar V: A proposal for a new method of evaluation of the newborn infant, *Anesth Analg* 32:260, 1953.
7. Association of Women's Health, Obstetric and Neonatal Nurses: *Near-term infant initiative*, Washington DC, 2005, The Association.
8. Barrington K, Vallerand D, Usher R: Frequency of morbidities in near-term infants, *Pediatr Res* 55:372A, 2004.
9. Behring A, Vezeau T, Fink R: Timing of the newborn first bath: a replication, *Neonatal Netw* 22:39, 2002.
10. Bhutani V, Johnson L: Kernicterus in late preterm infants cared for as healthy infants, *Semin Perinatal* 30:89, 2006.
11. Blackmon L: The role of the hospital of birth on survival of extremely low birth weight, extremely preterm infants, *NeoReviews* 4:e147, 2003.
12. Brazelton TB: *Neonatal behavioral assessment scale*, ed 2, Philadelphia, 1984, JB Lippincott/Spastics International Medical Publishers.
13. Browne J: Early relationship environments: physiology of skin-to-skin contact for parents and their preterm infants, *Clin Perinatol* 31:287, 2004.
14. Carbajal R, Veerapen S, Couderc S, et al: Analgesic effect of breastfeeding in term infants: randomized trial, *Br Med J* 326:13, 2003.
15. Carbaugh S: Understanding shaken baby syndrome, *Adv Neonatal Care* 4:105, 2004.
16. Casey B, McIntire D, Leveno K: The continuing value of the Apgar score for assessment of newborn infants, *N Engl J Med* 344:467, 2001.
17. Centers for Disease Control and Prevention (CDC): Prevention of perinatal group B streptococcal disease: revised guidelines from CDC, *MMWR* 51(RR-11):1, 2002.
18. Chien L, Whyte R, Aziz K, et al: Improved outcome of preterm infants when delivered in tertiary care centers, *Obstet Gynecol* 98:247, 2001.
19. Christensson K, Bhat GJ, Amadi BC, et al: Randomized study of skin-to-skin versus incubator care for rewarming low-risk hypothermic neonates, *Lancet* 352:1115, 1998.
20. Christensson K, Cabrera T, Christensson E, et al: Separation distress call in the human neonate in the absence of maternal contact, *Acta Paediatr* 84:468, 1995.
21. Clayton PE, Cianfarani S, Czernichow P, et al: Management of the child born small for gestational age through to adulthood: a consensus statement of the International Societies of Pediatric Endocrinology and the Growth Hormone Research Society, *J Clin Endocrinol Metab* 92:804, 2007.
22. Cordero L, Giannone P, Rich J: Mean arterial blood pressure in very low birth weight (801-1500 g) concordant and disconcordant twins during the first day of life, *J Perinatol* 23:545, 2003.

23. Crossland D, Furness J, Abu-Harb M, et al: Variability of four limb blood pressures in normal neonates, *Arch Dis Child Fetal Neonatal Ed* 89:F325, 2004.
24. Davidoff MJ, Dias T, Damus K, et al: Changes in the gestational age distribution among US singleton births: impact on rates of late preterm birth, 1992 to 2002, *Semin Perinatol* 30:8, 2006.
25. Donovan EF, Tyson JE, Ehrenkranz RA, et al: Inaccuracy of Ballard scores before 28 weeks' gestation, *J Pediatr* 135:147, 1999.
26. Dubowitz L, Dubowitz V, Mercuri E: The neurologic assessment of the preterm and full-term newborn infant, *Clinics in Developmental Medicine,* No. 148, London, 1999, University Press.
27. Engle W: A recommendation for the definition of "late preterm" (near-term) and the birth weight-gestational age classification system, *Semin Perinatol* 30:2, 2006.
28. Engle W, Kominiarek M: Late preterm infants, early term infants, and timing of elective deliveries, *Clin Perinatol* 35:325, 2008.
29. Engle W, Tomashek KM, Wallman C, and the Committee on Fetus and Newborn: "Late-preterm" infants: a population at risk, *Pediatrics* 120:1390, 2007.
30. Erlandsson K, Dsilna A, Fagerberg I, et al: Skin-to-skin care with the father after cesarean birth and its effect on newborn crying and prefeeding behavior, *Birth* 34:105, 2007.
31. Escobar G, Clark R, Greene J: Short-term outcomes of infants born at 35 and 36 weeks gestation: we need to ask more questions, *Semin Perinatol* 30:28, 2006.
32. Feldman R: Mother-infant skin-to-skin contact (kangaroo care): theoretical, clinical and empirical aspects, *Infants Young Child* 17:145, 2004.
33. Feldman R, Eidelman A: Mother-infant skin-to-skin contact (kangaroo care) accelerates autonomic and neurobehavioral maturation in premature infants, *Dev Med Child Neurol* 45:274, 2003.
34. Feldman R, Eidelman A, Sirota L, et al: Comparison of skin-to-skin (kangaroo) and traditional care: parenting outcomes and preterm infant development, *Pediatrics* 110:16, 2002.
35. Feldman R, Weller A, Eidelman A, et al: Testing a family intervention hypothesis: the contribution of mother-infant skin-to-skin (kangaroo care) to family interaction and touch, *J Fam Psychol* 17:94, 2003.
36. Feldman R, Weller A, Sirota L, et al: Skin-to-skin (kangaroo care) promotes self regulation in premature infants: sleep-wake cyclicity, arousal modulation, and sustained exploration, *Dev Psychol* 38:194, 2002.
37. Ferber S, Makhoul I: The effect of skin-to-skin contact (kangaroo care) shortly after birth on the neurobehavioral responses of the term newborn: a randomized, controlled trial, *Pediatrics* 113:858, 2004.
38. Ferreira E, Carcellar AM, Agogue C, et al: Effects of selective serotonin reuptake inhibitors and venlafaxine during pregnancy in term and preterm neonates, *Pediatrics* 119:52, 2007.
39. Fohe K, Kropf S, Avenarius S: Skin-to-skin contact improves gas exchange in premature infants, *J Perinatol* 5:311, 2000.
40. Gardner SL: Late-preterm ("near-term") newborns: a neonatal nursing challenge, *Nurse Currents* 1:1, 2007. Accessed January 2009 from www.abbottnutritionlearningcenter.com.
41. Gardner SL, Brown VD: *Clinical Practice Tool: "Nursing process applied to the late preterm ("near-term") infants (34 0/7 to 36 6/7 weeks)"* ©NPDPA, 2007. Accessed January 2009 from www.npdpa.com.
42. Gardner SL, Brown VD: *Clinical Practice Tool: "How will I know if my baby is sick?"*, ©NPDPA, 2008. Accessed January 2009 from www.pdpa.com.
43. Reference deleted in proofs.
44. Geerts CC, Grobbee DE, van der Ent CK, et al: Tobacco smoke exposure of pregnant mothers and blood pressure in their newborns: results from the wheezing illnesses study Leidsche Rijn birth cohort, *Hypertension* 50:572, 2007.
45. Gray L, Watt L, Blass E: Skin-to-skin contact is analgesic in healthy newborns, *Pediatrics* 105:110, 2000.
46. Hansen AK, Wisborg K, Uldbjerg N, et al: Elective caesarean section and respiratory morbidity in the term and near-term neonate, *Acta Obstet Gynecol Scand* 86:389, 2007.
47. Hernandez JA, Thilo E: Routine care of the full-term newborn. In Osborn LC, DeWitt TG, First LR, et al: *Pediatrics*, St Louis, 2005, Mosby.
48. Institute of Medicine: *Preterm birth: causes, consequences, and prevention*, Washington, DC, 2006, National Academies Press.
49. Johnston C, Stevens B, Pinelli J, et al: Kangaroo care is effective in diminishing pain response in preterm neonates, *Arch Pediatr Adolesc Med* 157:1084, 2003.
50. Kaminski J, Hall W: The effect of soothing music on neonatal behavioral states in the hospital newborn nursery, *Neonatal Netw* 15:45, 1996.
51. Kawakami K, Takai-Kawakami K, Kurihara H, et al: The effect of sounds on newborn infants under stress, *Infant Behav Dev* 19:375, 1996.
52. Keefe M: Comparison of neonatal nighttime sleep-wake patterns in nursery vs. rooming-in environments, *Nurs Res* 36:114, 1987.
53. Kennell J, McGrath S: Commentary: what babies teach us—the essential link between baby's behavior and mother's biology, *Birth* 28:20, 2001.
54. Koeingsberger R: Judgment of fetal age. I. Neurologic evaluation, *Pediatr Clin North Am* 13:823, 1966.
55. Kumar M, Paes B: Epidural opioid analgesia and neonatal respiratory depression, *J Perinatol* 23:425, 2003.

56. Leckman J, Herman A: Maternal behavior and developmental psychopathology, *Biol Psychiatry* 51:27, 2002.
57. Lee S, McMillian D, Ohlsson A, et al: The benefit of preterm birth at tertiary care centers is related to gestational age, *Am J Obstet Gynecol* 188:617, 2003.
58. Leuthner S: Fetal palliative care, *Clin Perinatol* 31:649, 2004.
59. Lubchenco L: *The high-risk infant*, Philadelphia, 1976, Saunders.
60. Reference deleted in proofs.
61. Lubchenco LO, Searls DT, Brazie JV, et al: Neonatal mortality risk: relationship to birthweight and gestational age, *J Pediatr* 81:814, 1972.
62. Ludington-Hoe S, Anderson G, Swinth J, et al: Randomized controlled trial of kangaroo care: cardiorespiratory and thermal effects on healthy preterm infants, *Neonatal Netw* 23:39, 2004.
63. Ludington-Hoe S, Cong X, Hashemi F: Infant crying: nature, physiologic consequences, and select interventions, *Neonatal Netw* 21:29, 2002.
64. Madar J, Richmond S, Hey E: Surfactant-deficient respiratory distress after elective delivery at 'term', *Acta Paediatr* 88:1244, 1999.
65. Meberg A, Brugmann-Pieper S, Due R, et al: First day of life pulse oximetry screening to detect congenital heart defects, *J Pediatr* 152:761, 2008.
66. Medves J: Three infant care interventions: reconsidering the evidence, *J Obstet Gynecol Neonatal Nurs* 31:563, 2002.
67. Medves J, O'Brien B: The effect of bather and location of first bath on maintaining thermal stability in newborns, *J Obstet Gynecol Neonatal Nurs* 33:175, 2004.
68. Mercer JS, Erickson-Owens DA, Graves B, et al: Evidence-based practices for the fetal to newborn transition, *J Midwifery Womens Health* 52:262, 2007.
69. Minkoff H, Chervenak F: Elective primary cesarean delivery, *N Engl J Med* 348:946, 2003.
70. Moore ER, Anderson GC: Randomized controlled trial of very early mother-infant skin-to-skin contact and breastfeeding status, *J Midwifery Womens Health* 52:116, 2007.
71. Moore ER, Anderson GC, Berman N: Early skin-to-skin contact for mothers and their healthy infants, *Cochrane Database Syst Rev* Jul 18(3):2007 CD003519.
72. Morrison J, Rennie J, Milton P: Neonatal respiratory morbidity and mode of delivery at term: influence of timing of elective caesarean section, *British J Obstet Gynaecol* 102:101, 1995.
73. Moses-Kolko EL, Bogen D, Perel J, et al: Neonatal signs after late in utero exposure to serotonin reuptake inhibitors: literature review and implications for clinical applications, *JAMA* 293:2372, 2005.
74. National Institutes of Health (NIH), National Institute of Child Health and Human Development (NICHD): Workshop: *Optimizing care and long-term outcome of near-term pregnancy and near-term newborn infants*, July, 2005. Accessed July 2007 from www.nichd.nih.gov/.
75. Nelson A: Transition to motherhood, *J Obstet Gynecol Neonatal Nurs* 32:465, 2003.
76. Oberlander TF, Warburton W, Misri S, et al: Neonatal outcomes after prenatal exposure to selective serotonin reuptake inhibitor antidepressants and maternal depression using population-based linked health data, *Arch Gen Psychiatry* 63:898, 2006.
77. Pados B: Safe transition to home: preparing the near-term infant for discharge, *Neonatal Infant Nurs Rev* 7:106, 2007.
78. Peters K: Dinosaurs in the bath, *Neonatal Netw* 15:71, 1996.
79. Reich JD, Connolly B, Bradley G, et al: The reliability of a single pulse oximetry reading as a screening test for congenital heart disease in otherwise asymptomatic newborn infants, *Pediatr Cardiol* 29:371, 2008.
80. Schwartz R: Effect of position on oxygenation, heart rate, and behavioral state in the transitional newborn infant, *Neonatal Netw* 12:73, 1993.
81. Shealy KR, Li R, Benton-Davis S, et al: *The CDC guide to breastfeeding interventions*, Atlanta GA, 2005, US Department of Health and Human Services, Centers for Disease Control and Prevention. Accessed July 2008 from www.cdc.gov/breastfeeding.
82. Tita A, Landon M, Spong C, et al: Timing of elective cesarean delivery at term and neonatal outcomes, *N Engl J Med* 360:111, 2009.
83. Tomashek KM, Shapiro-Mendoza CK, Davidoff MJ, et al: Differences in mortality between late-preterm and term singleton infants in the United States, 1995-2002, *J Pediatr* 151:450, 2007.
84. Usher R, McLean F, Scott KE, et al: Judgment of fetal age. II. Clinical significance of gestational age and an objective method for its assessment, *Pediatr Clin North Am* 13:835, 1966.
85. Varda K, Behnke R: The effect of timing of initial bathing on newborns temperature, *J Obstet Gynecol Neonatal Nurs* 29:27, 2003.
86. Walters MW, Boggs KM, Ludington-Hoe SM, et al: Kangaroo care at birth for full term infants: a pilot study, *MCN Am J Matern Child Nurs* 32:375, 2007.
87. Wang M, Dorer D, Fleming M, et al: Clinical outcomes of near-term infants, *Pediatrics* 114:372, 2004.
88. Warner B, Musial M, Chenier T, et al: The effect of birth hospital on the outcome of very low birth weight infants, *Pediatrics* 113:35, 2004.
89. Widstrom A, Ransjo-Arvidson AB, Christensson K, et al: Gastric suction in healthy newborn infants: effects on circulation and developing feeding behavior, *Acta Paediatr Scand* 76:566, 1987.

90. Yorifuji J, Yorifuji T, Nagai S, et al: Craniotabes in normal newborns: the earliest sign of subclinical vitamin D deficiency, *J Clin Endocrinol Metab* 93:1784, 2008.
91. Zanardo V, Simbi A, Franzoi M, et al: Neonatal respiratory morbidity risk and mode of delivery at term: influence of timing of elective caesarean delivery, *Acta Paediatr* 93:643, 2004.

RESOURCE MATERIALS FOR PROFESSIONALS

Academy of Neonatal Nursing: *Physical exam of the newborn* (video): www.academyonline.org

Association of Women's Health: Obstetric and Neonatal Nurses (AWHONN): *Late-preterm (near-term) infant assessment guide and optimizing health for the preterm infant*, Washington, DC, 2007, The Association. Available at www.awhonn.org

Gardner SL: Late-preterm ("near-term") newborns: a neonatal nursing challenge, *Nurse Currents* 1:1, 2007. Available at www.abbottlearningcenter.com

Gardner SL: *Clinical practice tool: NO rectal temperatures in the neonate—evidence-based practice*, Nurse's Professional Development & Practice Association, LLC™, 2007. Available at www.npdpa.com

Gardner SL, Brown VD: *Clinical practice tool: Nursing process applied to the late preterm ("near-term") neonate (34 0/7 to 36 6/7 weeks)*, Nurse's Professional Development & Practice Association, LLC™, 2007. Available at www.npdpa.com

Gardner SL, Brown VD: *"Near-term" deliveries and "near-term" infants: when almost isn't quite good enough!!*, Nurse's Professional Development & Practice Association, LLC™, 2007. Available at www.npdpa.com.

Gardner SL, Brown VD: *How will I know if my baby is sick?* Nurse's Professional Development & Practice Association, LLC™, 2008. Available at www.npdpa.com.

Hernandez JA, Fashaw L, Evans R: Adaptation to extrauterine life and management during normal and abnormal transition. In Thureen PJ, Deacon J, Hernandez JA, et al, editors: *Assessment and care of the well newborn*, ed 2, Philadelphia, 2004, Saunders.

Hernandez JA, Glass SM: Physical assessment of the newborn. In Thureen PJ, Deacon J, Hernandez JA, et al, editors: *Assessment and care of the well newborn*, ed 2, Philadelphia, 2004, Saunders.

Karlsen K: *S.T.A.B.L.E Program: physical examination and gestational age assessment* (CDROM): www.stableprogram.org..

March of Dimes Continuing Education Nursing Modules at www.marchofdimes.com/nursing.
Assessment of risk in the term newborn
Cultural competence in the care of childbearing families
Understanding the behavior of term infants

March of Dimes: Prematurity Awareness Campaign, Available at www.marchofdimes.org.

Tappero E, Honeyfield M: *Physical assessment of the newborn*, ed 4, Santa Rosa, Calif, 2009, NICU Ink.

RESOURCE MATERIALS FOR PARENTS

American Academy of Pediatrics: Parent Education Materials
Care of the uncircumcised penis—Fact Sheet
Circumcision: information for parents
Diaper rash
Early arrival: Information for parents of premature infants
Infant sleep positioning and SIDS—Fact sheet

American Academy of Pediatrics Shelov S, editor: *Your baby's first year*, ed 2, Elk Grove Village, Ill, 2005, The Academy.

American Academy of Pediatrics, Shelov S, Hannemann R, editors: *Caring for your baby and young child: birth to age 5*, ed 4, Elk Grove Village, Ill, 2004, The Academy.

Brazelton TB: *Baby basics* (video) and *Home before you know it* (video), Cambridge, Mass, 2004, Vida Health Communications.

Gardner SL, Brown VD: *"How will I know if my baby is sick?"*©. Nurse's Professional Development & Practice Association, LLC™, 2008. Available at www.npdpa.com.

Newborn Channel: www.newborn.com.

6 HEAT BALANCE

VIVIAN D. BROWN AND SUSAN LANDERS

Optimal care of sick newborn and premature infants requires meticulous attention to detail. The consequences of overlooking some details may not be readily apparent, whereas other details may affect the very survival of the neonate. Such was the case late in the nineteenth century when French authorities sought to decrease infant mortality as one way to increase the population and provide the needed manpower to support industrialization and the armies of the expanding French empire. Dr. Stephane Tarnier, Chairman of Obstetrics of the University of Paris, was distressed with the plight of the "weaklings" and applied earlier concepts of incubators to the regular care of premature and sick infants, believing that maintaining thermal stability was a key factor for their survival.

The ***first incubator for neonates*** was introduced in 1835 by Von Ruehl in St. Petersburg, Russia, and in 1857, the incubator was described by Denunce as a double-walled box that circulated warmed water within the interspace.[2] The care of newborns was delegated to Madame Henry, Midwife-in-Chief, who oversaw the building of a pavilion specifically for the care of these weakling newborns.[20] This pavilion housed 12 incubators in which fragile newborns were warmed over a hot-water reservoir attached to an external source of heat. These were impressive first steps in attempting to control the fragile heat balance of weak preterm infants and contributed to the reported decreased mortality rate from 66% to 38% in babies with birth weights between 1200 and 2000 g. Dr. Tarnier's successor, Dr. Budin, continued this important early practice of neonatology, focusing on the home care of these high-risk babies. Alexandre Lion improved the design of incubators and charged spectators a fee to see them in action, which led to a very popular show at the Berlin Exposition of 1896. An associate of Lion, Martin Couney, brought the incubator shows to the United States, where Dr. Joseph DeLee adopted the technology and opened an "incubator station" in 1900 at the Chicago Lying-in Hospital. Nearly all of the large expositions in America hosted "Incubator Baby Side Shows." These began in 1898 with the Trans-Mississippi Exposition and continued on to the New York World's Fair in 1939.

Dr. Couney's display of incubators at Luna Park on Coney Island and at a second park named *Dreamland* hosted premature babies from New York hospitals that lacked the facilities to care for them. These infants were lined up under heaters in incubators, and they breathed filtered air. At least 8000 babies passed through these incubators, and at least 6000 were saved. Servocontrolled radiant heat in incubators was initially reported by Agate and Silverman in 1963.[2]

Today's ***radiant warmer*** is an evolution from the original idea of Agate and Silverman. Radiant energy as the sole source of heat from an overhead panel was described in 1969 by Due and Oliver. Widespread use of the warmer in the delivery room was readily accepted and soon led to its use in the neonatal intensive care unit. The factors that effect heat loss and heat production were elucidated. As intensive care became more readily available, easy accessibility to the infants became increasingly necessary and the open warmer became more readily used.[12]

Changes in the radiant warmer have included introduction of incubators that are interchangeable with and convert to radiant warmers. The use of humidification in the incubators has also been improved to allow for varying humidification based on the infant's gestational age and weight. These new beds allow the caregiver to rotate the mattress 360 degrees for easy patient access and provide an in-bed scale. Recent studies have encouraged the introduction of ***polyethylene plastic bags*** and wraps for use with babies born at approximately 30 weeks'

Please note that the PURPLE type in each chapter is intended to make it easier to identify clinically applicable material.

gestation or less.[13] This type of warming is ideal for a preterm infant (at birth and the immediate hours following) awaiting transportation to a tertiary care facility or indeed a baby born in a tertiary care facility. The baby is placed on a warm towel (but not dried) and placed under a radiant warming heating device. The baby (excluding his or her head) is placed fully in the polyethylene bag or is wrapped in the polyethylene sheet. The baby should remain under the radiant warmer as the heat, acting through the covering on the baby's moist skin, creates a warm thermal environment. Cutting an appropriate-size hole through the covering over the area of insertion can facilitate the introduction of any catheter or cannula. Polyethylene bags for warmth have been adopted by the Neonatal Resuscitation Program (NRP) (see Chapter 4).

NRP guidelines emphasize how hypothermia may reduce the extent of brain injury after hypoxia and that hyperthermia may worsen the extent of brain injury during reperfusion after hypoxic events. The recommended goal is to maintain normothermia for the infant and avoid iatrogenic hyperthermia in resuscitated newborns (see Chapter 26).

Building on these early findings and occasional misguided efforts over the next several decades,[17,18] researchers have gained insight into the physiology of thermoregulation and developed the technology to maintain thermal neutrality in the tiniest and sickest neonates. Although the staffs of modern neonatal intensive care units (NICUs) have the expertise and equipment to avoid the consequences of inadequate thermoregulation, determining the most appropriate ways of attaining the best temperature balance is the subject of ongoing investigation. This chapter discusses the current knowledge of the physiology and pathophysiology of neonatal thermoregulation and techniques used not only to prevent heat loss but also to manage heat balance.

PHYSIOLOGY

Animals that maintain their body temperature within a narrow range through a wide range of environmental temperatures are known as ***homeotherms.*** Humans, as homeotherms, maintain a "normal" body temperature by balancing the amount of heat lost from the body with the amount of heat generated from within the body. Our ability to cope with changing thermal environments improves physically and physiologically with age. Eventually we are physically able to move to a different place with a more suitable environment or dress more appropriately when the temperature is uncomfortable.

Babies, especially preterm or small-for-gestational-age (SGA) babies, of course cannot physically respond as older children would, and even their physiologic responses are different and limited. Adults lose some thermoregulatory control during rapid-eye-movement sleep. Because newborns spend much time in active sleep, loss of their ability to compensate for changes in environmental temperatures may be detrimental to their well-being. Recent evidence suggests that thermoregulation is not impaired during active sleep in the neonate, which indicates the developmental importance of both thermoregulation and active sleep in the maturation of newborn infants.

Physiologic responses to a cold environment include metabolic reactions that consume substrate and oxygen and result in heat production. **A neutral thermal temperature is the body temperature at which an individual baby's oxygen consumption is minimized.** Thus a minimal amount of the baby's energy is expended for heat maintenance, and energy is conserved for other basic functions and for growth. Minimal metabolic activity is possible within a narrow range of temperatures, so temperatures that are too high or too low add stress and increase metabolic rate. Extreme deviations from this range overwhelm the thermoregulatory mechanisms, leading to body temperature changes and potentially death.

CAUTION: All studies used to develop Figures 6-1 and 6-2 were conducted under specific, controlled environments that may not exist in the clinical setting. The ideal temperature varies with the particular baby and environmental variables such as relative humidity, type of incubator, and clothing used.

The goal in controlling a neonate's environment is to minimize energy expended by him or her to maintain a "normal" temperature, thus eliminating thermal stress. This neutral thermal environment is the sum total of factors at which a baby with a normal body temperature has a minimal metabolic rate and therefore minimal oxygen consumption. Both traditional indirect calorimetry and the more accurate and sensitive direct calorimetry are used to study the production

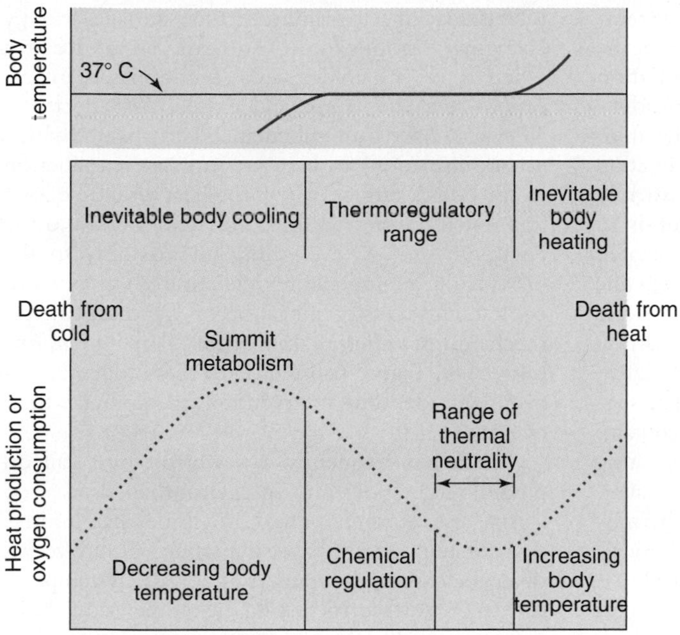

FIGURE 6-1 Temperature versus oxygen consumption. Effect of environmental oxygen consumption and body temperature. (From Klaus M, Fanaroff A: *Care of the high-risk neonate*, ed 2, Philadelphia, 1979, Saunders.)

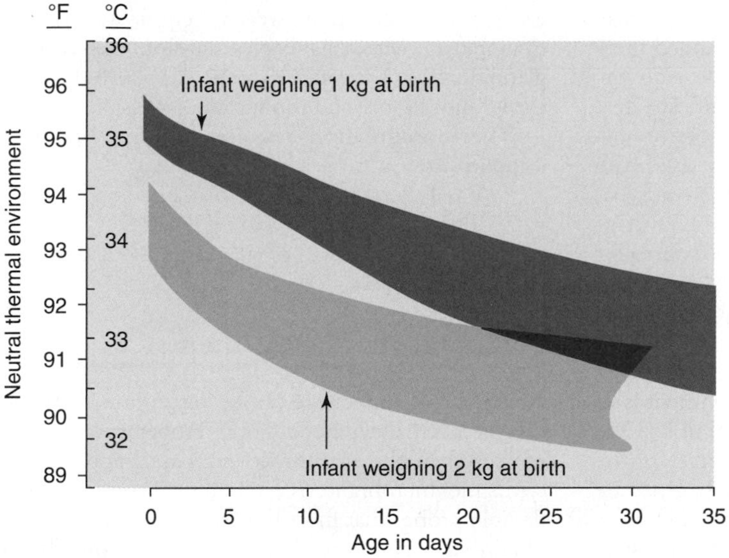

FIGURE 6-2 Neutral thermal environments. Range of temperature to provide neutral environmental conditions for infant lying naked on warm mattress in draft-free surroundings of moderate humidity (50% saturation) when mean radiant temperature is same as air temperature. *Shaded areas* show average neutral temperature range for healthy infant weighing 1 kg *(dark)* or 2 kg *(light)* at birth. Optimal temperature probably approximates to lower limit of neutral range as defined here. Approximately 1° C (1.8° F) should be added to these operative temperatures to derive appropriate neutral air temperature for single-walled incubator when room temperature is less than 27° C (80° F) and more if room temperature is much less. (From Hey EN, Katz G: The optimum thermal environment for naked babies, *Arch Dis Child* 45:328, 1970.)

and expenditure of heat in newborns. Factors such as ambient air temperature, airflow velocity, relative humidity, and temperature and composition of objects in direct contact with the infant or to which heat may be radiated compose the infant's thermal environment.

When exposed to a cold environment, a neonate senses the reduced skin surface temperature (using sensors in the skin, primarily the face) and senses core body temperature (using sensors along the spinal cord and in the hypothalamus). Information from these various sensors is processed (probably in the posterior hypothalamus), including average temperature, rate of temperature change, and size of the stimulated area. **Cold stress results in the initiation of a series of reactions to increase heat production and decrease heat loss.** In adults, the most significant involuntary method of heat production is shivering. **Neonates rarely shiver and must rely on nonshivering, or chemical, thermogenesis to produce the needed heat.** This process is initiated in the hypothalamus and transmitted through the sympathetic nervous system, leading to the release of norepinephrine at the site of brown fat. ***Brown fat,*** found mostly in the nape of the neck, axillae, and between the scapulae of newborns, is a specialized type of fat. It is unique in that it contains thermogenin, which is the key enzyme regulating nonshivering thermogenesis. Norepinephrine causes the release of free fatty acids, which with thermogenesis undergo combustion in the mitochondria of brown fat cells, releasing heat. Lipoprotein lipase also provides further triglyceride substrate for heat production.

Oxygen and glucose also are consumed during nonshivering thermogenesis. Thus an infant who already has low oxygen or glucose levels may become hypoxemic or hypoglycemic if added thermal stress occurs. Preterm babies do not develop sufficient brown fat stores to mount a significant heat production response to compensate for even minimal cold stress.[7] **When servocontrol is used, the thermistor must not be placed over an area of brown fat, which may directly heat the overlying skin, causing a decrease in servocontroller heat output.**

Heat generated within the body is transferred by conduction through tissues along a gradient from warmer to cooler areas such as the skin surface. An initial response to a cold environment is to constrict superficial blood vessels to minimize the transfer of heat from the core to the surface of the body. Superficial vasoconstriction, which gives the skin a mottled appearance in response to cold stimulus, results in a lower skin temperature reading to the thermocontroller and consequently causes an increase in the incubator temperature. **The smaller the body size, the less effective vasoconstriction is in conserving heat.**

Compared with adults, newborns have a very large surface area to body mass ratio and therefore have a relatively large area exposed to the environment from which heat can be lost. More mature infants may try to minimize their surface area by changing positions to decrease exposed surface area when faced with cold stimulus, but immature infants cannot flex the trunk and extremities effectively. They also have little subcutaneous fat tissue (which acts as insulation) to help prevent heat conduction to the body's surface, where the heat would be lost.

Heat is transferred from the infant's body to the environment (i.e., everything in proximity to the baby) along a temperature gradient from warmest to coolest. This transfer of heat occurs by four principal mechanisms: ***radiation, conduction, evaporation, and convection.*** Figure 6-3 illustrates these four mechanisms and identifies interventions to minimize their effects.

Much less frequently, a newborn must call on physiologic responses to an environment that is too warm, and these responses are somewhat limited. As skin temperature rises, superficial blood vessels dilate, increasing the transfer of core body temperature to the surface. Increasing the temperature gradient between the skin and the environment increases heat loss from the body. When exposed to elevated environmental temperatures, preterm babies generally cannot generate sweat to eliminate heat by evaporation. Maturing babies develop this eccrine gland function first on the forehead, followed by the chest, upper arms, and more caudal areas.

Thermoregulation requires energy (caloric) expenditure:

- Basal metabolic rate: 50 kcal/kg/day
- Thermoregulation: 10 kcal/kg/day
- Thermic effects of feeding: 8 kcal/kg/day[7] (see Chapter 17)

Temperature Management

A neonate's temperature can be determined by various methods. Deep body (core) temperature may be measured in the rectum or esophagus and on the tympanic membrane. Rectal thermistors are thin, flexible probes that must be inserted at least 5 cm to obtain an accurate reading. Insertion to this depth runs the risk for perforation, because the sigmoid colon makes a right-angle turn approximately 3 cm from the anal opening. Esophageal and tympanic readings are difficult to obtain and usually impractical. Noninvasive infrared thermometry, a rapid and painless method of determining tympanic membrane or axillary temperature in children, is not recommended for use in newborns at this time.

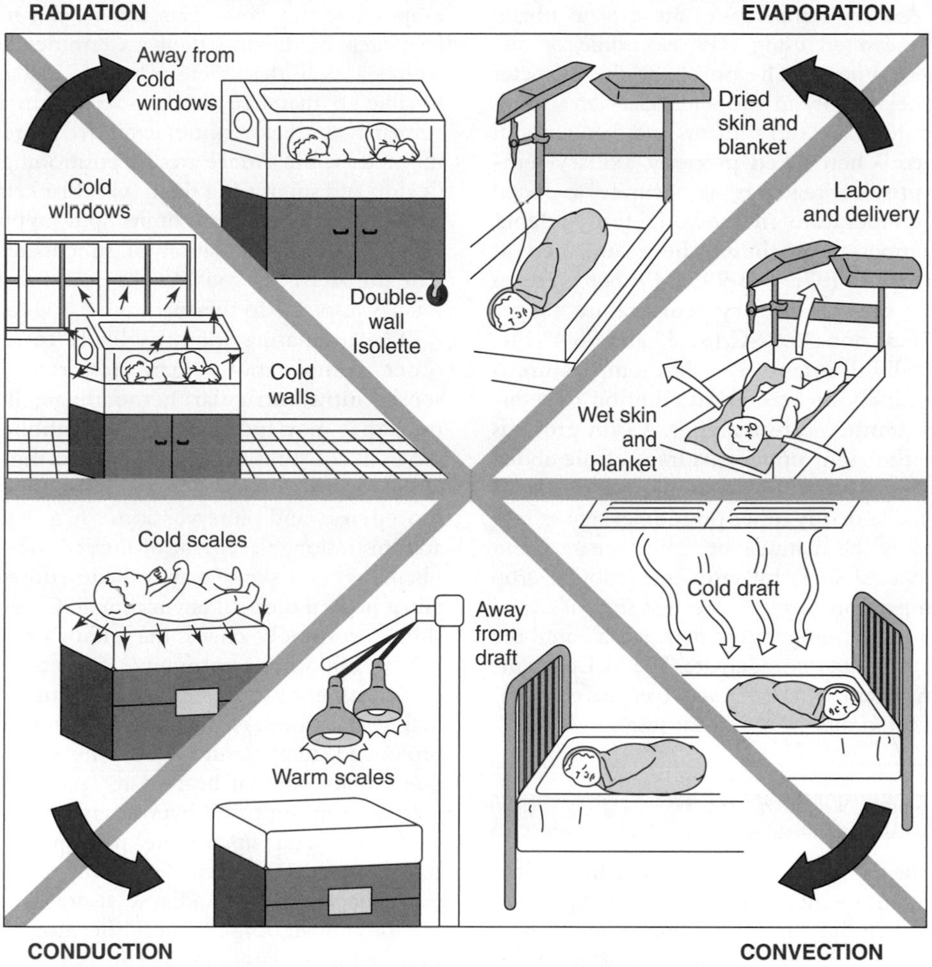

FIGURE 6-3 *Radiation*, or heat loss in the form of electromagnetic photons, occurs from warm skin surfaces to a cooler object not in contact with the newborn (e.g., inside the incubator wall, nursery wall, window). Radiant heat loss is independent of ambient air temperature and is the main source of heat loss because of the infant's large exposed body surface area. *Conduction* is the loss of heat to a cooler object in direct contact with the newborn (e.g., cold scale, unwarmed bed, stethoscope, examiner's hand). *Convection* is the loss of heat to moving air at the skin surface and depends on the air's velocity and temperature. *Evaporation* of water from the skin and mucous membranes also causes heat loss, especially in the delivery room. The thinner stratum corneum layer of skin of very-low-birth-weight infants makes evaporative heat and water loss and fluid management ongoing problems. (Courtesy Lynn Jones, RN.)

Studies have failed to demonstrate an accurate correlation between infrared thermometer readings and axillary or rectal temperature readings in newborn infants. Continuous monitoring of abdominal skin temperature with the newborn lying supine is a noninvasive method that has been reported to show good correlation with rectal temperatures. It is impractical to keep babies in a supine position constantly, so research to find the best practice to monitor and servocontrol infants' temperatures continues.[12] Correlation with this method and core temperature requires further study, and whether its use with servocontrol is appropriate is yet to be determined, because incubators are programmed to respond to insulated skin temperature, not core temperature.

Because of the risks involved, rectal temperatures should not be taken on a routine basis in

neonates. Axillary temperatures are easy to obtain and safely measured using glass, electronic, or disposable thermometers. The tip of the thermometer should be held firmly in the midaxillary area for at least 3 minutes in preterm infants and 5 minutes in term infants. **When taken properly, axillary temperatures provide readings as accurate as rectal and core temperature methods. In term infants, axillary temperatures should be maintained at 36.5° to 37.5° C (97.7° to 99.5° F). For preterm infants, the normal axillary temperature ranges between 36.3° and 36.9° C (97.3° and 98.4° F).**[2]

In critically ill infants, the skin temperature is usually routinely monitored in addition to regular axillary temperature readings. A skin probe is secured to the right upper quadrant of the abdomen. The temperature probe should not be placed under the axilla or any other position except as recommended by the manufacturer. Because an infant responds to cold stress by vasoconstriction, a drop in skin temperature may be the first sign of hypothermia. The core temperature may not fall until the infant can no longer compensate. The axillary temperature may remain normal (or even be elevated) because of proximity to brown fat stores.

ETIOLOGY

The ambient temperature range in which a healthy full-term infant maintains a stable core temperature is narrower than the temperature range in which an adult maintains a normal temperature. When measures are taken to provide a neutral thermal environment for the neonate, excessive heat losses or gains are avoided and heat balance is maintained. Recognition of infants at risk for heat imbalance is essential in the prevention of thermal stress.

Premature infants have a limited ability to control body temperature and are extremely susceptible to hypothermia. Factors that contribute to temperature instability include very thin skin, large surface area relative to body mass, limited substrate for heat production, decreased subcutaneous tissue, and an immature nervous system. These infants often have multiple health problems that necessitate frequent interventions by health care providers with consequent disruption of the infant's neutral thermal environment.

A premature infant's very thin skin and larger surface area to body mass ratio allow for increased evaporative heat loss. Term infants can reduce surface area by flexing their extremities onto their trunk, a skill that increases with gestational age. Unable to maintain flexion, a preterm infant lies primarily with extremities extended. Care providers may reduce the surface area by positioning infants in flexion and supporting them with blankets and rolls. The shortened gestation limits lipid supplies, brown fat, and the accumulation of subcutaneous tissue. The immature nervous system delays or mutes the infant's response to thermal stress.

The premature infant is likely to experience other complications (e.g., respiratory distress, sepsis, intraventricular hemorrhage, hypoglycemia) that may increase basal metabolic rate and oxygen consumption, thus interfering with the ability to maintain thermal stability. Numerous procedures and interventions (e.g., medication administration, placement of intravascular catheters, obtaining vital signs) may impede efforts to maintain a neutral thermal environment. **Care providers should routinely check the infant's temperature before initiating treatments.** If the temperature is low, treatment should be delayed until a more normal temperature is obtained. If interventions are prolonged, temperature should be monitored frequently, an external heat source provided, and the intervention stopped if hypothermia occurs.

Late-preterm infants are predisposed to morbidities because of their developmental immaturity (see Chapter 5). Less adipose tissue for insulation, less brown fat for chemical thermogenesis, more heat loss, and a larger ratio of surface area to weight contribute to problems with heat balance in these infants. Morbidity associated with heat balance in the late-preterm infant is 10% compared with 0% for term infants.[3]

Low-Birth-Weight Newborns

Low-birth-weight (LBW) (<2500 g) infants can be divided into two groups: the very-low-birth-weight (VLBW) infant (<1500 g) and the extremely-low-birth-weight (ELBW) infant (<1000 g). Preterms in each of these groups have specific needs for thermoregulation. Heated incubators, radiant warmers, and skin-to-skin care are all methods for maintaining the temperature and promoting weight gain of the VLBW infant. Infants weighing more than 1500 g may be weaned to an open crib if all criteria are met. (See Figure 6-5 for weaning criteria.)

During the first 12 hours of life, ELBW preterms become hypothermic with procedures such as intubations, chest x-ray examinations, IV line placement and manipulation, suctioning, repositioning, and vital signs. Like the late-preterm and the LBW infant, ELBW infants have even less brown and subcutaneous fat for maintaining body temperature. Their thin skin also contributes to increased insensible water loss.

SGA infants, like preterm infants, have a large surface area relative to body mass and decreased subcutaneous tissue, brown fat, and glycogen stores, all of which contribute to heat imbalance. Decreased placental blood flow frequently contributes to the small size. The relatively large surface area of an SGA infant increases evaporative and radiant heat loss, whereas limited brown fat stores and subcutaneous tissue contribute to a decreased ability to produce and conserve body heat. Some flexion of the extremities may be present because flexion depends on gestational age and not weight. SGA infants have a higher metabolic rate compared with infants at similar weights who are appropriate for gestational age. This is believed to be caused by the larger brain size relative to body weight. **Hypoxia in utero may depress the infant's central nervous system (CNS) and alter the ability to regulate temperature.** Increased energy requirements coupled with limited glycogen stores may result in hypoglycemia and limited ability to produce heat. SGA infants may require numerous interventions that disrupt the neutral thermal environment. **Care providers should ensure that the infant has a normal and stable temperature before initiation of treatments. If treatments are prolonged, temperature should be monitored frequently, an external heat source provided, and treatments stopped if hypothermia occurs.**

Infants with neurologic damage or depression may experience difficulty maintaining a stable temperature. Hypoxia before, during, or after delivery, neurologic defects, and exposure to drugs such as analgesics and anesthetics may depress the infant's neurologic response to thermal stress. Hypoxia decreases the effect of norepinephrine on nonshivering thermogenesis, the main route of thermal regulation in the newborn infant. Hypoxia also may reduce the oxidative capacity of the mitochondria in brown fat and skeletal muscles, which are involved in thermogenesis. Infants who have experienced hypoxia in utero may have increased norepinephrine concentrations, which result in peripheral vasoconstriction. This may cause a delayed metabolic response to cold stress and delayed vasodilation in response to heat stress.

Neurologic defects that affect the hypothalamus also may interfere with heat balance. The ***hypothalamus*** coordinates temperature input from various sensors. Drugs such as analgesics and anesthetics cause CNS depression and reduce the infant's ability to respond to thermal stress. Neuromuscular blocking agents inhibit the infant's ability to maintain a flexed position, increasing exposed body surface and heat loss. **Care providers must be alert to the effect of drugs on the CNS and the infant's ability to regulate temperature.**

Infants with sepsis may have hypothermia or hyperthermia. In a newborn, an elevated temperature may begin as a response to cold stress, with peripheral vasoconstriction and thermogenesis. Heat production continues as the infant attempts to achieve a higher core body temperature. Exogenous and endogenous pyrogens may enhance thermogenesis.

Initially, an infant with sepsis may feel cool to the touch and may have a low body temperature. As fever progresses, temperature may rise and the infant feels warm to the touch. **Infants nursed in servocontrolled incubators may not have an elevated temperature. The lower heater output in response to increasing skin temperature (by manual or servocontrol adjustment) may mask a fever by keeping the baby's temperature within normal limits. The care provider should be alert to a sudden decreased need for incubator heat support in a previously stable infant.**

Hyperthermia may be iatrogenic, caused by inappropriate control of the neonate's environmental temperature. The most common cause is the inappropriate use of external heat sources. Dehydration also may contribute to hyperthermia. **Infants nursed with the use of external heat sources should have their temperatures monitored frequently. Phototherapy, sunlight, and the use of excessive clothing and blankets contribute to overheating.** Dehydration may be avoided by early recognition of infants at risk for increased fluid loss. Increased insensible water loss occurs in preterm infants because of increased skin permeability and the use of phototherapy and radiant warmers. Vomiting, diarrhea, gastric suction, and ostomy drainage also increase fluid loss. These infants should receive additional fluids to replace the increased losses (see Chapter 14).

PREVENTION OF HEAT/COLD STRESS

Heat balance is determined by the amount of heat lost to the baby's environment offset by the amount of heat generated by the body plus the amount of heat supplied from outside sources. Because a smaller, more immature, and sicker baby is less able to regulate body temperature, it is crucial that care providers understand the physical and physiologic principles of heat balance and be able to maintain a neutral thermal environment. **Two broad categories of interventions foster thermal neutrality[1]: blocking avenues of heat loss; and providing external heat and environmental support to maintain temperature within the normal range of 36.5° to 37.5° C (97.7° to 99.5° F).**[4] The theoretical neutral thermal environment necessary for neonates of 1 and 2 kg at a given age is graphed in Figure 6-2. **Newborns of less than 800 g are not adequately addressed in currently available tables but should have a starting environmental temperature setting of 36.5° C (97.7° F).**

Attention to the details of these interventions begins in the delivery room, in which the first step is to adjust the ambient delivery room temperature higher than ordinary operating rooms or patient rooms. **The air temperature in newborn care areas should be kept at 23.8° to 26.1° C (75° to 79° F), and humidity should be kept at 30% to 60%.**[2] Warming the room and placing the resuscitation table away from doors or drafts minimize convective heat loss. The newborn's skin temperature may drop by as much as 0.3° C/min, with core temperature dropping more slowly after delivery. At birth, most heat loss results from evaporation of amniotic fluid from the baby's skin surface. Drying the infant with prewarmed towels and immediately replacing used ones with dry, warm towels minimize evaporative heat loss. Dry towels conduct heat poorly when contacting the neonate's skin. However, cold examiner hands, stethoscopes, scales, and bare mattresses are good heat conductors and can add significant cold stress if not warmed before coming in contact with the newborn.

Another means of preventing heat loss in very preterm infants in the delivery room is to wrap them in a ***polyethylene bag or sheet*** immediately after delivery. Resuscitation then proceeds as usual, and the baby is unwrapped after placement in a warmed incubator. Admission temperatures were higher in the wrapped group and did not drop after unwrapping when the infants were compared with babies who were dried but not wrapped.[21] **Treating hypothermia in the newborn prevents serious and life-threatening complications. In an attempt to maintain heat balance, the neonate increases cellular metabolism and oxygen consumption, which increases the risk for hypoxia, cardiorespiratory problems, and acidosis. Hypoglycemia is also a risk factor, since the infant must consume more glucose for heat production.** Other complications include clotting disorders, neurologic problems, hyperbilirubinemia, and even death if the untreated hypothermia progresses.

Resuscitation should take place on a preheated radiant warmer so that the adverse consequences of hypothermia are avoided. Because a significant amount of heat is lost through the surface area of the head, with its abundant blood supply and the brain's high heat production, covering the infant's head with some insulating material conserves heat during transfer to the nursery or NICU and afterward. Stockinet material is relatively ineffective for this purpose and provides poor insulation. The best material is thick, maintains its shape with use, and has a high percentage of air volume trapped in the fibers. Knitted wool caps or Thinsulate material may provide the best results.

There are a variety of ways to maintain thermal neutrality. Accessibility, insensible water loss, servocontrol versus manual control of temperature, and safety are major considerations when determining the method to use for an individual neonate.

Incubators

Incubators provide a controlled, enclosed environment that is heated convectively with warm air. The temperature in an incubator may be ***servocontrolled*** to maintain a desired skin temperature or air temperature. As the temperature varies from the desired "set point," proportional control units gradually increase or decrease heat output to maintain a constant temperature (without the wider temperature fluctuations seen with simple on-off controllers). **In setting the servocontrolled incubator to the desired skin temperature, the sensor should be attached to the right upper quadrant of the abdomen with insulated temperature patches. The sensor should not be placed over areas of brown fat deposits,**

because the higher-than-expected temperature information to the controlling unit will result in a lower-than-desired heat output.

Inadvertent cooling may take place if the sensor is covered with clothes or a blanket or if the baby lies on it. If the sensor becomes disconnected from the skin, unwanted heating may occur because an erroneously low temperature reading causes an unwanted increase in heat output. One also must consider that when an insulated patch is used to cover the thermistor, skin temperature is sensed as being higher than if tape covers the thermistor, resulting in decreased heat output by the warming device. **The desired skin temperature used for skin servocontrol is generally 36.0° to 36.5° C (96.8° to 97.7° F).**[15] Modern incubators also can be servocontrolled to a desired air temperature. This mode has been shown to provide a more stable thermal environment and less temperature variation when compared with skin servocontrol.

Air servocontrol maintains a constant ambient air temperature when other factors such as phototherapy, external radiant heat, unstable room temperature, or direct sunlight are not confounding variables. **Recently it has been shown that infants who had been managed with skin servocontrol had more variable but higher air temperatures and spent more time in a neutral thermal environment. Babies managed with air servocontrol had less variability in air temperatures but more variability in infant body temperature. A review of published trials concluded that VLBW babies whose skin servocontrol is set at 36° C had a lower mortality rate than those managed with air servocontrol at 31.8° C.**[19] The question of air versus skin servocontrol or manual control is still debatable for any given situation, and probably neither is the perfect solution for all babies. Figure 6-4 is a research-based algorithm for weaning from servocontrol to air control in an incubator.[9]

Radiant heat loss to cooler incubator walls, especially in single-walled incubators, is a significant source of heat loss. The use of ***double-walled incubators*** (with the inner wall warmed to the ambient air temperature inside the incubator) results in less radiant heat loss from the baby. With a skin-set servocontrol temperature, the decreased radiant heat loss (because of warmer incubator walls) is offset by increased convective heat loss (because the ambient air temperature necessary for the desired skin temperature is lower). Consequently, there is no net change in the mean environmental temperature. Double-walled incubators provide less temperature fluctuation when doors are open, thus providing a more stable caregiving environment. Evaporative heat loss is not appreciably different with single- and double-walled incubators. One may increase the humidity in incubators to decrease the infant's metabolic rate only if a neutral thermal environment cannot be achieved by increasing the ambient temperature.

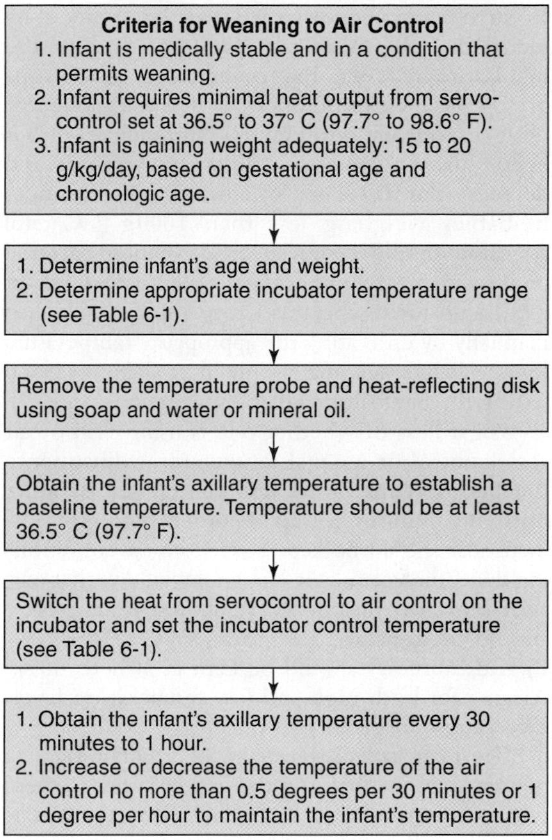

FIGURE 6-4 Research-based algorithm for weaning from servocontrol to air control mode in an incubator ©NPDPA™, 2008. (Modified from Brown V, Gardner SL: *Neonatal thermoregulation: clinical practice tools and policy/procedure/protocol packets*, 2008, Nurse's Professional Development & Practice Association, LLC. Accessed August 5, 2009, from www.npdpa.com.)

The tiniest neonate has a large evaporative heat loss, and maximum air temperature is limited by the incubator controls, thus making it difficult to reach an air temperature high enough for thermal support.

In such cases, hypothermia can be avoided by increasing the ambient humidity within the incubator by using the water reservoir or supplying warmed humidified air into the incubator with respiratory humidifiers. Humidification has been shown to decrease fluid requirements and decrease the incidence of electrolyte imbalances in babies weighing less than 1000 g.[10] Careful attention should be given to preventing bacterial growth in the humidification system (see Chapter 23). Incubator temperatures may also be controlled manually by estimating the appropriate temperature for the baby's age and weight from Table 6-1 and setting the incubator to that temperature.

Regardless of whether one is using skin or air servocontrol or manual temperature adjustments, the baby's temperature and the air temperature must be monitored and recorded regularly. The incubator should be kept away from air conditioning ducts, direct sunlight, and cool windows that may cool or warm the incubator. **Room temperature should be kept at 23.8° to 26.1° C (75° to 79° F) and humidity should be kept at 30% to 60%.**[4] **Alarms for both high and low temperature levels always should be turned on.**

The principal disadvantage of maintaining sick newborns in incubators is the limited access to them when extensive procedures are necessary. Incubators also may be perceived by mothers as a barrier between them and their infants and prolong feelings of fear and insecurity, compared with heating methods that provide easier access to the baby. Holding their baby for short periods outside the incubator may help promote bonding and relieve some of their fears. Stable preterm infants dressed in a diaper, shirt, and cap and wrapped in two blankets can maintain a normal temperature when held close to their parent's body. Keeping the skin probe attached to the infant and plugged into the incubator allows frequent monitoring of the infant's temperature. We also now have an increasing awareness of and concern about the high noise levels within incubators. Such noise poses a potential deleterious effect on the hearing development of preterm infants (see Chapter 13). Improved alarm technology minimizes the risk for inappropriate heating, but malfunctions still occur occasionally. When experienced nurses provide care, infants can be appropriately managed in incubators using any of the three modes of temperature control. Box 6-1 outlines dos and don'ts when using an incubator to provide heat and humidity.[9]

Weaning an infant from an incubator to an open crib is an important step in preparing for discharge but may result in an increase in the resting metabolic rate for LBW infants.[7] **Indicators that an infant may be successfully weaned include weight of at least 1500 g, 5 days of consistent weight gain, an absence of medical complications, and tolerance of enteral feeds. Weaning may occur over several days and involves dressing the infant in a shirt, hat, and diaper and swaddling with a blanket.** The incubator temperature is manually lowered while monitoring the infant's temperature. **Abdominal skin temperature should be 36° to 37° C (96.8° to 98.6° F).** Figures 6-5 and 6-6 are research-based algorithms for weaning infants to open cribs.[9] After weaning has been successful, the crib should be placed in a draft-free environment. **If an infant cannot maintain his or her temperature in an open crib, he or she is returned to the incubator. An attempt at weaning should be considered again by 48 hours after the initial weaning if all criteria for weaning have been met.** The temperature in the neonatal unit should be evaluated, as well as the location of the crib in relation to air conditioner vents or drafts. There may also be other medical reasons (e.g., infection) that the infant cannot maintain his or her temperature in the open crib if all other conditions have been ruled out.[1]

Humidification and Topical Ointments

Many studies and clinical trials have demonstrated the clinical application of the uses of both humidity and topical ointment therapy (see Chapter 19) in preterm infants. **The optimal humidity level for the neonate is 50% relative humidity (RH).** This is achieved by a variety of methods such as closed humidified incubators and humidity "tents." **In the first 2 weeks of life, extremely premature infants may require up to 85% RH.** Box 6-2 describes the advantages and disadvantages of using heated, humidified air for ELBW infants while in an incubator.[9]

Radiant Warmers

Radiant warmers provide infrared energy to heat the baby's skin while he or she lies naked on an open bed. The radiant warmer must generate enough energy to offset the tremendous amount of radiant

TABLE 6-1

NEUTRAL THERMAL ENVIRONMENTAL TEMPERATURES

AGE AND WEIGHT	STARTING TEMPERATURE (°C)	RANGE OF TEMPERATURE (°C)
0-6 hr		
Under 1200 g	35.0	34.0-35.4
1200-1500 g	34.1	33.9-34.4
1501-2500 g	33.4	32.8-33.8
Over 2500 g (and >36 wk)	33.9	32.0-33.8
>6-12 hr		
Under 1200 g	35.0	34.0-35.4
1200-1500 g	34.0	33.5-34.4
1501-2500 g	33.1	32.2-33.8
Over 2500 g (and >36 wk)	32.8	31.4-33.8
>12-24 hr		
Under 1200 g	34.0	34.0-35.4
1200-1500 g	33.8	33.3-34.3
1501-2500 g	32.8	31.8-33.8
Over 2500 g (and >36 wk)	32.4	31.0-33.7
>24-36 hr		
Under 1200 g	34.0	34.0-35.0
1200-1500 g	33.6	33.1-34.2
1501-2500 g	32.6	31.6-33.6
Over 2500 g (and >36 wk)	32.1	30.7-33.5
>36-48 hr		
Under 1200 g	34.0	34.0-35.0
1200-1500 g	33.5	33.0-34.1
1501-2500 g	32.5	31.4-33.5
Over 2500 g (and >36 wk)	31.9	30.5-33.3
>48-72 hr		
Under 1200 g	34.0	34.0-35.0
1200-1500 g	33.5	33.0-34.0
1501-2500 g	32.3	31.2-33.4
Over 2500 g (and >36 wk)	31.7	30.1-33.2
>72-96 hr		
Under 1200 g	34.0	34.0-35.0
1200-1500 g	33.5	33.0-34.0
1501-2500 g	32.2	31.1-33.2
Over 2500 g (and >36 wk)	31.3	29.8-32.8
>4-12 days		
Under 1500 g	33.5	33.0-34.0
1501-2500 g	32.1	31.0-33.2
Over 2500 g (and >36 wk)		
4-5 days	31.0	29.5-32.6
5-6 days	30.9	29.4-32.3
6-8 days	30.6	29.0-32.2
8-10 days	30.3	29.0-31.8
10-12 days	30.1	29.0-31.4
>12-14 days		
Under 1500 g	33.5	32.6-34.0
1501-2500 g	32.1	31.0-33.2
>2-3 wk		
Under 1500 g	33.1	32.2-34.0
1501-2500 g	31.7	30.5-33.0
>3-4 wk		
Under 1500 g	32.6	31.6-33.6
1501-2500 g	31.4	30.0-32.7
>4-5 wk		
Under 1500 g	32.0	31.2-33.0
1501-2500 g	30.9	29.5-32.2
>5-6 wk		
Under 1500 g	31.4	30.6-32.3
1501-2500 g	30.4	29.0-31.8

From American Academy of Pediatrics and American College of Obstetricians and Gynecologists: *Guidelines for perinatal care*, ed 2, Evanston, Ill, 1988, American Academy of Pediatrics and American College of Obstetricians and Gynecologists. Data from Scopes JW, Ahmed I: Minimal rates of oxygen consumption in sick and premature infants, *Arch Dis Child* 41:407, 1966; Scopes JW, Ahmed I: Range of critical temperatures in sick and premature newborn babies, *Arch Dis Child* 41:417, 1966.

Note: For their table, Scopes and Ahmed had the walls of the incubator 1° to 2° C warmer than the ambient air temperatures. Generally, the smaller infants in each weight group require a temperature in the higher portion of the temperature range. Within each time range, the younger the infant, the higher the temperature required.

BOX 6-1 USE OF AN INCUBATOR: DOS AND DON'TS

Dos

1. Place temperature probes according to manufacturer recommendations.
2. Change the incubator once a month.
3. Use sterile water for humidification.
4. Keep the incubator clean and free of spills.
5. Adequately humidify the incubator according to BW and GA of the infant.
6. Keep walls locked in place to prevent falls and provide a safe environment for the infant.
7. Clean incubators after each use and between patients with recommended cleaner, by trained staff.
8. Use servocontrol for infants when first placing them in an incubator.
9. Follow weaning guidelines when changing from servocontrol to air control, using the weight and age chart (see Table 6-1).
10. Change the temperature probe site as directed by manufacturer and hospital procedure.
11. Frequently monitor and record the infant's temperature, and observe for changes in clinical condition.

Don'ts

1. Don't place the temperature probe in the infant's axilla.
2. Avoid pinching lines/tubes when opening/closing portholes and sides.
3. Avoid placing noisy equipment inside or on top of the incubator.
4. Avoid tapping, hitting, or knocking the incubator when the infant is in the bed.
5. Avoid keeping portholes open except for care and handling.
6. Avoid epidermal stripping (see Chapter 19) when applying/changing temperature probe sites.
7. Avoid pulling out lines or extubating the infant when moving/taking him or her out of the incubator.
8. Don't wean the servocontrol temperature less than 36.5° C (97.7° F).
9. Don't wean the temperature on the air control any faster than 0.5° per 30 minutes or 1° per hour.
10. Avoid cleaning the incubator with alcohol or acetone.
11. Do not keep the incubator in an unlocked position when in use. Do not position the incubator next to an air conditioner duct or in direct sunlight from a window.

Modified from Brown V, Gardner SL: *Neonatal thermoregulation: clinical practice tools and policy/procedure/protocol packets,* 2008, Nurse's Professional Development & Practice Association, LLC. Accessed August 5, 2009, from www.npdpa.com.

BW, Birth weight; *GA,* gestational age.

heat lost to the room by a naked baby lying in an open environment. Heat output can be servocontrolled or manually controlled. Because with manual control no feedback from the infant is used, this poses a greater risk for overheating or overcooling. **Therefore manual control should not be used routinely except for short periods (e.g., while initiating resuscitation).** The servocontrol sensor measuring skin temperature must be protected from the infrared heat source, or the probe will sense a temperature higher than the skin temperature and decrease radiant heat output, leading to cold stress. Conversely, insulating the sensor with an aluminum reflective patch protects the underlying skin from the radiant heat and keeps the protected skin cooler than the surrounding skin. When the skin under the patch is warmed to the desired temperature, the rest of the skin may be overheated. Vasodilation then may increase convective heat loss, resulting in an effective, although precarious, heat balance. **Caregivers must use caution to ensure that the sensor does not become detached from the skin; otherwise the baby could be exposed to excess heat and become hyperthermic.**

Insensible water loss (IWL) for babies cared for under radiant warmers is increased by 40% to 50% compared with losses in incubators. Directly related to the amount of heat necessary from the warmer, this loss also is influenced by other factors (e.g., low relative humidity and convective air currents) on an open bed. Even though transepidermal water loss is increased under radiant warmers, there is evidence that the hydration of the stratum corneum is not affected; therefore the barrier function of the skin remains the same.[15] With very premature infants, severe dehydration may occur if water intake is not increased to replace the inordinate IWL (see Chapter 14). Plexiglas heat shields and polyethylene blankets (plastic wrap) have been used in an attempt to prevent large IWLs. Studies have shown these to be somewhat effective for this purpose; however, the microenvironment created by these blankets undergoes drastic

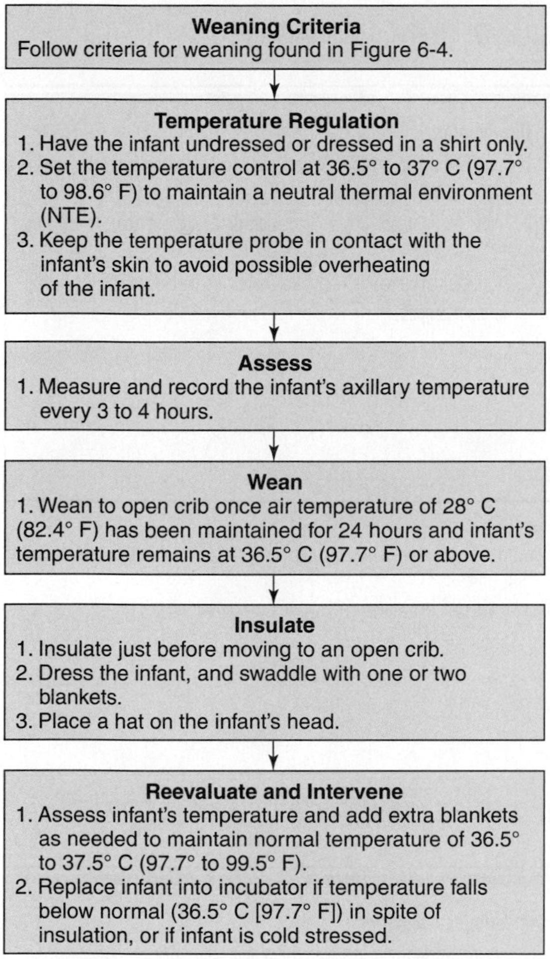

Weaning Criteria
Follow criteria for weaning found in Figure 6-4.
Temperature Regulation
1. Have the infant undressed or dressed in a shirt only.
2. Set the temperature control at 36.5° to 37° C (97.7° to 98.6° F) to maintain a neutral thermal environment (NTE).
3. Keep the temperature probe in contact with the infant's skin to avoid possible overheating of the infant.
Assess
1. Measure and record the infant's axillary temperature every 3 to 4 hours.
Wean
1. Wean to open crib once air temperature of 28° C (82.4° F) has been maintained for 24 hours and infant's temperature remains at 36.5° C (97.7° F) or above.
Insulate
1. Insulate just before moving to an open crib.
2. Dress the infant, and swaddle with one or two blankets.
3. Place a hat on the infant's head.
Reevaluate and Intervene
1. Assess infant's temperature and add extra blankets as needed to maintain normal temperature of 36.5° to 37.5° C (97.7° to 99.5° F).
2. Replace infant into incubator if temperature falls below normal (36.5° C [97.7° F]) in spite of insulation, or if infant is cold stressed.

FIGURE 6-5 Research-based algorithm for servocontrolled weaning from an incubator to an open crib. ©NPDPA™, 2008. (Modified from Brown V, Gardner SL: *Neonatal thermoregulation: clinical practice tools and policy/procedure/protocol packets*, 2008, Nurse's Professional Development & Practice Association, LLC. Accessed August 5, 2009, from www.npdpa.com.)

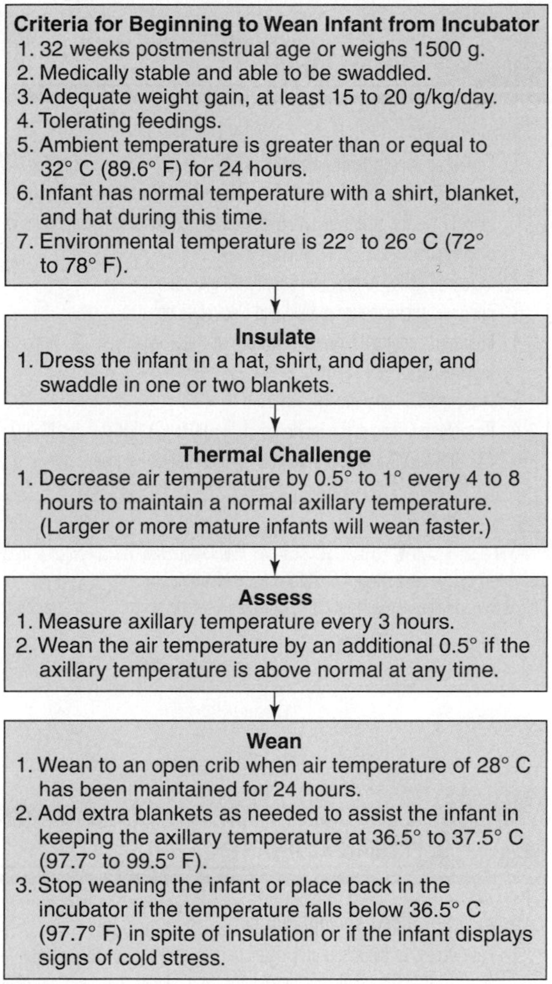

Criteria for Beginning to Wean Infant from Incubator
1. 32 weeks postmenstrual age or weighs 1500 g.
2. Medically stable and able to be swaddled.
3. Adequate weight gain, at least 15 to 20 g/kg/day.
4. Tolerating feedings.
5. Ambient temperature is greater than or equal to 32° C (89.6° F) for 24 hours.
6. Infant has normal temperature with a shirt, blanket, and hat during this time.
7. Environmental temperature is 22° to 26° C (72° to 78° F).
Insulate
1. Dress the infant in a hat, shirt, and diaper, and swaddle in one or two blankets.
Thermal Challenge
1. Decrease air temperature by 0.5° to 1° every 4 to 8 hours to maintain a normal axillary temperature. (Larger or more mature infants will wean faster.)
Assess
1. Measure axillary temperature every 3 hours.
2. Wean the air temperature by an additional 0.5° if the axillary temperature is above normal at any time.
Wean
1. Wean to an open crib when air temperature of 28° C has been maintained for 24 hours.
2. Add extra blankets as needed to assist the infant in keeping the axillary temperature at 36.5° to 37.5° C (97.7° to 99.5° F).
3. Stop weaning the infant or place back in the incubator if the temperature falls below 36.5° C (97.7° F) in spite of insulation or if the infant displays signs of cold stress.

FIGURE 6-6 Research-based algorithm for air mode/manual weaning from an incubator. ©NPDPA™, 2008. (Modified from Brown V, Gardner SL: *Neonatal thermoregulation: clinical practice tools and policy/procedure/protocol packets*, 2008, Nurse's Professional Development & Practice Association, LLC. Accessed August 5, 2009, from www.npdpa.com.)

change every time the blanket is removed for procedures or routine nursing care. Even without such blankets, the baby may experience wide swings in heat balance when the infrared heat is blocked from reaching him or her by hands, heads, or drapes during a procedure. These blankets should not be used while the infant is in an incubator, since the purpose is to have the humidity and heat reach the infant.

Both incubators and radiant warmers are effective in maintaining an appropriate thermal balance in sick and preterm infants. Evidence is insufficient to show a clear advantage of one method over the other with the caveat that IWL is significantly higher under radiant warmers.[8] The method chosen should be individualized to the infant and to the situation. Experience, skill, and nurse preference often influence the choice of heating methods. These factors also influence the extent to which incubators are perceived to interfere with the performance of care providers' tasks. Basic principles of care (e.g., keeping bed linens dry to prevent evaporative heat loss) apply to use of both heating methods. Box 6-3 lists advantages and disadvantages of open radiant

BOX 6-2 RESEARCH-BASED ADVANTAGES AND DISADVANTAGES OF HEATED HUMIDITY IN THE INCUBATOR OF ELBW INFANTS

Advantages

1. Decreased transepidermal water loss (TEWL) (e.g., insensible water loss [IWL], evaporative water loss, and epidermal heat loss) from the skin of infants less than 31 weeks' gestation. IWL is inversely proportionate to the gestational age of the infant.
2. Increased ability to maintain infant's temperature.
3. Improved maintenance of fluid and electrolyte balance.
4. Improved energy balance—fewer calories expended in temperature maintenance.
5. Improved skin integrity.
6. Possible reduction in the incidence of (1) PDA, (2) IVH (grades III/IV), and (3) BPD because of improved fluid and electrolyte balance.

Disadvantages

1. Increased risk for infection associated with contamination of the humidifier reservoir with bacteria.
2. Moist environment impairs adhesion of equipment (e.g., electrodes, ETT, dressings).
3. Unstable temperatures when procedures are performed and the incubator door is open.

Modified from Brown V, Gardner SL: *Neonatal thermoregulation: clinical practice tools and policy/procedure/protocol packets*, 2008, Nurse's Professional Development & Practice Association, LLC. Accessed August 5, 2009, from www.npdpa.com.

BPD, Bronchopulmonary dysplasia; *ELBW*, extremely low birth weight; *ETT*, endotracheal tube; *IVH*, intraventricular hemorrhage; *PDA*, patent ductus arteriosus.

BOX 6-3 ADVANTAGES AND DISADVANTAGES OF OPEN RADIANT WARMER VERSUS INCUBATOR USE FOR PREMATURE INFANTS

Advantages: Open Radiant Warmer

1. Easy access to the infant and larger surface on which to work
2. Useful for initial admission procedures (e.g., intubation, line placement, x-ray examination)
3. Decreased risk for infection without the use of humidity
4. Decreased risk for unplanned extubation and lines being pulled out
5. Better access by parents and staff

Disadvantages: Open Radiant Warmer

1. Increased insensible water loss (without humidification or plastic blanket)
2. Increased stimulation from external noise and light
3. Decreased growth and weight gain patterns
4. Decreased ability to wean the infant slowly from the heat source
5. Better access by parents and staff

Advantages: Incubator

1. Less insensible water loss with use of humidity
2. Acts as a barrier with more difficult access that decreases tactile contact. Easier to use minimal stimulation
3. Increased weight gain
4. Heat provided by two methods: convection and conduction
5. Ability to wean temperature control from servocontrol to air control, and from air control to an open crib
6. Ability to cover the incubator to decrease exposure to light

Disadvantages: Incubator

1. Decreased access for treatments, line placements, intubations, and laboratory draws
2. Increased chance of infection with humidity
3. Increased risk for extubation or accidental clamping of lines

Modified from Brown V, Gardner SL: *Neonatal thermoregulation: clinical practice tools and policy/procedure/protocol packets*, 2008, Nurse's Professional Development & Practice Association, LLC. Accessed August 5, 2009 from www.npdpa.com.

warmers and incubators for temperature management in premature infants.[15]

Radiant warmers provide easy access for performing procedures—a definite advantage over incubators, in which procedures must be done through portholes. Advances in equipment technology now make it possible to convert a single unit from radiant mode to convection mode without moving the baby from one platform to another. This seems to be an efficient way to provide the improved access needed when a baby's condition changes while maintaining appropriate warming without the potential risks of moving the baby.[11] Fluid management is easier for infants in incubators because humidity is easily added to the enclosed environment and there are fewer losses from radiation and convection. The large flux of heat exchange between radiant heat source, the baby, and the environment makes wide fluctuations in heat balance more likely when compared with the more easily controlled temperature within an incubator. Many variables influence oxygen consumption using these two heating methods. The metabolic rate and oxygen consumption of infants under radiant warmers are slightly higher than in incubators; however, the clinical significance of this finding is uncertain. Infection rates are comparable between the two methods.[16] Regardless of the type of heat supplied, care must be taken to minimize thermal instability during nursing interventions. **Radiant warmers may be able to rewarm a baby faster than an incubator with convective heating after a procedure.** Organizing interventions so their frequency and duration limit as much as possible the exposure to a thermally unstable environment can minimize this instability. Box 6-4 outlines dos and don'ts when using a radiant warmer for providing heat.[9]

Other Methods

In the tiniest preterm infants, a conductive heat source (e.g., a heating pad) may also be needed to raise and maintain body temperature. Heated water mattresses provide a neutral thermal environment for less critically ill babies lying in open cribs (making access easier than in closed incubators). This may also provide a feasible and effective means of rewarming hypothermic infants. Heated, water-filled mattresses are most useful in the newborn units of developing countries.

Electric warming mattresses filled with water provide additional moist heat when caring for the infant in surgery, to use for rewarming techniques, or when caring for the LBW or ELBW infant. Manufacturer's recommendations should be followed, and the **temperature is usually set at**

BOX 6-4 USE OF OPEN RADIANT WARMER (RW): DOS AND DON'TS

Dos

1. Use the automatic mode (skin probe/servocontrol) for continuous thermal support.
2. Use the manual mode for short-term warming *only;* check the infant's condition and temperature at least every 15 minutes.
3. Place the sensor on the skin surface exposed to the warmer and never beneath the infant. (Follow manufacturer's recommendations.)
4. Check sensor attachments frequently. Poor skin contact causes poor temperature control.
5. Change temperature probe sites according to unit policy and manufacturer's recommendations.
6. Adjust fluid replacement to compensate for increased insensible water loss (IWL).

Don'ts

1. Don't forget to switch from manual to servocontrol after weighing the infant. When removing the infant from the RW, keep the bed on servocontrol and silence the alarm until the infant is returned to the RW.
2. Never use a rectal temperature probe for warmer control. Before normal core temperature is reached, the infant's skin may be burned.
3. Don't place anything flammable on top of or under the radiant warmer.
4. Never just reset alarms; instead, determine the cause of any alarms.
5. Never use your hand to estimate the amount of heat reaching the infant. Set temperature control point at 36.5° C.
6. Avoid use of thermal blankets (e.g., bubble wrap); may cause incorrect skin temperature sensing and overheating.

From Brown V, Gardner SL: *Neonatal thermoregulation: clinical practice tools and policy/procedure/protocol packets,* 2008, Nurse's Professional Development & Practice Association, LLC. Accessed August 5, 2009, from www.npdpa.com.

100° F. Heat is provided by conduction; therefore a linen layer should be placed between the mattress and the infant to avoid skin burns. The temperature of these mattresses should be weaned prior to weaning any temperature of the open warmer or incubator.

Some **portable, disposable, warming mattresses** containing a gel that is chemically activated by squeezing may be used for initial stabilization of the infant and for transport. Because heat is provided by conduction, a linen layer is placed between the infant and the mattress surface. **The usual temperature for these mattresses is 100° F.**

Heel warmers, which are pads that are chemically activated by squeezing, are used to warm the heels of infants before obtaining blood and are especially necessary when obtaining capillary blood gases. The temperature should never exceed 104° F.

Swaddling materials include various types of infant wrappings (e.g., blanket, clothing, foil, or bubble wrap). The use of swaddling materials makes observation of the infant more difficult and blocks heat from overhead radiant warmers. **Before one wraps the infant in insulating materials, the infant must be warm, because these merely retain body warmth and do not generate heat.**

Oxygen and air delivered to the neonate should be warmed and humidified to minimize convective and evaporative heat loss (see Chapter 23).

Skin-to-skin (kangaroo) care provides a safe and effective alternative method of caring for premature infants. Both appropriate-for-gestational-age (AGA) and SGA infants experience a beneficial warming effect and a stable skin and core temperature when held skin to skin.[14] **Mothers exhibit thermal synchrony with the infants so that their body temperature increases or decreases to maintain the infant's thermal neutrality.** Regardless of the care provider (e.g., father, adoptive parent, grandparent) during skin-to-skin care, heat loss does not occur and temperature rises and can be maintained in acceptable parameters (see Chapter 5). In one study, each mother's skin temperature met the neutral thermal environmental zone of her particular infant. Mothers also preferred this method for holding their infant, compared with the traditional method of wrapping the infant in a blanket and the infant being cradled in the parent's arms. Heat loss may occur during the transfer process from bed to parent. Having a protocol in place that uses one or more staff to help with the transfer and covering the infant with a blanket will reduce the transfer time and subsequent heat loss[14] (see Chapter 13).

Skin-to-skin contact between mother and infant reduces conductive and radiant heat loss and is an excellent way to maintain a neutral thermal condition for the healthy newborn. If the infant remains with the parents for an extended time, temperature should be monitored. In the case of a preterm infant in stable condition, the use of an additional heat source (e.g., a radiant warmer) enables parents to spend more time with their infant before transfer to the NICU. Skin-to-skin contact should be delayed at least until week 2 of life in extremely premature infants, because they have been shown to lose heat during skin-to-skin contact during the first week of life.

Bathing is important for removing blood and body fluids from the newborn's skin, to prevent the transmission of infections, and to promote bonding. Sponge bathing is traditionally done in the NICU and newborn nursery and can result in significant heat loss. **Immersing the stable infant in a tub of water reduces evaporative heat loss and helps maintain a normal temperature.**[6,8]

Transport

The same principles of heat balance that apply to infants in a NICU apply to infants during transport. Infants should have a normal and stable temperature before transport. The infant should be transferred from nursery to transport incubator rapidly to prevent prolonged exposure to an uncontrolled thermal environment. Transport incubators that can provide thermal stability inside the transport vehicle must be used. Oxygen provided during transport also should be warmed and humidified. The infant's temperature should be monitored continuously or at least every 30 minutes. Thin plastic wrap may be useful in decreasing IWL and convective and radiant heat loss. Chemically heated mattresses can also be used to provide a short-term heat source.

After Cesarean Delivery

Most cesarean section (C-section) deliveries are performed using an epidural or spinal anesthesia so the mother is awake and able to hear her infant as soon as he or she is born. Once the baby is assessed after birth, he or she is then placed skin-to-skin on the mother's chest and both are wrapped with a warm blanket. When the infant recovers in the same room as the mother, skin-to-skin contact and bonding are facilitated.[16] If the mother is unable, the father may provide skin-to-skin care and keep the baby warm after C-section (see Chapter 5).

Providing Thermoregulation for the Surgical Patient

The chilled environment of the surgical suite poses extra challenges to the newborn for thermoregulation. Heat losses occur by (1) evaporation during surgery, (2) conduction when placed on cold surfaces, (3) convection with cold drafts around the infant,[19] and (4) radiation of heat from opened body cavities. Coordination between neonatal and surgical staff will be necessary to prevent heat imbalance, as follows:

- Prewarm transport incubator.
- Use portable, disposable mattresses in the incubators and on the operating table.
- Use radiant heat in the operating suite.
- Wrap the infant's extremities in warmed soft cotton material.
- Prewarm all surfaces, as well as all fluids for cleansing and irrigation of body cavities.
- IV fluids should be at room temperature and prewarmed if stored in refrigeration.
- Temperatures should be monitored/documented before, during, and after surgery.

DATA COLLECTION

Anticipation and early recognition of the infant at risk for temperature instability are important in the management and prevention of complications associated with both hypothermia and hyperthermia. The perinatal history and ongoing neonatal evaluation identify events and early risk factors of temperature instability.

History

Events during pregnancy and the early neonatal period may increase an infant's risk for thermal instability. Review of the maternal history should include estimated date of confinement because preterm infants at delivery are at increased risk for hypothermia. Exposure to viral agents (e.g., herpes), as well as vaginal and cervical colonization, increases the risk for acquiring an infection before or during delivery (see Chapter 22). Intrapartal use of analgesics and anesthetics may depress the infant's CNS and mute the thermoregulatory ability.

Fetal stress manifested as fetal decelerations, meconium-stained fluid, or low Apgar scores may suggest an impaired thermoregulatory response. Neonatal interventions that may depress the CNS and thermal response include resuscitation and administration of analgesics, anesthetics, or neuromuscular blocking agents. Invasive procedures (e.g., endotracheal intubations, umbilical catheterization) increase the infant's risk for infection and need for prolonged use of antibiotics. Poor handwashing by care providers also may contribute to infectious nursery outbreaks, such as outbreaks of necrotizing enterocolitis (see Chapters 22 and 28).

Physical Examination: Signs and Symptoms

Physical assessment of the infant should include not only gestational age but also appropriateness of size. Evaluation of the infant's neurologic status (e.g., tone, activity, alertness) may give the caregiver an indication of the extent of neurologic impairment. Hypotonia results in decreased flexion, with an increased exposed surface area and resultant heat loss.

TEMPERATURE DETERMINATIONS

Temperature determinations may need to be made as often as every 30 minutes until thermostability is achieved. After that, temperatures should be recorded every 1 to 3 hours in LBW and preterm infants and every 4 hours in the healthy term infant. Critically ill infants should have continuous monitoring of skin temperature, with axillary determinations every 1 to 2 hours.[4] Documentation should include environmental temperature (e.g., air temperature in the incubator or radiant warmer settings). Measuring the skin and core temperatures simultaneously may help differentiate fever as a result of disease versus environmental overheating. Noting that the baby's servocontrolled skin temperature is relatively stable but that the environmental temperature has dropped also may be indicative of fever as the incubator responds to the high probe reading by cooling the infant's environment.

HYPOTHERMIA

As the infant attempts to conserve heat by vasoconstriction, he or she may be pale, appear mottled, and feel cool to touch, particularly on the extremities. Acrocyanosis and respiratory distress may occur as the infant increases oxygen consumption in an attempt to increase heat production. If hypothermia continues, apnea, bradycardia, and central cyanosis may occur. The hypothermic infant initially may be irritable but may become lethargic as cold stress continues. Other changes that may occur include hypotonia, weak cry, weak suck, increased gastric residuals, abdominal distention, and emesis. Infants generally do not shiver in response to cold stress, but shivering may occur in more mature babies in the presence of severe hypothermia. Chronic hypothermia may result in poor weight gain. (See the Critical Findings box below.)

HYPERTHERMIA

The hyperthermic infant may feel warm to touch, and skin color may be ruddy as the infant attempts to increase heat loss by vasodilation. Sweating may occur in a term infant but generally is not present in infants of less than 36 weeks' gestation. Sweating may first appear on the forehead, followed by the chest, upper arms, and lower body. Hyperthermia is manifested by irritability, lethargy, hypotonia, apnea, a weak or absent cry, or poor feedings. Tachypnea or tachycardia may be seen as the infant attempts to increase heat loss.

Infants with thermal instability should be closely watched for changes in behavior, feeding patterns, and respiratory status. Temperatures should be monitored frequently in any infant exhibiting these symptoms or who feels cool or warm to touch. Early recognition of thermal instability may prevent further consequences and possibly permanent injury or death. (See the Critical Findings box below.)

Laboratory Data

The following may be used to evaluate metabolic derangements associated with thermal instability:

- Arterial blood gases (to assess for hypoxemia and metabolic acidosis)
- Complete blood count (to assess for sepsis)
- Blood glucose level (to assess for hypoglycemia)
- Electrolytes, blood urea nitrogen (BUN), serum and urine osmolality (to assess hydration, acid-base balance, and renal function)

Critical Findings

HYPOTHERMIA

Critical assessment findings for hypothermia are as follows:

- Pale, mottled skin that is cool to touch
- Acrocyanosis
- Respiratory distress
- Apnea, bradycardia, central cyanosis
- Irritability initially
- Lethargy developing as hypothermia worsens
- Hypotonia
- Weak cry and suck
- Gastric residuals, abdominal distention, emesis
- Shivering in more mature babies
- Metabolic acidosis
- Hypoglycemia

TREATMENT AND INTERVENTION

Hypothermia

To avoid the complications of hypothermia, rewarming of cold infants should begin immediately by providing external heat. However, rewarming too rapidly may further compromise the already cold-stressed infant and result in apnea. Oxygen consumption is minimal when

Critical Findings

HYPERTHERMIA

Critical assessment findings for hyperthermia are as follows:

- Reddened skin that is warm to touch
- Tachypnea
- Tachycardia
- Irritability, lethargy, hypotonia, weak cry
- Poor feeding
- Apnea
- Sweating in more mature babies
- Dehydration

the difference between the skin and the ambient air temperature is less than 1.5° C (2.7° F). Avenues of heat loss should be blocked, temperatures should be monitored, and iatrogenic or pathologic causes should be investigated.

If hypothermia is mild, slow rewarming is preferred. External heat sources should be slightly warmer than the skin temperature and gradually increased until the neutral thermal environmental temperature range is attained. Efforts to block heat loss by convection, radiation, evaporation, and conduction should be initiated. Skin, axillary, and environmental temperatures should be measured and recorded every 30 minutes during the rewarming period. For more extreme hypothermia (i.e., core temperatures less than 35° C [95° F]), more rapid rewarming with radiant heaters (servocontrol 37° C [98.6° F]) or heated water mattresses prevents prolonged metabolic acidosis or hypoglycemia and decreases mortality.

Hyperthermia

The usual approach to treating the hyperthermic infant is to cool by removing external heat sources and by removing anything that blocks heat loss. The most common causes of hyperthermia in intensive care nurseries are iatrogenic. Check the heating controls for proper function and thermistors for proper position. Consider other sources of heat (e.g., direct sunlight, heaters, lights) as possible causes of hyperthermia. Excessive bundling with blankets and a hat and elevated environmental temperature can cause a newborn's body temperature to rise into the febrile range. When evaluating the treatment options in the hyperthermic infant, one should consider removing extra blankets or swaddling materials.[9] Nonenvironmental causes of hyperthermia (e.g., infection, dehydration, CNS disorders) should be considered. During the cooling process, skin, axillary, and environmental temperatures should be monitored and recorded every 30 minutes.

COMPLICATIONS

Hypothermia

Acute cold stress results in the release of norepinephrine, which causes vasoconstriction to reduce heat loss and initiate thermogenesis. As glycogen stores are depleted and oxygen consumption increases, the infant uses anaerobic metabolism to increase heat production, resulting in lactic acid production (metabolic acidosis). Pulmonary vasoconstriction, accentuated by metabolic acidosis, is associated with hypoxia, decreased surfactant production, and further acidosis (see Chapter 23). Blood flow to vital organs is diminished, and pulmonary hemorrhage and death may occur if hypothermia continues.

Hyperbilirubinemia and kernicterus may occur as non-esterified free fatty acids from brown fat metabolism compete with bilirubin for albumin-binding sites. Acidosis not only decreases the affinity of albumin for bilirubin but also increases the permeability of the blood-brain barrier, allowing bilirubin to enter brain tissue. If hypothermia continues, carbohydrate, protein, and fat supplies will be used for heat production instead of growth.

Close monitoring of the hypothermic infant is essential for early identification and prevention of complications. Evaluation of vital signs, arterial blood gases, and oxygen saturation may give early indication of hypoxia and metabolic acidosis. The infant's skin may be dusky or bright red because failure of dissociation of oxyhemoglobin occurs at low body temperatures. Respirations may be rapid, shallow, and grunting and accompanied by bradycardia. Oxygen and ventilation should be initiated as needed to reduce hypoxia. Sodium bicarbonate may be given to correct metabolic acidosis. Seizures may occur as a result of hypoxia, requiring the administration of anticonvulsants.

Intravenous glucose may be necessary to prevent or correct hypoglycemia. Blood glucose levels should be monitored hourly until stable (see Chapter 15). Blood pressure and urine output should be measured to evaluate hydration and kidney function. An elevated BUN and hyperkalemia may be indicators of decreased renal perfusion and impaired renal function. As fluid is retained, edema of the extremities and face may occur.

Bilirubin should be monitored on a regular basis, and phototherapy may be initiated at a lower-than-usual level to prevent kernicterus. Adequate nutrition to promote growth should be given either intravenously or enterally. While the infant is hypothermic, nipple feedings should be avoided to conserve calories and energy for heat production and growth and to avoid aspiration.

During the rewarming process, the hypothermic infant should be observed for hypotension as vasodilation occurs. Volume expanders may be needed to maintain an adequate blood pressure. Apnea and seizures may occur as a result of hypoxia or decreased cerebral blood flow after vasodilation. Hypothermia as a strategy to minimize adverse outcomes from hypoxic-ischemic-encephalopathy continues to be the focus of considerable research to determine safety and efficacy (see Chapter 26).

Hyperthermia

Vasodilation to increase heat loss may cause hypotension and dehydration as a result of increased IWL. Seizures and apnea may also occur as a result of high core temperature. Fluid status should be monitored by assessing intake, output, electrolytes, serum and urine osmolality, skin turgor, and mucous membranes. Fluids should be adjusted to account for IWL. Blood pressure should be assessed to detect hypotension, and volume expanders should be administered as needed.

Cardiorespiratory monitoring to detect apnea should be used. Ventilation may be needed if apnea persists or is unresponsive to stimulation. Subtle signs of seizures may include facial grimacing, nystagmus, tremors, apnea, opisthotonus posturing, tongue thrusting, or staring (see Chapter 26).

PARENT TEACHING

While the neonate is in the NICU, parents should be taught the importance of maintaining the newborn's normal body temperature. Temperature should be taken before parents touch the infant through the portholes of the incubator or hold their infant. While the infant is outside the incubator, monitor the skin temperature continuously with a telethermometer. Unwrapping the infant to check the temperature exposes him or her to cold stress. Additional heat sources (e.g., radiant warmer, hat, extra blankets) may be needed while parents hold the infant. Teach parents to monitor their infant's temperature and notify the nurse if it rises or falls. (See the Parent Teaching box above.)

Before discharge, teach parents to take an accurate axillary temperature and to notify their physician if it drops below 36° C (96.8° F) or rises above 37.8° C (100° F). A parent should not routinely take a rectal temperature. The temperature should be taken whenever the infant feels cool or warm to the touch. The nurse should observe the parents taking the infant's axillary temperature before discharge.

The home environment should be kept at a temperature that prevents heat and cold stress. A room temperature that is comfortable for the parent usually is suitable for the infant. The infant should be in clothing appropriate for the room temperature. For example, if the parent requires a sweater to be comfortable, then the infant probably also requires a sweater. Parents often overdress the infant or overheat the home, and this may cause hyperthermia. Parents should be given written instructions before discharge on how and when to take an axillary temperature, when to call the physician, and how to maintain a comfortable environment for their infant.

Parent Teaching

- Teach parents how to take an axillary temperature on their newborn and maintain the axillary temperature between 36.5° and 37.4° C (97.7° and 99.3° F).
- Teach parents how to dress their infant with clothes and blankets and use an appropriate environmental temperature to maintain the baby's temperature in the above range.
- Teach parents appropriate safety precautions, which include verbal and written information about recognizing signs and symptoms of a sick/ill infant, how the infant acts, including temperatures either higher than or, more commonly, lower than the range of 36.5° to 37.4° C (97.7° to 99.3° F).
- Teach parents to notify their infant's primary health care provider immediately or to take the infant to the nearest emergency department for temperatures out of the above range, especially if the baby's feeding pattern changes.

REFERENCES

1. Adamkin D, Carlo W, Dreyer G, et al: Thermoregulation. In *Neonatal clinical management guidelines*, ed 5, Upper Saddle River, NJ, 2007 Paradigm Health. Accessed August 5, 2009, from www.paradigmhealth.com.
2. Philip AG: The evolution of neonatology, *Pediatr Res* 58(4):799, 2005. Epub ahead of print, February 2005.
3. American Academy of Pediatrics: "Late-Preterm" infants: a population at risk, *Pediatrics* 120:1390, 2007.
4. American Academy of Pediatrics and American College of Obstetricians and Gynecologists: *Guidelines for perinatal care*, ed 6, Elk Grove Village, Ill, 2007, The Academy.

5. Reference deleted in proofs.
6. Bryanton J, Walsh D, Barrett M, et al: Tub bathing versus traditional sponge bathing for the newborn, *J Obstet Gynecol Neonat Nurs* 33(6):704-712, 2004.
7. Dollberg S, Mimouni FB, Weintraub V: Energy expenditure in infants weaned from a convective incubator, *Am J Perinatal* 21:253-256, 2004.
8. Flenady VJ, Woodgate PG: Radiant warmers versus incubators for regulating body temperature in newborn infants, *Cochrane Database Syst Rev* 4: CD000435 2005.
9. Gardner SL, Brown VD: *Clinical practice tools and policy, procedure, protocol packets: neonatal thermoregulation*, NPDPA, 2008. Accessed August 5, 2009, from www.npdpa.com.
10. Gaylord MS, Wright K, Lorch K, et al: Improved fluid management utilizing humidified incubators in extremely low birth weight infants, *J Perinatal* 21:438, 2001.
11. Greenspan JS, Cullen AB, Touch SM, et al: Thermal stability and transition studies with a hybrid warming device in neonates, *J Perinatal* 21:167, 2001.
12. Knobel R, Holditch-Davis D: Thermoregulation and heat loss prevention after birth and during neonatal intensive care unit stabilization of extremely low-birth weight infants, *J Obstet Gynecol Neonatal Nurs* 36:280, 2007.
13. Lenclen R, Mazaraani M, Jugie M, et al: Reducing heat loss in preterm infants at delivery with polyethylene bags, *Arch Pediatr* 9:238, 2002.
14. Ludington-Hoe SM, Morgan K, Abouelfettoh A: A clinical guideline for implementation of kangaroo care with premature infants of 30 or more weeks' postmenstrual age, *Adv Neonatal Care* 8:S3, 2008.
15. Maayan-Metzger A, Yosipovitch G, Hadad E, et al: Effect of radiant warmer on transepidermal water loss (TEWL) and skin hydration in preterm infants, *J Perinatal* 24:372, 2004.
16. Mellien A: Incubators versus mothers' arms: Body temperature conservation in very-low-birth-weight premature infants, *J Obstet Gynecol Neonatal Nurs* 30:157, 2001.
17. Motil KJ, Blackburn MG, Pleasure JR, et al: The effects of four different radiant warmer temperature set-points used for rewarming neonates, *J Pediatr* 84:546, 1974.
18. Sheldon B: An encapsulated history of thermoregulation in the neonate, *Neo Reviews* 5:78, 2004.
19. Sinclair JC: Servo-control for maintaining abdominal skin temperature at 36° C in low birth weight infants, *Cochrane Database Syst Rev* 1: CD001074, 2002.
20. Toubas PL, Nelson R: The role of the French midwives in establishing the first special care units for sick newborns, *J Perinatal* 22:75, 2002.
21. Vohra S, Roberts R, Zhang B, et al: Heat loss prevention (HELP) in the delivery room: a randomized controlled trial of polyethylene occlusive skin wrapping in very preterm infants, *J Pediatr* 145:750, 2004.

7 PHYSIOLOGIC MONITORING

WANDA TODD BRADSHAW AND DAVID T. TANAKA

Significant advances in the management of the ill newborn have been made in the past 50 years. The clinical usefulness of the umbilical vein was first demonstrated by Diamond in 1947 to perform an exchange transfusion to prevent kernicterus. Later, James used the umbilical artery for acid-base determination. In most neonatal intensive care units (NICUs), use of these catheters has become the standard of care to assess blood gases, measure arterial and central venous pressures, administer medications and fluids, and obtain laboratory samples. The development of small indwelling peripherally inserted central catheters provides a route for administering the above mentioned items and may be used for laboratory sample withdrawal if no other method of obtaining blood is available. Because of the frequency and clinical significance of complications, alternatives to these intravascular routes have been vigorously sought. The development of noninvasive physiologic monitoring devices has been a major step toward this goal. In addition, the use of point-of-care testing for various laboratory values is evolving in neonatal care. This chapter reviews the procedures and advances in physiologic monitoring.

PHYSIOLOGY

Pulmonary Physiology

Gas exchange takes place in the alveoli of the lung. Ventilation is the movement of air into and out of these air spaces. Diffusion is the movement of oxygen (O_2) from the alveolar space into the pulmonary capillary and the movement of carbon dioxide (CO_2) from the pulmonary capillary into the alveolar space for eventual exhalation. Pulmonary perfusion is the flow of blood through the pulmonary capillaries that surround the alveolar spaces. Once oxygen diffuses through the alveolar lining cells and into the capillaries, it is bound to hemoglobin within the red blood cell. Oxygen content in the arterial blood is the sum of the amount of oxygen dissolved in the plasma and the amount bound to hemoglobin. Approximately 3% of the oxygen content is dissolved in the plasma, with the remaining 97% bound to hemoglobin. $Pa{O_2}$ is the partial pressure of the oxygen dissolved in the plasma. Fetal hemoglobin has a higher affinity for oxygen than does adult hemoglobin; therefore, at any given $Pa{O_2}$, more oxygen is bound to adult hemoglobin (Figure 7-1).

Oxygen saturation ($Sa{O_2}$) is the percentage of oxygen bound to hemoglobin. $Pa{CO_2}$ is the partial pressure of carbon dioxide in the blood.

Noninvasive Blood Gas Monitoring

OXYGEN

Noninvasive monitoring of oxygenation can be accomplished by using two monitoring technologies. ***Oxygen saturation monitoring*** is the most common and widely used method for assessing oxygenation status. Transmission technology relies on a pulsating arterial vascular bed between a dual light source and a photoreceptor.[30] As blood passes between the light source and the photoreceptor, different amounts of red and infrared light are absorbed, depending on the amount of oxyhemoglobin and reduced hemoglobin. With reflectance oximetry, the emitter and receptor are located beside each other. Emitted light is reflected back to the photoreceptor. This method uses the core body to obtain oxygen saturation and is useful when the patient's peripheral blood flow is diminished. **With both methods, the difference in light absorption is electronically processed and displayed by the monitor as the percentage of**

Please note that the PURPLE type in each chapter is intended to make it easier to identify clinically applicable material.

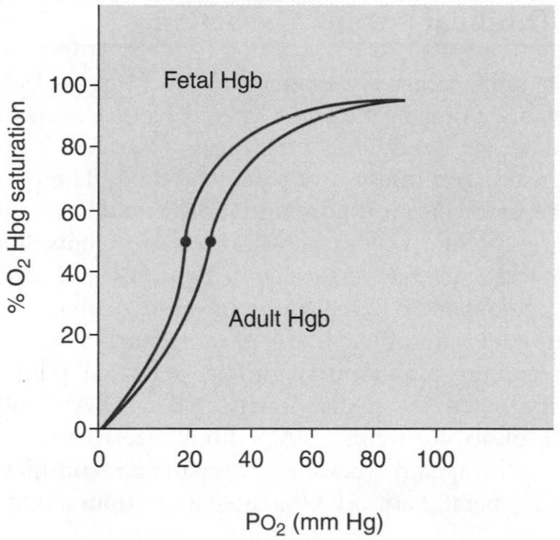

FIGURE 7-1 Oxygen dissociation curves for fetal hemoglobin *(Hgb) (left)* and adult hemoglobin *(right)*.

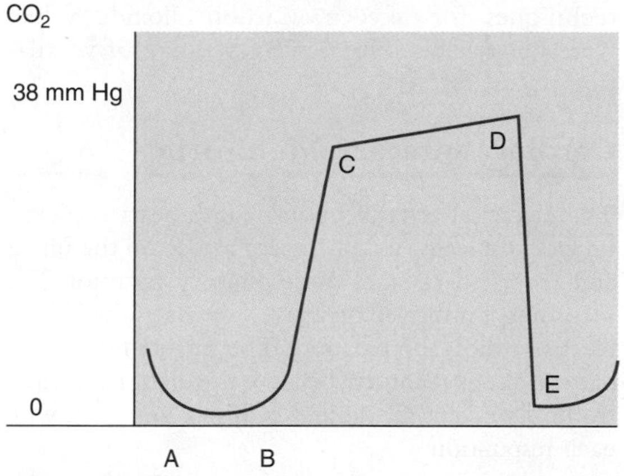

FIGURE 7-2 Variations in the content of carbon dioxide during phases of the respiratory cycle. **A,** End of inspiration. **B,** Beginning of exhalation. **C,** End of mixed gases washout (dead space and alveolar gases). **D,** End of expiration of alveolar gases. **E,** Inspiration.

arterial hemoglobin oxygen saturation expressed as ***Spo₂***.[30] **Pulse oximetry probes are easy to apply and require no calibration or application of heat.**

The second method of noninvasive monitoring of oxygenation is ***transcutaneous oxygen tension,*** which relies on the principle of oxygen diffusing from the skin capillaries through the dermis to the surface of the skin. To measure the oxygen, it is necessary to have adequate perfusion of the site, to intermittently calibrate the sensor, and to heat the skin, which then dilates the local capillaries and arterializes the capillary bed, as well as promotes faster diffusion of the oxygen from the skin.[31]

CARBON DIOXIDE

As with noninvasive monitoring of oxygen, carbon dioxide also can be assessed using two types of monitors. ***Transcutaneous carbon dioxide ($Ptcco_2$)*** monitoring works under similar principles as for transcutaneous oxygen monitoring. The probe is a glass pH electrode that detects changes in pH caused by CO_2. Heating of the probe enhances CO_2 diffusion, providing a better correlation between the probe value and the $Paco_2$ value.[20] The second method used to measure the content of the carbon dioxide in the respiratory gases during the respiratory cycle is ***end-tidal carbon dioxide ($Petco_2$)*** monitoring, also called ***capnometry.*** With capnometry, an infrared light absorption determines the amount of CO_2 present in the sample.[22] **Capnography provides a visual graphic curve of $Petco_2$.**[42] The carbon dioxide content varies widely with the phase of the respiratory cycle. During inspiration, there are minimal amounts of carbon dioxide, whereas at the end of expiration, the carbon dioxide values are at their maximum level (Figure 7-2). Until recently, the relatively fast respiratory rate of newborns, combined with the small tidal volumes, resulted in inaccurate values when measured by end-tidal carbon dioxide monitors. Advances in technology have improved the reliability of this monitoring technique for newborn infants.

COMBINED OXYGEN–CARBON DIOXIDE MONITORING

$Spo_2/Ptcco_2$ sensors combining pulse oximetry and transcutaneous carbon dioxide monitoring have been developed. The heated sensor is attached to the patient's ear. It provides rapid Spo_2 values followed by carbon dioxide information within minutes as the site is warmed and arterialized. A single probe, designed to withstand motion artifact and low perfusion states, leads from the patient to the monitor. Because the probe is attached to the ear, its removal for chest radiographs or prone positioning is not necessary. Studies on normal volunteers, neonates, and very-low-birth-weight (VLBW) infants have shown acceptable correlation with both invasive and noninvasive monitoring techniques for oxygen. Carbon dioxide values were less reliable but allowed trending of ventilation status.[4,25,40]

Cardiorespiratory Monitoring

The electrical activity of an infant's heart is picked up by chest leads (usually three) placed on the infant and recorded by a cardiorespiratory monitor. The recording is displayed on a visual screen as the infant's electrocardiographic pattern. The infant's respiratory pattern also is recorded, because the chest leads electronically detect movement of his or her chest with each respiration.

Blood Pressure Monitoring

Systolic blood pressure (measured in millimeters of mercury [mm Hg]) is the pressure at the height of the arterial pulse and coincides with left ventricular systole. Diastolic blood pressure (measured in mm Hg) is the lowest point of the arterial pulse and coincides with left ventricular diastole. Mean arterial pressure is the diastolic pressure plus one-third the pulse pressure. Central venous pressure is the pressure in the right atrium and may be approximated by the blood pressure (volume) in any of the large central veins.

Point-of-Care Testing

Point-of-care testing (POCT) involves testing performed at or near the patient rather than in a laboratory. This process has steadily evolved from crude blood glucose determinations to numerous types of monitoring. Currently, whole blood glucose values, transcutaneous bilirubin, fecal occult blood, Nitrazine and gastric pH, urine dipstick, activated clotting time, hematocrit, some electrolyte values, and arterial blood gases are part of POCT for the neonatal population.

DATA COLLECTION

The indications for using the various techniques for physiologic data collection depend on the infant's clinical situation. When umbilical artery and venous catheters cannot or should not be inserted or when such devices need to be removed, other devices may be considered.

Umbilical Artery Catheters

An umbilical artery catheter (UAC) is placed in those infants requiring frequent arterial blood gas determinations, continuous monitoring of arterial blood pressure, and infusion of parenteral fluids. The practice of medication administration through a UAC varies.[37] Infants who are candidates for indwelling catheters include critically ill neonates and those with congenital heart disease or disorders that cause respiratory insufficiency (e.g., surfactant deficiency, meconium aspiration syndrome, persistent pulmonary hypertension, diaphragmatic hernia). Although use of an indwelling UAC allows arterial pressure monitoring and accessibility for parenteral infusions, it is generally not used for these indications alone.

Umbilical Vein Catheters

Umbilical vein catheters (UVC) are useful for exchange transfusions, central venous pressure monitoring, emergency administration of fluids or chemicals in delivery room resuscitation, and administration of parenteral fluids and medications in the NICU, as well as obtaining blood for laboratory analysis. More complications are associated with umbilical venous lines than with umbilical arterial lines, but the complications are less severe.[3] UVCs are being used with increasing frequency for initial management of extremely-low-birth-weight (ELBW) infants. Catheters used as umbilical lines are available as both single-lumen and double-lumen items. Double-lumen catheters permit the simultaneous administration of infusates and medications. A Cochrane review supported the reduced need for peripheral lines when multi-lumen UVCs were used.[23]

Noninvasive Oxygen–Carbon Dioxide Monitoring

Oxygen monitoring is indicated in infants receiving oxygen for any reason (see Chapter 23). Acute monitoring is used as a part of the management of acute respiratory disorders. Long-term monitoring is used to wean infants with chronic lung disease from oxygen therapy. Noninvasive oxygen monitoring is useful during transport, in emergency situations, and during procedures. However, this method provides no information on hemoglobin level, adequacy of ventilation, and oxygen delivery to the tissues and should be used as one part of total oxygenation and ventilation assessment. Even though oxygen saturation monitoring is used more, less variability in oxygen tension has been demonstrated when transcutaneous oxygen monitoring has been employed.[31] Carbon dioxide monitoring is useful for verifying that the endotracheal tube is in the trachea (end-tidal CO_2 monitoring) and for the infant with a respiratory disease in which retention of carbon dioxide may become clinically significant (end-tidal CO_2 and transcutaneous CO_2 monitoring).[12]

Cardiorespiratory Monitoring

Cardiorespiratory monitoring should be used in any infant who requires intensive or intermediate care or is at risk for apnea or rhythm disturbances.

Blood Pressure Monitoring

Blood pressure monitoring should be used in the infant requiring surgery and in the acutely ill infant with cardiorespiratory distress or any other illness in which hypotension may be a significant contributor to the pathologic state. Central venous pressure should be monitored in infants who may experience an excess or loss of blood volume.

INTERVENTIONS

Umbilical Artery Catheter Placement

PROCEDURE

Determine the size and length of the catheter to be inserted. For infants weighing more than 1250 g, use a 5 Fr catheter, and for infants weighing less than 1250 g, use a 3.5 Fr catheter. Figures 7-3 and 7-4 correlate total body length with the length of the catheter to be inserted. Whereas these charts have worked reasonably well in larger preterm and term infants, a new formula (4 × birth weight in kilograms + 7) resulted in significantly better placement in VLBW infants.[41]

Place the infant in a supine position on a radiant heater or in an incubator. Ensure continuous temperature monitoring. Skin temperature should remain between 36° and 37° C (96.8° and 98.6° F). Provide appropriate oxygenation and ventilation. Ensure cardiorespiratory and oxygen saturation monitoring. Restrain the infant's hands and feet to

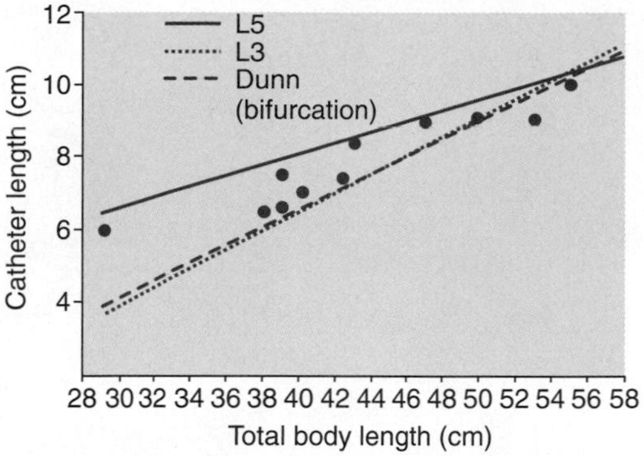

FIGURE 7-3 Graph for distance of catheter insertion from umbilical ring for low placement. (From Rosenfeld W, Biagtan J, Schaeffer H, et al: A new graph for insertion of umbilical artery catheters, *J Pediatr* 96:735, 1980.)

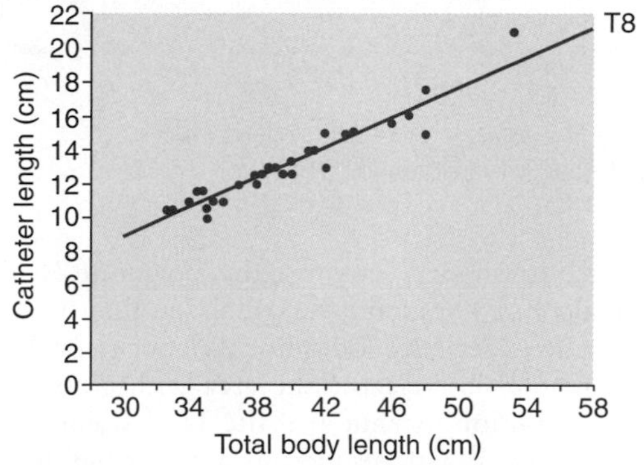

FIGURE 7-4 Graph for distance of catheter insertion from umbilical ring for high placement (T8). (From Rosenfeld W, Estrada R, Jhaveri R, et al: Evaluation of graphs for insertion of umbilical artery catheters below the diaphragm, *J Pediatr* 98:627, 1981.)

prevent him or her from contaminating the sterile field and interfering with the placement procedure. Wear a hat and mask. Wash hands before and after the procedure. Open the catheterization tray; most units now use commercially available disposable trays. Catheterization tray contents are shown in Figure 7-5. Put on sterile gown and gloves.

Connect the catheter to the stopcock, and flush and fill the entire system, including the catheter, with flush solution. Turn off the stopcock to the catheter to prevent fluid from draining out of the catheter during insertion and securing of the catheter. Cleanse the cord and base of the umbilicus with a povidone-iodine swab three times, and allow

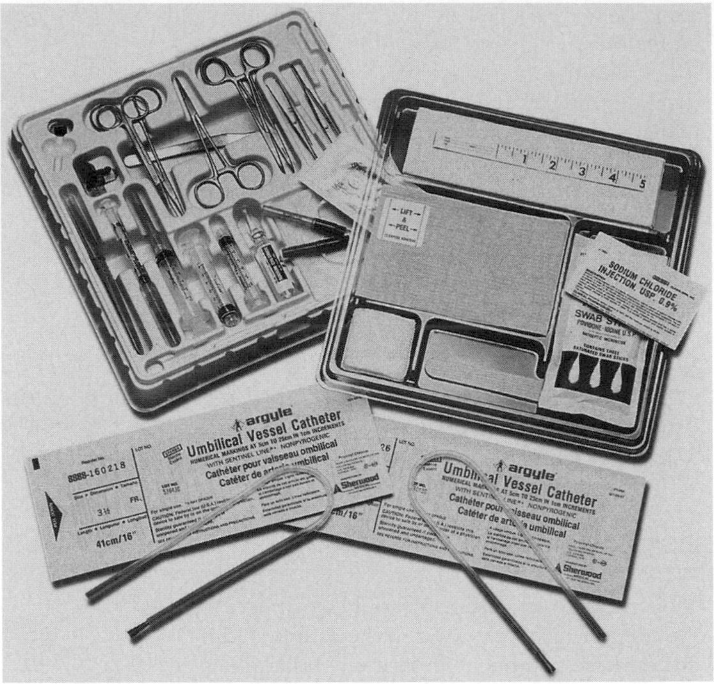

FIGURE 7-5 Argyle umbilical vessel catheter insertion tray. (Courtesy Tyco/Healthcare Kendall-LTP.)

the site to air-dry. Remove the povidone-iodine with alcohol. For infants weighing less than 1000 g, who may experience iodophor skin burns, or those with fragile skin, cleanse the area with povidone-iodine solution, permit the site to dry, and then remove the povidone-iodine with sterile water. Avoid using an excess of povidone-iodine solution so the infant is not lying in the solution during the procedure. Any residual iodophor should be washed off the infant carefully after the procedure is completed.

Drape the infant by placing an eye sheet over the umbilicus. An alternative method is to use sterile drapes, as follows:

1. Hold the diagonal corners of one drape, and allow the top half to fold over the bottom half. The result is a V shape.
2. Place the tips of the V on either side of the umbilicus.
3. Repeat with another drape and place on the other side of the umbilicus. The umbilical stump is now visible, yet surrounded by drapes.

After the UAC is inserted, the drapes can be removed easily without the need to pass the stopcock and catheter through an eyehole of a drape or cut or tear the eyehole drape. Ensure that the infant's head and feet remain visible during the procedure to assess his or her color. A small eye drape with adhesive backing (Steri-Drape) has the advantage of being transparent, so that the infant's color can be seen and temperature can be maintained. Towel drapes may interfere with a radiant heat source used for temperature regulation.

Place an umbilical cord tie (e.g., umbilical cord tape) around the base of the cord to control bleeding. A single overhand knot is preferred because it allows tightening as needed. Using tissue forceps, pick up the cord and cut it with a scalpel about 1 to 1.5 cm above the base. Arterial spasm allows only minimal bleeding. Identify the vessels. There are usually two arteries and one vein. **The arteries are small, thick walled, and constricted. The vein is larger, thin walled, and usually gaping open.** If the vein is at the 12 o'clock position, the arteries are usually at the 4 and 8 o'clock positions (Figure 7-6).

Stabilize the umbilical stump by grasping the cord between the thumb and index finger or grasping the edge of the stump with a mosquito hemostat. Ensure that the hemostat does not crush the umbilical vessels. With iris forceps, dilate one of

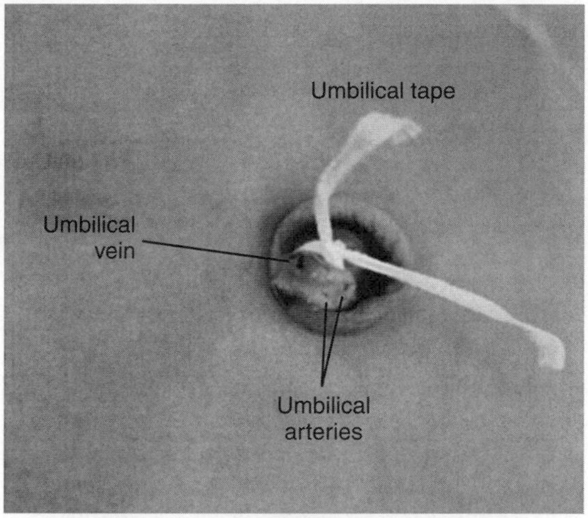

FIGURE 7-6 Umbilical tape and position of umbilical vessels.

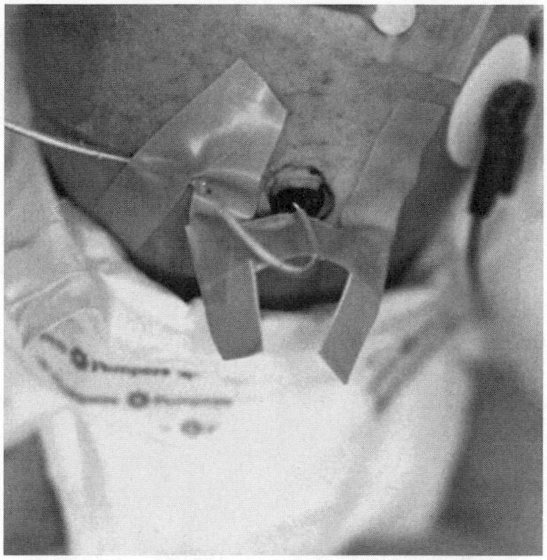

FIGURE 7-7 Umbilical artery catheter secured in "goalpost" design.

the arteries by placing the tips of the forceps in the artery and gently allowing them to spring open. This procedure may need to be repeated several times. In ELBW infants, the artery may be so small that it may be necessary to initially insert one forceps tip and then both to dilate the artery. While grasping one side of the wall of the dilated artery with small forceps, gently insert the catheter. An alternative method is to insert the catheter between the open prongs of the forceps used to dilate the artery. Instructional aids such as Baby Umb (Medical Plastics Laboratory, Inc., Gatesville, Tex.) and the Umbilical Artery Catheterization Slide-Tape Neonatal Educational Program (Charles R. Drew Postgraduate Medical School, Los Angeles, Calif.) are helpful. As the catheter passes into the artery, resistance may be encountered at several points, as follows:

- At the umbilical cord tie (tape): The tie (tape) may be tied too tightly. Loosen slightly.
- At the point at which the umbilical artery turns downward (caudal) into the abdomen: Steady, gentle pressure is important because forceful pressure may cause the catheter to perforate the artery wall and create a false channel.
- At the point at which the umbilical artery joins the external iliac artery: Once again, steady gentle pressure is important.

Insert the catheter to the predetermined length. Aspiration on the syringe should provide immediate blood return. Lack of blood return may indicate the following:

- The catheter is not inserted far enough. Insert farther.
- The vessel wall has been perforated, or a false channel has been created. If the catheter has pierced the vessel wall, repeat the procedure using the other artery.
- The catheter is kinked. Pull back slightly and then advance.
- The stopcock is turned off. Correct the stopcock position. Return aspirated blood to the infant; then clear the catheter with flush solution.

Observe the infant's lower extremities and buttocks for signs of vascular compromise. If any blanching or blueness is seen, follow the steps outlined in the Complications section (see pp. 148-149). Secure the catheter by suturing it to the umbilical stump and by the use of an adhesive-type tape after using skin prep to protect the skin. The most common taping method is the "goalpost" (Figure 7-7). Connect the stopcock to the intravenous (IV) solution, and set the prescribed infusion rate on the infusion pump. Ensure that no air is in the tubing, stopcock, or catheter. All connections must be secure. Automatic infusion pumps must be used for UACs because arterial pressure must be overcome to permit IV fluid infusion. Determine catheter placement

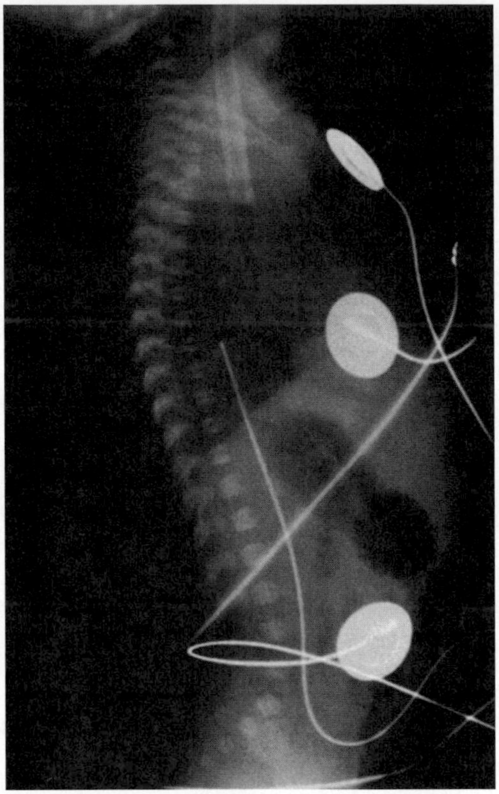

FIGURE 7-8 High catheter demonstrating "leg loop."

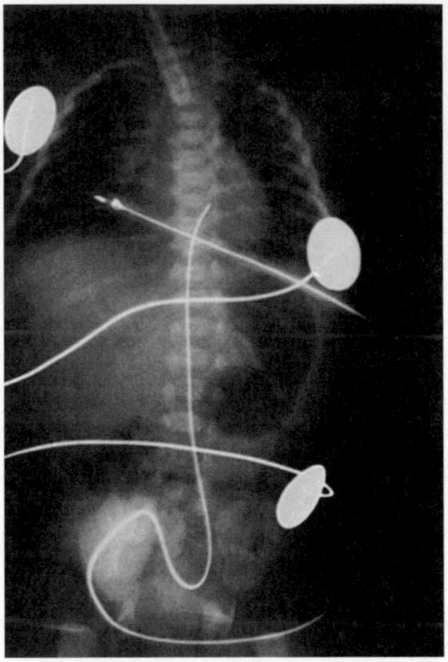

FIGURE 7-9 Umbilical artery catheter in high position (T8).

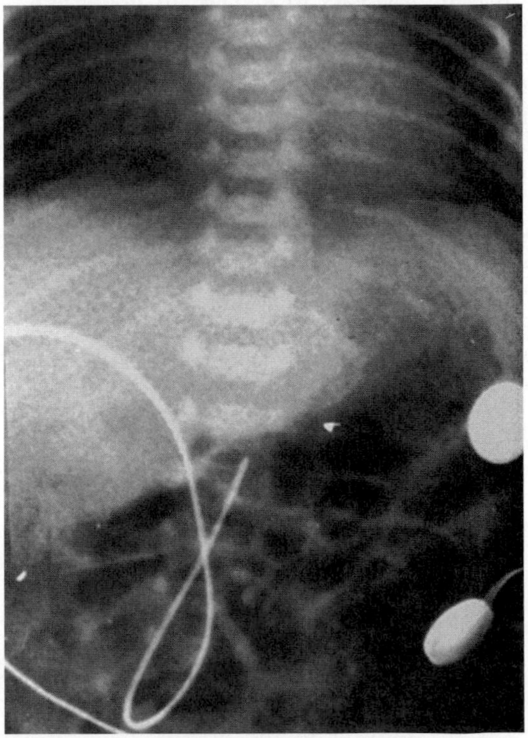

FIGURE 7-10 Umbilical artery catheter in low position (L3).

by an x-ray examination (abdominal, chest, or "babygram" depending on placement of the catheter). Figure 7-8 shows how the UAC appears on a lateral x-ray film.

Note that the catheter enters the umbilicus and travels inferiorly before turning superiorly. This "leg loop" is characteristic of an arterial catheter. A UAC follows the aorta and is positioned slightly to the left of the patient's vertebral column. **Optimal placement is below the renal arteries and above the aortic bifurcation (L3 to L4) for a low catheter and below the left subclavian artery and above the diaphragm (T7 to T9) for a high catheter.**[3] Exclusive use of high UACs is supported by Cochrane review because ischemia is significantly less frequent and duration of catheter use is prolonged with high catheter position.[3] Figure 7-9 shows high catheter placement, and Figure 7-10 shows low catheter placement.

If the catheter is too high, measure on the x-ray film the distance from the tip of the catheter to the desired level and pull the catheter back the appropriate distance. Some clinicians multiply this length by 0.8 to account for the magnifying effect of the x-ray film. If the catheter is placed too low, the catheter cannot be advanced but must be removed and replaced because the external portion of the original catheter is no longer sterile. Remove the umbilical cord tie (tape) or maintain the tie very loosely so as not to obstruct blood flow to the umbilical area.

TEACHING MODEL

The umbilical cord can be used for teaching the procedure of both arterial and venous catheterization. Many of the steps can be effectively carried out using a fresh placenta.

Special UACs and monitors are available for continuous Pao_2 or oxygen saturation monitoring.

NURSING CARE AND USE OF UMBILICAL ARTERY CATHETERS

Infants can be positioned on their sides or their backs. The abdominal position may be avoided because accidental slipping, kinking, and removal of the catheter may occur without being immediately apparent. If the abdominal position is used, the catheter should be monitored continuously; ensure pressure alarms are on with parameter settings that would rapidly detect pressure changes. Care needs to be taken so that the infant is positioned to prevent dislodgement of the catheter. Diapers are effective for preventing the feet and toes from becoming entangled in the catheter. The diaper is folded below the umbilicus. If the infant is receiving phototherapy and thus is not diapered, leg restraints or positioning aids may be indicated. A mitten or positioning aids are useful to prevent hands and fingers from contacting the catheter. Positioning the catheter away from the extremities lessens the chance of accidental dislodgement. **A dressing over the umbilicus is unnecessary; dressings inhibit inspection of the umbilicus and evaluation of the catheter.** The IV tubing, connecting tubing, and stopcock should be changed daily. Clots form in the stopcock, so changing it daily prevents the likelihood of embolus formation. Blood backing into the catheter can be caused by the following:

- Increased intraabdominal pressure, commonly caused by vigorous infant crying
- Disconnection of tubing or a loose connection
- Stopcock turned in wrong direction
- Infusion pump malfunction
- A leak in the filter or tubing or a crack in the stopcock

Drawing blood samples from an umbilical catheter is a sterile procedure. Samples may be obtained for blood gas analysis and to obtain laboratory specimens. Necessary items include a syringe for initially aspirating IV fluid and blood from the catheter, a heparinized blood gas syringe (if a blood gas sample is to be obtained), a syringe for aspirating laboratory samples (if laboratory samples are to be obtained), and a syringe containing flush solution.

PROCEDURE FOR DRAWING AN ARTERIAL BLOOD GAS SAMPLE

The reinfusion method of obtaining blood samples is described. This practice involves returning the "discard" blood and, in theory, minimizes patient blood loss.[16] Remove the stopcock cap and place it down so that sterility will be maintained. Attach the empty aspiration syringe to the stopcock. Turn off the stopcock to the IV solution so that the IV solution stops flowing. Aspirate 1 to 2 mL from the catheter into the dry aspiration syringe (Figure 7-11). The IV fluid is prevented from infusing, and aspiration clears the catheter of its IV fluid. Turn the stopcock to the neutral position (Figure 7-12), remove the syringe keeping the tip sterile, and replace it with the heparinized blood gas syringe or laboratory sample syringe. The neutral position of the stopcock

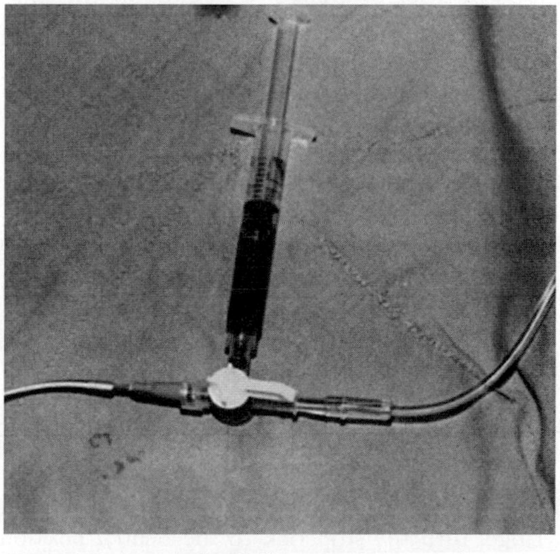

FIGURE 7-11 Stopcock off to IV solution; 1 to 2 mL aspirated into syringe.

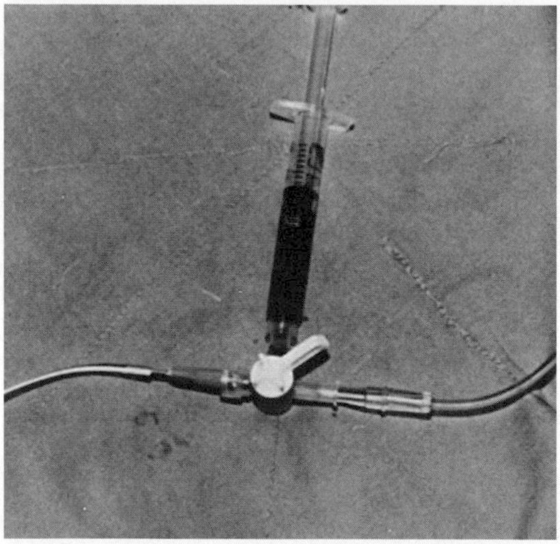

FIGURE 7-12 Stopcock in neutral position.

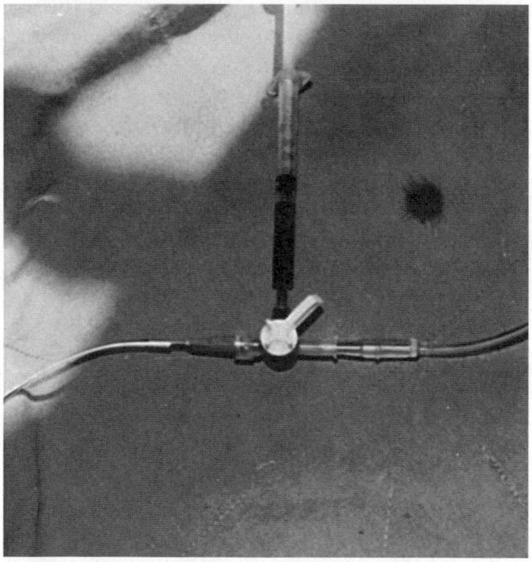

FIGURE 7-13 After blood is aspirated into heparinized 1-mL syringe, stopcock is placed in neutral position before syringe is removed.

prevents contaminating the sample with IV fluid and prevents blood loss from the infant.

CAUTION: Never allow blood to drip from an open stopcock. Turn the stopcock off to the IV fluid. Using steady, even pressure, aspirate blood into the heparinized blood gas or laboratory sample syringe. Turn the stopcock to the neutral position, and remove the syringe (Figure 7-13).

For blood gas samples, remove any air from the syringe, cap the end, and chill it to preserve values. Attach the aspiration syringe containing the aspirated blood and IV fluid. Slightly aspirate to remove any air in the stopcock, and then slowly infuse the aspirated blood and IV fluid. Turn the stopcock to the neutral position, and remove the aspiration syringe. Replace the now-empty aspiration syringe that had aspirated blood and IV fluid in it with the syringe filled with flush solution. Turn the off stopcock to the IV fluid. Slightly aspirate to remove any air in the stopcock, and then slowly infuse the flush solution until the catheter is clear. Return the stopcock to the off position, allowing the IV fluid to now infuse. Replace the stopcock cap. Record the amount of blood removed from the infant and the amount of flush solution used to clear the catheter.

To ensure the integrity of all connections, the stopcock and other connections must be visible at all times. Do not place the stopcock and other connections under linen, because this would hamper the immediate detection of an accidental disconnection that would cause severe blood loss in the infant. Immediately remove any air in the tubing or catheter, because air is a potential embolus. It is best removed through the stopcock. If the air has passed the stopcock, it can be aspirated back into a syringe easily.

Obtaining an arterial blood gas specimen from a high UAC is better tolerated in premature infants when the entire procedure is done slowly. Research indicates that obtaining the gas within 20 seconds resulted in decreased cerebral oxygenated hemoglobin and tissue oxygenation index. This alteration was not seen when the procedure was carried out over a 40-second period.[18]

Umbilical Vein Catheter Placement

PROCEDURE

Determine the size and length of the catheter to be inserted. A 5 Fr catheter is normally used in the UVC placement procedure. The ELBW infant may require a 3.5 Fr catheter. To determine the length of the catheter to be inserted, the distance from the umbilicus to the sternal notch should be measured and multiplied by 0.6. Complete steps for the placement procedure are found in the Umbilical Artery Catheter Placement section on pp. 137-142. The only difference is that the vein is used instead of the artery. The vein is usually gaping open and does not require dilation. The catheter can be advanced to the desired position easily. The catheter should lie in the inferior vena cava with the UVC above the diaphragm but below the right atrium of the heart. Catheter position must be ensured. Historically, position confirmation was by radiologic examination, using the anteroposterior (AP) or lateral views. Echocardiography is useful in determining correct catheter tip placement and prevention of complications such as pericardial effusion and tamponade.[34] **UVCs do not have the "leg loop" found on the lateral x-ray film of UACs.** An umbilical venous catheter follows the inferior vena cava and is positioned slightly to the right of the patient's vertebral column. The catheter should be secured in the same manner as for an umbilical arterial catheter.

Peripherally Inserted Central Catheter

Peripherally inserted central catheters (PICCs) typically are inserted for the following:

- **Neonates who require intravenous access that is expected to be necessary for an extended period**
- **Neonates with limited access**
- **As a transition from umbilical catheters for neonates weighing less than 1000 g**
- **As a first-line catheter for neonates weighing 1000 to 1500 g**
- **Neonates with gastrointestinal anomalies, necrotizing enterocolitis, or gastrointestinal diseases that will require surgical correction**

PICCs have long been used to provide highly concentrated parenteral nutrition and hyperosmolar medications.[29] These catheters are relatively easy to insert, affordable, low maintenance, and preclude surgical placement of central venous catheters. Because of extensive dwell time, they significantly reduce or eliminate the need for repeated painful procedures such as peripheral venipunctures, thus improving patient and parent satisfaction. PICC lines that are placed in central veins have complication rates lower than those placed in noncentral veins. Complications include infection, extravasation, catheter migration, catheter breakage, and occlusion. Establishment of a PICC team to insert and manage these devices, catheter tip placement in the superior or inferior vena cava, and heparinized solutions have been shown to reduce complications.[26]

The insertion sites for PICC lines include the brachial cephalic veins, the axilla, the scalp vessels, and the saphenous veins. This sterile procedure can be performed when the neonate is on a radiant warmer or in an incubator.

PROCEDURE

For an arm or hand insertion, measure the distance from the insertion site to the axilla and then to 1 cm above the nipple line. If the catheter is to be inserted in the scalp, measure from the insertion site to 1 cm above the nipple line, and for a leg insertion, measure from the insertion site to 1 cm above the umbilicus or to the level of the inferior vena cava.

Determine the size and length of the catheter to be inserted—PICC and introducer: 24-gauge, 8-, 10-, or 30-cm catheter (Figure 7-14). Trimming the catheter is not recommended. Trimming removes the tapered tip that facilitates insertion. A eutectic mixture of lidocaine and prilocaine (EMLA) anesthetic cream or a local anesthetic can be used before the procedure is begun (see Chapter 12). Place the infant in a supine position on a radiant heater or in an incubator. Ensure continuous temperature monitoring. Skin temperature should remain between 36° and 37° C (96.8° and 98.6° F). Provide appropriate oxygenation and ventilation. Ensure cardiorespiratory and oxygen saturation monitoring. Restrain the infant's hands and feet to prevent him or her from contaminating the sterile field and interfering with the placement procedure, or swaddle the infant, with the site to be used exposed. For hand or arm insertion sites, turning the infant's head toward the insertion site will cause a slight occlusion of the jugular vein so that, as the catheter is passed into the subclavian vein, the risk for the catheter advancing upward into the jugular is diminished. Wear a hat and mask. Wash hands before and after the procedure. Open the PICC insertion tray; most units now use commercially available disposable trays. PICC insertion tray contents are shown in Figure 7-15. Open the PICC and introducer (if packaged separately from the PICC insertion tray). Put on a sterile gown and gloves. Connect a lipid-compatible T-connector extension tubing to a syringe of flush solution, and fill the entire apparatus.

Grasp the extremity to be used with sterile gauze so that an occlusive dressing can be applied to the distal part of the extremity, thus allowing manipulation of the extremity and precluding contamination of the insertion site by bacteria from distal sites. Cleanse

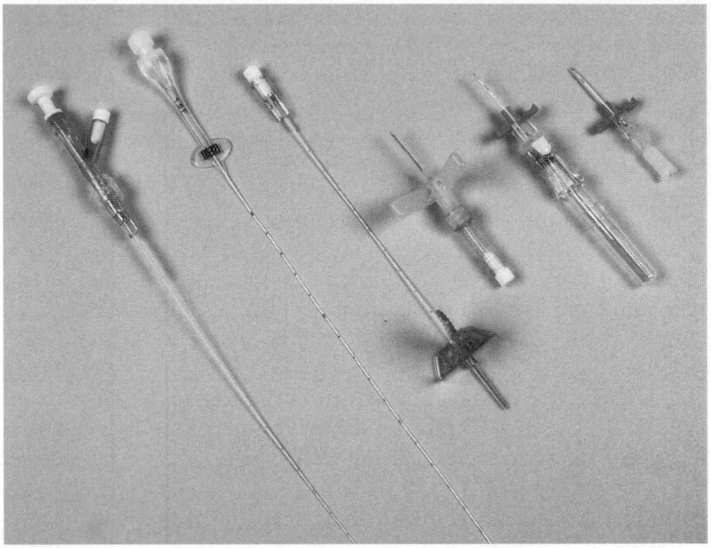

FIGURE 7-14 Peripherally inserted central catheters and introducers. (Courtesy Becton, Dickinson and Company, Franklin Lakes, NJ.)

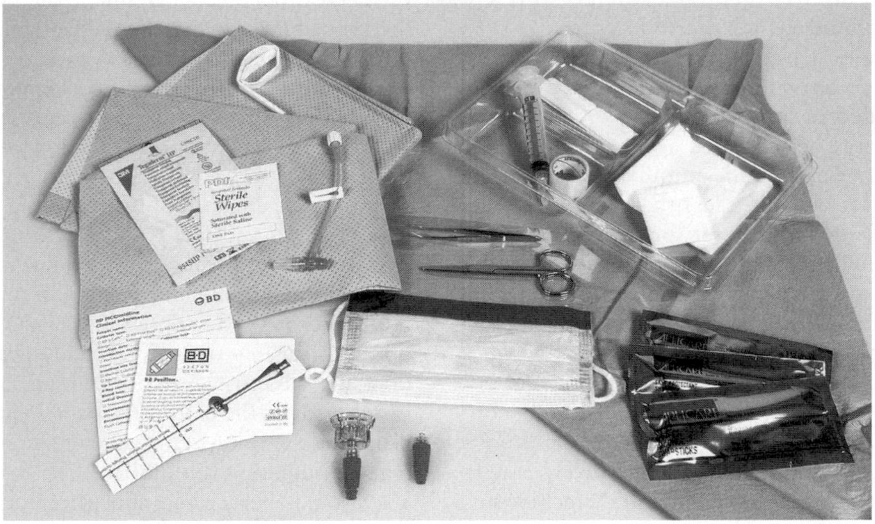

FIGURE 7-15 Disposable tray used for PICC insertion. (Courtesy Becton, Dickinson and Company, Franklin Lakes, NJ.)

the site with a povidone-iodine swab three times, and allow the site to air-dry. Remove the povidone-iodine with alcohol. For infants weighing less than 1000 g, who may experience iodophor skin burns, or for those with fragile skin, prepare the area with povidone-iodine solution, permit the site to dry, and then remove the povidone-iodine with sterile water. Avoid using an excess of povidone-iodine solution so the infant is not lying in the solution during the procedure. Any residual iodophor should be carefully washed off the infant after the procedure is completed. Place sterile drapes under the exposed insertion site. Re-glove with new sterile gloves. Place the introducer, catheter with stylet, syringe, and sterile forceps on the sterile field near the planned insertion site. Insert the catheter with stylet into the introducer, being cautious not to let the catheter with stylet extend beyond the tip of the introducer.

Insert the introducer tip at a flat angle to access the vein. The introducer is *not* advanced into the vein; it is used only as an introducer. At this point, there will probably be no blood return. Once the introducer is in the vein, pick up the catheter with stylet with the sterile forceps and gently advance the catheter with stylet to the premeasured length. Blood should fill the catheter. If the catheter is not advancing, pull the catheter back beyond the point of the introducer and reattempt to cannulate the vein. Once the catheter with stylet is advanced to the premeasured length, remove the stylet and attach an empty sterile syringe. Blood should be aspirated easily with a syringe. Flush the catheter with 0.5 to 1 ml of flush solution. Secure the catheter using sterile tape or nonfiber Steri-Strips at the insertion site. Wrap extra catheter material into a coil above or below the joint to prevent occlusion. Attach the lipid-compatible T-connector extension set, and secure it to the extremity. Dress the insertion site, extra catheter loops, and the PICC catheter to T-connector area with a sterile, clear, occlusive dressing. Ensure that the dressing does not completely encircle the extremity causing a tourniquet effect. Label the dressing with the gauge and length of the catheter, the line type (PICC), and the initials of the insertion person. **The occlusive dressing should be changed only when the integrity of the dressing has been lost.** A small amount of blood at the insertion site is not a reason to change the occlusive dressing. **Maintaining integrity of the occlusive dressing is instrumental in decreasing the risk for infection.**

Catheter position must be ensured by AP and lateral x-ray films, ultrasonography, or echocardiography.[28] For PICC lines inserted in the upper extremities, axillae, or scalp vessels, the catheter should lie in the superior vena cava above the right atrium of the heart. Catheters placed in other vessels have a significantly higher rate of thrombus formation and infection. For PICC lines inserted in the lower extremities, the catheter should lie in the inferior vena cava below the right atrium of the heart. Catheter placement in the right atrium can lead to complications of dysrhythmias, pleural effusion, and perforation with cardiac tamponade.[7]

PICC LINE DRESSING CHANGE

Changing the current dressing is indicated when it is no longer occlusive. The occlusive dressing is changed under sterile conditions. The person performing the dressing change wears a hat, mask, and sterile gloves. Changing the dressing entails removing the transparent film covering the area, cleaning the insertion site with povidone-iodine solution, allowing this to dry, and then cleaning the site with sterile water to remove the preparation agent from the skin. If the Steri-Strips or tape is no longer adhesive, they are replaced. Dress the insertion site, extra catheter loops, and the PICC catheter to T-connector area with a sterile, clear, occlusive dressing.[36] Ensure that the dressing does not completely encircle the extremity causing a tourniquet effect. Label the dressing with the gauge and length of the catheter, the line type (PICC), and the initials of the insertion person.

Removing Umbilical Arterial, Venous, and Peripheral Catheters

When the UAC, UVC, or PICC is no longer needed, it is removed. For UAC catheter removal, make certain the cord tie is snug. Sterile gauze is needed, and a suture removal kit should be available if the catheter was sutured in place. Turn off the stopcock to the patient and the IV fluid. Withdraw the catheter to 3 cm, and leave it in place for 30 minutes before withdrawing it completely. This procedure works well for infants with respiratory or abdominal issues because it avoids the application of external pressure to the abdomen. Alternatively, withdraw the catheter slowly over several minutes, allowing for the artery to spasm. Pinch the umbilical stump with the sterile gauze for 5 minutes until hemostasis is achieved. Observe the umbilicus for active bleeding or oozing. Observe the lower extremities and buttocks for diminished perfusion secondary to a thrombus or embolus. The procedure is similar for UVCs, with the exception that the catheter can be slowly withdrawn in one step. Pinch the umbilical stump with the sterile gauze for 5 minutes until hemostasis is achieved. Observe the patient for respiratory distress secondary to a pulmonary embolus. For PICC line removal, clamp the catheter, turn off the IV fluid infusion, and withdraw the catheter slowly and steadily. Apply pressure over the insertion site with the sterile gauze for 5 minutes until hemostasis is achieved. Ensure that the entire catheter was removed. Catheters that cannot be removed by traction necessitate invasive intervention for removal.[35] **All three types of lines require observation of the insertion site for bleeding.**

Noninvasive Oxygen–Carbon Dioxide Monitoring

END-TIDAL CARBON DIOXIDE MONITORING

End-tidal CO_2 monitors use either sidestream or mainstream analysis.[22] For sidestream analysis, the endotracheal tube has a second narrow lumen that opens at the end of the endotracheal tube. Gases are analyzed from samples taken from the end of the tube. The advantages of this system are that there is no increased dead space in the ventilator circuit and less chance of inspiratory gases contaminating the sample. The disadvantage to this method is that secretions may pool at the tip of the endotracheal tube and occlude the sampling port. The response time to changes in carbon dioxide content is slower than when mainstream analysis is used.

Mainstream analysis of carbon dioxide samples gases in the ventilator circuit. These gases are thought to be reflective of gases at the tip of the endotracheal tube. This method requires a separate chamber attached to the end of the endotracheal tube adapter, thus adding increased dead space and additional weight at the endotracheal tube adapter.

When sidestream and mainstream analyses of end-tidal CO_2 were compared, it was found that distal values were higher than proximal values and that distal values correlated more closely with $Paco_2$ values. This discrepancy was thought to result from the mixing of end-tidal gases with fresh gases in the ventilator circuit. In an infant with a large alveolar-arterial (A-a) gradient, $Petco_2$ monitoring cannot be relied on for accuracy. In premature infants, it may be useful if the lung disease is mild to moderate; in infants with normal lung function, this method is reliable.[5]

The waveform output of the end-tidal CO_2 monitor can be used clinically if the clinician understands how the waveform corresponds to the exchange of gases in the lung. **The waveform has a sharp rise on expiration that reflects the carbon dioxide content of various lung areas. This expiration is followed by a plateau that reflects the cessation of dead space gases and the measurement of alveolar gas. At the end of the plateau is a sharp drop that reflects the inspiration of fresh gases with minimal carbon dioxide content.** When using the monitor, the clinician should recognize that a sharp rise indicates compromised exhalation, such as in reactive airway disease. Partially plugged and dislodged endotracheal tubes will change the angle of rise on the capnogram. The plateau phase of the capnogram can be altered by severe hypotension or decreased cardiac output secondary to an altered minute ventilation-perfusion ($\dot{V}/\dot{Q}$) mismatch (as in pulmonary embolus, cardiac arrest, persistent pulmonary hypertension, atelectasis). No waveform or failure of the waveform to change indicates ineffective respiration (dislodged endotracheal tube).

TRANSCUTANEOUS OXYGEN–CARBON DIOXIDE MONITORING

Skin oxygen tension ($TcPo_2$) and carbon dioxide tension ($TcPco_2$) are measured by using one or two electrodes, depending on the model and brand of the monitor. The electrodes, once positioned on the skin, heat the area under the probe and cause certain physiologic changes as discussed. Oxygen and carbon dioxide that diffuse through the heated skin are measured by the electrode, and the value is digitally displayed on the monitor. **If intervals between calibration are longer than 4 hours, the readings are subject to drift.** The calibration procedures vary with the instruments used. Inherent in the calibration process is the necessity to change the position of the skin electrode on the infant. **Better correlations are found when the instrument is calibrated every 4 hours, the temperature is set correctly, and the infant is well perfused and normothermic.** If the temperature of the probe cannot be maintained at 43° to 44° C (109.4° to 111.2° F), a lower temperature should be selected to avoid possible burns. At a lower temperature, the $TcPo_2$ monitor can be used to monitor trends but should not be interpreted as actual Pao_2 values. The range of accuracy of $TcPo_2$ monitors is limited; hypoxia (<40 mm Hg) and hyperoxia (>120 mm Hg) may not be accurately reflected.

In an infant with suspected significant right-to-left shunting through a patent ductus arteriosus such as in persistent pulmonary hypertension, two transcutaneous oxygen electrodes can be placed on him or her: one preductally (right shoulder) and the other postductally (lower abdomen or legs). Significant right-to-left shunting through the patent ductus arteriosus is present when the preductal oxygen tension is significantly higher than the postductal oxygen tension.

The disadvantages of the use of transcutaneous monitoring are that the instrument requires frequent calibration, requires the use of a heated electrode, requires a 15-minute period after calibration to heat the skin to the correct temperature, and has a 15- to 20-second delay in the readings as compared with the patient's real-time values. The advantages are that it is not invasive, does not require the removal of blood for analysis, and displays a continuous readout of skin oxygen–carbon dioxide tensions.

NURSING CARE OF INFANTS WITH NONINVASIVE TRANSCUTANEOUS OXYGEN AND CARBON DIOXIDE MONITORS

The electrode can be placed on any portion of the infant's body as long as good contact between the electrode and the skin is maintained. Uneven areas of skin such as over bones and joints should be avoided because of poor contact between the membrane and the skin surface. The infant should not lie on the electrode. Placing the infant on top of the electrode increases the pressure on the underlying capillaries, thus affecting the flow of blood under the probe and resulting in a drop in $TcPo_2$ values. Because of the heat generated by the electrode (43° to 44° C [109.4° to 111.2° F]), small red areas resembling first-degree burns are produced on the infant's skin. **To minimize trauma to the infant's skin, the electrode should be repositioned every 2 to 4 hours, depending on his or her skin sensitivity.** Grouping of nursing interventions has resulted in minimizing the time that the infant receives less-than-optimal oxygenation.

Oxygen Saturation Monitoring by Pulse Oximetry

Oxygen saturation monitoring by pulse oximetry involves placing a small sensor on the infant in such a manner that his or her finger, toe, foot, or wrist comes between the light source and the photoreceptor. The light source emits wavelengths of light in the red and infrared spectrums. The difference between the absorption of the light is picked up by the receptor that is placed directly opposite the light source. The calculation of the ratio of oxyhemoglobin and deoxyhemoglobin is displayed as the percent of oxygen saturation. Key to accuracy of the monitor is that the light source and the receptor must be directly opposite each other over an area in which a pulse can be detected.

The monitor does not require any heat source or warm-up period, nor does it require calibration or changing of the probe position. Oxygen saturation monitoring provides continuous and instantaneous readout of the oxygen saturation in the infant. In comparison with a blood gas analyzer, which calculates the relative oxygen saturation based on established nomograms, **the oxygen saturation monitor measures the actual saturation of the hemoglobin.** Calculated values using standard nomograms do not reflect shifts in the affinity of oxygen for hemoglobin based on changes in the patient's temperature, pH, Pco_2, or 2,3-DPG.

The oxygen saturation monitor relies on adequate perfusion to the site and the ability to detect arterial pulsations; thus if it is placed distal to a blood pressure cuff, the reading will be inaccurate while the cuff is inflated. Newer models of pulse oximetry reduce the artifact that results from motion and low perfusion.[39] These newer models also are indifferent to ambient light, whereas older models were affected by light sources such as phototherapy. Newer neonatal probes have built-in external light source protectors. Pigmentation of the patient's skin may produce artificially high reading in pigmented individuals, especially at lower oxygen levels.[6,15]

Oxygen saturation is more indicative of the total oxygen content of the blood than is Pao_2 and is the most sensitive to hypoxemia when it is on the steep part of the oxygen dissociation curve (see Figure 7-1). **Keeping the Sao_2 at 90% to 92% keeps the infant in a normoxemic state under most conditions.** Oxygen saturation monitoring by pulse oximetry generally is considered reliable and practical for use in infants over a wide range of birth weights and postnatal ages.[1] Pulse oximetry saturation (Spo_2) values vary significantly from measured arterial tension values obtained with an arterial blood gas specimen.[32] A contributing factor may be that the calibration of pulse oximeters typically has been performed on healthy adult volunteers. A compelling argument for the use of both transcutaneous oxygen monitoring and pulse oximetry monitoring in critically ill neonates can be made, because each monitor has its own shortcomings.

Another consideration is the length of time an oximeter probe can be used. Because pulse oximetry monitoring is common in neonatal care and many infants in NICUs require prolonged monitoring, a long-lasting oximeter probe could offer a substantial cost savings.

No complications are associated with the use of oxygen saturation monitoring other than the potential for skin trauma caused by adhesive on the probe.

Newer probes held in position by gentle elastic pressure have no adhesive touching the infant's skin.

Cardiorespiratory Monitoring

The chest leads are applied in a triangular pattern on the infant's chest. Integrity of the leads must be ensured. Allowing the contact gel to dry or inadvertently dislodging the lead during procedures such as x-ray examination, echocardiography, and lumbar puncture may account for inaccurate tracings. Various components of the electrocardiogram (ECG) pattern may be diagnostically helpful. The QRS complex should be monitored for baseline height. **A sudden decrease in QRS complex height that is not caused by artifact may be an indication of pneumothorax.** The QT interval is helpful in diagnosing hypocalcemia in some infants. Other portions of the strip may be evaluated for electrolyte imbalance and possible cardiac ischemia. Changes registered on the visual display or strip recorder should be verified by a 12-lead ECG.

Blood Pressure Monitoring

Arterial pressure monitoring may be accomplished via the UAC attached to a transducer and monitor. Newer transducers require calibration only once daily. Central venous pressure (CVP) monitoring may be carried out in the same manner using the UVC. The same type of transducer may be used for either arterial or venous pressure recording.

Event Monitoring

The advancement of physiologic monitors with memory capability has enhanced the ability of the practitioner to review the physiologic status of the infant as measured by multiple physiologic parameters for the past 24 to 48 hours. In many NICUs, the monitor output is integrated into the electronic or computerized chart. This integration allows the care provider to "pull" the data from the monitors into the chart at preselected times, either prospectively or retrospectively. When the monitors are programmed with critical value ranges, any deviation outside these ranges is noted as an "event," which can then be reviewed, tallied, or otherwise annotated. For care providers at the bedside, the challenge is to keep iatrogenic events (e.g., lead removal, excessive activity of the infant, a stopcock turned the wrong direction) minimized such that the infant's record is as valid a reflection of actual physiologic status as possible. Any circumstances noted at the time of the event that may produce false readings should be recorded so that when the infant's record is reviewed, these events can be placed in context of the circumstances at the time.

Point-of-Care Testing

The Centers for Medicare and Medicaid Services regulate POCT through the Clinical Laboratory Improvement Act (CLIA).[10,11] These federal regulations require initial education about POCT procedures, as well as annual reassessment of competency. The quality of these tests is imperative to ensure proper diagnosis and treatment, and the CLIA regulations strive to ensure quality testing.

The accuracy of whole blood glucometers when compared with laboratory values may vary depending on hypoxia, hematocrit, and elevated triglyceride values. Accuracy also depends on the product that is being measured, because some glucometers measure glucose only, whereas others measure total sugars including glucose, galactose, maltose, and xylose. In addition, the clinician must remember that an **approximately 11% difference exists between plasma glucose (laboratory sample) and whole blood glucose (POCT device). The POCT value should be multiplied by 1.11 to determine a more approximate plasma value.**[14] A variance of accuracy also exists with bedside electrolyte assessment devices.[13] Transcutaneous neonatal bilirubin assessments require correlation between the serum bilirubin value and each device, institution, and patient population for which it is used.[9] As neonatal care advances, rapid availability of patient information will become more and more crucial. Expect expanded POCT in the future.

COMPLICATIONS

UACs act as foreign bodies, causing fibrin deposition and thrombus formation around the catheter. Although most catheters are associated with thrombus formation, it is of clinical significance in fewer than 10% of patients. (See the Critical Findings box on p. 149). **The most common problem associated with major complications of UACs is ischemic disease resulting from emboli or arterial spasms.**[17]

In such cases, the catheter should be removed immediately and antithrombin therapy should be considered. Although vasospasm is quite common, usually it does not require immediate removal of the catheter. Blue discoloration, commonly called "catheter toes," is seen, rather than blanching. Obviously, a hemorrhage may occur when the catheter slips out or when any of the various connections loosen. For reasons such as these, UACs **require constant attention.** If the lower extremities or buttocks blanch, the catheter should be removed immediately and antithrombin therapy considered. The benefit of antithrombin therapy must be balanced against the increased risk for intracranial hemorrhage. To prevent bleeding once the catheter is removed, pressure should be applied immediately below the umbilicus. When the color has returned to the affected area and the infant is stable, replacement of the catheter can be considered. **If vasospasm occurs in one leg or foot, apply warm wraps (diapers wetted with warm water or chemical heel warmers) to the opposite leg or apply wraps to the upper extremities, thereby producing a reflex vasodilation to the legs.** However, inherent in this action is the hazard of obscuring recognition of compromise in that extremity. The wraps should be reheated every 10 to 15 minutes until the spasm has resolved. The skin temperature of the infant must be greater than 36° C (96.8° F) for wraps to be effective.

UVCs may cause thrombus formation. Thrombi can result in pulmonary embolisms. Clots may form in the portal vessels, resulting in portal hypertension. Hepatic necrosis, gut ischemia, and hemorrhage have been associated with UVCs.[8] Other complications include dysrhythmias, myocardial perforation, pericardial effusion, and endocarditis. PICC lines are associated with occlusion, clotting, sepsis, malposition, cardiac tamponade, breakage, clotting, leaking, phlebitis, and peripheral edema.[28] Bacteremia, always a major concern, will require the removal of the catheter if the blood culture remains positive for more than 24 hours. Occlusion sometimes may be treated with clot-dissolving agents.[19] Clotting may be prevented with heparin or low-molecular-weight heparin.[27] **Transcutaneous blood gas monitoring may burn the skin.**

CONTROVERSIES

Clinicians continue to disagree on the optimal placement site for UACs. However, a Cochrane review and subsequent update determined that high UACs resulted in fewer vascular complications than did low UACs and recommended the exclusive use of high placement for UACs.[3] Prophylactic administration of antibiotic agents is not indicated. Use of the UAC for infusion of antibiotic agents, calcium, hyperalimentation solutions, or blood varies, and no

Critical Findings

COMPLICATIONS OF INDWELLING CATHETERS

- UACs
  - Ischemia from thrombi, emboli, or arterial spasms
  - Hemorrhage caused by catheter dislodgement or loose connections
  - Infection
  - Malposition
- UVCs
  - Thrombus formation leading to pulmonary embolization
  - Thrombus formation in portal vessels
  - Hepatic necrosis
  - Intestinal ischemia
  - Hemorrhage caused by catheter dislodgement or loose connections
  - Cardiac complications: dysrhythmias, myocardial perforation, pericardial effusion
  - Infection
- PICC lines
  - Occlusion
  - Clotting
  - Infection
  - Malposition
  - Cardiac complications: dysrhythmias, myocardial perforation, pericardial effusion
  - Breakage and leaking
  - Phlebitis
  - Peripheral edema

PICC, Peripherally inserted central catheter; *UAC,* umbilical artery catheter; *UVC,* umbilical vein catheter.

BOX 7-1 WHAT'S NEXT IN PHYSIOLOGIC MONITORING?

1. Esophageal pulse oximetry: Reflectance monitoring for patients undergoing prolonged procedures when Spo_2 monitoring is critical.[24]
2. Integration of biomedical sensors into textiles: Plastic optical fibers are integrated into common fabrics making data collection part of what is worn.[33]
3. An implantable pulse oximeter placed during an occurring surgical procedure to encircle an artery: It could provide surveillance of premature infants and optimize the timing for surgery in children with congenital heart defects.[32a]
4. Cerebral oximetry with near infrared spectroscopy to detect alterations in oxygenation before pulse oximetry.[38]

definitive studies are available. Blood cultures can be drawn from the UAC for up to 6 hours after insertion. The use of heparin in the infusate has been controversial, but a recent Cochrane review determined that use of heparin decreases catheter occlusion but not aortic thrombosis. In addition, heparin use in a flush solution alone is not beneficial in preventing catheter occlusion.[2] Enteral feeding with an umbilical line in place lacks definitive studies; however, this practice is more common than was previously thought. A recent study showed that **superior mesenteric blood flow in infants with an umbilical arterial catheter was not affected by trophic enteral feeding.**[21] Select NICUs provided trophic and more substantial enteral feedings with umbilical lines in place. **Routine monitoring of all infants is the standard of care.** Indwelling catheters for blood pressure monitoring have the advantage of continuous readout, but external cuffs are less invasive. There is a continued need for research into the efficacy and safety of umbilical catheters. Box 7-1 cites new research into future possibilities for neonatal physiologic monitoring.

PARENT TEACHING

Important elements of parent teaching are listed in the Parent Teaching box above. As with the many other invasive procedures in neonatology, the clinician obtains permission from the parents for umbilical vessel catheterization. This may be the clinician's first contact with the family and thus sets the atmosphere for future contacts. Although parents initially are hesitant about umbilical catheter placement, generally they are comforted to learn that it will result in a painless way of drawing blood; there are no nerves in the umbilical cord to sense pain. Before visiting the infant, providers need to inform parents about the technology that is being used to monitor their infant (i.e., umbilical catheter, transcutaneous monitors, cardiorespiratory monitors, blood pressure monitors) including what the technology is registering. Often parents are confused about where the catheter goes once it enters the umbilicus and the purposes of other monitoring devices.

Parents need to be instructed on how to hold their infant while an umbilical catheter is in place, because manipulating the infant may accidentally dislodge the catheter, resulting in blood loss and potential for infection. When the infant is being held out of the incubator and wrapped in blankets, the integrity of the catheter and connections are not easily evaluated. The parents' vigilance around the technology used on their infant could avoid these potential incidents.

Parent Teaching

1. Placement of umbilical lines is invasive. Educate parents about the following:
   - Placement is painless: the umbilical cord contains no nerves.
   - The point of catheter insertion and where the tip of the catheter is located.
   - The umbilical catheter can be used for numerous functions: administering IV fluid, medications, and blood products; monitoring; and obtaining laboratory specimens.
   - Care should be taken when holding or manipulating the infant to prevent catheter dislodgement and blood loss.
   - Holding the infant out of the incubator and wrapped in blankets obscures visualization of the catheter and connections.
2. The NICU environment can be frightening. Educate parents about the following:
   - The baby is being monitored by various methods including cardiorespiratory, blood pressure, and transcutaneous monitors.
   - The purpose and a short description of each monitor.

REFERENCES

1. Ahrens T: Monitoring carbon dioxide in critical care: the newest vital sign, *Crit Care Nurs Clin North Am* 16:445, 2004.
2. Barrington KJ: Umbilical artery catheters in the newborn: effects of heparin, *Cochrane Database Syst Rev* 4: CD00005072008 DOI:10.1002/14651858.CD000507.
3. Barrington KJ: Umbilical artery catheters in the newborn: effects of position of the catheter tip, *Cochrane Database Syst Rev* 4: CD0005052008 DOI:10.1002/14651858.CD000505.
4. Bernet V, Doll C, Cannizzaro V, et al: Longtime performance and reliability of two different $Ptc{CO_2}$ and $Sp{O_2}$ sensors in neonates, *Paediatr Anaesth* 18(9):872, 2008.
5. Bhat YR, Abhishek N: Mainstream end-tidal carbon dioxide monitoring in ventilated neonates, *Singapore Med* 49(3):199, 2008.
6. Bickler PE, Feiner JR, Severinghaus JW: Effects of skin pigmentation on pulse oximeter accuracy at low saturation, *Anesthesiology* 102(4):715, 2005.
7. Bowe-Geddes LA, Nichols HA: *An overview of peripherally inserted central catheters*, 2005. Accessed August 6, 2009, from www.medscape.com/viewarticle/508939.
8. Bradshaw WT, Furdon SA: A nurse's guide to early detection of umbilical venous catheter complications in infants, *Adv Neonatal Care* 6(3):127, 2006.
9. Carceller-Blanchard A, Cousineau J, Delvin E: Point of care testing: transcutaneous bilirubinometry in neonates, *Clin Biochem* 42(3):143–149, 2008. Accessed August 6, 2009, from www.ncbi.nlm.nih.gov/pubmed/18929553?ordinalpos=1&itool=EntrezSystem2.PEntrez.Pubmed.Pubmed_ResultsPanel.Pubmed_DefaultReportPanel.Pubmed_RVDocSum.
10. Centers for Medicare and Medicaid Services: *Clinical laboratory improvement amendments*, 2006. Accessed September 22, 2008, from www.cms.hhs.gov/clia.
11. Centers for Medicare and Medicaid Services: *Clinical laboratory improvement amendments*, 2006. Accessed November 12, 2008, from www.cms.hhs.gov/clia.
12. DeBoer S, Seaver M: End-tidal CO_2 verification of endotracheal tube placement in neonates, *Neonatal Netw* 23(3):29, 2004.
13. Dimeski G, Barnett RJ: Effects of total plasma protein concentration on plasma sodium, potassium and chloride measurements by an indirect ion selective electrode measuring system, *Crit Care Resusc* 7(1):12, 2005.
14. D'Orazio P, Burnett RW, Fogh-Anderson N, et al: Approved IFCC recommendations on reporting results for blood glucose, *Clin Chem Lab Med* 44(12):1486, 2006.
15. Feiner JR, Severinghaus JW, Bickler PE: Dark skin decreases the accuracy of pulse oximeters at low oxygen saturation: the effects of oximeter probe type and gender, *Anesth Analg* 105(Suppl 6):S18, 2007.
16. Frey AM: Drawing blood samples from vascular access devices: evidence-based practice, *J Inf Nurs* 26:285, 2003.
17. Furdon SA, Horgan MJ, Bradshaw WT, et al: Nurse's guide to early detection of umbilical arterial catheter complications in infants, *Adv Neonatal Care* 6(5):242, 2006.
18. Gordon M, Bartruff L, Gordon S, et al: How fast is too fast? A practice change in umbilical arterial catheter blood sampling using the Iowa Model for Evidence-Based Practice, *Adv Neonatal Care* 8(4):198, 2008.
19. Haire WD, Deitcher SR, Mullane KM, et al: Recombinant urokinase for restoration of patency of occluded central venous access devices: a double-blind, placebo-controlled trial, *Thomb Haemost* 92(3):575, 2004.
20. Hansen TN, Corbet A, Gest A, et al: Principles of respiratory monitoring and therapy. In Taeusch HW, Ballard RA, Gleason CA, editors: Avery's diseases of the newborn, ed 8, Philadelphia, 2005, Saunders.
21. Havranek T, Johanboeke P, Madramootoo C, et al: Umbilical artery catheters do not affect intestinal blood flow responses to minimal enteral feedings, *J Perinatol* 27(6):375, 2007.
22. Jaffe MB: Infrared measurement of carbon dioxide in the human breath: "Breathe-through" devices from Tyndall to the present day, *Anesth Analg* 107:890, 2008.
23. Kabra N, Kumar M, Shah S: Multiple versus single lumen umbilical venous catheters for newborn infants, *Cochrane Database System Rev* 20(3):2005 CD004498.
24. Kyriacou PA, Jones DP, Langford RM, et al: A pilot study of neonatal and pediatric esophageal pulse oximetry, *Anesth Analg* 107:905, 2008.
25. Lacerenza S, DeCarolis MP, Fusco FP, et al: An evaluation of a new combined $Sp{O_2}$/$Ptc{CO_2}$ sensor in very low birth weight infants, *Anesth Analg* 107(1):125, 2008.
26. Linck DA, Donze A, Hamvas A: Neonatal peripherally inserted central catheter team, *Adv Neonatal Care* 7(1):22, 2007.
27. Monagle P, Chalmers E, Chan A, et al: Antithrombotic therapy in neonates and children: American College of Chest Physicians evidence-based clinical practice guidelines, ed 8, *Chest* 133(Suppl 6):S887, 2008.
28. Paulson PR, Miller KM: Neonatal peripherally inserted central catheters: recommendations for prevention of insertion and postinsertion complications, *Neonatal Netw* 27(4):245, 2008.
29. Pettit J: Technological advances for PICC placement and management, *Adv Neonatal Care* 7(3):122, 2007.

30. Popovich DM, Richiuso N, Danek G: Pediatric health care providers' knowledge of pulse oximetry, *Pediatr Nurs* 30(1):14, 2004.
31. Quine D, Stenson BJ: Does the monitoring method influence stability of oxygenation in preterm infants? A randomised crossover study of saturation versus transcutaneous monitoring, *Arch Dis Child Fetal Neonatal Ed* 93(5):F347, 2008.
32. Quine D, Stenson BJ: Pao_2 values in infants <29 weeks of gestation at currently targeted saturations, *Arch Dis Child Fetal Neonatal Ed* 94(1):F515–F553, 2008. Epublished February. DOI:10.1136/adc.2007.135285.
32a. Reichelt S, Fiala J, Werber A, et al: Development of an implantable pulse oximeter, *IEEE Trans Biomed Eng* 55(2 Pt 1):581, 2008.
33. Rothmaier M, Selm B, Spichtig S, et al: Photonic textiles for pulse oximetry, *Opt Express* 16(17):12973, 2008.
34. Sehgal A, Cook V, Dunn M: Pericardial effusion associated with an appropriately placed umbilical venous catheter, *J Perinatol* 27(5):317, 2007.
35. Serrano M, Garcia-Alix A, Lopez JC, et al: Retained central venous lines in the newborn: report of one case and systematic review of the literature, *Neonatal Netw* 26(2):105, 2008.
36. Sharpe EL: Tiny patients, tiny dressings: a guide to the neonatal PICC dressing change, *Adv Neonatal Care* 8(3):150, 2008.
37. Smith L, Dills R: Survey of medication administration through umbilical arterial and venous catheters, *Am J Health Syst Pharm* 60:1569, 2003.
38. Tobias JD: Cerebral oximetry monitoring with near infrared spectroscopy detects alterations in oxygenation before pulse oximetry, *J Intensive Care Med* 23(6):384–388, 2008. Epublished September. Accessed August 6, 2009, from www.ncbi.nlm.nih.gov/pubmed/18794168?ordinalpos=3&itool=EntrezSystem2.PEntrez.Pubmed.Pubmed_ResultsPanel.Pubmed_DefaultReportPanel.Pubmed_RVDocSum.
39. Townshend J, Taylor BJ, Galland B, et al: Comparison of new-generation motion resistant pulse oximeters, *J Paediatr Child Health* 42:359, 2006 DOI:10.1111/j.1440-1754.2006.00873.x.
40. Weaver LK: Transcutaneous oxygen and carbon dioxide tensions compared to arterial blood gases in normals, *Respir Care* 52(11):1490, 2007.
41. Wright IM, Owers M, Wagner M: The umbilical arterial catheter: a formula for improved positioning in the very low birth weight infant, *Pediatr Crit Care Med* 9(5):498, 2008 DOI:10.1097/PCC.0b013e318172d48d.
42. Zwerneman K: End-tidal carbon dioxide monitoring: a vital sign worth watching, *Crit Care Nurs Clin North Am* 18(2):217, 2006.

8 ACID-BASE HOMEOSTASIS AND OXYGENATION

AMY M. WOOD AND M. DOUGLAS JONES, JR.

Examination of arterial blood gases and interpretation of acid-base balance are essential to proper diagnosis, management, and outcome in an ill neonate.[3,17,28] The measurement of arterial blood gases allows analysis of two interrelated but separate processes: acid-base homeostasis and oxygenation.[1,16,21] This chapter describes the parameters that designate these processes, their measurements, and the effects of proposed treatment on homeostasis.[1,28] Common abbreviations and their meanings are listed in Box 8-1.

Components of arterial blood gases include (1) actually measured values (Pao_2, $Paco_2$, and pH) and (2) calculations from these values (oxygen saturation, bicarbonate concentration, and base excess). Some analyzer systems also estimate hemoglobin concentration. The pH, $Paco_2$, base excess, and bicarbonate components are used to assess acid-base homeostasis,[16,21,31] whereas Pao_2, saturation (Sao_2), and hemoglobin[1,3] are used to assess adequacy of oxygenation (Table 8-1).

PHYSIOLOGY

Acid-Base Homeostasis

To review basic chemistry, an acid is a hydrogen ion donor and a base is a hydrogen ion receptor. The pH refers to the concentration of hydrogen ions $[H^+]$ in blood and reflects the acid-base balance in blood.[31] The quantity of hydrogen ions is minute, approximately 0.0000001 mole/L. Therefore the negative log of the hydrogen ion concentration is used to define pH and create a positive, workable number (pH = 7) (Equation 1). A pH of 7 represents a neutral solution, a pH of less than 7 represents acidity, and a pH greater than 7 represents alkalinity:

(1)

$$pH = -\log\left[H^+\right]$$
$$pH = -\log\left[0.0000001\right]$$
$$pH = -\left[-7\right]$$
$$pH = 7$$

The Henderson-Hasselbalch equation describes pH as equal to a constant (pK) plus the logarithm of the ratio of the base-to-acid concentration (Equation 2).[3,17] Thus if there is an increase in the concentration of hydrogen ions (reflected in the denominator), the blood pH value decreases and acidemia results. Conversely, if there is less acid or more base, pH increases and alkalemia results.[3]

(2)

$$pH = pK + \log\frac{\text{base}}{\text{acid}}$$

The first step in determining acid-base homeostasis is measurement of pH. Normal human pH is between 7.35 and 7.45. Acidemia and acidosis are often used interchangeably, but strictly speaking, pH of less than 7.35 is acidemia and the process that caused it is acidosis; a pH of greater than 7.45 is alkalemia and the process that caused it is alkalosis.[17] **Arterial carbon dioxide ($Paco_2$) and bicarbonate $[HCO_3^-]$ values represent the two main components of acid-base homeostasis: (1) respiratory contribution ($Paco_2$) controlled by alveolar ventilation,[1,8,11] and (2) nonrespiratory or metabolic contribution controlled primarily by renal excretion, retention, or production of $[HCO_3^-]$.[1,15,26] Other factors that affect nonrespiratory components of**

Please note that the **PURPLE** type in each chapter is intended to make it easier to identify clinically applicable material.

BOX 8-1 ABBREVIATIONS

A	Alveolar
a	Arterial
D	Difference
F	Fraction
I	Inhalation, inspired
P	Partial pressure (tension, driving force)
pH	Negative log of hydrogen ion concentration

Combined Abbreviations

PaO_2	Partial pressure of arterial oxygen
FIO_2	Fraction of inspired oxygen
PIO_2	Partial pressure of inspired oxygen

TABLE 8-1 NORMAL (ARTERIAL) BLOOD GAS VALUES

BLOOD GASES	VALUES
pH	7.35-7.45
$PaCO_2$	35-45 mm Hg
HCO_3^-	18-26 mEq/L
Base excess	(−5) to (+5)
PaO_2	60-80 mm Hg
O_2 saturation	92%-94%

acid-base balance cause a change in [HCO_3^-]; thus [HCO_3^-] is an indicator of the nonrespiratory component.[15,19,26]

RESPIRATORY CONTRIBUTION

Carbon dioxide is produced by each cell as a product of metabolism.[1,23] As carbon dioxide is produced, it dissolves in intracellular fluid and can be measured as the partial pressure (P) of the dissolved gas (CO_2). As the pressure of the dissolved gas increases inside the cell, carbon dioxide moves out of the cell into the blood. Blood transports dissolved carbon dioxide (some combined with hemoglobin as carboxyhemoglobin, most as bicarbonate) to the lung, where the partial pressure in the pulmonary capillary is greater than in the alveoli,[21] causing carbon dioxide to move into the alveoli. **Ventilation is the only method of removing carbon dioxide.** The amount of carbon dioxide in the blood is the net result of the body's metabolism (production) and alveolar ventilation (clearance). Because metabolism does not change greatly and CO_2 diffuses easily across membranes, the only clinically important limitation to CO_2 removal is at the lungs. **Thus $PaCO_2$ reflects alveolar ventilation.**[3,8,11,17]

In the red blood cell, the enzyme ***carbonic anhydrase*** promotes combination of a fraction of dissolved CO_2 with water to form carbonic acid (H_2CO_3), which then dissociates into a hydrogen ion [H^+] and a bicarbonate ion [HCO_3^-][1,23]:

$$\textbf{(3)}\quad CO_2 + H_2O \rightleftharpoons H_2CO_3 \rightleftharpoons [H^+] + [HCO_3^-]$$

Therefore an increase in $PaCO_2$ causes pH to fall. Hypoventilation causes an increase in carbon dioxide. **This is called *respiratory acidosis* because the respiratory system is responsible for regulating $PaCO_2$ as the lung regulates the amount of carbon dioxide in the body.**[8] A decrease in $PaCO_2$ results in less acid in the blood and causes pH to rise. **A pathophysiologic process that causes hyperventilation and reduces dissolved carbon dioxide is known as *respiratory alkalosis*.**

NONRESPIRATORY (METABOLIC) CONTRIBUTION

Nonrespiratory (metabolic) derangements can also disturb acid-base homeostasis. Normal metabolism produces hydrogen ions. Blood pH is maintained within normal limits by renal mechanisms for excreting hydrogen ions. **Increased production of [H^+] may occur in conditions such as shock with poor perfusion of the gastrointestinal system or genetically determined aberrations of metabolism.**[27] The hydrogen ions produced must be eliminated to avoid a fall in blood pH. Derangements also occur when hydrogen ions are lost (e.g., in gastric juice) or when bicarbonate is lost (e.g., in diarrheal fluid or ileostomy drainage).[28]

Authorities differ as to the best way to describe nonrespiratory derangements in acid-base status. The traditional approach relies on measurement of pH, PCO_2 and [HCO_3^-]. The alternative is description of acid-base status in terms of (1) strong ions (Na^+, K^+, Ca^{2+}, Mg^{2+}, Cl^-), strong because they remain dissociated at body pH, and (2) weak acids (hemoglobin, albumin, inorganic phosphate), weak because they are partially dissociated at body pH. **Blood pH in this conceptualization is a function of the**

	Respiratory parameter P_{CO_2}	Metabolic parameter HCO_3^-	Cause
Respiratory acidosis	⬆	↑	Hypoventilation
Respiratory alkalosis	⬇	↓	Hyperventilation
Metabolic acidosis	↓	⬇	Add acid or lose base
Metabolic alkalosis	↑	⬆	Add base or lose acid

FIGURE 8-1 Acid-base derangements. *Large arrow* indicates primary process that produces change in pH. *Small arrow* indicates compensatory process.

difference between strong cations and strong anions, the strong ion difference (SID). As an example, the alkalosis associated with loss of gastric fluid would be described exclusively in terms of loss of [Cl^-] with loss of [H^+] making no independent contribution to the resulting alkalemia. Advocates maintain that measurement of SID leads to greater understanding of the causes of nonrespiratory and mixed acid-base derangements.[7,12,14,23] Others favor staying with the traditional bicarbonate-center model.[6,18] The present discussion focuses on the traditional bicarbonate-centered approach. Readers are referred to recent reviews for comparisons of the two methods.[14,18]

A fall in blood [HCO_3^-] might indicate that bicarbonate, a base and therefore a hydrogen ion acceptor, has been used up by the addition of [H^+]. As shown in Equation 3, a change in [HCO_3^-] might also reflect a change in P_{CO_2}. This difficulty is overcome in blood gas analyzers by correcting the P_{CO_2} (graphically) to 40 mm Hg, yielding a "standard bicarbonate" concentration.[23] The standard bicarbonate concentration and the buffering properties of hemoglobin are combined in the concept of base excess (BE). A positive value suggests a deficit of fixed (i.e., not volatile as with H_2CO_3) acid or an excess of base; a negative value indicates an excess of fixed acid or a deficit of base.[23] An abnormality of the standard bicarbonate concentration or base excess indicates a process of nonrespiratory (metabolic) alkalosis[15] or nonrespiratory (metabolic) acidosis.[26]

In the Henderson-Hasselbalch equation (Equation 2), the pH is equal to a constant, pK, plus the logarithm of the base/acid ratio.[1,17,23] If we substitute [HCO_3^-] for the base and dissolved CO_2 for the acid,[8,23] multiplying CO_2 by its solubility coefficient (0.03 mEq/L/mm Hg), the equation becomes the following:

(4) $$\mathrm{pH} = \mathrm{pK} + \log\left(\frac{HCO_3^-}{(P_{CO_2} \times 0.03)}\right)$$

The value of pK is 6.1; normal [HCO_3^-] is 24 mEq/L, and normal Pa_{CO_2} is 40 mm Hg.

Substituting, we obtain the following:

(5) $$\mathrm{pH} = 6.1 + \log\left(\frac{20}{1.2}\right)$$

or

$$\mathrm{pH} = 6.1 + 1.3 = 7.4$$

Changes in the 20:1.2 ratio have profound effects on the pH.[1,17] The following are two examples:

1. Hypoventilation of sufficient degree that Pa_{CO_2} is doubled from 40 to 80 (respiratory acidosis) results in a ratio of 24:2.4, or 10. The logarithm of 10 is 1, and the pH would be 6.1 + 1, or 7.1.
2. If a metabolic acidosis reduced [HCO_3^-] from 24 mEq/L to 12 mEq/L, the ratio would be 12:1.2 or 10:1, and the pH would be 7.1.

MIXED CONTRIBUTIONS

Thus far, these derangements (Figure 8-1) have been discussed as if they happened in isolation, but combined respiratory and nonrespiratory problems often occur, depending on pathologic processes in the body. Besides the four single acid-base derangements, there are combined acid-base derangements: (1) respiratory acidosis and metabolic acidosis, (2) respiratory acidosis and metabolic alkalosis, (3) respiratory alkalosis and metabolic acidosis, and (4) respiratory alkalosis and metabolic alkalosis. The combined acidoses or combined alkaloses have a cumulative effect on the pH, whereas an acidosis and alkalosis combination tends to negate the effects of each on the pH value.[16,17,21,31]

COMPENSATION

Acid-base homeostasis maintains pH near the normal range. **Thus if either the respiratory or nonrespiratory acid-base system is "deranged," the other system will become "unbalanced" in the opposite direction to counterbalance the primary process.** The body attempts to maintain equilibrium by balancing a pathologic process with a physiologic process or predictable buffering response.[3,17,28] For example, any respiratory process that leads to retention of carbon dioxide (respiratory acidosis) stimulates a nonrespiratory system, in this case the renal system, to return pH toward normal. This occurs by renal retention of bicarbonate and corresponding excretion of hydrogen ions. Given sufficient time, this may increase blood bicarbonate by as much as 3 to 4 mEq/L for each 10 mm Hg increase in carbon dioxide. Thus a neonate with a chronically increased $Paco_2$ and a compensatory rise in bicarbonate may attain a near-normal pH.[17]

Metabolic compensations to respiratory processes can go to remarkable extremes, but respiratory compensations to metabolic processes are limited. Hyperventilation cannot lower the $Paco_2$ much below 10 mm Hg in compensation for a metabolic acidosis. Similarly, hypoventilation is limited in compensation for a metabolic alkalosis by the onset of hypoxemia.[28] Hypoxemia stimulates respiratory drive, overriding compensatory hypoventilation, limiting correction of alkalemia.[17]

CORRECTION

Correction of an acid-base disturbance occurs when the health care provider detects the pathophysiologic process and directs therapy at the primary pathologic process, rather than counterbalancing it with a second pathologic process.

For example, if a respiratory acidosis is present, the clinician assesses the patient to discover the cause of the carbon dioxide retention and directs therapy at improving the ventilatory capacity of the lung, rather than attempting to increase the retention of bicarbonate.

Oxygenation

The remaining components of the blood gas analysis are the Po_2, hemoglobin, and oxygen saturation.[21] Oxygenation is related to but also distinct from ventilation.[3] **The two main factors contributing to oxygenation at the tissue level are oxygen delivery and oxygen consumption.** Oxygen delivery is the product of the cardiac output and the oxygen carrying capacity of blood, whereas oxygen consumption is determined by the metabolic needs of the body's tissues. **Tissue hypoxia may be caused by many different factors that derange the balance between oxygen delivery and tissue needs. Inability of the lung to oxygenate the blood** would decrease oxygen delivery because of arterial hypoxemia. Another cause of tissue hypoxia is interference with blood flow, as in heart failure. The Pao_2 may be normal, but because of **heart (pump) failure,** oxygenated blood is not delivered in sufficient quantity. Treatment should be directed toward improving delivery by the pump (see Chapter 24). A third cause of tissue hypoxia is **decreased blood oxygen–carrying capacity as with anemia.** In this instance, the heart and lungs work adequately, so Pao_2 is normal but hemoglobin is insufficient to provide adequate oxygen. Finally, tissue hypoxia may result from an **abnormally high affinity of oxygen for hemoglobin.** Because oxyhemoglobin affinity is increased, oxygen will not dissociate from hemoglobin unless the venous, and therefore tissue, Po_2 falls to an unusually low level.[5]

Because Pao_2 measures only the partial pressure of oxygen in arterial blood (i.e., measures the amount of dissolved oxygen gas in the blood), it reflects lung function but not tissue oxygenation. Despite this, measurement of Pao_2 together with measurement of hemoglobin and clinical assessment of tissue perfusion is usually sufficient.[3] Two situations merit special comment. First, in a preterm infant whose retinal development is incomplete, high Pao_2 can lead to retinopathy of prematurity, especially at Pao_2 greater than 100 mm Hg (see Chapter 23). Second, in cyanotic congenital heart disease, there is a right-to-left intracardiac shunt that does not allow Pao_2 to rise despite administration of supplemental oxygen because a portion of venous return goes directly to the left side of the heart, bypassing the lungs. Low PaO_2 in these patients is not related to lung disease, although lung disease may complicate the picture.

Theoretically, in a **normal lung with perfectly matched ventilation and perfusion, the alveolar (PAO_2) and the arterial oxygen tension (PaO_2) should be equal.** This is not achieved. **A difference (gradient) exists between the PAO_2 and the PaO_2.** Minor mismatching of ventilation and perfusion leads to a functional intrapulmonary shunt. This creates an alveolar-arterial oxygen gradient (D[A-a] O_2).[3,8] However, a D(A-a)O_2 greater than 20 mm Hg indicates pulmonary disease.[3]

OXYHEMOGLOBIN SATURATION

Oxyhemoglobin saturation is the percentage of hemoglobin that is combined with oxygen. Oxygen binding with hemoglobin increases as the partial pressure of oxygen increases, but not linearly.[3,31] The oxygen dissociation curve is a measure of the affinity that hemoglobin has for oxygen (Figure 8-2).

The "30-60-90 rule" is useful in remembering percent saturation and reconstructing the adult hemoglobin dissociation curve if necessary (see Figure 8-2). At a PaO_2 of 30 mm Hg, the oxygen saturation is 60%; at a PaO_2 of 60 mm Hg, saturation is 90%; and at 90 mm Hg PaO_2, the hemoglobin is 95% saturated. At the normal venous oxygen tension of 40 mm Hg, the oxygen saturation is 75%. Factors that affect this affinity include temperature, pH, and hemoglobin structure. Hypothermia, alkalemia, hypocapnia, and fetal hemoglobin increase the affinity of hemoglobin for oxygen (shift the curve to the left), whereas fever, acidemia, and hypercapnia decrease the affinity of hemoglobin for oxygen (shift the curve to the right).

At a given tissue PO_2, an increased affinity for oxygen releases less oxygen at the tissue level, whereas a decreased affinity releases more oxygen to the tissue. Alternately, the PO_2 at which the oxygen-binding sites of hemoglobin are 50% saturated (the P_{50}) is low when the hemoglobin affinity is great and higher when the hemoglobin affinity is low.[3] **The affinity of fetal hemoglobin for oxygen is higher than adult hemoglobin (see Figure 7-1). The P_{50} of fetal hemoglobin is 19 mm Hg compared with a P_{50} of 27 mm Hg for adult hemoglobin. Approximately 70% of hemoglobin in term infants, and more in preterm infants, consists of fetal hemoglobin.[5] As a result, hemoglobin in a term infant with a PaO_2 of 35 mm Hg will be 80% saturated, and a "pink" newborn infant may have a very low PaO_2.**

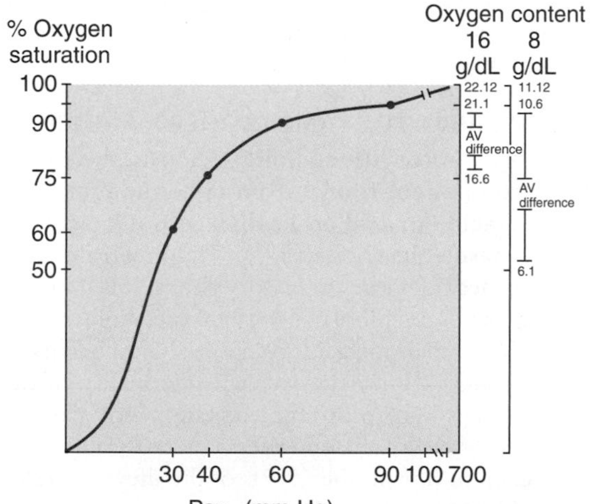

FIGURE 8-2 Oxygen hemoglobin dissociation curve; the 30-60-90 rule is demonstrated. *Right,* The oxygen content for a hemoglobin concentration of 16 and 8 g/dL is given, demonstrating the effect of anemia on venous saturation and tissue oxygenation.

OXYGEN CONTENT

Oxygen content is calculated from the hemoglobin saturation and hemoglobin concentration. One gram of hemoglobin binds 1.39 mL of oxygen. The oxygen content in milliliters per deciliter is the product of the saturation percentage and the hemoglobin in grams per deciliter plus the amount of dissolved oxygen. For clinical purposes, we can neglect the amount of dissolved oxygen in plasma, because it is only 0.003 mL/dL/mm Hg.

Oxygen content becomes critical in anemia, which can cause a significant derangement in tissue oxygenation unless organ blood flow and cardiac output increase to maintain the delivery of oxygen.[3,31] The blood of an infant with a hemoglobin of 8 g/dL will have half the oxygen content of that of an infant with a hemoglobin of 16 g/dL at an equivalent percentage saturation. In Figure 8-2, an infant with 16 g hemoglobin that is 95% saturated (PaO_2 = 90 mm Hg) carries 21.1 mL/dL oxygen, whereas the infant with 8 g hemoglobin carries 10.6 mL/dL oxygen. Tissues require approximately 4 to 5 mL/dL oxygen for metabolism. With normal cardiac output, venous blood contains 4 to 5 mL/dL oxygen less than the arterial blood. The venous oxygen content in an infant with 16 g hemoglobin would be between 16 and 17 mL/dL, which corresponds to approximately 75% saturation, or a Pvo_2 of 40 mm Hg. However, unless cardiac output increases, the venous oxygen content in an infant with 8 g hemoglobin would be 6.1 mL/dL oxygen. The saturation is 55%, which corresponds to a Po_2 of less than 30.

BLOOD FLOW AND SHUNTS

The product of oxygen content and blood flow returning from the lungs determines the total amount of oxygen in arterial blood. Total pulmonary blood flow can be divided into the amount of blood in pulmonary capillaries and the amount that is shunted through or around (i.e., through an intracardiac shunt) the lungs.

A right-to-left shunt occurs when blood passes from the systemic venous to the systemic arterial circulation without receiving oxygen. This can occur because of anatomic defects in the heart (e.g., cyanotic congenital heart disease) or because of blood perfusing alveoli that are not ventilated (e.g., intrapulmonary shunts). Shunts lower the final arterial oxygen saturation. The usual degree of shunt in a newborn is 15% to 20% of the cardiac output.

Acid-Base and Oxygenation Disorders

Ventilation is defined as the amount of gas leaving the mouth per unit of time (e.g., minute ventilation). Minute ventilation is equal to the product of the tidal volume and respiratory frequency in breaths per minute. Tidal volume can be divided into (1) gas in the airway plus the gas in nonperfused alveoli (this is called ***physiologic dead space***) and (2) gas in the alveolar space involved in gas exchange.[3,8] ***Alveolar ventilation*** is defined as the ratio of CO_2 production by the body to the $Paco_2$. **$Paco_2$ indicates the magnitude of alveolar ventilation and is inversely related to it such that if $Paco_2$ doubles, alveolar ventilation is one half of the original value. If the $Paco_2$ triples, alveolar ventilation in one third of the original value, and so forth.**[1]

RESPIRATORY ACIDOSIS

When the lungs become less effective at removing carbon dioxide, $Paco_2$ increases and respiratory acidemia ensues. Causes of respiratory acidosis can be separated into pulmonary and nonpulmonary causes.[8] The most common pulmonary cause of respiratory acidosis is obstructive lung disease, such as meconium aspiration[30] and transient tachypnea[20] of the newborn. Obstructive lung disease is also found in the recovery phase of uncomplicated respiratory distress syndrome (RDS) and in bronchopulmonary dysplasia.[24] Also, included in the pulmonary causes of hypoventilation are conditions that interfere with expansion of the lungs, such as diaphragmatic hernia, phrenic nerve paralysis, or pneumothorax. These limit tidal volume.[8]

A nonpulmonary cause of carbon dioxide retention is poor respiratory effort. Decreased respiratory drive may be secondary to narcosis because of maternal anesthesia before delivery, depressed respiratory drive because of sepsis, intracranial hemorrhage, including intraventricular hemorrhage, and metabolic disturbances, such as hypoglycemia, affecting the respiratory center.[8]

RESPIRATORY ALKALOSIS

In respiratory alkalosis, carbon dioxide clearance is increased and thus $Paco_2$ is below normal.[11] Respiratory alkalosis occurs as a result of hyperventilation, which may be caused by (1) overly vigorous ventilator therapy; (2) central nervous system (CNS) stimulation of the respiratory drive (e.g., hyperammonemia from a genetic abnormality of the urea cycle)[4]; and (3) hypoxemia, which stimulates respiratory centers through chemoreceptors.[11]

NONRESPIRATORY (METABOLIC) ACIDOSIS

In nonrespiratory (metabolic) acidosis, the metabolic component results from either adding nonvolatile acid (an acid other than carbonic acid) or losing base (bicarbonate).[19,25,28] Nonvolatile acids include lactic acid in circulatory shock and hypoxia, organic acids in inborn errors of metabolism, and ketoacids in diabetic acidosis. Loss of base occurs in renal tubular acidosis (a defect in the ability of the renal tubules to reabsorb bicarbonate), with diarrhea with loss of bicarbonate in the feces, or through urinary excretion from the effects of the diuretic ***acetazolamide*** (Diamox).[26,27,29]

Measurement of the anion gap helps identify the mechanism of metabolic acidosis.[6,9,14,29] The anion gap is variably calculated as the serum sodium concentration minus the serum chloride concentration minus the serum bicarbonate concentration,[17,29] or, alternately, sodium plus potassium minus chloride minus bicarbonate.* The upper limit of the normal anion gap with the first method is given as 14 mEq/L[29] and with the second method as 15 mEq/L.[13] Addition of nonvolatile acids is associated with an increased anion gap. Loss of base or excess chloride [Cl^-] is the likely mechanism of acidosis with a normal anion gap.[23,29] An advantage of measuring the anion gap in understanding the effect of excessive chloride administration is clear. Given that there must be balance between blood cations and anions to preserve electroneutrality, [Cl^-] in excess simply displaces [HCO_3^-], resulting in metabolic acidosis.[29] In normal anion gap acidosis, low serum potassium indicates loss of base (e.g., diarrhea) and high serum potassium points to a renal defect (e.g., renal tubular acidosis).[17]

Albumin is a major component of the anion gap. Hypoalbuminemia, common in critically ill neonates and children, may mask the presence of the anions of lactic and organic or other nonvolatile acids.[6,7,9,13,17] A "normal" anion gap in combination with low serum albumin indicates that a nonvolatile acid anion is making up the difference for "absent" anions that albumin would ordinarily provide. Thus hypoalbuminemia may hide a metabolic acidosis. Correcting the anion gap for hypoalbuminemia is accomplished by adding 2.5 mEq/L to the anion gap for every g/dL that the concentration of serum albumin is reduced below the normal value of approximately 3.5 g/dL.[6,27]

NONRESPIRATORY (METABOLIC) ALKALOSIS

Nonrespiratory (metabolic) alkalosis is caused by either a loss of acid or addition of base, principally bicarbonate.[15] Bicarbonate addition is probably iatrogenic secondary to administration of sodium bicarbonate. Alkalosis also occurs when excessive amounts of acetate, citrate, or lactate are given; metabolism of these anions in the liver generates bicarbonate. Loss of acid occurs with nasogastric suctioning or prolonged vomiting with pyloric stenosis. Acid loss by renal mechanisms can occur through the influence of diuretics, digitalis, and corticosteroids.[11] Urine electrolytes, especially chloride, are useful in the differential diagnosis of metabolic alkaloses. Low urine Cl^- (<20 mEq/L) is associated with chloride (saline)-responsive metabolic alkalosis from acid loss (e.g., vomiting, nasogastric suction), whereas high urine Cl^- is associated with chloride (saline)-unresponsive metabolic alkalosis from renal acid loss (e.g., diuretics).[9,17]

OXYGENATION

Although delivery system failure (heart failure), anemia, abnormal hemoglobin affinity for oxygen, and hypoxemia (decreased Pa_{O_2}) may cause tissue hypoxia, hypoxemia results only from lung disease or cyanotic congenital heart disease. **The most common lung abnormality is mismatched ventilation and perfusion.**[3] Perfect matching of ventilation and perfusion would occur if all alveoli were perfectly oxygenated and ventilated and supplied with an appropriate amount of pulmonary capillary blood. This ideal situation rarely applies. There is always some degree of ventilation and perfusion mismatch. **Two extreme examples are (1) ventilated and oxygenated alveoli without perfusion (e.g., pulmonary emboli) and (2) perfused but nonventilated alveoli (atelectasis).** The former is an example of wasted ventilation, and the latter represents an intrapulmonary shunt. Either extreme is incompatible with life. Clinically relevant degrees of ventilation-perfusion mismatch lie somewhere between those extremes.[3]

Hypoxemia resulting from ventilation-perfusion mismatch can be overcome with supplemental inspired oxygen. An increased inspired oxygen concentration will eventually displace nitrogen from even the most poorly ventilated alveoli, and alveolar and then arterial oxygen tension will increase. However, an extrapulmonary shunt bypasses the lungs. Pa_{O_2} cannot increase. This is why placing a neonate in 100% oxygen helps separate lung disease from cyanotic congenital heart disease as a cause of hypoxemia.

To perform the ***"shunt test,"*** the caretaker should place the hypoxemic neonate in 100% oxygen; if Pa_{O_2} rises to more than 150 mm Hg, cyanotic congenital heart disease is very unlikely.

Central hypoventilation from narcosis may cause hypoxemia. As alveolar carbon dioxide rises, $P_{A_{O_2}}$ falls and Pa_{O_2} decreases. This condition should be clinically evident and should not be confused with lung or congenital heart disease. Other causes of hypoxemia are sufficiently rare in the infant that we need only mention them: decreased inspired oxygen tension, as with increasing altitude, and oxygen

*References 3,7,9,12,13,23.

diffusion limitation. Diffusion limitation is not clinically important in neonatology.

PREVENTION

Prevention of acid-base and oxygenation disturbances and maintenance of acid-base homeostasis require attention to detail. Prevention of premature births or transport of pregnant women who may deliver a high-risk infant to tertiary care centers for treatment can minimize perinatal asphyxia and its consequences.

With respiratory disturbances, immediate assessment and prompt therapy, including supplemental inspired oxygen and assisted ventilation, help avoid oxygenation and respiratory component of acid-base disturbances (see Chapter 23). Careful monitoring of fluid and electrolyte intake and output, minimizing blood loss, and observing for sepsis help the clinician prevent development of nonrespiratory acid-base disturbances (see Chapter 14).

DATA COLLECTION

Monitoring inspired oxygen concentrations and arterial oxygen tension and supplying appropriate concentrations of additional inspired oxygen will prevent hypoxemia (see Chapter 23). Monitoring may be accomplished intermittently through indwelling arterial catheters or continuously by transcutaneous oxygen monitors and pulse oxygen saturation devices (see Chapter 7). Monitoring hemoglobin concentrations and blood loss, with appropriate replacement, helps ensure adequate blood oxygen content.

Reviewing the patient's history, performing a physical examination, and evaluating laboratory data augment each other in the assessment of disturbances in acid-base homeostasis and oxygenation (Box 8-2).

BOX 8-2 EVALUATION OF ACID-BASE DISTURBANCES AND OXYGENATION PROBLEMS IN NEONATES

1. History
    a. Obstetric and perinatal
    b. Neonatal
    c. Family
2. Physical examination
    a. Vital signs
    b. General appearance
    c. Respiratory effort
    d. Pulmonary examination
    e. Cardiac examination
    f. Abdominal examination
    g. Neurologic examination
3. Laboratory
    a. Chest x-ray film
    b. Arterial blood gases
    c. Urinalysis
    d. In selected cases: sepsis evaluation, serum electrolytes, serum albumin, urine electrolytes, and urine osmolality

History

An adequate obstetric and perinatal history may warn of potential acid-base and oxygenation disturbances:

- Premature delivery predisposes the infant to shock and respiratory distress.
- Meconium staining may portend respiratory difficulties.
- Prolonged rupture of membranes, maternal diabetes, or abnormal maternal bleeding may be associated with either metabolic or respiratory acid-base disturbances and hypoxemia.
- A neonatal history of vomiting, diarrhea, or other gastrointestinal disturbances can cause acid-base disturbances.
- The infant's general appearance, feeding habits, and activity level may indicate sepsis or CNS injury, both of which promote acid-base disturbances and hypoxemia.
- Nosocomial infections and pneumonia may significantly influence acid-base and oxygenation disturbances.
- A family history of inherited renal problems such as tubular acidosis may suggest an acid-base disturbance.
- A family history of salt-losing endocrinopathies may produce an acid-base disturbance.

Physical Examination

SIGNS AND SYMPTOMS

Signs of acid-base disturbance vary widely and often go undetected. Hypothermia and low blood pressure should alert caretakers to the possibility of metabolic acidosis. **Altered respiratory rate and pattern, grunting respirations, nasal flaring, and chest wall retractions raise the possibility of respiratory acidosis or respiratory compensation for metabolic acidosis or may indicate abnormal oxygenation.** Abnormalities on auscultation of the heart may point to congenital heart disease and resulting acid-base and oxygenation abnormalities. Lethargy, seizures, and abnormal neurologic signs increase concern for acid-base disturbances or hypoxemia.

Laboratory Data

Chest Radiograph: A chest x-ray examination may identify a respiratory cause for acid-base disturbance and hypoxemia.

Urinalysis: The routine urinalysis records urine specific gravity and demonstrates that urine is being produced. Urine electrolytes are helpful in differentiating among the pathophysiologic mechanisms of metabolic derangements.

Arterial Blood Gases: Interpretation of the arterial blood gases will point to the primary acid-base derangement and may reveal a secondary compensation and define the degree of hypoxemia.[3,16,21,31] Presently, methods for monitoring the components of acid-base analysis comprise both invasive and noninvasive techniques. Intermittent arterial punctures or indwelling catheters in various vessels (often the umbilical artery or vein) supply data. However, we can continuously measure transcutaneous PO_2 or O_2 saturation. Monitors can continuously measure expired end-tidal CO_2, which corresponds to the alveolar CO_2. (Alveolar and arterial CO_2 are equivalent unless respirations are excessively rapid.) In addition, skin electrodes are available that measure PaO_2 and $PaCO_2$ (see Chapter 7).

Although the pathophysiologic condition of the acid-base disturbance is determined through the analysis of arterial blood gases, further assessment of the infant is necessary, as follows:

- Respiratory alkalosis or acidosis should be suggested by physical examination, arterial blood gas analysis, and chest x-ray examination.
- Metabolic acidosis often accompanies shock and septicemia. The anion gap and urine electrolytes may provide additional information to delineate causes. Blood pressure measurement, a complete blood cell count, serum and urine electrolytes, serum albumin and glucose determinations, and assessment of intake and output of fluids are often needed to identify the source of a metabolic acidosis.
- Oxygenation disturbances may be analyzed from the preceding laboratory tests, and when indicated, electrocardiogram and arterial blood gas response to increased inspired oxygen concentrations are used to evaluate the possibility of congenital heart disease.

Another calculation, the ***oxygenation index (OI),*** is used to assess critically ill neonates receiving ventilator therapy. The OI is ($FIO_2 \times 100 \times$ mean airway pressure) $\div$ PaO_2. An OI of 25 or greater has been considered an indication for extraordinary ventilatory support, such as inhaled nitric oxide or extracorporeal membrane oxygenation (ECMO).

TREATMENT

In respiratory acidosis, the pathophysiologic mechanism is decreased alveolar ventilation. Treatment is directed at the underlying cause.[8] **Hypoxemia caused by ventilation-perfusion mismatch is treated with increased inspired oxygen concentration.** Techniques that may be of benefit include continuous positive airway pressure (CPAP), standard ventilation, high-frequency ventilation, ECMO, inhaled nitric oxide, and others (see Chapter 23). **Treatment of respiratory alkalosis usually consists of reducing ventilator settings.** One of the few causes of central hyperventilation is hyperammonemia caused by an inborn error of urea cycle metabolism[4] (Chapter 27). Prompt recognition is crucial to early diagnosis and treatment.

Asphyxia often leads to combined respiratory and metabolic acidosis. Ventilation will resolve the respiratory acidosis. Improved oxygenation usually allows lactic acidosis to resolve without bicarbonate therapy. In narcosis, temporary ventilator support may be necessary. **The narcosis may be reversed with administration of naloxone (Narcan) at a dose of 0.1 mg/kg if the possibility of maternal opiate drug abuse has been ruled out.** (Repeated doses may be necessary; see Chapter 4.)

With any acidosis and alkalosis, a careful search must be instituted for causes. If the cause of metabolic acidosis is septicemia, intestinal necrosis, or poor cardiac output severe enough to result in metabolic acidosis, successful treatment of the cause is of far more importance than buffer therapy for acidosis.* **Sodium bicarbonate administration was once thought to be vitally important to management of metabolic acidosis. Use in neonatal intensive care has decreased dramatically as shortcomings have emerged, especially the possibility that "push" administration may cause intraventricular hemorrhage.[19,22] It should not be used if severe lung disease restricts carbon dioxide elimination (see Equation 3).**

COMPLICATIONS

The outcome of unrecognized and untreated acid-base or oxygenation disturbances may be an increased mortality or an increased morbidity in the survivors. Complications of the correction of the acid-base and oxygenation disturbance vary according to the disturbance and treatment provided.

One effect of acidosis is CNS depression. In metabolic acidosis, the rate and depth of respiration are increased, whereas in respiratory acidosis, respiration may be labored or depressed. An effect of alkalosis is increased excitability of the CNS and tetany (often of the respiratory muscles).[8,9,15,26] Complications associated with sodium bicarbonate therapy for metabolic acidosis are discussed above.

Treatment of respiratory acidosis by assisted ventilation can produce all of the complications of assisted ventilation, including infection, trauma, oxygen toxicity, sepsis, air leak, and subglottic stenosis (see Chapter 23).

Complications of oxygen therapy include hypoxemia and hyperoxemia. **Severe hypoxemia may cause pulmonary vasoconstriction, a change from aerobic to anaerobic metabolism (with eventual metabolic acidosis), cyanosis, bradycardia, hypotonia, and decreased CNS and cardiac function.** Prolonged high inspired oxygen concentrations can result in pulmonary oxygen toxicity and contribute to retinopathy of prematurity. If ventilatory support is necessary to achieve adequate oxygenation, one must deal with the additional complications of ventilator therapy (see Chapter 23).

*References 2,9,12,19,23,25.

PARENT TEACHING

Obtaining blood for blood gas analysis by invasive techniques (arterial punctures and heel sticks) is stressful for parents and their infant. Explaining the rationale for the test, eliciting parental assistance (if they are present), and encouraging them to comfort their crying baby involve parents as primary caregivers. Explaining the results of the analysis and needed changes in therapy keeps parents apprised of their baby's progress. Many parents become quite adept at blood gas interpretation and are able to anticipate therapeutic alterations: "Did you change the FIO_2? The ventilator rate?" This helps parents master a difficult situation. Beyond sharing technical information, the care provider should also personalize the infant to his or her parents (see Chapter 29).

REFERENCES

1. Adrogué HE, Adrogué HJ: Acid-base physiology, *Respir Care* 46:328, 2001.
2. Boyle M, Lawrence J: An easy method of mentally estimating the metabolic component of acid/base balance using the Fencl-Stewart approach, *Anaesth Intensive Care* 31:538, 2003.
3. Breen PH: Arterial blood gas and pH analysis: clinical approach and interpretation, *Anesthesiol Clin North Am* 19:885, 2001.
4. Brusilow SW: Hyperammonemic encephalopathy, *Medicine* 81:240, 2002.
5. Delivoria-Papadopoulos M, Roncevic NP, Oski FA: Postnatal changes in oxygen transport of term, premature, and sick infants: the role of red cell 2,3-diphosphoglycerate and adult hemoglobin, *Pediatr Res* 5:235, 1971.
6. Dubin A, Menises MM, Masevicius FD, et al: Comparison of three different methods of evaluation of acid base disorder, *Crit Care Med* 35:1264, 2007.
7. Durward A, Mayer A, Skellett S, et al: Hypoalbuminaemia in critically ill children: incidence, prognosis, and influence on the anion gap, *Arch Dis Child* 88:419, 2003.
8. Epstein SK, Singh N: Respiratory acidosis, *Respir Care* 46:366, 2001.
9. Fencl V, Jabor A, Kazda A, et al: Diagnosis of metabolic acid-base disturbances in critically ill patients, *Am J Respir Crit Care Med* 162:2246, 2000.
10. Finer NN, Barrington KJ: Nitric oxide for respiratory failure in infants born at or near term, *Cochrane Database Syst Rev* 4: CD000399, 2006.
11. Foster GT, Vaziri ND, Sassoon CS: Respiratory alkalosis, *Respir Care* 46:384, 2001.
12. Gunnerson KJ, Kellum JA: Acid-base and electrolyte analysis in critically ill patients: are we ready for

the new millennium? *Curr Opin Crit Care* 9:468, 2003.

13. Hatherill M, Waggie Z, Purves L, et al: Correction of the anion gap for albumin in order to detect occult tissue anions in shock, *Arch Dis Child* 87:526, 2002.
14. Kellum JA: Clinical review: reunification of acid-base disorders, *Crit Care* 9:500, 2005.
15. Khanna A, Kurtzman NA: Metabolic alkalosis, *Respir Care* 46:354, 2001.
16. Kirksey KM, Holt-Ashley M, Goodroad BK: An easy method for interpreting the results of arterial blood gas analysis, *Crit Care Nurs* 21:49, 2001.
17. Kraut JA, Madias NE: Approach to patients with acid-base disorders, *Respir Care* 46:392, 2001.
18. Kurtz I, Kraut J, Ornekian V, et al: Acid-base analysis: a critique of the Stewart and bicarbonate-centered approaches, *Am J Physiol Renal Physiol* 294:F1009, 2008.
19. Levraut J, Grimaud D: Treatment of metabolic acidosis, *Curr Opin Crit Care* 9:260, 2003.
20. Sandberg K, Sjöqvist BA, Hjalmarson O, et al: Lung function in newborn infants with tachypnea of unknown cause, *Pediatr Res* 22:581, 1987.
21. Shoulders-Odom B: Using an algorithm to interpret arterial blood gases, *Dimens Crit Care Nurs* 19:36, 2000.
22. Simmons MA, Adcock EW, Bard H, et al: Hypernatremia and intracranial hemorrhage in neonates, *N Engl J Med* 291:6, 1974.
23. Sirker AA, Rhodes A, Grounds RM, et al: Acid-base physiology: the 'traditional' and the 'modern' approaches, *Anaesthesia* 57:348, 2002.
24. Sivieri EM, Bhutani VK: Pulmonary mechanics. In Sinha SK, Donn SM, editors: *Manual of neonatal respiratory care*, Armonk, NY, 2000, Mosby.
25. Story DA, Morimatsu H, Bellomo R: Strong ions, weak acids and base excess: a simplified Fencl-Stewart approach to clinical acid-base disorders, *Br J Anaesthesiol* 92:54, 2004.
26. Swenson ER: Metabolic acidosis, *Respir Care* 46:342, 2001.
27. Van Gosen L: Organic acidemias: a methylmalonic and propionic focus, *J Pediatr Nurs* 23:225, 2008.
28. Whittier WL, Rutecki GW: Primer on clinical acid-base problem solving, *Dis Mon* 50:122, 2004.
29. Wilson WC: Clinical approach to acid-base analysis: importance of the anion gap, *Anesthesiol Clin North Am* 19:907, 2001.
30. Wiswell TE, Srinivasan P, Roberton NRC: Aspiration syndromes. In Greenough A, Milner AD, editors: *Neonatal respiratory disorders*, London, 2003, Arnold.
31. Woodrow P: Arterial blood gas analysis, *Nurs Stand* 18:45, 2004.

9 DIAGNOSTIC IMAGING IN THE NEONATE

JOHN D. STRAIN AND JULEY C. JENKINS

Imaging has become an important part of the diagnosis and workup of medical problems of newborns. The ability to use a noninvasive means to diagnose disease, screen for potential pathologic conditions, monitor the effects of therapy, and assist in defining prognosis for counseling has made imaging an essential part of health care. With refinements in diagnostic equipment and capabilities, the role of imaging has expanded significantly in recent years. There are many ways to assess any problem, and the vast potential of the new imaging modalities makes appropriate imaging a constant challenge (Table 9-1). New modalities have been introduced, and advancement in computer technology has added sophistication to established modalities. Nearly 60% of diagnostic imaging involves modalities that were not even available 20 years previously.

There are many excellent reference books and textbooks on neonatal imaging, and specific questions can be addressed most adequately through these resources. This chapter reviews the various imaging modalities available for diagnosis and intervention. A short summary of each imaging modality includes background information, a discussion of image acquisition, and the risks and benefits of each. We have provided a thumbnail description of each modality; however, for clarity, we have taken significant liberty and license in discussing the physics of image acquisition. Each section addresses the most common usage of the modality in neonates, followed by a focused discussion of one or two aspects of image interpretation.

Because there may be more than one appropriate way to evaluate any given problem, it is essential to understand the inherent advantages and limitations of each modality to decide which might be most effective. We have pointed out some of the challenges associated with diagnostic imaging. A focused problem-solving approach with appropriate collaboration and consultation can yield positive results.

RADIOGRAPHY

Background

The 1896 introduction of the roentgenogram was met with great enthusiasm, and x-ray examination quickly became an indispensable diagnostic tool in clinical settings throughout the world. Until 25 years ago, the field of radiology was based almost exclusively on use of the x-ray.

A beam of ionizing radiation from a source (x-ray tube) passes through the patient, and various structures within the body interact to attenuate the x-ray before it is received on the other side. The x-rays pass through the patient and then expose a film, just as light exposes a negative in black-and-white film photography. The film is developed, and the resultant image (radiograph) is a map that corresponds to the transmitted x-ray (that portion of the x-ray not attenuated by absorption or scattered as it passes through the patient). Somewhat analogous to the shadows that result from objects in the sun, the images from x-ray are a shadow of the object being radiographed. (Hence the slang term "shadow doctor" came into use in reference to early radiologists.) Bone attenuates a greater amount of the x-ray (or allows the penetration of fewer x-rays) than lung tissue does; this results in a film on which the rib is white and the lung black. In some ways, this can be compared with the different shadows cast

Please note that the **PURPLE** type in each chapter is intended to make it easier to identify clinically applicable material.

TABLE 9-1 COMPARATIVE ANALYSIS OF IMAGING MODALITIES

	IONIZING RADIATION	SPATIAL RESOLUTION	CONTRAST RESOLUTION	COST	SEDATION	MISCELLANEOUS
X-ray	Very low	Excellent	Fair	Low	Never	Very fast acquisition eliminates motion
Fluoroscopy	Low	Excellent	Fair	Moderate	Never	Evaluates motion real-time
Ultrasonography	None	Good	Fair	Moderate	Never	Portable; evaluates motion real-time
Computed tomography	Low	Good	Good	Moderate to high	Sometimes	Cross-sectional imaging
Magnetic resonance imaging	None	Good	Excellent	High	Frequent	Multiplanar (i.e., in multiple planes) imaging, flowing blood without contrast
Nuclear medicine	Very low	Poor	Excellent	Moderate to high	Sometimes	Physiologic imaging

by the trunk of a tree and by its leaves. With radiography, the spatial resolution is exquisite although the contrast resolution is lacking. One can capture 10 to 20 line pairs per millimeter with film radiography, although **only five different densities can be distinguished routinely: air, fat, water (which includes all solid viscera—liver, spleen, kidney, pancreas, and heart), bone, and metal.**

More recent developments in x-ray technology include computed radiography (CR) and digital radiography (DR). Although the physics of x-ray generation is essentially the same, the receiver has changed. With CR, a phosphorescent plate replaces film and the latent image can be either exposed to film or captured digitally. With DR, the image is directly captured in a digital mode. The introduction of these products was driven by the desire to capture, archive, distribute, and display digital images. Almost all medical imaging is now digital, and a picture archiving and communication system (PACS) has become an essential component of any imaging department.

Clinical Utility in the Neonatal Intensive Care Setting

Radiography is the simplest and most reliable way to define tube and line position. Radio-opaque markers are incorporated into most of these devices. **From peripherally inserted central catheters (PICC) to endotracheal, thoracostomy, and feeding tubes, a simple radiograph can help eliminate the complications of suboptimal line or tube placement (Table 9-2). Chest radiographs are most commonly used to evaluate the heart and lungs. Abdominal imaging allows one to assess the solid viscera (the liver, spleen, and kidneys), as well as the bowel gas pattern, useful in evaluating a neonate with a feeding intolerance (Figure 9-1). Bones of the trunk and extremities are assessed easily with plain film radiology.**

TABLE 9-2 POSITION OF LINES AND TUBES

LINE/TUBE	POSITION
Endotracheal tube	1 cm above the level of the carina
Umbilical artery catheter	Descending aorta between T8 and T10
Umbilical venous catheter	Junction inferior vena cava and right atrium
Central line	Junction superior vena cava and right atrium
PICC line	Junction superior vena cava and right atrium
Nasogastric tube	Antrum of the stomach

PICC, Peripherally inserted central catheter; *T8 and T10*, thoracic vertebrae 8 and 10.

In addition to helping determine a specific diagnosis, imaging is frequently a valuable means for assessing patient response to therapy. For instance, lung compliance and volume, as assessed by x-ray studies, help determine the patient's response to various ventilator rates and pressures; therefore the x-ray findings can be very useful in the selection of the most appropriate ventilator settings.

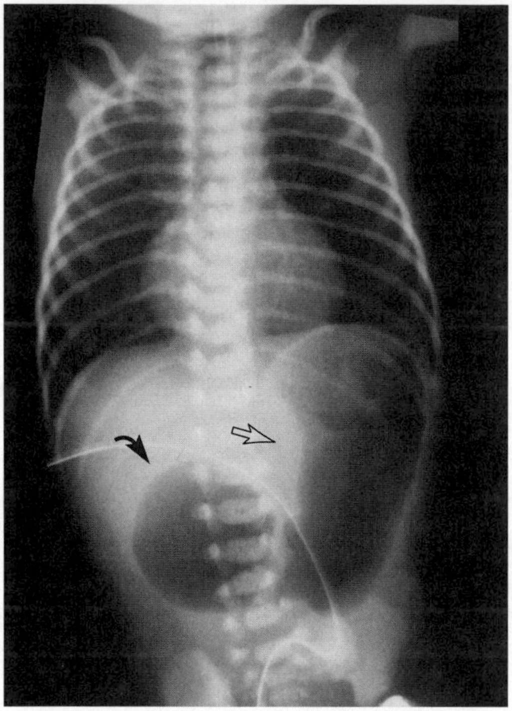

FIGURE 9-1 Frontal chest and abdomen show gaseous distention of the stomach *(open arrow)* and duodenal bulb *(curved arrow)*, the classic double bubble seen in duodenal atresia. Incidental note is made of thirteen pairs of ribs in this patient with Down syndrome.

Focused Discussion: Chest Radiographs

The most common use of x-ray imaging in the neonatal unit is for evaluation of the chest to help define abnormalities that might contribute to respiratory distress. Respiratory distress in newborns can be divided into three categories: conditions that are managed medically, those that are managed surgically, and iatrogenic respiratory distress.

MEDICALLY MANAGED RESPIRATORY DISTRESS

Table 9-3 summarizes plain film diagnosis of respiratory distress in newborns. Use of this approach takes advantage of the fact that only a limited number of changes can be identified radiographically, and a constellation of findings can define a specific group of etiologic factors. A systematic analysis of these various characteristics helps determine a specific group that has a fairly limited differential diagnosis (Box 9-1).

SURGICALLY MANAGED RESPIRATORY DISTRESS

Respiratory conditions that are managed surgically can be subdivided into three groups: (1) those associated with aspiration, such as cleft palate,

TABLE 9-3 PLAIN FILM DIAGNOSIS OF MEDICALLY MANAGED CAUSES OF RESPIRATORY DISTRESS IN THE NEWBORN (CHIMP DIFFERENTIAL)

		GESTATIONAL AGE	HEART SIZE	LUNG VOLUME	NATURE OF INFILTRATE	PROGRESSION	ANCILLARY FINDINGS
C	Congenital heart disease		Increased	Normal or increased	Increased pulmonary vascularity or edema	Stable or progressive	Abnormal situs, aortic discordance
H	Hyaline membrane disease*	<36 weeks		Decreased	Diffuse granularity with air bronchograms	Progressive over first 24 hours	No pleural effusions or body wall edema
I	Immature lung	<26 weeks	Normal	Decreased	Diffuse granularity	Progressive	Absent thymus from stress
M	Meconium aspiration	≥39 weeks	Normal	Increased	Streaky and patchy	Stable	Air leak (i.e., pneumothorax)
P	Neonatal pneumonia		Normal or increased		Either diffuse or focal		Pleural effusions and body wall edema

*Idiopathic respiratory distress syndrome (IRDS).

laryngeal cleft, or tracheoesophageal fistula; (2) those that compromise functional lung volume, including congenital diaphragmatic hernia (CDH), congenital lobar emphysema (Figure 9-2), and congenital cystic adenomatoid malformation (CCAM); and (3) those associated with tracheal or bronchial narrowing, such as a double aortic arch, congenital tracheal stenosis, and bronchogenic cyst (Box 9-2).

IATROGENIC RESPIRATORY DISTRESS

Most iatrogenic respiratory distress results from either a misplaced catheter or tube or from barotrauma. An endotracheal tube (ETT) can be placed too deep and will preferentially ventilate only a single lung. An ETT may even be inadvertently placed into the esophagus, resulting in inadequate ventilation (Figure 9-3), which is further compromised by distention of the esophagus and small bowel, limiting lung expansion.

Air leaks are considered to be the result of barotrauma (Figure 9-4). Although barotrauma occurs much less frequently since the introduction of exogenous surfactant and high-frequency ventilation, air leaks continue to be a problem that causes significant concern. Appropriate ventilation management requires timely and accurate diagnosis. One goal in review of a chest x-ray film is to define the location of the extrapulmonary gas. Abnormal extrapulmonary gas can include any one or a combination of the following: pulmonary interstitial emphysema, subcutaneous emphysema, pneumomediastinum, pneumothorax, pneumopericardium, pneumocardia, and portal venous gas.

BOX 9-1 CHIMP DIFFERENTIAL

Congenital heart disease
- Transient tachypnea of the newborn (resolves over first 24 hours)
- Extracardiac shunts

Hyaline membrane disease*
- Diffuse atelectasis

Immature lung
- Represents anectasis rather than atelectasis

Meconium aspiration
- Amniotic fluid aspiration

Pneumonia
- Diffuse
  - Birth asphyxia
- Focal
  - Pulmonary hemorrhage

Bronchopulmonary dysplasia represents the chronic lung disease that may result from any of the causes of respiratory distress.

*The use of exogenous surfactant modifies the picture of hyaline membrane disease (idiopathic respiratory distress syndrome [IRDS]) significantly. The irregular distribution after endotracheal administration causes a much less uniform infiltrate, and the patchy pattern that results has a look similar to that in meconium aspiration, which might be seen in a term or postterm infant.

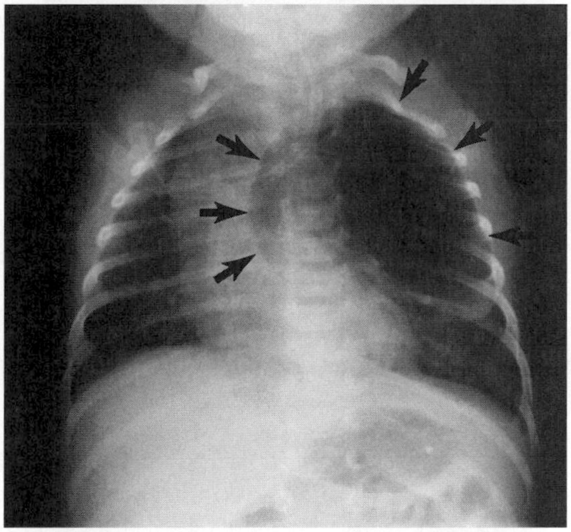

FIGURE 9-2 Frontal view of the chest shows a hyperaerated lucent left upper lobe *(arrows)* associated with mediastinal shift from left to right and is characteristic of congenital lobar emphysema.

BOX 9-2 SURGICALLY MANAGED RESPIRATORY DISTRESS

1. Associated with aspiration
   a. Cleft palate
   b. Laryngeal cleft
   c. Tracheoesophageal fistula
2. Compromised functional lung volume involvement
   a. Congenital diaphragmatic hernia
   b. Congenital lobar emphysema
   c. Congenital cystic adenomatoid malformation
3. Cause tracheal or bronchial narrowing
   a. Double aortic arch
   b. Tracheal stenosis
   c. Bronchogenic cyst

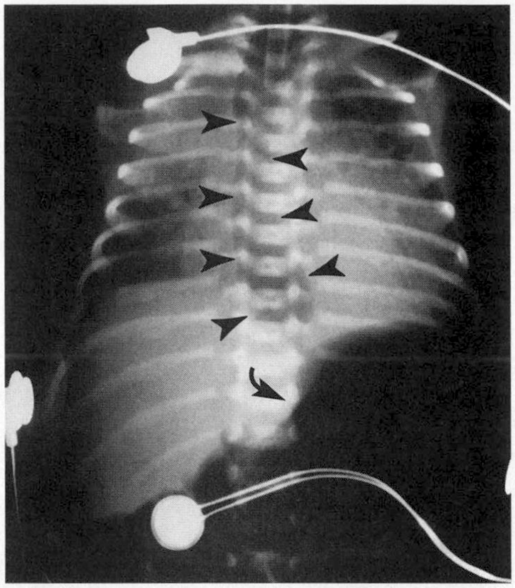

FIGURE 9-3 Frontal chest film. Although the endotracheal tube projects over the midline mediastinum near the thoracic inlet, the dilated esophagus *(arrowheads)* and distended stomach *(arrow)* associated with right upper lobe and left lower lobe atelectasis suggested esophageal intubation, which was diagnosed in this patient.

FLUOROSCOPY

Background

In fluoroscopy, an x-ray tube similar to that used for plain film radiography is used. The x-ray is generated in the same manner as in plain radiography, but it is received in most cases by a device that is similar to a TV camera or VCR. Fluoroscopy allows real-time evaluation of a patient and can be performed with or without contrast material. Spatial resolution in fluoroscopy is not as good as that in plain film radiography, but it is still excellent. Contrast resolution is about the same: air, fat, water, bone, and contrast are about the only densities that can be separated. Contrast media can be given orally or per rectum, instilled into the urinary bladder, or given intravenously. The contrast attenuates the radiation beam to a variable extent related to physical properties and thickness of the attenuator. Most contrast agents are compounds that use either inert barium or iodine as the attenuator of the radiation beam. **The most important characteristic of fluoroscopic imaging is the ability to evaluate motion in real time. This is essential in the**

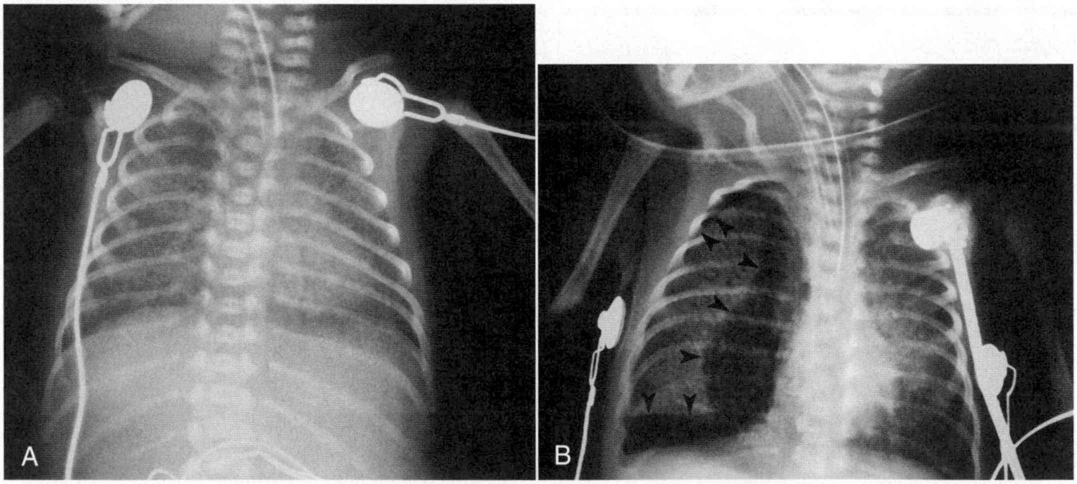

FIGURE 9-4 **A,** Frontal chest film. Hyaline membrane disease in this patient is defined by the diffuse symmetric granular infiltrates with small lung volumes. This patient required intubation, and the endotracheal tube tip projects in satisfactory position. **B,** Follow-up examination in the same patient demonstrates linear lucencies within the right lung resulting from pulmonary interstitial emphysema. A tension pneumothorax *(arrowheads)* is identified on the right with mild mediastinal shift from right to left. The lack of atelectasis on the right is the result of extremely poor lung compliance that accompanies pulmonary interstitial emphysema. The endotracheal tube tip projects in satisfactory position, but the nasogastric tube is in the midesophagus.

evaluation of swallowing function, gastrointestinal (GI) peristalsis, and diaphragmatic motion.

Clinical Utility in the Neonatal Intensive Care Setting

The most common fluoroscopic examinations requested for neonates include the upper GI (UGI) series, the contrast enema, and voiding cystourethrography. The UGI series is useful in the evaluation of swallowing, aspiration, feeding intolerance, vomiting, and abdominal distention with possible bowel obstruction.

A contrast enema can be diagnostic in Hirschsprung's disease (Figure 9-5). It can be both diagnostic and therapeutic in meconium plug syndrome and meconium ileus.

A voiding cystourethrogram is used to evaluate the urinary bladder and the urethra and to look for vesicoureteral reflux (Figure 9-6), which is associated with urinary tract infection. Vesicoureteral reflux is a common cause of hydronephrosis, which is now frequently identified during prenatal ultrasonography. Ureteroceles, periureteral diverticula, and posterior urethral valves all can be associated with hydronephrosis in the neonatal period and demonstrated with cystourethrography.

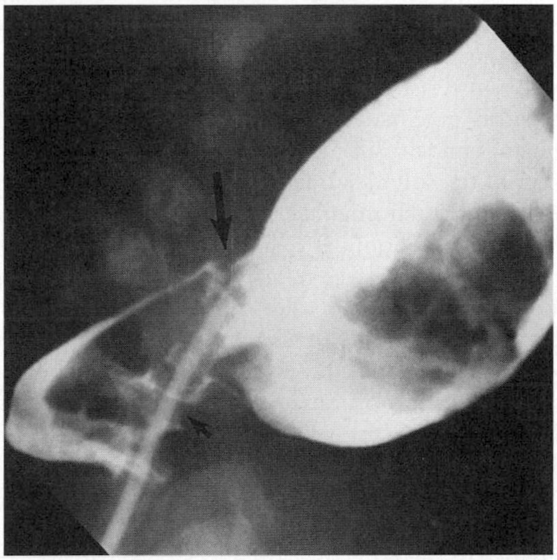

FIGURE 9-5 A lateral film from the early filling phase of a barium enema demonstrates spasm of the distal rectal segment *(short arrow)* with a transition zone to dilated colon *(long arrow)*. These findings are characteristic of colonic Hirschsprung's disease.

Air works as a fine contrast agent, and the nasal and oral airway, as well as the trachea and proximal bronchus, can be easily evaluated fluoroscopically. Because the diaphragm is immediately adjacent to aerated lung, diaphragmatic motion and its relationship to inspiratory effort help in the evaluation of phrenic nerve injury and diaphragmatic paralysis. Eventration of the diaphragm also can be evaluated fluoroscopically but, at times, can be indistinguishable from diaphragmatic hernia.

Focused Discussion: Upper Gastrointestinal Series

Indications for performing a UGI series include swallowing dysfunction, aspiration, vomiting, choking, and apnea. An appropriately performed UGI series offers a systematic approach to the upper GI tract. Starting with the patient in a left-side-down recumbent position, deglutition is evaluated. Tongue action, transport, nasopharyngeal regurgitation, aspiration, and laryngeal penetration all can be assessed. The right-side-down position

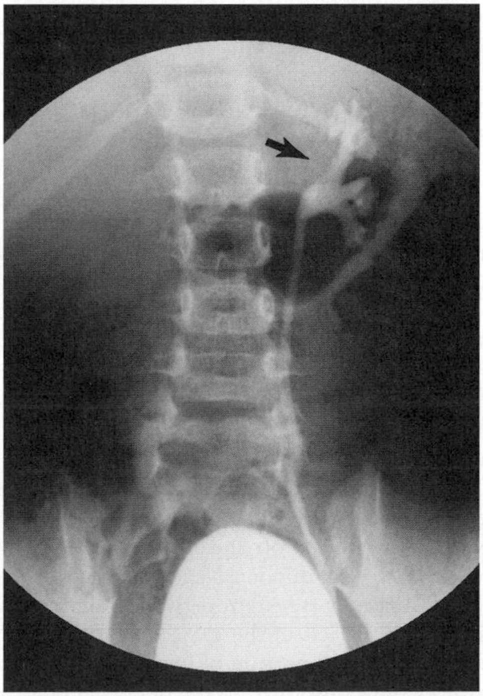

FIGURE 9-6 Frontal view from a voiding cystourethrogram demonstrates grade II vesicoureter on the left *(arrow)*.

better separates the esophagus and the tracheal air column. However, if this position is used initially and the evaluation of the deglutition is prolonged, the stomach may empty, filling the proximal small bowel and obscuring the location of the ligament of Treitz. The left-side-down position allows one to evaluate swallowing without concern that the stomach may empty prematurely. Once deglutition is satisfactorily evaluated, one can concentrate on the esophagus. Vascular rings and slings are evaluated in both the frontal and lateral positions.

Esophageal atresia usually is diagnosed clinically; plain film observation of intraluminal bowel gas defines the most common form, which is associated with a distal tracheoesophageal fistula. The benefit of a proximal pouch study in esophageal atresia is controversial. There is a small incidence of fistula from the proximal pouch to the trachea; this incidence is independent of the presence or absence of a distal fistula. If the surgical approach to esophageal atresia repair includes direct visualization of the proximal pouch, the pouch contrast study is superfluous. If, on the other hand, esophagoscopy is not routinely performed, there is some value in evaluating the proximal pouch before surgery. In the absence of esophageal atresia, the location of the fistula (H type) is at the thoracic inlet. This is higher than the fistula that occurs in the most common form of esophageal atresia, in which the fistula is at the level of the carina.

The caliber of the esophagus is informative, because it is usually dilated in association with significant gastroesophageal reflux. Esophageal contour, mucosal detail, and peristalsis are assessed. The configuration of the gastroesophageal junction can indicate gastroesophageal reflux, and rare hiatal hernias can be diagnosed. Gastric emptying is evaluated and gastric peristalsis examined. Because the rotation and fixation of the bowel have important consequences in the newborn period, this is an important part of a complete examination. The duodenal bulb, C-loop, and ligament of Treitz are defined. The lateral film is essential in localizing the ligament of Treitz. For proximal bowel rotation and fixation to be considered normal, the duodenal-jejunal junction (ligament of Treitz) must be retroperitoneal and therefore posterior, to the left of the spine, and at the level of the retroperitoneal portion of the second portion of the duodenum (just distal to the duodenal bulb).

The rotation of the proximal bowel may be independent of the rotation of the hindgut. **Therefore if the clinical question is malrotation and possible volvulus, the UGI series is the examination of choice.** The caliber, contour, and fold pattern of the proximal bowel are evaluated and the transit time observed. This simple, systematic, yet comprehensive approach to a UGI series yields a tremendous amount of information.

ULTRASONOGRAPHY

Background

One of the most prominent mass media introductions of ultrasound (US) technology came when Dr. Robert Ballard located the wreckage of the Titanic using US to explore the ocean floor of the North Atlantic. Medical ultrasonography has its roots in sound navigation and ranging (sonar) developed during World War II.

In medical ultrasonography, a transducer (essentially a piezoelectric crystal) converts electrons into mechanical vibration that creates high-frequency sound waves within the body. The same transducer serves as both the transmitter of the sound wave and the receiver of the reflected sound. Within the body, these high-frequency sound waves propagate through the soft tissues until they meet a reflective surface that reflects some of those fluid waves back to the transducer. The percent of the sound beam reflected relates to the difference in the acoustic impedance of the material being evaluated. When the acoustic impedances of materials are similar, as is the case with the abdominal wall musculature (e.g., liver, kidney), most of the sound is transmitted and a small percent reflected at each interface. As the sound wave travels through the abdominal wall to the liver, the abdominal wall–liver interface reflects a portion of the beam and transmits most of the sound through the liver to the liver-kidney interface. The small difference in acoustic impedance between the liver and kidney causes reflection of some of the beam and transmission of most to the posterior abdominal wall. This allows the visualization of multiple interfaces that are deep to the first structure encountered. If the velocity of the sound beam in tissue is known, the distance to the reflective surface can be estimated by measuring the time it takes for the pulse to travel the distance to and from the object imaged.

Most of the tissues in the body have similar acoustic impedances; however, air has extremely

low impedance and bone extremely high impedance. This means that there is a big difference in the acoustic impedance between these substances and the organs most commonly imaged. For this reason, both bone and air reflect nearly all of the sound that reaches them. This is why a coupling gel is used on the skin surface to eliminate the air gap between the transducer and the skin. This is also why imaging through the liver gives a good acoustic window to deeper structures but bowel gas obscures imaging lower in the abdomen. For ultrasonographic imaging of the brain in a neonate, the anterior fontanel serves as the acoustic window because the bone of the skull acts as a reflective surface that limits through-transmission of US to deeper structures. Bulk fluids within the body, such as urine in the urinary bladder, bile in the gallbladder, or cerebrospinal fluid in the ventricles, have no internal interfaces and therefore are seen as solid black on conventional ultrasonography. Cysts have a sharp posterior wall and have increased through-transmission, because the sound wave penetrates the fluid without any reflections to block transmission of the sound.

Doppler ultrasonography takes advantage of the physical principle that the US reflection from a moving object distorts the wavelength, with the distortion related to the velocity of the object being measured. This is the principle that causes the pitch of a train's whistle to change from high to low as the train passes an observer. It is the same principle police use to monitor the speed of a car and the Judd gun uses to measure the velocity of a pitcher's fastball. In fact, this same principle is responsible for the "red shift" observed by astronomers in determining that we live in an expanding universe. The Doppler evaluation in medical ultrasonography uses the distortion of the wavelength caused by moving red cells to identify flowing blood.

One of the major advantages of US imaging is the lack of ionizing radiation. Although most diagnostic imaging that requires ionizing radiation is of low dose, any radiation exposure is a concern and should be avoided when possible. The portability of ultrasonographic equipment has made it a valuable adjuvant to diagnostic imaging in the neonatal intensive care setting.

Clinical Utility in the Neonatal Intensive Care Setting

Ultrasonography has had a major impact in the evaluation of the neonatal brain. Most of the early work focused on intracranial hemorrhage, which was a common occurrence in preterm neonates. Even though the incidence has decreased, intracranial hemorrhage remains an issue for which US imaging is extremely well suited. Ultrasonographic instrumentation has improved tremendously, and with the addition of color and pulse Doppler technology, great strides have been made in the refinement and sophistication of intracranial imaging. Numerous complex structural abnormalities can be recognized, and screening for developmental abnormalities can largely be accommodated with cranial ultrasonography. Because bone reflects most of the sound-limiting through-transmission, the open fontanel is the window to the brain. As the fontanel closes over time, ultrasonography becomes less and less useful for intracranial imaging. This same limitation affects the utility of ultrasonographic evaluation of the spine as the patient ages.

Renal imaging offers another major role for ultrasonography in the neonatal unit. The kidneys are well visualized ultrasonographically, either through a posterior approach or, more commonly, by using the liver or spleen as soft-tissue acoustic windows to the kidneys. Ultrasonography is an excellent way to evaluate hydronephrosis, which is now frequently picked up on routine prenatal evaluations. Ultrasonography has a role in the evaluation of a jaundiced patient because it is ideal for evaluating cystic structures, such as the gallbladder, and can readily identify dilated biliary ducts. Jaundice caused by biliary obstruction from a choledochal cyst, for instance, can be diagnosed readily ultrasonographically. Because of the reflectivity related to bone and bowel gas, US imaging is much more effective in the upper abdomen, in which the liver and spleen serve as the acoustic windows, or in the pelvis, in which the urinary bladder can function as the window.

Even though ultrasonography is reflected by bone, ultrasonographic imaging has a significant role in the evaluation of hips in the neonate. Because the capital femoral epiphysis of the newborn is cartilage, the hip can be well imaged in a neonate. Maternal estrogen causes ligamentous laxity. This changes significantly during the first weeks of life; therefore the accuracy of hip ultrasonographic examinations improves after the first 3 to 4 weeks. Ultrasonography is very good for the detection of developmental dysplasia of the hip and can be used to evaluate the degree of femoral head coverage, the acetabular angle, and any instability of the hip.

Focused Discussion: Cranial Ultrasonography

Ultrasonography is an ideal tool for evaluating the brain in a newborn. **In general, an ultrasonographic examination is the first step in the imaging evaluation for any neurologic question. Structural abnormalities, intracranial hemorrhage, sequelae of anoxic or ischemic events, and infection are all well assessed via US imaging.** The most common approach is through the anterior fontanel, but additional information can be gained with axial imaging through the squamosa of the temporal bone. The posterior fossa can be evaluated through the posterior lateral fontanel. Familiarity with the normal anatomy is essential. Coronal and parasagittal views are obtained generally. Normal structures can be recognized easily; their absence or deformity is necessary to define developmental abnormalities of the brain. The ventricular size and configuration are assessed. Characteristic ventricular configurations can define lobar or semilobar holoprosencephaly. In addition, the ventricular configuration can suggest septo-optic dysplasia or agenesis of the corpus callosum. The corpus callosum can be visualized directly; abnormalities of the corpus callosum are associated commonly with Chiari malformation and other structural abnormalities of the brain, such as Dandy-Walker malformation. Dilation of one or more of the ventricles can be an indication of a pathologic condition. An obstruction of cerebrospinal fluid (CSF) flow in the region of the aqueduct of Sylvius manifests with disparity in ventricular size. The third and lateral ventricles are enlarged, whereas the fourth ventricle remains normal in size. Dilation of one of the lateral ventricles, especially when associated with an area of porencephaly, is indicative of an in utero destructive event.

Seizures or apnea may indicate an anoxic or ischemic event in a neonate. Certain structural abnormalities can suggest a specific diagnosis; for instance, periventricular nodules and cortical tubers define tuberous sclerosis. US examination is less sensitive than computed tomography (CT) and magnetic resonance imaging (MRI) in defining subtle areas of gray matter heterotopia or focal pachygyria, examples of developmental abnormalities associated with seizures. **US imaging is very sensitive to intracranial hemorrhage, and areas of increased echogenicity can be demonstrated in areas of edema.** Increased sulcal echogenicity is suggestive of meningitis, and encephalitis results in increased parenchymal echogenicity, which is a manifestation of localized brain swelling. Intracranial hemorrhage generally is a concern in a premature neonate (Figure 9-7). It is classified into four grades, and each grade generally is associated with a prognosis. Grade I hemorrhage usually has a good outcome, whereas the prognosis with grade IV hemorrhage is frequently poor. Grade I hemorrhage is confined

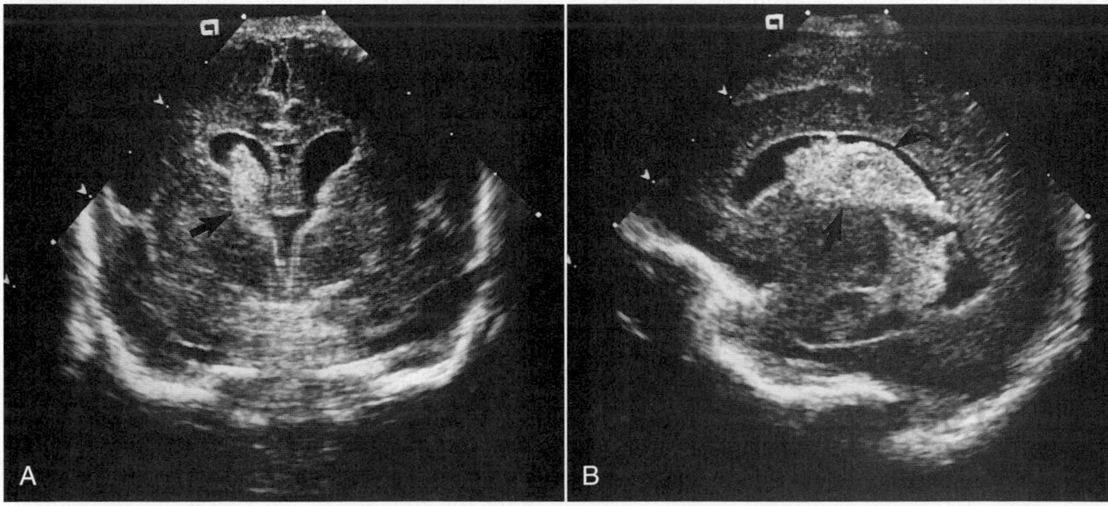

FIGURE 9-7 Coronal **(A)** and parasagittal **(B)** ultrasound images from a cranial ultrasound study demonstrate an echogenic clot *(arrows)* within the dilated right ventricle. The intraventricular clot with ventricular dilation defines a grade III hemorrhage.

to germinal matrix in the caudothalamic groove. This is the last fetal germinal matrix to mature and is prone to hemorrhage in preterm babies. Grade II intracranial hemorrhage has intraventricular blood. Grade III hemorrhage is associated with ventricular dilation as the intraventricular clot enlarges the lateral ventricles. Grade IV hemorrhage must demonstrate parenchymal extension. It has been hypothesized that grade IV hemorrhage may be the result of venous infarction that occurs from obstruction of the septal veins by the swollen germinal matrix hemorrhage. **Periventricular leukomalacia is a consequence of anoxic or ischemic injury to the brain that manifests as increased echogenicity in the deep periventricular white matter of the centrum semiovale. This may progress to cavitation and is then called *cystic leukoencephalomalacia*.** Ultrasonographic examination is a very sensitive way to detect this change, which is usually apparent within 2 weeks of birth.

COMPUTED TOMOGRAPHY

Computed axial tomography (CAT, or more frequently, CT) was initially developed in 1972 in Middlesex, England. Image acquisition takes place with a fairly sophisticated algorithm that interprets projections made by x-rays taken from multiple different positions around a single axial plane. These multiple projections are analyzed, and a composite image is developed. In essence, a series of x-rays from various angles are obtained in a single imaging plane. This renders a cross-sectional slice that can show all of the structures within that slice. For instance, a slice through the upper abdomen may show the liver, spleen, pancreas, both kidneys, and the spine, each separated by a plane of fat and each with a subtly different density.

Spiral CT imaging, which is most commonly used today, allows a gantry to continuously rotate while the table translates through the scanning plane. This generates a data set resembling a coil spring around the body. Multidetector arrays of 4, 8, 16, 64, and even 256 elements accommodated rapid acquisition of multiple slices in a single rotation of the tube. This renders high-resolution iso-voxel datasets (each volume element has the same width, height, and depth) that render spectacular multi-planer and 3-D reconstructions without the stair-stepping artifact that degraded prior reconstructions. Dual-source CT tubes have added to the speed, sensitivity, and differentiation of tissue in a way never before possible. Eliminating the mechanical movement of the tube and detectors allows the fastest image acquisition. In these systems, the x-ray beam is focused through all of the various angles of the slice by electromagnetic manipulation of the beam to a circular array of detectors. A single slice can be acquired in less than 0.2 second, in essence stopping motion from interfering with image acquisition.

These recent advances in CT technology have resulted in spectacular images and an explosion in CT utilization. The radiation dose in CT, however, is significantly higher than that in routine radiography. CT now accounts for more than 60% of the radiation exposure from medical imaging in the United States. Respect for the risk for radiation-induced malignancy has curbed the use of CT to some extent. Although CT remains a superb imaging tool, it should be used judiciously and only for appropriate indications. **Medical research suggests that the radiation dose currently used in diagnostic CT is associated with an increase in the risk for radiation-induced malignancy. Neonates, infants, and children are more susceptible to the effects of radiation than are adults.** In addition, their longer life expectancy puts them at greater long-term risk related to the potential ill effects of radiation. Caution is the key: (1) image only when indicated, (2) limit the scan to the region of concern, and (3) be cognizant of dose and use as low peak kilovoltage (kVp) and milliampere second (mAs) as possible while maintaining diagnostic quality examinations.

Clinical Utility in the Neonatal Intensive Care Setting

Cranial imaging is the most common use of CT in most neonatal intensive care settings. CT adds significant specificity to the abnormalities recognized with ultrasonography. Concern about ionizing radiation and the fact that CT equipment generally is not portable make obtaining a CT film more difficult than obtaining a sonogram. CT is more accurate in assessing the nature of extra-axial fluid collections and is very helpful in further defining structural abnormalities of the brain, particularly those associated with abnormal distribution of gray or white matter. It is also very good for evaluating intracranial hemorrhage and infection. Exquisite bone detail defines craniofacial anomalies, choanal atresia and stenosis, and abnormalities of the petrous bone associated with hearing loss. Chest imaging is becoming much more frequent in the neonatal intensive care unit (NICU). It is used to evaluate abnormalities detected during intrauterine ultrasonographic examination and for potential surgical lesions identified on chest x-ray films. Ultrasonography remains the first-line diagnostic tool for the evaluation of kidneys, liver, and spleen, but when a pathologic condition of the abdomen is a concern and a good acoustic window for US imaging is not available, CT is frequently the examination of choice. CT can be performed with significantly less sedation than that necessary for MRI. CT eliminates many of the artifacts, including those of vascular flow, respiratory motion, and even bowel peristalsis, that limit the utility of MRI. Skeletal lesions are well visualized with CT. Ultrasonography is the method of choice in the evaluation of congenital hip dysplasia, but CT can be very helpful in evaluating the position of the femoral heads after reduction and treatment of congenital hip dysplasia when the patient is immobilized in a plaster cast.

CT can be very helpful in identifying the organ of origin of a specific pathologic condition. This, of course, is the first step in narrowing a differential diagnosis. The addition of intravenous contrast is very useful in defining tumor thrombus in renal arteries and the inferior vena cava, which may affect surgical approach to renal and hepatic neoplasm. The nature of abnormalities seen on CT can frequently lead to a specific diagnosis. Although the spatial resolution of CT is inferior to that of plain film radiography, the contrast resolution is significantly better and CT has taken advantage of this trade-off. Acquisition time for CT is much slower than that of radiography, and therefore motion artifact is more of a problem. The cross-sectional rendition of anatomy, which allows deep structures to be distinguished from one another, is the most significant advantage that CT has over radiography.

Focused Discussion: Intracranial Blood

CT is extremely sensitive and specific for the detection and localization of intracranial blood (Figure 9-8). Blood from acute hemorrhage has a density (measured in Hounsfield numbers) higher than any normal structure except bone. The increased contrast resolution that is available through CT allows the separation of gray matter from white matter and lends itself to detailed structural evaluation of the brain. The ventricles are low in density (0 Hounsfield units of water), the white matter more dense, and the gray matter more dense still, followed by blood from acute hemorrhage and, finally, calcium and bone. Blood from acute hemorrhage is visualized as white as soon as a clot is formed, and this high density will slowly decrease over time. By 2 to 3 weeks, for instance, the blood in a subdural hematoma will become lower and lower in density until it is indistinguishable from water, which is equal to CSF density in the ventricular system. MRI can differentiate blood from a chronic subdural hematoma for a longer time than CT because the protein within a chronic subdural hematoma modifies the signal on MRI for an extended period. Although all intracranial blood does change density over time, the compartment in which the blood is found affects the rate of change to some extent. Therefore the timing of an event responsible for the blood cannot be precisely determined based on the density alone.

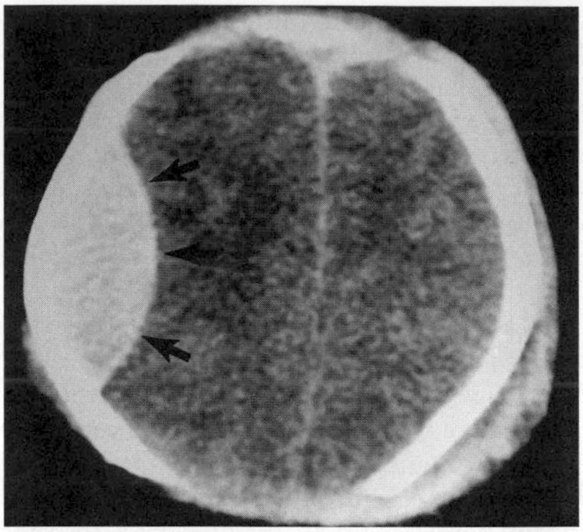

FIGURE 9-8 A single axial image near the vertex demonstrates a high-density lenticular mass *(arrows)* in the extra-axial space over the right cerebral cortex. The lenticular configuration is that of an epidural fluid collection and the high-density characteristic of blood from a chronic hematoma.

The location of the blood is the next issue. **CT is the most accurate imaging method for detection of subarachnoid blood.** The presence of subarachnoid blood postpartum is common even after a relatively nontraumatic birth. Unfortunately, on rare occasions, subarachnoid blood can cause vasospasm of vessels near the skull base, which can result in relative ischemia or hypoperfusion of the peripheral cortex. Areas of edema can be detected by looking for loss of the normal gray-white differentiation or by finding a focal area of brain edema characterized by relatively low density caused by the addition of low-density water to an otherwise normal area of brain.

The shape of a collection of blood is an important variable used in evaluating intracranial hemorrhage. Subarachnoid blood assumes a configuration that follows the arachnoid space. Therefore it is most frequently seen in the suprasellar cistern, the ambient cistern, the sylvian fissure, or the interhemispheric fissure, or layering on the tentorium. The most sensitive locations for identifying subarachnoid blood are in the region of the quadrigeminal plate cistern, the posterior aspect of the third ventricle, and the interpeduncular cistern. Subdural hematomas occur most frequently over the convexities or along the interhemispheric fissure. Those over the convexity can be differentiated from epidural hematomas by their crescentic configuration. This is opposed to the lenticular configuration of an epidural hematoma. The dura is the periosteum of the inner table of the skull; therefore an epidural hematoma is limited by the adhesion of the periosteum to the skull and hence the lenticular configuration. This is also why epidural hematomas are associated most often with higher-pressure arterial bleeding and why subdural hematomas frequently are associated with venous bleeding. Another key to differentiating the compartment is the relationship to cranial sutures. An epidural hematoma will not cross a suture line because of the anatomic limitation of the dura by the suture. A similar limitation by dural attachment at suture lines helps distinguish a cephalohematoma from a caput succedaneum. The direct sagittal imaging of MRI has made us more aware of the high prevalence of subdural blood in the posterior fossa.

MAGNETIC RESONANCE IMAGING

Background

MRI is a modality that images protons or hydrogen ions within the body. Rapid development of magnetic resonance was, in part, because of the transfer of some of the sophisticated reconstruction algorithms used in CT and the computer power developed in other fields, such as three-dimensional graphics used in cartoon animation, cartology, and seismology. These technologic advances allow tremendous amounts of information to be manipulated quickly enough to make image reconstruction a reality. MRI is essentially hydrogen imaging, and because the human body is 98% water, much hydrogen is available to image.

MRI is performed by placing a patient in a strong magnetic field, which varies slightly from the head to the foot. Each proton acts as a small magnet, and just as the needle on a compass orients itself in one direction when placed next to a magnet, the protons in the body align when placed into the magnetic field of the imaging magnet. This alignment of protons is essential to create an environment that has a net electromagnetic field effect or induces the movement of electrons. Without the alignment of protons by the magnetic field, the random orientation of protons would have no measurable net field effect when stimulated and therefore would create no signal to image.

Once the patient is in the magnet, a radiofrequency (RF) pulse is delivered. In current imaging systems, the pulse wave has a frequency of an FM radio wave. Less than 1 in 1 million hydrogen ions will absorb any energy, and only certain RFs will allow the transfer of energy from the RF pulse to a hydrogen ion.

An analogy of this energy transfer can be seen on a schoolyard playground. Visualize a child on a swing. If you push the swing in rhythm or resonance with the natural frequency of the motion of that swing, then the swing will absorb the energy and the child will swing higher and higher with each push. This natural rate of harmonic motion depends on the length of the rope on the swing and the mass of the swing and the child. If you were to push at a rate that was not synchronous with the swing's natural rhythm, pushing would not allow the energy to assist in propelling the swing higher and higher, and in fact, you would disrupt the normal rhythm of the swing.

In the memorable TV commercial in which Aretha Franklin was recorded by Memorex and the playback of her voice caused a goblet to break, the phenomenon being demonstrated was absorption of resonance frequency by the crystal in the goblet. That absorbed energy caused the goblet to shatter.

In MRI, FM RF energy is used to stimulate hydrogen ions or protons in the body.

Because the field strength of the magnet used for imaging varies slightly from one end of the patient to the other and the resonance frequency depends on the field strength of the magnet, one can selectively stimulate various locations within the patient. By changing the RF slightly, a different specific group of protons is stimulated. Protons stimulated by an RF pulse absorb that energy and move to an unstable higher energy state. They give up that energy as an RF pulse or "echo" of the pulse they received. The echo is received by an antenna just as with a radio receiver and converted to an image. The signals or echoes received are the result of T1 and T2 relaxation times, which are simply physical parameters that describe the environmental interactions that influence the signal released from a proton. Spin-echo pulse sequences are frequently used sequences in routine MRI.

A spinning top analogy can help to explain the T1 and T2 relaxation times that result in spin-echo imaging. Each hydrogen ion has a dipole moment (a positive pole and a negative pole) and therefore acts like a small magnet within the powerful magnetic field of the imaging magnet. These protons spin or precess with a precessional frequency that is related to the field strength of the magnet. Electromagnetic energy can be transferred to these protons if the energy is delivered at the resonance frequency. Once an RF pulse of resonance frequency is delivered, a certain number of protons (less than 1 in 1 million) absorb this energy and move to a higher energy state. The T1 relaxation time reflects the time it takes for these excited protons to give up their higher energy and return to baseline.

T2 relaxation times relate to a second parameter of physical interactions. Although the protons are rotating at a frequency proportionate to the magnetic field in which they exist, they are not in phase. In other words, there is no net direction of polarity from all of these spinning magnets. Once the RF pulse perturbs or stimulates these protons, they begin to spin synchronously and therefore create a net magnetic field. This spinning net magnetic field generates an electromagnetic wave that can be picked up by the RF antenna of the imaging system as an "echo" of the original RF pulse delivered. (The principle of a spinning magnet inducing an electromagnetic pulse is the basis for the turbines of hydroelectric generators.)

Because its immediate electromagnetic environment affects each proton differently, these protons will remain synchronous in their precession for a very short period. As they move out of phase or synchrony, the net magnetic field that was created dissipates; therefore the signal received by the RF antenna diminishes. The T2 relaxation time indicates the time it takes the protons to go from a state of synchronous rotation, when maximal signal is created, to random, out-of-phase precession, with zero net magnetic field and hence no signal. The requirement of a net magnetic field to create signal is used to evaluate flowing blood without the need for contrast. An RF pulse saturates the protons in the field being imaged. The saturated blood within the vessels of that field flow out of the field and are replaced with non-saturated blood from an adjacent slice. Consequently there is no signal from the vessel containing the blood flowing perpendicular to the slab being imaged.

Diffusion-weighted sequences have proven to be very sensitive in defining neonatal pathology. It is the most sensitive technique in the identification of early anoxic ischemic injury. Diffusion weighting takes advantage of random Brownian motion of molecules in fluid and the restriction of Brownian motion by anatomic barriers or edema. Water within the ventricular system will diffuse homogeneously in all directions (i.e., no restricted diffusion) and will be low signal on a diffusion-weighted sequence and high signal (white) on an apparent diffusion coefficient map (ADC map). Focal edema from an infarction, for instance, will cause restricted diffusion in the region of the infarction and be high signal on the diffusion sequence and low signal on the ADC map. Diffusion tensor imaging measures diffusion in at least six planes simultaneously. From that data, a map of the magnitude and direction of water movement can be generated. The axons within white matter tracts will allow diffusion in the direction of the axon but will restrict diffusion in any direction other than the course of the axon. This allows one to map the white matter tracts and has been studied in relation to developmental abnormalities in brain, the relationship of intracranial neoplasm to white matter tracts, and the plasticity of the developing brain in response to injury.

This is a simplified explanation of the physics necessary for image acquisition. **The key is that images are acquired without ionizing radiation. Therefore there is no risk from ionizing radiation with MRI, and this is particularly attractive in pediatrics.**

No known harmful effect of either magnetic exposure or RF exposure at the levels used in MRI has been observed. However, MRI is still relatively new, and one should be cautious in using fetal and newborn imaging. Energy deposition is a concern, and protocols have been established that limit patient exposure. Another concern is the effect a magnetic field might have on electronic instrumentation, such as pacing devices and metallic surgical clips. The torque on metallic implants can be quite high, but this is rarely of clinical significance. However, the artifact caused by the disturbance of the magnetic field can be significant. **The most important and real safety concern is that of the magnetic field attraction of ferromagnetic material. Pens, stethoscopes, or even oxygen canisters can act as projectiles when inadvertently brought too close to a magnetic field.** One also should be cautious about the effect that a magnetic field might have on magnetic strips of credit cards and identification badges, but this is more of a nuisance than a safety concern.

The main drawback of current MRI technology is the time it takes to acquire an image. Motion-free imaging is necessary for optimal image quality, and because image acquisition in MRI takes minutes, sedation frequently is necessary. Respiratory and cardiac gating can help for physiologic motion, but even physiologic motion can be problematic.

Focused Discussion: Practical Considerations

The physics of MRI is complex, and variables that influence the signal received are protean (Figure 9-9). These influences variably affect the T1 and T2 relaxation times in spin-echo imaging. Imaging sequences tend to be called ***T1*** or ***T2 sequences,*** depending on which physical parameter has the most influence on the appearance of the image. A simplified approximation of spin-echo imaging that can be helpful for the novice is that in T1-weighted spin-echo sequences, fluid is black and in T2-weighted imaging, fluid is white. **Most pathologic conditions are characterized either by the distortion of the normal anatomy or by edema, which is manifested by increased fluid in an otherwise normal structure or within the particular lesion.** Therefore if one looks for a fluid collection (e.g., CSF in the ventri-

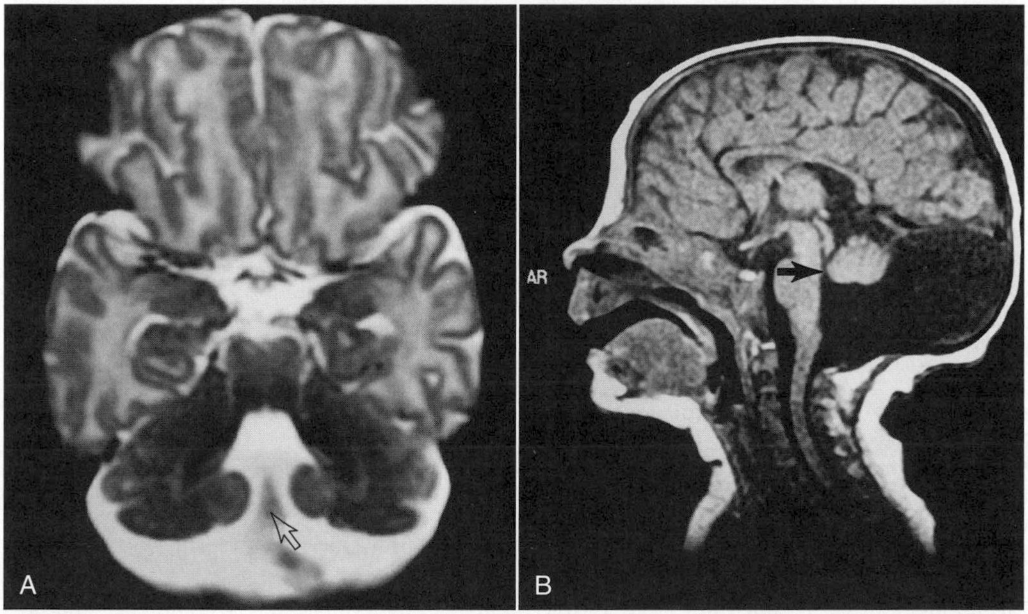

FIGURE 9-9 **A,** Axial T2-weighted image through the posterior fossa demonstrates the high-signal cerebrospinal fluid in the posterior fossa cyst, which communicates with the fourth ventricle more anteriorly *(open arrow).* **B,** Midsagittal T1-weighted image demonstrates a Dandy-Walker variant in this patient. The partial formation of the vermis seen best on the sagittal image defines a Dandy-Walker variant *(black arrow).*

cles of the brain, such as CSF in the subdural space around the cord; orbital fluid of the aqueous humor; or fluid in the heart or urinary bladder), one usually can determine whether the imaging sequence is T1 weighted, in which the fluid appears black, or T2 weighted, in which the fluid appears white. On T1-weighted sequences, a pathologic condition is seen as a black or lower signal, because a pathologic state is associated with increased water in the area of abnormality. In T2-weighted sequences, the pathologic lesion tends to be white.

NUCLEAR SCINTIGRAPHY

Nuclear scintigraphy is the most physiologic of the tools commonly used in neonatal imaging. A pharmaceutical is tagged with a radiotracer, which is a radioactive isotope that can be detected by a nuclear medicine camera. The pharmaceutical may be injected intravenously, given orally, or delivered directly into the urinary bladder. The pharmaceutical is distributed in the body based on the parent compound to which the radioisotope is chelated or bound. The patient then is imaged using a detector that maps the distribution of the tagged isotope in the body.

The radiation dose in scintigraphy is small. With the doses used for diagnostic purposes, there is no risk to the individual or anyone who is in immediate contact with the patient. The pharmaceutical agents have both a biologic half-life that is related to the natural elimination of the parent compound from the body and a radioactive half-life that is determined by the isotope used to label the pharmaceutical. The spatial resolution is poor, but contrast resolution is exquisite, because the radiopharmaceutical is distributed so specifically within the body.

Clinical Utility in the Neonatal Intensive Care Setting

Three common investigations for which nuclear medicine is well suited are renal scintigraphy, hepatobiliary imaging, and splenic imaging. In patients with the syndrome defined by vertebral, anal, cardiac, tracheal, esophageal, renal, and limb (VACTERL) anomalies, renal scans can be helpful in determining the number and location of the kidneys. Renal scintigraphy can be used to quantify relative renal function. Scintigraphy is a functional way to evaluate the degree of obstruction in hydronephrosis. Nuclear cystography has a very low radiation dose; therefore it is a good method for following vesicoureteral reflux. Fluoroscopic cystography usually is performed for the initial evaluation because the excellent spatial resolution can assist in defining anatomic abnormalities that may be responsible for reflux (e.g., that might be missed with the poor spatial resolution of nuclear imaging).

Hepatobiliary imaging can assist in the evaluation of the jaundiced patient. The radiopharmaceutical is extracted from the blood pool by the liver and excreted like bile, allowing one to determine transit time and flow of the bile from the liver into the gallbladder, through the common bile duct, and into the duodenum. Hepatobiliary imaging can help diagnose neonatal hepatitis, in which there is limited clearance of the pharmaceutical agent from the blood by the liver; therefore the liver shows little activity compared with the background. In biliary atresia, the clearance or extraction of the radiopharmaceutical agent from the blood is closer to normal, but the isotope never leaves the liver and therefore no activity is seen in the duodenum and small bowel, even on delayed images. A choledochal cyst accumulates radiotracer and is diagnosed by an intense area of focal activity and a dilated biliary system more proximally.

Splenic imaging can be performed with technetium sulfur colloid, which is taken up in the Kupffer cells in the liver and spleen. Alternatively, radiolabeling of red blood cells can be used for splenic images because damaged cells are sequestered in the spleen. Splenic imaging frequently is helpful in patients with complex congenital heart disease and situs abnormalities to diagnose asplenia or polysplenia.

Focused Discussion: Renal Scintigraphy

The radiopharmaceutical choices for renal imaging are either cortical agents that bind in the renal cortex, filtered agents that transit the cortex and then are excreted into the collecting system, or a combination of both cortical and filtered agents. Cortical agents are useful in defining size, number, location, and relative function of the kidneys when there are two. The US characteristics of multicystic dysplastic kidney (MDK) usually are diagnostic; however, renal scintigraphy (Figure 9-10) occasionally can help differentiate the hydronephrotic form of MDK

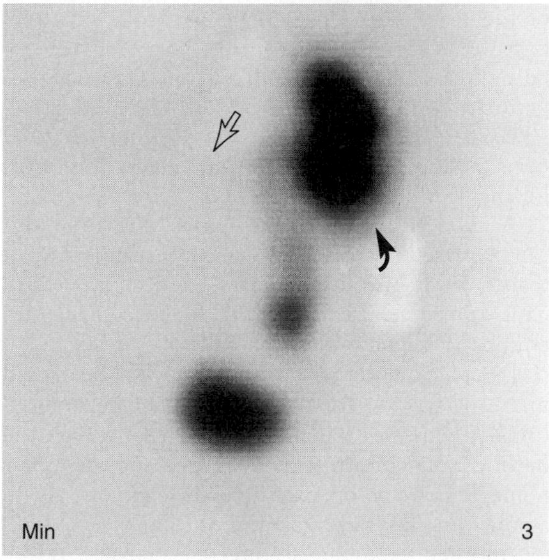

FIGURE 9-10 This posterior image from a diethylene triamine pentaacetic acid (DTPA) renal scan demonstrates the collecting system, ureter, and urinary bladder associated with the functioning right kidney *(black arrow)*. The multicystic dysplastic kidney on the left shows no functional renal tissue *(open arrow)*.

from severe ureteropelvic junction (UPJ) obstruction. A combination agent such as MAG3 is useful in the evaluation of hydronephrosis, because one can determine the relative function of each kidney and evaluate the degree of obstruction. Addition of the furosemide (Lasix) washout study augments the evaluation of hydronephrosis by rendering a washout curve that is indicative of the severity of obstruction. In evaluating hydronephrosis, generally it is helpful to place a catheter in the urinary bladder to prevent possible vesicoureteral reflux from confounding examination results. Although all of these tests can be performed in the newborn period, the concentrating ability of the newborn kidney is marginal. Therefore the tests often are reserved until the patient is 3 to 6 months of age to improve their accuracy and prognostic capability.

POSITRON EMISSION TOMOGRAPHY

Background

The radiation dose required for positron emission tomography (PET) is significant, and the utilization in neonates and young infants to this point has been limited. Nonetheless, the recent growth and interest in PET requires a section if for no other reason than for completeness.

The concept of PET was initially put forth in the early 1950s. Medical positron emission tomography was first attempted in the mid-1970s. The physics of PET involves introduction of a positron emitting radiopharmaceutical combined with a biologically active substance. These short half-life radiopharmaceuticals require a cyclotron to produce and are therefore less available than the technician kelate pharmaceuticals most commonly used in routine nuclear scintigraphy. A positron is a particle with the opposite charge of an electron that travels only a very short distance within the body until it hits an electron. The collision of the positron with an electron results in two annihilation electrons (gamma rays) of a specific energy 511 keV being emitted in opposite directions (≈180 degrees along a line) at equal velocity. The location in space of the point source of the electrons can be calculated from the fractional difference in the time it takes for the electron to reach the detector. The positron-emitting tracer attached to a metabolically active substance is introduced into the body intravenously, and the radiotracer is distributed throughout the body with the active metabolite. After 30 to 60 minutes of redistribution within the body, a scintillation scanning device detects the nearly coincident paired gamma rays. In the body, bones and other attenuators block some of the electrons from reaching the detector. Therefore a means of identifying the blockers is needed.

Computed tomography happens to be a very efficient means of locating bones and other blockers but has the added benefit of rendering anatomic images. This allows for more precise localization of signal and its relationship to internal structures. Because of the ability to acquire both anatomic and metabolic information simultaneously, the combination of PET and CT (PET/CT) has been responsible for the rapid growth of PET in recent years. Not only can one identify regions of high metabolic activity but also the location can be more precisely correlated with the internal anatomy with significant improvement in diagnostic accuracy. In humans, the most common pharmaceutical used is fluorodeoxyglucose (FDG), which is a glucose analog. FDG is distributed like glucose throughout the body. Regions of abnormal metabolic activity can be identified and, with CT, localized to a specific structure in the body. A metabolically active tumor, for instance, would demonstrate a focus of increased activity in a PET image. For example, if it were localized in the anterior mediastinum, it would be consistent with the diagnosis of lymphoma.

Clinical Utility in the Neonatal Intensive Care Setting

The relatively high radiation dose associated with PET has limited its use, but it has been effectively utilized in staging neonatal neoplasm. The role PET will play in the evaluation of hypoxic ischemic injury and the evaluation of neonatal seizures is yet to be determined.

INTERVENTIONAL RADIOLOGY

Intervention is one of the newest but most rapidly growing subspecialty areas in medical imaging. Interventional radiology has assumed an important role as a minimally invasive way to treat disease. Imaging is used to direct the surgical approach. From a practical standpoint, **there are four major areas of radiology intervention: (1) vascular access, (2) tissue sampling for minimally invasive diagnosis of neoplasm or infection, (3) catheter or needle drainage of fluid collections or abscesses, and (4) directed delivery of cells, chemotherapy, or embolic material, which may be used to diminish flow in a vascular lesion.**

Any of the imaging modalities may be used to guide the intervention, but the most commonly used are fluoroscopy, ultrasonography, and CT.

Clinical Utility in the Neonatal Intensive Care Setting

Vascular access is the most commonly requested radiologic intervention in most pediatric institutions. Ultrasonography or fluoroscopy can be used to visualize veins for venous access.

Most tissue sampling is performed to diagnose neoplasm. In general, a needle can be placed into an area of abnormal tissue and either a fine-needle aspirate is obtained or, in solid tumors, a core needle biopsy may be performed. The advantage of a core needle biopsy is that the tissue obtained is frequently of volume sufficient to complete many of the biologic studies necessary in the preoperative evaluation of the neoplasm. This can be particularly helpful in patients in whom a neoplasm, once defined, can be pretreated before definitive surgical resection is performed.

Cysts or abscesses can be drained, obviating the need for an open surgical procedure and thus minimizing morbidity and shortening recovery time.

A gastrostomy or gastrojejunostomy tube also can be placed in a minimally invasive manner, rather than a more invasive standard surgical procedure. This can be an ideal approach for placement of a temporary feeding tube.

Directed delivery of chemotherapy has been used in neonatal units for the treatment of hepatoblastoma. Chemotherapy can be directed through the hepatic artery into the involved lobe and the tumor reduced in size before excision. The technique allows a previously nonresectable tumor to be resected.

Another example of directed delivery is the embolization of hepatic hemangioendothelioma. Hemangioendothelioma is an infrequent cause of congestive heart failure resulting from an extracardiac shunt in the neonatal period. It is possible to embolize the benign neoplasm, thereby diminishing the shunt and correcting the heart's failure. Vein of Galen aneurysm is another extracardiac vascular shunt that frequently predisposes the patient to high-flow cardiac failure. A significant spectrum of disease is related to vein of Galen aneurysms, and the success of embolization is highly dependent on the degree of vascular insufficiency related to the steal associated with a high-flow lesion. In patients who present early and in florid heart failure, the outcomes are predictably less positive than in patients who present later with an abnormality discovered during a routine physical examination, in which an intracranial bruit might be identified.

Finally, directed delivery for cell implantation and genetic engineering shows great promise. These areas are early in their development, but the ability to direct a catheter to a specific organ for cell implantation or genetic engineering will clearly have a role in future applications of interventional radiology.

Focused Discussion: Vascular Access

The availability of ultrasonographic equipment can allow placement of peripherally inserted central catheters (PICCs) or central venous catheters in vessels as small as 2 mm. With US imaging, the vessel is visualized directly. Fluoroscopic guidance requires limited venography through a peripheral intravenous (IV) line. Indirect visualization of the venous system is possible because intravascular contrast defines the vascular lumen. After visualization with either ultrasonography or fluoroscopy, a 21-gauge needle is placed into the selected vessel. Once good blood return confirms the intraluminal position of the needle tip, a 0.18-wire is passed through the needle. The needle is removed, and the tract is dilated. Next, a peel-away sheath is placed over the wire. The catheter is sized and then passed through the peel-away sheath. The location of the catheter tip is confirmed fluoroscopically.

PICTURE ARCHIVING AND COMMUNICATIONS SYSTEMS

The widespread use of picture archiving and communications systems (PACSs) has had a significant impact on diagnostic imaging and medicine throughout the United States and the world. Simply put, a PACS is the process of image acquisition, display, distribution, and archive as it relates to radiology (Box 9-3). A PACS allows images obtained by CT, MRI, ultrasonography, nuclear imaging, and plain radiography to be obtained and distributed to any location for simultaneous access by any number of caregivers and specialists. Examination images can be distributed via a local network within a hospital, over a regional network to a group of providers, or over the Internet for viewing anywhere in the world. Systems have been developed that offer resources never before possible with film. Archives are protected for patient privacy and safety.

BOX 9-3 PICTURE ARCHIVING AND COMMUNICATION SYSTEM

- Acquires, displays, distributes, and archives patient images
- Displays digital images on computer monitors (soft copy)
- Enables manipulation of images to enhance visualization
- Provides brightness, contrast, magnification
- Makes simultaneous viewing at multiple sites possible
- Improves efficiency and accelerates results reporting
- Enhances decision support, which improves patient management

For a number of years, CT, MRI, and ultrasound images have been acquired digitally or, at a minimum, were handled digitally after an analog-to-digital conversion. Before computerized radiography (CR) and digital radiography (DR), x-rays obtained in a conventional manner could be converted into a digital format by scanning the image in a laser scanner. Fluoroscopic and x-ray images now can be captured digitally with CR or DR and thereby become immediately available for "soft copy reading." ***Soft copy reading*** is the term used to describe reading from a computer monitor as opposed to viewing a radiograph at a view box, known as ***hard copy reading.*** CR is very similar to conventional radiography except that film is replaced by a phosphorescent imaging plate that transfers the latent image into a digital format when developed. DR provides for direct conversion of the x-ray into an electronic digital format that requires no processing of the imaging plate.

The subtleties of CR and DR acquisition are beyond the scope of this chapter. Suffice it to say that the flexibility provided by digital imaging is incredible. The contrast and brightness (window and level) can be adjusted to optimize visualization of selected images or even portions of an image. These parameters can be changed when viewing an image to enhance a particular structure or finding. The window and level can be changed when viewing a chest x-ray, for example, to accentuate the lung, bones, a central catheter, an endotracheal tube, or a gastrostomy button. Images can be magnified, rotated, inverted (black to white and white to black), and even screened by sophisticated computer programs to improve detection of pathology. Radiology reports can be transcribed with voice recognition software, allowing the radiologist to edit and sign a report within minutes of acquisition. The reports then are associated with images from the examination. It is now common to have images and interpretations available on a computer monitor in the NICU by the time the patient returns from radiology. Reports and images then are assimilated into the patient's electronic medical record. The PACS is a powerful tool that improves medical management by translating bits of data into clinically relevant information. It enhances medical care and decision support by making images and interpretations available simultaneously in numerous locations in a fraction of the time previously necessary.

FAMILY EDUCATION AND INVOLVEMENT

The caregiver can have a positive impact on imaging by helping educate the parent. When the parents understand the procedure and know what to expect, they can be very helpful. Not only is the imaging made optimal but also the experience of the parent and patient is improved. An informed parent can effectively assist in the imaging process when included in the treatment plan.

An optimal study requires motion-free imaging. Even with fluoroscopy and ultrasonography in which motion is being recorded, the actual acquisition of the image must be motion free. With x-ray, this is done by shortening the acquisition time. Respiratory motion can be limited by taking the image at the end of inspiration. Some modalities cannot acquire the image data fast enough to eliminate motion. These examinations frequently require sedation. The most common modalities to require sedation are MRI, nuclear scintigraphy, and CT.

Sedation protocols vary from institution to institution, but certain aspects of sedation are universal. The patient must be given nothing by mouth (NPO) for a period of time before sedation. It is simply unsafe to sedate a patient who has eaten recently. Failure to keep a patient NPO is one of the most common reasons that a scheduled examination has to be canceled and rescheduled. Parents generally are informed of the need for sedation and asked for consent (verbal or written). The choice of sedation depends upon many factors. These include the length of the examination, the fragility of the patient, and the experience and training of the individual responsible for sedation. The route of administration also is variable and includes IV, intramuscular (IM), oral (PO), rectal, and inhalation. The sedated patient is monitored throughout the procedure and recovery. Recovery can occur in the imaging suite, a recovery area, or newborn center, but the patient must be monitored until fully recovered.

Some unique aspects of newborn care require special attention in the imaging suite that might not be as important in older patients. These important issues are of even more concern in the sedated patient. Thermoregulation is always of concern in the neonate. Imaging suites frequently are cold. Maintaining body heat is especially problematic in studies that require prolonged imaging times and in those in which the patient could get wet, such as cystography and fluoroscopic GI procedures. Blankets and heat lamps can mitigate the problem, but one must anticipate the issue.

Fluid administration also can be problematic in the neonate. Newborns need dextrose in their IV lines, especially if they are not feeding. Keep IV lines open and functioning. Most IV pumps are not compatible with MRI, and many cause interference that degrades image quality. However, it is not appropriate to suspend fluid administration for the duration of the study. The issue should be anticipated and addressed in a timely fashion.

SUMMARY

Care of a critical newborn in the imaging suite can be challenging. It requires cooperation between the NICU staff (nursing and medical) and the imaging staff. Parental education enables the parents to participate in the care of their newborn and has a positive impact on the care the newborn will experience.

Numerous imaging alternatives are available for the evaluation of any patient condition. The best imaging choice varies depending on local expertise and availability. A clear understanding of the differential diagnosis, along with a thoughtful and specific analysis of the clinical question, is essential for optimal imaging consultation. The pros and cons of each modality should be considered by the clinician, and consultation with a radiologist is advisable if there is any uncertainty as to the best method of imaging.

BIBLIOGRAPHY

Amplatz K, Moller JH: *Radiology of congenital heart disease*, St Louis, 1993, Mosby.

Barkovich AJ: *Pediatric neuroimaging*, ed 4, Philadelphia, 2005, Lippincott Williams & Wilkins.

Barrington KJ: Umbilical artery catheters in the newborn: effects of position of the catheter tip, *Cochrane Database Syst Rev* 2: CD000505, 2000.

Barrington SF, Maisey MN, Wahl RL: *Atlas of clinical positron emission tomography* (with Interactive DVD), ed 2, London, 2006, Hodder Arnold Publishers.

Brenner DJ, Elliston CD: Estimated radiation risks potentially associated with full-body CT screening, *Radiology* 232:735, 2004.

Brenner DJ, Elliston CD, Hall EJ, et al: Estimated risks of radiation-induced fatal cancer from pediatric CT, *AJR Am J Roentgenol* 176:289, 2001.

Brenner DJ, Hall EJ: Computed tomography: an increasing source of radiation exposure, *N Engl J Med* 357:2277, 2007.

Cohen M, Edwards M: *Magnetic resonance imaging of children*, Philadelphia, 1990, Decker.

Hall EJ, Brenner DJ: Cancer risks from diagnostic radiology, *Br J Radiol* 81:362, 2008.

Kirks DR: *Practical pediatric imaging: diagnostic radiology of infants and children*, ed 3, Boston, 1998, Little, Brown.

Kuhn JP, Slovis TL, Haller JO: *Caffey's pediatric diagnostic imaging*, ed 10, St Louis, 2003, Mosby.

Osborn AG: *Diagnostic neuroradiology*, St Louis, 1994, Mosby.

Purdy IB, Wiley DJ: Magnetic resonance imaging and the neonate, *Neonatal Netw* 22:9, 2003.

Rumack CM, Wilson SR, Charboneau JW: *Diagnostic ultrasound*, ed 2, St Louis, 1998, Mosby.

Siegel M: *Pediatric sonography*, ed 3, Philadelphia, 2001, Lippincott Williams & Wilkins.

Silverman FN, Kuhn JP: *Caffey's pediatric x-ray diagnosis: an integrated imaging approach*, ed 9, St Louis, 1993, Mosby.

Stark D, Bradley W Jr: *Magnetic resonance imaging*, ed 3, St Louis, 1999, Mosby.

Swaiman KF: *Pediatric neurology: principles and practice*, ed 3, St Louis, 1999, Mosby.

Swischuk LE: *Imaging of the newborn, infant, and young child*, ed 4, Baltimore, 1997, Williams & Wilkins.

Volpe JJ: *Neurology of the newborn*, ed 4, Philadelphia, 2001, Saunders.

10 PHARMACOLOGY IN NEONATAL CARE

MARY MILLER-BELL, C. MICHAEL COTTON, AND DEANNE BUSCHBACH

Optimal pharmacotherapy delivers the maximum intended beneficial effect with the minimum toxicity. Determining the optimal pharmacotherapy for neonates is problematic in that much of the data have been extrapolated from research in adults, children, and laboratory animals. Neonates show dramatic differences in the way they respond to drugs compared with older children and adults and within the neonatal population.[18] Gestational age, chronologic age, and disease state alter a neonate's ability to metabolize medications and affect the infant's response to the drug.

This chapter discusses pharmacology as it relates to the neonate and illustrates how rational medication decisions can be made for neonatal intensive care unit (NICU) patients. It also discusses strategies to avoid medication errors, strategies for drug delivery, and the new frontier of a genetic variation–based approach to pharmacotherapy.

PHYSIOLOGY

Pharmacodynamics and Pharmacokinetics

The drug-receptor theory states that the amount and duration of a drug's availability to a receptor determine its effectiveness. ***Pharmacodynamics*** describes what the drug does to the body, whereas ***pharmacokinetics*** describes what the body does to the drug, how much drug is available to the receptors, and for how long (Figure 10-1).[12] A drug's disposition can be described by four processes: drug entry (absorption), distribution, biotransformation, and elimination.

Pharmacodynamics relates the amount of available drug (or active metabolite) to the effect and depends on receptor availability, affinity of the drug for the receptor, and cellular function.

Antagonist drugs block a receptor's cellular and physiologic activity (e.g., naloxone), whereas agonist drugs elicit the receptor's action (e.g., cardiovascular agents such as dopamine and epinephrine). Some drugs act with receptors to increase or decrease gene expression (e.g., antenatal steroids), whereas others affect cell membrane permeability. Some drugs, such as methylxanthines, increase or decrease the amount or activity of "second messenger" molecules within cells. Antibiotics and antiviral agents act through some of these mechanisms to reduce the viability of pathogenic organisms by changing vital characteristics and functions. Readers should note that most drugs have more than one effect, so although the desired therapeutic effect may occur, the drug's other effects can limit its usefulness. Side effects, which can vary from the minor to the prohibitive, occur within the therapeutic range of concentration. Toxic effects result from drug overdose or serum concentrations higher than the recommended therapeutic range.

Individual infants may have idiosyncratic responses to medications, as well as expected responses. Infants who are low sensitivity responders exhibit a drug response less than that expected for a usual dose, whereas infants who are extreme sensitivity responders exceed the expected response for a given dose and drug level. Unpredictable adverse reactions differ from expected responses. Patients may become tolerant to a given drug dosage, as is commonly seen with opiates. ***Tachyphylaxis,*** a rapid decrease in drug response without a dosage change,

Please note that the **PURPLE** type in each chapter is intended to make it easier to identify clinically applicable material.

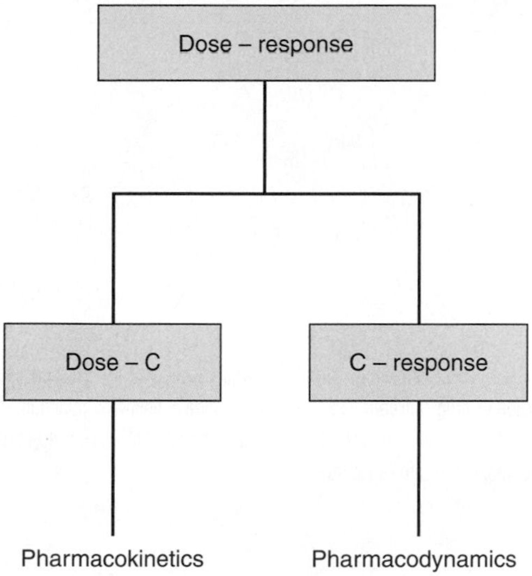

FIGURE 10-1 Variability in dose-response relationship can be the result of differences in pharmacokinetics or pharmacodynamics. *C*, Drug concentration (plasma or serum).

BOX 10-1 ABBREVIATIONS

C	Drug concentration (plasma or serum)	mg/L
Css	Steady state concentration (average)	mg/L
MEC	Minimum effective concentration	mg/L
MSC	Maximum safe concentration	mg/L
F	Extent of drug availability (0-1): how much active drug gets to the systemic circulation	Unitless
Vd	Volume of distribution: relates to loading dose	L/kg
Cl	Clearance: relates to maintenance dose	L/kg/hr
$t_{1/2}$	Drug elimination half-life: relates to the time course of changes in drug concentration	Hours

L, Liter = 1000 milliliters; *mg*, milligram = 1000 micrograms.

may be related to limited receptors or other intracellular mechanisms.[3,10]

Developmental differences in number and function of receptors and intracellular mechanisms are critical to estimating drug actions. An example of developmental effect on pharmacodynamics is the diminished sensitivity of the cardiovascular system to digitalis in the youngest patients; the receptor number increases with age. Changes in alpha- and beta-adrenergic receptors also occur with gestational and chronologic age and must be considered in determining dosage with pressors and inotropes.[12]

To elicit the desired therapeutic effect, the drug must be delivered to the receptor and remain available for an appropriate amount of time.[29]

***Pharmacokinetics* describes the delivery and removal of the drug to and from the body.** Doses and dose intervals are expressed mathematically by pharmacokinetic disposition parameters related to distribution, biotransformation, and elimination, such as clearance, volume of distribution, and half-life.

A clinician bases drug choice and dose regimen largely on the desired therapeutic response and toxic effect in "average" patients. *Plasma concentration* provides a surrogate for effect when the relationship between concentration (C) and effect has been demonstrated in similar patients. The ***minimum effective concentration (MEC)*** is that at which 50% of patients exhibit the desired response (Box 10-1). The ***maximum safe concentration (MSC)*** is that at which 50% of patients exhibit a toxic response (Figure 10-2). **To continue the desired effect, the clinician aims to obtain a target plasma concentration at "steady state" (Css), somewhere between the MEC and the MSC, where most patients exhibit the desired effect and few suffer toxic effects. With ideal maintenance therapy, drug input equals drug elimination. The variability around the Css depends on dose, dose interval, and drug disposition.**

The target Css is influenced by the amount of drug bound to plasma protein. In a newborn, free unconjugated bilirubin can displace numerous medicines of lower protein affinity, and numerous medicines can displace unconjugated bilirubin, increasing unconjugated bilirubin's serum concentration and its potential for toxicity. Intravenous (IV) lipid infusions also can affect protein binding of both bilirubin and some medicines. The drug concentration measured in most available assays is usually the total, both protein-bound and free; therefore the available concentration at the receptor usually is somewhat less than the total serum concentration.

DOSE-CONCENTRATION CONSIDERATIONS RELATED TO AGE

The reported therapeutic range for theophylline in adults is 10 to 20 mcg/mL for bronchodilation. In neonates, the drug has been used to treat apnea of

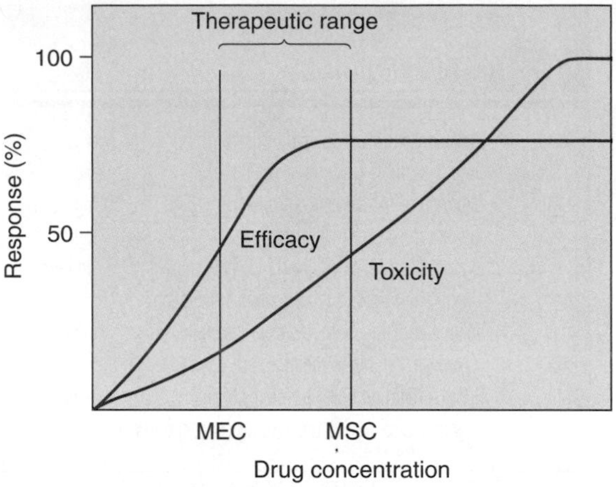

FIGURE 10-2 Percentage of patients with desired and toxic responses as a function of drug concentration. Therapeutic range is bound by minimum effective and maximum safe concentrations. *MEC,* Minimum effective concentration; *MSC,* maximum safe concentration.

prematurity, and the effective range for this disorder has been 4 to 12 mcg/mL.[29] Theophylline is reported to be 36% bound to plasma protein at a total concentration of 8 mcg/mL in newborns, compared with 70% bound in adults. A total theophylline concentration of 10 mcg/mL in an adult represents 3 mcg/mL free theophylline available to receptors, whereas in a neonate, a total of 4.7 mcg/mL equals 3 mcg/mL of free theophylline (also, the metabolism of theophylline in neonates leads to measurable free caffeine). Decreased bound theophylline in neonates could explain why therapeutic effect is achieved with lower total serum concentration in neonates.

In the NICU, doses and intervals must be adjusted based on changes in the dose-concentration and the concentration-response relationships. This enables a more accurate and precise response to changes in dose-concentration effects, especially total concentrations, but as with the theophylline case, we must watch for clinical effects and estimate other factors' influences to estimate the free concentration's effectiveness and the receptor and cellular responsiveness. Potential causes of changes in dose-concentration relationships unique to newborns are described for the pharmacokinetic processes that follow.

Absorption

The process of absorption defines the rate and amount of drug that enters the bloodstream. The parameter *F* indicates the percentage of dispensed drug available in the systemic circulation, with F = 1 indicating the drug is 100% available. We lack systematic studies of absorption in sick newborns, and differences in absorptive processes are expected but remain unmeasured generally. Some differences in newborns that potentially affect bioavailability include developmental changes in surface area and permeability of gastrointestinal (GI) mucosa, age-dependent changes in acid secretion in the stomach (higher pH than in older children and adults), changes in gastric emptying time and total GI transit time, and the characteristics of GI flora. Drugs such as ranitidine and metoclopramide also affect absorption of other medications by means of the same mechanisms.

"First-pass" pharmacokinetics means the drug is absorbed through the GI mucosa and travels directly to the liver, where it is metabolized and excreted in significant amounts, limiting bioavailability. Different drugs are absorbed at different rates, and different formulations of the same medication may be protected from first-pass metabolism. Drugs also may be given by inhalation, intranasally, intrarectally, topically, intramuscularly, subcutaneously, and intravenously.[12]

Distribution

Medications rely on blood flow and drug solubility for distribution to their sites of therapeutic effect. The *volume of distribution* for a drug is a parameter that relates total amount of drug distributed throughout the body to the serum or plasma concentration.[3] It is an attempt to quantify the space in which the drug can go. Strictly defined, it is the hypothetical volume of body fluid necessary to dissolve the total amount of drug as found in the serum. **Volume of distribution must be used to estimate the amount of a loading dose or a change in plasma concentration with any bolus dose:**

$$\text{Loading dose} \times F \text{ (the absorption parameter)} = \text{Change in concentration } (\Delta C) \times Vd \text{ (volume of distribution)}$$

Or, put another way:

$$\Delta C = F \times \text{Loading dose}/Vd$$

Volume of distribution usually is expressed as a function of body weight, with units of volume per kilogram. Major factors that affect distribution volume are plasma protein binding and body composition.[12,18,29] Changes in body composition happen throughout fetal and newborn life. Total body water decreases with increasing age: 85% in the smallest, most preterm infants; 70% in term infants; and 55% in most adults. Total body water may increase with such conditions as the syndrome of inappropriate antidiuretic hormone (SIADH) excretion, which increases total body water. Extracellular water composes about half this amount in a healthy term neonate. Large water-soluble molecules reach this compartment. Intravascular water composes about 10% of the body weight; protein-bound medications stay in this small compartment. Water-soluble drugs such as penicillins, aminoglycosides, and cephalosporins are distributed in a greater volume in smaller, more preterm infants, therefore requiring a higher loading dose per kilogram, if total body water were the only determinant of volume of distribution.

Plasma protein amounts and binding capacities also differ with gestational and chronologic age. Protein binding is decreased in newborns, because lower amounts of albumin are available than later in life, and fetal albumin has less capacity to bind some drugs. Acidic drugs such as ampicillin, phenytoin, and phenobarbital bind less well, thus increasing the free (available to receptor) fraction of the drug, with resultant increase in effect. Changes in pH also can affect a drug's affinity for albumin. Fat content varies with gestational age and degree of illness; increased fat content increases the volume of distribution. Lipid-soluble molecules also are distributed in this space.

Of particular concern in newborns is the interaction of circulating unconjugated bilirubin and protein-bound drugs. Several anionic compounds bind to albumin and can displace bilirubin, increasing free bilirubin, thus increasing its potential for toxicity. Bilirubin has a higher affinity for albumin than some other medications; it may displace them from albumin, increasing the medication's availability and potential to reach toxic levels.

Biotransformation

Biotransformation, or drug metabolism, occurs most commonly in the liver. Phase I metabolism describes the nonsynthetic metabolism of medications. Phase II, usually conjugation, or the addition of a substance to a medication, is synthetic metabolism. Oxidation, conjugation, glucuronidation, and hepatic blood flow change with gestational and chronologic age, diseased states, and use of certain medications. For example, oxidation and glucuronidation are decreased in newborns. Drugs such as acetaminophen, phenobarbital, and phenytoin, which require oxidation for elimination, remain available longer and may be transformed to other active metabolites (the neonatal liver metabolizes theophylline to caffeine), or the drug may remain at significant free concentrations for a prolonged period. The possibility of prolonged peak concentrations of available drug or active metabolites for many pharmaceuticals mandates careful monitoring of drug levels and clinical conditions to titrate dose intervals. To further the potential for confusion and trouble and further the argument for careful assessment of levels and clinical signs of effectiveness and toxicity, a decrease in plasma protein binding (or any other change in volume of distribution) may increase the hepatic clearance of a drug.

Clearance (Elimination)

Drug clearance or elimination occurs by excretion of unaltered drug or biotransformation to an inactive metabolite. Most drug elimination pathways can become saturated if the dose is high enough and dose intervals are too frequent. Most drugs in use in the NICU have therapeutic doses less than those necessary to saturate the elimination system. When clearance mechanisms are not saturated, the Css in plasma is proportional to the dose rate. Clearance equals the rate of drug elimination divided by the drug concentration.[19] Just as volume of distribution relates to loading dose and initial concentration, clearance relates to a maintenance dose that keeps a drug's concentration at steady state. So for an ideal drug maintained at steady-state concentration:

$$(\text{Dose/dose interval}) \times F = \text{Cl (clearance)} \times \text{Css}$$

Stated another way:

$$\text{Cl} = F \times \text{Dose}/(\text{Dose interval} \times \text{Css})$$

Or, to tailor the dose for a desired steady-state concentration:

$$\text{Dose rate} = (\text{Cl} \times \text{Css})/F$$

The appropriate dosing rate can be calculated if the clinician can specify the desired steady-state plasma concentration and knows the clearance and bioavailability of a drug (from peak and trough levels in a particular patient).

For example, clearance of theophylline in preterm infants is reported to be 0.017 L/kg/hr. If the desired Css = 8 mg/L, assuming F = 1, particularly if the dose is to be given intravenously:

$$\text{Dose rate} = (\text{Cl} \times \text{Css})/F = (0.017 \times 8)/1 = 0.136\ \text{mg/kg/hr or } 1.1\ \text{mg/kg q 8 hr}$$

RENAL EXCRETION

The kidney is the primary route of excretion for many drugs commonly used in the NICU. The kidney clears drugs through glomerular filtration and tubular secretion. Examples of medications eliminated through the kidney are aminoglycosides, digoxin, diuretics, and penicillins. Doses and dose intervals of drugs that have renal excretion must change with age and disease state. **The glomerular filtration rate (GFR) (i.e., the amount of blood filtered by the kidney in a unit of time) is low at birth and gradually increases over the first weeks. In preterm infants, the GFR starts even lower than in term infants, with a somewhat significant increase occurring at 34 weeks after conception.** Tubular secretion also matures with increasing gestational age and depends on tubular function. In adults, aminoglycosides may be dispensed based on creatinine clearance, but in neonates less than 1 week old, serum creatinine may reflect maternal levels, as well as renal impairment. Acidosis and a history of hypoxia or ischemia also may modify an infant's renal function, slowing excretion and altering pharmacokinetics. Again, measuring levels in cases of suspected renal impairment, whether from suspicious history or laboratory values, is important to determining an appropriate dosing strategy.

Half-Life

A drug's "half-life" ($t_{1/2}$) is the time necessary for the drug level to decline by 50%. Half-life is related to both volume of distribution (Vd) and clearance (Cl), so that:

$$t_{1/2} = 0.7 \times \text{Vd/Cl}$$

The $t_{1/2}$ is used to predict and interpret the time course of changes in plasma drug concentrations. For example, the time to steady state is 4 to 5 half-lives. The half-life is useful in selecting dose intervals. This concept is illustrated in Figure 10-3.

Loading doses help expedite reaching desired therapeutic concentrations, especially for drugs with long half-lives, in which a desired effect is needed immediately. For drugs with one-compartment distribution that stay in the circulation and are not stored in cells or tissue, the loading dose may be given as a simple single dose. Drugs that are fat soluble or stored intracellularly are more difficult to assess, and therapeutic levels must be included in the loading dose assessment.

$$\text{LD (loading dose)} = (\text{Vd} \times \text{Concentration [C]})/F$$

If the volume of distribution for theophylline in preterm infants is 0.7 L/kg, and 8 mg/L is the desired concentration, and F, for an intravenous dose, is assumed to be 1, a loading dose can be calculated.

$$\text{LD} = (\text{Vd} \times \text{C})/F = 0.7\ \text{L/kg} \times 8\ \text{mg/L} = 5.6\ \text{mg of theophylline/kg}$$

Pharmacogenetics and Pharmacogenomics

In the 30,000-plus known genes, there are over 4 million "common" variants (occurring in more than 1% of the population), many of which directly

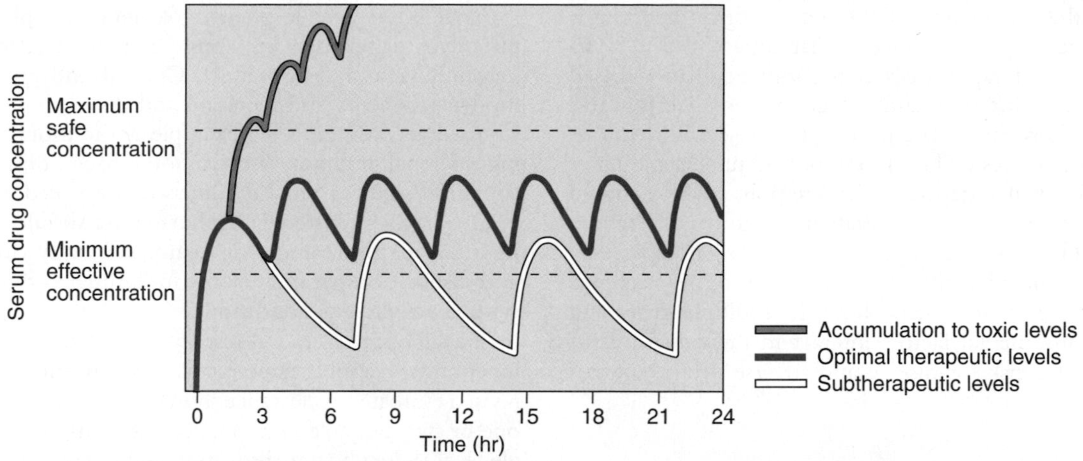

FIGURE 10-3 Effect on serum drug concentration of multiple dosing along with different time intervals between doses. (From Roberts RJ: *Drug therapy in infants,* Philadelphia, 1984, Saunders.)

affect the function of the coded protein. **In addition to the multiple factors like age, gender, disease, and concurrent medications, a patient's genetic code can cause variation in the response to a particular drug.** Once a drug is administered, it is absorbed and distributed to its site of action, then interacts with targets, and is finally metabolized and excreted. The enzymes and other compounds involved in each of these processes are subject to genetic variation that leads to variation in function. ***Pharmacogenetics*** is the study of the role of inheritance in the individual variation in drug response. ***Pharmacogenomics*** is the study of the influence of multiple genes and their interaction with each other and the environment on drug effects.[5,24,28]

The first description, over 40 years ago, of a genetically caused variation in drug metabolism was for the enzyme responsible for hydrolysis of succinylcholine. One in 3500 people are homozygous for a gene encoding an atypical form of the enzyme ***butyrylcholinesterase,*** which is quite slow to hydrolyze the succinylcholine, leading to prolonged muscle paralysis. Concurrently, an enzyme responsible for N-acetylation, another form of drug metabolism, was found to have a common genetic variant, so some patients are fast metabolizers and others are slow metabolizers of drugs such as hydralazine.

The cytochrome P-450 enzymes are important in phase I drug metabolism. One in particular, CYP-450 2D6, responsible for metabolism of many drugs, has been extensively studied. About 5% to 10% of the adult Caucasian population have genetic variants of the enzyme, leading to decreased activity and higher and more prolonged active drug levels.

Recently, a genetic variant in mitochondrial DNA, the A1555G mutation gene, has been linked to risk for hearing loss associated with aminoglycoside toxicity. The risk-additive variant's frequency in the general population is estimated between 1% and 3%, but among deaf subjects tested, concurrence of deafness with aminoglycoside treatment with this mutation is quite common. This could lead to future testing before use of aminoglycosides. It is unknown whether tight control of aminoglycoside levels would reduce risk for hearing loss. No recommendations can be made until more extensive, population-based studies are done. Such studies must include accounting for drug levels and duration and genotypes in assessment of risk for hearing loss.[21]

In addition to genetic variation in drug metabolism, the genetic polymorphisms of drug targets—including adrenergic and dopamine receptors and enzymes such as acetylcholinesterase—are likely to have effects on the response to drugs targeting these proteins. This may occur with the use of medications such as bronchodilators, pressors, and inotropes, and ACE-inhibitors such as enalapril and captopril.

The study of pharmacogenetics and pharmacogenomics is new, especially to neonatology, in which little is known about pharmacokinetics and pharmacodynamics of commonly used medications. The genetic revolution that has come with completion of the sequencing of the entire human genome is on its way to reaching neonatology with the availability of rapid analysis of large population-based samples for thousands of genes and their variants and how they relate to drug response. In the future, these studies will lead to improved understanding of individual variation in drug response, which should allow development of strategies to individualize care and help avoid complications resulting from heretofore unexplained genetic variations. The challenge will be to understand how the multiple genes and environmental factors interact in individual infants to alter risk for disease and adverse drug responses in fragile infants.

DATA COLLECTION

Clinicians should be aware of a medication's desired effects, side effects, and toxicities; know when they are expected to occur; and monitor for these effects. Whether a dose effect occurs or not should be noted. Dose–plasma concentration results should be recorded when therapeutic drug monitoring is done. If the drug's serum concentration relates to clinical response, the blood concentration should be followed in addition to clinical signs. To optimally use drug serum levels, the expected blood concentration is calculated from the dosing history, and patient variables that may affect pharmacokinetics with the timing of blood samples are considered. A comparison of expected values with measured values allows rational adjustment of future dosing.[4] Potential explanations for differences between measured and expected concentrations are listed in Box 10-2.

BOX 10-2 POTENTIAL EXPLANATIONS FOR DISCREPANCIES BETWEEN MEASURED AND EXPECTED DRUG CONCENTRATIONS

- Inadequate compliance
- Inadequate medication delivery
- Inappropriate timing of samples
- Laboratory error
- Revision in initial estimates of necessary pK required

pK, Pharmacokinetics.

Even if predictable pharmacokinetic and pharmacodynamic changes are considered, other factors may influence a drug's effect. Clinical end-points must be followed and recorded and dose regimens adjusted accordingly. One example is the monitoring of renal function with indomethacin dosing: If clinical signs of renal dysfunction are noted, the drug is not administered. **A pharmacist should be included in the caregiving team to clarify dose and disposition parameters for individual patients with their various conditions.**

If a suboptimal clinical response is noted in conjunction with a subtherapeutic plasma concentration, revised estimates of clearance should be adjusted with one or two available plasma concentrations. If a single level is drawn after absorption and distribution is complete or near steady state, then the maintenance dose formula can be rearranged to calculate the revised clearance. The common-sense approach suggests that if a patient has half the expected concentration of a drug, then perhaps the clearance is twice the initial estimate. If the patient has twice the expected concentration, the clearance likely is half the initial estimate. However, this technique is misleading if steady state has not been reached. **If a drug's level is higher than expected and higher than what is considered safe or if toxicity is noted, the drug should be discontinued until the concentration decays to the appropriate target.** If two concentrations are available after absorption and distribution, half-life is determined by plotting the concentrations on semilog paper. The revised clearance is calculated by rearranging the half-life formula:

$$\text{Clearance} = 0.7 \times \text{Vd}/t_{1/2}$$

Once the clearance and desired steady state are known, a new dose rate can be calculated:

$$\text{Dose rate} = (\text{Cl} \times \text{Css}_{\text{desired}})/\text{F}$$

Examples

The following examples illustrate the need to pay close attention to issues of drug delivery and clinical effects. The following examples are for caffeine citrate in neonates. The half-life of caffeine citrate in neonates is 3 to 4 days, the Vd is 0.8 to 0.9 L/kg, and clearance is 0.008 L/kg/hr.

EXAMPLE 1: A 15-day-old 1-kg preterm infant receives oral caffeine for apnea of prematurity.

After the loading dose of 20 mg/kg, the infant has received 5 mg every 24 hours for 5 days. At 8 AM on the fifth day, 4 hours after the last dose, the baby's heart rate is more than 180 beats/min but apnea has not been a problem. Clinical and laboratory evaluation of tachycardia includes consideration of caffeine toxicity. A blood sample for caffeine is sent to the laboratory. Estimate the concentration.

Necessary data:

Total body weight: 1 kg

Vd = 0.8 L/kg = 0.8 L in this patient

Cl = 0.008 L/kg/hr = 0.008 L/hr in this patient

$t_{1/2} = 0.7 \times Vd/Cl = 0.7 \times 0.8\ L/(0.008\ L/hr) = 70\ hr$

Time to steady state (Tss) = $4 \times t_{1/2} = 280$ hr

Assume F = 1; maximum safe concentration (MSC) = 30 mg/L; minimum effective concentration (MEC) = 20 mg/L

Therefore:

$$
\begin{aligned}
Css &= F \times Dose/(Dose\ interval \times Cl) \\
&= 1 \times 5\ mg/(24\ hr \times 0.008\ L/hr) \\
&= 26\ mg/L
\end{aligned}
$$

The Css was estimated using average Vd and Cl values reported in similar infants, adjusted for this infant's weight. If this infant has diminished clearance relative to "average," toxicity may result from the standard dose. Toxicity may not have been noted until day 5 because of the estimated time to steady state (Tss) of 115 hours.

EXAMPLE 2: At 4 AM, 24 hours after the last dose, when the next dose is due, caffeine concentration of 27 mg/L is reported. This is higher than the therapeutic range for caffeine in neonates and is most likely the result of decreased clearance. Using this concentration, estimate the time when the concentration will decline to 20 mg/L and determine a 24-hour dose schedule to maintain that concentration. The 4 AM dose is held, and the tachycardia resolves 24 hours later.

$$
Clearance\ revised = F \times Dose/(Interval \times Css) = 1 \times 5\ mg/(24\ hr \times 27\ mg/L) = 0.008\ L/hr
$$

$$
Revised\ t_{1/2} = 0.7 \times Vd/Cl_{revised} = 0.7 \times 0.7\ L/0.008\ L/hr = 70\ hr
$$

Therefore the concentration 70 hours later should be one half of the measured 27 mg/L, or about 13.5 mg/L. To maintain a concentration of 20 mg/L:

$$
\begin{aligned}
Dose &= (Interval \times Cl_{revised} \times Css)/F \\
&= 24\ hr \times 0.008\ L/hr \times 20\ mg/L)/1 \\
&= 3.8\ mg\ caffeine\ PO\ q\ 24\ hr
\end{aligned}
$$

EXAMPLE 3: Before the new oral regimen is initiated, another blood specimen is drawn 70 hours after the first and is 14 mg/L. Because tachycardia has resolved, an oral regimen based on the last two levels is begun to maintain a caffeine concentration of 20 mg/L. Estimate the necessary maintenance dose: The concentration fell 50%, from 27 to 13.5 mg/L in 70 hours, which confirmed our original estimate of half-life.

DRUG CATEGORIES

Antimicrobial Agents

Antimicrobial agents inhibit growth or kill microorganisms; they include antibacterial, antiviral, and antifungal agents. ***Bacteriostatic*** agents limit growth, allowing host defenses to control spread; this will not reliably eliminate a pathogen. ***Bactericidal*** agents kill the pathogen. Bactericidal agents at low concentrations may be bacteriostatic. ***Minimum inhibitory concentration (MIC)*** is the lowest concentration of an antimicrobial that stops the spread of an organism in laboratory culture media. This cannot be directly measured in an infected neonate and depends on tissue concentration and numbers of bacteria present. ***Minimum bactericidal concentration (MBC)*** is the lowest concentration of antimicrobial that reduces microbial number in laboratory media by 99.9%. Pathogens can develop ***resistance*** to antimicrobials by changing their cellular structures or producing enzymes that reduce antimicrobial activity.

For effective antimicrobial action, the drug must reach an adequate concentration in the infected tissue. The ideal concentration elicits maximum effect on the pathogen with minimum effects on the patient. Selection criteria for antimicrobials include the microorganism's sensitivity, the availability of the drug to the target tissue (some antibiotics do not cross the blood-brain barrier), bioactivity of the antimicrobial in the target tissue, the known MIC and MBC relative to side and toxic effect levels for the medication, and the individual infant's biologic state—that is, whether the systems of absorbance and elimination are working adequately for effective and safe drug delivery and removal. When the use of antimicrobial agents is planned in a seriously ill infant, as with other drugs, greater consideration must be given to clinical status than to the gestational or chronologic age.

Diuretics

Diuretics are used in the NICU to remove excessive extracellular fluid. Diuretics commonly cause a loss of electrolytes along with water. **Response to any diuretic depends on renal function and the drug's ability to reach its target in adequate amounts.** Most diuretics work within the tubule, but any drug that increases GFR can increase water loss. Drugs that increase cardiac output without decreasing renal perfusion and others that specifically increase renal blood flow also cause diuresis.

In infants, renal tubular function improves with increasing chronologic and gestational age. Because of poor absorption and response to aldosterone (especially in extremely preterm infants), electrolyte losses can be clinically significant with the addition of a loop diuretic such as furosemide or bumetanide. The ongoing losses may lead to hypochloremic metabolic alkalosis and less response to the diuretic.

Delivery of diuretics to the kidney loop increases with increasing chronologic and gestational age. Most diuretics rely on secretion from the proximal tubule and filtration through the glomerulus to reach their site of action. Both these functions improve with age. Enteral absorption of some diuretics is limited, so clinical effectiveness and electrolyte stability must be monitored closely to help determine safe and effective dosage regimens. The kidney also is responsible for diuretic excretion, again through tubular secretion and glomerular filtration. Because these functions are age dependent, the clinician must ensure that clearance time is adequate to avoid toxic levels.

Cardiovascular Drugs

Medicines used to improve cardiovascular function include digitalis and the sympathomimetic amines, which include drugs such as dopamine, dobutamine, and epinephrine. Antiarrhythmics, including digoxin, act to control the electrical conduction within the myocardium.

The sympathomimetic amines bind to β and G receptors; the number and availability of receptors determine response. **β_1 receptor response leads to constriction of vascular smooth muscle. β_2 receptors cause decrease in GI motility. G1 receptor stimulation stimulates cardiac contractility, and G2 response includes vascular and bronchial smooth muscle relaxation.** The response in any individual, and in any individual's specific organ system, depends on the relative amount of these receptors. Receptor numbers and their linked response elements within cells vary with gestation and clinical condition, and response must be monitored to aid in dosing decisions. Prolonged administration of sympathomimetic amines can lead to decreased response—an example of tachyphylaxis.

Antihypertensive agents occasionally are used in neonates for essential hypertension and occasionally to decrease afterload in neonatal patients with heart failure. These include volume reducers such as diuretics, inhibitors of physiologic regulators of blood pressure like enalapril, and drugs that decrease vascular resistance through β and G receptors.

The pathophysiology of neonatal disease should direct choice of cardiovascular agent. Extremely close monitoring of physiologic effects helps determine safety and efficacy of therapy. Monitoring must include very frequent, if not continuous, monitoring of blood pressure, heart rate, perfusion, and oxygen saturation (preductal and postductal in some cases). **Because other drugs are often given as a neonate receives cardiovascular medicines, thorough knowledge of possible drug interactions is mandatory.** Absorption of cardiovascular drugs is unpredictable. The sympathomimetic amines must be given by the intravenous route unless used in an emergency situation when endotracheal (ET) administration of epinephrine is indicated. Once dosed, the drug must be delivered to the target organ system. Infants in shock may not have the circulatory wherewithal to deliver the medication to elicit the desired therapeutic response. Because of the variability in β and G receptor development and distribution, undesired side effects in various organ systems may accompany desired responses. Rapid metabolism of the sympathomimetic amines demands continuous IV infusion, and infiltration of IV fluids may lead to significant tissue damage. Along with the physiologic effects, these IV lines must be carefully monitored.[19,29]

Central and Peripheral Nervous System Drugs

Nervous system drugs include ***analgesics,*** which decrease pain sensations; ***anesthetics,*** which control pain peripherally or in the central nervous system (CNS); ***sedatives/hypnotics*** including barbiturates (phenobarbital) and non-barbiturates (chloral hydrate, lorazepam), which do not control pain and can control some seizures; and ***antiepileptic*** agents, which are designed to control seizures (phenytoin, fosphenytoin). These drugs are associated with problems of addiction, tolerance, dependence, and withdrawal.

Addiction is a complex lifestyle change that involves drug-seeking behavior, which is not applicable to neonates. Tolerance occurs with many drug types. ***Tolerance*** exists when increasing doses and serum concentrations of a medicine are necessary to achieve a desired effect. A patient is ***dependent*** on a medication when regular drug administration is necessary for physical well-being. ***Withdrawal*** is a collection of physiologic and behavioral signs attributed to the absence of a medication in a dependent individual. Withdrawal has been identified for many medications, but it has been classified and described, along with weaning protocols, for opiate analgesics (see Chapter 11).[8]

The mechanism of action of most CNS medications is not clearly known. Again, careful monitoring of therapeutic effects relative to dose, duration, and serum concentrations is extremely important. **Significant respiratory depression can occur with most CNS medications, so appropriate resuscitation equipment must be available.** Variations in hepatic metabolism and volume of distribution are important in the ongoing assessment of dose-response. Some medications are highly fat bound and are slowly released into the circulatory system, causing prolonged effects, both therapeutic and undesired (e.g., respiratory depression, poor gastric motility, and abnormal neurologic function, such as feeding difficulties).

If hypothermia is used for infants with hypoxic-ischemic encephalopathy (HIE), evidence suggests that opiates accumulate in the circulation in excess of accumulation in similar infants with HIE who are not cooled. **Therefore, when using opiates in cooled infants with HIE, opiate levels are likely to be higher than expected for a given dose and expectations for neurologic examination must be modified given accumulation of high levels and delayed expectations.**[25]

PREVENTION OF THERAPEUTIC MISHAPS

More individuals die each year in the United States from medical error than from traffic accidents. Many medical errors are medication errors.[16] Even after making a correct choice of medication, one must pay attention to the appropriate dose and interval based on factors that affect a drug's pharmacokinetics and pharmacodynamics. Drug delivery must be ensured: This includes appropriate dose calculations; appropriately written and read orders; appropriate mixing with diluents; attention to drug interactions, incompatibilities, and contraindications; and drug delivery systems. In addition, effects of therapy at the chosen dose and systematic monitoring for therapeutic and toxic effects must be included in NICU care when medications are used.

Human error may occur, and it is in hospital areas of highest acuity, such as intensive care units and emergency departments, that the majority of medication errors have been described. In a review of medication errors in a large general hospital, pediatric medication errors occurred at a higher rate (5.89 errors per 1000 patients) than in the emergency department and medicine, surgery, and obstetric and gynecology (OB-GYN) units, with dosage calculation errors being the most common problem.[16] The authors suggested initiatives designed to prevent, detect, and avert problems associated with major factors associated with errors. In addition to calculation errors, problems included availability and information on drug therapy such as pharmacokinetic and drug interaction information, appreciation of patient characteristics that alter drug therapy, and confusing drug nomenclature.[1,2,6,15] In another review of hospital errors involving dosage equations,[17] antibiotics were the principal drug class involved. Errors in the equations used to calculate doses for all drug classes accounted for 29.5% of the errors.

Completing the "six rights" of medication administration (Box 10-3) in the NICU is complicated by the small doses and dosage adjustments based on infant weight or surface area. Investigators estimate that 8% of drug doses calculated and administered by competent NICU nurses are at least 10 times greater or less than

the ordered dose.[26] Another error risk arises from the fact that many drugs must be diluted because they are ordered in amounts that are not commercially available. The rate of drug entry, or absorption, also varies, depending on route of administration. **Calculations can be difficult and at least must be double-checked.** Examples should be readily available to those responsible for calculating doses. Other suggestions include the use of standardized drug preparations and dosing and standardized nomenclature or computer/digital order entry, with alerts for unusual doses. To avoid errors with emergency "code" medications, the doses of emergency medications should be calculated on admission, along with appropriate infusion rates (Figure 10-4). **The calculated doses for the most commonly administered medications should be posted at the bedside; these should be updated routinely with the passage of days and weight changes (as the pharmacokinetics and pharmacodynamics change).**

The ***Rule of Six*** was developed originally for use with vasopressor agents in code situations (its use has extended beyond that). The Rule, which allows nurses to estimate a pediatric dose by using a factor of 6, is prone to error. Standardized drug concentrations are less error prone and safer for patients than the Rule of Six.[22] **Because of medication errors, The Joint Commission (TJC) has required that standardized intravenous drug concentrations be used for pediatric patients receiving medications for which the Rule of Six was routinely used.** Another error-avoidance strategy, not mandated by TJC but strongly recommended, is to integrate a clinical pharmacist into patient care rounds with physicians and nurses, particularly in intensive care and oncology, to provide more direct patient care and consultation rather than the traditional role of drug preparation and dispensing. **Pharmacist interventions can reduce medication errors and adverse drug events.**[14,27] In addition, designing the ordering system to reduce complexity and provide rule-based order screening and double-checking of

BOX 10-3 THE "SIX RIGHTS" OF DRUG ADMINISTRATION

Right drug	Right dose
Right patient	Right time
Right route	Right response

NEONATAL RESUSCITATION MEDICATIONS

Name: ____________ Weight: ________ Suction depth: ________

Date of birth: ____________ ET tube size: ________

Drug	Strength	Dose	Route	Amount to administer
Epinephrine	1:10,000	0.1 mL/kg	IV, ET	____________
Atropine	0.1 mg/mL	0.1 mL/kg	IV	____________
Volume expanders		10 mL/kg	IV	____________

____

Signature of preparer

FIGURE 10-4 Calculations for neonatal resuscitation medications. Other drugs and dosages could be added (see Table 4-2). *ET*, Endotracheal; *IV*, intravenous.

calculations and developing effective information delivery may be more effective than traditional education or process-improvement efforts that target interventions after an error occurs.[9,16]

The American Academy of Pediatrics has published further recommendations for reducing medication errors for pediatric patients.[2] These include some hospital-wide actions, including the establishment of a clearly defined system for drug ordering, dispensing, and administration, with review of the original drug order before dispensing and administration. Confirmation of patient weight and drug dosage and strength is also recommended.[17] Avoiding the use of the terminal zero to the right of the decimal point (e.g., writing 5 instead of 5.0), and using a zero to the left of a dose less than 1 (e.g., using 0.1 rather than .1) will help reduce medication errors. Avoid abbreviations of drug names (e.g., MS may mean either morphine sulfate or magnesium sulfate), spell out dosage units rather than using abbreviations (e.g., units rather than U, or mcg for microgram rather than μg), and use generic medication names rather than trade names. Avoid verbal orders whenever possible.[22] See Box 10-4 for other interventions to reduce medication errors. For pediatric nurses, recommendations include the following:

- Familiarizing oneself with the medication ordering and use system
- Verifying drug orders before administration
- Confirming patient identity before each dose
- Verifying calculations with a second individual
- Verifying any unusually large volumes or dosage units for a single patient dose
- Verifying verbal orders by "reading back" the complete order to the prescriber
- Listening to the patient, parent, or other caregiver
- Asking questions as to whether a drug should be administered
- Maintaining familiarity with the operation of administration devices and the potential for errors with such devices

BOX 10-4 INTERVENTIONS TO REDUCE MEDICATION ERRORS

Strategy	*Examples*
Develop a neonatal and pediatric formulary	Neonatal/pediatric dilutions of pediatric formulary for gentamicin, hydrocortisone, magnesium sulfate
Develop age-specific dosing guidelines	All medications commonly used to treat neonatal and pediatric patients
Use technology	Computerized physician order entry
Develop protocols and procedures	Fluid management, skin care, insulin
Support nonpunitive error reporting	Medication incident reports
Provide up-to-date references	Neonatal and pediatric drug dosage handbooks

METHODS OF ADMINISTRATION

Once a clinician orders a medication and the drug and dose are found to be appropriate for that particular infant, the nurse's challenge is to administer the medication correctly. The following sections address some of the means of delivery that help improve accuracy of drug delivery.

Oral Administration

Variations in oral bioavailability and unanticipated and unmeasurable loss of drug complicate administering oral medications to newborns. Loss of medication occurs when infants regurgitate or require gastric suctioning and lose residual fluid that may include medication. If an infant is receiving orogastric (OG) or nasogastric (NG) feedings, medication should be placed into the center of the barrel of a syringe containing a small portion of the feeding. Medication may adhere to the plastic and decrease the amount of medicine delivered. The nurse must document drug administration attempts and any possible loss of drug, with an estimate of the amount lost. For infants receiving oral medications, documenting the color of the emesis or residual material helps determine presence of medications that have distinctive color.

If an infant is bottle fed, the nurse may put the medication in the full bottle. However, if the infant fails to take the whole volume, he or she has not received the full dose. One option is to finish the volume with gavage feeding. Another option is to gently introduce very small portions of a dose into the cheek pouch and wait for the infant to swallow.

Another method is to put 5 to 10 mL of a feeding, with the medication, in a small bottle and let the infant take that amount; then continue with the remainder of the feeding. Medication also may be placed into a nipple with a small volume of formula and offered to an infant. For breast-feeding infants, medication may be administered into the mouth as just described, with or without a small volume of expressed breast milk. As with all dosing of medicines, it is imperative to record doses and volume and characteristics of any residual material or emesis.

Intramuscular Injection

A newborn infant has relatively little muscle mass to receive injections. **When intramuscular (IM) injections are necessary, as with vitamin K, the anterior thigh is the site of choice. Comfort measures should be given before and after injection (see Chapters 5 and 12).** Clean the site with alcohol, insert a 22- to 25-gauge needle into the muscle, and for most medications, draw back on the syringe to ensure safe needle placement (unless specifically contraindicated); then inject the medication. After injection, the area is massaged. For an infant weighing less than 1500 g, the volume injected into one leg should not exceed 0.5 mL. Document the administration.

Intravenous Administration

IV medication can be given by push or antegrade injection, pump infusion, and retrograde injection. Retrograde injection is no longer recommended to administer IV medications to neonates.[3] Although drugs directly enter the bloodstream, the time necessary to complete drug delivery to receptors is a function of dosage volume, IV flow rate, and injection site (depending on particular IV methods).[23,29] Failure to recognize these potential time lags could result in inappropriate expectations of the timing of physiologic responses and peak and trough concentrations. The use of microbore IV tubing will facilitate rapid drug delivery because the volume of the fluid in the tubing is reduced. An example of a pediatric syringe infusion preparation and delivery chart for common neonatal drugs may be useful to the reader.[29] **Some drugs should never be administered into the umbilical vein or artery, and drug incompatibilities should be recognized before setting up multiple drug dosing through the same IV line. Careful monitoring for infiltrates and knowledge of drug-specific treatment for this complication are essential to safe IV drug administration. Continuous IV infusion of pressors is common in the NICU, and because of their rapid clearance and physiologic importance, these infusions should never be interrupted without orders.** Because of the sudden influx of potent medication, flushes to clear lines with continuous infusions of sympathomimetic amines should be avoided.

PUSH INJECTION

IV push medications must be mixed in appropriate volumes, delivered through appropriate-size syringes, and followed with an appropriate flush solution: heparin with normal saline solution (NS), 10% or 5% dextrose and water ($D_{10}W$ or D_5W). If numerous flushes are given, care must be taken with the osmolality of the flush solution.

To administer an IV push injection, prepare the IV port closest to the patient. Administer a small volume of appropriate flush solution, and then administer the medication over 1 to 2 minutes. Slow pushes are ordered sometimes, but the rate should be specified by the ordering medical care provider. A post-medication flush is given at the same rate as the medication to clear the line of remaining medication. **IV push administration of many medications used in the NICU is contraindicated because of the possibility of immediate adverse reactions associated with rapid bolus injections. Opiates and sedatives should be given with great care and with constant attention to respiratory and cardiovascular parameters.** Check a pharmacology reference if there is any uncertainty.

ANTEGRADE INJECTION

Antegrade injection is the introduction of medication into an entry port along the course of the IV tubing. The flow of maintenance fluid carries the medication to the patient at its rate. Because infusion rates in neonates are characteristically low, significant delays in drug delivery result. If rapid infusion is necessary, as with emergency resuscitation medications, more rapid infusion rates are necessary. This can lead to a significant medication error if, after drug delivery, the IV rate is not returned to baseline.

PUMP INFUSION

To avoid delay of drug delivery, two methods of pump infusion using a mechanical infusion device allow control of drug amount and delivery

rate. These devices consist of a pump that can be set to deliver a specific volume over a specific time, a syringe or other container that holds the medication or fluid to be delivered, and connecting tubing to connect the pump to a port for drug delivery. Because pumps vary by manufacturer and some may be used in a variety of ways, **each NICU should have a policy to ensure that each staff member carries out pump infusions in the same manner.** If different care providers start and end an infusion, the method used must be communicated.

Method 1. An exact ordered amount of medication is drawn into a syringe and diluted if necessary to provide the volume necessary for pump operation. This drug plus diluent fluid is flushed through the tubing, and the syringe is placed in the pump. After the pump finishes the infusion, some medication remains in the tubing and syringe hub. This medication needs to be flushed into the IV line with a flush solution to deliver the entire ordered dose.

Method 2. Medication is drawn into the syringe through the connecting tubing until the desired volume is in the syringe. The syringe then is placed on the pump, and a volume carrying the ordered amount of drug is infused. The tubing and syringe hub need not be flushed, because the infant has already received the entire ordered dose.

OTHER CONSIDERATIONS

Health care providers must remain attuned to additional concerns when administering IV medications. **Medications may require filters or protection from light sources or have significant specific gravity osmolarity. A 0.22-mcg filter may provide "cold sterilization"** (i.e., remove particulate matter and bacterial contamination). Some medications cannot be administered through a filter, because the filter removes the active ingredient. Medications with a specific gravity less than that of the IV fluid have a tendency to accumulate at high points in the IV tubing, whereas those with a higher specific gravity settle into low tubing loops, in both cases resulting in delayed and inaccurate drug delivery.

HOW TO GET INTRAVENOUS ACCESS: INSERTING PERIPHERAL INTRAVENOUS LINES

Common sites for IV placement in neonates include the hands, feet, arms, legs, or scalp veins. A transilluminator may help outline vessels in extremities. (When using a transilluminator, be mindful of potential burns from the high-intensity light source.)

Equipment

- Catheters with needles of appropriate size for the vessel
- Tape
- Alcohol
- Gauze
- Syringe with flush solution
- Tourniquet
- Arm board or leg board
- Restraints (as necessary)
- Gloves
- Comfort measures (see Chapter 12)

Procedure. Always consider comfort measures with any potentially painful procedure. Use of local anesthetic or other analgesic also should be considered (see Chapter 12). Assemble equipment at the bedside. Provide adequate temperature support. Tear two pieces of tape that are about 2 inches long and 1/2 inch wide; also tear three pieces that are 6 inches long. Select a vessel after confirming it is not an artery. Determine the direction of flow; veins fill toward the heart, arteries away from the heart.

Restrain the infant enough to avoid movement that prevents line placement. Some care providers place a leg board or arm board before the catheter is placed; others secure the limb after the catheter is in position. First flush the needle/catheter, and then remove the syringe. Place a tourniquet around the extremity, taking care to not pinch the skin. (Some caregivers prefer to not use a tourniquet and with practice may achieve success equal to that of caregivers using one.) Clean the site with alcohol, and allow it to dry. After gloving, insert the needle catheter into the vessel using your hand and fingers to anchor the skin surrounding the vessel. Insert the needle catheter at an acute angle and in the direction of blood flow. Observe for blood return or flashback into the tubing or cannula of the catheter. Some vessels do not provide blood return; babies in hemodynamic shock also may not have blood return. If the needle is thought to be in the vessel but no blood return is seen, then a small amount of flushing solution may be injected. If the needle is not in the vessel, the tissue will swell. If it blanches, the vessel is probably an artery. If blood return is seen, inject flushing solution to clear the needle, remove the needle, and gently advance the catheter.

Place a short piece of tape or small piece of transparent dressing across the catheter to secure it. Cross a longer piece of tape around the back of the catheter, and cross the ends across the front of the catheter. Check for proper position by disconnecting the IV catheter from the syringe to note blood return or by infusing a small amount of flushing solution. If necessary, use gauze under the IV catheter for support. Secure the IV catheter in place by using another long piece of tape. Cover the IV site to protect it. Leave adequate access to skin close to the IV site to allow monitoring for infiltrates.

If the medication is to be administered intermittently and the line is not otherwise used, it may be "heparin-locked" and flushed every shift with heparin solution (0.2 unit of heparin per milliliter of solution). Heparin solutions are available in several concentrations. It is good unit practice to standardize the volume and container type for each concentration and to individualize how each concentration-specific container looks and where it is kept. Controversy exists over the use of heparin versus NS for flushing lines. Two articles may be of interest: in one a rabbit model was used to determine the length of time for patency of catheters "locked" with heparin compared with those with NS; the second article examined the same issue in newborns and included a useful table comparing and contrasting the literature on the topic. Neither study found significant difference in length of time for catheter patency based solely on the infusate.[11,13]

Teaching Model. Models for teaching IV insertion with various needles and catheters vary from the highly sophisticated (and expensive) computerized human patient simulator to the "low-tech" and inexpensive human placenta. The computerized human patient simulator is available in three models: adult, pediatric, and neonatal. The simulator allows lines to be inserted in vessels; then barcoded syringes of "drugs" can be administered through the lines, and the simulator will respond with the appropriate physiologic response, which may include changes in blood pressure, heart rhythms, respiratory effort, and pupil dilation. Less advanced techniques include various models of neonate-size manikins with visible "vessels" in the scalp, arms, legs, and feet.

Critical Assessment

CRITERIA FOR INTRAVENOUS EXTRAVASATION

- Check all indwelling lines hourly for signs of extravasation.
- Look for phlebitis, edema, burns, adequacy of perfusion to site, hardness of tissue, or inflammation at needle site.
- For scalp veins, check dependent side of head for edema.

The fetal side of a human placenta is an inexpensive and easy-to-use model. The needed supplies and procedure follow.

Supplies

- Placenta
- Assorted needles and catheters
- Syringes with flush solution
- Gloves
- Tape

Procedure. After gloving, place the placenta fetal side up on drapes. Remove the fetal membranes, exposing the rich network of vessels. After re-gloving, insert IV needles with catheters into the larger vessels first and then into smaller vessels with improving technique. Tortuous or branching vessels can be used for various methods. Once catheters are in position, practice securing with various taping methods.

COMPLICATIONS OF INTRAVENOUS THERAPY

Complications of intravenous therapy include phlebitis, infiltration, hematomas, chemical burns, compartment syndrome, and emboli.[19] Long-term complications include disfigurement, contractions, and the need for surgical repair or amputation. Frequent (at least hourly) assessment of IV sites helps reduce, but does not absolutely prevent, IV complications (see the Critical Assessment box above). Swelling or discoloration of the extremity or skin at the needle tip is a sign of trouble, and the line should be removed. In the scalp, infiltration may be difficult to assess because swelling occurs not only at the IV site but also on the dependent side of the head. Scalp edema on the dependent side or a swollen eye is an indicator of scalp vein infiltration.

TABLE 10-1 **TREATMENT OPTIONS FOR EXTRAVASATION**

DRUG SUPPLIED	DOSAGE/ADMINISTRATION	COMMENTS
Hyaluronidase (Amphadase) 150 units/mL	1 mL (150 units) given as 4 or 5 intradermal 0.2 mL injections with a 25-gauge needle around the periphery of the IV extravasation site	Use with extravasation of hyperosmolar or extreme pH drugs. Administer within 1 hr of event. Not for use with vasoactive drugs.
Phentolamine (Regitine) 5 mg/mL in 1-mL vial	0.5 mg/mL given as 4 or 5 intradermal 0.2 mL injections with a 25-gauge needle around the periphery of the IV extravasation site	Prepare a dilution. Use with vasoactive drugs. May be given up to 12 hr after an event.

Modified from Roberts RJ: Intravenous administration of medication in pediatric patients: problems and solutions. *Pediatr Clin North Am* 28:23, 1981.

Footdrop[7] and compartment syndrome, in which nerves and vessels are damaged by swelling of tissue within a limited space, have been associated with positioning a footboard along the lateral aspect of the fibula, with or without an IV infiltration. The use of rolled washcloths as footboards or extensive padding of IV boards with cotton or gauze may prevent excessive pressure. Unnoticed infiltrations may result in significant tissue loss. **Warm soaks are contraindicated, because when extravasated fluid is warmed, it may exacerbate the burn, maceration, and necrosis.** In addition, heat increases oxygen demand in already compromised tissues.

Elevating the infiltrated area increases venous and lymphatic drainage, which helps decrease the edema. Hyaluronidase destroys extracellular barriers, allowing rapid diffusion and absorption of the extravasated fluid. For vasoconstrictive substances that extravasate, local use of vasodilators like phentolamine can aid in reperfusion.

Table 10-1 lists treatment approaches for extravasation.

Parent Teaching

INDWELLING LINES FOR PARENTS

Talk with parent about indwelling lines. Discuss:

- Type of line, purpose, and any limitations on holding, handling, or feeding the infant
- Pain control measures for the placement of lines
- That lines often need to be restarted

At discharge:

- The name of the medications, the dosages, purpose, routes, and any potential side effects
- Medication administration and what to do if the infant does not receive the full dose of medication

PARENT TEACHING

IV lines in newborns may frighten parents, especially scalp vein lines (see the Parent Teaching box above). Without information, parents may mistakenly believe the fluid or a needle is going directly into their baby's brain. It is helpful to reassure the parents that a needle, the fluid, and possibly medications are going into large veins. Also, reminding parents that although their infant has an IV line in place, they may still touch, hold, and feed him or her may help parents cope with interventions.

Parents should be made aware that pain assessment and control are part of the caregiver's ongoing efforts, and both are addressed during IV placement and maintenance. Encourage parents to assist in pain management strategies during IV placement (see Chapter 12). They should be told that a newborn's venous fragility, combined with the types of solutions used, makes restarting IV lines and multiple sticks per line relatively commonplace. **The potential for infiltration also should be addressed, and parents should be included in the effort to monitor the appearance of IV sites.**

As for an infant's medications, the parents should be made aware of treatment choices in the NICU. They need not know the details of medication dosing but should be made aware of significant medications in their infant's treatment regimen. **At discharge, parents must know the names of their infant's medications, their actions and the dosage, frequency of administration, and side effects, as well as where to obtain refills for each drug.** Some of the medications given for infants are not readily available at some of the smaller pharmacies. Caregivers must teach parents to administer prescribed medicines, and the parents must demonstrate their ability to safely and reliably give their infant the recommended doses. **The parents should receive written drug information instructions, which may be developed by the unit for their families or may be commercially available** from such companies as Micromedex Thomson Reuters Healthcare (www.micromedex.com). **Instructions must include actions, dosing amounts, routes of administration, dosing schedule, and potential side effects.**

REFERENCES

1. American Academy of Pediatrics: *Red Book: Report of the Committee on Infectious Diseases*, ed 27, Elk Grove Village, Ill, 2006, The Academy.
2. American Academy of Pediatrics: Committee on Drugs and Committee on Hospital Care: Prevention of medication errors in the pediatric inpatient setting, *Pediatrics* 112:431, 2003.
3. Brodsky D, Martin C: *Neonatology review*, Philadelphia, 2003, Hanley & Belfus.
4. Capparelli EV: Clinical pharmacokinetics in infants and children. In Yaffe SJ, Aranda JV, editors: *Neonatal and pediatric pharmacology*, Philadelphia, 2005, Lippincott Williams & Wilkins.
5. Evans WE, McLeod HL: Drug therapy: pharmacogenomics—drug disposition, drug targets, and side effects, *New Engl J Med* 348:538, 2003.
6. Fernandez CV, Gillis-Ring J: Strategies for the prevention of medical errors in pediatrics, *J Pediatr* 143:155, 2003.
7. Fischer AQ, Strasburger J: Footdrop in the neonate secondary to the use of footboards, *J Pediatr* 101:1003, 1982.
8. Franck L, Vilardi J: Assessment and management of opioid withdrawal in ill neonates, *Neonatal Netw* 14:39, 1998.
9. Glauber J, Goldmann DA, Homer CJ, et al: Reducing medical error through systems improvement: the management of febrile infants, *Pediatrics* 105:1330, 2000.
10. Hamzaui FH, Murakawa GJ: Topical medications. In Yaffe SJ, Aranda JV, editors: *Neonatal and pediatric pharmacology*, Philadelphia, 2005, Lippincott Williams & Wilkins.
11. Hanrahan KS, Kleiber C, Berends S: Saline for peripheral intravenous locks in neonates: evaluating a change in practice, *Neonatal Netw* 19:19, 2000.
12. Kauffman RE: Drug action and therapy in the infant and child. In Yaffe SJ, Aranda JV, editors: *Neonatal and pediatric pharmacology*, Philadelphia, 2005, Lippincott Williams & Wilkins.
13. Kyle LA, Turner BS: Efficacy of saline vs. heparin in maintaining 24-gauge intermittent intravenous catheters in a rabbit model, *Neonatal Netw* 18:49, 1999.
14. Leape LL, Cullen DJ, Clapp MD, et al: Pharmacist participation on physician rounds and adverse drug events in the intensive care unit, *JAMA* 282:267, 1999.
15. Lesar T, Briceland L, Stein DS: Factors related to errors in medication prescribing, *JAMA* 277:312, 1997.
16. Lesar TS: Errors in the use of medication and dosage equations, *Arch Pediatr Adolesc Med* 152:340, 1998.
17. Lucas AJ: Improving medication safety in a neonatal intensive care unit, *Am J Health Syst Pharm* 61:33, 2004.
18. Lugo R, Ward RM: Basic pharmacokinetic principles. In Polin R, Fox W, Abman S, editors: *Fetal and neonatal physiology*, Philadelphia, 2004, Saunders.
19. MacCara ME: Extravasation: a hazard of intravenous therapy, *Drug Intell Clin Pharm* 17:713, 1983.
20. McCurdy DE, Arnold MT: Development and implementation of a pediatric/neonatal IV syringe pump delivery system, *J Neonatal Nurs* 16:9, 1995.
21. Nance WE: The genetics of deafness, *Ment Retard Dev Dis Res Rev* 9:109, 2003.
22. *National Patient Safety Goals for 2005 and 2004*: n.d. Accessed August 12, 2004, from www.jcaho.org.
23. Nicholas P, Agius C: Toward safer IV medication administration: the normal safety margins of many IV medications make this route particularly dangerous, *J Infusion Nurs* 28:25, 2005.
24. Rioux PP: Clinical trials in pharmacogenetics and pharmacogenomics: methods and applications, *Am J Health Syst Pharm* 57:887, 2000.
25. Roka A, Melinda KT, Vasarhelyi B, et al: Elevated morphine concentrations in neonates treated with morphine and prolonged hypothermia for hypoxic ischemic encephalopathy, *Pediatrics* 121:e844, 2008.
26. Sakowski J, Newman JM, Dozier K: Severity of medication administration errors detected by bar-code medication administration system, *Am J Health Syst Pharm* 65:1661, 2008.
27. Scarsi KK, Fotis MA, Noskin GA: Pharmacist participation in medical rounds reduces medication errors, *Am J Health Syst Pharm* 59:2089, 2002.
28. Weinshilboum R: Genomic medicine: inheritance and drug response, *New Engl J Med* 348:529, 2003.
29. Yaffe SJ, Aranda JV, editors: *Neonatal and pediatric pharmacology*, Philadelphia, 2005, Lippincott Williams & Wilkins.

11 DRUG WITHDRAWAL IN THE NEONATE

SUSAN M. WEINER AND LORETTA P. FINNEGAN

The epidemic of maternal substance abuse over the past 35 years has continued to escalate at an alarming rate. The extent of drug use during pregnancy is often underestimated, as are the effects on the fetus and neonate. According to the National Survey on Drug Use and Health (Substance Abuse and Mental Health Services Administration [SAMHSA]),[80,86] an estimated 4% of pregnant women (ages 15 to 44 years) reported using illicit drugs in any given month. An estimated 11.8% of pregnant women reported current alcohol use with 2.9% reporting binge drinking and 0.7% reporting heavy drinking. Cigarette use was reported as 16.5% in pregnant women of the same age.[66] Using prevalence data from SAMHSA's National Survey on Drug Use and Health combined with live birth data from National Vital Statistics, out of the 4.1 million births in 2004, 160,370 pregnancies involved illicit drugs.[66] Data also showed that 8% of black pregnant women reported using an illicit drug in the past month, compared with 4.4% of white women and 3% of Hispanic women.[66]

The National Institute of Drug Abuse (NIDA)–funded 2007 Monitoring the Future study showed that 0.8% of 8th graders, 0.8% of 10th graders, and 0.9% of 12th graders had abused heroin at least once in the year before being surveyed.[58] As health care providers, we must recognize these data as a snapshot of affected young people who are future parents. **The sequelae of both licit and illicit substance abuse by the mother during pregnancy must be recognized and addressed to provide optimal medical care of the neonate.** Stereotypic biases should not interfere with the diagnosis or treatment. Drug dependence in pregnancy crosses all socioeconomic and racial barriers. **Therefore health care providers should not rule out drug exposure in any neonate who is exhibiting symptoms at birth related to withdrawal from or exposure to illicit or prescribed drugs.**

Opioid addiction in the mother during pregnancy has been studied in detail for decades in terms of its effects on the woman, the fetus, and the developing child.* An ***opioid*** is defined as any natural or synthetic drug that has pharmacologic properties similar to those of opium.[25] An opiate is derived from opium or contains opium. Because time, circumstances, and knowledge have changed, other factors now should be considered in treating neonates. **Diagnostic data can no longer be gathered on the assumption that one drug or substance was used. Polydrug use (the concurrent use of three or more drugs) is now the norm and not the exception.**[35] Polydrug use also can be the combination of illicit substances with those that are legal or found over the counter. The impact on the fetus and neonate is not necessarily minimized by the legality of the substance. Patterns of abuse, purity of the illicit drug, and sometimes potent or poisonous additions to them also may cause catastrophic sequelae in newborns.

Iatrogenic physical dependence has been documented in infants given intravenous fentanyl or morphine to maintain continuous analgesia and/or sedation during extracorporeal membrane oxygenation (ECMO) and mechanical ventilation.[83] Among the first to document this was Franck and Vilardi[29] in 1995 when neonatal abstinence syndrome (NAS) or neonatal opiate abstinence syndrome (NOAS)[66] was observed after abrupt withdrawal of sedation. The signs of withdrawal are much like those reported in infants born

Please note that the PURPLE type in each chapter is intended to make it easier to identify clinically applicable material.

*References 15-18,21-23,26,35,47,50,53.

to opioid-dependent mothers. Fifty to 84% of neonates removed from fentanyl within a 24-hour period exhibited withdrawal symptoms, and 48% exhibited signs and symptoms with morphine withdrawal.[83] Regardless of the agent(s) used for sedation, once the decision is made to start weaning the medication, **careful observation of the infant is crucial to monitor for signs and symptoms of withdrawal.**[83] A review of the literature points out the importance of initiatives for adequate analgesia in neonates, to the development of formal policies concerning intensive care sedation, and to treatment of the withdrawal[2,4,82,83] (see Chapter 12).

Osborn et al in a Cochrane Database Review of opiate treatment for newborn withdrawal discuss the use of the Lipsitz Tool (1975), the Finnegan Scoring System (1975), and the Neonatal Withdrawal Inventory by Zahorodny (1998) for the documentation of manifestations of withdrawal by various institutions.[59,62] The literature cites various pharmacologic agents that have been used to alleviate the symptoms of opioid withdrawal with methadone, buprenorphine, and oral morphine sulfate.[19,52,56,59,62] Advances in neonatology have continued to broaden the period of viability as many more premature infants are being kept alive. **What appears to be decreased severity of abstinence in preterm infants may be related to developmental immaturity of the central nervous system (CNS) or to differences in total drug exposure.** This proves to be a problem in evaluating the severity of abstinence signs in a preterm infant, because scoring tools were developed largely for use with term or near-term infants.[3,57]

This chapter presents current information about treatment issues surrounding drug-exposed neonates, with the main focus on opioid withdrawal. The effects of other substances such as stimulants, hallucinogens, selective serotonin reuptake inhibitors (SSRIs), tricyclic antidepressants, non-opioid CNS depressants, tobacco, methamphetamines, and alcohol are addressed when symptoms deviate from those of NAS.

PHYSIOLOGY

Because of their low molecular weight and lipid solubility, all drugs of abuse reach the fetal circulation by crossing the placenta, causing direct toxic effects on the fetus.* Although certain drugs may produce specific effects, many abused drugs produce similar manifestations of fetal and neonatal disease. In addition, the effects of legal drugs such as tobacco, caffeine, and alcohol may confound simple drug-effect relationships.[3] A hostile intrauterine environment also may be caused by adverse effects of the mother's drug addiction and must be considered when diagnosing the neonate's problems. **Examples of factors that could have an impact on neonatal outcome include lifestyle, homelessness, physical or sexual abuse, prostitution, poverty, poor or no prenatal care, polydrug abuse, intravenous drug abuse, binge and withdrawal cycles, anorexia, poor maternal nutrition, pica, dehydration, alcoholism, sexually transmitted diseases, dental abscesses, preexisting medical conditions requiring pharmacologic therapy, human immunodeficiency virus (HIV)–positive status or acquired immunodeficiency syndrome (AIDS), and hepatitis B and hepatitis C.**†

Opioid Substances

When drugs such as heroin, methadone, morphine, buprenorphine, and meperidine cross the placenta, the fetus may become passively dependent. Morphine, the major metabolite of heroin, methadone, as well as buprenorphine and its metabolite have been identified and measured in amniotic fluid, cord blood, breast milk,[1,30,33,51] neonatal urine, and meconium.[17,43,49,51,63] Non-opioid CNS depressants (e.g., benzodiazepines, barbiturates) and the other opiates/opioids (e.g., codeine, hydrocodone, oxycodone, hydromorphone, pentazocine, propoxyphene) all have been identified in neonatal urine and meconium.[19,47,92] Ethanol and its primary metabolite, acetaldehyde, have been identified in placental tissue and amniotic fluid.[10,11,73,77–79]

Human and animal studies have shown that use of opioids during pregnancy directly affects fetal growth. Heroin is associated with intrauterine growth restriction (IUGR), with only a slight reduction in gestational length, although the mechanism by which heroin inhibits growth is not known.[18] Although early speculation that maternal opiate (heroin) use during pregnancy was reported to accelerate fetal lung maturity, this has not been

*References 6,7,9,12,14,17,19,21-23,26,44.

†References 3,17,21,23,48,69.

borne out when formally studied and no plausible mechanism by which heroin exposure resulted in this was elucidated—even the associated growth restriction and chronic stress.[36] Older studies comparing methadone-exposed with non-exposed infants have found that methadone-exposed infants had lower birth weights. However, infants born to methadone-maintained women have been reported to have higher birth weights than those born to women using heroin. Decreased head circumference has been an inconsistent finding with these babies. Shempf conducted a meta-analysis looking at illicit drug use and neonatal outcomes and found birth weights of newborns born to mothers using heroin were lower than those of newborns whose mothers used methadone alone and those of newborns whose mothers used both heroin and methadone during their pregnancy.[69] A mean reduction of 483 g in birth weight and a relative risk for low birth weight were associated with any opiate use during pregnancy.[69] Neither heroin nor methadone has been associated with congenital malformations or any specific dysmorphic syndrome in offspring.

Methadone maintenance has been an accepted treatment strategy for opioid dependence for the past 40 years. Recently, several multi-site research studies have been studying buprenorphine instead of methadone, which was approved by the FDA for general use but not for the opiate-addicted pregnant woman.[57] The preliminary results of these studies have been inconclusive, although buprenorphine may offer some advantages for treatment of opiate dependence during pregnancy as seen in European studies.[27,28,44] It seems clear that patient preferences for methadone or buprenorphine seem to exist, so choices of medication should be considered now for non-pregnant women and perhaps in the future for pregnant women in the United States.

Neonatal withdrawal from psychoactive substances that the fetus is exposed to occurs in varying degrees. Because most opiates/opioids are short acting and not stored by the fetus in appreciable amounts, **neonatal abstinence is usually apparent within the first 24 to 72 hours of life.**[26] **The onset of clinical NAS symptoms depends on which opiates/opioids the pregnant women used.**[16,26] For example, with heroin, NAS may occur in the first 24 hours, whereas with methadone, it may not develop until after 48 hours.[16] **Symptoms of NAS in heroin-exposed infants occur earlier than in infants of methadone-maintained mothers because of heroin's shorter half-life.**[25] When compared with methadone, a lower incidence of NAS has been reported in buprenorphine-exposed neonates and it has been suggested that it is because of the limited placental transfer of this drug, thereby limiting fetal exposure and development of dependency.[37,40,42,44] A study by Ebner et al showed that a significant portion of neonates of buprenorphine-maintained mothers did not require pharmacologic treatment of their withdrawal.[16]

Non-opioid Substances

COCAINE

Although still controversial, the neonatal impact of maternal cocaine use, especially on fetal growth, is more consistently observed.[69] Researchers hypothesize that cocaine reduces fetal growth through maternal vasoconstriction, reduced uteroplacental transfer, and direct effect on fetal metabolism interfering with fat deposition.[69] Cocaine crosses the placenta by simple diffusion. This occurs because of its high lipid solubility, low molecular weight, and low ionization at physiologic pH. In addition, the low level of plasma esterases in the fetus and the relatively low pH of fetal blood (cocaine is a weak base) enhance the accumulation of cocaine in fetal compartments.[23] Taking advantage of the fact that cocaine and its metabolite ***benzoylecgonine (BE)*** accumulate and can be detected months after exposure in maternal and neonatal hair, an analytic test for cocaine and BE was developed by Garcia-Bournissen. These investigators looked at the characteristics of maternal and neonatal hair cocaine as biomarkers of fetal exposure.[32] They found that cocaine in hair and BE concentrations were not normally distributed, and they did not observe a correlation between maternal hair cocaine concentration and the baby-to-mother cocaine ratio, which ruled out a dose-dependent mechanism. However, the positive correlation between cocaine concentrations in maternal and neonates' hair corroborates previous reports showing transplacental transfer of cocaine.[32] Cocaine has a significant vasoconstrictive property, which decreases blood flow to the placenta and fetus, contributing to fetal growth restriction and hypoxia.[5,32]

Although direct teratogenic effects of cocaine have been dismissed by many authors and researchers on the basis of epidemiologic studies, available data appear to confirm an association between cocaine use and low birth weight, prematurity, placental abruption, and behavioral abnormalities.[32,37] In a recent review by Helmbrecht and Thiagarajah, it was posited that the mechanism by which cocaine induces placental abruption is via intense transient hypertension and vasoconstriction produced by the drug.[37] Several studies have shown that the placenta itself is a direct target for cocaine toxicity, which may play an important role in the pathogenesis of cocaine-induced complications in pregnancy.[32,37] Aside from generalized sympathetic effects, cocaine may more specifically impair fetal/neonatal cardiac function caused by apoptosis (programmed cell death) in fetal heart muscle.[1] This effect is attributed to the formation of oxygen free radicals.[5] The literature has suggested that these infants have an increased risk for prematurity, perinatal cerebral infarctions, abnormal electroencephalograms (EEGs) at birth, non-duodenal intestinal and anal atresias, necrotizing enterocolitis, terminal limb defects, cardiovascular effects, genitourinary anomalies, reduced head circumference, and, rarely, a pattern of congenital malformations termed ***fetal vascular disruption***.[39] Maternal cocaine abuse also has been shown to produce neuromotor deficits, which include impaired muscle tone leading to abnormal movement patterns and tremors.[5,37,69] The most important central action of cocaine is its stimulation of the central nervous system by inhibiting the reuptake of norepinephrine, serotonin, and dopamine. In the neonatal period, cocaine, unlike opiates, does not produce an abstinence syndrome but, rather, causes a direct neurotoxicity.[23,32,37] Initial signs of irritability and tremulousness are transient, usually lasting only a few days. This period of CNS irritability is followed by a more extended period of hyporeactivity, lethargy, and poor interaction with caregivers.[23]

As part of the Maternal Lifestyle Study, Bada et al used multivariate regression models with over 11,000 mother-infant dyads to try to estimate the effects of cocaine exposure on intrauterine growth and to investigate when fetal growth deviation would manifest itself in the woman's gestation.[6] After controlling for confounders, at 40 weeks' gestation, cocaine exposure was estimated to be associated with decreases of 151 g in birth weight, 0.71 cm in length, and 0.43 cm in head circumference. Investigators concluded that in utero cocaine exposure was associated with growth deceleration that becomes more pronounced as gestation advances.[6]

Lester et al compared auditory brain response (ABR) in 1-month-old infants exposed to cocaine and/or opiates and in those who were not exposed. Three previous published studies were conducted more than 20 years ago, before sophistication of research methodology and toxicology.[51] Their results both confirmed and expanded upon the earlier findings that perinatal cocaine or opiate exposure does affect neural transmission, which suggests delayed brainstem maturation in these infants.[51,91]

ALCOHOL

Alcohol has been shown to cause diminished deoxyribonucleic acid (DNA) synthesis, disruption of protein synthesis, and impaired cellular growth, differentiation, and migration. These cellular effects can be seen with both ethanol and acetaldehyde and are instrumental in inducing fetal malformations. It is unclear whether ethanol exerts its effects by interacting with neuronal membrane lipids or by interfering with membrane receptors and intracellular signaling systems.[23] The literature discusses altered embryonic cell organization, with IUGR and chronic fetal hypoxia as the result.[78,81]

The most serious effect to the infant of maternal alcohol use during pregnancy is fetal alcohol spectrum disorders (FASD). FASD is an umbrella term describing the range of effects that can occur in an individual who was prenatally exposed to alcohol. These effects may include physical, mental, behavioral, and/or learning disabilities with lifelong implications. FASD is not a diagnostic term. It refers to specific conditions such as fetal alcohol syndrome (FAS), alcohol-related neurodevelopmental disorder (ARND), and alcohol-related birth defects (ARBD).[75,79] Recent research documenting deleterious outcomes for children prenatally exposed to small amounts of alcohol (0.5 drink per day) has led to a realization that a threshold has not been adequately identified; therefore the woman should be counseled by her health care professional to not drink any alcohol while pregnant.[75,76]

When women consume cocaine and alcohol together, they compound the danger. Researchers have found that the human liver combines cocaine and alcohol to produce a unique metabolite, cocaethylene, which intensifies cocaine's euphoric effects. Cocaethylene is associated with a greater risk for sudden death than cocaine alone.[60] Discussions in the 1990s surrounding the use of cocaine and alcohol together suggested that cocaethylene was reported to be 10 times more potent than cocaine alone and more toxic to the growing fetus. This has not been discussed in more current literature; however, Vidaeff and Mastrobattista state that the expression of fetal cocaine effects or nonspecific anomalies could be expected to increase when the pregnant woman is combining cocaine with the teratogen ***ethanol,*** because the toxicity is augmented.[88]

AMPHETAMINES

Amphetamines and methamphetamines known as *crystal, ice,* or *crank* are abused by pregnant women in many geographic areas in the United States with the same frequency as cocaine. Like cocaine and "crack," the amphetamines are potent stimulants and effects on the fetus and neonate are similar; and like cocaine, the preponderance of available data would suggest little or no effect of amphetamine on organogenesis.[23,37] Early research has shown how in utero amphetamine exposure can lead to congenital brain lesions, including hemorrhage, infarction, or cavitary lesions. Investigators also described the sites of these lesions as frontal lobes, basal ganglia, posterior fossa, or generalized atrophy; the effects of the lesions are not exhibited until the child is older. In the neonatal period, neurologic abnormalities including decreased arousal, poor state control, difficulty with habituation, tremors, hyperactive neonatal reflexes, abnormal cry, increased stress, drowsiness, poor feeding, and seizures have been reported.[23,74] Outcome effects of prenatal exposure to amphetamines have yet to be isolated from the effects of alcohol and nicotine, the two drugs most often used with the methamphetamines.[60]

A review of the most recent literature documents lack of prenatal care as the hallmark of maternal cocaine and amphetamine use with an increase in maternal morbidity and mortality as its consequence.[3,70,77,78] **The use of these stimulants is reported to be toxic to the fetal brain, and there may be an increase in sudden infant death syndrome (SIDS).[3] Stimulants (amphetamines and cocaine) have been found in breast milk in extremely high levels and may produce an acute neurotoxic syndrome with hypertonia, tremors, apnea, and seizures.***

*References 6,32,36,38,51,68,74.

MARIJUANA

Marijuana, one of the most popular illicit drugs, has also been studied for many years.[31] de Moraes et al, in a prospective cross-sectional study that included full-term infants born to adolescent mothers who used marijuana, found that marijuana exposure was detected in both the mother's and the infant's hair and that the exposure during pregnancy altered the neurobehavioral performance of the term newborns when assessed with the neonatal intensive care unit (NICU) Network Neurobehavioral Scale (NNNS).[14] Other recent studies have highlighted the long-term impact of marijuana use in pregnancy on the neonate and child. These studies showed that prenatal marijuana use was "significantly related to increased hyperactivity, impulsivity, inattention symptoms, and delinquency" as the child grew older.[60]

INHALANTS

No well-controlled, prospective studies have been done on maternal inhalant use—often substances of abuse in poor and underprivileged communities and groups because they are widely available, legal, and relatively inexpensive.[89] Organic solvents are chemical compounds used to dissolve substances, and although their chemical structures widely differ, they share some common features: low molecular weight, lipophilia, and volatility at room temperature.[54,71] Inhalants are classified into four different groups: volatile solvents, aerosols, gases, and nitrites.[54,55,71]

Inhalants may produce a variety of rapid neuropsychiatric effects with euphoria or drowsiness coming on within seconds to minutes. Case reports and follow-up studies of children of inhalant/solvent–abusing mothers are available. Inhalant/solvent–abusing mothers give birth to babies who are small for gestational age (SGA) and who have developmental delays, craniofacial deformities, and an alcohol-like withdrawal syndrome.[41]

ANTIDEPRESSANT USE IN PREGNANT WOMEN AND NAS OCCURRENCE

Another area of concern is the psychopharmacology employed in the complex care needs of pregnant women with coexisting mental health diagnoses.[34] It has been estimated that up to 70% of pregnant women experience some symptoms of depression, with 10% to 16% of pregnant women meeting diagnostic criteria for a major depressive disorder.[84] The typical or atypical antipsychotic drugs and lithium all pass the blood-placenta barrier, with significant difference among compounds.[67] **Continuing treatment throughout the pregnancy may be necessary to prevent relapse, and the pharmacologic treatment for depressive disorders may be either the tricyclic antidepressants (TCAs) or the SSRIs.** A prospective study done by Kallen showed that both maternal TCA and SSRI use significantly increased the risk for neonatal respiratory distress, hypoglycemia, neonatal convulsions, and the occurrence of NAS.[45,46] Table 11-1 gives the signs and symptoms of withdrawal from TCAs and SSRIs.

Lithium. Lithium, often used for bipolar disorders, should be avoided during the first trimester of pregnancy. The placenta provides no protection to the developing fetus, and neonatal lithium toxicity is exhibited as hypotonia, cyanosis, lethargy, jaundice, hypothermia, poor sucking, poor respiratory effort, poor Moro reflex, reversible inhibition of thyroid function, and diabetes insipidus.[61]

ETIOLOGY OF NEONATAL ABSTINENCE SYNDROME

NAS is occurring in two ways: (1) by the passive exposure to opiates/opioids in utero as a consequence of maternal addiction to heroin, methadone, and other narcotic analgesics or to treatment of opiate/opioid addiction with methadone or buprenorphine; and (2) iatrogenically, by the administration of opiates/opioids such as fentanyl, morphine, and methadone to the neonate for analgesia and sedation.[29] Infants exposed in utero and born to heroin-, methadone-, or buprenorphine-dependent mothers have a high incidence of NAS (60% to 90%).[20] Less potent opioids or opioid-like agents have also been implicated in the development of NAS. (Box 11-1 gives a complete list.) **Neonatal abstinence is described as a generalized disorder characterized by CNS hyperirritability, gastrointestinal dysfunction, respiratory distress, and autonomic dysfunction manifesting as vague symptoms such as yawning, hiccups, sneezing, mottled skin color, and fever.**[16,22,48,50] When narcotics cross the placenta, equilibrium is established between maternal and fetal circulations. Before birth, the drug is cleared from the infant's circulation primarily by the mother's excretory and metabolic mechanisms.[25]

The onset of withdrawal symptoms varies from minutes or hours after birth to 2 weeks of age, but the majority of symptoms appear within 72 hours. Many factors influence the onset of NAS (Boxes 11-2 and 11-3).

Once the umbilical cord has been cut, the neonate is no longer exposed to the drug and monitoring of symptoms of withdrawal should commence. Because heroin is not stored in appreciable amounts by the fetus, signs of heroin withdrawal usually are apparent shortly after delivery and generally within 24 to 48 hours. However, methadone is stored in the fetal lung, liver, and spleen, facilitating the slow decline of methadone levels, but the rate of metabolic disposition varies for each infant, making the age at onset of NAS unpredictable. As mentioned on p. 203, the recent use of buprenorphine with maternal addiction is being studied. One such 5-year multi-site randomized study with early results is the Maternal Opioid Treatment Human Experimental Research (MOTHER) study. These data are not published yet; however, authors such as Fischer et al[27,28] have reported on the use of buprenorphine with pregnant women and neonates.

Buprenorphine

Buprenorphine, an opioid agonist/antagonist, has a wide safety profile (e.g., less respiratory depression, less risk for overdose), few autonomic symptoms with abrupt cessation, an occurrence of NAS at 20% to 60%, and a shorter duration of NAS and fewer symptoms, as evidenced by a decreased length of stay when compared with methadone-exposed neonates.[20,27,28,42]

Both methadone and buprenorphine are found in breast milk. Methadone appears in very low levels so that the mean daily methadone ingestion for an infant is 0.05 mg/day.[20] Buprenorphine's plasma-to–breast milk ratio approximates 1, and its poor oral bioavailability enables an infant to be exposed to one fifth to one tenth of the total available amount—the lowest amount of any opiate.[20] If a mother is compliant with methadone maintenance and is HIV negative, breast feeding is safely recommended (see Chapter 18). Further research and comparisons of the use of methadone and buprenorphine, especially in large randomized controlled trials such as the MOTHER study, are needed.[20,42]

Withdrawal may be mild, transient, and delayed in onset, or it may increase stepwise in severity. **Symptoms may be present intermittently or follow a biphasic course characterized by**

TABLE 11–1 NEONATAL SSRI AND TCA WITHDRAWAL SYMPTOMS

	CNS, SLEEP, ENERGY		GI SYSTEM		MOTOR		SOMATIC		RESPIRATORY/CARDIO	
	SSRI	TCA	SSRI	TCA	SSRI	TCA	SSRI	TCA	SSRI	TCA
Somnolence	X	X								
Irritability	X	X								
Convulsions	X	X								
Abnormal cry patterns	X									
Aberrant stool			X							
Poor suck/may need tube feedings			X	X						
Agitation					X	X				
Tremors, jitteriness, shivering					X	X				
Decreased tone					X	X				
Increased tone, rigidity, apathy					X	X				
Temperature instability							X	X		
Hypoglycemia							X			
Tachypnea									X	X
Dyspnea, respiratory distress									X	X
Dysrhythmias, unstable B/P, cyanosis									X	X

Modified from ter Horst PG, Jansman FG, van Lingen RA, et al: Pharmacological aspects of neonatal antidepressant withdrawal, *Obstet Gynecol Surv* 63(4):267, 2008.
B/P, Blood pressure; *CNS*, central nervous system; *GI*, gastrointestinal; *SSRI*, selective serotonin reuptake inhibitor; *TCA*, tricyclic antidepressant.

BOX 11-1 DRUGS ASSOCIATED WITH NEONATAL ABSTINENCE SYNDROME

Opioids

- Heroin
- Fentanyl
- Methadone/buprenorphine
- Morphine
- Meperidine (Demerol)

Less Potent Opioids and Opioid-like Agents

- Propoxyphene hydrochloride
- Codeine
- Pentazocine (Talwin)

Non-opioid Central Nervous System Depressants

- Tranquilizers and sedatives
- Bromides
- Chlordiazepoxide (Librium)
- Desipramine (Pertofrane, Norpramin)
- Diazepam (Valium)
- Ethchlorvynol (Placidyl)
- Glutethimide (Doriden)
- Hydroxyzine HCl (Atarax)
- Oxazepam (Serax)
- Alcohol
- Inhalant solvent abuse

BOX 11-2 FACTORS INFLUENCING THE ONSET OF PASSIVELY ACQUIRED NEONATAL ABSTINENCE SYNDROME

- Drugs used by the mother
- Both the timing and the dose of the drugs before delivery
- Character of labor
- Type of analgesia and/or anesthesia given during labor
- Maturity, nutritional status, and the presence of intrinsic disease in the neonate

acute NAS signs, followed by improvement and then the onset of a subacute withdrawal reaction.[18,21,23,49,90] Withdrawal seems to be more severe in infants whose mothers have taken large amounts of drugs for an extended period. **In general, the closer to delivery a mother takes the drug, the more severe the symptoms and the greater the delay in onset.**

BOX 11-3 FACTORS INFLUENCING THE ONSET OF IATROGENIC NEONATAL ABSTINENCE SYNDROME

- Prolonged opiate sedation for mechanical ventilation
- Duration of opioid analgesia use during extracorporeal membrane oxygenation
- Type of opiate used
- Maturity and presence of intrinsic disease in the neonate

Usually the origin of NAS lies in the abnormal intrauterine environment. A series of steps appear to be necessary for the onset of NAS and thus the recovery of the infant. The growth and ongoing survival of the fetus are threatened by the continuing or episodic transfer of addictive substances from the maternal to the fetal circulation. During this time, the fetus goes through a biochemical adaptation to the abnormal element. At delivery, abrupt removal of the drug is the catalyst needed to start the onset of symptoms. The newborn continues to metabolize and excrete the substance, so that withdrawal signs occur when critically low tissue levels have been reached. Recovery from NAS is gradual and occurs as the infant's metabolism is reorganized to adjust to the absence of the offending drug.[22,23]

Studies of the relationship between maternal dose of methadone and severity of NAS have yielded inconsistent results: 50% of the studies find a relationship, whereas 50% find no relationship.[8,13,20,72] Use of adequate maternal methadone for therapeutic effect may decrease concomitant drug use and fetal risk; there is no compelling evidence to reduce maternal dosing to avoid NAS.[20] Box 11-4 outlines the impact of maternal methadone maintenance on mother and newborn.

PREVENTION

Neonatal drug withdrawal is preventable if women do not use dependence-producing substances, licit or illicit, during pregnancy. Through intense educational efforts, the desirability and availability of drugs may be thwarted. Unfortunately, the psychosocial and socioeconomic milieu of modern society

BOX 11-4 IMPACT OF MATERNAL METHADONE MAINTENANCE ON MOTHER AND CHILD

- Reduces illegal opiate use as well as use of other drugs, diminishing the risk for hepatitis, HIV/AIDS, and other sexually transmitted diseases
- Helps remove the opiate-dependent woman from the drug-seeking environment
- Eliminates the illegal behavior including prostitution
- Prevents fluctuation of the maternal drug level that may occur throughout the day
- Decreases mortality and severe maternal morbidity
- Permits a more stable intrauterine environment for the fetus, decreasing chances of hypoxia; ***increases birth weight***
- Increases retention in substance abuse treatment
- Stabilized mothers on methadone more likely to retain custody of their children
- Children can be monitored by methadone clinic staff
- Provides opportunity for parenting education and other life skills
- No association between NAS severity and the following:
  - Maternal methadone dose
  - Trimester of methadone initiation
  - Duration and amount of methadone exposure
  - Duration of maternal drug use before pregnancy

Modified from Pregnant, Substance-Using Women (TIP2) BKD127 Guideline 4, SAMHSA, DHHS.

continues to propagate dysfunctional families, victimization of women, and an intergenerational cycle of substance abuse.

Therefore our goals must be to provide prenatal care for the pregnant drug-dependent woman and her fetus to diminish or eliminate the sequelae of passive addiction. The medical community is challenged to become more astute in its assessment and intervention for the problems of drug-dependent parturients. More treatment is necessary for these women and their neonates through inpatient residential care and outpatient interdisciplinary clinics that focus on the elimination, as well as the consequences, of addiction.

Franck and Vilardi, in addressing iatrogenic NAS, stated that guidelines for effective weaning of neonates from opiate analgesics and sedatives are becoming more established.[29] **Investigators encourage dose reductions of 10% to 20% per day.** For the prevention of iatrogenic NAS, discussions in recent literature include limiting total doses of fentanyl during ECMO therapy by administering morphine boluses or using continuous morphine infusions to replace fentanyl, substituting enteral methadone for morphine, or using sublingual buprenorphine.[48,56]

DIAGNOSIS

History

A comprehensive prenatal medical and drug history, especially with respect to polydrug abuse, is of prime importance. All pregnant patients who are substance abusers, regardless of the drug used, are considered high risk because of the effects of the drug, as well as complications arising from concomitant infections and lifestyle.[26] Fear of referral to child welfare agencies or the legal system in recent years has prompted women to conceal their drug abuse and/or pregnancy. This fear and denial may prevent the pregnant woman from seeking prenatal care. Thus she may appear at the emergency room of the hospital either in crisis or ready to deliver. In this instance, a prenatal history is absent, making neonatal assessment more difficult.

Signs and Symptoms of Neonatal Abstinence Syndrome

At birth, most infants exposed to narcotics appear physically and behaviorally normal with **symptoms of withdrawal beginning shortly after birth and up to 2 weeks of age, but the majority are exhibited within 72 hours.**[3,17,23] **Acute symptoms may persist for several weeks, whereas subacute symptoms (e.g., irritability, sleep problems, hyperactivity, feeding problems, hypertonia) may persist for 4 to 6 months.**[11,29]

The most common signs and symptoms of NAS are those of CNS hyperirritability, gastrointestinal dysfunction, respiratory distress, and autonomic instability (see the Critical Findings box on p. 210). A NAS scoring system is recommended and is discussed on pp. 212-214; however, for the convenience of referencing, the signs and symptoms discussed here are in the order in which they appear on the assessment sheet shown in Figure 11-2 on p. 213 (neonatal abstinence score sheet).

Initially, the infants appear only to be restless. Tremors develop, which are mild and occur only when the infants are disturbed, but these progress

Critical Findings

NEONATAL ABSTINENCE SYNDROME*

- Signs and symptoms of neonatal abstinence syndrome may not be exhibited for up to 72 hours.
- Most common signs and symptoms of neonatal abstinence syndrome are central nervous system hyperirritability, gastrointestinal dysfunction, respiratory distress, and autonomic instability.
- The closer to delivery a mother takes the drug, the more severe the symptoms and the greater the delay in onset.
- Acute signs and symptoms that may persist for several weeks:
  - Restlessness
  - Tremors (disturbed at first to undisturbed)
  - High-pitched cry
  - Increased muscle tone
  - Irritability and inconsolability
  - Increased deep tendon reflexes
  - Exaggerated Moro reflex
  - Seizures in about 1% to 2% of heroin-exposed neonates and approximately 7% of methadone-exposed neonates
- Subacute signs and symptoms that may persist for 4 to 6 months:
  - Irritability
  - Sleep pattern disturbance
  - Hyperactivity
  - Feeding problems
  - Hypertonia

*References 17, 18, 25, 35.

to the point at which they occur spontaneously without any external stimulation of the infant. A high-pitched cry, increased muscle tone, and further irritability to the point of inconsolability develop. When examined, the infant tends to have increased deep tendon reflexes and an exaggerated Moro reflex.*

One of the most serious but rare consequences of neonatal narcotic abstinence is the development of seizures. The relationship between maternal methadone dosage and the frequency or severity of the seizures has not been established. In addition, no significant differences were found between neonates with seizures and those without seizures in birth weight, gestational age, occurrence of their withdrawal symptoms, day of onset of withdrawal symptoms, or the need for specific pharmacologic treatment.[17,26] The mean age at seizure onset was 10 days. Generalized motor seizures, or myoclonic jerks, are the principal seizure manifestation, although in some infants the seizure manifestation can be complex. Seizures may occur even while the infant is being treated for NAS. Abnormal EEG tracings tend to occur only during the seizure itself, with normal interictal tracings.[3] The short-term prognosis for abstinence-associated seizures is favorable when compared with the prognosis after seizures associated with other causes. Finnegan and Kaltenbach suggested that this observed improvement in neurologic function may be based on the replenishment of neurotransmitters after transient depletion in the neonatal period.[22]

Infants with NAS frequently exhibit respiratory distress symptoms such as rhinorrhea, a stuffy nose, tachypnea, nasal flaring, chest retractions, intermittent cyanosis, and apnea. These symptoms may increase in severity when the infant regurgitates, aspirates, or develops aspiration pneumonia.

There is some evidence of transient abnormality of lung compliance and tidal volume in infants born to methadone- or heroin-abusing mothers, as well as tachypnea in NAS, suggesting that opioids may alter the fetal development of the respiratory system.[29] Infants with acute heroin withdrawal have shown increased respiratory rates associated with hypocapnia and an increase in blood pH during the first week of life. The observed respiratory alkalosis was thought to have a beneficial role in the binding of indirect serum bilirubin to albumin and possibly in the prevention of respiratory distress syndrome, which is rarely observed in infants of opioid-abusing mothers. However, alkalosis can decrease the levels of ionized calcium and lead to tetany.[24]

Infants undergoing narcotic withdrawal have seriously disturbed sleep patterns. Sisson et al studied EEG tracings and simultaneous electromyogram (EMG) recordings of eye and mouth movements before, during, and after treatment of withdrawal in 10 infants.[73] Rapid eye movement (REM), and non-REM sleep patterns were correlated with muscular and respiratory activity. This study concluded that narcotics obliterate REM sleep in neonates; withdrawal prevents normal adequate periods of deep sleep; proper therapy causes the return of REM and sleep cycles; and maintenance of therapy can be regulated better by use of polygraphic recordings

*References 17,26,47,59,64,69,87.

than by observed absence of gross signs and symptoms of withdrawal. Research has demonstrated the absence of quiet sleep in eight full-term infants whose mothers used heroin until delivery.[73] More recent studies by Pinto et al have substantiated the findings of previous sleep studies.[65]

The risk for sudden infant death syndrome (SIDS) should be considered when the neonate has an especially difficult course of NAS, when the mother supplemented her methadone with other substances (stimulants such as cocaine or amphetamine, nicotine), and when a combination of therapeutic agents is used for treatment. The rate of SIDS in these infants has been demonstrated to be 5 to 10 times over that in the general population. Research reports that the risk for SIDS is increased in opiate-exposed infants and varies from 2.5% to 4%.[40] Wingkun and other investigators studied carbon dioxide sensitivity in infants of substance-abusing mothers and found that these infants have abnormal sleep ventilatory patterns and "an impaired repertoire" of protective responses to hypoxia and hypercapnia during sleep cycles.[91] Infants undergoing withdrawal from narcotics have disturbed sleep patterns and exhibit excessive spontaneous generalized sweating, which may result from the predominantly central-neurogenic stimulation of sweat glands induced by heroin withdrawal.[23] Other autonomic nervous system signs include yawning, elevation of temperature, sneezing, and skin mottling. The rooting reflex is exaggerated. It is not surprising then that these infants frequently suck their fists or thumbs; yet when fed, their suck and swallow reflexes are uncoordinated and ineffectual. Therefore they tend to regurgitate or vomit in a projectile manner. The infant also may develop loose stools and is susceptible to dehydration and electrolyte imbalance.[21,26,29]

These symptoms are exhibited as a result of exposure to opioids, as well as to non-opioid CNS depressants. However, with non-opioid CNS depressant exposure, symptoms tend to begin at a later age, with malnourishment at birth an unusual feature. Because barbiturate withdrawal may not develop until an infant has been discharged from the nursery, it may not be treated unless suspicion has been aroused by the mother's symptoms or actions. Furthermore, **there is a greater risk for seizure activity in neonates withdrawing from barbiturates than in those withdrawing from opioids.**[3,20,22,26]

Symptoms exhibited by stimulant-exposed newborns differ significantly from those associated with maternal opiate use, unless the mother was using cocaine or amphetamines along with the opiates. Recent literature describes cocaine-exposed infants as tremulous, irritable, lethargic, unable to respond appropriately to stimuli, and having abnormal state control and cry patterns.* Also described are abnormalities in orientation, motor ability, state regulation, muscular hypertonia, and abnormal reflexes. Infants may show symptoms of lethargy intermittently with irritability, poor sucking patterns, and sleep disturbances. When cocaine has been the primary drug of abuse, most clinicians have not seen symptoms severe enough to treat the infant pharmacologically.[24,26] Most would refer to the symptoms associated with cocaine not as withdrawal but, instead, as a manifestation of toxicity.

Laboratory Data

Before initiating medication for treatment of NAS, one must rule out common neonatal metabolic alterations that can mimic or compound withdrawal, such as hypocalcemia, hypomagnesemia, hypoglycemia, and hypothermia. Serum glucose and calcium tests may be indicated. If the mother has had no prenatal care, it would be prudent to thoroughly assess the infant at birth, including testing for occult disease, sepsis, and intracranial bleeding. A ***urine test for toxicology*** should also be obtained. ***Meconium testing,*** although expensive and not readily available in all institutions, appears to be more accurate and can detect a longer period of drug exposure.[3,63,92] Recent studies support meconium drug analysis, because the test is noninvasive, highly accurate, and can detect prior drug use over a 20-week period.[63,92]

Hair analysis of the mother and infant shows some promise; however, this approach is still in the investigative stages and problems exist with regard to hair color, texture, and acceptability to postpartum women. Drugs of abuse are retained in hair for prolonged periods, and, unlike urine, hair samples cannot be adulterated. Unfortunately, hair sampling is invasive and the sample may be insufficient in newborns.[32,63] However, depending on the confidentiality laws of the state and whether members of the medical team are responsible by law for report-

*References 3,5,6,38,69,85.

ing the results of any drug testing to child protection agencies, informed consent may be needed from the mother. Health care professionals caring for infants of mothers who have received no prenatal care should check their own state laws and institutional policies for clarification about this procedure.[66,82]

TREATMENT AND INTERVENTION

To determine whether an infant will need pharmacologic treatment for withdrawal, appropriate assessment of symptoms is essential. **Because only 50% to 60% of exposed infants have symptoms significant enough to require medication, an assessment tool is helpful.**

We have used a ***scoring system*** to monitor the neonate in a ***comprehensive and objective*** way. With this score, one can assess the onset, progression, and resolution of symptoms. The score is used also to **monitor the infant's clinical response to pharmacotherapy for the control of NAS symptoms.** Titration of therapeutic agents is thus based on the degree of withdrawal symptoms that correspond to a specific score (Figure 11-1). **Although a number of scores have been used in both clinical and research settings, in our experience, the 21-item Finnegan neonatal abstinence score has been useful.** The nurse is vital in the assessment of withdrawal symptoms, because he or she will administer and record the score and any other activities that may affect the infant's progress. Therefore it is essential that interrater reliability be developed among all nurses responsible for the infant.

The ***Finnegan abstinence scoring sheet*** uses a weighted scoring of 31 items most commonly observed in an opioid-exposed neonate.[3] Signs and symptoms are recorded as single entities or in several categories if they occur in varying degrees of severity. Each symptom, with its associated degree of severity, has been assigned a score. Higher scores are assigned to symptoms found in infants with more severe withdrawal. The total score is determined by adding the scores assigned to each symptom observed throughout the entire scoring interval. The scoring system is dynamic rather than static; all of the signs and symptoms observed during the 4-hour intervals at which infant symptoms are monitored are point-totaled for that interval. **Infants are assessed 2 hours after birth and every 4 hours afterward.**

If medication is not warranted, the infant is scored for the first 4 days of life at the prescribed intervals. If the symptoms are severe enough

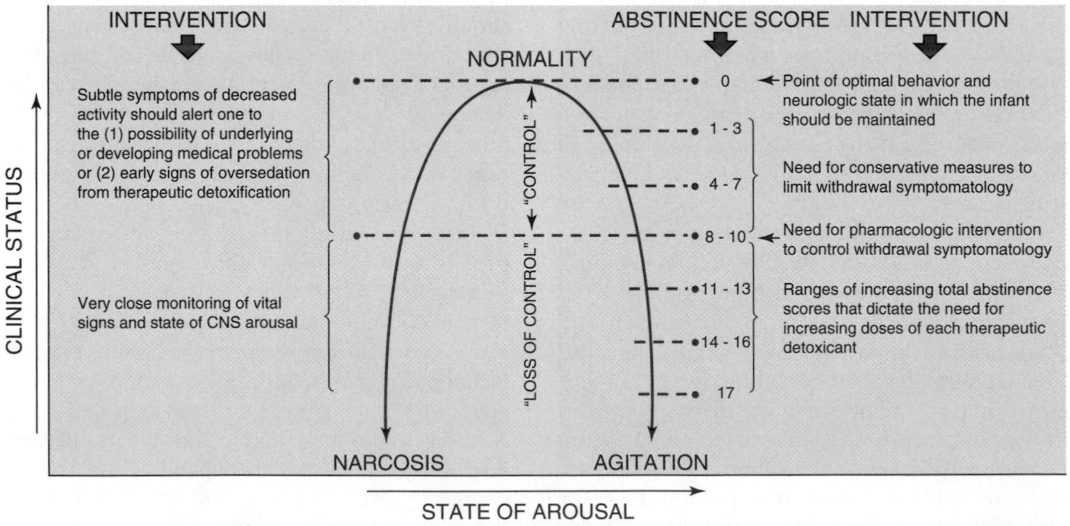

FIGURE 11-1 Management of the neonatal abstinence syndrome. *CNS*, Central nervous system. (From Finnegan LP: Neonatal abstinence syndrome. In Nelson N, editor: *Current therapy in neonatal-perinatal medicine*, ed 2, Ontario, 1990, Decker.)

to require medication, the infant is scored at 2- or 4-hour intervals, depending on whether the score is 8 OR LESS or 8 OR HIGHER, as described previously, throughout the duration of the therapy. Once medication is discontinued, if there is no resurgence of the total score to 8 or higher after 3 days, scoring may be discontinued. However, if there is a resurgence of symptoms with scores consistently equaling 8 or higher, scoring should be continued for a minimum of 4 days after discontinuation of medication to ensure that the infant is not discharged prematurely, with the consequent development of symptoms at home.

Figure 11-2 shows the NAS scoring system. Symptoms are listed on the left, scores to the right. Times of each evaluation are listed at the top, and the total score is listed for each evaluation. A new sheet should be started at the beginning of each day. A "Comments" column has been provided for nursing and medical staff to record important notes about the infant's progress.

The first score should be recorded approximately 2 hours after the neonate's admission to the nursery. This score reflects all infant behaviors from admission to that first point in time when the scoring interval is complete. The times designating the end of the scoring intervals (whether every 2 or 4 hours) have been left blank to permit the nursing staff to choose the most appropriate times for scoring intervals in relation to effective planning and implementation of nursing care.

NEONATAL ABSTINENCE SCORE

Date:________________ Weight: ________________

System	Signs and Symptoms	Score	Time AM PM	Comments
Central nervous system disturbances	Excessive high-pitched cry	2		
	Continuous high-pitched cry	3		
	Sleeps <1 hour after feeding	3		
	Sleeps <2 hours after feeding	2		
	Sleeps <3 hours after feeding	1		
	Hyperactive Moro reflex	2		
	Markedly hyperactive Moro reflex	3		
	Mild tremors when disturbed	1		
	Moderate - severe tremors disturbed	2		
	Mild tremors when undisturbed	3		
	Moderate - severe tremors undisturbed	4		
	Increased muscle tone	2		
	Excoriation (specific area)	1		
	Myoclonic jerks	3		
	Generalized convulsions	5		
Metabolic/vasomotor/ respiratory disturbances	Sweating	1		
	Fever <101° F (37.2° - 38.2° C)	1		
	Fever 38.4° C and higher	2		
	Frequent yawning (>3 - 4 times/interval)	1		
	Mottling	1		
	Nasal stuffiness	1		
	Sneezing (>3 - 4 times/interval)	1		
	Nasal flaring	2		
	Respiratory rate >60/min	1		
	Respiratory rate >60/min with retractions	2		
Gastrointestinal disturbances	Excessive sucking	1		
	Poor feeding	2		
	Regurgitation	2		
	Projectile vomiting	3		
	Loose stools	2		
	Watery stools	3		
	TOTAL SCORE			
	Initials of Scorer			

FIGURE 11-2 Neonatal abstinence score sheet. Check sign or symptom observed at various time intervals and add scores for total at each evaluation. (Modified from Finnegan LP, Kaltenbach K: The assessment and management of neonatal abstinence syndrome. In Hoekelman RA, Nelson N, editors: *Primary pediatric care*, ed 3, St Louis, 1992, Mosby.)

Salient points to consider in using the scoring system are as follows:

- **All infants should be scored at 4-hour intervals unless high scores indicate a need for more frequent scoring.**
- **All symptoms exhibited during the entire scoring interval, not just a single point in time, should be included.**
- **The infant should be awakened to elicit reflexes and specified behavior, but if the infant is awakened to be scored, one should not score him or her for diminished sleep after feeding.** Sleeping should never be recorded for a scoring interval except when the infant has been unable to sleep for an extended period: more than 12 to 18 hours. If the infant is crying, he or she must be quieted before assessing muscle tone, respiratory rate, and the Moro reflex.
- **Respirations are counted for 1 full minute.**
- **The infant is scored if prolonged crying is exhibited, even though it may not be high pitched in quality.**
- Temperatures should be taken (mild pyrexia is an early sign indicating heat production by increased muscle tone and tremors).
- If the infant is sweating solely because of conservative nursing measures (e.g., swaddling), a point should not be given. **Medication is not indicated if consecutive total scores or the average of any three consecutive scores continues to be 7 or less during the first 4 days of life.**

The total scores dictate the specific dose of medication, such as morphine, paregoric, or phenobarbital, and all subsequent doses are determined by and titrated against the total score. In the phenobarbital loading dose approach, an initial dose of 20 mg/kg is administered in an attempt to achieve an expected therapeutic serum level with a single dose. **Current recommendations are an opiate.** Phenobarbital is used only in resistant polydrug exposures.

The need for medication is indicated when the total score is 8 or higher for three consecutive scorings (e.g., 9-8-10) or when the average of any three consecutive scores is 8 or higher (e.g., 9-7-9). Once an infant's score is 8 or higher, the scoring interval automatically becomes 2 hours, so that the infant exhibits symptoms that are out of control for no longer than 4 to 6 hours before therapy is initiated. If subsequent 2-hour scores continue to be 7 or less for 24 hours, 4-hour scoring intervals may be resumed.

If the infant's total score is 12 or higher for two consecutive intervals or the average of any two consecutive scores is 12 or higher, therapy should be initiated at the appropriate dosage for that score before more than 4 hours elapse.

The longer the delay in initiating an appropriate medication dose, the greater the risk for increased infant morbidity. ***Comfort measures*** employed for the infant should include the following[12]:

- **Swaddling**
- **Offering a pacifier** for nonnutritive, excessive sucking
- **Aspirating nasal secretions** when needed
- **Changing the diaper frequently;** exposing hyperemic buttocks in severe cases for air-drying
- **Providing soft sheets or sheepskin** to decrease excoriations
- **Positioning on right side-lying** to reduce aspiration if vomiting or regurgitation is a problem
- **Protecting the infant from face scratching** by using mitten cuffs on the undershirt or tying a rubber band to the end of the shirt sleeves
- **Considering demand feedings** if weight-change patterns are an issue
- **Modifying the infant's environment (noise and light control);** for severe cases, some literature recommends self-activated non-oscillating waterbeds as a useful adjunct to supportive care of narcotic-exposed neonates.

Table 11-2 describes the symptoms of withdrawal and appropriate nursing interventions.

The pharmacologic agents most commonly used in the treatment of withdrawal include morphine sulfate, paregoric (camphorated tincture of opium), and tincture of opium (10 mg/mL) with the latter preferred over the paregoric. The American Academy of Pediatrics (AAP) supports the use of a 25-fold dilution of tincture of opium, which contains the same concentration of morphine equivalent as paregoric 0.4 mg/mL morphine equivalent without the additives (camphor) or high alcohol content found in paregoric.[3] A review of recent literature finds that some NICUs are treating NAS with an oral morphine solution because of concerns about the contents of the paregoric mixture: morphine or

TABLE 11-2 CREATING A SUPPORTIVE ENVIRONMENT FOR THE DRUG-EXPOSED NEONATE

INFANT BEHAVIOR	OBSERVATIONS	INTERVENTIONS
High-pitched cry	Note onset. Note length of time the cry persists: Is it continuous? Is it high pitched and piercing as though infant were in pain? Observe infant for other causes of abnormal crying patterns (e.g., meningitis, intracranial bleed, pain): Is anterior fontanel full or bulging? Are cranial sutures widely separated? Is head circumference increased? Does infant stare without blinking; exhibit tongue darting? Is cry aggravated or alleviated when infant is picked up?	Soothe infant by swaddling, holding firmly and close to your body; soft-pack baby carrier; smooth, slow rocking. Nonnutritive sucking. Decrease feeding intervals or implement a demand-feeding schedule. Reduce environmental stimuli (noise, light). Use waterbeds, lambskin.
Inability to sleep	Note how long infant sleeps after feeding. Note general sleep/wake patterns. If drug therapy has been initiated, note changes in sleep patterns, ability to rest, and any decreased activity indicative of drug overdose.	Decrease environmental stimuli (noise, light). Swaddle or use soft-pack baby carrier. Feed small amounts at frequent intervals. Use waterbeds, lambskin. Organize care to minimize handling.
Frantic sucking of fists	Note onset and amount of fist sucking. Observe for blisters on fingertips and knuckles. If blistering occurs, observe sites for signs of infection.	Use infant shirts with sewn-in sleeves for mitts to prevent skin trauma. Offer pacifier for nonnutritive sucking. Keep skin area clean; use aseptic technique.
Yawning	Note onset and frequency.	None.
Sneezing	Observe onset and frequency.	Aspirate nasopharynx as needed.
Nasal stuffiness	Note severity of nasal stuffiness and determine whether it hinders breathing and feeding; if mucus is excessive, consider possibility of other underlying problems, such as esophageal atresia, tracheo-esophageal fistula, and congenital syphilis.	Allow more time for feeding with rest between sucking. Aspirate trachea if tracheal mucus is increased. Check rate and character of respirations frequently. Use cardiorespiratory monitor with alarms set.
Poor feeding	Note sucking pattern: Is infant uncoordinated in attempt to suck, swallow, and breathe? Observe for other possible causes of poor feeding (e.g., sepsis, hypoglycemia, immaturity, bowel obstruction, pyloric stenosis).	Weigh daily. Decrease environmental stimuli. Feed small amounts at close intervals. Wrap securely. Maintain fluid and caloric intake required for infant's weight. Consider demand feedings. Use alternative feeding methods (e.g., gavage). Avoid rocking; may be helpful for some babies. Avoid talking or eye contact during feeding.

Modified from Finnegan LP, MacNew BA: Care of the addicted infant, *Am J Nurs* 74:685, 1974.

Continued

TABLE 11-2 CREATING A SUPPORTIVE ENVIRONMENT FOR THE DRUG-EXPOSED NEONATE—cont'd

INFANT BEHAVIOR	OBSERVATIONS	INTERVENTIONS
Regurgitation	Note when regurgitation or vomiting occurs: Is there a precipitating factor (e.g., medication, handling, manipulation, position)? Observe for signs of dehydration: Specific gravity >1.015 Urinary output <1 mL/kg/hr Dry mucous membranes Marked weight loss Poor skin turgor Sunken anterior fontanel Note time, color, consistency, and quantity of vomitus or stool. When stools are loose, estimate amount of water loss with stools. Note whether vomiting is forceful (projectile) or not. Observe for electrolyte imbalance.	Measure intake and output closely, and correlate with infant's general condition, progress, and therapy. Offer supplementary fluids if signs of dehydration appear. Weigh frequently if weight loss, vomiting, and diarrhea persist. Maintain IV at prescribed rate. Maintain infant in side-lying position. Head of bed may be elevated. Give skin care to prevent excoriation of neck folds, buttocks, and perineum. Change diaper frequently; expose hyperemic buttocks for air-drying. Consider barrier dressings on knees, elbows, etc.
Hyperactive Moro reflex	Is reflex moderately or markedly exaggerated? If drug therapy has been started, is Moro reflex diminished or absent? Is there asymmetry of the reflex? Asymmetry may indicate underlying pathophysiology (Erb's palsy, fractured clavicle, intracranial hemorrhage).	None
Hypertonicity	Note degree (mild, moderate, or severe) of increased muscle tone by: Attempting to straighten arms and legs and recording degree of resistance Picking infant up by hands and noting body rigidity with degree of head lag (a withdrawing infant often exhibits trunk rigidity and holds the head on a plane with the body for a prolonged time) Raising infant by arms and letting baby stand (a withdrawing neonate exhibits marked leg rigidity and can support body weight for considerable periods) Correlate mother's obstetric history and delivery with infant's condition; observe baby for other pathophysiology—hypocalcemia, hypoglycemia, meningitis, asphyxia, and intracranial hemorrhage. Observe for reddened areas over heels, occiput, sacrum, and knees. Observe temperature frequently; increased activity may cause hyperthermia.	Change infant's position often because prolonged or marked rigidity predisposes the infant to develop pressure areas. Use sheepskin to reduce pressure and for relaxation and comfort. Decrease environmental temperature if infant's temperature is >37.6° C (99.7° F).

TABLE 11-2 CREATING A SUPPORTIVE ENVIRONMENT FOR THE DRUG-EXPOSED NEONATE—cont'd

INFANT BEHAVIOR	OBSERVATIONS	INTERVENTIONS
Tremors, convulsions	Note whether tremors occur when infant is disturbed or undisturbed. Note location of tremors: Upper extremities Lower extremities Generalized Note whether degree of tremors is mild, moderate, or severe. Observe skin over nose, elbows, fingers, toes, knees, and heels for excoriation. Observe face for scratches. Observe for underlying pathology mentioned in the "Hypertonicity" section. Check temperature often for hyperthermia. Observe for seizures; if they occur, note onset, length, origin, body involvement, type (tonic, clonic, or both), eye deviation, and infant's color.	Change position frequently to prevent excoriation. Give frequent skin care (cleansing, ointment, and exposure to air and/or a heat lamp). Use sheepskin. Observe excoriations for healing, worsening, and infection. Decrease environmental temperature if infant exhibits hyperthermia. If infant convulses, maintain patent airway and prevent self-trauma. If infant is apneic after seizure, stimulate appropriately and be prepared to resuscitate. Decrease environmental stimuli. Organize nursing care to decrease handling. Support movements during caregiving. Swaddle as much as possible during caregiving.

Modified from Finnegan LP, MacNew BA: Care of the addicted infant, *Am J Nurs* 74:685, 1974.

opioid alkaloids, camphor, alcohol (46%), anise oil, and benzoic acid. Oral morphine solution contains only 10% alcohol.[11,23,29,50] Some recent literature describes using enteral methadone or sublingual buprenorphine.[48,56]

Table 11-3 outlines drug treatment for NAS. Any infant who exhibits a precipitous drop in a total score of 8 points or higher should be monitored for vital signs immediately. It is important to determine whether any underlying medical problems are developing, such as sepsis, meningitis, hypocalcemia, or hypoglycemia. **Detection of underlying medical problems may be difficult, because poorly controlled abstinence may mimic and/or disguise many common neonatal conditions.**

An infant may become increasingly depressed by a medication that is not used specifically for withdrawal. This situation may be seen in the infant's gradual development of depression and simultaneous poorly controlled withdrawal, requiring reevaluation for appropriateness of the medication (Box 11-5).

The efficacy of the medication always must be assessed. Two common situations indicate the need for reassessment: (1) **CNS depression,** and (2) **failure to achieve "control"** despite aggressive pharmacologic intervention and/or near-toxic serum levels of the agents. In these situations, the following measures are indicated:

- **Evaluate the infant for metabolic derangements, sepsis, and CNS disturbances to detect an occult problem compounding the clinical picture.** Evaluate laboratory data, including serum calcium, electrolytes, glucose determinations, and blood cultures.
- **Review maternal drug history along with both maternal and infant urine toxicology results to ensure appropriate medication.**
- **If a single medication is ineffective, consider a combination of therapeutic agents.** Phenobarbital may be used in conjunction with an opiate in cases of ***maternal*** polydrug abuse.

TABLE 11-3 DRUGS USED FOR NEONATAL ABSTINENCE SYNDROME

DRUG	DOSAGE	COMMENTS
Tincture of opium (1 mL is added to 24 mL sterile water) Final concentration equal to 0.4 mg morphine sulfate	Starting dose is 0.4 mg PO in 6 to 8 divided doses. Dose should be increased by 0.04 mg/kg/day or 0.1 mL as needed as frequently as every 4 hours until control is achieved. Weaning: decrease infant's dose by 10% daily, or as tolerated until daily dose is 0.2 mg/kg/day; then discontinue.	Control is evidenced by an NAS average score <8, rhythmic feeding/sleep cycles, optimal weight gain, same opium dose for 72 hours, pharmacologic weaning. Continue to score for NAS. Scores must remain <8.
Morphine	0.08-0.2 mg/dose PO q 3-4 hr. Use a 0.4 mg/mL dilution: 1 mL of the 4 mg/mL injectable solution added to 9 mL preservative-free normal saline solution. Protect from light; stable for 7 days, refrigerated.	Advantages: Diminishes bowel motility and loose stools; 20% to 40% bioavailability when administered orally; lower doses and shorter dosing interval are associated with shorter hospital stays in infants with NAS resulting from maternal methadone treatment. Disadvantages: Respiratory depressant, hypotension, delayed gastric emptying, ileus, urine retention.
Phenobarbital	Loading dose: 20 mg/kg to achieve an expected therapeutic level in a single dose. If score is ≥8, give 10 mg/kg every 12 hours until control or signs of toxicity appear. Maintenance dose (once under control): 2-6 mg/kg/day for 3 to 4 days. Decrease dose to 3 mg/kg/day. Discontinue: serum levels <15 mcg/mL.	Daily serum levels can be obtained. Advantages: Drug of choice for polydrug use; especially effective in controlling irritability and insomnia; controls symptoms in 50% of infants. Disadvantages: Does not prevent loose stools. Infant should be in a nursery where he or she can be monitored closely.

NAS, Neonatal abstinence syndrome; *PO*, by mouth.

BOX 11-5 COMPLICATIONS OF EXCESSIVE PHARMACOLOGIC TREATMENT

- Diminished or absent reflexes: Moro, sucking, swallowing, Galant, Perez, tonic neck, corneal, grasp (palmar, plantar)
- Truncal (central) or circumoral cyanosis or persistent mottling not associated with ambient temperature decreases
- Decreased muscle tone with passive resistance to extension of extremities, or decreased neck or trunk tone
- Altered state of arousal (e.g., obtunded, comatose)
- Diminished response to painful stimuli
- Failure of visual following
- Hypothermia
- Altered respirations: irregular (periodic breathing in full-term infants), shallow (decreased air entry), decreased respiratory rate (<20/min), apnea
- Cardiac alterations: irregular rate, distant heart sounds with weak peripheral pulses, heart rate of 80-100 beats/min, poor peripheral perfusion (pale, gray, mottled skin), cardiac arrest

PARENT TEACHING

It is important for primary caretakers to understand that infants exposed to narcotics through maternal addiction have been found to be more irritable and less cuddly, exhibit more tremors, and have increased tone (see the Parent Teaching box on p. 219). These infants are also less responsive to visual stimulation and are less likely to maintain an alert state. **Some symptoms of withdrawal may persist for 2 to 6 months, and the nurse should discuss this possibility with the caregivers well before discharge so that they may begin building the skills they will need under the watchful eye of supportive staff.** The infant may continue to feed poorly and regurgitate, yet vigorously suck fists and hands. Mothers frequently misread this continued, exaggerated rooting reflex as hunger and therefore may overfeed the infant. Loose stools may continue.

Parent Teaching

CARING FOR AN INFANT EXPOSED TO NARCOTICS

Some symptoms may persist for 2 to 6 months

- Infants exposed to narcotics in utero are more irritable, less cuddly, and tremulous and have increased tone: **Parent(s) may interpret these behaviors as signs of rejection; infant may not want to be held or cuddled as other babies**
- Less responsive to visual stimulation
- Less likely to maintain a quiet-alert state: **Let parent know symptoms are time limited**
- Poor feeding habits, continue to regurgitate yet show vigorous sucking of fists or pacifier: **Constant sucking and exaggerated rooting reflex may lead to overfeeding the infant**
- Continuation of loose stools: **Important to stress good diaper hygiene to prevent infection from excoriated skin**
- Infants easily disturbed by sounds: **Parent may decrease stimuli in house**
- Sweat more than other newborns: **Dress infant appropriately to avoid overheating**
- High-pitched cry: **Not easily consoled, parents need someone to share infant care and give them some rest from an irritable infant to prevent neglect or abuse**
- Hypertonia
- Less eye-to-eye contact, which decreases social interaction

These infants are easily disturbed by normal household sounds and do not sleep well. They sweat more than other infants and, when crying, continue to have a high-pitched cry. Hypertonia may continue, and the mother may interpret this as a sign of rejection. Nursing support, including thorough descriptions of the potential symptoms and their management and the fact that they are time limited, is vital if maternal-infant attachment is to occur and potential neglect and abuse are to be avoided.

In recent studies, drug-dependent mothers and their infants were assessed for patterns of interaction. Both drug-dependent mothers and their newborns demonstrated poor performance on a measure of social engagement. The drug-dependent mothers demonstrated significantly less positive affect and greater detachment, and the drug-exposed infants presented fewer behaviors promoting social involvement. Drug-exposed infants and their mothers experience a difficult early period during which both are less available, less likely to initiate, and less responsive to social involvement.[88] Therefore parents of the drug-exposed infant may need assistance in recognizing important symptoms that signal problems and cues necessary for caregiving.

All drugs of abuse pass through the breast milk. However, breast feeding in the methadone-maintained mother need not be discouraged, because it does not appear to shorten or worsen the course of withdrawal.[20,38] On the other hand, women using stimulants and other drugs, as well as those who are infected with HIV, should not be encouraged to breast feed because of the potential toxic and negative effects on the neonate. **Finally, secondary crack smoke, crystal methamphetamine smoke, marijuana smoke, and tobacco smoke can be detrimental to the health of the newborn; therefore parents should be warned of the consequences of using these substances around their infant.**

Although much has been learned over the past several decades from research in the field of perinatal substance abuse, continued evidence-based studies are essential if we are going to determine the intricacies of neonatal abstinence syndrome and the overall immediate and long-term effects of in utero substance exposure.

REFERENCES

1. Abdel-Latif ME, Pinner J, Clews S, et al: Effects of breast milk on the severity and outcome of neonatal abstinence syndrome among infants of drug-dependent mothers, *Ann Pharmacother* 117:6, 2006.
2. American Academy of Pediatrics, Committee on Fetus and Newborn: Prevention and management of pain in the neonate: An update, *Pediatrics* 118:2231, 2006.
3. American Academy of Pediatrics, Committee on Substance Abuse: Neonatal drug withdrawal, *Pediatrics* 101:1079, 1998.
4. Anand KJS and the International Evidence-based Group for Neonatal Pain: Consensus statement for the prevention and management of pain in the newborn, *Arch Pediatr Adolesc Med* 155:173, 2001.
5. Askin DF, Diehl-Jones B: Cocaine: effects of in-utero exposure on the fetus and neonate, *J Perinat Neonatal Nurs* 14:83, 2001.
6. Bada HS, Das A, Bauer CR, et al: Gestational cocaine exposure and intrauterine growth: maternal lifestyle study, *Am J Obstet Gynecol* 100:916, 2002.
7. Bandstra ES: Assessing acute and long-term physical effects of in utero drug exposure on the perinate, infant, and child. In Kibley MM, Asghar K,

editors: *Methodological issues in epidemiological, prevention, and treatment and research on drug-exposed women and their children*, NIDA Research Monograph 117, Washington, DC 1992.

8. Berghella V, Lim PJ, Hill MK, et al: Maternal methadone dose and neonatal withdrawal, *Am J Obstet Gynecol* 189:312, 2003.
9. Boucher N, Bairam A, Beaulac-Baillargeon L: A new look at the neonate's clinical presentation after in utero exposure to antidepressants in late pregnancy, *J Clin Psychopharm* 28:3, 2008.
10. Church MW, Abel EL: Fetal alcohol syndrome: hearing, speech, language, and vestibular disorders, *Obstet Gynecol Clin North Am* 25:85, 1998.
11. Coyle MG, Ferguson A, Lagasse L, et al: Diluted tincture of opium (DTO) and phenobarbital versus DTO alone for neonatal opiate withdrawal in term infants, *J Pediatr* 140:561, 2002.
12. D'Apolito K, Hepworth JT: Prominence of withdrawal symptoms in polydrug-exposed infants, *J Perinatal Neonatal Nurs* 14:46, 2001.
13. Dashe JS, Scheffield JS, Olscher DA, et al: Relationship between maternal methadone dosage and neonatal withdrawal, *Obstet Gynecol* 100:1244, 2002.
14. de Moraes Barros MC, Guinsburg R, Araujo Peres C, et al: Exposure to marijuana during pregnancy alters neurobehavior in the early neonatal period, *J Pediatr* 149:6, 2006.
15. Desai SA, HsiehEbling H, Greenspan J: *Modified Finnegan scoring system for the management of infants with neonatal abstinence syndrome*, Unpublished abstract, Philadelphia, 2004, Department of Pediatrics-Neonatology, Thomas Jefferson University & duPont Hospital for Children.
16. Ebner N, Rohrmeister K, Winklbaur B, et al: Management of neonatal abstinence syndrome in neonates born to opioid maintained women, *Drug Alc Dependence* 87:2, 2007.
17. Finnegan LP: Clinical perinatal and developmental effects of methadone. In Cooper JR, Altman F, editors: *Research on the treatment of narcotic addiction: state of the art*, Washington, DC, U.S. Department of Health and Human Services, National Institute of Drug Abuse.
18. Finnegan LP: Neonatal abstinence syndrome: assessment and pharmacology. In Rubaltelli FF, Granati B, editors: *Neonatal therapy: an update*, New York, 1986, Elsevier.
19. Finnegan LP: Influence of maternal drug dependence on the newborn. In Kacew S, Lock S, editors: *Toxicologic and pharmacologic principles in pediatrics*, Washington, DC, 1988, Hemisphere.
20. Finnegan L, Amass L, Jones H, et al: *Addiction and pregnancy*, Paper presented at the EUROPAD conference, Paris, 2004.
21. Finnegan LP, Kaltenbach K: Neonatal abstinence syndrome. In Hoekelman RA, Nelson N: *Primary pediatric care*, ed 2, St Louis, 1992, Mosby.
22. Finnegan LP, Kaltenbach K: The assessment and management of neonatal abstinence syndrome. In Hoekelman RA, Friedman SB, Nelson NM, et al, editors: *Primary pediatric care*, ed 3 St Louis, 1997, Mosby.
23. Finnegan LP, Kandall SR: Neonatal abstinence syndromes. In Yaffee SJ, Aranda JV, editors: *Neonatal and pediatric pharmacology: therapeutic principles in practice*, ed 3, Philadelphia, 2004, Lippincott Williams & Wilkins.
24. Finnegan LP, Kron RE, Connaughton JF, et al: Assessment and treatment of abstinence in the infant of the drug-dependent mother, *Int J Clin Pharmacol Biopharmacol* 12:19, 1975.
25. Finnegan LP, Macnew B: Care of the addicted infant, *Am J Nurs* 74:685, 1974.
26. Finnegan L, Wapner RJ: Drug use in pregnancy. In Neibyl JR, editor: *Narcotic addiction in pregnancy*, Philadelphia, 1987, Lea & Febiger.
27. Fischer G, Etzersdorfer P, Eder H, et al: Buprenorphine maintenance in pregnant opiate addicts, *Euro Addict Res* 4(Suppl):32, 1998.
28. Fischer G, Johnson RE, Eder H, et al: Treatment of opioid-dependent pregnant women with buprenorphine, *Addiction* 95(2):239, 2000.
29. Franck L, Vilardi J: Assessment and management of opioid withdrawal in ill neonates, *Neonatal Netw* 14:39, 1995.
30. Franssen EJF, Meijs V, Ettaher F, et al: Citalopram serum and milk levels in mother and infant during lactation, *Therapeut Drug Monitor* 28:1, 2006.
31. Fried PA, Buckingham M, Von Kulmiz P: Marijuana use during pregnancy and perinatal risk factors, *Am J Obstet Gynecol* 146:992, 1983.
32. Garcia-Bournissen F, Rokach B, Karaskov T, et al: Cocaine detection in maternal and neonatal hair: implications to fetal toxicity, *Therapeut Drug Monitor* 29:1, 2007.
33. Gardiner SJ, Kristensen JH, Begg EJ, et al: Transfer of olanzapine into breast milk, calculation of infant drug dose, and effect on breast-fed infants, *Am J Psychiatry* 160:8, 2003.
34. Gjere NA: Psychopharmacology in pregnancy, *J Perinat Neonatal Nurs* 14:12, 2001.
35. Green CM, Goodman MH: Neonatal abstinence syndrome: strategies for care of the drug-exposed infant, *Neonatal Netw* 22:4, 2003.
36. Hanlon-Lundberg KM, Williams M, Lund T, et al: Accelerated fetal lung maturity profiles and maternal cocaine exposure, *Obstet Gynecol* 87:128, 1996.
37. Helmbrecht GD, Thiagarajah S: Management of addiction disorders in pregnancy, *J Addict Med* 2:1, 2008.

38. Huffman DM, Price BK, Langel L: Therapeutic handling techniques for the infant affected by cocaine, *Neonatal Netw* 13:9, 1994.
39. Hume RF Jr, Martin LS, Bottoms SF, et al: Vascular disruption birth defects and history of prenatal cocaine exposure: a case control study, *Fetal Diagn Ther* 12:292, 1997.
40. Hytinantti T, Kahila H, Renlund M, et al: Neonatal outcome of 58 infants exposed to maternal buprenorphine in utero, *Acta Paediatr* 97:8, 2008.
41. Jones HE, Balster RL: Inhalant abuse in pregnancy, *Obstet Gynecol Clin North Am* 25:153, 1998.
42. Jones H, Johnson R, Jasinsky D, et al: Buprenorphine versus methadone in the treatment of pregnant opioid-dependent patients: effects on the neonatal abstinence syndrome, *Drug Alc Depend* 79:1, 2005.
43. Kacinko S, Jones H, Johnson R, et al: Correlations of maternal buprenorphine dose, buprenorphine, and metabolite concentrations in meconium with neonatal outcomes, *Clin Pharmacol Ther* 84(5):604, 2008 Epub ahead of print: Aug 13, 2008.
44. Kakko J, Helig M, Sarman I: Buprenorphine and methadone treatment of opiate dependence during pregnancy: comparison of fetal growth and neonatal outcomes in two consecutive case series, *Drug Alc Depend* 96:1, 2008.
45. Kallen B: Neonate characteristics after maternal use of antidepressants in late pregnancy, *Arch Pediatr Adolesc Med* 158:312, 2004.
46. Kallen B, Olaussan PO: Maternal use of selective serotonin reuptake inhibitors and persistent pulmonary hypertension of the newborn, *Pharmacoepidemiol Drug Saf* 17:8, 2008.
47. Kandall S, Gartner LM: Late presentation of drug withdrawal symptoms in newborns, *Am J Dis Child* 127:58, 1974.
48. Kraft WK, Gibson E, Dysart K, et al: Sublingual buprenorphine for treatment of neonatal abstinence syndrome: a randomized trial, *Pediatrics* 122:3, 2008.
49. Kreek MJ: Opioid disposition and effects during chronic exposure in the perinatal period in man. In Stimmel B, editor: *Advances in alcohol and substance abuse*, New York, 1982, Haworth.
50. Lainwala S, Brown ER, Weinschenk NP, et al: A retrospective study of length of hospital stay in infants treated for neonatal abstinence syndrome with methadone versus oral morphine preparations, *Adv Neonatal Care* 5:5, 2005.
51. Lester BM, LaGasse L, Seifer R, et al: The maternal lifestyle study: effects of prenatal cocaine or opiate exposure on auditory brain response at one month, *J Pediatr* 142:279, 2003.
52. Lohmann AB, Smith FL: Buprenorphine substitution ameliorates spontaneous withdrawal in fentanyl-dependent rat pups, *Pediatr Res* 49:1, 2001.
53. Maichuk GT, Zahorodny W, Marshall R: Use of positioning to reduce the severity of neonatal narcotic withdrawal syndrome, *J Perinatol* 19:510, 1999.
54. McGuinness TM: Nothing to sniff at: inhalant use and youth, *J Psychosocl Nurs* 22:8, 2006.
55. Medina-Mora ME, Real T: Epidemiology of inhalant use, *Curr Opin Psychiatry* 21:247, 2008.
56. Meyer MT, Berens RJ: Efficacy of an enteral 10-day methadone wean to prevent withdrawal in fentanyl-tolerant pediatric intensive care unit patients, *Pediatr Crit Care Med* 2:4, 2001.
57. Minozzi S, Amato L, Vecchi S, et al: Maintenance agonist treatments for opiate dependent pregnant women (Review), *The Cochrane Collaboration* 4, 2008.
58. Monitoring the future: Accessed November 10, 2008, from www.monitoringthefuture.org/.
59. Nandakumar N, Sankar VS: What is the best evidence based management of neonatal abstinence syndrome? *Arch Dis Child-Fetal Neonat Ed* 91:F463, 2006.
60. National Institute on Drug Abuse (NIDA): *Infofacts*, Accessed November 6, 2008, from www.drugabuse.gov/infofacts/cocaine.html.
61. Newport DJ, Viguera AC, Beach AJ, et al: Lithium placental passage and obstetrical outcome: implications for clinical management during late pregnancy, *Am J Psychiatry* 162:2162, 2005.
62. Osborn DA, Jeffery HE, Cole M: Opiate treatment for opiate withdrawal in newborn infants, *Cochrane Database Syst Rev* 3:CD002059, 2005.
63. Ostrea EM: Understanding drug testing in the neonate and the role of meconium analysis, *J Perinat Neonatal Nurs* 14:61, 2001.
64. Pichini S, Garcia-Algar O: In-utero exposure to smoking and newborn neurobehavior: how to assess neonatal withdrawal syndrome? *Therapeut Drug Mon* 28:3, 2006.
65. Pinto F, Torrilli M, Casella G, et al: Sleep in babies born to clinically heroin-addicted mothers: a follow-up study, *Drug Alcohol Dep* 1:43, 1998.
66. Prenatal Substance Exposure, National Abandoned Infants Assistance Resource Center, 2008, Accessed November 10, 2008, from http://aia.berkley.edu 2008.
67. Reis M, Kallen B: Maternal use of antipsychotics in early pregnancy and delivery outcome, *J Clin Psychopharmacol* 28:3.
68. Sawnani H, Jackson T, Murphy T, et al: The effect of maternal smoking on respiratory and arousal patterns in preterm infants during sleep, *Am J Respir Crit Care Med* 169:733, 2004.
69. Schempf AH: Illicit drug use and neonatal outcomes: a critical review, *Obstet Gynecol Survey* 62:11, 2007.
70. Schempf AH, Strobino DM: Illicit drug use and adverse birth outcomes: is it drugs or context? *J Urban Health* 85:858, 2008.

71. Schwerha JJ: Solvent exposure: a wolf in sheep's clothing? Recognition and assessment from a clinical perspective, *JOEM* 49:813, 2007.
72. Seligman NS, Salva N, Hayes EJ, et al: Predicting length of treatment for neonatal abstinence syndrome in methadone-exposed neonates, *Am J Obstet Gynecol* 199:4, 2008.
73. Sisson TRC, Wickler M, Tsai P, et al: Effect of narcotic withdrawal on neonatal sleep patterns, *Pediatr Res* 8:451, 1974.
74. Smith LM, Lagasse LL, Derauf C, et al: Prenatal methamphetamine use and neonatal neurobehavioral outcome, *Neurotoxicol Teratol* 30:1, 2008.
75. Sokol RJ, Delaney-Black V, Nordstrom B: Fetal alcohol spectrum disorder, *JAMA* 290:2996, 2003.
76. Sood B, Delaney-Black V, Covington C, et al: Alcohol exposure and childhood behavior at age 6 to 7 years. I. Dose-response effect, *Pediatrics* 108:e34, 2001.
77. Streissguth AP: Alcohol and motherhood: physiological findings and the fetal alcohol syndrome. In *Women and alcohol: health related issues*, Research Monograph No. 16 Washington, DC, 1986, U.S. Department of Health and Human Services.
78. Streissguth AP, Finnegan LP: Effects of prenatal alcohol and drugs. In Kinney J, editor: *Clinical manual of substance abuse*, ed 2, St Louis, 1996, Mosby
79. Streissguth AP, LaDue RA: Fetal alcohol syndrome: teratogenic causes of developmental disabilities. In Schroeder S, editor: *Toxic substances and mental retardation*, Washington, DC, 1987, American Association on Mental Deficiency.
80. Substance Abuse and Mental Health Services Administration: *Results from the 2006 National Survey on Drug Use and Health: national findings*, 2007. Accessed November 10, 2008, from www.oas.samhsa.gov.
81. Substance Abuse and Mental Health Services Administration, U.S. Department of Health and Human Services: *Summary of findings from the 2007 National Household Survey on Drug Abuse*, 2008. Accessed November 24, 2008, from www.oas.samhsa.gov.
82. Substance Exposed Infants: *Noteworthy policies and practices: National Abandoned Infants Assistance Resource Center*, 2006, Accessed November 10, 2008, from http://aia.berkeley.edu.
83. Tobias JD: Tolerance, withdrawal, and physical dependency after long-term sedation and analgesia of children in the pediatric intensive care unit, *Crit Care Med* 28:6, 2000.
84. ter Horst PG, Jansman FG, van Lingen RA, et al: Pharmacological aspects of neonatal antidepressant withdrawal, *Obstet Gynecol Surv* 63(4):267, 2008.
85. Tronick EZ, Beeghly M: Prenatal cocaine exposure, child development, and the compromising effects of cumulative risk, *Clin Perinatol* 26:151, 1999.
86. U.S. Department of Health and Human Services, Substance Abuse and Mental Health Services Administration, Center for Substance Abuse Prevention: DHHS Publication No. (SMA) 06-4236, 2007, Accessed November 3, 2008, from www.samhsa.gov.
87. Vagnarelli F, Ammarri S, Scaravelli G, et al: TDM grand rounds: neonatal nicotine withdrawal syndrome in an infant prenatally and postnatally exposed to heavy cigarette smoke, *Therapeut Drug Mon* 28:5, 2006.
88. Vidaeff AC, Mastrobattista JM: In utero cocaine exposure: a thorny mix of science and mythology, *Am J Perinatol* 20:165, 2003.
89. Wick R, Gilbert JD, Felgate P, et al: Inhalant deaths in South Australia: a 20-year retrospective autopsy study, *Am J Forensic Med Path* 28:4, 2007.
90. Wilbourne P, Wallerstedt C, Dorato V, et al: Clinical management of methadone dependence during pregnancy, *J Perinat Neonat Nurs* 14:26, 2001.
91. Wingkun JG, Knisely JS, Schnoll SH, et al: Decreased carbon dioxide sensitivity in infants of substance-abusing mothers, *Pediatrics* 95:864, 1995.
92. Zenewicz D, Kuhn PJ: Routine meconium screening versus drug screening per physician order: detecting the true incidence of drug-exposed infants, *Pediatr Nurs* 24:543, 1998.

12 PAIN AND PAIN RELIEF

SANDRA L. GARDNER, MARY ENZMAN-HINES, AND LORRAINE A. DICKEY

Pain is a complex phenomenon whose nature is, at best, elusive in the neonate. Rationalization for inadequate treatment of pain has resulted in unnecessary suffering for these fragile infants. Research has shown that the "unchecked release of stress hormones by untreated pain may exacerbate injury, prevent wound healing, lead to infection, prolong hospitalization, and even [lead] to death."[198] These fragile neonates are simply too sick to ***not*** have their pain treated. Health care professionals are responsible for influencing positive change in clinical practice about neonatal pain.[3,6-10,133,192,236]

In the past, neonates have not been given analgesia and/or anesthesia agents for surgery because of the controversy as to whether they feel pain and whether they are physiologically stable enough to tolerate the effects of these drugs. The rationale for withholding analgesia and/or anesthesia agents included the following beliefs:

- Neonates have an immature central nervous system (CNS) with nonmyelinated pain fibers and are thus incapable of perceiving pain.
- Neonates have no memory of pain.
- Pain is a highly subjective experience that is difficult to objectively assess in nonverbal neonates.
- Anesthetics and analgesics are dangerous when administered to neonates, and neonates are safer being unmedicated.

There is increasing evidence from over 20 years of research that neonates, including preterm infants, have a CNS that is much more mature than previously thought.[7,23,71] Pain pathways are myelinated in the fetus during the second and third trimesters and are completely myelinated by 30 to 37 weeks' gestation. Even thinly myelinated or nonmyelinated fibers carry pain stimuli. Incomplete myelination implies only a slower transmission, which is offset in the neonate by the shorter distance the impulse must travel.[23]

Even though pain is not expressed verbally in semiconscious patients, nonverbal adults (e.g., intubated, mute), or infants, this does not negate their experience of pain. In response to the question of whether the neonate's responses are reflexive or express a perception of pain, research has focused on measuring the infant's pain experience. The infant's capacity for memory is far greater than was previously thought,[7,14,15,26,227] and a neuropsychologic complex of altered pain threshold and pain-related behavior has been identified.*

Concern has been expressed that giving potent medications to an already critically ill infant might be dangerous. Local and systemic drugs now available, as well as new techniques and devices for monitoring, enable neonates (including preterm infants) to be safely anesthetized and provide safe and effective analgesia while maintaining a stable condition.[23]

Neonates, including premature infants, exhibit (1) physiologic, (2) hormonal, (3) metabolic, and (4) behavioral responses to invasive procedures that are similar to, but more intense than, adult responses.[11,13,17,23,103] Exposure to multiple painful procedures may increase the vulnerability of preterm infants to gross neurologic damage (intraventricular hemorrhage, periventricular leukomalacia).[12-14,16,96] Pain relief benefits the neonate by decreasing physiologic instability, hormonal and metabolic stress, and the behavioral reactions accompanying painful procedures.† The Committee on Fetus and Newborn of the American Academy of Pediatrics (AAP) has recommended the administration of local or systemic drugs for anesthesia or analgesia to neonates undergoing surgical procedures.[7] The committee further states that any decision to withhold these drugs should not be based solely on the infant's age or perceived degree of cortical maturity but should be based on the same criteria used in older patients.[7,17]

Please note that the **PURPLE** type in each chapter is intended to make it easier to identify clinically applicable material.

*References 72,101,168,183,193,221,222,227.

†References 11,12,23,24,101,168,243.

The AAP, in the latest version of the guidelines, cites that prolonged exposure to untreated pain increases morbidity and alters subsequent behavioral and physiologic responses to pain.[8] National associations have promulgated standard-of-care guidelines or position statements about neonatal pain management.[3,6-10,17,192,236] The focus of these documents is on the proactive assessment and management of pain in the neonate. The National Association of Neonatal Nurses (NANN) guidelines outline the following recommendations.[236]

- Parents should be informed of pain relief as an important part of the neonate's health care plan and should be encouraged to actively participate in their neonate's assessment and management of pain.
- ***Every*** institution must mandate clinical practice guidelines that ensure access and safe administration of pain control to the neonate. Institutions also should develop guidelines for assessing and monitoring pain management practices that include parental input with the goal of measuring the adequacy of pain relief and control in the neonate.
- Institutions should support interdisciplinary research and ongoing education that includes a description of neonatal pain, accurate pain assessment, interventions to improve patient care and reduce morbidity, as well as guidelines ensuring adequate administration of analgesics and sedatives for the neonate.

All neonatal health care providers have an ethical and legal obligation to practice the standard of care* in assessing and intervening to relieve the neonate's pain, as well as to reevaluate the safety and efficacy of the pharmacologic and comfort interventions used to treat pain.[17,76,115,157,175]

PHYSIOLOGY AND PATHOPHYSIOLOGY

"Pain is an unpleasant sensory and emotional experience associated with actual or potential tissue damage, or described in terms of such damage."[123] The neonate's expression of pain does not fit the self-report aspect of this definition, which often results in the health care provider's failure to recognize and treat pain. Because self-report is absent in the preverbal neonate, nonverbal behavioral information needs to be assessed and used to determine the treatment options for neonates. **The definition of pain has been amended. "The inability to communicate in no way negates the possibility that an individual is experiencing pain, and is in need of appropriate pain-relieving treatment."**[123] Although we cannot assess the emotional experience associated with pain in these babies, the necessary sensory pathways are now better understood. Neonates have a developing, incompletely myelinated nervous system at birth; however, all the components of the nociceptive (pain) pathways are present.[71,108] As background for an understanding of neonatal responses and their differences from adult responses, the basic mechanisms of adult pain transmission are presented in Figure 12-1.

Types of pain experienced by the neonate have been identified as (1) physiologic, caused by tissue injury, (2) inflammatory, caused by inflammation of tissues, (3) neuropathic, caused by nerve inflammation/damage, and (4) visceral, caused by distention, inflammation, and contraction of viscera.[19,20] Sources of neonatal pain are either acute, established, or chronic/prolonged.[19,20]

NEUROANATOMY

Peripheral Nervous System

Peripheral nerves can be classified into three broad categories based on fiber diameter and velocity (Table 12-1). Pain receptors (nociceptors) are the A-delta fibers (A-δ) and C fibers that are widely spread in the superficial layers of the skin, periosteum, fascia, peritoneum, joints, muscle, pleura, dura, and tooth pulp. Most visceral tissues have fewer nociceptors, and these transmit to the spinal cord through the sympathetic, parasympathetic, and splanchnic nerves. Tissue damage and inflammation cause the release of arachidonic acid and other chemicals that can sensitize nerve endings and cause vasodilation and plasma extravasation. This causes pain, swelling, and hyperalgesia.[64]

A-δ fibers are myelinated and therefore capable of fast impulse conduction. These nerves are responsible for "fast" or "first" pain. They are also known as ***high-threshold mechanoreceptors (HTMs)*** because they respond to strong pressure or tissue

*References 3,6-10,17,76,133,138,192.

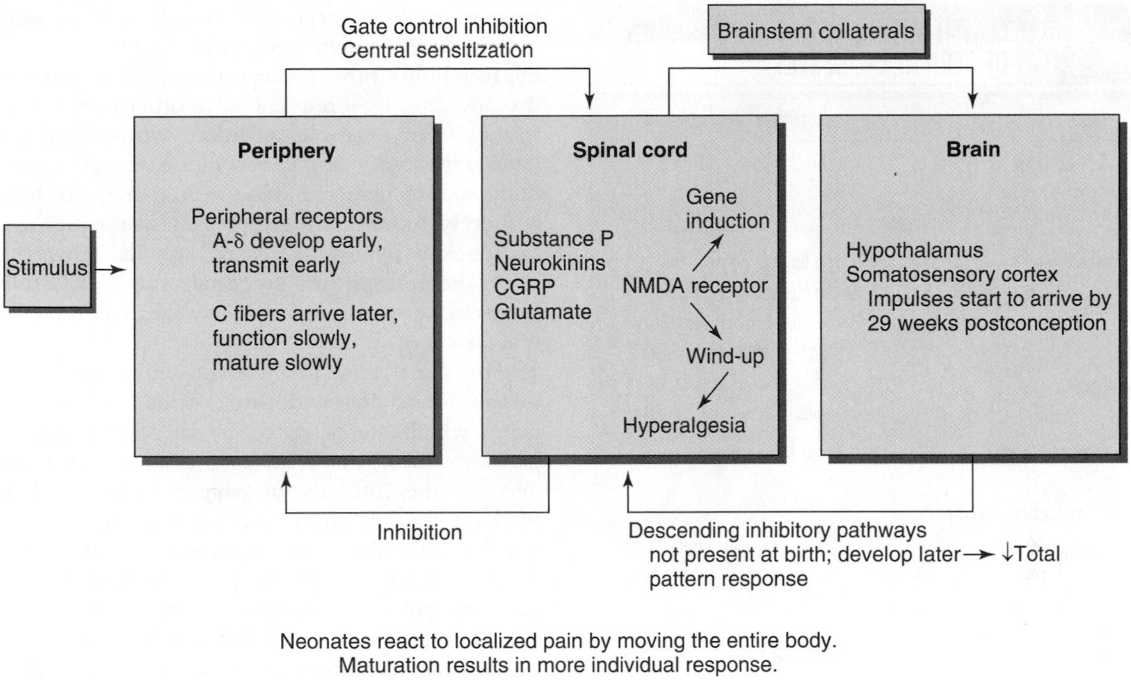

FIGURE 12-1 Schematic representation of transmission of noxious stimuli from the periphery to the brain. *CGRP*, Calcitonin gene–related peptide; *NMDA*, *N*-methyl-D-aspartate.

injury. The C fibers (polymodal nociceptors) are unmyelinated, conduct impulses more slowly, and are the main nociceptors for transmitting chemical, thermal, and mechanical noxious stimuli to the spinal cord.[160] The A-δ fibers develop ahead of the C fibers in the skin and the spinal cord. A-δ fibers are involved in the cutaneous flexion reflex. This reflex is exaggerated in the preterm. Thresholds to mechanical skin stimulation (which may or may not be perceived as pain in a newborn) are lower and responses last longer. Complete myelination occurs during the second and third trimesters. Lack of myelination had been thought to indicate the inability of a neonate to perceive pain; however, incomplete myelination leads only to slower conduction, which is offset by the shorter distances traversed in the infant.[23,108]

Reflex responses to somatic stimuli begin at 7½ weeks post-conceptual age (PCA) in the perioral skin and continue to develop in the palms of the hands before finally reaching the hind limbs by 13 to 14 weeks. Peripheral pain receptors are in place throughout the body by 20 weeks' gestation.[208] It is likely that both A-δ fibers (touching) and A-δ fibers (pinching) transmit painful stimuli in the human fetus. In rat pups, the C fibers reach the spinal cord but do not start to stimulate dorsal horn cells until the end of the first postnatal week. They subsequently continue to mature for several weeks. This slow maturation in rats may be caused by low levels of neuropeptides such as substance P (SP), neurotransmitters, or immature receptor sites. These changes in rat pups appear to correlate with the third trimester and the early neonatal period in humans.[71]

Spinal Cord

The pain transmission system begins with the peripheral pain receptors (nociceptors). Once a noxious stimulus is detected by the nociceptors, the signal is transmitted via the primary afferents to the dorsal root ganglia and from there to the dorsal horn of the spinal cord.[64] Neurotransmitters and their receptors amplify or attenuate the signal in the dorsal horn before sending the signal to the brain.

Excitatory neurotransmitters such as SP and other neurokinins are increased after acute inflammation and may be necessary for the transmission of painful

TABLE 12-1 CLASSIFICATION AND CHARACTERISTICS OF PERIPHERAL NERVES

NAME/CHARACTERISTICS	FUNCTION
A-alpha (A-α) d: 10-20 μ v: 70-120 m/sec myelinated	Innervate skeletal muscle
A-beta (A-β) d: 12-20 μ v: 30-70 m/sec myelinated	Light touch or pressure may be involved in peripheral sensitization and allodynia; in the premature and newborn infant, may be involved in the transmission of noxious stimuli
A-gamma (A-γ) d: 3-6 μ v: 15-30 m/sec myelinated	Muscle tone
A-delta (A-δ) d: 2-5 μ v: 12-30 m/sec myelinated	Fast, well-localized pain; high threshold mechanoreceptors
B d: 3 μ v: 3-15 m/sec myelinated	Preganglionic autonomic fibers may be involved in sensory or sympathetic coupling
C d: 0.4-1.2 μ v: 0.5-2 m/sec unmyelinated	Slow pain, touch, temperature, post-ganglionic sympathetic fibers, polymodal nociceptors

d, Nerve diameter; *v,* nerve velocity.

stimuli to the brain.[128] Glutamate and aspartate are amino acids that appear to be involved in central hypersensitivity and wind-up.[22] ***Wind-up*** **is a phenomenon in which repetition of the same noxious stimulus leads to an exaggerated response. This response continues even after the noxious stimulus ceases.** Wind-up also may be responsible for converting a low-level, pain-related activity to a high-level, pain-related activity.[64,227] The preterm experiences increased stress and activity in the nociceptive pathways after prolonged periods of exposure to painful stimuli. After prolonged exposure, the preterm exhibits similar pain responses when exposed to other caregiving activities (e.g., handling, suctioning the endotracheal tube, positioning).[69]

An additional factor in the development of **hypersensitivity (e.g., decreased pain threshold) and hyperalgesia** is the presence of nociceptive specific receptors,[108] which respond only to pain. In the presence of peripheral inflammation, the threshold of these receptors is decreased so that they are capable of responding to other nonnoxious stimuli.[64] **For example, an infant whose heel has been repeatedly stuck for blood samples may demonstrate pain behavior, even when the heel is merely touched. Many of these responses can be blocked by low doses of opioids. However, once these responses are established, a tenfold increased dose of opioids may be necessary to reverse them.**[72,243]

The spinal cord also contains inhibitory neurotransmitters (γ-aminobutyric acid [GABA], glycine), which are activated by descending neural pathways (from the brain to the spinal cord) and decrease the intensity of pain transmission. This results in modulation of pain transmission from the spinal cord to the cortex. Descending inhibition is necessary to modulate the pain response and yet allow for specific pain responses (e.g., withdrawal from a needle stick). **Delayed maturation of the descending inhibitory fibers results in a higher pain threshold in the upper extremities and lower in the lower extremities, resulting in more pain sensitivity in the lower extremities.**[19] Lack of inhibition produces exaggerated, generalized, but definite responses to pain such as body wriggling, facial grimacing, and excessive crying. These pathways, in contrast to the excitatory ones, are not fully developed at birth in "rat pups and probably in preterm infants"[108]; therefore the neonatal spinal cord is more excitable.[71] **The pain transmission system of the premature infant (<36 weeks) is more developed than the pain modulation system; therefore preterm infants are *more* sensitive to pain than are term or older infants.**[108,208]

Neurotransmitters in the developing nervous system may be expressed early but are not necessarily located in areas normally found in an adult. This is particularly true of SP and glutamate, which may contribute to the unorganized responses noted with pain stimuli in the newborn (e.g., the whole body moves when an intravenous [IV] line is started).

Brain

Much less is known about the development of the pathways to the higher brain centers, such as the hypothalamus and cortex. Once again, there is evidence of immaturity of the inhibitory pathways.[71]

Development in the human cortex continues for many years after birth. **Contrary to prior beliefs that newborns do not feel pain, it appears that, in fact, cutaneous responses are exaggerated and occur at much lower thresholds and reflex muscle contractions last longer in newborns than in mature individuals.** Using real-time near-infrared spectroscopy in 18 preterm infants (25 to 45 weeks post-menstrual age [PMA]), an increase in cerebral oxygenation over the somatosensory cortex was measured in response to heel stick blood draws[206] and in response to venipuncture in another study.[32] From these findings, researchers concluded that **pain is transmitted to the cerebral cortex of preterm infants from 25 weeks PMA.**[206] Other recent research has found that low biobehavioral responsiveness to pain at 32 weeks post-conceptual age (PCA) is associated with poorer quality of motor function at 8 months PCA; therefore pain reactivity in the neonatal intensive care unit (NICU) may be a marker of neuromotor development in later infancy.[102] In summary, the newborn's nervous system, although still developing, is fully capable of transmitting, perceiving, responding to, and probably remembering noxious stimuli.

PHYSIOLOGIC RESPONSES

Acute pain in adults is associated with increased sympathetic stimulation, heart rate, respiratory rate, blood pressure, cardiac output, myocardial oxygen consumption, peripheral resistance, anxiety, emotional distress, and hormonal imbalance and greater morbidity and mortality. **Numerous studies have shown that both premature and full-term infants express the same physiologic responses to pain and noxious stimuli (e.g., intubation) as adults do (see the Critical Findings box on p. 228).**[7,23,237] **Infants undergoing circumcision without the use of pain medication demonstrated higher pain scores, increased irritability after the procedure, an altered sleep-wake state, and abnormal feeding patterns for up to 22 hours. These responses can be attenuated or blocked with the appropriate use of analgesics.**[187] Despite research about infants' pain response to circumcision and recommendations to use anesthetics or analgesics during circumcision, a recent survey in a large academic medical center showed that only 30% of infants being circumcised by obstetricians received any pain relief and there was no documentation of discussion with parents about pain management.[143]

Pain reactivity varies by gestational age (GA) and prior experience with pain.[222] Studies on pain reactivity in very-low-birth-weight (VLBW) infants at 32 weeks PCA found that younger gestational ages and increased numbers of invasive procedures at birth resulted in a "dampening" of normal pain reactions and cortisol response.[97] These infants had higher baseline heart rates, which may have indicated that they were in a perpetual state of stress or pain. A longitudinal comparison of 81 preterm infants' pain responses to repeated heel sticks found that both a higher severity of illness and number of prior heel sticks lowered pain scores (this may be one reason that venipuncture is less painful than heel sticks in the neonate).[68] Previous exposure to morphine was associated with a "normalization" of responses to painful stimuli. More recent studies of the pain response in extremely-low-birth-weight (ELBW) preterms (<27 weeks GA) found (1) similar responses to older infants but also "dampened" responses[83,84] and (2) lower cortisol levels representing down-regulation of the hypothalamic-pituitary-adrenal axis that is not counteracted by morphine use.[97] Two other studies have compared the biobehavioral pain responses of ELBW infants with term controls. The studies found that (1) at 4 months corrected age, behavioral and cardiac autonomic responses were similar, with less parasympathetic withdrawal and more sustained sympathetic response during recovery in the ELBW group[168] and (2) at 8 months corrected age, behavioral response was similar to that in term infants but less sustained (i.e., faster dampening); baseline heart rate was significantly higher in those born at ELBW.[101] The number of previous painful experiences in the NICU was significantly related to subsequent pain reactivity in the ELBW infants, and those ELBW infants exposed to more morphine had heart rate recovery more similar to that of the term infants.[101]

ETIOLOGY

Invasive Procedures

Pain is produced with any invasive procedure (Table 12-2).[17,107,203] One study found that the number of invasive procedures in 54 neonates during admission to the NICU was 3283.[31] The most common (56%) was heel stick, followed by endotracheal suctioning (26%) and intravenous cannula insertion (8%). The most premature infants underwent the

Critical Findings

NEONATAL PAIN RESPONSE*

Physiologic

- Increase in
  - Heart rate
  - Blood pressure (also fluctuations)
  - Intracranial pressure/cerebral blood flow,[153] which leads to higher risk for intraventricular hemorrhage
  - Respiratory rate
  - Mean airway pressure
  - Muscle tension
  - Carbon dioxide (↑$TcPco_2$; Pco_2)
  - Pulmonary vascular tone
  - Oxygen consumption
- Decrease in
  - Depth of respiration (shallow)
  - Oxygenation (↓Po_2; Sao_2), which leads to apnea or bradycardia
  - Vagal tone
- Pallor or flushing
- Diaphoresis or palmar sweating
- Dilated pupils

Behavioral

- Vocalizations
  - Crying (higher-pitched, tense, and harsh)
  - Whimpering
  - Moaning
- Facial expressions
  - Grimacing
  - Furrowing or bulging of the brow
  - Quivering chin
  - Eye squeeze
  - Nasal flaring
  - Curling/curving of the tongue
  - Facial twitching
- Body movements
  - General diffuse body activity (flexing/extending extremities; extending legs; finger splay, hand on face)
  - Limb withdrawal, swiping, thrashing
- Changes in tone
  - Hypertonicity, rigidity, fist clenching
  - Hypotonicity, flaccidity
- Touch aversion
- States
  - Sleep-wake cycle changes, wakefulness
  - Activity level changes: increased fussiness, irritability, listlessness, lethargy
  - Feeding difficulties
  - More difficult to comfort, soothe, quiet
  - Disruption of interactive ability with parents

Hormonal/Catabolic Stress Response

- Increase in
  - Plasma rennin activity
  - Catecholamine levels (epinephrine and norepinephrine)
  - Cortisol levels (serum and hair[245])
  - Nitrogen excretion/protein catabolism
  - Release of
    - Growth hormone
    - Glucagons
    - Aldosterone
  - Serum levels of
    - Glucose
    - Lactate
    - Pyruvate
    - Ketones
    - Non-esterified fatty acids
- Decrease in
  - Insulin secretion
  - Prolactin

*References 11,12,23,61,85,99,103,106,115,131,164,166,167,212,218,238,240.

highest number of procedures, with one infant undergoing 488 procedures! Two more recent studies of the first 14 days in the NICU found (1) an average of 196 procedures per neonate with 14 invasive procedures per day per infant[203] and (2) a median of 115 procedures per neonate with 16 invasive procedures per day per infant.[52] In the most recent study, treatment for painful procedures included the following[52]:

1. Pharmacologic-only therapy (2.1%)
2. Nonpharmacologic-only therapy (18.2%)
3. Combination therapy (both No. 1 and No. 2) (20.8%)
4. Without specific analgesia (79.2%)
5. Performed while the neonate was receiving concurrent analgesia/anesthesia for other purposes (34.2%)

TABLE 12-2 SELECTED COMMON CAUSES OF PAIN IN NEONATES

INVASIVE PROCEDURES	SURGICAL PROCEDURES	OTHERS
Intravenous cannulation	Central line placement	Clavicle, rib fracture
Venipuncture	PDA ligation	Extremity fracture
Heel stick	TEF repair	Chest pain
Intramuscular injection	Gastroschisis repair	Central pain syndrome (i.e., pain derived from CNS damage)
Arterial line, blood gas	Omphalocele repair	Spasticity
Umbilical catheterization	CDH repair	Abdominal pain resulting from short gut syndrome, multiple abdominal surgeries
Chest tube insertion or removal	Inguinal hernia repair	Necrotizing enterocolitis
Bone marrow aspiration	Cardiac surgery	Bowel obstruction
Lumbar puncture	Circumcision	Prolonged and/or improper positioning
Paracentesis	Broviac catheter insertion or removal	Position changes
Endotracheal intubation/removal	ECMO catheter insertion or removal	NG tube placement
Endotracheal suction		Flushing lines
Mechanical ventilation		Dressing changes
Nasal continuous positive airway pressure (NCPAP)		Eye examination for ROP
Bladder catheterization		IV administration of medications
Suprapubic aspiration		Addition/withdrawal of fluid from umbilical catheter
Ventricular tap		Transient mechanical birth trauma (e.g., cephalic hematoma, molding, bruising, forceps marks, petechiae)
Endoscopy		Cryo/laser surgery for ROP
Bronchoscopy		Chest physiotherapy
PICC line insertion/removal		Changing tape/suture removal
Cutdown (arterial/venous) for access		

Data from Anand KJ and the International Evidence-Based Group for Neonatal Pain: Consensus statement for the prevention and management of pain in the newborn, *Arch Pediatr Adolesc Med* 155:173, 2001; Barker D, Rutter N: Exposure to invasive procedures in neonatal intensive care unit admissions, *Arch Dis Child Fetal Neonatal Educ* 72:F47, 1995; Bauchner H, May A, Coates E: Use of analgesic agents for invasive medical procedures in pediatric and neonatal intensive care units, *J Pediatr* 4:647, 1992; Belda S, Pallas C, Dela Cruz J, et al: Screening for retinopathy of prematurity: is it painful? *Biol Neonate* 86:195, 2004; Evans JC, Vogelpohl DG, Bourguignon CM, et al: Pain behaviors in LBW infants accompany some "nonpainful" caregiving procedures, *Neonatal Netw* 16:33, 1997.

CDH, Congenital diaphragmatic hernia; *CNS*, central nervous system; *ECMO*, extracorporeal membrane oxygenation; *IV*, intravenous; *NG*, nasogastric; *PDA*, patent ductus arteriosus; *PICC*, peripherally inserted central catheter; *ROP*, retinopathy of prematurity; *TEF*, tracheoesophageal fistula.

Another study examining the use of analgesics for "minor" procedures in NICUs and pediatric intensive care units (PICUs) found that analgesics were rarely used for the placement of IV catheters, suprapubic bladder aspiration, urinary bladder catheterization, venipuncture, arterial line placement, lumbar puncture, and paracentesis in NICUs. **Analgesics were used approximately 60% of the time in NICUs for the placement of chest tubes, central lines, and bone marrow aspiration.**[34] By contrast, analgesics were used in the majority of patients in PICUs undergoing arterial line placement, lumbar puncture, and paracentesis and in more than 90% of chest tube insertions, central line placements, and bone marrow aspirations. Possible reasons for these differences were that (1) neonates were more often critically ill and the use of analgesics may have prolonged the procedure or exacerbated the infants' medical problems, (2) the use of neuromuscular blocking agents prevented the physical response to pain, and (3) not all infants respond to pain by crying loudly, withdrawing, or otherwise "protesting." A study of painful procedures in NICUs found that 239 patients were subjected to 2134 invasive procedures in 1 week and an analgesic was administered in only 0.8% of these procedures.[129] More recent studies have found that only one third of the neonates received an analgesic for painful procedures,[203] no pain guidelines were present in 25% of surveyed NICUs, and the majority of these NICUs had no guideline for pain relief for routine invasive procedures.[158] Health care providers underestimate the pain caused by procedures,[65] and even when they believe that most NICU procedures are painful, relief is provided only 33% of the time.[139,203] A recent study of neonates at increased risk for neurologic impairment found that these infants had the highest number of invasive procedures but received the least amount of analgesic in the first day of life.[213] These studies indicate that considerable work is needed to educate practitioners about the safety, efficacy, and benefits of appropriate pain management in neonates. Use of "better practices" strategies and proven quality improvement methods has resulted in better pain management for neonates in the NICU.[66,201]

Endotracheal intubation has been associated with hypoxia, catabolism, increased intracranial pressure, intraventricular hemorrhage/periventricular leukomalacia (IVH/PVL), blood pressure, and stress hormones.[139,161,181] Recent research has shown that use of premedication for elective, nonurgent intubations is safer and more effective than awake intubations (see p. 598 in the Endotracheal Intubation section in Chapter 23). Unmedicated endotracheal intubation in the neonate should be reserved for emergency resuscitation in the delivery room.

Benefits of pain management in the ventilated neonate include (1) improved ventilator synchrony, (2) improved pulmonary function, (3) less neuroendocrine (cortisol, beta-endorphins, catecholamine) response, and (4) potentially ameliorated adverse effects (Figure 12-2) of mechanical ventilation in the preterm.[28,110] Researchers have shown that even a single dose of fentanyl during mechanical ventilation decreases pain scores, heart rate, blood pressure, and serum cortisol levels and increases clinical stability of the infant.[106] Other researchers have documented the possible protective role of continuous low-dose analgesic on the neurologic outcome in certain infants.[21,144] Furthermore, studies have compared fentanyl with morphine for analgesia

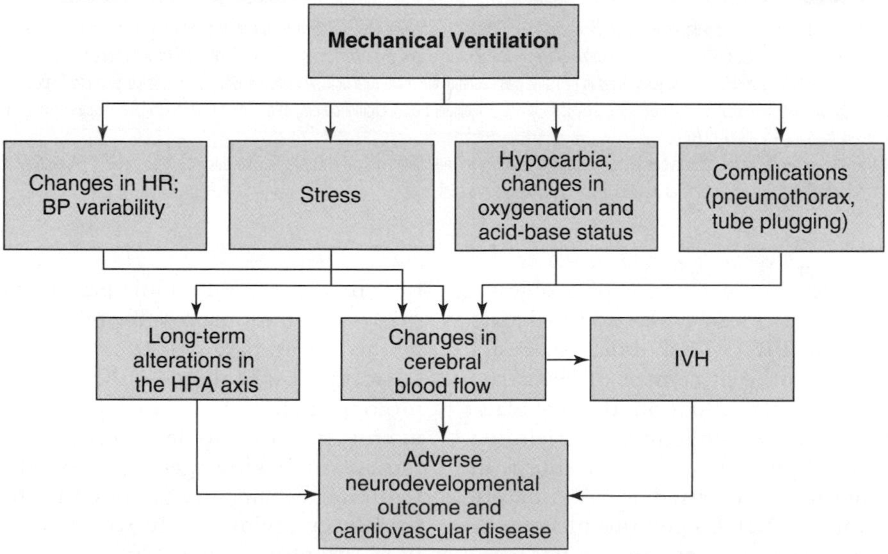

FIGURE 12-2 Potential mechanisms leading to adverse effects from mechanical ventilation in preterm neonates. *BP*, Blood pressure; *HPA*, hypothalamic-pituitary-adrenal; *HR*, heart rate; *IVH*, intraventricular hemorrhage. (Modified from Hall RW, Boyle E, Young T: Do ventilated neonates require pain management? *Semin Perinatol* 31:289, 2007.)

during mechanical ventilation in neonates and found that fentanyl was equianalgesic with fewer side effects, thus leading to decreased plasma adrenaline and noradrenaline concentrations.[195] Therefore both morphine and fentanyl reduce the pain and stress of preterms being mechanically ventilated but may prolong the duration of ventilation.[28]

Although use of analgesia in ventilated infants is recommended,[8,17] a recent meta-analysis concluded that there is insufficient evidence for "routine use" of opioids during mechanical ventilation.[37] The meta-analysis states that opioids should be selectively used for individual neonates based on clinical judgment and pain assessment.[37] The findings of two studies question the use of morphine for analgesia in certain ventilated preterm infants. A randomized, double-blind, placebo-controlled trial of morphine infusion for ventilated preterms showed that (1) the analgesic effect was similar between the treated and placebo group, (2) routine morphine infusion decreased the incidence of IVH but did not influence poor neurologic outcome, and (3) the impact of fewer IVHs on neurologic development needs to be evaluated in long-term neurobehavioral follow-up.[204] The most recent study, an international, multicenter (16 NICUs), blinded, randomized trial found that (1) use of morphine decreased the clinical signs of pain, (2) preemptive use of morphine infusions in ventilated preterms did not reduce the frequency of severe IVH, periventricular leukomalacia (PVL), or death, and (3) use of intermittent boluses of morphine was associated with an increased rate of severe IVH, PVL, and death.[22] Based on several study findings, multiple authors conclude the following[39,45,111,159,204]:

- Use of continuous morphine infusions does not reduce early neurologic injury in ventilated preterms.
- Preemptive morphine infusions, additional morphine, and lower gestational age are associated with hypotension.
- Severe IVH, any IVH, and death were associated with preexisting hypotension, but morphine therapy did not contribute to these outcomes.
- Although morphine infusions cause hypotension, they can safely be used for most preterm neonates but should be used cautiously for 23- to 26-week preterms and those with preexisting hypotension.
- Short-term pulmonary outcomes are not improved, and use of additional morphine doses (in the sickest infants) was associated with worsening pulmonary outcomes in ventilated preterms.
- Morphine delays the start of and the full attainment of enteral feedings but does not increase gastrointestinal (GI) complications.
- Clinical markers of persistent pain in ventilated infants receiving morphine include high activity, facial expressions of pain, poor responses to "routine" care, and poor synchrony with the ventilator.

Surgery

Painful stimuli, surgery, and traumatic injuries have been shown in adults to trigger the "stress response," which causes the release of a variety of hormones, including epinephrine, norepinephrine, corticosteroids, glucagon, and growth hormones. These hormones prepare the body for a fight-or-flight response and cause, among other things, an increase in heart rate, respiratory rate, glucose production, and muscle and fat breakdown. This response allows the body to deal with an insult in the short term. If the insult continues or is untreated, the ongoing catabolic stress response may become deleterious to the body's well-being by promoting more tissue breakdown while preventing growth and tissue repair. **Both premature and full-term infants have a decreased stress response with the use of appropriate analgesia both during and immediately after surgery.*** Physiologic indicators (e.g., heart/respiratory rate, blood pressure) of postoperative pain may be unreliable or confounded by illness severity and use of analgesics and neuromuscular blocking agents.[48,74]

Use of adequate operative anesthesia[7,8] and postoperative analgesia is mandatory, even if its use might prolong postoperative ventilatory support.[4]

A special example of untreated operative pain is newborn circumcision. In addition to

*References 10,12,17,21,23,24.

the previously mentioned short-term effects of not treating the pain associated with circumcision, male infants who have undergone circumcision without analgesia have an increased pain response to vaccination at 4 to 6 months of age.[221,223] When these infants were pretreated for their immunizations with a topical anesthetic, their pain response was lessened.[223] Another recent study of 14- and 45-month-old children who had major surgery with appropriate analgesia (in their first 3 months of life) found that their biobehavioral pain response to immunizations was not altered compared with a matched group of toddlers who had not had surgery.[177] However, prolonged exposure to early hospitalization did contribute to an altered pain response (in areas of prior tissue damage) that "recovered" over time.[177,178] Although early painful memories may not be consciously recalled, experiences of pain are "remembered" by the developing nervous system.[14,15,26,178] Newborns have a much greater capacity for memory than was previously thought!

Other Causes

Rib, clavicular, and extremity fractures are not uncommon and should be considered in the presence of prolonged crying and failure to move the affected extremity.

Bronchopulmonary dysplasia is a common problem in infants who were premature and may cause chest pain, a syndrome known to occur in some older patients with chronic lung disease. Neurologic dysfunction can leave patients with ongoing pain from central pain syndrome or excessive spasticity. One study showed that 27% of former ELBW infants who were now teenagers had neurosensory impairment and 9% reported moderate or severe pain.[196]

PREVENTION

Prevention of pain in the neonate and preterm infant begins with a proactive plan of care aimed at preventing the pain cycle.[139] The key approaches in this plan include (1) anticipation, (2) comprehensive and ongoing assessment of the variables, (3) distinguishing agitation and irritability from pain expressions and responses of the preterm infant, (4) ongoing communication among health care providers, using input from the parents, (5) advocating and implementing timely and effective treatment for irritability, agitation, and pain (e.g., pharmacologic and comfort measures), (6) reducing the number of painful procedures,[33,52] and (7) ongoing reevaluation of this proactive plan of care.[3] **Different types of common procedures in the NICU can be anticipated to be painful.** ***Diagnostic procedures*** include arterial puncture, heel stick, lumbar puncture, and retinopathy of prematurity (ROP) examination. ***Therapeutic procedures*** include tracheal intubation and extubation, tracheal suctioning, chest tube insertion, mechanical ventilation, suture removal, and removal of adhesive tape. Some of the ***common surgical procedures*** are circumcision, patent ductus arteriosus ligation, and insertion of central venous catheters.[139] **Anticipation and prevention of pain during such procedures can markedly affect the success of the procedure and the condition of the infant. Preventing, reducing, and relieving neonatal pain constitute an essential health care provider goal to maintain the sick neonate's behavioral, physiologic, and biochemical homeostasis.**[17,242]

Individualized behavioral and developmental care is another important area in preventing stress and sensory overload, which often contribute to an ongoing pain cycle.[205] These approaches help prevent disorganization in the neonate. Several recent studies have shown that clustering care, a common practice in the NICU (see Chapter 13), actually results in an increase in behavioral responses and cortisol secretion for preterms of younger gestational ages when exposed to a painful procedure.[116-118] To facilitate stability and self-regulation before and during an invasive painful procedure, (1) do not cluster care and provide a period of rest before the procedure, (2) assess the infant's state and facilitate a change to an alert state, (3) contain extremities (see Chapter 13), (4) provide a pacifier and an opportunity to grasp (a finger, hand, or blanket), and (5) use another person (e.g., parent, caregiver) to support, contain, and observe for stress. After the procedure, provide support, comfort, and slow withdrawal so that the infant remains calm.

The suffering of neonates can be avoided. Needless suffering is prevented by an established plan of care for assessment, management, and evaluation of pain and attempts to relieve pain. Neonates depend on the skilled observations, assessments, and interventions of care providers for prompt, safe, and effective relief.[174] **A cooperative effort among health care providers and the parents in the form of pain management teams[155] and well-established pain protocols prevents unnecessary suffering of both neonates and their families.** Controlling environmental stimuli (e.g., dimming lights, controlling noise level, turning off radios, speaking softly when near the incubator or warmer, performing rounds outside of the unit), although often difficult in the NICU, is crucial for decreasing stress and preventing unnecessary agitation. Use of an individualized, developmentally appropriate plan of care reduces the need for sedation in severely ill, VLBW neonates.[11,205] Quieting techniques are also a useful way to help control pain response in the neonate; these include nonnutritive sucking, containment interventions, and rocking (see Chapter 13).

DATA COLLECTION

History

Neonates experiencing procedural, surgical, and/or chronic pain must be provided measures to alleviate pain. Neonatal irritability and agitation (see the Critical Findings box below) secondary to chronic conditions (e.g., bronchopulmonary dysplasia, necrotizing enterocolitis [NEC], short bowel syndrome, neurologic deficits) **and/or environmental overstimulation also may require a combination of environmental interventions and sedation.**[8]

Critical Findings

INDICATORS OF IRRITABILITY AND AGITATION

Physiologic

- Increase in
  - Heart rate and blood pressure only with activity
  - Oxygenation (↑$TcPco_2$; Po_2; Sao_2)
  - Respiratory rate and effort
- Decrease in
  - Oxygenation (↓Po_2; Sao_2) after prolonged agitation
  - Heart rate (bradycardia)
  - Respirations (apnea)
- Alterations in skin color: cyanosis, mottling, duskiness, pallor
- Diaphoresis
- Vomiting
- Poor pattern of weight gain

Behavioral

- Vocalizations
  - Whining cry
  - Intense, urgent cry
  - High-pitched cry
  - Resumes fussiness when consolation ceases
- Facial expressions
  - Frowning
  - Worried facies
  - Gaze aversion
  - Closes eyes to tune out
- Body movements
  - Random movements of head and body
  - Hypertonic, rigid posturing; arching; hyperextended neck
  - Flailing, thrashing, frantic activity of extremities during fuss or cry
  - Decreased activity
  - Tremulousness
- States
  - Hyperalert—easily aroused from sleep; startles easily
  - Rapid and frequent state changes to fuss or cry
  - Sleep-wake cycles unpredictable
  - Feeding difficulties
  - Difficult to console, soothe
  - High level of persistence
  - Needs environmental structure to fall asleep; takes a long time to fall asleep
  - Ineffective in self-consoling; requires vestibular stimulation or body containment to console; responds inconsistently to consolation
  - Non-cuddly

Modified from Broome ME, Tanzillo H: Differentiating between pain and agitation in premature neonates, *J Perinat Neonat Nurs* 4:53, 1990; Burdeau G, Kleiber C: Clinical indicators of infant irritability, *Neonat Netw* 9:23, 1991; Franck LS: A national survey of the assessment and treatment of pain and agitation in the NICU, *J Obstet Gynecol Neonat Nurs* 16:387, 1987.

Signs and Symptoms

Assessment of pain in neonates is often challenging because they cannot verbalize their subjective experience.[61] The four objectives in the assessment of pain are (1) detecting the presence of pain, (2) assessing the impact of pain, (3) providing pain-relieving interventions, and (4) evaluating the effectiveness of interventions.[182] **Guidelines for the assessment of pain are listed in Box 12-1. Expression of pain through behavior is one of the neonate's only means of communicating about pain.** Behavioral cues may include diffuse or localized motor activity (e.g., pulling extremity away, hypotonia), facial grimacing, crying, agitation, and change in level of activity (see the Critical Findings box on p. 233). In both preterm and term neonates, gender differences in pain expression may exist. Female infants show more facial expressions of pain when compared with male infants.[105] In an analysis of the responses of 149 infants to a painful event, facial actions were found 40% of the time to account for pain indicators in vulnerable neonates.[209] **Assessment of pain in the neonate is further complicated by the infant's state and level of neural development.**[61,82,103,164,185]

BOX 12-1 GUIDELINES FOR ASSESSING PAIN

- Assess and document pain, with vital signs every 4 to 6 hours or as indicated by pain scores and/or the clinical condition of the neonate.
- Use standardized pain assessment tools and methods with evidence of validity, reliability, and clinical utility.
- Use pain assessment tools that are sensitive and specific for infants of different gestational ages and/or with acute, chronic, or continuous pain (e.g., postoperative pain, inflammatory conditions).
- Use pain assessment tools that are comprehensive and multidimensional (e.g., measure behavioral, physiologic, and hormonal/biochemical indicators of pain) within the context of pain experience.
- Assess the neonate's pain after each potentially painful clinical intervention.
- Reassess and reevaluate neonate's pain to assess the efficacy of pharmacologic, behavioral, and environmental interventions.

Modified from Anand KJ and the International Evidence-Based Group for Neonatal Pain: Consensus statement for the prevention and management of pain in the newborn, *Arch Pediatr Adolesc Med* 155:173, 2001; Prince W, Horns K, Latta T, et al: Treatment of neonatal pain without a gold standard: the case for caregiving interventions and sucrose administration, *Neonatal Netw* 23:33, 2004.

The younger gestational age, more immature CNS, more limited autonomic and self-regulatory abilities to deal with pain and stress, and disorganized ineffective responses make it more difficult to communicate pain.[61,82,185] A more immature, fragile neonate may manifest alterations in sleep-wake cycles and habituate to the overwhelming stimuli of the NICU (see Chapter 13) and thus cannot exhibit any response to pain.[185]

Behavioral expressions of pain by the neonate are further hampered by intubation, use of restraints, and neuromuscular blockers.[61,167] Similarly, chronically ill infants who have been exposed to repeated painful procedures have difficulty generating a pain response and exhibit a "dampened" pain response.[83,84,97] Recent research shows that several body movements (e.g., fisting, flexing/extending extremities, finger splay, hand on the face) commonly assessed in the Newborn Individualized Care and Assessment Program (NIDCAP) developmental care program (see Chapter 13) are associated with acute pain response in preterms[164] (see the Critical Findings box on p. 228). Preterm infants who have experienced more invasive procedures, who are lower in GA at birth, and who have spent more days on ventilators have a diminished behavioral and cardiac autonomic pain response (i.e., a blunted response) to acute pain at 32 weeks PCA.[82,96,98] Another study indicates that neonates (both preterm and term) who undergo handling and immobilization may exhibit exaggerated behavioral and physiologic response to later painful procedures.[82] VLBW infants with parenchymal brain injury exhibit a biobehavioral response to pain that is unaltered from that in VLBW infants without brain injury.[166]

Physiologic parameters also may indicate pain (e.g., increased heart and respiratory rates, elevated blood pressure, desaturation, apnea, palmar sweating). These symptoms are the result of sympathetic nervous system activation (see the Critical Findings box on p. 228). A recent study found that some physiologic responses to pain (e.g., facial activity and state) moderately correlated to heart rate changes, whereas other behavioral expressions (e.g., finger splay) did not correlate with any autonomic changes.[163] However, in the same study, specific measures of cardiac autonomic modulation did not correlate with behavioral change, suggesting that cardiac alterations are influenced by a multitude of factors[167] and may be independent measures of pain in the preterm.[163] **Some preterm infants respond to pain with more behavioral changes,**

whereas others respond with more physiologic changes.[212] In the first week of life, all infants of different gestational ages (e.g., <28 to 36 weeks) can differentiate between mild and more invasive procedures.[184] At 36 weeks, these same infants exhibited differing physiologic pain responses based on their GA at birth (e.g., those born closer to term had lower increases in heart rate than those born at a younger gestational age).[184] Other research studies show that (1) preterms between 27 and 32 weeks GA respond physiologically to pain, (2) some older GA preterms had diminished responses, and (3) the physiologic and behavioral pain responses of other preterms became more robust over time.[82,237]

When pain is repetitive or persists for hours or days, there is a decompensatory response, resulting in hormonal and metabolic alterations (Figure 12-3; see also the Critical Findings box on p. 228. The fight-or-flight mechanism of the sympathetic nervous system can no longer compensate, so an adaptation syndrome begins with a return to baseline physiologic parameters. The return of the heart rate, respirations, and blood pressure to baseline parameters makes assessment of the infant's pain more difficult and does not mean that the infant has "adjusted" to or is no longer experiencing pain.[48]

The lack of an expression of pain through physiologic and behavioral responses also does not mean that the neonate is not experiencing pain.[61,123] Pain responses may be delayed, cumulative, or absent. In the preterm infant, sustained elevations in vital signs and decreased oxygenation confirm the persistence of physiologic alterations after painful stimuli.[61,211] Very critically ill neonates and immature preterm infants may be so weak and overwhelmed that they have completely exhausted their energy and cannot respond.[73,100] **The incidence of crying in response to painful or noxious stimuli is less than 50% in the preterm infant.**[211] Depending on gestational age, a preterm infant's behavioral responses (e.g., facial changes, bodily movements) to pain are similar to those of the term infant. The responses of the very preterm infant are highly variable (a reflection of continuous maturation of the CNS) and less robust.[61,82,211,237] Preterm infants exhibit significant variability in behavioral and physiologic responses to preparatory procedures and handling, making it unclear if these responses are related to stress, behavioral disorganization, or a conditioned response and/or pain perception.[14,61,100,211] **A recent prospective cohort study comparing full-term infants (e.g., of diabetic mothers who were exposed to repeated heel sticks in the first 1 to 2 days of life) showed that these infants learned by conditioning to anticipate pain after their heel was swabbed with alcohol and exhibited a more intense pain response to a later venipuncture than infants who had not been exposed to repeated painful procedures.**[227]

Pain responses of the neonate are also influenced by the number and timing of painful procedures, the technique used, and the degree of professional expertise.[8,227] Lack of a response to a painful stimulus occurs more frequently in younger newborns (both gestational age and post-conceptual age) who are asleep and who have recently

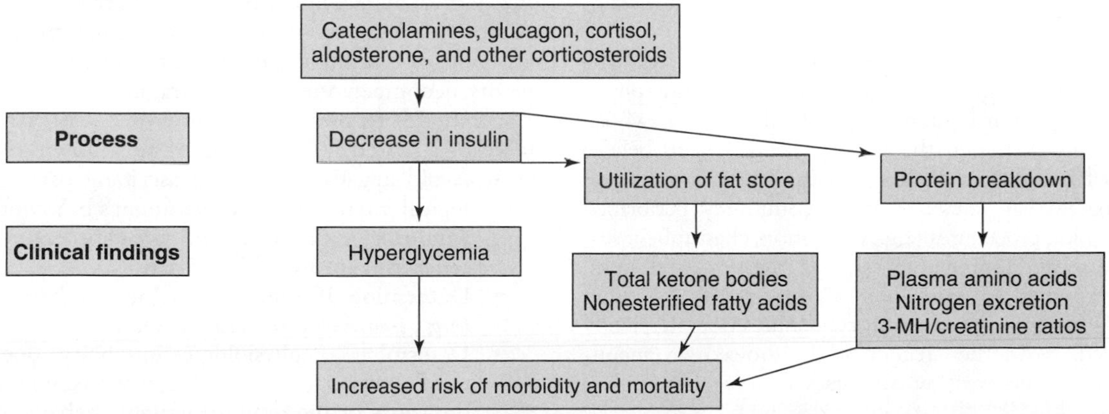

FIGURE 12-3 Hormonal response to pain in infants. *3-MH*, 3-methylhistidine. (From Johnston C, Stevens B: Pain in infants. In Watt-Watson J, Donovan M, editors: *Pain management: nursing perspective*, St Louis, 1992, Mosby.)

undergone another painful procedure.[132,167,184] Pain scores may be lowered in preterms with higher severity of illness and higher number of prior invasive procedures[68] while there is a larger heart rate response to repeated pain.[180] Use of mechanical lancets rather than manual lancets results in less behavioral and physiologic distress, fewer repeat punctures, and less bruising.[68,234] **Venipuncture has been shown to be associated with less pain in the neonate than heel stick,**[170,199] and a new blood glucose device using the forearm has been found to be less painful for term infants than heel sticks.[197]

Assessment of neonatal pain is influenced by the attitudes and beliefs of care providers, amount of time spent observing for and having knowledge of pain responses, discrepancy between attitudes and practice, knowledge and education of parents and professionals about pain, and prioritization of pain recognition and relief in the NICU and the social community.* Professional attitudes of (1) denial of newborn pain, (2) desensitization to the newborn's pain experience and the professional as the "inflictor" of pain on the most vulnerable of society, and (3) rationalizations for why pain is not assessed or treated and about individual professional responsibility and accountability for relief of pain and suffering hamper change in neonatal pain assessment and management.[17,61,157,230] Numerous other social factors influencing pain recognition and relief include (1) appearance/behavior/responsiveness of a sick neonate that varies markedly from the usual expectations about newborns, (2) lack of knowledge about analgesia and belief that pain is secondary in importance to the focus on survival, and (3) lack of knowledge about the impact on morbidity, mortality, and long-term consequences.[17,61,157]

Researchers have examined the beliefs and management techniques of 374 clinicians (both physicians and nurses) about procedural pain in newborn infants. Although the majority of clinicians believe that infants experience pain in the same or greater degree than adults, 9 of 12 commonly performed bedside procedures (e.g., intubation, chest tube insertion, arterial or venous catheter insertion, heel sticks) were rated as "moderately to very painful." Neither pharmacologic nor comfort measures were frequently used.[184] Another recent study showed an inconsistency between what nurses believe about infant pain assessment and the documentation practices in the NICU.[190] Even though nurses believed that pain assessment was important to provision of effective pain relief, there was a lack of knowledge about neonatal pain and a corresponding lack of documentation (e.g., 62% of day shift and 56% of night shift had no documented pain assessment; 74% of postoperative neonates had no documented pain assessment).[190] A multisite (n = 10) observational study of postoperative pain assessment and management found 88% of pain assessments documented by nurses and 9% documented by physicians; pain documented by physicians was the most significant predictor of the neonate receiving postoperative analgesia.[230] **Despite over 20 years of research into pain and pain control in neonates, "clinical use of pain-control measures in neonates undergoing invasive procedures remains sporadic and suboptimal."**[25]

*References 17,61,65,78,107,112,135,157,171,190,210,230.

IRRITABILITY AND AGITATION

Differentiation between pain and irritability or agitation is a challenge (Figure 12-4).[61] **Agitation is a behavioral symptom of many problems, including environmental overstimulation, respiratory insufficiency, neurologic irritability, and pain. Factors influencing chronic irritability and agitation in neonates in the NICU are shown in Figure 12-5.** Causes of agitation other than pain should be eliminated before pain management and/or sedation is initiated. Assessment of environmental stimuli should be a routine part of the neonate's care. The neonate may associate certain stimuli with unpleasant events over time, and repeated exposure (e.g., ventilator alarms, placement of heel warmer, the odor of an alcohol wipe) may trigger agitation. Although these stimuli are inevitable, identifying, avoiding, or limiting them will help prevent anticipatory decompensation in these fragile infants.[235]

Strategies to prevent and intervene with irritable or agitated infants include the following:

- **Avoid negative labels and ascribing psychological intentionality to the infant's behavior.**
- **Minimize caregivers, and provide consistency in care by staff and family.**
- **Determine if there is a "locus of pain" (e.g., pain-related irritability).**
- **Determine if physiologic instability (e.g., needs suction/position change; hypoxemia) is the cause or the result of irritable behaviors.**
- **Use developmental care (see Chapter 13).**
- **Use sedatives judiciously.**[235]

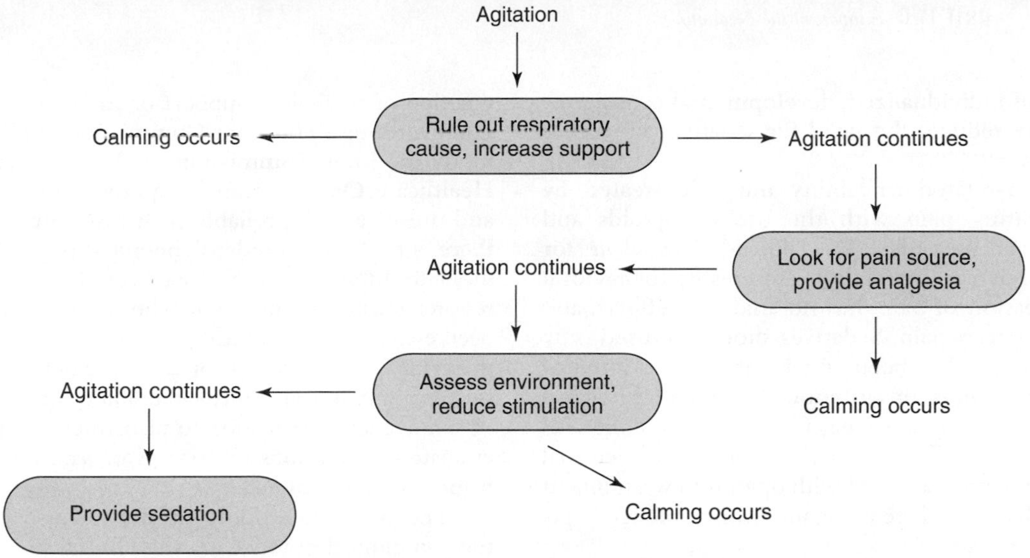

FIGURE 12-4 Decision tree for assessing and managing pain and/or agitation. (From Gordin P: Assessing and managing agitation in the critically ill infant, *Matern Child Nurs* 15:26, 1990.)

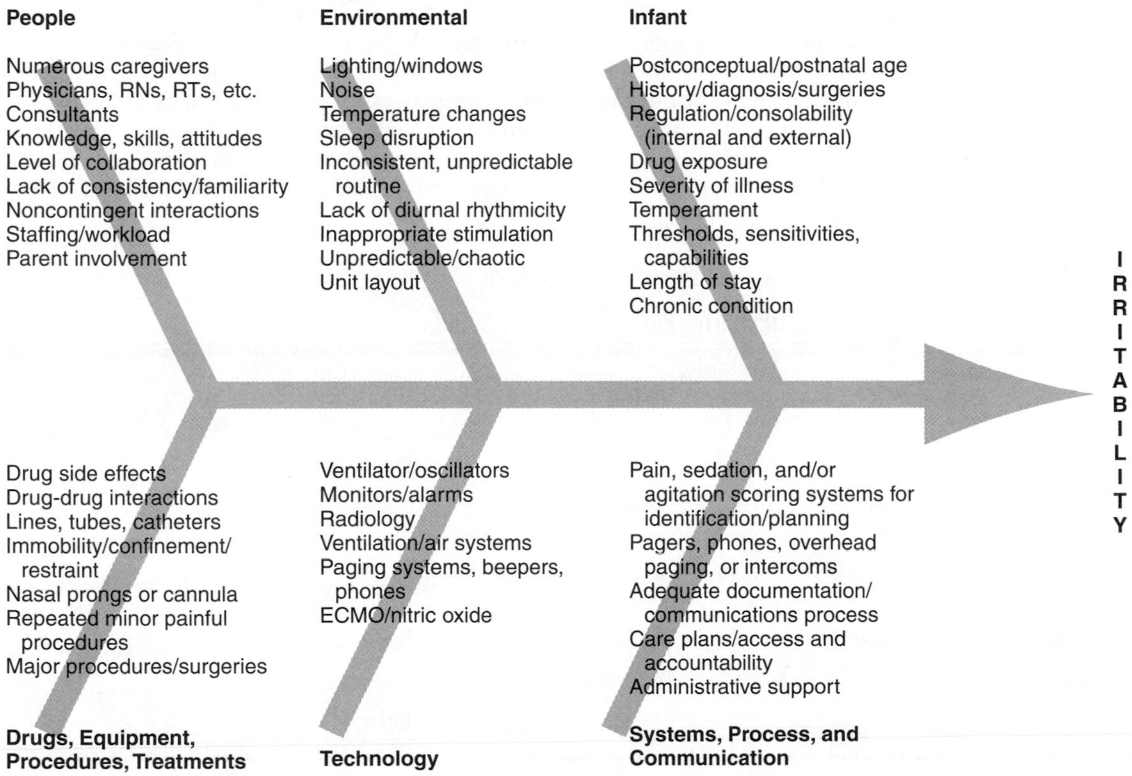

FIGURE 12-5 Fishbone diagram of factors influencing irritability. *ECMO*, Extracorporeal membrane oxygenation; *RNs*, registered nurses; *RT*, respiratory therapist. (From Walden M, Carrier C: Sleeping beauties: the impact of sedation on neonatal development, *J Obstet Gynecol Neonatal Nurs* 32:393, 2003.)

Use of individualized, developmental care significantly reduces the need for sedatives in VLBW infants.[235]

Pain-related irritability must be treated by alleviating pain with the use of opioids and comfort measures. Use of sedatives *alone* for pain-related irritability suppresses behavioral expression of pain, has no analgesic effects, and may *increase* pain. Sedatives should be used only when pain has been ruled out as the source of the irritability or agitation. Although no research documents the safety or efficacy of combining sedatives and analgesics for the treatment of neonatal pain, sedatives are used with opioids to wean infants who have developed tolerance from prolonged opioid therapy.[235]

Assessment Tools

To quantify and objectify a neonate's pain experience and to facilitate health care professionals' recognition of the presence and severity of pain in neonates, ongoing research is aimed at tool development. A recent retrospective analysis in an NICU showed that systematic evaluation of pain, using a pain scale, resulted in (1) increased awareness of treating and preventing pain in the newborn, (2) increased use of pharmacologic analgesics, and (3) no increase in the duration of respiratory support or parenteral nutrition.[4] **Although The Joint Commission (TJC, formerly the Joint Commission on Accreditation of Healthcare Organizations) requires the selection and use of a valid, reliable pain assessment tool, there is no "gold standard" neonatal pain assessment tool.**[18,133] Pain tools have been developed for research purposes; limited reliability and validity have been established for clinical practice,[210] especially in the critically ill newborn or the extremely premature infant. Clinical utility—the ability of users to obtain needed information to plan, implement, and evaluate interventions or services of pain tools—is beginning to be studied.

The most commonly used pain assessment tools in clinical practice are the CRIES Neonatal Postoperative Pain Assessment Score, Premature Infant Pain Profile (PIPP), and Neonatal Pain, Agitation, and Sedation Scale (N-PASS). All of these pain tools (except the N-PASS) assess *only* acute, not chronic/prolonged, pain.[20] **The CRIES assessment tool (Table 12-3), developed to measure physiologic and behavioral pain responses of term babies postoperatively, is used hourly with vital sign assessment.** CRIES uses a scoring system similar to the Apgar score: A score of 4 or above indicates pain and requires intervention.[40] CRIES requires the calculation of a percentage of change

TABLE 12-3 CRIES: NEONATAL POSTOPERATIVE PAIN ASSESSMENT SCORE

	SCORING CRITERIA FOR EACH ASSESSMENT			
	0	1	2	INFANT'S SCORE
Crying	No	High-pitched	Inconsolable	______
Requires O_2 for saturation greater than 95%	No	<30%	>30%	______
Increased vital signs*	HR and BP within 10% of preoperative value	HR or BP 11%-20% higher than preoperative value	HR or BP 21% or more above preoperative value	______
Expression	None	Grimace	Grimace/grunt	______
Sleepless	No	Wakes at frequent intervals	Constantly awake	______
			Total score†	______

From Krechel SW, Bildner J: Neonatal pain assessment tool developed at University of Missouri-Columbia.

BP, Blood pressure; *HR*, heart rate.

*BP should be done last.

†Add scores for all assessments to calculate total score.

from the infant's baseline physiologic values and relies on continuous cardiorespiratory monitoring. Validity and reliability to measure postoperative pain and pain relief after administration of an analgesic have been established,[142] whereas use of CRIES to measure procedural pain has not been validated.[40]

The PIPP (Table 12-4) is a multidimensional (physiologic and behavioral) assessment tool intended for use within clinical practice.[212] The PIPP is a seven-item, four-point scale whose maximum score depends on the infant's GA and behavioral state of the premature at baseline. The PIPP has been validated with both full-term and preterm neonates and can distinguish between procedural and postoperative pain and nonpain (e.g., noxious) events.[30] The PIPP has not been validated for assessment of the efficacy of analgesia nor for its usefulness in the assessment of continuous pain.

TABLE 12-4 PREMATURE INFANT PAIN PROFILE (PIPP)

Infant Study Number: ______________________

Date/Time: ______________________

Event: ______________________

PROCESS	INDICATOR	0	1	2	3	SCORE
Chart	Gestational age	36 wk and more	32-35 wk, 6 days	28-31 wk, 6 days	Less than 28 wk	
Observe infant 15 sec	Behavioral state	Active/awake; eyes open; facial movements	Quiet/awake; eyes closed; no facial movements	Active/asleep; eyes closed; facial movements	Quiet/asleep; eyes closed; no facial movements	
Observe baseline Heart rate Oxygen saturation						
Observe infant 30 sec	Heart rate (max)	0-4 beats/min increase	5-14 beats/min increase	5-24 beats/min increase	25 beats/min or more increase	
	Oxygen saturation (min)	0%-2.4% decrease	2.5%-4.9% decrease	5.0%-7.4% decrease	7.5% or more decrease	
	Brow bulge	None 0%-9% of time	Minimum 10%-39% of time	Moderate 40%-69% of time	Maximum 70% of time or more	
	Eye squeeze	None 0%-9% of time	Minimum 10%-39% of time	Moderate 40%-69% of time	Maximum 70% of time or more	
	Nasolabial	None 0%-9% of time	Minimum 10%-39% of time	Moderate 40%-69% of time	Maximum 70% of time or more	

Scoring method for the PIPP:

1. Familiarize yourself with each indicator and how it is to be scored by looking at the measure.
2. Score gestational age (from the chart) before you begin.
3. Score behavioral state by observing the infant for 15 seconds immediately before the event.
4. Record baseline heart rate and oxygen saturation.
5. Observe the infant for 30 seconds immediately after the event. You will have to look back and forth from the monitor to the infant's face. Score physiologic and facial action changes seen during that time and record immediately after the observation period.
6. Calculate the final score.

From Stevens B, Johnston C, Petroshen P, et al: Premature Infant Pain Profile: development and initial validation, *Clin J Pain* 12:13, 1996.

The N-PASS (Table 12-5) is an easily used clinical scale to assess, document, and manage pain and sedation.[121] NICU infants being mechanically ventilated or in the immediate postoperative period were assessed with the N-PASS before and after pharmacologic intervention. N-PASS is only one of three tools that measure not only acute but also prolonged/chronic pain.[185] N-PASS is a reliable and valid assessment tool for pain/agitation and sedation in postoperative and/or ventilated neonates (0 to 100 days of age) at 23 or more weeks' gestation.[122]

The Neonatal Facial Coding System (Table 12-6) is an assessment tool based on nine facial expressions of term newborns in four sleep-wake states while experiencing the discomfort of heel rub and the pain of heel lance. Quiet, awake neonates demonstrate the most facial activity, whereas those in quiet sleep demonstrate the least.[99,103] Facial activity also increases with gestational age, so both infant state and GA must be considered when using this scale. Because this tool is sensitive to changes in pain intensity, it is also useful for evaluating the effectiveness of interventions. There is recent evidence of reliable clinical use of this tool in term and preterm infants and for postoperative pain assessment, although it is time consuming and unidimensional and requires experienced coders.[100,114]

The Neonatal Infant Pain Scale (NIPS) (Table 12-7) is a behavioral assessment tool for preterm and term neonates responding to a needle puncture. NIPS scores reveal an increase in behavioral response during the procedures and a decline in response scores after the procedure (Figure 12-6). Thus NIPS provides a measurement of intensity of infant responses to a painful procedure during and after the event.[146] NIPS scores have been correlated with GA (e.g., maturity, level of behavior) and Apgar scores. NIPS provides an objective measure of pain-relieving interventions and their effectiveness.[146] The NIPS is objective and nonintrusive and assesses only behavioral response to pain; in comparison with other pain scales, it has been found to be easy and quick to use.[120,146] The clinical utility of the NIPS has not been established.[207] Flow sheets also have been designed to facilitate the documentation of pain scores and behaviors.[146]

The National Practice Guidelines provides a list of assessment questions to ask when assessing pain management in the neonate (Box 12-2). Lack of validated assessment tools may leave health care providers wondering if behaviors are indicators or responses to pain. The Acute Pain Management Guideline suggests that "if care providers are unsure whether a behavior indicates pain, and if there is reason to suspect pain, an analgesic trial can be diagnostic, as well as therapeutic."[3]

Assessment of pain and delivery of effective pain-relieving interventions in daily clinical practice must not be delayed while adequate, objective assessment tools are developed.[211] All health care providers must use their highly developed assessment skills, along with input from the parents, to gather information about infant behavioral, physiologic, and hormonal or catabolic stress responses before, during, and after painful stimuli. These same assessment skills enable care providers and parents to evaluate the effectiveness of pharmacologic and comfort interventions and institute more and/or different interventions as necessary to relieve pain and suffering.

Laboratory Data

Hormonal and metabolic changes are listed in the Critical Findings box on p. 228. Serum glucose levels and reagent test strips monitor for hyperglycemia, which may result in increased serum osmolality and increase the risk for IVH. Glucosuria, ketonuria, and proteinuria result in elevated specific gravity. Metabolic acidosis may result from increased serum levels of lactate, pyruvate, ketones, and non-esterified fatty acids. These data also may be indicative of other serious neonatal problems (e.g., sepsis, acute tubular necrosis).

TREATMENT

The neonate relies on the skilled observations, assessment, and interventions of care providers for prompt, safe, and effective relief of pain. Pain management is an interactive, relationship-based process that comprises the (1) environment of pain management, (2) preparation of the newborn for a procedure, (3) pain relief during a procedure, and (4) restoring safety and security to the infant after a procedure.[36,107] Limiting factors in providing adequate analgesia in these patients include an unfamiliarity with medication doses and with regional techniques and concern over increased drug sensitivity in neonates. Because routine care can be irritating to newborns, differentiating between agitation, which may respond well

Text continued on p. 246

TABLE 12-5 NEONATAL PAIN, AGITATION, AND SEDATION SCALE (N-PASS)

ASSESSMENT CRITERIA	SEDATION		SEDATION/PAIN	PAIN/AGITATION	
	−2	−1	0/0	+1	+2
Crying Irritability	No cry with painful stimuli	Moans or cries minimally with painful stimuli	No sedation/No pain signs	Irritable or crying at intervals Consolable	High-pitched or silent, continuous cry Inconsolable
Behavior state	No arousal to any stimuli No spontaneous movement	Arouses minimally to stimuli Little spontaneous movement	No sedation/No pain signs	Restless, squirming Awakens frequently	Arching, kicking Constantly awake ***or*** Arouses minimally/no movement (not sedated)
Facial expression	Mouth is lax No expression	Minimal expression with stimuli	No sedation/No pain signs	Any pain expression intermittent	Any pain expression continual
Extremities Tone	No grasp reflex Flaccid tone	Weak grasp reflex ↓ muscle tone	No sedation/No pain signs	Intermittent clenching toes, fists, or finger splay Body is not tense	Continual clenched toes, fists, or finger splay Body is tense
Vital signs HR, RR, BP, Sa_{O_2}	No variability with stimuli Hypoventilation or apnea	<10% variability from baseline with stimuli	No sedation/No pain signs	↑↓ 10%-20% from baseline Sa_{O_2} 76%-85% with stimulation, quick recovery	↑↓ >20% from baseline Sa_{O_2} ≤75% with stimulation, slow recovery Out of sync with vent

Continued

TABLE 12-5 NEONATAL PAIN, AGITATION, AND SEDATION SCALE (N-PASS)—cont'd

Assessment of Sedation

- Sedation is scored in addition to pain for each behavioral and physiologic criterion to assess the infant's response to stimuli.
- Sedation does not need to be assessed/scored with every pain assessment/score.
- Sedation is scored 0 → −2 for each behavioral and physiologic criterion, then summed and noted as a negative score (0 → −10).
  - A score of 0 is given if the infant has no signs of sedation, does not underreact.
- Desired levels of sedation vary according to the situation:
  - "Deep sedation" → goal score of −10 to −5
  - "Light sedation" → goal score of −5 to −2
  - Deep sedation is not recommended unless an infant is receiving ventilatory support, related to the high potential for hypoventilation and apnea.
- A negative score without the administration of opioids/sedatives may indicate:
  - The premature infant's response to prolonged or persistent pain/stress
  - Neurologic depression, sepsis, or other pathology

Assessment of Pain/Agitation

- Pain assessment is the fifth vital sign. Assessment for pain should be included in every vital sign assessment.
- Pain is scored from 0 → +2 for each behavioral and physiologic criterion and then summed:
  - Points are added to the premature infant's pain score based on his or her gestational age to compensate for his or her limited ability to behaviorally communicate pain.
  - Total pain score is documented as a positive number (0 → +11).
- Treatment/interventions are indicated for scores >3.
  - Interventions for known pain/painful stimuli are indicated before the score reaches 3.
- The goal of pain treatment/intervention is a score ≤3.
- More frequent pain assessment indications:
  - Indwelling tubes or lines that may cause pain, especially with movement (e.g., chest tubes) → at least every 2-4 hours
  - Receiving analgesics and/or sedatives → at least every 2-4 hours
  - 30-60 minutes after an analgesic is given for pain behaviors to assess response to medication
  - Postoperative → at least every 2 hours for 24-48 hours and then every 4 hours until off medications

Paralysis/Neuromuscular Blockade

- It is impossible to behaviorally evaluate a paralyzed infant for pain.
- Increases in heart rate and blood pressure at rest or with stimulation may be the only indicator of a need for more analgesia.
- Analgesics should be administered continuously by drip or around-the-clock dosing.
  - Higher, more frequent doses may be required if the infant is postoperative, has a chest tube, or has other pathology (e.g., NEC) that would normally cause pain.

Scoring Criteria

Crying/Irritability

−2 → No response to painful stimuli:

- No cry with needle sticks
- No reaction to ETT or nares suctioning
- No response to care giving

−1 → Moans, sighs, or cries (audible or silent) minimally to painful stimuli (e.g., needle sticks, ETT, or nares suctioning, care giving)

0 → No sedation signs or No pain/agitation signs

+1 → Infant is irritable/crying at intervals, but can be consoled

- If intubated, intermittent silent cry

+2 → Any of the following:
- Cry is high pitched
- Infant cries inconsolably
- If intubated, silent continuous cry

Behavior/State

−2 → Does not arouse or react to any stimuli:
- Eyes continually shut or open
- No spontaneous movement

−1 → Little spontaneous movement; arouses briefly and/or minimally to any stimuli:
- Opens eyes briefly
- Reacts to suctioning
- Withdraws to pain

0 → No sedation signs or No pain/agitation signs

+1 → Any of the following:
- Restless, squirming
- Awakens frequently/easily with minimal or no stimuli

+2 → Any of the following:
- Kicking
- Arching
- Constantly awake
- No movement or minimal arousal with stimulation (not sedated, inappropriate for gestational age or clinical situation)

Facial Expression

−2 → Any of the following:
- Mouth is lax
- Drooling
- No facial expression at rest or with stimuli

−1 → Minimal facial expression with stimuli

0 → No sedation signs or No pain/agitation signs

+1 → Any pain face expression observed intermittently

+2 → Any pain face expression is continual

Extremities/Tone

−2 → Any of the following:
- No palmar or planter grasp can be elicited
- Flaccid tone

−1 → Any of the following:
- Weak palmar or planter grasp can be elicited
- Decreased tone

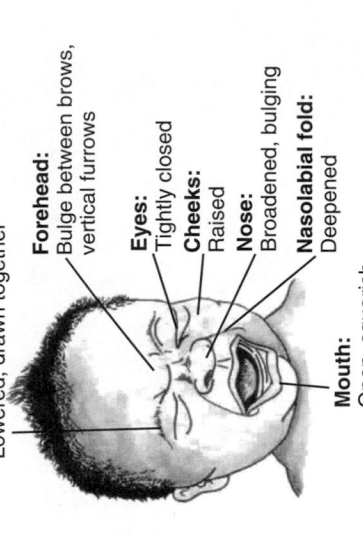

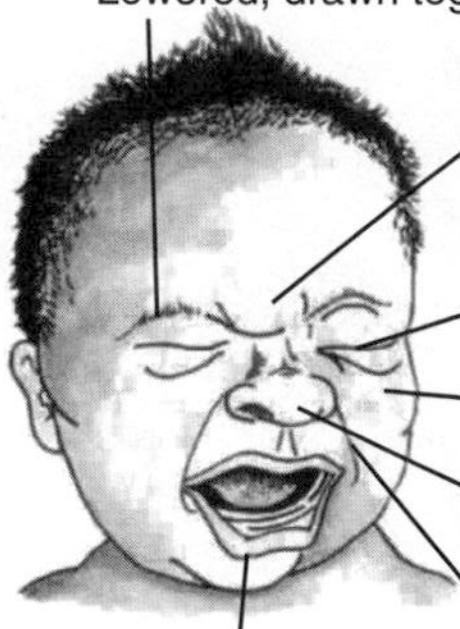

Facial expression of physical distress and pain in the infant

Continued

TABLE 12-5 NEONATAL PAIN, AGITATION, AND SEDATION SCALE (N-PASS)—cont'd

Extremities/Tone—cont'd

0 → No sedation signs or No pain/agitation signs

+1 → Intermittent (<30 seconds' duration) observation of toes and/or hands as clenched or fingers splayed

- Body is ***not*** tense

+2 → Any of the following:

- Frequent (≥30 seconds' duration) observation of toes and/or hands as clenched or fingers splayed
- Body is tense and stiff

Vital Signs: HR, BP, RR, and O_2 Saturations

−2 → Any of the following:

- No variability in vital signs with stimuli
- Hypoventilation
- Apnea
- Ventilated infant—no spontaneous respiratory effort

−1 → Vital signs show little variability with stimuli—less than 10% from baseline

0 → No sedation signs or No pain/agitation signs

+1 → Any of the following:

- HR, RR, and/or BP are 10%-20% above baseline
- With care/stimuli, infant desaturates minimally to moderately (Sao_2 76%-85%) and recovers quickly (within 2 minutes)

+2 → Any of the following:

- HR, RR, and/or BP are >20% above baseline
- With care/stimuli, infant desaturates severely (Sao_2 <75%) and recovers slowly (>2 minutes)
- Out of sync/fighting ventilator

We value your opinion
Pat Hummel,
MA, APN, NNP, PNP
Phone/voice mail: 708-327-9055
Email: phummel@lumc.edu
Website: www.n-pass.com

BP, Blood pressure, *ETT*, endotracheal tube; *HR*, heart rate; *NEC*, necrotizing enterocolitis; *RR*, respiratory rate; *Sao_2*, oxygen saturation.

TABLE 12-6 NEONATAL FACIAL CODING SYSTEM

ACTION	DESCRIPTION
Brow bulge	Bulging, creasing, and vertical furrows above and between brows occurring as a result of the lowering and drawing together of the eyebrows
Eye squeeze	Identified by the squeezing or bulging of the eyelids; bulging of the fatty pads about the infant's eyes is pronounced
Nasolabial furrow	Primarily manifested by the pulling upward and deepening of the nasolabial furrow (a line or wrinkle that begins adjacent to the nostril wings and runs downward and outward beyond the lip corners)
Open lips	Any separation of the lips
Stretch mouth (vertical)	Characterized by a tautness of the lip corners coupled with a pronounced downward pull on the jaw; seen when an already wide-open mouth is opened a fraction further by an extra pull at the jaw
Stretch mouth (horizontal)	Appears as a distinct horizontal pull at the corners of the mouth
Lip purse	Lips appear as if an "oo" sound is being pronounced
Taut tongue	Characterized by a raised, cupped tongue with sharp tense edges; the first occurrence of taut tongue usually is easy to see, often occurring with a wide-open mouth; after this first occurrence, the mouth may close slightly; taut tongue is still scorable on the basis of the still visible tongue edges
Chin quiver	An obvious high-frequency up-down motion of the lower jaw

Data from Grunau RVE, Craig KD: Pain expression in neonates: facial action and cry, *Pain* 28:399, 1987; Grunau R, Craig K: Facial activity as a measure of neonatal pain expression. In Tyler DC, Krane EJ, editors, *Advances in pain, research and therapy*, vol 15, New York, 1990, Raven.

TABLE 12-7 NEONATAL INFANT PAIN SCALE (NIPS) OPERATIONAL DEFINITIONS

FACIAL EXPRESSION	
0—Relaxed muscles	Restful face, neutral expression
1—Grimace	Tight facial muscles; furrowed brow, chin, jaw (negative facial expression—nose, mouth, and brow)
CRY	
0—No cry	Quiet, not crying
1—Whimper	Mild moaning, intermittent
2—Vigorous cry	Loud scream; rising, shrill, continuous (**NOTE:** Silent cry may be scored if baby is intubated as evidenced by obvious mouth and facial movement)
BREATHING PATTERNS	
0—Relaxed	Usual pattern for this infant
1—Change in breathing	Indrawing, irregular, faster than usual; gagging; breath-holding
ARMS	
0—Relaxed/restrained	No muscular rigidity; occasional random movements of arms
1—Flexed/extended	Tense, straight arms; rigid and/or rapid extension, flexion
LEGS	
0—Relaxed/restrained	No muscular rigidity; occasional random leg movement
1—Flexed/extended	Tense, straight legs; rigid and/or rapid extension, flexion
STATE OF AROUSAL	
0—Sleeping/awake	Quiet, peaceful sleeping or alert and settled
1—Fussy	Alert, restless, and thrashing

From Lawrence J, Alcock D, McGrath P, et al: Children's Hospital of Eastern Ontario, 1993.

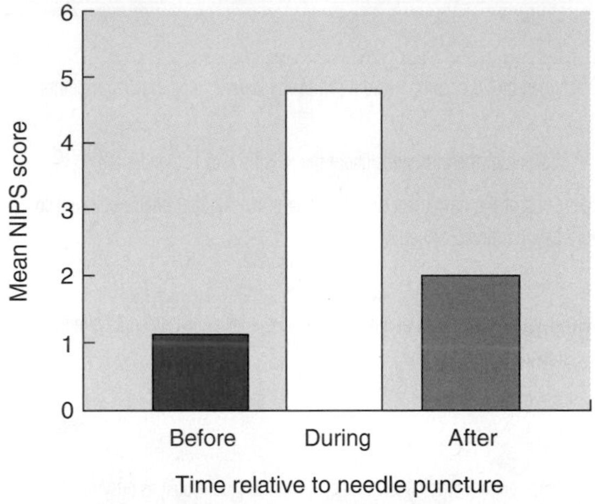

FIGURE 12-6 Mean Neonatal Infant Pain Scale (NIPS) scores over time in 22 infants. (From Lawrence J, Alcock D, McGrath P, et al: The development of a tool to assess neonatal pain, *Neonat Netw* 12:62, 1993.)

BOX 12-2 CRITICAL QUESTIONS TO ASK ABOUT PAIN MANAGEMENT IN NEONATES

- Is the infant being adequately assessed at appropriate intervals?
- Are analgesics ordered for prevention and relief of pain?
- Is the analgesic strong enough for the pain expected or the pain being experienced?
- Is the timing of the drug administration appropriate for the pain expected or being experienced?
- Is the route of administration appropriate (preferably oral or intravenous) for the infant?
- Is the infant adequately monitored for side effects?
- Are side effects appropriately managed?
- Has the analgesic regimen provided adequate comfort and satisfaction from the family's perspective?

Questions to Consider About Nonpharmacologic Strategies

- Is the strategy appropriate for the infant's developmental level, condition, and type of pain?
- Is the timing of the strategy sufficient to optimize its effects?
- Is the strategy adequately effective in preventing or alleviating the infant's pain?
- Is the family satisfied with the strategy for prevention or relief of pain?

From Acute Pain Management Guideline Panel: *Acute pain management: operative or medical procedures and trauma—clinical practice guideline*, AHCPR Pub No 92-0032, Rockville, Md, 1992, Agency for Health Care Policy and Research, Public Health Service, USDHHS.

to comfort measures, and pain, which will not, is mandatory. **Opioids are the mainstay of pharmacologic treatment; however, other useful medications and techniques may be used for pain relief.[8] Guidelines for managing pain in the neonate are listed in Box 12-3. Commonly performed painful procedures and recommended management strategies based on the consensus statement of the International Evidence-Based Group for Neonatal Pain[17] are listed in Table 12-8.**

Pharmacologic Measures

Absorption, metabolism, distribution, and clearance of drugs in the neonate differ from those in the older child and adult (see Chapter 10). These differences are summarized in Table 12-9.

OPIOIDS AND BENZODIAZEPINES

Opioids have their primary effect on the μ-receptor in the brain and spinal cord. High-affinity μ-receptors are associated with analgesia, and low-affinity μ-receptors are associated with respiratory depression. **There may be fewer high-affinity μ-receptors in the newborn that are less sensitive to the analgesic effects of opioids.**

BOX 12-3 GUIDELINES FOR PAIN MANAGEMENT IN THE NEONATE

- Use strategies to prevent pain (e.g., avoid recurrent painful stimuli).
- Use developmental care and environmental interventions to reduce noxious stimuli and stress in the NICU (see Chapter 13).
- Use comfort measures (e.g., sucrose, nonnutritive sucking, containment with swaddling or facilitated tucking).
- Sucrose administration recommendations:
  - Preterm infants: 0.1 to 0.4 mL; dipping a pacifier into sucrose results in 0.1 mL intake
  - Term infants: 2 mL
  - Administer 2 minutes before a painful procedure
  - Analgesic effect lasts about 5 minutes
- Use pharmacologic therapy for preemptive analgesia (see Table 12-10).
- Use pharmacologic therapy for ongoing pain.
- Use of a combination of pain interventions (e.g., sucking, containment, medication) may have an additive or synergistic clinical effect.

Modified from Anand KJ and the International Evidence-Based Group for Neonatal Pain: Consensus statement for the prevention and management of pain in the newborn, *Arch Pediatr Adolesc Med* 155:173, 2001; Prince W, Horns K, Latta T, et al: Treatment of neonatal pain without a gold standard: the case for caregiving interventions and sucrose administration, *Neonatal Netw* 23:33, 2004.

TABLE 12-8 SUGGESTED MANAGEMENT OF PAINFUL PROCEDURES COMMONLY PERFORMED IN THE NEONATAL INTENSIVE CARE UNIT

PROCEDURES	PACIFIER WITH SUCROSE	SWADDLING, CONTAINMENT, OR FACILITATED TUCKING	EMLA CREAM/AMETHOCAINE GEL/LIPOSOMAL LIDOCAINE	SUBCUTANEOUS INFILTRATION OF LIDOCAINE	OPIOIDS	OTHER
DIAGNOSTIC PROCEDURES						
Arterial puncture	✓	✓	✓	✓		
Heel lancing	✓	✓				Consider venipuncture, skin-to-skin contact with mother, mechanical spring-loaded lance
Lumbar puncture	✓		✓	✓		Use careful physical handling
Venipuncture	✓	✓	✓		✓	
THERAPEUTIC PROCEDURES						
Central venous line placement	✓	✓	✓	✓	✓	Consider general anesthesia or benzodiazepines
Chest tube insertion	✓			✓	✓	Anticipate need for intubation and ventilation in neonates spontaneously breathing; consider short-acting anesthetic agents; avoid midazolam
Gavage tube insertion	✓	✓				Use gentle technique and appropriate lubrication
Intramuscular injection	✓	✓	✓			Give drugs intravenously whenever possible
Peripherally inserted central catheter placement	✓	✓	✓		✓	
Endotracheal intubation				Consider ***topical*** lidocaine spray	✓	Consider various combinations of atropine, ketamine, thiopental sodium, succinylcholine chloride, morphine, fentanyl, non-depolarizing muscle relaxant
Endotracheal suction	Sucrose optional	✓			✓	
SURGICAL PROCEDURES						
Circumcision	✓		✓	Dorsal penile block, ring block, or caudal block using plain or buffered lidocaine		Mogen clamp is preferred over Gomco clamp; consider acetaminophen for postoperative pain

Adapted from Walden M, Franck L: Identification, management, and prevention of newborn/infant pain. In Kenner C, Lott J, editors: *Comprehensive neonatal nursing* (ed 3, p. 853), Philadelphia, 2003, Saunders; Anand KJ, Johnston CC, Oberlander TF, et al: Analgesia and local anesthesia during invasive procedures in the neonate, *Clin Ther* 27:844, 2005.

TABLE 12-9 PHARMACOLOGIC DIFFERENCES BETWEEN NEWBORNS AND ADULTS

DIFFERENCES	CAUSE	EFFECTS
Altered gastric activity	Presence of alkaline amniotic fluids at birth Immature gastric mucosa Consumption of alkaline milk	Variable drug absorption
Decreased gastric emptying time		Increased absorption of some drugs
Decreased protein binding	Lower levels of albumin, α-acid glycoprotein Increased competition for binding sites by endogenous substances (bilirubin)	Increased levels of free drug (opioids, local anesthetics)
Increased volume of distribution	Larger volume of body water in the newborn	Larger initial dose may be needed for effect (e.g., neuromuscular blocking agents, local anesthetics)
Decreased drug metabolism	Immature liver enzyme systems	Prolonged effect of some medications (e.g., morphine, fentanyl, neuromuscular blockers)
Decreased drug clearance	Immature renal system and decreased glomerular filtration rate	Prolonged effect of some medications (morphine)

From Rovee-Collier C, Hayne H: Reactivation of infant memory: implications for cognitive development, *Adv Child Dev* 10:185, 1987.

Higher initial doses of opioids may therefore be necessary for effect, which may in turn increase the risk for respiratory depression. A randomized, double-blind study of postoperative (e.g., thoracic or abdominal surgery) pain relief in full-term newborns receiving either continuous or intermittent morphine found an age-related difference in morphine requirements and metabolism.[42,43] Younger infants (e.g., 7 days or younger) needed less morphine postoperatively (e.g., loading dose [50 mcg/kg], continuous dose [5 to 10 mcg/kg/hr], and need for additional "break through" doses) than neonates older than 7 days (e.g., loading dose [100 mcg/kg] and continuous dose [10 mcg/kg/hr]). This study also found that neonates being mechanically ventilated had slower morphine metabolism and clearance.[42] A more recent retrospective analysis of the postoperative use of morphine in 82 full-term neonates after thoracic and/or abdominal surgery found the following[67]:

- 76% received morphine as a continuous IV infusion.
- Both dosage (i.e., increased morphine rate by 10 mcg/kg/hr, prolonged mechanical ventilation by 24 hours) and duration (increased morphine duration by 1 hour, prolonged mechanical ventilation by 38 minutes) were significantly associated with longer mechanical ventilation.
- After extubation, there was no apnea or hypotension associated with morphine use.

Decreased protein binding, drug metabolism, and drug clearance may contribute to higher plasma and CNS concentrations and prolonged drug effect. Effective drug doses and metabolism or use by the individual neonate (preterm and full-term neonates) depend on weight, gestational age, postnatal age, genetic variation, and the corresponding pharmacokinetics and pharmacodynamics, which may change in the first days of life.[220,231,233] Therefore all doses must be titrated to the individual neonate's needs and current clinical circumstances.[231]

All the opioids have similar mechanisms of action; however, there are a few important differences in side effects (Table 12-10). Morphine is the most commonly used opioid and may cause hypotension in dehydrated patients or when used in high doses; it provides more sedation than fentanyl.[139] Recent research on the blood pressure effects of morphine administration showed (1) no hypotensive effects on ventilated newborns[194] or on preterms[233] given analgesic doses[15] and (2) occurrence of hypotensive effects with loading and higher dosages.[22,233] **However, morphine should be used with caution in preterms of 23 to 26 weeks' gestation and those with preexisting hypotension.**[111] For acute procedural pain (e.g., heel stick), a loading dose of morphine followed by continuous IV infusion does not provide adequate analgesia for invasive procedures in ventilated preterms.[51]

TABLE 12-10 ANALGESICS, SEDATIVES, AND REVERSAL AGENTS FOR THE NEONATE

DRUG	DOSAGE	COMMENTS
NARCOTIC		
Morphine	0.05-0.1 mg/kg/dose q 4-6 hr PRN IV, IM, or Sub-Q Continuous IV infusion: 10-15 mcg/kg/hr (up to 30-40 mcg/kg for ventilator therapy and major surgery)[231] Mean onset of action: 5 min Peak effect: 15 min Duration: 4-5 hr	CNS and respiratory depressant; bronchospasms; peripheral vasodilation with hypovolemic infants; hypotension, decreases gastric/intestinal motility; intestinal obstruction; risk for NEC; increases intracranial pressure; seizures; urinary retention; easily reversed with naloxone; slower onset but longer duration than for fentanyl; withdrawal symptoms may occur. Ceiling effect (after reaching a therapeutic level, higher doses result in more adverse rather than analgesic effects) reached by using doses up to 0.5 mg/kg.[19]
Fentanyl (Sublimaze)	0.3-2 mcg/kg/dose q 1-2 hr PRN IV or Sub-Q Continuous IV infusion: 0.3-5 mcg/kg/hr Onset of action: 2-3 min Peak effect: 3-4 min Duration: 30-60 min	Same as for morphine. Rapid onset of action; decreases motor activity; does not increase intracranial pressure in the absence of respiratory depression; easily reversed with naloxone; short duration of action; may cause bradycardia, hypotension, apnea, seizures, or rigidity if given too rapidly; hypothermia; withdrawal symptoms occur with prolonged use.
Sufentanil citrate (Sufenta)	0.5-1 mcg/kg/dose q 30 min to 1 hr Peak effect: 5-6 min Duration: 30 min	Ten times more potent than fentanyl; has a quicker onset and shorter duration of action than fentanyl. Use with caution in neonates with intraventricular hemorrhage, hepatic or renal impairment, or pulmonary disease. Same side effects as for fentanyl, above. Bolus and continuous infusion affects electroencephalogram (EEG) results in very-low-birth-weight/extremely-low-birth-weight infants; use of sufentanil must be considered in EEG interpretation.[232]
Meperidine (Demerol)		***Not*** recommended in preterm or term infants. The active metabolite, normeperidine, accumulates in tissues and causes CNS stimulation (e.g., tremors, muscle twitching, hyperactive reflexes, dilated pupils) and also lowers the seizure threshold level.[8]
NONNARCOTIC		
Acetaminophen (Tylenol)	Oral loading dose: 20-25 mg/kg PO; then 12-15 mg/kg PO q 8 hr	May cause hepatotoxicity in overdose. Potentiates effects of narcotics but alone does ***not*** relieve surgical pain or heel lance pain.[4] Do not use in patients with G6PD deficiency.
Ibuprofen (Advil, Motrin)	4-10 mg/kg/dose q 6-8 hr PO	Gastric irritant—administer with or after feeding; use with caution in neonates with necrotizing enterocolitis, impaired renal function, hypertension, or compromised cardiac function.
LOCAL ANESTHETICS		
Lidocaine	0.5%-1% solution (to avoid systemic toxicity, volume should be less than 0.5 mL/kg of 1% lidocaine solution—5 mg/kg)	Local infiltration anesthesia for invasive procedures; use solution ***without epinephrine*** to avoid vasoconstriction. Use topical creams (EMLA/amethocaine) before needle insertion; warm solution to body temperature; inject slowly to reduce the pain of injection.[148]

CBF, Cerebral blood flow; *CNS*, central nervous system; *EMLA*, eutectic mixture of lidocaine and prilocaine; *G6PD*, glucose-6-phosphate dehydrogenase; *IM*, intramuscular; *IV*, intravenous; *IVH*, intraventricular hemorrhage; *NEC*, necrotizing enterocolitis; *NICU*, neonatal intensive care unit; *PO*, per os; *PR*, per rectum; *PRN*, as needed; *PVL*, periventricular leukomalacia; *Sub-Q*, subcutaneous.

*Not yet approved by the Food and Drug Administration for use in the United States.

Continued

TABLE 12-10 ANALGESICS, SEDATIVES, AND REVERSAL AGENTS FOR THE NEONATE—cont'd

DRUG	DOSAGE	COMMENTS
LOCAL ANESTHETICS—cont'd		
Bupivacaine Levobupivacaine Ropivacaine	2.5 mg/kg one-time epidural dose Continuous IV infusion: 0.2 mg/kg/hr (maximum dose)	Monitor for CNS (e.g., seizures, irritability) and cardiotoxic (e.g., ventricular dysrhythmias) side effects. Monitor catheter integrity. Epidural infusion is titrated to effect but ***must not*** exceed maximum dose. Levobupivacaine and ropivacaine are less cardiotoxic than bupivacaine.
EMLA (lidocaine and prilocaine)	2.5-5 g to site for at least 60 min Peak effect: 2-3 hr Duration: 1-2 hr after removal	Vasoconstriction at the site. Site must be covered with water-impermeable dressing (e.g., Tegaderm). Single doses have not been shown to cause methemoglobinemia in preterm or term neonates.[225] Does not relieve pain of heel lance.[8] The possibility of toxicity is increased when EMLA is applied to (1) open skin and (2) a larger area than recommended by manufacturer.[172] Cannot be used on abraded skin or mucous membranes.[139]
Amethocaine gel* (4%) (liposome-encapsulated tetracaine) (Ametrope)	1.5 g to site for 30 min to 1 hr	Site must be covered with water-impermeable dressing (e.g., Tegaderm). Vasodilation at the site—mild transient (≈20 min) erythema or blanching.[126,148,169,224]
Liposomal lidocaine (4%) cream	Onset of action: 20-30 min	Available in United States without a prescription. Does not cause methemoglobinemia, can be applied without an occlusive dressing, and has fewer vasoactive effects.
SEDATIVE-HYPNOTICS		
Barbiturates		Do ***not*** provide pain relief; help reduce agitation precipitated by painful events. Frequently produce hyperalgesia and increased reaction to painful stimuli; contraindicated for neonates who have pain and also require sedation.
Phenobarbital	Loading: 10-20 mg/kg IV to maximum 40 mg/kg Maintenance: 5-7 mg/kg in two divided doses beginning 12 hr after last loading dose	Prolonged sedation possible once therapeutic levels achieved (20-25 mg/mL); depresses CNS—motor and respiratory; slow onset of action; little or no pain relief; not easily reversed; withdrawal symptoms may occur; incompatible with other drugs in solution.
NON-BARBITURATES		
Chloral hydrate	25-75 mg/kg/dose q 6 hr PRN PO or PR Onset: 10-15 min Duration: 2-4 hr	Gastric irritant—administer with or after feeding; paradoxic excitement; prolonged use associated with direct hyperbilirubinemia[145]; not to be used for analgesia; respiratory depressant; in repeated doses to premature infants—adverse effects—CNS depression, dysrhythmias, and renal failure.[86] For occasional procedural sedation, although not recommended. Recovery from chloral hydrate accompanied by a "hangover."
Benzodiazepines		Do ***not*** provide pain relief. Produce sedation, muscle relaxation, amnesia, anxiolysis, and anticonvulsant effects.
Diazepam (Valium)	0.02-0.3 mg/kg IV, IM, or PO q 6-8 hr	Do ***not*** dilute injection; venous sclerosing; may displace bilirubin and result in kernicterus; respiratory depression; hypotension; may cause agitation; induces sleep; relaxes muscles; withdrawal symptoms may occur; no analgesic effect; this drug should be used with caution in the neonate because of its long half-life, long-acting metabolites, and preservative (benzyl alcohol).[8]

TABLE 12-10 ANALGESICS, SEDATIVES, AND REVERSAL AGENTS FOR THE NEONATE—cont'd

DRUG	DOSAGE	COMMENTS
NON-BARBITURATES—cont'd		
Lorazepam (Ativan)	0.05-0.1 mg/kg/dose (give over >3 min) q 4-8 hr	Respiratory depressant, partial airway obstruction, drowsiness; respiratory depression potentiated when narcotics or barbiturates also being given; infuse slowly to avoid apnea, bradycardia, and hypotension. Rhythmic myoclonic jerking in preterms.
Midazolam (Versed)	0.05-0.15 mg/kg/dose IV (give over ≥5 min) q 2-4 hr PRN Continuous IV infusion: <32 wks: 0.03 mg/kg/hr or 0.5 mcg/kg/min >32 wks: 0.06 mg/kg/hr or 1 mcg/kg/min PO: 0.25 mg/kg/dose of oral syrup Onset: IV—1-2 min; PO—15-30 min Duration: 1 hr after single IV dose For procedural sedation: Give 0.05 mg/kg IV and repeat ×1 PRN for procedure	Same as for lorazepam; continuous IV infusion enables precise titration until sedative effect is obtained; calms agitated infant on ventilator. Rapid bolus delivery and/or use with fentanyl is associated with (1) myoclonus—rhythmic twitching of all extremities that ceases with discontinuation of drug and does not return, and (2) respiratory depression and hypotension—caution use in hypotensive and hypovolemic neonates.[125,152] A systematic review shows (1) increased incidence of adverse neurologic outcomes (e.g., grade 3-4 IVH; PVL), altered CBF); (2) longer duration of NICU stay with midazolam use; and (3) conclusion that there is insufficient evidence to support IV midazolam use as a sedative for neonates in NICU.[165]
REVERSAL AGENTS		
Naloxone (Narcan)	1-10 mcg/kg	Reverses effects of opioids (both side effects and analgesia).
Flumazenil (Mazicon)	10 mcg/kg	Reverses the effects of benzodiazepines (e.g., midazolam, diazepam, lorazepam).

CBF, Cerebral blood flow; *CNS*, central nervous system; *EMLA*, eutectic mixture of lidocaine and prilocaine; *G6PD*, glucose-6-phosphate dehydrogenase; *IM*, intramuscular; *IV*, intravenous; *IVH*, intraventricular hemorrhage; *NEC*, necrotizing enterocolitis; *NICU*, neonatal intensive care unit; *PO*, per os; *PR*, per rectum; *PRN*, as needed; *PVL*, periventricular leukomalacia; *Sub-Q*, subcutaneous.
*Not yet approved by the Food and Drug Administration for use in the United States.

Fentanyl is the preferred drug in many NICUs because of its cardiovascular stability and its ability to decrease pulmonary vascular resistance. It can, however, cause chest wall rigidity and decreased lung compliance if administered too quickly. Neuromuscular blocking agents or slow administration of the drug will prevent this problem. Fentanyl also is commonly used in patients on extracorporeal membrane oxygenation (ECMO) to provide sedation and analgesia and to prevent increases in pulmonary vascular resistance and pressure.[149] Fentanyl is used also for artificial ventilation, persistent pulmonary hypertension of the newborn (PPHN), diaphragmatic hernia, and postoperative pain.[231] Because of its rapid onset and short duration, fentanyl relieves procedural pain.[231] **Sufentanil is 10 times more potent than fentanyl** and significantly more expensive. It is shorter acting and can have even greater effects on lung and chest wall compliance.

Administering drugs by as-needed (PRN) schedule may result in peaks and valleys of pain relief and increases in side effects. Because an analgesic is most effective if given before the peak of pain (wind-up), continuous infusions or regular administration can help prevent undue neonatal suffering.[8,220]

Benzodiazepines are commonly used in the NICU for sedation. Midazolam (Versed) has been used increasingly to provide sedation in mechanically ventilated neonates. However, according to Khurana et al,[139] **recent concern over the safety of**

midazolam has been reported because of adverse neurologic effects including severe intraventricular hemorrhage, periventricular leukomalacia, abnormal movements, and hemodynamic effects.[139] A meta-analysis of the research on midazolam concluded that there are significant adverse effects and no clinical benefit to the use of midazolam; there is insufficient evidence to justify the use of midazolam for ventilated neonates in the NICU (see Table 12-10).[28,165] Benzodiazepines potentiate the effects of opiates.[208] Therefore when they are used in combination (e.g., fentanyl and midazolam), lower doses of each medication may be used to gain the same effect as would be attained if either one was used separately. It is very important to note that while benzodiazepines provide sedation, they have *no* analgesic effect.[208] Therefore if pain is a concern for the patient, an analgesic should be given as well.

The long-term effects of analgesic use on the developing brain are poorly understood because of a paucity of data on neurodevelopmental outcomes. Several researchers have found a protective effect of analgesic use on neurodevelopmental outcomes, perhaps because of decreased fluctuation in blood pressure, cerebral blood flow, oxygenation, respiratory synchrony with ventilation, and stress hormones.* More recent studies on the long-term neurologic effects of morphine analgesia in ventilated preterm infants caution against the lack of protective effects and have documented an increase in severe IVH/PVL[22,204] (see the Invasive Procedures section on pp. 228-231) and subtle neurobehavioral differences in preterm infants exposed to morphine analgesia.[186]

*References 14,21,26,144,153,168,183.

LOCAL ANESTHETICS

Local anesthetics have a variety of uses and provide analgesia by preventing the transmission of noxious stimuli at either the peripheral receptor site or the spinal cord. Bupivacaine and lidocaine are the two most commonly used local anesthetics (see Table 12-10). A recent study showed that bupivacaine confers better analgesia for neonatal circumcision than that achieved with lidocaine.[216]

Bupivacaine is longer acting but more cardiotoxic than lidocaine. Both are more toxic in neonates than in adults because of increased organ sensitivity and free fraction of drug. The cardiovascular toxicity may be enhanced if epinephrine-containing local anesthetics are used. The new long-acting local anesthetics ***levobupivacaine*** and ***ropivacaine*** are as effective as bupivacaine but are less cardiotoxic.[244]

Regional Technique. Regional techniques provide adequate analgesia, thus reducing the need for higher doses of opioids (Table 12-11). Advantages include the following[63]:

- Stress responses are significantly decreased.
- Normal respiratory patterns return more quickly.
- The need for postoperative ventilation may be avoided or shortened.
- Intestinal motility recovers more quickly.
- Morbidity decreases, particularly with the use of epidural blocks.

TABLE 12-11 TYPES OF REGIONAL BLOCKADE: POTENTIAL USES

BLOCK	POTENTIAL USES	COMPLICATIONS
Spinal	In place of general anesthesia for surgery below the umbilicus; decreased incidence of postoperative apnea	Inability to access space; incomplete block or inadequate duration of anesthesia
Caudal/epidural	Intraoperative and postoperative analgesia for thoracic, abdominal, perineal, and lower extremity surgery	Inadequate block; local or opioid-related toxicity; nerve damage, paralysis
Dorsal penile nerve/ring block	Circumcision, analgesia for any penile surgery	Hematoma formation; end-organ damage if epinephrine-containing solutions are used
Intercostal nerve block	Rib fractures, thoracic surgery	Pneumothorax; local anesthetic toxicity (highest rate of absorption)

Dorsal Penile Nerve/Ring Block.[141] Dorsal penile nerve block is extremely easy to perform with a high degree of success that can provide surgical anesthesia for circumcision.[141] The block is performed by injecting 1% lidocaine 3 to 5 mm below the skin at the 2 o'clock and 10 o'clock positions on the dorsum of the penis (Figure 12-7). In a full-term neonate, 0.5 mL/side is used, and 0.2 mL/kg/side is used in premature infants. An alternative technique less likely to cause hematoma is to inject a subcutaneous ring of 0.5% or 1% lidocaine around the base of the penis. All solutions should be without epinephrine, and a "wait time" of 5 to 8 minutes is necessary to achieve adequate anesthesia.[147]

A recent study of pain responses to circumcision using dorsal penile nerve block/ring block, topical ELA-Max, and 24% oral sucrose solution found that infants receiving a combination of dorsal block/sucrose or ring block/sucrose had lower pain scores than those with use of ring block or sucrose alone.[187] Infants receiving topical ELA-Max had pain scores that were not significantly different from those in the infants receiving dorsal penile or ring block. Both dorsal and ring nerve blocks resulted in similar pain scores. As a result of this nursing research, the institutional policy was changed so that newborn circumcision is performed only with the use of analgesic and not oral sucrose alone. Liposomal lidocaine was compared with a eutectic mixture of lidocaine and prilocaine (EMLA) and dorsal penile block in a study of 54 full-term infants being circumcised; liposomal lidocaine was found to be a safe and effective topical anesthetic.[147] Another recent video study found that the dorsal penile nerve block was significantly more effective for pain relief during circumcision than use of topical EMLA cream.[80]

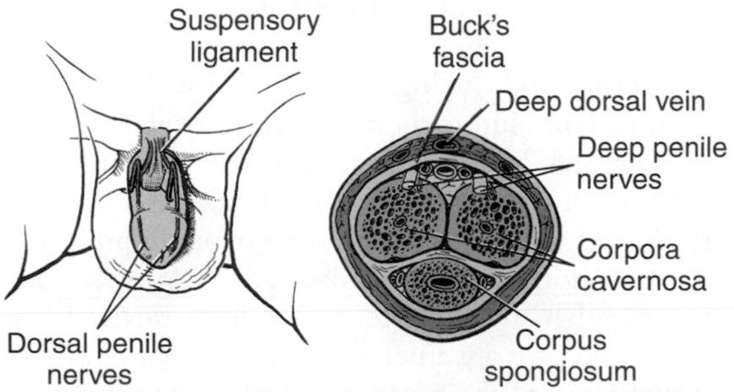

FIGURE 12-7 Anatomic landmarks for placement of a dorsal penile nerve block. (From McClain B, Anand KS: Neonatal pain management. In Deshpande J, Tobias J, editors: *The pediatric pain handbook*, St Louis, 1996, Mosby.)

Epidural Block. The epidural space is an area surrounding the dura of the spinal cord. This space can be accessed from the caudal, lumbar, or thoracic region. An epidural block is performed by a skilled pediatric anesthesiologist, often with the patient under general anesthesia.[156] A small catheter can be left in the space, or a one-time dose of medication can be given. Local anesthetics act by anesthetizing either the local nerve roots or the spinal tracts at the level of the spinal cord where they are placed. The most commonly used medications are the local anesthetics ***lidocaine*** and ***bupivacaine.*** They are often used in combination with low doses of opioids, which have both local and systemic action. The major advantages of these techniques are the ability to provide continuous pain relief and the potential to minimize respiratory depression, facilitate extubation, and hasten recovery.

Eutectic Mixture of Local Anesthetic and Infiltration. Eutectic mixture of local anesthetic (EMLA) is a local anesthetic cream that anesthetizes the skin and has been used for a variety of procedures (e.g., lumbar puncture, venipuncture).[1,240] A recent study of EMLA, applied 60 to 90 minutes before lumbar puncture, showed a significant decrease in pain response during needle insertion and withdrawal but not during positioning/handling of the newborn.[137] EMLA has been used for analgesia with circumcisions in newborns and has been shown to be efficacious.[240] However, its analgesic properties are not as effective as those of dorsal penile blocks in relieving postoperative circumcision pain.[119] Use of combined modalities (i.e., EMLA, penile block, a sucrose pacifier, and acetaminophen) has been shown to provide the greatest analgesia and comfort during invasive procedures.* A meta-analysis of the efficacy of EMLA for a variety of procedures in neonates found that EMLA diminishes pain during circumcision, venipuncture, arterial puncture, and placement of a peripheral/central IV line.[139,225,240] For maximum effectiveness, EMLA should be applied and left on for at least 1 to 2 hours before starting an invasive procedure. Unfortunately, EMLA does not appear to alleviate pain resulting from heel sticks.[75,139,225,240] Infiltration of local anesthetic can also help decrease pain for such procedures as placement of percutaneous central lines,

*References 107,115,141,187,215,226,240.

removal of Broviac catheters, and circumcision. Methemoglobinemia does not appear to be a problem when single daily doses of 0.5 g EMLA are left in place for 60 minutes,[225] but studies are ongoing to address this issue.

Amethocaine gel (lysosome-encapsulated tetracaine) is a topical local anesthetic preparation that provides more effective superficial analgesia than EMLA in adults. Amethocaine has demonstrated similar efficacy to EMLA when appropriate application times are used and has a more rapid onset and longer duration of action than EMLA.[169] Studies have documented its effectiveness in neonates as follows:

- It relieves pain during venipuncture,[126,150] IV insertion, and injections of vitamin K.[200]
- It does not relieve pain from heel sticks[176] or peripherally inserted central catheter (PICC) insertion, unless combined with morphine use.[224]
- It relieves circumcision pain.[240]
- It does not cause methemoglobinemia.
- It is effective within 30 to 40 minutes of application.

OTHER MEDICATIONS

Acetaminophen and nonsteroidal anti-inflammatory drugs (NSAIDs) can be helpful in providing analgesia for mild to moderate pain (see Table 12-10). These medications are more effective when administered on a regular schedule, augment the effects of narcotics, and may be delayed in effect because of the rate of gastric emptying.[27,233] **Acetaminophen given 2 hours before circumcision does not reduce pain during the procedure but is effective in postoperative pain relief; repeated doses every 4 to 6 hours for the first 24 hours after circumcision are recommended.** The analgesic effects of intravenous NSAIDs have not been studied in preterms, and the adverse effects of prolonged NSAID use may lead to renal, circulatory, hepatic, gastrointestinal, and hematologic complications.[20,25]

Sedatives can help decrease agitation and improve comfort but do *not* by themselves provide analgesia. Use of developmental care significantly reduces the need of VLBW infants for sedative drugs.[235] Sedatives are appropriate to induce sleep for diagnostic procedures (e.g., computed tomography [CT] scan, magnetic resonance imaging [MRI]), to calm chronically irritable infants whose physiologic stability or ventilatory status is compromised by agitation, and for pain-related agitation.[21,235] Sedatives have potential toxicities, effect behavioral changes, and affect consciousness, which deprive neonates of their ability to communicate and interact with their parents, caregivers, and the environment.[236] Furthermore, the short-term and long-term effects of frequent or continuous use of sedatives on the developing brain are unknown.

Comfort Measures

Comfort measures alone do not relieve pain; however, their use reduces agitation, which indirectly reduces pain by promoting behavioral organization, relaxation, general comfort, and sleep.[8,139] **Although comfort measures may prevent the intensification of pain (e.g., guarding an abdominal incision by positioning is less painful than four-point restraint), they may not relieve moderate to severe pain. Comfort measures are helpful but inadequate by themselves, considering the intensity of the noxious stimuli causing moderate to severe pain.**[8,60,139]

As partners in care, parents should be encouraged and facilitated to engage in providing comfort measures for their infants having painful procedures. Recent research studies show the efficacy of parental involvement. Initiation of skin-to-skin contact,[93] taste, and suckling was described in the first study as full-term infants receiving heel sticks for genetic screens experienced less crying (91%) and grimacing (84%) when being held and breast fed by their mothers.[53,92] **Several studies show that both very preterm, healthy preterm and term newborns (between 28 and 36 weeks PMA) receiving heel sticks experienced diminished pain response, less crying, and quicker recovery when being held skin-to-skin (e.g., kangaroo care) by their mothers for 15 to 30 minutes before and during the procedure.**[55,93,130,140,151] A study combining sucrose, nonnutritive sucking, and parental holding for multiple immunizations in 2-month-old infants resulted in significantly less crying and this approach became strongly preferred by parents for future immunizations.[189] Animal studies show that the short-term and long-term effects of repeated pain are ameliorated by the presence and ministrations of the mother[238]; perhaps the presence of the human mother or parent provides the same protection for the human neonate.[36]

Developmental care not only prevents pain but also decreases behavioral and physiologic pain scores in preterm infants.[56,68,139,205] A recent study of a simple diaper change in VLBW preterms showed less physiologic response (e.g., alteration in heart rate, hypoxia, bradycardia, desaturation events) and less pain response (measured with two pain scales) when developmental care was used before and during the procedure.[205] In this study, developmental supports such as opportunities for grasping, hand swaddling, decreasing light and noise, nonnutritive sucking, and body support and containment were used.

NONNUTRITIVE SUCKING

Nonnutritive sucking (e.g., the infant's own fingers or hands or a pacifier) soothes by reducing the infant's level of arousal and duration of cry while promoting the quiet alert state.[49] Nonnutritive sucking is effective in reducing pain in preterm infants during heel stick, circumcision, and immunizations and during retinopathy of prematurity (ROP) screening eye examinations.[44,139] The effect of nonnutritive sucking is immediate, but the effect ceases immediately on cessation of sucking/removal of the pacifier.[139]

ORAL SUCROSE/GLUCOSE

Distressed infants offered oral sucrose calmed quickly, stayed calm longer, and spent more time in a quiet alert state than did infants offered only a pacifier.[41] Sucking soothes, reduces heart and metabolic rates, induces hand-to-mouth behavior, and elevates the pain threshold through opioid and non-opioid systems.[41] **Administration of sucrose (into the mouth) within 2 to 3 minutes before an invasive procedure (e.g., heel stick/venipuncture; bladder catheterization; eye examinations for ROP) has been shown to decrease crying duration, heart rate, facial activity, and electroencephalogram (EEG) changes associated with pain in full-term and preterm infants.*** In these studies, the amount (0.05 to 2 mL) and concentrations (24% to 50%) of sucrose varied but even the smallest dose administered once to preterm infants of 26 to 34 weeks' gestation reduced pain behaviors.[38,215] The small doses of concentrated sucrose solution used to treat neonatal pain have not been shown to cause hyperglycemia in preterm infants.[46]

When sucrose is paired with developmental interventions such as rocking, carrying,[89] **nonnutritive sucking,**[59,82,189] **prone positioning, or parental holding,**[107,139,189] **sucrose is more effective in decreasing behavioral pain responses.** Use of oral sucrose alone has been shown to result in higher pain scores than use of any other form of analgesia during circumcision; sucrose is an adjunct to pain control during circumcision and should not be the only analgesic used for this operative procedure.[187] **In a systematic meta-analysis of 21 studies of sucrose use for analgesia, sucrose was found to be safe, effective, and cost effective for single painful procedures (e.g., heel stick/venipuncture).**[215] Despite being aware that sucrose relieves pain, only 10% of recently surveyed NICUs used sucrose before a heel stick and only 11% used sucrose before venipuncture.[94] Another recent survey showed only 33% of responding NICUs using sucrose before routine painful procedures.[158]

A recent randomized controlled trial of 2 mL of 25% oral sucrose solution given to healthy preterms (e.g., <37 weeks GA) 2 minutes before a venipuncture significantly decreased heart rate and crying during the venipuncture.[2] The safety and efficacy of "routine use" (e.g., use for every invasive procedure in the first week of life; administered a maximum of three times, 2 minutes apart) of sucrose (0.1 mL of 24% solution) in preterms less than 31 weeks PCA were studied in a randomized controlled trial.[131] In the group of preterms receiving sucrose, the higher number of doses of sucrose predicted poorer neurobehavioral development (e.g., scores on motor development, vigor, alertness, and orientation at 36 weeks; lower motor development and vigor at 40 weeks) and poorer physiologic outcomes.[131] Other recent studies have found that repeated sucrose use is safe (no side effects) and effective for pain relief from repeated procedural pain in the NICU.[81,214]

Several studies have compared use of glucose versus sucrose for pain relief, with conflicting results. A comparison of oral glucose versus sucrose showed that glucose solution (e.g., 33% to 50%) was more effective in reducing pain response in term newborns having heel sticks.[104] Another study found that 30% sucrose solution was more effective in reducing crying time than 10% to 30% glucose solutions.[124] When oral glucose (30% solution) was given to full-term newborns undergoing venipuncture compared with (1) EMLA cream[91] and (2) subcutaneous injections,[50] the infants treated with glucose had significantly lower pain scores. Future studies of glucose and sucrose for pain relief should

*References 1,38,70,79,107,124,162,191,215,228.

examine (1) the most effective method of administration, (2) the optimal dose and solution strength, (3) the effectiveness when paired with other behavioral and pharmacologic interventions, (4) the long-term effects of repeated administration, and (5) the use in the VLBW infant (e.g., at risk for necrotizing enterocolitis [NEC]; nil per os [NPO] status; unstable; ventilated).[38,82,131,215]

TACTILE INTERVENTIONS

A reassuring human presence (of parents or caregivers) during painful procedures for all neonates in the NICU is mandatory.[36] Body containment of extremities in a flexed position (e.g., holding, swaddling, nesting; providing an opportunity to grasp a finger or pacifier) decreases gross motor movements that contribute to the infant's increased level of arousal, reduces physiologic and behavioral stress, and facilitates energy conservation in the preterm.[49,229] Improper body position contributes to discomfort and pain. **Facilitated tucking—gentle containment of flexed extremities in the midline on the trunk while side-lying or supine—during a painful procedure (e.g., heel stick) results in lower heart rate, shorter crying time, less sleep disruption, and fewer sleep-state changes.**[60] A study of facilitated tucking (provided by parents for endotracheal tube [ETT] suctioning) showed that participation by parents was a safe, effective pain-management strategy that provided parents with an active role in their infant's pain care and was also preferred by parents.[29] Use of a 2-minute massage of the ipsilateral leg before heel stick in preterm infants was safe and resulted in a decreased pain response (decreased pain score and heart rate) when compared with non-massaged preterms.[127]

Motoric boundaries (e.g., containment of extremities) assist a preterm infant to maintain a more secure, controlled response and facilitate self-regulation. **Therapeutic interventions include the use of positions that support flexion and restraint in physiologic position, periodic release of restraint and exercise of extremities, gentle change in body position, and positioning to guard operative sites.** Along with comfort measures, minimizing stimulation in the NICU environment enables a neonate who is agitated or in pain to use internal and external resources in organizing his or her behavior and develop self-soothing strategies (see Chapter 13). Individualizing care and handling to the infant's likes and dislikes and listing these at the bedside help maintain consistency of care and build trust in these developing neonates.

Picking up, holding, and rocking provide tactile soothing, vestibular stimulation, and the calming effect of rhythmic, repetitive movement. Use of massage, rocking, and water mattresses provides tactile, vestibular, and kinesthetic stimuli that modify and accelerate behavioral, state control, and decreased stress behaviors (see Chapter 13).

COMPLEMENTARY HEALING MODALITIES

Complementary healing (e.g., therapeutic touch [TT], acupressure, acupuncture, Reiki) is gaining increasing interest among neonatal health care providers. Little research exists, but clinical reports have depicted the benefits of pain relief with integration of these modalities. Recent research conducted with registered nurses (RNs) who provided TT to preterm infants (25 to 37 weeks' gestation) revealed that the infants' responses to TT included (1) decreased heart and respiratory rates, (2) enhanced restful periods, (3) improved sucking, swallowing, and breathing, and (4) a greater ability to interact with the environment.[113] Acupuncture and acupressure may be safely used to treat pain, agitation, and drug withdrawal in the neonate.[88] A recent pilot study of the use of acupuncture in 10 infants for withdrawal symptoms found a significant reduction in the amount of drug therapy (with benzodiazepines and opioids) within 48 hours of beginning the acupuncture treatments.[87] Research in this area is desperately needed to validate the use of these modalities for pain management.[136]

Activation of cutaneous sensory nerves with a transcutaneous electrical nerve stimulation (TENS) unit and application of thermal (topical skin refrigerant) blocks inhibit transmission of peripheral pain impulses from procedural pain. Low-frequency, monotonous sounds (e.g., heartbeat, vacuums) quiet and increase behavioral organization. Use of music (see Chapter 13) and recordings of family voices soothes term and preterm infants, resulting in fewer state changes, less time in the arousal state, and increased behavioral organization. However, during circumcision, music (with or without a pacifier) is not an effective distraction or soothing strategy for relief of the pain of the procedure. Another recent study showed that preterm infants presented with a familiar odor during venipuncture exhibited significantly less crying and grimacing, compared with the preterms presented with an unfamiliar odor or no odor.[90]

END-OF-LIFE CARE

When the decision is made to terminate or not begin aggressive medical intervention, the neonate receives end-of-life care, also known as *comfort care* or *palliative care* (see Chapter 32). Neonates who receive end-of-life care are at the threshold of viability, have multiple congenital anomalies that are incompatible with life, or are not responding to NICU interventions (e.g., deterioration in condition despite medical efforts).[179,188]

End-of-life care should combine comfort measures, pharmacologic management, developmental care (see Chapter 13),[218] and spiritual and psychosocial support for the neonate and family (see Chapters 29 and 30).[54,57,179,217,218] The family is provided a quiet, private, homelike area in which to touch, hold, and interact with their terminally ill neonate. Use of skin-to-skin care (kangaroo care), soft, soothing music, dimmed lighting, infant massage, holding, and rocking provides both a comforting environment for the infant and family, as well as parenting and comforting opportunities.[218] Parents, siblings, and extended family members remain with their infant during and after death. Clergy are present for family support and may perform a religious service, such as baptism or blessing.

For comfort care, all invasive procedures, including measurement of vital signs, monitors, machines, and artificial feeding, are discontinued. The infant, cleaned and wrapped in a warm blanket, is held by the family. Intravenous access may remain in place for administration of pain medications or sedatives. **Medication is administered in sufficient doses to provide comfort, relieve pain, and ensure that the infant does not suffer at the end of his or her life.**

In the only study that documents use of analgesia for dying infants whose life support is withdrawn or withheld, 165 deaths in a university-based NICU were reviewed.[173] Opioid analgesia was administered to 84% of infants when life support was withdrawn or withheld. Infants with major congenital anomalies (93%) and NEC (100%) were more likely to receive opioids than were ELBW infants (66% to 83%). Overall, opioid analgesia was administered to at least 65% of infants. Reasons for life support discontinuation also influenced administration of opioids: (1) futility of treatment (84% medicated), (2) severe lifelong impairment (85% medicated), and (3) suffering caused by treatment (100% medicated). The median dose of opioids was within the usual pharmacologic range in 64% and greater in 36%. Of the infants receiving a higher dose, 94% had previously been receiving an analgesic and may have needed a higher dose as a result of tolerance. The median time until death from the discontinuation of life support was 18 minutes for those who received the standard dose and 20 minutes for those who received the higher dose.

A survey of hospital staff providing pediatric palliative care found that 50% of physicians and 30% of nurses reported feeling inexperienced in pain management.[58] Providers also shared how personally distressing it is to witness a child's suffering, especially when pain relief was possible but not available or delivered. In the same study, families also described their anguish in watching their child experience and suffer any amount of pain and discomfort. Unlike the health care providers, families thought that everything had been done to alleviate their child's pain. Another recent study found that insufficient education in pain and palliative care of pediatric care providers was a barrier to use of palliative care in children.[62]

COMPLICATIONS

A neonate's complex behavioral response to pain has both short-term and long-term ramifications (Box 12-4).* These behavioral changes may disrupt parent-infant interaction and attachment, adaptation to the postnatal environment, and feeding behaviors.[23,242] An alteration in brain development and maldevelopment of sensory systems can occur when distorted or inappropriate sensory input occurs during a critical period in development.† Because of a neonate's memory, painful experiences increase his or her sensitivity to subsequent medical encounters.‡ These initial experiences may affect the development of attitudes, fears, anxiety, conflicts, wishes, expectations, and patterns of interactions with others.[72,154,242]

Younger infants are more susceptible to long-term consequences (see Box 12-4) because there is heightened sensitivity at earlier developmental

---

*References 14,15,21,23,101,109,168,177,183,227,242.
†References 13-15,21,26,72,108,109,183,193,242.
‡References 13,101,109,168,177,183,193,222,225,227.

BOX 12-4 LONG-TERM CONSEQUENCES OF REPETITIVE PAIN*

- Less physiologic stability (e.g., alterations in heart and/or respiratory rates and blood pressure)
- Alterations in cerebral blood flow[153] increasing the risk for intraventricular hemorrhage and periventricular leukomalacia
- Inappropriate sensory input (pain) disrupts neural activity, and chronic activation of neuroendocrine system results in abnormal brain development
- Hyperinnervation (e.g., neural reorganization in the periphery and the spinal cord) associated with increased pain behaviors such as allodynia and hypersensitivity
- Altered pain responsiveness:
  - Heightened responsiveness to pain (hyperalgesia)/lower pain threshold
  - Decreased responsiveness to pain (associated with more exposure to painful experiences) in the NICU and later in infancy and childhood
- Neurodevelopmental and behavioral sequelae of prematurity (see Chapter 31)
- Alteration of parent-infant interactions and relationships; temperament and pain expression

*References 13–21,26,72,95,96,101,108,109,154,168,177,184,193,221–225, 227,238,242.

stages.[108,109] In the most immature preterm infants, lower pain thresholds and the lack of inhibitory controls (both develop with increasing gestational age) influence hypersensitivity.[95] **When tissue injury occurs early in development, increased pain sensitivity develops both at the site of the damage (primary hyperalgesia) and in the surrounding skin (secondary hyperalgesia) because of hyperinnervation at the site.**[95,178] The lower pain threshold of the more preterm infant is also influenced (i.e., decreased further) by repeated exposures.[95] The consequences of this altered excitability include (1) perceiving nonnoxious tactile stimuli as noxious,[5] depending on the number of invasive procedures in the previous 24 hours,[98] (2) systemic responses of chronic pain and discomfort, (3) associating earlier pain with decreased behavioral responses to pain, (4) variable physiologic responses,[95] and (5) lower tenderness thresholds and more tender points in adolescence.[47] **Ongoing studies demonstrate the importance of infant and family factors (Figure 12-8) in ameliorating developmental alterations initiated by early and repeated pain exposures.**[95] Studies to evaluate the long-term effects of pharmacologic and comfort interventions are also needed.[95]

As mentioned, unanesthetized surgery and/or unrelieved pain causes suffering that might itself be a risk to life.[23] Maintaining metabolic homeostasis by the appropriate use of anesthetics and analgesics improves postoperative outcome by preventing (1) protein wasting, (2) electrolyte imbalance, (3) impaired immune function, (4) sepsis, (5) metabolic acidosis, (6) pulmonary and cardiac insufficiency, (7) hypermetabolic state, and (8) death.[11,24,63,85] Increasing evidence confirms that exposure to prolonged, severe, or untreated pain increases morbidity and alters brain development and subsequent behavioral and physiologic responses to pain.★

Narcotic analgesics may produce respiratory depression severe enough to require mechanical ventilation. Naloxone (0.1 mg/kg IV or intramuscular [IM]) is the specific antidote for narcotic overdose (see Table 12-10). Lower doses of naloxone (0.001 to 0.01 mg/kg IV or IM) can be used for moderate respiratory depression. Complete opioid reversal with 0.1 mg/kg naloxone increases agitation and stress response in neonates with ongoing pain. Subsequently it is more difficult to manage the neonate's pain until the effects of the naloxone wear off. Lower doses of naloxone should be used and the dose titrated to prevent this outcome. **An ampule of neonatal naloxone should always be immediately available with the appropriate dose precalculated on the infant's emergency card. Flumazenil is a specific antagonist for the benzodiazepines and should be used to treat respiratory depression (see Table 12-10). Respiratory depression may produce hypoxemia, so a pulse oximeter should be standard equipment along with cardiorespiratory monitoring.**[8,139,220] **All equipment for assisted ventilation should be at the bedside.**[8]

An overdose of local anesthetics can cause seizures, ventricular tachycardia, bradycardia, and cardiovascular collapse. Toxic doses for neonates should be carefully calculated, and lower doses should be administered. Benzodiazepines or phenobarbital can be used to treat refractive seizures; cardiopulmonary resuscitation (CPR) and defibrillation

★References 8,10,14,15,17,23,72,96,154,242.

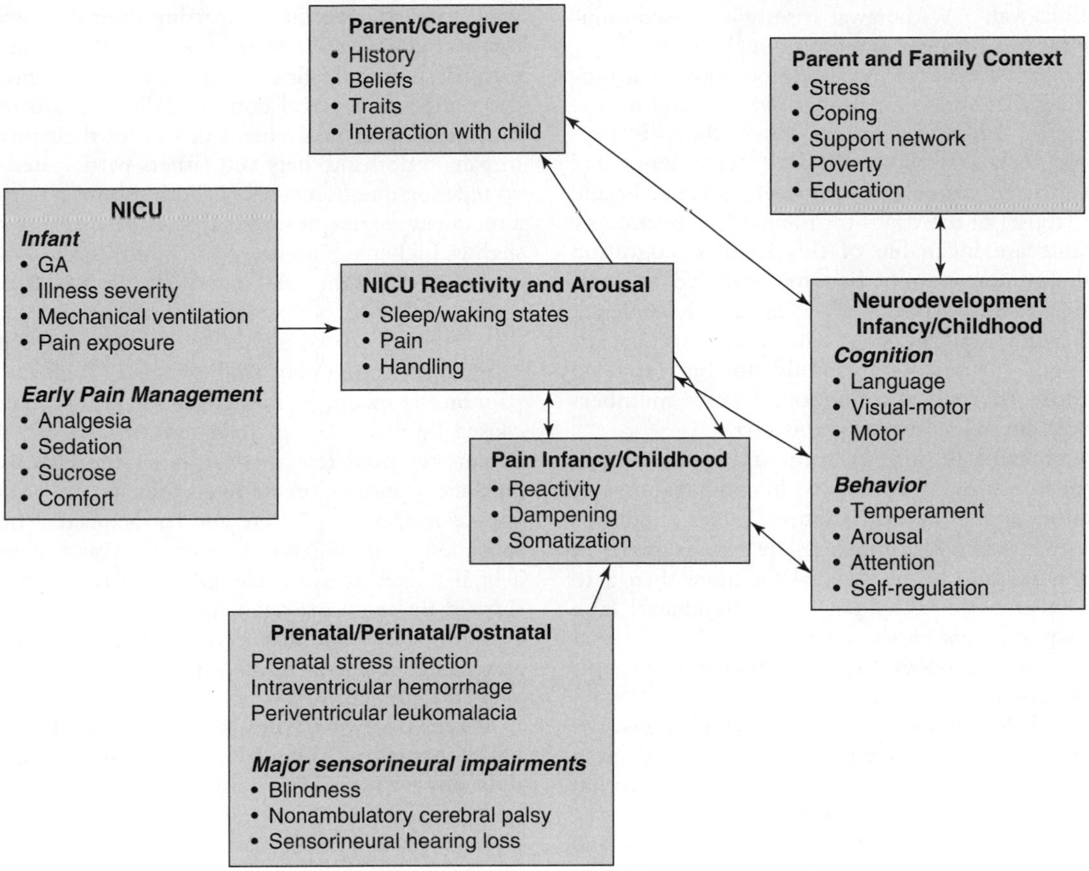

FIGURE 12-8 Model of long-term effects of pain showing complex, interactive, bidirectional relationships among multiple biologic and environmental factors. *GA*, Gestational age; *NICU*, neonatal intensive care unit. (From Grunau R: Early pain in preterm infants: a model of long-term effects, *Clin Perinatol* 29:376, 2002.)

may be necessary to treat the cardiovascular complications. **Patients who are receiving epidural analgesia for postoperative pain control should be monitored for signs of potential CNS toxicity** (e.g., irritability, jitteriness, twitching, myoclonic jerking). If an opioid is being administered with the local anesthetic infusion, then respiratory depression is also a possibility and patients should be monitored as described. Other extremely rare complications of epidurals are nerve injury and/or paralysis.

Hematoma formation can occur (1.2%) with the placement of a dorsal penile nerve block. Using a ring block usually avoids this problem. **Epinephrine-containing solutions must *never* be used, because this can lead to compromise of the blood supply to the penis and severe tissue damage.**

Tolerance and Withdrawal

Tolerance is the need for escalating doses of drug to achieve the same effect. Tolerance (1) occurs more often with the use of synthetic opioids (e.g., fentanyl) than with naturally occurring opioids (e.g., morphine), (2) is related to the duration of use—the longer the use (>5 days),[20] the more likely tolerance is to develop and use for less than 72 hours usually is not associated with tolerance, (3) develops more rapidly with continuous infusions versus intermittent therapy, (4) may develop more rapidly in preterm neonates than in term neonates, and (5) occurs more often in males than in females.[19,219,220,233]

Physical dependence is the state wherein continued drug is needed to prevent the signs of

withdrawal.[233] Withdrawal arises when discontinuing the drug causes symptoms such as irritability, diarrhea, tachycardia, hypertension, insomnia, restlessness, diaphoresis, or palmar sweating and muscle twitches. **Addiction occurs when there is psychological, as well as physical, dependence** and is associated with active drug-seeking behavior and use (abuse) of the drugs for nonmedical conditions. **Infants are incapable of this level of cognition and therefore cannot become addicted to analgesics and sedatives.**[88,208] Tolerance, dependence, and withdrawal can occur with opioids and benzodiazepines. **Medications should not be restricted because of fear of addiction. Family members should be made aware of this fact.**

Critically ill infants sometimes need long-term infusions of opioids or benzodiazepines to provide analgesia and sedation. ECMO and prolonged mechanical ventilation are two examples of this situation. Use of fentanyl for more than 5 to 7 days can lead to tolerance and withdrawal (also known as ***opioid abstinence syndrome***) (see Chapter 11). **Tapering doses to wean neonates off opioids depends on the duration of the medication's use and the infant's response to the changes.** For short-term use, decrease by 25% to 50% of the drug dose per day, so that the drug is discontinued within 2 to 3 days. For longer opioid use, decrease doses by no more than 10% to 20% every 1 to 3 days, and infusion regimens can be changed to intermittent administration before the drug is discontinued.[220] Shorter-acting medications such as fentanyl and midazolam can be switched to methadone and lorazepam, which have the advantage of being longer acting and being available in an oral form. **Addition of oral clonidine 1.5 to 3 mcg/kg two times daily (BID) can help alleviate withdrawal symptoms. The dose of clonidine can be titrated up to 5 to 10 mcg/kg BID as tolerated.** The side effects of clonidine include bradycardia, hypotension, and sedation. In addition, minimal handling and a quiet, darkened environment help decrease external stimuli. A pacifier, swaddling, and holding are effective comfort measures.

PARENT TEACHING

Mothers of neonates in the NICU report dissatisfaction with pain management, worry about their infant's pain and pain management, and want to participate in comforting their distressed infants.[75,77,227] A multicenter (i.e., 11 NICUs) international study is the first to provide a comprehensive description of parental concerns, distress, information needs, and involvement in care of their infant in pain.[75] Both mothers and fathers participated in completing questionnaires: (1) both parents reported a moderate degree of stress, (2) stress responses were slightly higher for mothers, (3) mothers' stress was related to the sights and sounds of the NICU and their inability to perform their maternal role, and (4) mothers reported higher anxiety levels. Specific parental concerns about pain included (1) effects of pain on the infant, (2) immediate medical problems caused by pain, and (3) long-term effects of pain. Parents reported few worries about the effects of pain medications. Parents rated their infant's worst pain as moderate to severe and had expected there to be less pain and that their infant would receive a high degree of pain relief. A more recent study showed that pain management was a priority concern for parents and that seeing their babies in pain and being unable to protect them from pain was very stressful.[134]

Parents in two studies received primarily verbal information (i.e., 81%[77] and 58%[75]) rather than any written (4%)[75] information about pain and pain relief. Nurses (41%) more commonly than physicians (28%) provided information about pain to parents.[75] Although parents usually were satisfied with the pain information they received, 30% indicated that they wished they had received more information about infant pain.[75] Fifty percent of parents reported that they were shown how to recognize if their infant was in pain and how to provide comfort.[77] In the more recent study, 18% of parents were shown how to assess pain in their infant and 55% were shown how to comfort the infant.[75]

In the multicenter study, 57% of parents reported that they would prefer to be with their infant during procedures.[75] Yet most parents had never (52%) or not often (24%) been asked their preference about being present for procedures. Parents who would have preferred to be absent during procedures reported higher stress levels, anxiety, and current worry about pain for their infant than did parents who preferred to be present. Eighty-seven percent of parents stated that they wanted greater involvement in their infant's pain care. Generally, the parents in this survey reported a high level of satisfaction with their infant's pain care.[75]

Parental stress was related to (1) their estimation of infant pain, (2) their worries about infant pain, and (3) their degree of satisfaction about information about infant pain care.[75] The influences of these factors on the degree of parental stress were "strikingly consistent" among the diverse NICUs in the study. More research is needed to determine if (1) more parental information, involvement, and satisfaction with pain care reduces parental stress, (2) greater parental involvement in pain care improves parent-infant attachment, interaction, competence, and confidence after discharge, (3) culturally and socially diverse families respond similarly, and (4) barriers exist to providing more parental information and facilitating more involvement.[75]

The lack of information (see the Parent Teaching box below) and passive involvement of parents in pain care for their infant[75,202] should be addressed in the NICU. Parents are excellent observers of their infant and often recognize when the infant is experiencing pain even before the care provider does.[19] The health care provider loses credibility and parental trust when he or she does not acknowledge and effectively treat the infant's pain.[157] Listening to parents' concerns about their infant's pain, including the parents' report of their assessment, communicating the plan of care about analgesia or sedation, and offering the rationale behind the medication decision making help the parents become active participants in the management of their infant's pain.

Parents of medically fragile infants have identified specific sources of stress in the NICU: (1) parental role alterations, especially inability to comfort the infant, and (2) infant appearance and behavior, especially pain and difficulty breathing. **The most common fear expressed by parents is that their infant will experience undue pain while being cared for in the NICU.** Three years after their infant's NICU experience, mothers can still recall the pain and procedures that their infants endured.[241] The care provider's sensitivity to the neonate's pain and advocating for pain relief are comforting for parents.[75,157,239] Teaching parents to report their assessments and encouraging parents to comfort their infants will help them in the attachment process and foster a trusting relationship with the health care team. **Comfort measures are ideally provided by parents, who may then actively participate in their infant's pain relief.[36]**

Parent Teaching

- The body that is in pain is "stressful" to the infant.
- The body that is in pain cannot grow, cannot heal, and may not survive.
- Newborn infants, both full-term and preterm, feel pain in the NICU. Remember that pain (and repeated pain) may have long-term consequences.
- Newborns in the NICU deserve to have their pain assessed, adequately treated with medications and comfort measures, and reevaluated to determine if the therapies have relieved their pain.
- Newborn infants, both full-term and preterm, DO NOT become "addicted" to medications that are used for pain relief, although they may develop tolerance and withdrawal, which can be managed by the health care provider.
- Comforting distressed infants and children is basic to the maternal/paternal role.
- No research or reports have ever documented a newborn forming a negative association with the mother/parent while she or he was providing comfort during a painful event.
- Research shows that skin-to-skin contact with mother before, during, and after a painful procedure decreases the pain response in preterm and full-term infants.[93]
- Research shows that breast feeding full-term newborns before, during, and after a painful procedure markedly decreases their pain response (e.g., crying, grimacing, less tachycardia).[92]

REFERENCES

1. Abad F, Diaz-Gomez N, Domenech E, et al: Oral sucrose compares favorably with lidocaine-prilocaine cream for pain relief during venipuncture in neonates, *Acta Paediatr* 90:160, 2001.
2. Acharya A, Annamali S, Taub N, et al: Oral sucrose analgesia for preterm infant venipuncture, *Arch Dis Child Fetal Neonatal Educ* 89:F17, 2004.
3. Acute Pain Management Guideline Panel: *Acute pain management: operative or medical procedures and trauma, clinical practice guideline*, AHCPR Pub No 92-0032. Rockville, MD, 1992, Agency for Health Care Policy and Research, Public Health Service, USDHHS.
4. Allegaert K, Tibboel D, Naulaers G, et al: Systematic evaluation of pain in neonates: effect on the number of intravenous analgesics prescribed, *Eur Clin Pharmacol* 59:87, 2003.
5. Alvares D, Torsney C, Beland B, et al: Modeling the prolonged effects of neonatal pain, *Prog Brain Res* 29:365, 2000.
6. American Academy of Pediatrics Committee on Fetus and Newborn: Circumcision policy statement, *Pediatrics* 103:686, 1999.

7. American Academy of Pediatrics Committee on Fetus and Newborn: Committee on Drugs, Section on Anesthesiology, and Section on Surgery: Neonatal anesthesia, *Pediatrics* 80:446, 1987.
8. American Academy of Pediatrics and Canadian Paediatric Society: Prevention and management of pain in the neonate, *Pediatrics* 118:2231, 2006.
9. American College of Obstetricians and Gynecologists: Committee opinion (#260): Circumcision, *Obstet Gynecol* 98:707, 2001.
10. American Society of Pain Management Nurses: *Position statement: Neonatal circumcision pain relief,* Pensacola, Fla, 2001, The Society.
11. Anand KJ: Neonatal stress responses to anesthesia and surgery, *Clin Perinatol* 17:207, 1990.
12. Anand KJ: Relationship between stress responses and clinical outcomes in newborns, infants and children, *Crit Care Med* 21(Suppl):358, 1993.
13. Anand KJ: Clinical importance of pain and stress in preterm neonates, *Biol Neonate* 73:1, 1998.
14. Anand KJ: Effects of perinatal pain and stress, In Mayer E, Saper C, editors: *Progress in brain research,* Amsterdam, 2000, Elsevier.
15. Anand KJ: Pain, plasticity, and premature birth: a prescription for permanent suffering? *Nat Med* 6:971, 2000.
16. Anand KJ: Systemic analgesic therapy, In Anand KJ, Stevens B, McGrath P, editors: *Pain in neonates*, ed 3, Amsterdam, 2007, Elsevier.
17. Anand KJ and the International Evidence-Based Group for Neonatal Pain: Consensus statement for the prevention and management of pain in the newborn, *Arch Pediatr Adolesc Med* 155:173, 2001.
18. Anand KJS: Pain assessment in preterm infants, *Pediatrics* 119:605, 2007.
19. Anand KJS: Pharmacologic approaches to the management of pain in the neonatal intensive care unit, *J Perinatol* 27(Suppl):S4, 2007.
20. Anand KJS, Aranda JV, Berde CB, et al: Summary proceedings from the neonatal pain-control group, *Pediatrics* 117:S9, 2006.
21. Anand KJ, Barton BA, McIntosh N, et al: Analgesia and sedation in preterm neonates who require ventilatory support: results from the Neonatal Outcome and Prolonged Analgesia in Neonates (NOPAIN) trial, *Arch Pediatr Adolesc Med* 153:331, 1999.
22. Anand KJ, Hall R, Desai N, et al, for the NEOPAIN Trial Investigators Group: Effects of morphine analgesia in ventilated preterm neonates: primary outcomes from the NEOPAIN randomised trial, *Lancet* 363:1673, 2004.
23. Anand KJ, Hickey PR: Pain and its effect in the human neonate and fetus, *N Engl J, Med* 317:1321, 1987.
24. Anand KJ, Hickey PR: Halothane-morphine compared with high-dose sufentanil for anesthesia and postoperative analgesia in neonatal cardiac surgery, *N Engl J Med* 326:1, 1992.
25. Anand KJ, Johnston CC, Oberlander TF, et al: Analgesia and local anesthesia during invasive procedures in the neonate, *Clin Ther* 27:844, 2005.
26. Anand KJ, Scalzo FM: Can adverse neonatal experiences alter brain development and subsequent behavior? *Biol Neonate* 77:69, 2000.
27. Anderson B, Van Lingen R, Hansen T, et al: Acetaminophen developmental pharmacokinetics in premature neonates and infants, *Anesthesiology* 96:1336, 2002.
28. Aranda JV, Carlo W, Hummel P, et al: Analgesia and sedation during mechanical ventilation in neonates, *Clin Ther* 27:877, 2005.
29. Axelin A, Salantera S, Lehtonen L: "Facilitated tucking by parents" in pain management of preterm infants: a randomized crossover trial, *Early Human Dev* 82:241, 2006.
30. Ballantyne M, Stevens B, McAllister M, et al: Validation of the premature infant pain profile in the clinical setting, *Crit J Pain* 15:297, 1999.
31. Barker D, Rutter N: Exposure to invasive procedures in neonatal intensive care unit admissions, *Arch Dis Child Fetal Neonatal Ed* 72:F47, 1995.
32. Bartocci M, Bergqvist LL, Lagercrantz H, et al: Pain activates cortical areas in the preterm newborn brain, *Pain* 122:109, 2006.
33. Batton DG, Barrington KJ, Wallman C: Prevention and management of pain in the neonate: an update, *Pediatrics* 118:2231, 2006.
34. Bauchner H, May A, Coates E: Use of analgesic agents for invasive medical procedures in pediatric and neonatal intensive care units, *J Pediatr* 4:647, 1992.
35. Reference deleted in proofs.
36. Bellieni C, Bagnoli F, Buonocore G: Alone no more: pain in premature children, *Ethics Med* 19:5, 2003.
37. Bellu R, de Waal KA, Zanini R: Opioids for neonates receiving mechanical ventilation, *Cochrane Database Syst Rev* 1: CD004212, 2008.
38. Benis M: Efficacy of sucrose as analgesia for procedural pain in neonates, *Adv Neonatal Care* 2:93, 2002.
39. Bhandari V, Bergqvist LL, Kronesberg SS, et al: Morphine administration and short-term pulmonary outcomes among ventilated preterm infants, *Pediatrics* 116:352, 2005.
40. Bildner J, Krechel S: Increasing staff nurse awareness of post operative pain management in the NICU, *Neonatal Netw* 15:11, 1996.
41. Blass EM, Watt L: Suckling- and sucrose-induced analgesia in human newborns, *Pain* 83:611, 1999.
42. Bouwmeester N, Hop W, van Dijk M, et al: Postoperative pain in the neonate: age-related differences in morphine requirements and metabolism, *Intensive Care Med* 29:2009, 2003.

43. Bouwmeester N, van den Anker J, Hop W, et al: Age- and therapy-related effects on morphine requirements and plasma concentrations of morphine and its metabolites in postoperative infants, *Br J Anaesthesiol* 90:642, 2003.
44. Boyle E, Freer Y, Khan-Orakzai Z, et al: Sucrose and non-nutritive sucking for the relief of pain in screening for retinopathy of prematurity: a randomized controlled trial, *Arch Dis Child Fetal Neonatal Ed* 91:F166, 2006.
45. Boyle EM, Freer Y, Wong CM, et al: Assessment of persistent pain or distress and adequacy of analgesia in preterm ventilated infants, *Pain* 124:87, 2006.
46. Bucher H, Moster T, Siebenthal K, et al: Sucrose reduces pain reaction to heel lancing in preterm infants: a placebo-controlled, randomized and masked trial, *Pediatr Res* 38:332, 1995.
47. Buskila D, Neumann L, Zmora E, et al: Pain sensitivity in prematurely born adolescents, *Arch Pediatr Adolesc Med* 157:1079, 2003.
48. Buttner W, Finke W: Analysis of behavioral and physiological parameters in the assessment of postoperative analgesia demand: a comprehensive report of seven consecutive studies, *Pediatr Anesthes* 10:303, 2000.
49. Campos RG: Soothing pain-elicited distress in infants with swaddling and pacifiers, *Child Dev* 60:781, 1989.
50. Carbajal R, Lenclen R, Gajdos V, et al: Crossover trial of analgesic efficacy of glucose and pacifier in very preterm neonates during subcutaneous injections, *Pediatrics* 110:389, 2001.
51. Carbajal R, Lenclen R, Jugie M, et al: Morphine does not provide adequate analgesia for acute procedural pain among preterm neonates, *Pediatrics* 115:1494, 2005.
52. Carbajal R, Rousset A, Danan C, et al: Epidemiology and treatment of painful procedures in neonates in intensive care units, *JAMA* 300:60, 2008.
53. Carbajal R, Veerapen S, Couderc S, et al: Analgesic effect of breast feeding in term neonates: randomized trial, *BMJ* 326:13, 2003.
54. Carter B, Howenstein M, Gilmer M, et al: Circumstances surrounding the deaths of hospitalized children: opportunities for pediatric palliative care, *Pediatrics* 114:361, 2004.
55. Castral TC, Warnock F, Leite AM, et al: The effects of skin-to-skin contact during acute pain in preterm newborns, *Eur J Pain* 12:464, 2008.
56. Catelin C, Tordjman S, Morin V, et al: Clinical, physiologic, and biologic impact of environment and behavioral interventions in neonates during a routine nursing procedure, *J Pain* 6:791, 2005.
57. Catlin A, Carter B: Creation of a neonatal end-of-life protocol, *J Perinatol* 22:184, 2002.
58. Contro N, Larson J, Scofield S, et al: Hospital staff and family perspective regarding quality of pediatric palliative care, *Pediatrics* 114:1248, 2004.
59. Corbo M, Mansi G, Stagni A, et al: Nonnutritive sucking during heelstick procedures decreases behavioral distress in the newborn infant, *Biol Neonate* 77:162, 2000.
60. Corff K, Seideman R, Venkataraman PS, et al: Facilitated tucking: a nonpharmacologic comfort measure for pain in preterm neonates, *J Obstet Gynecol Neonatal Nurs* 24:143, 1995.
61. Craig K, Korol C, Pillai R: Challenges of judging pain in vulnerable infants, *Clin Perinatology* 29:445, 2002.
62. Davies B, Shering SA, Partridge JC, et al: Barriers to palliative care for children: perceptions of pediatric health care providers, *Pediatrics* 121:282, 2008.
63. Desborough J: The stress response to trauma and surgery, *Br J Anaesth* 85:109, 2000.
64. Devor M: Pain mechanism and pain syndromes. In Campbell J, editor: *Pain 1996: an updated review*, Seattle, 1996, IASP Press.
65. Dodds E: Neonatal procedural pain: a survey of nursing staff, *Paediatr Nurs* 15:18, 2003.
66. Dunbar AE, Sharek PJ, Mickas NA, et al: Implementation and case-study results of potentially better practices to improve pain management of neonates, *Pediatrics* 118:S87, 2006.
67. El Sayed MF, Taddio A, Fallah S, et al: Safety profile of morphine following surgery in neonates, *J Perinatol* 27:444, 2007.
68. Evans JC, McCartney EM, Lawhon G, et al: Longitudinal comparison of preterm pain responses to repeated heelsticks, *Pediatr Nurs* 31:216, 2005.
69. Evans JC, Vogelpohl DG, Bourguignon CM, et al: Pain behaviors in LBW infants accompany some "nonpainful" caregiving procedures, *Neonatal Netw* 16:33, 1997.
70. Fernandez M, Blass E, Hernandez-Reif M, et al: Sucrose attenuates a negative EEG response to an aversive stimulus for newborns, *Dev Behav Pediatr* 24:261, 2003.
71. Fitzgerald M, Beggs S: The neurology of pain: developmental aspects, *Neuroscientist* 7:246, 2001.
72. Fitzgerald M, deLima J: Hyperalgesia and allodynia in infants. In Anand KJ, Stevens B, McGrath P, editors: *Pain in neonates*, Amsterdam, 2001, Elsevier.
73. Franck L: Identification, management, and prevention of pain in the neonate. In Kenner C, Brueggemeyer A, Gunderson L, editors: *Comprehensive neonatal nursing: a physiologic perspective*, Philadelphia, 1998, Saunders.
74. Franck L, Boyce W, Gregory G, et al: Plasma norepinephrine levels, vagal tone index, and flexor reflex threshold in premature neonates receiving intravenous morphine during the postoperative period: a pilot study, *Clin J Pain* 16:95, 2000.
75. Franck L, Cox S, Allen A, et al: Parental concern and distress about infant pain, *Arch Dis Child Fetal Neonatal Ed* 89:F71, 2004.

76. Franck L, Lefrak L: For crying out loud: the ethical treatment of infants' pain, *J Clin Ethics* 12:275, 2002.
77. Franck L, Scurr K, Couture S: Parent views of infant pain and pain management in the NICU, *Newborn Infant Nurs Rev* 1:106, 2001.
78. Franck LS: A national survey of the assessment and treatment of pain and agitation in the NICU, *J Obstet Gynecol Neonatal Nurs* 16:387, 1987.
79. Gal P, Kissling GE, Young WO, et al: Efficacy of sucrose to reduce pain in premature infants during eye examinations for retinopathy of prematurity, *Ann Pharmacother* 39:1029, 2005.
80. Garry DJ, Swoboda E, Elimian A, et al: A video study of pain relief during newborn male circumcision, *J Perinatol* 26:106, 2006.
81. Gaspardo CM, Miyase CI, Chimello JT, et al: Is pain relief equally efficacious and free of side effects with repeated doses of oral sucrose in preterm neonates? *Pain* 137:16, 2008.
82. Gibbins S, Stevens B: The influence of gestational age on the efficacy and short-term safety of sucrose for procedural pain relief, *Adv Neonatal Care* 3:241, 2003.
83. Gibbins S, Stevens B, Beyene J, et al: Pain behaviors in extremely low gestational age infants, *Early Hum Dev* 84:451, 2008.
84. Gibbins S, Stevens B, McGrath PJ, et al: Comparison of pain responses in infants of different gestational ages, *Neonatology* 93:10, 2008.
85. Goldman R, Koren G: Biologic markers of pain in the vulnerable infant, *Clin Perinatol* 29:415, 2002.
86. Goldsmith J: Ventilation management casebook: chloral hydrate intoxication, *J Perinatol* 14:74, 1994.
87. Golianu B, Dooley T, Ratner E, et al: Acupuncture and acupressure minimizes symptoms of withdrawal in neonates in the intensive care unit, (in press).
88. Golianu B, Krane E, Seybold J, et al: Non-pharmacologic techniques for pain management in neonates, *Semin Perinatol* 31:318, 2007.
89. Gormally S, Barr R, Wertheim L, et al: Contact and nutrient caregiving effects on newborn infant pain responses, *Dev Med Child Neurol* 43:28, 2003.
90. Goubet N, Rattaz C, Pierrat V, et al: Olfactory experience mediates response to pain in preterm newborns, *Dev Psychobiol* 42:171, 2003.
91. Gradin M, Erikkson M, Holmqvist G, et al: Pain reduction at venipuncture in newborns: oral glucose compared with local anesthetic cream, *Pediatrics* 110:1053, 2002.
92. Gray L, Miller L, Philipp B, et al: Breastfeeding is analgesic in healthy newborns, *Pediatrics* 109:590, 2002.
93. Gray L, Watt L, Blass E: Skin-to-skin contact is analgesia in healthy newborns, *Pediatrics* 105:110, 2000.
94. Gray PH, Trotter JA, Langbridge P, et al: Pain relief for neonates in Australian hospitals: a need to improve evidence-based practice, *J Paediatr Child Health* 42:10, 2006.
95. Grunau R: Early pain in preterm infants: a model of long-term effects, *Clin Perinatol* 29:373, 2002.
96. Grunau R: Long-term consequences of pain in human neonates. In Anand K, Stevens B, McGrath P, editors: *Pain in neonates*, ed 3, Amsterdam, 2007, Elsevier.
97. Grunau R, Holsti L, Haley DW, et al: Neonatal procedural pain exposure predicts lower cortisol and behavioral reactivity in preterm infants in the NICU, *Pain* 113:293, 2005.
98. Grunau R, Holsti L, Whitfield M, et al: Are twitches, startles, and body movements pain indicators in extremely low birth weight infants? *Clin J Pain* 16:37, 2000.
99. Grunau R, Johnston C, Craig K: Neonatal facial and cry responses to invasive and non-invasive procedures, *Pain* 42:295, 1990.
100. Grunau RE, Oberlander T, Holsti L, et al: Bedside application of the neonatal facial coding system in pain assessment of premature neonates, *Pain* 76:277, 1998.
101. Grunau RE, Oberlander TF, Whitfield M, et al: Pain reactivity in former ELBW infants at corrected age 8 months compared with term born controls, *Infant Behav Dev* 24:41, 2001.
102. Grunau RE, Whitfiled MF, Fay T, et al: Biobehavioral reactivity to pain in preterm infants: a marker of neuromotor development, *Dev Med Child Neurol* 48:471, 2006.
103. Grunau RVE, Craig KD: Pain expression in neonates: facial action and cry, *Pain* 28:395, 1987.
104. Guala A, Pastore G, Liverani M, et al: Glucose or sucrose as an analgesic for newborns: a randomized controlled blind trial, *Minerva Pediatr* 53:271, 2001.
105. Guinsburg R, deAraujo Peres C, Almeida B, et al: Differences in pain expression between male and female newborn infants, *Pain* 85:127, 2000.
106. Guinsburg R, Kopelman BI, Anand KJ, et al: Physiological, hormonal and behavioral responses to a single fentanyl dose in intubated and ventilated preterm neonates, *J Pediatr* 132:954, 1998.
107. Halimaa S: Pain management in nursing procedures on premature babies, *J Adv Nurs* 42:587, 2003.
108. Hall R, Anand KJS: Physiology of pain and stress in the newborn, *NeoReviews* 6:e61, 2005.
109. Hall R, Anand KJS: Short- and long-term impact of neonatal pain and stress: more than an ouchie, *NeoReviews* 6:e69, 2005.
110. Hall RW, Boyle E, Young T: Do ventilated neonates require pain management?, *Semin Perinatol* 31:289, 2007.
111. Hall RW, Kronsberg SS, Barton BA, et al: Morphine, hypotension, and adverse outcomes among preterm neonates: who's to blame? Secondary results from the NEOPAIN trial, *Pediatrics* 115:1351, 2005.

112. Hancock S, Newell S, Brierley J, et al: Premedication for neonatal intubation: current practice in Australia and the United Kingdom, *Arch Dis Child Fetal Neonat Ed* 82:A29, 2000.
113. Hanley M: Therapeutic touch with preterm infants: composing a treatment, *Explore* 4:4:249, 2008.
114. Harrison D, Evans C, Johnston L, et al: Bedside assessment of heel lance pain in the hospitalized infant, *J Obstet Gynecol Neonatal Nurs* 31:551, 2002.
115. Henry P, Haubold K, Dobrzykowski T: Pain in the healthy full-term neonate: efficacy and safety of interventions, *Newborn Infant Nurs Rev* 4:106, 2004.
116. Holsti L, Grunau R, Oberlander T, et al: Prior pain indices heightened motor responses during clustered care in preterm infants in the NICU, *Early Hum Dev* 81:293, 2005.
117. Holsti L, Grunau R, Whitfield M, et al: Behavioral responses to pain are heightened after cluster care in preterm infants born between 30 and 32 weeks gestational age, *Clin J Pain* 22:757, 2006.
118. Holsti L, Weinberg J, Whitfield MF, et al: Relationships between adrenocorticotropic hormone and cortisol are altered during clustered nursing care in preterm infants born at extremely low gestational age, *Early Hum Dev* 83:341, 2007.
119. Howard C, Howard FM, Fortune K, et al: A randomized controlled study of a eutectic mixture of local anesthetic cream versus penile hemiblock for pain relief during circumcision, *Am J Obstet Gynecol* 181:1506, 1999.
120. Hudson-Barr D, Capper-Michel B, Lambert S, et al: Validation of the Pain Assessment in Neonates (PAIN) scale with the Neonatal Infant Pain Scale (NIPS), *Neonatal Netw* 21:15, 2002.
121. Hummel P, Puchalski M: *The N-PASS: Neonatal Pain, Agitation, and Sedation Scale.* Chicago, 2000, Loyola University Health Systems.
122. Hummel P, Puchalski M, Creech SD, et al: Clinical reliability and validity of the N-PASS: neonatal pain, agitation and sedation scale with prolonged pain, *J Perinatol* 28:55, 2008.
123. International Association for the Study of Pain: Task Force on Taxonomy: modification of pain definition, *IASP Newsletter* 2:2, 2001.
124. Isik U, Ozek E, Bilgen H, et al: Comparison of oral glucose and sucrose solutions on pain response in neonates, *J Pain* 1:275, 2000.
125. Jacqz-Aigrain E, Daoud P, Burton P, et al: Placebo-controlled trial of midazolam sedation in mechanically ventilated newborn babies, *Lancet* 344:646, 1994.
126. Jain A, Rutter N: Local anaesthetic effect of topical amethocaine gel in neonates: randomised controlled trial, *Arch Dis Child Fetal Neonatal Ed* 82:F42, 2000.
127. Jain S, Kumar P, McMillan DD: Prior leg massage decreases pain response to heel stick in preterm babies, *J Paediatr Child Health* 42:505, 2006.
128. Ji R, Hiroshi B, Brenner G, et al: Nociceptive-specific activation of ERK in spinal neurons contributes to pain hypersensitivity, *Nat Neurosci* 2:1114, 1999.
129. Johnston CC, Collinge J, Henderson S, et al: A cross-sectional survey of pain and pharmacological analgesia in Canadian NICUs, *Clin J Pain* 13:308, 1997.
130. Johnston CC, Filion F, Campbell Yeo M, et al: Kangaroo mother care diminishes pain from heel lance in very preterm neonates: a crossover trial, *BMC Pediatr* 8:13, 2008.
131. Johnston CC, Filion F, Snider L, et al: Routine sucrose analgesia during the first week of life in neonates younger than 31 weeks' postconceptual age, *Pediatrics* 110:523, 2002.
132. Johnston CC, Stevens B, Franck L, et al: Factors explaining lack of responses to heel stick in preterm newborns, *J Obstet Gynecol Neonatal Nurs* 28:587, 1999.
133. Joint Commission on Accreditation of Healthcare Organizations (JCAHO): *Know your tools: read pain signs in the youngest ones with evidence based tools.* Joint Commission Benchmark 2001 (3). Accessed August 14, 2009, from www.jcrinc.com.
134. Joseph RA, Mackley AB, Davis CG, et al: Stress in fathers of surgical neonatal intensive care unit babies, *Adv Neonatal Care* 7:321, 2007.
135. Kahn DJ, Richardson DK, Gray JE, et al: Variation among neonatal intensive care units in narcotic administration, *Arch Pediatr Adoles Med* 152:844, 1998.
136. Kassity N, Jones J, Kenner C, et al: Complementary therapies. In Kenner C, Lott J, editors: *Comprehensive neonatal nursing*, ed 3, Philadelphia, 2003, Saunders.
137. Kaur G, Gupta P, Kumar A: A randomized trial of eutectic mixture of local anesthetics during lumbar puncture in newborns, *Arch Pediatr Adolesc Med* 157:1065, 2003.
138. Kennedy-Schwarz J: Pain management: a moral imperative, *Am J Nurs* 100:49, 2000.
139. Khurana S, Hall R, Anand KJS: Treatment of pain and stress in the neonate: when and how, *NeoReviews* 6:e76, 2005.
140. Kostandy RR, Ludington-Hoe SM, Cong X, et al: Kangaroo care (skin contact) reduces crying response to pain in preterm neonates: pilot study, *Pain Manag Nurs* 9:55, 2008.
141. Kraft N: A pictorial and video guide to circumcision pain, *Adv Neonatal Care* 3:50, 2003.
142. Krechel SW, Bildner J: CRIES: a new neonatal postoperative pain measurement score—initial testing of validity and reliability, *Paediatr Anaesth* 5:53, 1995.
143. Kumar P: *Analgesia underused for management of circumcision pain*, San Francisco, 2004, Poster session presented at the American Academy of Pediatrics National Conference and Exhibit October 9.

144. Lago P, Benini F, Agosto C, et al: Randomised controlled trial of low dose fentanyl infusion in preterm infants with hyaline membrane disease, *Arch Dis Child Fetal Neonatal Ed* 79:F194, 1998.
145. Lambert GH, Muraskas J, Anderson CL, et al: Direct hyperbilirubinemia associated with chloral hydrate administration in the newborn, *Pediatrics* 86:277, 1990.
146. Lawrence J, Alcock D, McGrath P, et al: The development of a tool to assess neonatal pain, *Neonatal Netw* 12:59, 1993.
147. Lehr VT, Cepeda E, Frattarelli DAC: Lidocaine 4% cream compared to lidocaine 2.5% and prilocaine 2.5% or dorsal penile nerve block for circumcision, *Am J Perinatol* 22:231, 2005.
148. Lehr VT, Taddio A: Topical anesthesia in neonates: clinical practices and practical considerations, *Semin Perinatol* 31:323, 2007.
149. Leuschen MP, Willard LD, Hoie EB, et al: Plasma fentanyl levels in infants undergoing extracorporeal membrane oxygenation, *J Thorac Cardiovasc Surg* 105:885, 1993.
150. Long C, McCafferty D, Sittlington N, et al: Randomized trial of novel tetracaine patch to provide local anesthesia for neonates undergoing venipuncture, *Br J Anaesth* 91:514, 2003.
151. Ludington-Hoe S, Hosseini R, Torowicz DL: Skin-to-skin contact (kangaroo care) analgesia for preterm infant heel stick, *AACN Clin Issues* 16:373, 2005.
152. Magny JF, d'Allest AM, Nedelcoux H, et al: Midazolam and myoclonus in neonate, *Eur J Pediatr* 153:389, 1994.
153. Mainous RO, Looney S: A pilot study of changes in cerebral blood flow velocity, resistance, and vital signs following a painful stimulus in the premature infant, *Adv Neonatal Care* 7:88, 2007.
154. Maroney D: Recognizing the potential effect of stress and trauma on premature infants in the NICU: how are outcomes affected? *J Perinatol* 23:679, 2003.
155. McCleary L, Ellis J, Rowley B: Evaluation of the pain resource nurse role: a resource for improving pediatric pain management, *Pain Manag Nurs* 5:29, 2004.
156. McGown R: Caudal analgesia in children: 500 cases for procedures below the diaphragm, *Anaesthesia* 37:806, 1982.
157. McGrath P, Unruh A: The social context of neonatal pain, *Clin Perinatol* 29:555, 2002.
158. McKechnie L, Levene M: Procedural pain guidelines for the newborn in the United Kingdom, *J Perinatol* 28:107, 2008.
159. Menon G, Boyle EM, McIntosh N, et al: Morphine analgesia and gastrointestinal morbidity in preterm infants: secondary results from the NEOPAIN Trial, *Arch Dis Child Fetal Neonatal Ed* 93:F362–F367, 2008.
160. Meyer R, Campbell J, Raja S: Peripheral neural mechanisms of nociception. In Wall P, Melzack R, editors: *Textbook of pain*, Edinburgh, 1994, Churchill Livingstone.
161. Millar C, Bissonnetter B: Awake intubation increases intracranial pressure without affecting cerebral blood flow velocity in infants, *Can J Anaesth* 41:281, 1994.
162. Mitchell A, Stevens B, Mungan N, et al: Analgesic effects of oral sucrose and pacifier during eye examinations for retinopathy of prematurity, *Pain Manag Nurs* 5:160, 2004.
163. Morison S, Grunau R, Oberlander T, et al: Relations between behavioral and cardiac autonomic reactivity to acute pain in preterm neonates, *Clin J Pain* 17:350, 2001.
164. Morison S, Holsti L, Grunau R, et al: Are there developmentally distinct motor indicators of pain in preterm infants? *Early Hum Dev* 72:131, 2003.
165. Ng E, Taddio A, Ohlsson A: Intravenous midazolam infusion for sedation of infants in the neonatal intensive care unit, *Cochrane Database Syst Rev* 1: CD002052, 2003.
166. Oberlander T, Grunau R, Fitzgerald C, et al: Does parenchymal brain injury affect biobehavioral pain responses in VLBW infants at 32 weeks' postconceptual age? *Pediatrics* 110:570, 2002.
167. Oberlander T, Saul JP: Methodological considerations for the use of heart rate variability as a measure of pain reactivity in vulnerable infants, *Clin Perinatol* 29:427, 2002.
168. Oberlander TF, Grunau RE, Whitfield MF, et al: Biobehavioral pain responses in former extremely low birth weight infants at 4 months' corrected age, *Pediatrics* 105:e6, 2000.
169. O'Brien L, Taddio A, Lyszkiewicz DA, et al: A critical review of the topical anesthetic amethocaine (Ametop) for pediatric pain, *Paediatr Drugs* 7:41, 2005.
170. Ogawa S, Ogihara T, Fujiwara E, et al: Venepuncture is preferable to heel lance for blood sampling in term neonates, *Arch Dis Child Fetal Neonatal Ed* 90:F432, 2005.
171. Ohlsson A, McMillan D, Schmidt B, et al: Variations in use of narcotics, benzodiazepines and pancuronium in newborn babies with assisted ventilation, *Pediatr Res* 45:313A, 1999.
172. Parker J, Vats A, Bauer G: EMLA toxicity after application for allergy testing, *Pediatrics* 113:410, 2004.
173. Partridge JC, Wall SN: Analgesia for dying infants whose life support is withdrawn or withheld, *Pediatrics* 99:76, 1997.
174. Pasero C: Pain relief for neonates, *Am J Nurs* 104:44, 2004.
175. Pasero C, McCaffery M: The undertreatment of pain: are providers accountable for it? *Am J Nurs* 101:62, 2001.

176. Patel A, Czerniawski B, Gray S, et al: Does amethocaine gel reduce pain from heel prick blood sampling in premature infants? A randomized double-blind cross-over controlled study, *Paediatr Child Health* 8:222, 2003.
177. Peters J, Koot H, deBoer J, et al: Major surgery within the first 3 months of life and subsequent biobehavioral pain responses to immunizations at later age: a case comparison study, *Pediatrics* 111:129, 2003.
178. Peters JW, Schouw R, Anand KJ, et al: Does neonatal surgery lead to increased pain sensitivity in later childhood? *Pain* 114:444, 2005.
179. Pierucci R, Russell K, Leuthner S: End-of-life care for neonates and infants: the experience and effects of a palliative care consultation service, *Pediatrics* 108:653, 2001.
180. Pineles BL, Sandman CA, Waffarn F, et al: Sensitization of cardiac responses to pain in preterm infants, *Neonatology* 91:190, 2007.
181. Pokela M, Koivisto M: Physiological changes, plasma beta-endorphin and cortisol responses to tracheal intubation in neonates, *Acta Paediatr* 83:151, 1994.
182. Porter F: Pain assessment in children and infants. In Schecter N, Bende C, Yaster M, editors: *Pain in infants, children and adolescents*, ed 2, Philadelphia, 2002, Lippincott Williams & Wilkins.
183. Porter F, Grunau R, Anand KJ: Long-term effects of neonatal pain, *J Behav Dev Pediatr* 20:253, 1999.
184. Porter FL, Wolf CM, Miller JP, et al: Procedural pain in newborn infants: the influence of intensity and development, *Pediatrics* 104:105, 1999.
185. Ranger M, Johnston CC, Anand KJ: Current controversies regarding pain assessment in neonates, *Semin Perinatol* 31:283, 2007.
186. Rao R, Sampers JS, Kronsberg SS, et al: Neurobehavior of preterm infants at 36 weeks postconception as a function of morphine analgesia, *Am J Perinatol* 24:511, 2007.
187. Razmus I, Dalton M, Wilson D: Pain management for newborn circumcision, *Pediatr Nurs* 30:414, 2004.
188. Rebagliato M, Cuttini M, Broggin L, et al: Neonatal end-of-life decision-making: physicians' attitudes and relationship with self-reported practices in 10 European countries, *JAMA* 284:2451, 2000.
189. Reis E, Roth E, Syphan J, et al: Effective pain reduction for multiple immunization injections in young infants, *Arch Pediatr Adolesc Med* 157:1115, 2003.
190. Reyes S: Nursing assessment of infant pain, *J Perinat Neonatal Nurs* 17:291, 2003.
191. Rogers AJ, Greenwald MH, Deguzman MA, et al: A randomized, controlled trial of sucrose analgesia in infants younger than 90 days of age who require bladder catheterization in the pediatric emergency department, *Acad Emerg Med* 13:617, 2006.
192. Royal College of Nursing: *Clinical practice guidelines: recognition and assessment of acute pain in children*. RCN, 1999, Bristol, England.
193. Ruda M, Ling Q, Hohmann A, et al: Altered nociceptive neuronal circuits after neonatal peripheral inflammation, *Science* 289:628, 2000.
194. Rutter N, Evans N: Cardiovascular effects of an intravenous bolus of morphine in the ventilated preterm infant, *Arch Dis Child Fetal Neonatal Ed* 83:F101, 2000.
195. Saarenmaa E, Huttenun P, Leppaluoto J, et al: Advantages of fentanyl over morphine in analgesia for ventilated newborn infants after birth: a randomized trial, *J Pediatr* 134:144, 1999.
196. Saigals S, Feeny D, Rosenbaum P, et al: Self-perceived health status and health related quality of life of extremely low-birth-weight infants at adolescence, *JAMA* 276:453, 1996.
197. Sato Y, Fukasawa T, Hayakawa M, et al: A new method of blood sampling reduces pain for newborn infants: a prospective, randomized controlled trial, *Early Hum Dev* 83:389, 2007.
198. Schecter N, Berde C, Yaster M: *Pain in infants, children and adolescents*, ed 2, Philadelphia, 2002, Lippincott Williams & Wilkins.
199. Shah V, Ohlsson A: Venipuncture versus heel lance for blood sampling in term neonates, *Cochrane Database Syst Rev* 4: CD001452, 2007.
200. Shah V, Taddio A, Hancock R, et al: Topical amethocaine gel 4% for intramuscular injection in term neonates: a double-blind, placebo-controlled, randomized trial, *Clin Ther* 30:166, 2008.
201. Sharek PJ, Powers R, Koehn A, et al: Evaluation and development of potentially better practices to improve pain management of neonates, *Pediatrics* 118:S78, 2006.
202. Simons J, Franck L, Robertson E: Parent involvement in children's pain care: views of parents and nurses, *J Adv Nurs* 36:591, 2002.
203. Simons S, vanDijk M, Anand KS, et al: Do we still hurt newborn babies? A prospective study of procedural pain and analgesia in neonates, *Arch Pediatr Adolesc Med* 157:1058, 2003.
204. Simons S, van Dijk M, van Lingren R, et al: Routine morphine infusion in preterm newborns who received ventilatory support: a randomized controlled trial, *JAMA* 290:2419, 2003.
205. Sizun J, Ansquer H, Browne J, et al: Developmental care decreases physiologic and behavioral pain expression, *J Pain* 3:446, 2002.
206. Slater R, Cantarella A, Gallella S, et al: Cortical pain response in human infants, *J Neuroscience* 26:3662, 2006.
207. Spence K, Gillies D, Harrison D, et al: A reliable pain assessment tool for clinical assessment in the NICU, *J Obstet Gynecol Neonatal Nurs* 34:80, 2005.

208. Stevens B: Pain in infants. In McCaffery M, Pasero C, editors: *Pain: clinical manual*, ed 2, St Louis, 1999, Mosby.
209. Stevens B, Franck L, Gibbins S, et al: Determining the structure of acute pain responses in vulnerable infants, *Can J Nurs Res* 23:32, 2007.
210. Stevens B, Gibbins S: Clinical utility and clinical significance in the assessment and management of pain in vulnerable infants, *Clin Perinatol* 29:459, 2002.
211. Stevens B, Johnston C, Hurton L: Factors that influence the behavioral pain responses of premature infants, *Pain* 59:101, 1994.
212. Stevens B, Johnston C, Petroshen P, et al: Premature Infant Pain Profile: development and initial validation, *Clin J Pain* 12:13, 1996.
213. Stevens B, McGrath P, Gibbins S, et al: Procedural pain in newborns at risk for neurologic impairment, *Pain* 105:27, 2003.
214. Stevens B, Yamada J, Beyene J, et al: Consistent management of repeated procedural pain with sucrose on preterm neonates: is it effective and safe for repeated use over time?, *Clin J Pain* 21:543, 2005.
215. Stevens B, Yamada J, Ohlsson A: Sucrose for analgesia in newborn infants undergoing painful procedures, *Cochrane Database Syst Rev* 3: CD001069, 2004.
216. Stolik-Dollberg O, Dollberg S: Bupivacaine versus lidocaine analgesia for neonatal circumcision, *Pediatr Res* 55:518A, 2004.
217. Stringer M, Shaw V, Savani R: Comfort care of neonates at the end of life, *Neonatal Netw* 23:41, 2004.
218. Sudia-Robinson T: Palliative care. In Kenner C, McGrath J, editors: *Developmental care of newborns and infants*, St Louis, 2004, Mosby.
219. Suresh S, Anand KJ: Opioid tolerance in neonates: a state of the art review, *Paediatr Anaesth* 11:511, 2001.
220. Taddio A: Opioid analgesia for infants in the neonatal intensive care unit, *Clin Perinatol* 29:493, 2002.
221. Taddio A, Goldbach M, Ipp M: Effect of neonatal circumcision on pain responses during vaccination in male infants, *Lancet* 345:291, 1995.
222. Taddio A, Katz J: The effects of early pain experience in neonates on pain responses in infancy and childhood, *Paediatr Drugs* 7:245, 2005.
223. Taddio A, Katz J, Ilersich AL: Effects of neonatal circumcision on pain response during subsequent vaccination, *Lancet* 349:599, 1997.
224. Taddio A, Lee C, Yip A, et al: Intravenous morphine and topical tetracaine for treatment of pain in (corrected) neonates undergoing central line placement, *JAMA* 295:793, 2006.
225. Taddio A, Ohlsson A, Einarson TR: A systematic review of lidocaine-prilocaine cream (EMLA) in the treatment of acute pain in neonates, *Pediatrics* 101:el. 1998.
226. Taddio A, Pollock N, Gilbert-MacLeod C, et al: Combined analgesia and local anesthesia to minimize pain during circumcision, *Arch Pediatr Adolesc Med* 154:620, 2000.
227. Taddio A, Shah V, Gilbert-MacLeod C, et al: Conditioning and hyperalgesia in newborns exposed to repeated heel lances, *JAMA* 288:857, 2002.
228. Taddio A, Shah V, Hancock R, et al: Effectiveness of sucrose analgesia in newborns undergoing painful medical procedures, *CMAJ* 179:37, 2008.
229. Taquino L, Blackburn S: The effects of containment during suction and heelstick on physiological and behavioral responses of preterm infants, *Neonatal Netw* 13:55, 1994.
230. Taylor BJ, Robbins JM, Gold JI, et al: Assessing postoperative pain in neonates: a multicenter observational study, *Pediatrics* 118:e992, 2006.
231. Tibboel D, Anand KJ, van der Anker JN: The pharmacologic treatment of neonatal pain, *Semin Fetal Neonatal Med* 10:195, 2005.
232. Tich S, Vecchierini M, Debillon T, et al: Effects of sufentanil on EEG in VLBW and ELBW preterm infants, *Pediatrics* 111:123, 2003.
233. Van Lingen R, Simons S, Anderson B, et al: The effects of analgesia in the vulnerable infant during the perinatal period, *Clin Perinatol* 29:511, 2002.
234. Vertanen H, Fellman V, Brommels M, et al: An automatic incision device for obtaining blood samples from the heels of preterm infants causes less damage than a conventional lancet, *Arch Dis Child Fetal Neonatal Ed* 84:F53, 2001.
235. Walden M, Carrier C: Sleeping beauties: the impact of sedation on neonatal development, *J Obstet Gynecol Neonatal Nurs* 32:393, 2003.
236. Walden M, Gibbins S: *Pain assessment and management: guideline for practice*, ed 2, Glenview, Ill, 2008, National Association of Neonatal Nurses.
237. Walden M, Penticuff J, Stevens B, et al: Maturational changes in physiologic and behavioral responses of preterm neonates to pain, *Adv Neonatal Care* 1:94, 2001.
238. Walker C, Kudreikis K, Sherrard A, et al: Repeated neonatal pain influences maternal behavior, but not stress responsiveness in rat offspring, *Dev Brain Res* 140:253, 2003.
239. Ward K: Perceived needs of parents of critically ill infants in a NICU, *Pediatr Nurs* 27:281, 2001.
240. Weise K, Nahata M: EMLA for painful procedures in infants, *J Pediatr Health, Care* 19:42, 2005.
241. Wereszczak J, Miles M, Holditch-Davis D: Maternal recall of the neonatal intensive care unit, *Neonatal Netw* 16:33, 1997.
242. Whitfield M: Psychosocial effects of intensive care on infants and families after discharge, *Semin Neonatol* 8:185, 2003.
243. Whitfield M, Grunau R: Behavior, pain perception and the extremely LBW survivor, *Clin Perinatol* 27:363, 2000.

244. Wilder R: Local anesthetics for the pediatric patient, *Pediatr Clin North Am* 47:545, 2000.
245. Yamada J, Stevens B, de Silva N, et al: Hair cortisol as a potential biologic marker of chronic stress in hospitalized neonates, *Neonatology* 92:42, 2007.

RESOURCE MATERIALS AND WEBSITES:

American Chronic Pain Association: at www.theacpa.org or 1-916-632-0922.

American Pain Foundation: at www.painfoundation.org or 1-888-615-PAIN.

American Pain Society: at www.ampainsoc.org or 1-847-375-4715.

Anand KJS, Stevens BS, McGrath PJ: *Pain in neonates and infants*, ed 3, Philadelphia, 2007, Elsevier.

Brune K, Handwerker H, editors: *Hyperalgesia: molecular mechanisms and clinical implications*, Seattle, 2004, International Association for the Study of Pain Press.

Carter B, Levetown M, editors: *Palliative care for infants, children, and adolescents*, Baltimore, 2004, Johns Hopkins University Press.

City of Hope/Palliative Care Resource Center: at www.cityofhope.org/prc/.

Dannemiller Memorial Education Foundation: at www.pain.com.

Dworkin R, Breitbart W, editors: *Psychosocial aspects of pain: a handbook for health care providers*, Seattle, 2004, International Association for the Study of Pain Press.

End-of-Life Nursing Education Consortium (ELNEC): *ELNEC Pediatric Palliative Care Training Program—a comprehensive national program to improve end-of-life care for neonatal and pediatric patients*, Website: www.aacn.nche.edu/ELNEC.

Field M, Behrman R: *When children die: improving palliative and end-of-life care for children and their families*, Washington, DC, 2003, Institute of Medicine, National Academies Press.

Finley GA, McGrath P, editors: *Acute and procedure pain in infants and children*, Seattle, 2003, International Association for the Study of Pain Press.

Folk LA: Guide to capillary heelstick blood sampling in infants, *Adv Neonatal Care* 7:171, 2007.

Gardner SL: *Clinical Practice Tool: Nursing strategies to relieve neonatal pain—evidence-based nursing practice*, 2008, Nurse's Professional Development and Practice Association, LLC, Accessed August 14, 2009, www.npdpa.com.

Gregory G: *Pediatric anesthesia*, ed 4, St Louis, 2001, Elsevier.

McCaffery M, Pasero C: *Pain: clinical manual*, ed 2, St Louis, 1999, Mosby.

McGrath P, Finley GA, editors: *Pediatric pain: biological and social context*, Seattle, 2003, International Association for the Study of Pain Press.

Meldrum M, editor: *Opioids and pain relief: a historical perspective*, Seattle, 2003, International Association for the Study of Pain Press.

Mogil J, editor: *The genetics of pain*, Seattle, 2004, International Association for the Study of Pain Press.

Partners for Understanding Pain: At www.theacpa.org or 1-800-533-3231.

Pediatric Pain Sourcebook: At http://painsourcebook.ca/index.html.

Stellwagen L, Wang M: *Local analgesia for neonatal circumcision (video)*, Boston, 2000, Massachusetts General Hospital. Available at www.aap.org/bookstore.

Website for continuing education for professionals: www.painedu.org.

13 THE NEONATE AND THE ENVIRONMENT: IMPACT ON DEVELOPMENT

SANDRA L. GARDNER AND EDWARD GOLDSON

For centuries the newborn baby has been considered a ***tabula rasa***—a blank slate on which parents and the world "write" to create the individual. In the first half of the twentieth century, research emphasized the contributions of the environment in shaping the infant and child. Only recently has the individuality of the infant been recognized as a powerful shaper of the caregiver, the care given, and thus the environment.

This chapter explores the psychosocioemotional development of term and preterm neonates. Infant development is a reflection of the dynamic relationship between endowment and environment. Along the continuum of development, development of the infant is the beginning of the child's and, ultimately, the adult's competence in the world. Understanding the dynamic relationship between endowment and environment is enhanced by a review of the principles of development in Box 13-1. First, the developmental tasks of infancy are presented, along with the influences of endowment and environment on mastery. Home and family life, in which most infants are raised, is then contrasted with the experiences of babies in the neonatal intensive care unit (NICU). Intervention strategies to normalize the NICU environment also are presented, along with strategies for parent teaching. The developmental and social outcomes of infants exposed to the NICU are then presented.

DEVELOPMENTAL TASKS OF THE NEONATE AND INFANT

Neonates begin extrauterine life able to attend with their sensory capabilities and communicate with their environment through a complex repertoire of behaviors. They are able to accumulate experience in memory. Infancy (birth to 12 months) is the time of further development and maturation of these capabilities through self-mastery and adaptation to the extrauterine environment.

Biorhythmic Balance: The Primary Developmental Task of Newborns

In utero, the fetus depends on the mother's physiologic systems to regulate its own systems. At birth, the neonate's basic physiologic needs (i.e., feeding, elimination, cleaning, heat balance, stroking, communicating) are met in new and different ways. The process of emerging from a physiologically dependent state as a fetus into a physiologically independent neonate introduces new variables for both mother and infant in the development of their extrauterine relationship.

The primary task of newborns is to establish independent biorhythmic balance by stabilizing the function of sleep-wake cycles, respiratory and heart rates, blood chemistry levels, metabolic processes, and eating patterns.

Although biorhythmic balance is internally determined, caregiving interaction between newborn and parent or caregiver either facilitates or disturbs this transition.[213] After birth, this balance is facilitated by contact with familiar surroundings (the mother's body) (see Chapter 5).

When immediate recontact between the neonate and the mother is not possible (e.g., when the mother refuses or is ill) or when the neonate is preterm or sick and requires immediate emergency medical intervention or transport, the primary "mothering" role is

Please note that the PURPLE type in each chapter is intended to make it easier to identify clinically applicable material.

BOX 13-1 PRINCIPLES OF DEVELOPMENT

- Development is a continuous process from conception to maturation (i.e., development also occurs in utero).
- Growth and development are influenced by genetic traits and environmental experiences.
- Development occurs in an orderly sequence, largely determined by readiness or maturation.
- The sequence of development is the same in all children; the rate of development is individual.
- Development is cephalocaudad (head → foot) and from gross to specific (e.g., peripheral → central → lateralization).
- The first 5 years are marked by a rapid period of growth of all body systems. During this time, behavior patterns are developed and are greatly influenced by the environment.
- Environmental stimulation influences conceptual development and has an impact on cognitive function.
- Learning occurs when behavioral change does not result solely from maturation; learning is facilitated by reinforcement of the behavior through experience.
- Development of the infant occurs within the framework of interaction with a caregiver and the family.
- Equifinality postulates multiple paths to the same developmental outcome: complex developmental patterns rather than simple development milestones.

Modified from Barnard K, Erikson M: *Teaching children with developmental problems,* ed 2, St Louis, 1976, Mosby; Illingworth RS: *The development of the infant and the young child,* ed 5, Edinburgh, 1972, Churchill-Livingstone.

temporarily transferred to professional (medical and nursing) care providers. Interactional dynamics necessary for reestablishing biorhythmic balance and fostering the psychosocioemotional development of the newborn also are transferred into the NICU.

Just as in a home or family setting, the infant's personality and behavioral development are affected by the nature and dynamics of the stimuli and relationships encountered with the staff in a nursery or NICU setting.[105] The level of function or dysfunction in the biorhythmic balance affects the neonate's long-range outcomes and is interwoven with the development of a sense of self and a basic trust.

Sense of Self

In utero, the fetus has continuous tactile-kinesthetic stimulation that contributes to the development and maturation of the central nervous system (CNS) and establishes kinesthesis as the most natural pathway for growth and development. The interaction between infants and the extrauterine environment also is kinesthetic. However, tactile contact and vestibular stimulation are also essential for (1) the development of a physical identity (body image), (2) organization and sorting of stimuli, (3) coordination of sensorimotor skills, (4) a psychologic and social sense of self, (5) normal neurophysiologic development (mental and cognitive abilities), and (6) emotional stability and temperament.[33]

Daily caregiving and interactions such as feeding, diapering, holding, and playing with the parent or caregiver provide infants with reciprocal stimuli for further developing their identity. Through the manner in which the infant is handled, he or she receives messages about how the caregiver feels about him or her.

Response cues given by an infant affect the caregiver's response to and interaction with the infant.[4,33] As the infant quiets in response to caregiving, the parent is positively reinforced to continue nurturing and soothing behavior. Withdrawal, irritability, or continuous crying is perceived by the caregiver as rejection and may result in parental frustration, withdrawal, and decreased interaction. Repeated exposure to the caregiver's style and nonverbal messages thus enables the infant to adapt to these patterns of caregiving. **The self of the infant is formed through interaction with people and objects within the environment.**

Because the nature (amount and type) of the kinesthetic interaction between infants and caregivers influences how infants develop and mature, a lack of appropriate stimulation can have long-term negative consequences. **Stimulus deprivation results in impairment or retardation of, or deviancy in, skill development for productive living.** The degree or extent of impairment depends on the severity of the restrictions and limitations encountered. Studies have demonstrated that infants who were well cared for physically (e.g., fed, diapered, cleaned) but did not receive tactile or kinesthetic stimulation either died or were seriously impaired mentally, emotionally, and socially.[33,251] Institutionally reared infants who had minimal contact and no social interaction with their caregivers displayed significant developmental delays.[224] The effect of kinesthetic deprivation was seen in the minimal expression of social skills (e.g., cooing, babbling, crying), minimal interest in objects in the environment, increased self-stimulation (rocking), touch aversion, flat or withdrawn affect, and retarded mental and motor development. **Environmental deprivation may also affect the physical growth of the infant.** Montagu[196] stated that infants can overcome mental and nutritional deprivation so long as they are not deprived of tactile stimulation.

The Psychosocial Task: Trust Versus Mistrust

Trust versus mistrust in self and the environment is solidified during infancy.[4] The response of the environment from the moment of birth is the means by which neonates continue to develop trust in themselves and decide on the reliability of their new environment. **Two major factors influence the development of trust versus mistrust: (1) the infant's ability to communicate needs to the environment and (2) the reliability and contingency of the responding environment.**

In the course of routine caregiving, an infant associates the caregiver with either comfort and trust or lack of need satisfaction and mistrust. The infant cries to communicate a need (e.g., "I'm hungry"; "I'm wet"). The caregiver responds to the infant and meets the need—the infant is fed; the diaper is changed. Thus the newborn learns to communicate when the need arises again, because the environment or caregiver has responded and will respond. This ***contingent response*** of the caregiver to the infant's need is the necessary reinforcement for the development of trust in self, others, and ultimately humankind. As a result, the infant develops a sense of mastery over his or her world and a sense that it is okay to experience needs and that they will be met.

Caregiving that ignores or delays needs gratification is ***noncontingent*** to the infant's cues for care. Need meeting that is externally defined by the caregiver's agenda (e.g., feeding schedule, rigid or inflexible routines, medical or nursing procedures in the NICU) discourages the infant from being aware of and experiencing needs and communicating them. Such infants eventually detach themselves (emotionally and kinesthetically) from the sensation of their needs, thus no longer experiencing or communicating them.[34]

As a result, these infants conclude that they and their needs (which they perceive as one and the same) are not important and that they have no effect on their environment. They do not cultivate their sense of self or their own existence, physically (where their boundaries end and another's begin) or psychologically (their identity, which exists independent of another).

Survival depends on the caregiver's meeting the newborn's needs. Need meeting is either contingent on the infant's cues or noncontingent on an external agenda. The degree of the mother's emotional investment and connectedness with the newborn will determine the nature and quality of the caregiving. Likewise, the temperament and responsiveness of the infant will affect the mother's feelings of competence, success, and emotional connectedness to her infant.[34] Parents who relate to the newborn as an individual (i.e., a person with feelings, wants, and needs; a person who knows what these are) will be sensitive and responsive to the infant's needs and interact with the baby during caregiving. This relationship facilitates the ongoing development of a good sense of self (e.g., esteem, confidence, emotional security) and mastery of the world. Caregivers who do not perceive infants as individuals do not respond to their "need cry" or interact with them during caregiving. This style fosters the development of mistrusting, suspicious, helpless, emotionally insecure, and isolated children and adults.

ENDOWMENT

Infants possess innateness and individuality. **Primitive reflex behaviors, higher cognitive abilities, temperament, and sensorimotor competencies are the endowment of the individual infant.** Individual variation and use of these endowments are influenced by the environment of the newborn.

Even before conception, the genetic endowment of the parents and preceding generations affects the fetus or newborn. Everything that the individual will inherit from his or her parents is determined at the moment of conception. Of the vast number of possible combinations of chromosomes, chance determines which characteristics the individual receives. Thus each individual, except monozygotic twins, is genetically and biologically different from every other person. Either a faulty gene (e.g., sickle cell anemia) or an altered number of chromosomes (e.g., Down syndrome) is responsible for inherited defects (see Chapter 27).

Although after the moment of conception, hereditary endowment can never be changed, it is influenced by the intrauterine environment. Some birth defects are caused by teratogens or poisons—any environmental agent (e.g., drugs, virus, chemical, pollutant) that interferes with normal fetal development. An individual's potential for growth and development is limited by his or her genetic endowment. As Montagu[196] stated, "Genetic endowment determines what we can do—environment what we do do."

The exception to individual genetic endowment is identical twins, who share the same heredity. Identical twins have been extensively studied because it is hypothesized that any differences between them are the result of environmental effects. Identical twins raised apart have been found to be more similar in intelligence, temperament, and personality characteristics than are fraternal twins raised together.

Genetic endowment imposes limits on a child's potential. Studies show that children resemble their parents both physically and mentally more than they differ from them. Parental expectations that are unrealistic or beyond the child's capacity may set the child up for disappointment when he or she fails to meet these expectations. Too often, abilities and potential are stifled within this environment, so that the child cannot achieve what is within his or her capability.

The exact influence of genetics for most psychologic traits is unknown. Introverted (timid, shy, withdrawn) and extroverted (active, friendly, outgoing) personality types may be partially genetically controlled. The degree to which intelligence is inherited is currently unknown, although the intelligence of children is most often similar to parental intelligence (i.e., intelligence is more similar between child and biologic mother than between child and adoptive mother).

Freedman[97] studied newborns of many ethnic groups to see if there were any similarities in disposition within the group or differences from other ethnic groups. He found that Chinese-American newborns were more adaptable, less irritable, and easier to console than Caucasian-American newborns. Maneuvers such as the Moro and covering the face with a cloth elicited very different responses, depending on the newborn's ethnic origin.

The same environmental stimuli elicit very different behavioral responses, which are individual and genetically influenced. These genetically influenced behaviors are also influenced by environment—both internal and external. Thus an individual may be more vulnerable to or more resilient in a specific environment. Therefore we are totally endowment and totally environment (100% endowment + 100% environment = An individual).[97]

Temperament

Parents often notice behavioral differences in their children from the first day. These differences are obvious in motor activity, irritability, and passivity. Some infants are quiet and placid, others are irritable and easily upset, and others are somewhere in between (see the Critical Findings box on p. 274). These temperamental qualities enable the following three basic types of infants to be identified:

- The "easy" child who is seen as regular, pleasant, and easy to care for and love
- The "difficult" child who is difficult to rear and reacts with protest and withdrawal to strange events or people
- The "slow to warm" child who reacts with withdrawal or passivity to new events

Neurologic Development

Brain growth of the fetus and newborn occurs in two stages.[68]

STAGE I

Stage I is from 10 to 18 weeks of pregnancy. The number of nerve cells that the individual has develops during this period. Any environmental perturbation (e.g., maternal malnutrition, medications, infections) that affects brain growth during this stage also may affect neonatal behavioral responses.

STAGE II

Stage II is from 20 weeks' gestation to 2 years of age. This period marks a brain growth spurt and is the most vulnerable period of growth of the dendrites of the human cortex.

The maturity of an infant is reflected in his or her behavior. Infants of a younger gestational age have less mature responses than infants of an older gestational age. A neurologic assessment of the newborn includes evaluation of (1) newborn reflexes, (2) neonatal states, (3) psychosocial interaction, and (4) sensory capabilities. The neonate is born with behaviors

Critical Findings

BEHAVIORAL CATEGORIES DESCRIPTIVE OF INDIVIDUAL TEMPERAMENT

TEMPERAMENTAL QUALITY	RATING
Activity level	*Low*—Decreased movement when dressed or during sleep *High*—Increased movement when asleep; increased wiggling and activity when diaper changed
Rhythmicity	*Regular*—Establishes own feeding; sleep and bowel movement patterns are fairly predictable *Irregular*—Amounts of sleep, feeding variable; "no 2 days are alike"; no pattern established
Approach and withdrawal	*Positive*—Eagerly tries new foods, interested in new surroundings and people *Negative*—Rejects new foods, new toys, and new environments; apprehensive, cries with new people
Adaptability	*Adaptive*—Little resistance to first bath; may enjoy bath *Nonadaptive*—Startles easily; resists diapering, bathing, and other manipulating
Quality of mood	*Positive*—Pleasant, easygoing disposition; easy to comfort; smiles *Negative*—Fussy; cries easily and is not easily comforted by external stimuli; unable to comfort self easily
Intensity of mood	*Mild*—No crying when wet; frets instead of crying when hungry *Intense*—Vigorously cries; rejects food
Sensory threshold (intensity of stimulus necessary to elicit a response)	*High*—Not startled or interested by noise or other stimuli *Low*—Noise, activity, or other stimuli enough to interrupt infant's behavior
Distractibility	*Distractible*—Rocking, pacifier, toy, voice, music decrease fussing *Nondistractible*—No stimuli decrease distress until need is met—food; stop changing diaper; bath over
Attention span and persistence	*Short*—Cries when awakened but stops immediately, mild objection if needs are not immediately met *Long*—Repeatedly rejects substitutions for perceived needs (no pacifier until diaper is changed; no water if milk is wanted)

Data from Thomas A, Chess S: *Temperament and development*, New York, 1977, Brunner-Mazel.

that are unlearned, instinctual, and of an adaptive and survival nature. They reflect the state of the nervous system and the level of neonatal maturation (see Figure 5-3; see the Critical Findings box on p. 275). Serial testing of reflex behavior gives more reliable data than one observation. Observations indicative of major deviations include asymmetry—total absence or no response on one side or in upper versus lower extremities.

Psychologic Interaction and Neonatal States

For years, newborn behavior was thought to occur only on a reflexive, instinctual level. **Through the work of Brazelton[38] and others, newborns have been shown to have the ability to interact with and shape their environment. With the Neonatal Behavioral Assessment Scale (NBAS),[38] care providers can observe and score the interactive behavior of newborns.** The NBAS enables assessment of the infant's individual capabilities for social relationships rated on the infant's best performance. Interest in the best performance is based on the belief that newborns may briefly respond to external stimuli from higher centers of the nervous system (i.e., the cerebrum). Six categories of abilities are considered in evaluating an infant's performance: habituation, orientation to auditory and visual stimuli, motor maturity, state changes, self-quieting ability, and social behaviors.

Response decrement (i.e., habituation) is the protective mechanism by which an infant decreases responsivity to external stimuli. Habituation represents the cerebral behavior of memory—the infant stores the memory of the stimulus and, with repeated presentation, learns not to respond. Infants who are able to habituate can "tune out" mild to moderate stimuli in the environment and protect themselves from overstimulation.

Infants who become "bored" with their toys have habituated to them—infants like variety. **Dishabituation represents increasing attention to a new stimulus (e.g., new mobile, toy, face) after**

Critical Findings

NEONATAL REFLEX BEHAVIORS

BEHAVIOR	BEGINS (IN UTERO) (WK)	INTEGRATES
Protection		
Moro reflex	28	At 6-8 mo to allow sitting and protective extension of the hands
Palmar grasp	28	At 5-6 mo to allow voluntary grasping of objects
Plantar grasp	28	At 7-8 mo with foot rubbing on objects; complete at 8-9 mo for standing and walking
Babinski reflex	28	Same as for plantar grasp
Tonic neck reflex	35	At 4 mo, so rolling over and reaching or grasping may occur
Gag* reflex	36	Protects against aspiration—does ***not*** disappear
Blink reflex	25	Does ***not*** disappear
Crossed extension	28	Disappears around 2 mo of age
Survival		
Rooting*	28	At 3 mo; decreased response if baby is sleepy or satiated
Sucking*	26-28	Not yet synchronized with swallowing
Swallowing*	12	32-34 wk, stronger synchronization with sucking; perfect by 34-37 wk

*Although isolated components of feeding behaviors are all present before 28 weeks gestational age, they are not effectively coordinated for oral feedings before 32 to 34 weeks gestational age.[101,182,243] Coordination of respiration with sucking and swallowing during bottle feeding is consistently achieved by infants more than 37 weeks post-conceptual age.[45]

habituation to an old stimulus. The infant thus "recognizes" the novelty of the new stimulus and chooses to respond.

An infant who is unable to habituate will continue to react vigorously to repeated stimuli. Compared with term infants, preterm infants are more reactive (e.g., less able to control their level of excitation) and less able to self-regulate (e.g., modulate reactivity, reflected in habituation rate and self-soothing abilities).[77] **Very-low-birth-weight (VLBW) infants are less able to (1) modulate attention, (2) take brief breaks from processing information, and (3) habituate to stimuli.[77] Thus the preterm is easily overstimulated and less able to deal with multiple sources of stimuli.[2]**

Neonates are able to imitate the facial and manual gestures of adults.[184] Infants as young as 12 days imitate gestures such as mouth opening and tongue protrusion. Because a neonate has never seen his or her own face, this innate ability to match behaviors to those of another is a remarkable use of the cerebral cortex. Imitation may operate as a positive feedback mechanism to caregivers; thus it is significant in parent-infant reciprocity and represents early learning behaviors.

Learning, a function of the cerebral cortex, occurs with habituation and imitation. Early cognitive development is important to later learning and future cognitive function. Knowledge of the cognitive ability of the neonate enables care providers to provide opportunities for learning. Learning occurs in the context of experience and influences structural development; there is increased CNS development during the first 2 years of life.[38,68]

The state of consciousness influences the reactions of a newborn to internal and external stimuli. The infant's state at the time of observation must be considered in interpretation of the findings (see the Critical Findings box on pp. 276-277).

Clinical application of the NBAS includes evaluation of infant capabilities after illness, prematurity, or maternal medications. The most important application of the NBAS is in anticipatory guidance for parents. Demonstration of parts of the examination for parents enables them to become familiar with their infant's individual patterns of behavior, temperament, and states. Thus parents can more accurately assess and interpret their infant's cues for interaction and need for quiet.

Critical Findings

NEWBORN STATES AND CONSIDERATIONS FOR CAREGIVING

NEWBORN STATE	COMMENTS
Sleep States	
Deep sleep (non–rapid-eye-movement [REM] or quiet sleep): Slow state changes Regular breathing Eyes closed; no eye movements No spontaneous activity except startles and jerky movements Startles with some delay and suppresses rapidly Lowest oxygen consumption	Infant is very difficult if not impossible to arouse. Infant will not breast feed or bottle feed in this state, even after vigorous stimulation. Infant is unable to respond to environment, which is frustrating for caregivers. Term infants may exhibit a "slow" heart rate (80-90 beats/min), which may trigger heart rate alarms and result in unnecessary stimulation by NICU staff. At birth, preterm infants have altered states of consciousness. Early dominant states are light sleep, quiet, and active alert. "Protective apathy" enables the preterm to remain inactive, unresponsive, and in a sleep state to conserve energy, grow, and maintain physiologic homeostasis.[273] As maturation occurs, there is an increase in quiet alert.
Light sleep (REM or active sleep): Low activity level Random movements and startles Respirations irregular and abdominal Intermittent sucking movements Eyes closed, REM Higher oxygen consumption	Full-term infants begin and end sleep in active sleep; preterm infants are more responsive (than term infants) to stimuli in active sleep. Infant may cry or fuss briefly in this state and be awakened to feed before truly awake and ready to eat. Lower and more variable oxygenation states.
Awake States	
Drowsy or semi-dozing: Eyelids fluttering Eyes open or closed (dazed) Mild startles (intermittent) Delayed response to sensory stimuli Smooth state change after stimulation Fussing may or may not be present Respirations are more rapid and shallow	Infants may awaken further or return to sleep (if left alone). Quietly talking and looking at the infant or offering a pacifier or an inanimate object to see and listen to may arouse the infant to the quiet, alert state. Less mature infants (30 weeks) demonstrate a more drowsy than quiet alert state than more mature infants (36 weeks).
Quiet alert, with bright look: Focuses attention on source of stimulation Impinging stimuli may break through; may have some delay in response Minimal motor activity	Immediately after birth, term newborns exhibit a period of quiet alert, which is their first opportunity to "take in" their parents and the extrauterine environment. Dimmed lights, quiet talking, and stroking optimize this time for parents. Best state for learning to occur, because infant focuses all of attention on visual, auditory, tactile, and sucking stimuli; best state for interaction with parents—infant is maximally able to attend and reciprocally respond to parents.

Circadian Rhythm

Circadian rhythms are cyclic variations in function that occur daily at about the same time. Humans cycle their bodily functions (e.g., temperature, hormonal changes, blood pressure, urine volume, sleep-wake cycles) in a 24-hour period.[228,229] These daily fluctuations are innately controlled by the individual's "biologic clock" in the suprachiasmatic nuclei (SCN) in the anterior hypothalamus. The SCN are located at the base of the third ventricle, above the optic chiasm.[228] The circadian

Critical Findings—cont'd

NEWBORN STATE	COMMENTS
Awake States—cont'd	
Active alert—eyes open: Considerable motor activity—thrusting movements of extremities; spontaneous startles	Infant has decreased threshold (increased sensitivity) to internal (hunger, fatigue) and external (wet, noise, handling) stimuli. Infant may quiet self, may escalate to crying, or with consolation by caregiver, may become quiet alert or go to sleep.
Reacts to external stimuli with increase in movements and startles (discrete reactions difficult to differentiate because of general higher activity level)	Infant is unable to maximally attend to caregiver or environment because of increased motor activity and increased sensitivity to stimuli.
Respirations irregular	
May or may not be fussy	
Crying—intense and difficult to disrupt with external stimuli; Respirations rapid, shallow, and irregular	Crying is the infant's response to unpleasant internal or external stimulation—infant's tolerance limits have been reached (and exceeded). Infant may be able to quiet self with hand-to-mouth behaviors; talking may quiet a crying infant; holding, rocking, or putting infant upright on caregiver's shoulder may quiet infant.

Data from Blackburn S: *JOGN Nurse* 12(suppl 3):76S-86S,1983; and Brazelton TB: *Neonatal behavioral assessment scale*, ed 2, Philadelphia, 1984, International Medical Publishers/Lippincott.

pacemaker must be reset daily by the relay of photic (light) information from the retina to the SCN, along the direct pathway from the retinohypothalamic tract (RHT) to the SCN.[228] During the 18th week of prenatal life, the SCN form and continue maturation after birth. In utero, the fetus expresses endogenous circadian rhythms (in heart/respiratory rates and steroid secretion) that are influenced by the mother.[191,228] The RHT has been identified in human newborns of 36 weeks' gestation; SCN are functionally innervated by the retina at stages equivalent to 25 weeks after conception in human infants.[228]

In infants, the development of circadian rhythm is influenced by genetic factors, brain maturation, and the environment.[91,228-230] Because there are individual differences in the development of circadian rhythms, in both preterm and full-term infants, the influences of prenatal rhythms or postnatal environmental influences are being studied.[191,228-230] Research and experimental outcomes in the development of circadian rhythms in the neonate are influenced by feeding, environmental lighting, and chronologic/post-conceptual age.[191,228-230] Intrauterine growth influences the development of circadian rhythms; in one study, more appropriate-for-gestational-age (AGA) than small-for-gestational-age (SGA) infants developed body temperature and heart rate rhythms.[102] More mature infants (i.e., greater post-conceptual age) of 35 to 37 weeks' gestation have a higher amplitude on body temperature rhythm when compared with infants of 32 to 34 weeks' gestation.[102] Infant biorhythms have been studied in the areas of temperature, heart and respiratory rates, blood pressure, sleep-wake cycles, rest-activity patterns, endocrine secretion, and feeding frequency.[102,191,228-230]

Active (or light) sleep is characterized by rapid eye movements (REM), whereas quiet (or deep) sleep has no rapid eye movements (i.e., non-REM sleep) (see the Critical Findings box on p. 276 and above). At birth and for the first few weeks of life, term newborns generally distribute sleep over a 24-hour period and sleep from 16 to 19 hours a day. As sleep begins, a term infant enters active, rather than quiet, sleep and spends more time in active sleep than does an adult.[72]

Active sleep durations vary from 10 to 45 minutes, whereas quiet sleep lasts about 20 minutes.[72] An infant's sleep cycle is 50 to 60 minutes, as compared with an adult's 90- to 100-minute cycle. Although day-night rhythms are difficult to detect in the neonatal period, some infants exhibit such rhythms as early as 1 week of age.[228,229]

Maturation of infant sleep is characterized by (1) increased organization of sleep states, (2) decrease in total sleep time, (3) increase in quiet sleep, (4) decrease in active sleep, and (5) increase in active and quiet waking.[72,262] Arousability from sleep is altered by gestational and postnatal age.

In term infants, arousal thresholds are significantly elevated in quiet sleep compared with active sleep (at 2 to 3 weeks and at 2 to 3 months of age), so that spontaneous arousal is greater in active than in quiet sleep.

Infants have their own "clock" for sleep-wake, hunger, and feeding or fussy times. This clock often does not coincide with the family's rhythms and may cause disruption and conflict. Sleep-wake states reflect the underlying status of the neurologic system. The infant's maturity at birth greatly affects his or her rhythms and development of normal circadian rhythm. Rhythmicity of sleep-wake cycles is influenced more by brain maturation than by environmental influences. Early relationships with caregivers provide the organization and stabilization necessary for sleep regulation, as well as other biologic functions. At 6 weeks, infants are awake more during the day than at night; by 12 weeks, more sleep occurs at night as daytime sleep duration continues to decrease. A term newborn has innate rhythms and, over a period of time (about 16 to 18 weeks), develops adult regularity (e.g., more sleep at night than in the daytime).

In preterm infants, active and quiet sleep cycles are less organized and of shorter duration (a sleep cycle is about 30 to 40 minutes) than in term infants.[71] Active sleep is "lighter" than quiet sleep—there is more response to stimuli in active sleep.[71] Quiet sleep is a more controlled state and occurs more frequently in term infants than in premature infants. Quiet sleep does not become significant in the preterm until approximately 36 weeks' gestation. Hence a third sleep state, transitional sleep, has been identified for premature infants.[209] This state is characterized by quiet sleep with periods of closed eyes, regular or periodic respirations, no body movements, and no REM. Before 36 weeks' gestation, a preterm infant's predominant sleep state is transitional sleep. As the preterm infant matures, he or she spends progressively less time in transitional sleep, has more quiet than active sleep, and has more awake, alert time. However, a preterm of 40 weeks post-conceptual age does not have sleep patterns that are as organized as those of a term newborn.[209] Spontaneous arousal from sleep is greater in active sleep compared with quiet sleep (at 2 to 3 weeks and at 2 to 3 months post-term age). During quiet sleep, spontaneous arousals at 2 to 3 weeks do not differ in preterm infants compared with term infants; however, at 2 to 3 months of age, preterm infants have significantly fewer spontaneous arousals compared with term infants. Long-term follow-up studies fail to show a difference in sleep distribution between preterm and term infants when corrected for age.[246] Both preterm and full-term infants who are exposed to an appropriate light intensity at home develop day-night rhythmicity by 44 and 48 weeks of post-conceptual age, respectively.[191,229,230,246]

As day and night rhythms in sleep-wake cycles develop, diurnal rhythm in hormone production also develops: (1) melatonin production is detectable at 12 weeks of age; and (2) variations in cortisol levels appear between 3 and 6 months of age.[228] **Sleep disruption may interfere with growth and development by altering neuronal maturation and growth hormone secretion. Human growth hormone has a rhythmic pattern associated with sleep-wake cycles. The highest peaks of growth hormone in infants occur during REM (active) sleep.** A fetus (29 to 32 weeks' gestation) spends 80% of the time in utero in REM sleep; a term newborn's sleep is 50% REM sleep.[71,72] **Because growth hormone secretion depends on the regular recurrence of sleep, any disturbance of the sleep-wake cycle results in irregular spikes of growth hormone during a 24-hour period.**

Although infant circadian rhythms are synchronous with those of the mother, desynchronous rhythms at birth may occur.[209,228] An infant whose cycles are discrepant from his or her family's may be perceived as "difficult." Because this behavior does not fit parental expectations of regular eating, sleeping, or eliminating, the parent-infant interaction is off to a rocky start. Gradually, through caregiving, parents teach the infant synchronization with family rhythms. By 9 months of age, most term infants develop day-night fluctuations that are similar to adult patterns.

Sensory Capabilities

At birth, a neonate's senses are developed and functioning. Sensory development proceeds in a specific order: tactile/vestibular, olfactory/gustatory, and auditory/visual. Stimuli (e.g., type, timing) to one sense affect the development of other senses. Sensory enhancement or deprivation of a later developing sensory system (e.g., vision) could either accelerate or decelerate the development of behavior mediated by earlier developing sensory systems (e.g., tactile and olfactory). A newborn is able to communicate—react to and initiate a response from those in the environment. Through the neonate's sensory perception, learning occurs by (1) habituating to some stimuli while attending to other stimuli, (2) discriminating between related and unrelated sensory events, and (3) integrating multisensory stimuli. As the neonate takes in the sensory information, he or she associates features of the environment that occur together (e.g., sound, smell, sight, touch of "mother" or "father"), demonstrating complex and intermodal abilities for handling the sensory input from the environment.

TACTILE/KINESTHETIC

Touch is the major method of communication for neonates and infants. Touch is the first sense to develop (at about 7½ weeks gestational age) and the last sense to fade. In utero, a fetus's existence has been primarily one of movement—floating within the amniotic fluid and experiencing rhythmic maternal movements. The senses of touch, temperature, and pressure are all well developed, and receptors lie in the newborn's skin. **The sensitivity to touch is especially well developed in the face, around the lips (root reflex), and in the hands (grasp reflex).** Because newborns are nonverbal, they pick up messages through the manner in which they are held and handled—by the adult's "body language." Infants are often barometers for adult feelings; if the adult is tired and irritable, the infant knows and may respond with irritability and crying.

Infants love to be held, rocked, and carried; note the soothing effects on a crying infant. Adults do not spoil infants by providing these important stimuli. Increased carrying of infants contributes to less crying at 6 weeks of age.[27] In response to being held, infants adjust their body posture to the body of the caregiver. Adults describe an infant as "cuddly" (assumes a comfortable, relaxed curl; snuggles to adult body; and attempts to root or suck) or "noncuddly" (sprawls; tenses or stiffens; and pushes away). The most comforting position for a crying infant is upright on an adult's shoulder.[138] Responsiveness to tactile stimulation has been found to be greater in female than in male neonates.[138]

HEARING

The fetus in utero has heard the voices of mother, father, and siblings beginning in the 22nd to the 24th week of intrauterine life.[163] These voices are "familiar" to newborns, so they "know" their family and are able to differentiate them from the voices of strangers.[62,63] Neonates prefer their mother's voice and the maternal language that they heard in utero.[198] Studies have suggested that fetuses and neonates exhibit memory.[62,63,198] Newborns who had been read a particular story while in utero responded to the story reread to them after birth with a recognition and attentiveness that was not exhibited in response to unfamiliar stories.[62,63,198] The ability to hear the outside world, particularly the spoken word, is a prerequisite to further verbal language development.

Fetal responses to sound include increases in breathing, body movements, fetal heart rate, cerebral blood flow, and glucose use and changes in behavior states. Neonates with an intact CNS are able to orient and respond to the auditory environment. In response to a sound, the neonate will demonstrate the following:

- Change in motor activity (eye blink, decrease in activity, limb movements, head turn)
- Change in heart rate (if the infant is quiet, the heart rate increases with stimuli; if the infant is crying, the heart rate decreases with stimuli) and/or change in respiration (increase in rate; decrease in amplitude; or decrease in respiratory cycle rate)
- Smile
- Startle or grimace
- Alert or arouse
- Cry or cease to cry
- Stop sucking

The response to sound depends on the sound's quality. The intensity of intrauterine noise is approximately 85 dB. When frequency and pitch are low, the infant is soothed and distress is decreased; high frequency and pitch alert and distress the infant and disturb sleep. Therefore monotonous low-frequency sounds are an auditory soother and induce sleep.

Frequencies below 4000 Hz (the range of human speech is 500 to 3000 Hz) produce the most newborn response. Infants are maximally reactive to the human voice in typical speech patterns (rather than disconnected syllables). Infants prefer the high-pitched (e.g., female) voice over the low-pitched (e.g., male) voice.

Note that adults and children instinctively pitch their voices higher when talking to an infant. The higher-pitched voice elicits sustained attention from newborns. Presented with a female and a male voice, the infant always turns toward the female voice. Parents who talk with their infants elicit increasing eye contact with the infant.

Experience with sound improves an infant's behavioral responses to sound. Stimuli presented for 5 to 15 seconds elicit the best reaction. Stimuli lasting longer than several minutes are less effective, because the term infant habituates to the sound and ceases responding. **The ability to habituate to sound is indicative of an intact CNS. Full-term newborns habituate to sound better and faster than do preterm infants.** Infants exhibit startle behavior if the stimulus rapidly reaches maximal loudness. A slower time to reach maximal loudness is associated with infant alerting and searching for the stimulus. Infant state is important in evaluation of response to auditory stimuli; light sleep is the optimal state. Infants quiet and soothe in response to rhythmic sounds (rather than dysrhythmic ones). Neonates move their bodies in rhythmic synchrony ***(entrainment)*** with the spoken word.

VISION

Eye development begins 22 days after conception. The eyelids fuse at about 10 weeks' gestation and remain fused until about 26 weeks' gestation. Eyelid opening is a function of maturity—more mature neonates open their eyes more than younger gestation neonates. At birth, photoreceptors are already developed, but maturation is not complete for several months. The fetus can distinguish light from dark and recoils from a bright light shone at the mother's abdomen. Even at term birth, the visual system is immature; significant development occurs over the next 6 months to a year. **The ability to fix, follow, and alert is indicative of an intact CNS.[190]**

At birth, infants can see an object within 8 to 10 inches of the face (visual acuity of 20/140).[82] Within seconds after birth, the neonate can recognize his or her mother's face. The cradled-in-the-arms position of feeding is the exact distance from the adult's face that the newborn can see. In response to an interesting visual stimulus, neonates stop sucking to look, alert, and attend to the object; horizontally scan the object; and fix and follow a moving object in a 90-degree arc.

Infants prefer the human face as a visual stimulus, prefer a patterned over a nonpatterned stimulus, and attend longer to larger patterns with more complex patterns and angles.[82] Infants prefer black and white because of the greater contrast and will focus on the outside of a figure where the contrast is the greatest[190]; color discrimination occurs around 2 to 3 months. Newborns are sensitive to bright light and will tightly close their eyes in its presence. They prefer moderate, diffuse lighting. Newborns exposed to cycled light (e.g., day-night changes) open their eyes more than those exposed to continuous bright light. Presentation of visual stimuli enables development of the neural pattern for vision. During the infant's first year of life, visual investigation of the environment is a primary mode of learning.

SMELL AND TASTE

The fetus increases its amniotic fluid consumption when saccharine is added to the fluid and decreases consumption with the injection of distasteful substances. Taste may be a way the fetus monitors the intrauterine environment. **Olfaction is well developed at birth.[241] Olfactory cues guide the full-term newborn to the maternal nipple.** Flavors in the mother's diet are present in amniotic fluid, and infants show a preference for these familiar flavors later in infancy.[186] Many of the flavors in amniotic fluid are the same in mother's breast milk.[186] At 5 days of age, a neonate can differentiate his or her mother's breast pad and demonstrates a preference for the smell over that of a "stranger"; full-term newborns stop crying and increase their mouthing behaviors when exposed to their mother's odor.[255] The infant's response to pleasant odors is to arouse and suck. After several presentations of the stimulus, the infant will habituate to the odor. Infants withdraw from unpleasant odors such as vinegar and ammonia. They are also able to differentiate tastes, preferring sweet solutions and refusing, by turning the head away, bitter, acid, and sour substances. Asphyxiated infants demonstrate a loss of olfaction that parallels the suppression of brainstem reflexes and activities.

COMMUNICATION SKILLS

A neonate's ability to communicate is a naturally endowed survival skill. Crying is an infant's language to communicate needs.[157] Crying also may be a response to the environment: noisy, cold, overstimulating, multiple caregiving, or lack of synchrony. Because the cry brings someone to meet the need, the infant soon learns that the caregiver gives attention and the world is a trustworthy place. The more responsive the caregiver is to the infant's crying, and thus the infant's needs, the less crying behavior is necessary.[27,157] Learning occurs as the infant associates comfort with the caregiver. The temperament of the individual infant and his or her ability to habituate to disturbing stimuli influence the amount of crying behavior. Tension in the caregiver or the environment is communicated nonverbally to the infant and may potentiate or contribute to the infant's crying.

The amount and tone of the newborn's cry are influenced by birth weight, gestational age, and the events of birth. **Types of cries include birth cry, hunger cry, pain cry, and pleasure cry.[52,53] Infants separated from their mothers in the first 90 minutes after birth exhibit a "separation distress call" (also seen in other mammal species) that ceases at reunion.[52,53]** The newborn's cry physiologically affects the mother: her breasts change and prepare to nurse. Neonates possess a repertoire of self-quieting behaviors when in a fussy state: (1) hand-to-mouth efforts; (2) sucking on fist or tongue; and (3) use of visual or auditory stimuli from the environment.[38]

After birth, crying develops a diurnal pattern: term infants cry more during the day than at night. Persistent crying (>3 hours a day) is more likely by breast-fed babies, whereas early evening crying is more likely by formula-fed infants. Postnatal age is a significant predictor of crying. Crying decreases with increasing chronologic age.[263] The neonatal cry may be a signal of robustness or wellness, a signal of pain, or diagnostic of existing conditions or trauma. CNS insult often results in a high-pitched, shrill cry.

A smiling infant is a joy to the caregiver. Smiling may be either spontaneous (from birth) or a response to the social human face (at 4 to 12 weeks of life). A smile is most easily elicited by the stimulus of a moving, smiling human face. The ability to smile begins before 40 weeks in a preterm infant, as observed during REM sleep. The social implications of the smile include positive feedback to the caregiver that the infant is happy and contented, which results in parental feelings of adequacy and competence.

ENVIRONMENT

Prenatal Environment

In utero, the fetus depends totally on the mother's emotional and physical health and well-being for his or her own. It is through the mother that the fetus receives the nurturance, housing, and stimulation to develop the body, the sensory organs, and the rudiments of personality and temperament.

Conditions present at birth may not be congenital but, rather, the result of the impact of uterine environmental conditions on development. Maternal-fetal programming, known as the ***Barker hypothesis,***[23] postulates that the maternal prenatal environment influences the developing fetal brain and also the long-term permanent effects on health and susceptibility to disease.[39,200]

Recent studies have documented the relationship between increased antepartal maternal anxiety and the susceptibility of the child to the development of attention deficit–hyperactivity disorder (ADHD), self-reported anxiety, and externalizing problems.[275] Brain substrates in animals and maybe humans may influence a wide variety of affiliative behaviors, including infant-mother attachment.[194] The racial discrepancy in preterm birth may be the result of stressful life events in black mothers.

Intrapartal Environment

Birth is a major transition from physiologic dependence to physiologic independence. At term, a neonate's physiologic systems are developed, sensory organs function, and the foundation of personality and temperament is established. Birth is disorienting and disruptive. The amount of disruption depends on the degree of trauma incurred during the labor and birth processes. Not having a social support system compounds the stress, often escalating it beyond the mother's tolerance and coping skills. Anxious and fearful women have longer labors and more delivery complications than women who are confident about themselves and their infants.[239] The recent shift toward family-centered birth enables mothers to receive support from their families, be an active participant in the birth process, and have immediate contact with their newborns.

A neonate also is influenced by medications and the events of labor and birth (see Chapter 2).

Maternal medications for analgesia and anesthesia affect neonatal behaviors, resulting in decreased sucking ability, lethargy, and decreased habituation. Medicated infants are less able to evoke caregiver behaviors such as smiling, touching, and vocalization. They also give less feedback to their parents than do unmedicated infants. The parents may feel rejected, tend to stimulate the infant less, and thus begin a pattern of aberrant interaction.

Postnatal Environment

Home and family are the primary media through which newborns (1) reestablish their biorhythmic balance, (2) stabilize themselves in the extrauterine world, (3) develop a sense of self and mastery in the world, and (4) become socialized as human beings. Socialization teaches the adaptive psychosocial skills necessary for survival and functioning in society. Cultural and family values, behavioral expression, and ways of meeting social and emotional needs are learned within the family. Thus the home and family environment is considered to be a "normalizing" environment for human development.

CAREGIVER FACTORS

The dyadic relationship continues postpartally between the caregiver and the infant—the behavior of one reinforces the behavior of the other. The infant's physical and emotional needs are satisfied by caregivers. The infant's response to the caregiver depends on how the infant perceives and receives ministrations; this response affects the level of emotional satisfaction the caregiver receives from the interaction. Parental expectations have a major effect on their perceptions and their behavior and ultimately affect the child's development. Parents must work out the discrepancy between the wished-for and the actual child, especially if the infant is preterm or ill or has an anomaly. How attached the parents are to the infant influences their relationship with and ability to care for their infant (see Chapter 29). If the pregnancy has failed to produce a normal, healthy infant, the parents must grieve the loss of their expectations. Parents are unable to attach to and care for the infant until they have completed their grief work (see Chapter 30).

A caregiver and an infant have a reciprocal interaction when their cycles and signals are synchronized with each other. The biorhythmic cycle of the newborn has been in synchrony with one person (mother) in utero, and the infant is accustomed to her cycles and rhythms for developing adaptive behavior. Consistent maternal caregiving enables a newborn to regulate his or her rhythms to those of the mother and begin adapting to the postnatal environment. From her, they expand their adaptation to the family and the larger world of society.

Experience in relating to infants influences the caregiver's efficiency in interpretation of and sensitivity to infant cues. Multiparous women have more sensitivity to infant cues than do primiparous mothers. Mothers with little or no experience exhibit more difficulty in quieting a crying infant. The competence of parents may be improved through acquisition of knowledge about infants, so that the quality of interaction between parent and infant is enhanced. In one study, prenatally, first-time mothers received videotaped education about infant behavior, states, and communication cues that resulted in significant differences in sensitivity to infant cues and social and emotional growth fostering behaviors in early (first 24 hours) mother-infant interaction.[290]

Consistency in maternal responses is especially important as the infant continues to learn the accepted patterns of cues from the caregiver. Cared for by one or two people, an infant is able to develop synchrony with and expectations of the parents. Single caregiving improves establishment of biorhythms for sleep-wake cycles, feeding, and visual attentiveness. Consistent cues soon elicit a consistency of response from the infant. Consistency and promptness of maternal response result in less infant crying during the first year of life. A predictable and responsive environment enables the infant to progress to varied types of communication (not just crying). Care by parents provides for mutual cueing and mastery of the environment through interaction. Inconsistent cues distress and confuse the infant. **Multiple caregivers confuse the infant, increases distress with feeding, causes irritability, and upsets visual attention.**

Regardless of how stable or unstable, consistent or inconsistent it is, family life has a rhythm, synchronicity, and predictability of its own. Through interaction with parents and siblings, infants further develop their ability to form relationships. From these primary relationships, the foundation and format for other relationships are established. The quality of subsequent relationships depends on the quality of the relationship experienced within the primary family from birth throughout infancy.[103]

NEONATAL FACTORS

The neonate is not a passive recipient of the environment of the family but, rather, is an active participant in shaping that environment. Infants send cues about their ability and readiness for interpersonal interactions. In their first 4 months of life, infants' interactions with persons differ from their interactions with inanimate objects (Figure 13-1). The excitement generated by interpersonal interaction is seen in an infant's arm and leg movements, bodily movement toward the other person, smiling, vocalizing, and increased visual attention. Because of the infant's immaturity, he or she is unable to maintain a continuous interaction. The infant attends for short periods and then turns away to decrease excitement, protect himself or herself from bombardment by overwhelming stimuli, and process the experience. **Maternal or care provider sensitivity to the attention-withdrawal cycle of interaction enables the adult to modulate his or her behavior in synchrony with the infant's cues.** Successful interaction with an infant includes reading the infant's cues, responding appropriately, and not overwhelming the infant with too much stimulation (thus overstepping the infant's tolerance for interaction). Overwhelming the infant results in withdrawal for progressively longer periods to protect himself or herself from overstimulating and insensitive others.

Just as the parent has expectations, the infant also has physiologic needs that require care. The infant needs relief or protection from painful experiences,

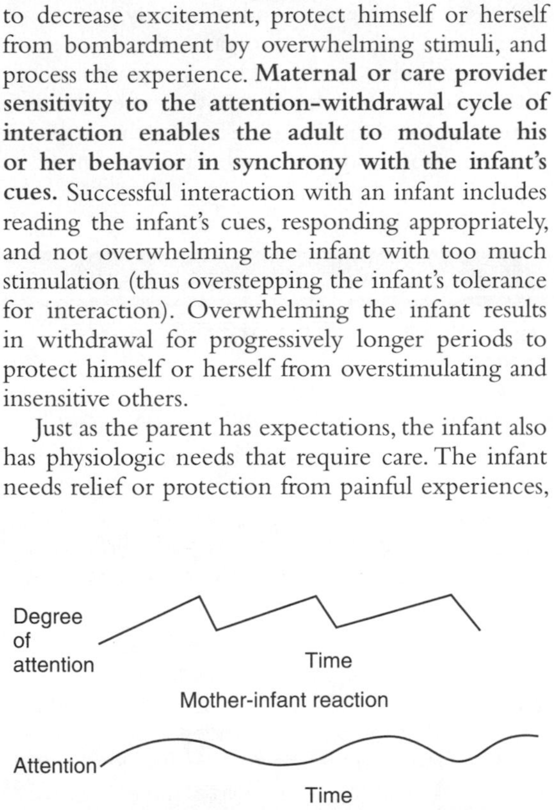

FIGURE 13-1 Interaction pattern with object and with mother. Object interaction is characterized by abrupt attention and excitement phases followed by sudden and abrupt looking away. Interaction with person is cyclic and involves initiation of interaction, orientation to person, acceleration of excitement, peak of excitement, deceleration of excitement, and withdrawal or turning away. (From Brazelton TB, Koslowski B, Main M: The origins of reciprocity: the early infant-mother interaction. In Lewis M, Rosenblum LA, editors: *The effect of the infant on its caregiver*, New York, 1974, John Wiley & Sons.)

maintenance of comfort, and homeostasis. Relief from the discomforts of hunger, cold, sleeplessness, and boredom enables the infant to respond positively to the care provider.

Care-eliciting behaviors are those neonatal cues used to signal the caregiver that attention is needed. Crying, visual following, and smiling are care-eliciting behaviors. Newborn responses to care include quieting, suckling, clinging and cuddling, looking, smiling, and vocalizing. These social interactions positively reward the care provider and encourage and promote continued care. Infant characteristics that modify maternal attitudes include (1) a healthy or sickly infant, (2) an attractive, pretty infant or an infant with obvious congenital anomaly, (3) a premature infant, (4) a calm and contented or a fussy and irritable infant, and (5) an infant responsive to or rejecting of maternal care. A maternal or care provider ability to soothe the infant reinforces a feeling of success (or failure) in his or her feelings of competence.

The infant's gender also affects the cues and the caregiver's response. Male infants exhibit more startles, more muscle activity, and more physical strength. In response, caregivers hold them more as a means of soothing.[138] Females exhibit more tactile and oral sensitivity, more smiling, and more responsivity to sweet taste. As a result, girls are more often soothed by talking, eye-to-eye contact, and a pacifier.[138]

The infant's level of neurophysiologic development influences the appropriateness of maternal and caregiving behaviors. The neurologically mature term infant who has already mastered autonomic, motoric, and state regulation is able to actively elicit and respond to caregiving behaviors.[38] **Because of the immaturity of the CNS, a preterm infant lags behind a term infant in care eliciting and responsivity to the care provider[177,283,291] (see the Critical Findings box on p. 284).** Because a young preterm infant's priority is mere survival, interaction with the environment and care providers will occur at the expense of physiologic stability.[273] Because a preterm infant sends cues different from those of a term infant, knowledge of these stages enables caregivers to modulate their behavior and the environment.[136] Although overwhelming the term infant results in withdrawal from interaction, overwhelming the preterm infant results first in a real threat to physiologic survival and then to withdrawal from interaction.

The ability of an infant to be a social partner and to respond in a social interaction is developmentally determined and influenced by the infant's physical condition. The response of preterm infants (weight <1500 g) to social stimulation (e.g., talking and talking combined with touching) develops over time: (1) at 29 to 32 weeks' gestation, respond with distress (e.g., eye closing) to all forms of social stimuli; (2) at approximately 33 weeks' gestation, begin to respond with increased attention to talking; they remain distressed with combined stimuli; and (3) at approximately 35 to 36 weeks' gestation, pay more attention to talking; more distress at combined stimuli is seen in high-risk infants (e.g., preterms <1500 g) and better habituation seen in healthier infants.[76] Sicker preterm infants have a more difficult time attending to and modulating their response to social interactions than do healthier preterm infants.[75-77,283,291] Although VLBW preterm infants respond to talking with increased attention and eye opening, the addition of touch results in increased eye closing and facial grimacing.[77] Sicker infants demonstrate the same pattern of response but in a more exaggerated way that reflects their increased reactivity (i.e., level of excitation) and decreased ability for self-regulation (i.e., modulate reactivity).[75,77,273]

Because preterm infants are not as neurologically mature as term infants, the NBAS has little value with this population. **A behavioral assessment scale for preterm infants, Assessment of Preterm Infant's Behavior (APIB), has been developed that evaluates the preterm infant's behavioral organization along five subsystems of functioning: autonomic, motor, state, attentional-interactive, and self-regulatory.**[6] Although subsystems are observed independently, they are interdependent because disorganization in one system affects other systems. This examination delineates the quality and duration of the preterm infant's response, the difficulty in eliciting the response, and the effort and cost to the preterm infant of

Critical Findings

STAGES AND CHARACTERISTICS OF BEHAVIORAL ORGANIZATION IN PRETERM INFANTS

ALS, BRAZELTON*	GORSKI†
Physiologic homeostasis—stabilizing and integrating temperature control, cardiorespiratory function, digestion, and elimination. Characteristics: become pale, dusky, cyanotic; heart and respiratory rates change—all symptoms of disorganization of autonomic nervous system.	"In-turning"—physiologic stage of mere survival characterized by autonomic nervous system responses to stimuli (rapid color changes caused by swings in heart and respiratory rates); no or limited direct response; inability to arouse self spontaneously; jerky movements; asleep (and protecting the central nervous system from sensory overload) 97% of the time. Preterms (<32 weeks) are easily physiologically overwhelmed by stimuli.
Motor development may infringe on physiologic homeostasis resulting in defensive strategies (e.g., vomiting, color change, apnea, bradycardia). State development becomes less diffuse and encompasses full range: sleep, awake, crying. States and state changes may affect physiologic or motor stability.	"Coming out"—first active response to environment may be seen as early as 34-35 weeks (provided some physiologic stability has been achieved). Characteristics: remains pink with stimuli, has directed response for short periods, arouses spontaneously and maintains arousal after stimulus ceases; if interaction begins in alert state: maintains quiet alert for 5-10 min, tracks animate or inanimate stimuli, spends 10%-15% of time in alert state with predictable interaction patterns.
Alert state is well differentiated from other states; may interfere with physiologic or motor stability.	"Reciprocity"—active interaction and reciprocity with environment at 36-40 weeks. Characteristics: directs response, arouses and consoles self, maintains alertness, interacts with animate/inanimate objects, copes with external stress.

*Data from Als H, Brazelton TB: A new model of assessing the behavioral organization in preterm and full-term infants: two case studies, *J Am Acad Child Psychiatry* 20:239, 1981.
†Modified from Gorski PA: Stages of behavioral organization in the high-risk neonate: theoretical and clinical considerations, *Semin Perinatol* 3:61, 1979.

achieving and maintaining a response. Because it, too, is an interactive test, the nature and amount of organization provided by the care provider is an indication of the preterm infant's lack of integrative skill. As the preterm infant matures and advances in development of organization, he or she is more able to interact with the environment (animate and inanimate). However, it must be remembered that this maturation process is "uneven"; as the preterm infant advances in one area of development, he or she may become, at least temporarily, more vulnerable (i.e., experience difficulties) in other areas such as physiologic stability.[103]

Another recently developed examination, the Neonatal Intensive Care Unit Network Neurobehavioral Scale (NNNS), assesses neurologic integrity and behavioral factors of high-risk infants (e.g., preterms, drug-exposed infants) by evaluating neurobehavioral organization, neurologic reflexes, motor development, muscle tone (active/passive), and signs of (drug) withdrawal and stress.[150] The NNNS differs from the NBAS in that the NNNS (1) was developed for at-risk populations, not for the normal newborn, (2) is more structured and standardized than the NBAS, and (3) gives results more reflective of infant capabilities rather than infant-examiner interaction.[150] The NNNS is performed on medically stable infants, between more than 30 weeks' gestation and 46 to 48 weeks post-conceptual age, for research purposes and for clinical practice.[32,150] Clinical applications include the following[32]:

- Evaluates the infant's personality and temperament as capacities for state regulation of arousal, response to stimuli, self-soothing, and tolerance of handling
- Documents the physiologic and behavioral manifestations of drug withdrawal or stressors in the environment
- Documents the capacity to habituate, orient to stimuli, and respond to handling, muscle tone, and quality of movement
- Evaluates infants withdrawing from in utero drug exposure and those being weaned from analgesia in the NICU
- Determines when the infant is ready for discharge
- Is used as a teaching and care-planning tool when the examination includes parents and other care providers
- Is a tool that bridges the assessment from early gestation/neonatal period to 2 months corrected age when other tools are unreliable

INTERVENTIONS

Life in a special care nursery is characterized by sensory deprivation of normal stimuli that the preterm infant would have experienced in the womb and that term infants would experience at home with their families. However, the NICU is also an environment of sensory bombardment—constant noise, light, and tactile stimulation; intrusive, invasive procedures; upset of sleep-wake cycles; and multiple caregivers. **Rather than too much or too little stimulation, infants in the NICU receive an inappropriate pattern of stimulation (e.g., noncontingent, nonreciprocal, painful [rather than pleasant], and multiple stimuli).**[3,7,43,103,105] Because the immature CNS of the premature infant cannot tolerate these stimuli, the easily overstimulated preterm infant protects himself or herself by physiologic and interactional defensive maneuvers that threaten survival and social ability and may lead to lifelong maladaptations. Long-term physiologic instability is linked with poor outcomes in preterm infants. Exposure to acute and chronic stress may lead to enduring alterations in the individual's threshold for activation and arousal and increase the risk for stress-related diseases.[28,165,291]

Research has shown medical, developmental, and cost benefits to low-birth-weight infants from individualized behavioral and environmental care in the NICU (Table 13-1). The most effective interventions (1) follow the Newborn Individualized Developmental Care and Assessment Program (NIDCAP®),[5,258] **(2) are contingent on the infant's responses, (3) balance protection from sensory overload with provision of enough stimulation to promote emerging capabilities, and (4) involve the parents.***

The first randomized controlled trial (RCT) of individualized developmental care (NIDCAP®)[5] **for VLBW (inborn and transported) infants conducted in three diverse NICUs showed improvement in medical well-being and neurobehavioral and family function.**[5] Medical benefits to the VLBW infants receiving individualized

*References 3,5,7,43,135,293.

TABLE 13-1 OUTCOMES OF INDIVIDUALIZED DEVELOPMENTAL INTERVENTION IN THE NICU*

PHYSIOLOGIC BENEFITS	DEVELOPMENTAL BENEFITS	COST SAVINGS
Decrease in:	Improvement in:	Shorter length of stay
Incidence of IVH or pneumothorax and severity of BPD, ROP, NEC	Behavioral organization of autonomic, motor, attention modulation, and self-regulatory abilities	Earlier discharge at younger age
Ventilator/CPAP use	Interactive capability of infant with staff and parents	Decrease in hospital charges
Need for supplemental oxygen	Quality of parent-infant interaction	
Need for gavage feedings/IV nutrition	Feelings of closeness with preterm	
Number of apneic episodes	Cognitive function/IQ	
Need for sedation/analgesia	Development of feeding skills (earlier full oral feedings)	
Increase in:	Fewer behavioral problems and attentional difficulties	
Daily weight gain; head growth/length	Continuation of maternal ability to read and respond to infant behavioral cues/appreciation of the infant	
Stability of cardiorespiratory function		
Sleep states/sleep duration		
Significant electrophysiologic differences in frontal, temporal, central, occipital, and parietal lobes of the brain		

*References 3,5,7,28,43,92,135,136,258,286,287,293.

BPD, Bronchopulmonary dysplasia; *CPAP*, continuous positive airway pressure; *IQ*, intelligence quotient; *IV*, intravenous; *IVH*, intraventricular hemorrhage; *NEC*, necrotizing enterocolitis; *NICU*, neonatal intensive care unit; *ROP*, retinopathy of prematurity.

developmental care included (1) fewer days of parenteral nutrition because of shorter transition to full enteral nutrition, (2) improved average daily weight gain and better growth, (3) fewer cases of necrotizing enterocolitis (NEC), and (4) younger age at discharge, decreased NICU/hospital stay, and lower hospital costs.[5] Neurobehavioral benefits included better autonomic or motor system regulation and self-regulation and reduced need for facilitation.[5] Benefits to family functioning included maternal perceptions of (1) their infant being better regulated, more gratifying, and more autonomous, (2) less personal stress, and (3) enhanced competence in their parental roles.[5] Given the diversity of the NICU settings and populations, the biggest differences in beneficial outcomes were appreciated in the most challenged settings (e.g., NICUs initially using the least developmental care, families with multiple social and cultural vulnerability, the sickest infants).[5]

A separate, more recent RCT studied the effectiveness of NIDCAP®, initiated within 72 hours of NICU admission in 30 preterms (28 to 33 weeks gestational age [GA]) on brain structure and function.[3] **The group of preterms receiving NIDCAP® showed significantly better neurobehavioral functioning at 2 weeks and 9 months corrected age on mental and psychomotor development than that of the control group.** Changes in the brain included a more mature brain fiber structure between brain regions (e.g., frontal to occipital; frontal to parietal) than is consistent with enhanced neurobehavioral functioning. **The study's conclusion is that the quality of early experiences (e.g., before term) significantly alters brain structure and function.**[3]

Preterm infants are not the only infants at risk from the stress of overstimulation in the NICU. **Acutely ill infants and chronically ill infants with prolonged hospitalization also experience stress.** A term infant with persistent pulmonary hypertension (see Chapter 23) is particularly vulnerable to repeated handling, procedures, and interventions that decrease PaO_2. Thus these infants are managed on a minimal intervention regimen: care is organized, coordinated, and individualized to decrease noxious stimuli and physical manipulations. Even when a "minimal handling" (i.e., parents and staff are discouraged from providing any unnecessary tactile stimulation) protocol[144] is encouraged for the sickest neonates, one study documented no difference in the amount of handling the infant endured.[285] The chronically ill infant with bronchopulmonary dysplasia (BPD) has been shown to improve when behavioral or environmental changes were initiated. The term SGA infant is sleepy and not alert in the first few weeks of life, which may result in the infant's being left alone or overstimulated to awaken for interaction. After a few weeks, these infants become very irritable, fussy, and disorganized in spontaneous and social behaviors. Anticipatory guidance, reassurance that the disorganization is in the infant rather than a result of parental care, and practical intervention strategies enable the parents to shape the environment and the infant's response.[103]

The ultimate goal of intervention strategies in the NICU is to facilitate and promote infant growth and development and thus task mastery.[213] In the NICU, this goal is achieved by the following:

- **Altering the environmental and caregiving stressors that interfere with physiologic stability**
- **Promoting individual neurobehavioral organization and maturation by identifying and facilitating stable behaviors and reducing stressful behaviors**
- **Conserving energy**
- **Teaching parents to interpret infant behavior**
- **Promoting infant-parent interaction and caregiving**

Establishing biorhythmic balance and physiologic homeostasis is necessary for survival and is enhanced by a sensitive, responsive NICU environment.[262] **An unresponsive environment may so stress the preterm infant that apnea, bradycardia, and other physiologic instabilities severely compromise and prolong recovery.**[46,103,147,213,273] For the hospitalized infant, development of the sense of self and trust is undermined by noncontingent stimulation that prevents establishing a sense of competence and control of the environment.[105] When the ventilated infant experiences hunger or is wet, he or she cannot signal the care provider with a cry because of the tube. Thus the infant experiences a need but cannot signal and bring care and relief. The infant soon learns that he or she is not in control of the situation. Another intubated infant may be quietly asleep and not experiencing a need; however, it is "care time," so the nurse moves, wakes, changes, and generally disturbs the infant. This infant also soon learns about not being in control of the situation.

Hospitalized infants, especially those with prolonged stays, may exhibit the classic signs of institutionalized infants or infants suffering from maternal deprivation (see the Critical Findings box on p. 288).[251] It is the goal of "environmental neonatology"[105] to prevent this maladaptive behavior by altering the NICU to be more developmentally appropriate and responsive to infants. Normalizing the environment begins with an assessment of the stimulation to which the individual infant is exposed. The type (i.e., noxious versus pleasant; contingent versus noncontingent), amount, and timing of stimulation should be noted. To decrease noxious stimuli, no infant should have "routine" care (e.g., all infants are suctioned every 2 hours; all infants have a glucose test every 4 hours).[103] Care should be individualized by asking these questions: "Why are we doing this procedure?" and "Is this procedure necessary for this infant's care?" Overstimulation in the NICU occurs when 81% to 94% of all contacts are medical or nursing procedures, an average of 40 to 132 of which are performed per day.[79,285] The frequency, pattern, and trends of caregiver encounters and disturbance have not changed over the past 20 years,[18,213] although caregivers grossly underestimate the amount of handling to which NICU infants are exposed. Nurses, who are best able to control overstimulation, provide the majority of handling, excessive disturbance, and noncontingent interaction to these fragile infants (number of contacts ranging from 79 to 164 times, evenly distributed over a 24-hour period).[18] Painful, invasive procedures that are not vital to the individual infant are stress-producing events that should be eliminated. A recent study demonstrated that in three very different NICUs, highly individualized, sensitive, and responsive care by NICU nurses was commonly given to the most fragile infants by following the preterm's cues for when intervention was most appropriate.[262]

Rest may be the most important environmental change.[28,117,213] In a study of ventilated extremely-low-birth-weight (ELBW) infants, the relationship between hypoxemia and state revealed that sleep disruption with its accompanying motor activity was associated with hypoxemia more often than when these infants were in active/quiet sleep.[147] Recommendations of this study include (1) using strategies (e.g., clustering care, kangaroo care [KC]) to promote sleep in ventilated infants and (2) sleep cycling analogous to in utero patterns (e.g., more quiet sleep) to improve ventilatory stability, decrease hypoxemia, and improve oxygenation.[147] Although rest periods are necessary for normal growth and development and optimal immune function,[232] care continues to be evenly distributed over 24 hours without adequate periods of undisturbed rest.[213] **Rest periods of less than 60 minutes are ineffective and insufficient for the preterm to complete a normal sleep cycle.**[213] The length of rest periods in most NICUs has not changed (Table 13-2), and institution of a rest period (even only 1 hour in length) does not necessarily decrease the amount of disturbance.[122]

A fetus in utero and a term infant at home relate to a minimum of caregivers and thus need to learn one or only a few sets of cues. **Consistency of caregivers is essential for an infant's developmental agenda.**[41] **Multiple caregivers in the NICU confuse the infant by providing many care-related cues for the infant to learn—many techniques of handling and many emotional, nonverbal messages to decode. Primary nursing minimizes the number of care providers, because the primary nurse and one or two associates always (or as much as possible) care for the infant; assess, revise, and write the care plan; and coordinate care.** Primary nursing also adds consistency and continuity for parents.

The infant's state or level of arousal provides an appropriate context for caregiving. Some infants exhibit a low threshold for stimuli; they are easily overwhelmed and fatigued. Others with a higher threshold are quieter, more difficult to arouse, initiate less, and thus receive less interaction.[6] **Organizing care to be reciprocal to the infant's state reinforces the infant's competence in signaling a need (sense of self) and having it met (sense of trust and mastery).** As the infant matures, feeding on demand rather than on a schedule not only

TABLE 13-2 REST PERIODS FOR NICU INFANTS: RESEARCH BASIS

AUTHOR/YEAR	LENGTH OF REST PERIOD
Korones, 1976[139]	Range of mean rest periods 5.6-19.2 min
Duxbury, 1984[74]	Average time of 30.2 min
Evans, 1994[79]	Time between handling: 1-38.45 min in first nursery 1-60 min in second nursery
Appleton, 1997[18]	2-59 min

NICU, Neonatal intensive care unit.

Critical Findings

CLASSIC SIGNS OF "HOSPITALITIS"

Asocial Behavior

- Gaze aversion—fleeting glances at caregiver with inability to maintain eye contact
- Flat affect—social unresponsiveness (little fixing and following; little smiling) to caregiver
- Little or no quiet alert state—infant abruptly changes state and often is described as "either asleep or awake and crying" (crying is only "awake" state); out-of-control crying

*Touch Aversion**

- Becomes hypotonic or hypertonic with caregiving or attempts at socialization
- Fights, flails, and resists being cared for or held
- Aversive responses (see the Critical Findings box on p. 291) to caregiving or holding

Feeding Difficulties

- Have multiple origins, including delayed onset of oral feedings; touch aversion around mouth secondary to invasive procedures; multiple caregivers; feeding on schedule, rather than demand
- Rumination syndrome—voluntary regurgitation, a form of self-comfort and gratification when environment is not nurturing or gratifying

Failure to Thrive

- Poor or no weight gain despite adequate caloric intake
- Develops mental delays (language, motor, social, emotional)

*Infant associates human touch with pain.

teaches this valuable lesson but also increases absorption and use of caloric intake.[103,175,247] If the infant is asleep, ask: "Should we do this now? Would another time be better?"[262] In some centers, physicians make an appointment with the nurse to examine the infant, at a time that is optimal for the infant.

Because preterm infants exhibit short duration of state cycles until around 38 weeks, they have decreased tolerance for stimuli. **The smaller, sicker, and less mature the infant, the less he or she is able to handle stimuli.** Some preterm infants tolerate all care done at once and long periods of rest; others do not and need care spread out to decrease overstimulation and decompensation. **Clustering of care—performance of several procedures together in a short period of time**—may result in more physiologic alterations (changes in cardiorespiratory stability, changes in blood pressure, increased cortisol levels, and heightened pain responses) than a single care-taking event or the actual length of the handling episode.[119,120,274] Recent studies show increased and prolonged behavioral motor responses and increased cortisol levels indicative of stress during clustered care; **clustered care is especially stressful for preterms less than 28 weeks gestational age.**[118,120] Clustering care may not ensure long rest periods, because 50% of all rest periods in several NICUs were shorter than 10 minutes (see Table 13-2).[79] If the practice of clustering care, with its prolonged disturbance of the preterm infant, results in alterations of vital signs, oxygen saturation, and infant stress and fatigue, then care should be individualized and provided to minimize physiologic and behavioral disturbances.[111,119,147,213] A study of medically stable preterms found that after nursing interventions, these infants generally sleep—either from satiety or from the significant energy expenditure associated with caregiving.[257]

Even "preterm growers" may be unable to tolerate more than one stimulus at a time—they feed best if visual, auditory, and social stimuli are not provided until after the feeding. As the infant matures and is able to tolerate integrated experience, multimodal stimuli are provided.[289] Studies of multimodal stimuli (e.g., auditory, tactile, vestibular, visual) provided to preterms demonstrate (1) increased alertness, (2) earlier discharge, (3) faster progression to full oral feedings, (4) improved organization of behavioral states, (5) stable respiratory rate and oxygen saturation, and (6) a significant decrease in resting heart rate.[289,290]

Alterations in the individual infant's daily schedule are made to accommodate a more flexible or structured schedule—whichever is better for the infant.[105,262] **Assessing the infant before, during, and after an interaction or intervention guides the care provider in adapting care and the environment to the individual infant (Table 13-3).**

An organized infant is able to interact with the environment without disrupting his or her physiologic and behavioral functioning.[6] **When a disorganized preterm interacts with the environment, signs of physiologic and behavioral stress may occur (see the Critical Findings box on p. 291), in which case the interaction should cease.**[111,138] The potential effects of stress and trauma to fragile preterm infants may have not only short-term but also long-term effects on their outcomes.[165] An intubated preterm infant cared for in a NICU with a strict suction "routine" every 2 hours responds with profound cyanosis, lowered $TcPo_2$ and pulse oxygenation, and bradycardia and requires bagging after every suction (with no secretions obtained), an obviously unnecessary and stressful intervention. In a less rigid, more individualized care setting, that same infant may signal the need for suction by becoming restless, by a decrease in oxygenation, or by heart rate changes (tachycardia or bradycardia). Suctioning improves the infant's condition—the infant lies quietly and has improved oxygenation, and the heart pattern stabilizes. This infant has signaled his or her need, and the care providers have read the cues and responded with a stabilizing intervention—the infant has not been stressed by an unnecessary procedure. A recent study showed that stress cues and motor activity (e.g., multiple extremity movements) often are related to oxygen desaturations; recommendations include caretaker vigilance of behavioral stress and motor activity cues in response to caregiving and minimizing stimuli that evoke these responses.[111]

Knowledgeable professionals are able to role model for and teach parents how to relate to their premature infant.[46,136,165] Parents are taught to recognize and use infant states to maximize appropriate interaction.[136,148,165] The drowsy premature infant may be unable to engage in eye-to-eye contact with the parents or be able to sustain it for too short (for the parents) a period. Waiting until the infant is more awake to initiate eye contact is more rewarding for the parent and less stressful for the infant. Role model for parents that this infant is an individual and,

TABLE 13-3 PARAMETERS FOR ASSESSING INTERACTION AND INTERVENTION WITH NEONATES

TIME FRAME	ASSESSMENT
BEFORE	
Gather baseline data ***before*** touching the infant	Gestational age and post-conceptual age Diagnosis Level of physiologic homeostasis: Previous vital signs Oxygenation state—continuous pulse oximetry or transcutaneous monitor Neonatal state: Sleep—deep, light, drowsy Awake—quiet, active alert, crying Self-regulatory versus stress behaviors (see the Critical Findings box on p. 291)
DURING	
Gently and as unobtrusively as possible assess physiologic and behavioral signs ***during*** intervention	Level of (current) physiologic homeostasis—vital signs and changes: Observation (without touching infant)—color, posture, general appearance, respiratory rate, temperature (skin, incubator), blood pressure (transducer), oxygenation (from continuous monitor) Quiet (with minimal disturbance)—auscultate heart, lungs, and abdomen; axillary temperature, blood pressure (cuff); head-to-toe assessment; oxygenation (saturation decreases with distressful, disturbing stimuli) Neonatal state change: Sleep—deep, light, drowsy Awake—quiet alert, active alert, crying Self-regulatory versus stress behaviors (see the Critical Findings box on p. 291)
AFTER	
Assess physiologic and behavioral signs ***after*** intervention (delayed reactions may occur minutes after care)	Level of physiologic homeostasis Vital signs—Returned to baseline values? More stable or less stable than baseline values? Neonatal state change—Return to baseline state? To a higher state? Unable to be consoled? More consolable left alone?

although premature, can signal for more or less stimulation (see the Critical Findings box on p. 291).

A preterm infant who is lightly touched may startle, jerk, or withdraw from parental touch. In response, the parent suddenly and sadly pulls his or her hand away and is reticent to touch the infant again. Intervention includes helping parents read cues and learn appropriate responses to their infant. The infant may be interpreted to the parents: "Jamie likes firm touch...like this." Teach parents how to recognize a stressed infant and how to intervene. **At the same time, be sure to acknowledge the parents' knowledge of the infant and support them. Above all, do not patronize. Professionals have much to learn from parents, who are "professionals" in their own right. The prime rule of relating to infants is this: The infant leads; the adult follows.**

Feeding a premature infant may be difficult, because the infant "goes to sleep" during feedings. The usual parental ministrations of talking to the infant, soothing with touch, or holding upright on the shoulder may not work with a fussy, irritable preterm infant.

The preterm infant's behavior may be so disorganized, unpredictable, or misunderstood by the parents that an appropriate response is not possible.[2,103]

Critical Findings

SELF-REGULATORY VERSUS STRESS BEHAVIORS

ORGANIZATION	DISORGANIZATION
Physiologic	
Cardiorespiratory: stable heart and/or respiratory rate; regular, slow respirations	Cardiorespiratory: increase or decrease in respiratory rate; irregular respirations; apnea; gasping; bradycardia; blood pressure instability; sneezing, hiccoughs, coughing, sighing
Color: pink, stable	Color: mottling, duskiness; cyanosis—central or generalized; pallor or plethora
Gastrointestinal: tolerates feedings	Gastrointestinal: abdominal distention; spitting up; vomiting; gagging; stooling
Behavioral	
Body movements smooth and synchronous: consistent tone of all body parts; arms and legs flexed with smooth movements	Tremors, jittery and jerking movements; hypotonia or hypertonia (flaccid trunk, extremities; movements arching, flailing, extended extremities; finger splays, fisting)
States: well-defined sleep-wake	Unable to modulate states: sudden state changes; more active than quiet sleep; awake states with gaze aversion, frowning, grimacing, staring, irritability, wide-eyed "help me" look
Self-quieting behaviors: hand-to-mouth, hand or foot clasping, finger folding or grasping, sucking, foot or leg bracing	Limited use of self-quieting behaviors (may need assistance from caregiver)
Attentive behaviors: alert gaze; fixes and follows visual stimuli; ceases to suck or slows suck rate, turns toward auditory stimuli, smiles; imitates; opens mouth, extends tongue; vocalizes: coos, babbles, habituates to stimuli	May demonstrate any of above stress signals when attempting to interact with one or more modes of stimuli (e.g., rocking, talking) simultaneously in environment (either animate or inanimate)

Data from Als H, Brazelton TB: A new model of assessing the behavioral organization in preterm and full-term infants: two case studies, *J Am Acad Child Psychiatry* 20:239, 1981; Gorski PA: Stages of behavioral organization in the high-risk neonate: theoretical and clinical considerations, *Semin Perinatol* 3:61, 1979.

Thus parents often become exhausted, bewildered, and frustrated in their encounters with their preterm infant's behavioral response to their care as rejecting and unloving: "My baby doesn't like me." **Teach parents that their infant's disorganization with stimuli is related to prematurity (i.e., an immature CNS) and not to parent ministrations.** Reassure them that as the premature infant grows and evidences maturational changes, he or she will be able to tolerate more stimulation and will be more responsive to their care.

Just as parent-infant interaction is responsible for normal development of the term infant, parent-infant interaction is crucial in the development of at-risk infants.[46,165] Many parents of premature infants have been observed making heroic efforts, over long periods, to interact with their less alert, active, and responsive infants.[75,103,177] Parenting the preterm has been described as "more work and less fun." **"Setting parents up to succeed" involves placing parents in situations in which they will experience positive feedback from their infants.** Suggesting and role modeling intervention strategies show parents what and how to play and interact with their infants. Parent participation in intervention strategies is ensured by stressing how important it is to infant development, that professionals are too busy to provide all the necessary interventions, and that parents are in a unique position to provide developmental care in the hospital and at home after discharge. **Parents, with help from professionals, are the ideal planners and providers of developmentally appropriate intervention strategies.**[46] The beneficial effects of parent involvement in developmental care of VLBW infants include better interaction with and perception of the infant and improved cognitive development (see Table 13-1).

A rooming-in setting for parents and their at-risk newborns is the best environment for cues to be learned and care given according to these cues. **Unlimited and unrestricted contact of parents and newborns should be the policy in every normal, medium-risk, and high-risk nursery (see Box 29-2).** Providing a family room, bonding room, or apartment in which parents and their soon-to-be-discharged newborn can room-in helps the transition from hospital to home care. Rooming-in before discharge gives mothers and fathers an opportunity to assume full responsibility for their infant's care, tests the reality of caregiving, helps them learn caregiving activities and their infant's behavior patterns, and confirms their readiness for independent parenting and the infant's readiness for discharge.

Intervention Strategies

Because infants experience their environment through sensory processes, intervention strategies are based on tactile/kinesthetic, auditory, visual, olfactory/gustatory, and communication skills. Interventions must be individualized according to the infant's state, sensory threshold, physiologic homeostasis, and stability or stress cues.[79,109,119,147]

CIRCADIAN RHYTHMS

In utero, the states of the fetus are regulated by the sleep-wake cycles of the mother. **In the NICU, multiple intrusions disrupt regulation.[228-230] How this affects an infant is not fully known, although limited energy may be drained, the infant may be subjected to further stress,[2,105] and outcomes of therapeutic interventions may not be optimized.** To minimize interruptions and excessive handling, infants should not be awakened when asleep; if they must be awakened for care, it should be during active sleep by talking softly and stroking gently.[71,262] Appointments for examinations should be made before feeding to decrease unnecessary disturbance of sleep but with enough rest time (if needed) before actual feeding.

Adequate numbers of caregiving encounters—physical assessment, vital signs, diaper or linen change, and procedures—must be balanced against constant manipulations.[103] **Because essentially all NICU (levels II and III) infants are continuously monitored, "laying on of hands" every 1 to 2 hours is often unnecessary. Thorough physical assessment and vital sign recording every 4 hours is easily alternated with recordings from the monitors every 4 hours. Thus the infant is evaluated every 2 hours but not disturbed that often.** An acutely ill infant may need closer observation, but alternating "hands-on" with monitor readings accomplishes the goal without overwhelming an infant with few reserves.

Sleep-wake patterns are influenced by feeding method,[263] temperature, position,[162] CNS maturation,[191] birth weight, caregiving practices,[262] and environmental effects (e.g., ambient light, noise).[191,228-230] Sleep-wake patterns in breast-fed and bottle-fed infants differ. Full-term breast-fed infants awaken more and sleep less during the night.[99] In one study, preterm breast-fed infants cried approximately 1 hour more during the day than preterm infants being bottle fed with formula.[263] Although being held in skin-to-skin contact, babies sleep 50% to 75% of the time with no change in the amount of quiet sleep.[162]

Day-night cycles are facilitated by afternoon nap time and nighttime in which the dimming of lights or covering of incubators and cribs with blankets and quieting of NICU noise enable infants to sleep. Deep, quiet sleep is facilitated by quiet and dark, soft (classical) music, gentle stroking of the head, and self-regulated tasks (self-sought proximity of infant to "breathing bear").[261] Maintaining daily nap time and nighttime hours helps infants reset their diurnal rhythms and become accustomed to sleeping in dim light and a quiet environment (something that babies discharged from the hospital for even short stays have difficulty doing). Among convalescing preterm infants (<34 weeks gestational age), four standard rest periods per day resulted in (1) increased daily weight gain, (2) increased sleep, (3) less-active states during nap time, (4) decreased occurrences of apnea, and (5) by 3 weeks, less quiet waking time and longer uninterrupted sleep episodes.[117,271] Uninterrupted sleep and diurnal rhythmicity also are associated with improved state organization in VLBW infants.[229,230]

TACTILE AND KINESTHETIC INTERVENTION

Because the sense of touch is highly developed in utero, even a very immature preterm has acute tactile sensitivity. **For newborns, human touch is the most important tactile stimulation.** Not all touch is equal, however, nor is it responded to equally by term or preterm infants who are well, critically ill, or recovering from illness. One study has shown the effect of the vulnerability of low-birth-weight (LBW) infants in their response to the nurturing touch of their mothers. Nurturing maternal touch was associated with a secure attachment in robust infants; in highly vulnerable, sick LBW infants, this same nurturing touch was associated with a less secure attachment.[283] Any type of tactile stimulation is composed of six factors: duration, location, action, intensity, frequency, and sensation. **Tactile sensation both arouses and quiets. Gentle but firm handling quiets infants because they feel more secure; light, uncertain touch often results in agitation and withdrawal. Handling for routine care (e.g., vital signs, changing the diaper or position, venipuncture for blood draws or placement of IV lines, feeding, heel sticks, suction, and physical or neurologic examinations) can result in hypoxia, increased intracranial pressure, episodes of apnea/bradycardia, agitation, and increased or decreased heart rate and blood pressure.***

Handling. **How a neonate is handled during care affects his or her physiologic and behavioral response. Use of body containment during suction decreases the physiologic and behavioral responses to this stressful procedure.**[260] Comparing preterm responses to swaddled and unswaddled weighing, unswaddled infants exhibit more physiologic distress, more motor disorganization, poorer self-regulation, and more need for caregiver facilitation than when they were swaddled for weighing.[204] Transferring preterm infants from the incubator to the parent for holding or KC is stressful. One study evaluated physiologic disorganization in preterms based on the method of transfer from the incubator for KC (e.g., nurse picking up the baby and transferring him or her to the parent versus the parent picking the baby up directly from the incubator).[205] Both transfer methods resulted in increased physiologic and motor disorganization (i.e., oxygen desaturation, tachycardia, cyanosis/pallor, hypotonia, decreased self-regulation, and increased need for caregiver facilitation to maintain physiologic stability during transfer). In both methods of transfer (which lasted 6 to 9 minutes), the ventilator was disconnected (for 5 seconds). Both the infant's desaturation readings and tachycardia recovered to baseline levels faster with the parent transfer; during and after KC, oxygen saturation and heart rate returned to baseline values.[205]

Excessive handling of preterm or sick neonates results in significant physiologic consequences, such as blood pressure changes, alterations in cerebral blood flow, and hypoxia and other stress behaviors.[155,248] A particularly vulnerable group of preterm infants, those with periventricular leukomalacia (PVL), react to handling and multisensory stimulation (e.g., auditory, tactile, visual, vestibular) with an increase in heart rate above their already higher resting heart rate.[290] These CNS-injured preterms require close observation and monitoring during handling, stressful procedures, and interventions.[290]

A total body position change is not considered a painful procedure, but in LBW preterm infants with endotracheal tubes and umbilical artery catheters, the handling necessary to change the infant's position elicits pain behaviors.[81] Nonpainful tactile stimulation (e.g., routine nursery handling) of preterm infants has been shown to produce equal or higher levels of physiologic stress activation than does a painful stimulus (e.g., heel stick).[114] In the same study, the relatively low behavioral activation during "routine handling" led the researchers to conclude that this tactile stimulus was not unpleasant to the infants, even though it produced a high level of physiologic stress response. Perhaps the low behavioral response to being handled is analogous to the variable behavioral pain responses of the preterm infant and the lack of a behavioral response does not mean that the preterm neonate is not experiencing pain (see Chapter 12). Another study of diaper change (with and without developmental support in VLBW preterms) showed a significant decrease in pain scores and hypoxic events with developmental care.[248]

In the NICU, infants who are repeatedly subjected to painful, intrusive procedures develop touch aversion—the association of human touch with pain. Tactile vulnerability has also been found in infants who require multiple postnatal medical interventions, who are exposed to illicit drugs in utero, and whose mothers had their own predisposition regarding being touched (a genetic component?).[282] These infants cry uncontrollably, squirm

*References 59,60,80,114,155,211,248,257.

away, flail arms and legs, and recoil when touched, knowing that pain will soon follow. An infant who has received ventilatory therapy may have touch aversion around the mouth: the infant is averse to facial stroking and rooting, has a hypersensitive gag reflex, and refuses to nipple feed. **Painful procedures should be minimized to those absolutely (medically) indicated—no infant should be subjected to "routine" painful procedures. During those necessary procedures, it is essential to provide body containment, comfort measures (e.g., a pacifier), and adequate pain relief (see Chapter 12).**

Touch. Touch that is not related to caregiving (i.e., social contact) should be provided by parents and professionals when the preterm infant is aware, alert, and receptive. When parents touch their babies, the amount and types of touch vary widely—most frequently, holding, stroking, rubbing, or placing a finger in the infant's hand. Preterm infants respond individually and physiologically to their parents' touch; there is more variation in heart rate and oxygen saturation levels compared with baseline values. These variations depend on gestational age, infant state, and the amount of handling before parent handling.[110] **Less touching by the nurse within the 2 hours before parental holding results in less mean decrease in heart rate during parental holding.**[110] Parents provide more positive touch (kissing and stroking); preterm infants are more likely to smile and sleep for their parents when compared with the increase in sleep-wake transitions, larger body movements, and jitters exhibited after a nurse's touch. In animal studies, increased parental touching in infancy results in changes in brain structure, decreased levels of stress hormones, and better ability to survive a stressful environment.[181,280] Perhaps parental touch of preterm humans enables them to withstand the stress of illness and the NICU environment.[83]

Nonpainful touch such as stroking (the head, trunk, or hands) during care may calm, soothe, and prevent touch aversion. **Stroking of physiologically stable preterm infants has been associated with increased activity and alertness, a faster regaining of birth weight, more rapid weight gain, less crying and apnea, enhanced developmental status, and better social scores.**[109] **In studies of ventilated preterms, stroking resulted in no adverse effects on oxygenation and respiratory and heart rates.**[64] **However, in preterm infants (26 to 30 weeks' gestation) who are *not* physiologically stable, stroking results in decreased oxygen saturation, signs of behavioral stress (e.g., grasping, grunting, gaze aversion), and more avoidance cues (e.g., grimacing, yawning, fussing or crying, tongue protrusion).** Other behavioral and physiologic effects include heart rate and blood pressure changes, changes in respiratory rate and rhythm, increase in avoidance signals (e.g., increased startle reflex, agitation, crying), increase in activity and movement, and decreased visual responsivity.[60,110,155,205]

If the preterm infant becomes agitated with stroking, a hand firmly placed on the head and lower back, buttocks, or abdomen often quiets.[57,108] **Hand placement without stroking does not decrease oxygen saturation or alter heart rate and has a soothing effect (i.e., decreases active sleep, increases quiet sleep, and decreases motor activity and behavioral distress) on small preterm infants.**[112,193] **Handle gently to avoid stressful reactions (e.g., flailing, arching, oxygen desaturation) and enable the infant to become calm and rest between caregiving.** Parents should be taught and encouraged to provide their preterm with "gentle human touch"[108,193] in the form of supportive containment with their hands, use of gradual and rhythmic action, observation of infant responses (see the Critical Findings box on p. 291), and modification, alteration, or cessation of touch when necessary.[41,108,109,111] Maternal use of stimulating touch over the first year of life in preterm LBW infants results in improved infant development of visual-motor and language expression, and frequency of touch improves gross motor development.[284]

Massage. The touching and stroking of massage stimulate nerve pathways and aid myelinization by increasing hypothalamic activity and production of the growth hormone ***somatotropin.*** In animal studies, touch deprivation decreases growth hormone secretion, which results in undergrowth of all organ systems; a return to normal secretion occurs with tactile stimulation.[242] More recently, a growth gene that responds to tactile stimulation has been discovered; this suggests a genetic origin for the touch-growth relationship.[89] Because touch stimulation of the inside of a neonate's mouth increases the release of gastrointestinal food absorption hormones (i.e., gastrin, insulin), it is postulated that the tactile stimulation of massage leads to a similar hormone release. Current assays of glucose and insulin levels in heel-stick samples of preterm infants suggest that massaged infants show increased levels of insulin.[89]

Research on massage therapy with preterm infants has been conducted on medically stable growing infants (i.e., preterm growers) (Table 13-4). Massage therapy provides social touch rather than painful touch, prevents or treats touch aversion, and should be taught to and provided by parents in the hospital and at home.[88,180] Confidence in parenting skills and tactile communication between parents and infant are encouraged when parents massage their infant. **Because massage has not been studied**

TABLE 13-4 BENEFITS OF MASSAGE WITH PRETERM INFANTS: RESEARCH BASIS

STUDY	RESULTS
40 preterm "growers" (31 wk GA; 1280 g BW; 20 days of NICU care) massaged for 15 min, 3 times/day for 10 days[89]	Gained 47% more weight (no difference in caloric intake) More awake/active time Better performance on habituation, orientation, and motor activity; regulation of state behavior Hospitalized 6 days less (cost saving $3000/infant) Infant preferred some degree of pressure (rather than light stroking) 1 year later: weight advantage, better performance on developmental scales—higher mental and motor scores
Three times/day massage of preterms with physiologic and biochemical measurements[240]	21% increase in daily weight gain Discharged 5 days earlier Superior performance on habituation Fewer stress behaviors (mouthing, grimacing, clenched fists) Increase in catecholamine secretion in neonatal period (analogous to the normal developmental increase after birth) Increase in vagal activity
10 healthy preterm "growers": 3 times/day massage for 15 min in a randomized sequence of 5 days of massage and 5 days without massage[142]	Energy expenditure significantly lower after 5 days of massage than after 5 days without massage in metabolically and thermally stable preterms Decreased energy expenditure may contribute to enhanced growth caused by massage
Massaged for 15 min three times/day for 5 days:	Fewer stress behaviors and less activity from first to last day of the study
68 preterms (mean GA = 30 wks) with either light-pressure or moderate-pressure massage[90]	Moderate-pressure group: significantly more daily weight gain; more relaxed, less aroused than light-pressure group
80 preterms randomized to moderate-pressure massage or standard care[65]	Increase in vagal activity and gastric motility, which may contribute to greater weight gain in massaged preterms
72 preterms randomized to massage or control therapy[66]	Greater increase in body temperature in massage versus control preterms (even though incubator portholes were open for the massage but not for the control group)
MOTHER MASSAGE	
57 healthy preterm "growers" (6-34 wks GA; 600-2200 g) massaged for 15 min, three times/day, for 10 days by mother and a trained professional[88]	Gained 21%-47% more weight (no difference in caloric intake) Mother-massaged babies gained as much weight (about 6 g/day) as babies massaged by professionals (about 8 g/day) when compared with the control group who were not massaged Significant weight gain occurred across a wide range of gestational ages Cost-effective parental intervention
104 VLBW infants (≥750 to ≤1500 g; ≤32 wks GA) randomized to control or standard care with maternal massage four times/day of face and limbs with passive limb exercises[185]	Significantly lower incidence of late-onset sepsis Discharged from the hospital 7 days earlier

BW, Birth weight; *GA*, gestational age; *NICU*, neonatal intensive care unit; *VLBW*, very low birth weight.

in acutely ill preterm infants, its use should be confined to preterm growers.[41,89,277] Chronically ill infants (e.g., babies with BPD or congenital heart disease) may exhibit physiologic and behavioral disorganization with massage, so the risk-benefit ratio must be assessed carefully.[41]

Varying sensations and touch patterns keep infants interested in stroking and massaging. As a preterm infant matures and is able to tolerate variety, he or she should be introduced to different textures (e.g., lambskins, stuffed toys, cotton, satin). Baby clothes provide various textures, decrease heat loss (especially hats), and make the infant more attractive ("He looks like a real baby!"; "She looks like a girl, because her shaved head is covered!").

Holding. **When the infant is preterm or a sick term baby, holding him or her, an essential step of parent attachment, is disrupted.** Some NICUs promote parental holding as soon as possible, whereas others have specific protocols about weight criteria and extubation before parents are able to hold their infant.[94] A national survey on holding policies found (1) written protocols for conventional holding (26%) and for KC (40%), (2) for extubated infants: 73% offered KC, 99% conventional holding, and (3) for holders of extubated babies: mothers 73% KC, fathers 68% KC, and 99% conventional holding for both parents.[94] Potential benefits of enhanced parent-infant interaction and attachment,[137] closeness of parents to their infant, increased lactation, and improved parental self-esteem are factors that influence staff to facilitate holding.[94]

KC (Figure 13-2), skin-to-skin contact between parents and infant by placing the infant in a vertical position between the maternal or paternal breasts, benefits both parents and neonates (Box 13-2). KC improves physiologic self-regulation, reduces stress and crying, reduces pain, and facilitates neurodevelopment and maturation for the neonate.[83-87] For the mother, KC functions to reverse the negative effects of preterm birth and separation and enhances both early and long-term maternal-infant interactions.[1,83,85,86]

KC for the healthy preterm has been used in the delivery room, in the transitional period (see Chapter 5), for adoptive parents,[208] and for transport.[250] National surveys of holding/KC have been conducted and have found that KC is practiced more commonly in subspecialty (level III) than in specialty (level II) care NICUs.[78,94] One of the surveys

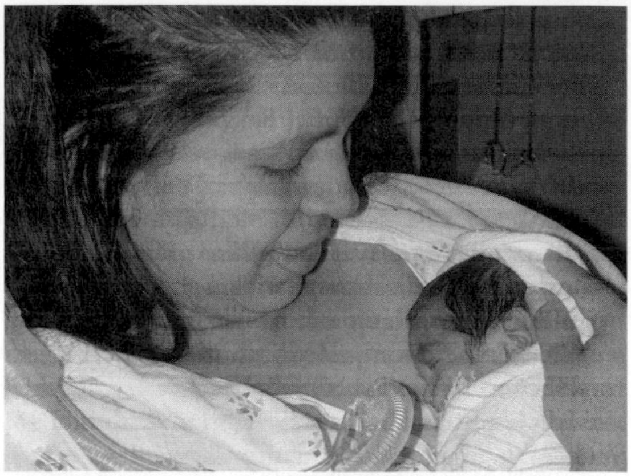

FIGURE 13-2 Kangaroo care. (From Ballweg D: Individualized care: actions for individualized staff member. In Kenner C, McGrath J, editors: *Developmental care of newborns and infants*, St Louis, 2004, Mosby.)

found that 82% of the respondent NICUs practice KC, generally upon parental request (87%); nurses were knowledgeable about KC; and most (93%) did not know that transfer of the infant to the parent's chest is the most stressful aspect of KC.[78]

KC is well tolerated in the first week of life by preterm infants with current or resolving neonatal illness. A recent RCT in healthy preterms (33 to 35 weeks GA) found that KC for 3 hours improved breathing patterns and resulted in no apnea or bradycardia or periodic breathing or temperature instability.[156] KC improves gas exchange in preterm infants of less than 1800 g. The smallest infants (<1000 g) remained more clinically stable (i.e., smallest increase in heart rate, highest decrease in respiratory rate and increase in oxygen saturation, no hypothermia) when compared with infants larger than 1000 g.[93]

When KC was compared with conventional cuddling care (i.e., mother holding her swaddled, clothed infant), there was no difference in maintenance of vital signs, oxygenation, parental stress/expectation, or breast feeding.[231] In another study, the total time spent in KC was less than was expected because of (1) cultural constraints, (2) interruptions for routine care, and (3) desire of the mother for others to hold the infant.[17] Recommendations from this study include provision of privacy, support and education to mothers about the benefits of KC, minimization of interruptions, and adjustment of care to promote longer periods of continuous holding.[17]

BOX 13-2 BENEFITS OF KANGAROO CARE/SKIN-TO-SKIN CONTACT*

Parental

- Activates maternal processes of search for meaning and mastery of the experience of premature birth
- Increases maternal self-confidence, competence, and self-esteem
- Enhances parent-infant attachment
- Initiates and maintains maternal behavior
- Positively affects mother's mood/behavior; less maternal depression; calming
- Positive and personally beneficial experience
- Positively affects parental identity and knowledge of infant[234]
- Increases confidence in meeting infant's needs
- More frequent visiting
- Parental eagerness for infant's discharge
- Long term:
  - More consistent/contingent maternal responses at 15 months of age
  - More sensitive, less intrusive, more reciprocal interactions from 6 months to 2 years from both mothers and fathers
  - More affectionate touch, more adaptive to infant signals, and infants more alert during interactions at 3 to 6 months
  - Less maternal separation anxiety at 6 months
  - Improved family cohesiveness

Neonatal

- Thermal synchrony: mother's body temperature rises and falls to maintain infant in neutral state (see Chapter 6)
- Cardiopulmonary:
  - Adequate or improved oxygenation
  - Fewer/no episodes of periodic breathing, apnea, and bradycardia
  - Lower heart rate/stable respiratory rate
  - Higher vagal tone: indicative of quicker maturation of the autonomic nervous system
- Breast feeding:
  - Increased incidence and length
  - Increased milk supply
- Behavioral:
  - Increased alert activity
  - Increased deep sleep
  - Improved self-regulation: sleep-wake cycles, arousal, sustained exploration
  - Better emotional regulation and arousal modulation for interaction and rest
  - Decreased stress response: decrease in beta-endorphin and cortisol levels
  - Decreased or no crying[80,81]
  - Increased ***en face*** positioning
  - Better orientation and habituation
  - Less pain response to painful procedure (e.g., heel lance) in both preterm and term infants[128,140,159]
- Earlier discharge:
  - Increased weight gain
  - No increased infection/fewer infections; decreased severity of infection and mortality
  - Out of incubator earlier
- Regulatory interaction:
  - Behavioral
  - Sucking
  - Neurochemical
  - Metabolic
  - Sleep-wake cycles/improved sleep organization[160]
  - Cardiovascular
  - Endocrine
  - Immune
  - Circadian
- Long-term:
  - Increased length and head circumference at 9 months and 1 year of age
  - Less crying at 6 months of age
  - Higher psychomotor scales at 6 months and higher mental scales at 6 months to 2 years
  - Enhanced mental and psychomotor development at 1 year

*Data compiled from references 1,42,49,55,83-87,93,107,156,158,162,178,183,206,233,234.

Parental holding is often (17% to 33%) limited or not supported by nurses and physicians.[94] Barriers to holding infants include (1) infant safety concerns (e.g., accidental extubation, loss of arterial/venous lines, vital sign or oxygenation instability) and (2) reluctance of professionals and families to initiate or participate in KC (e.g., adding to workload, difficulty providing care, lack of experience, used for babies who are not developmentally ready, belief that technology is better than KC).[78,94] More than 60% of NICUs responding to one survey stated that low birth weight and gestational age were not contraindications for KC; many NICUs did not permit KC for babies on high-frequency

BOX 13-3 SELECTION CRITERIA FOR KANGAROO CARE WITH VENTILATED INFANTS

- Birth weight >600 g; ≥30 weeks GA
- Ventilator for at least 24 hr before first kangaroo care
- SIMV: <35 breaths/min; FIO_2 <0.50 (50%)
- Stable vital signs (TPR; B/P) and oxygen saturation
- Stable blood gases, bilirubin level
- No signs/symptoms of sepsis
- Not receiving vasopressors; no chest tube
- Lines (Broviac, umbilical, arterial, IVs) well secured

Modified from Ludington-Hoe S, Morgan K, Abouelfrettoh A: A clinical guideline for implementation of kangaroo care with premature infants of 30 or more weeks' postmenstrual age, *Adv Neonatal Care* 8:S3, 2008.

B/P, Blood pressure; *FIO_2*, fraction of inspired oxygen; *GA*, gestational age; *IV*, intravenous; *SIMV*, synchronous intermittent mandatory ventilation; *TPR*, temperature, pulse, respiration.

oscillator ventilation (HFOV) or vasopressors.[78] **All infants being held either conventionally or by KC should be continuously monitored for vital signs and oxygen saturation.**[156]

"Risky populations" for KC include infants who are intubated, have arterial/venous lines and chest tubes, are on pressors to maintain blood pressure, and are on HFOV. One of the national surveys found that 64% of NICUs offered conventional holding to parents of intubated infants and 45% offered KC of intubated infants.[94] The survey does not indicate if the 36% of NICUs that do not offer holding of an intubated infant "enforce the rule" if the infant requires prolonged intubation (1 to 2 weeks). The other survey found that 60% of NICU nurse managers think that intubated infants should not receive KC.[78] Several small case studies of ventilated infants receiving KC show increase in quiet sleep, decrease in oxygen requirement, higher or stable oxygen saturations, stable body temperature, fewer apnea episodes, and decrease in airway resistance during KC. Only one case study showed a need for higher oxygen concentration (14%), possibly because of an increase in body temperature during KC. None of these studies discuss selection criteria or the procedure for KC or are multicenter RCTs.

Based on a 3-year study in five NICUs of mechanically ventilated infants receiving KC, selection criteria (Box 13-3) and a safe protocol (Box 13-4) for KC in this population have been developed.[158,161] During this study, no adverse physiologic or behavioral events or accidental extubations occurred. None of these babies was agitated, and all slept and tolerated KC well. Previously reported parental perceptions of KC with ventilated babies include the following:

- Ambivalence toward KC: yearning to hold the infant yet being apprehensive about it
- The necessity of a supportive environment
- The special quality of parent-infant interaction: intense connectedness and active parenting

Perhaps these parental concerns, as well as staff concerns, may be overcome with careful selection of infants, a consistent procedure for transfer, increase in confidence of the staff assisting parents in KC, and a clinical guideline for implementing KC.[158,161]

Parents and staff need education about KC, and staff can offer KC to parents instead of waiting for parents to request this intervention.* Recommendations about KC include the following:

- It is an important therapeutic intervention for healthy preterms (gestational age ≥34 weeks) and their mothers in a modern, well-equipped NICU[156,288] as recommended by the World Health Organization (WHO).[295]
- It is a simple, safe, cost-effective intervention that reduces severe infant morbidity without serious side effects, and more well-designed randomized controlled trials are needed.[55]
- Mothers need a trusting relationship and individualized support from health care providers to be comfortable with KC.[203]

One should also note that fathers can also participate in KC without endangering the infant. Aside from the positive effects on the baby, paternal KC very often enhances the engagement and attachment of the father to the infant and includes him in the infant's care.

Bathing. **There is a lack of evidence of the safety and efficacy of sponge bathing preterm babies in the NICU on a daily or every-other-day schedule.**[95] **Sponge bathing critically ill preterm infants (28 to 34 weeks gestational age) results in significant increases in behavior state and activity levels (i.e., motor stress behavior, stability, reorganization), increase in stress cue**

*References 17,42,67,78,83,156.

BOX 13-4

PROTOCOL FOR KANGAROO CARE WITH VENTILATED INFANTS

In Preparation for Transfer

1. Record baseline vital signs, oxygen saturation, and ventilator settings. Secure and maintain continuous monitoring of these parameters during kangaroo care (KC) to determine infant's tolerance of KC.
2. Place infant supine on a clean blanket (folded in fourths) with assistance of second person, and note changes in vital signs, saturations, or ventilator settings.
3. Auscultate chest and evaluate breath sounds, suction endotracheal tube, and change diaper.
4. Drain water from ventilator tubings to decrease resistance, maintain airflow, and prevent retrograde water flow toward infant when moved or positioned lower than or at the level of the ventilator.
5. Assess infant's responses: Wait 15 minutes to enable physiologic adaptation (e.g., return of baseline vital signs/oxygenation for 3 minutes). If still unstable at 15 minutes, the infant is probably not stable enough for KC at this time.
6. Position the reclining chair near the ventilator, making sure there is ample tubing length.
7. Two or three staff members will assist the parent in transfer of the infant:
   - One person gathers lines to one side of the infant.
   - One person transfers and secures the ventilator tubing.
   - One person assists the parent.

Transfer Procedure

1. After a staff member disconnects the endotracheal tube (ETT) from the ventilator, the parent slides his or her hands under the blanket and infant, lifts both, and places the infant prone against his or her chest in one movement. Reconnect the ventilator tubing, and let the infant stabilize. (If the infant was not placed on a clean blanket or it was soiled before transfer, the parent can lift the baby and a clean blanket is placed over the infant when he or she is prone on the parent's chest.)
2. Disconnect ventilator tubing from ETT and move parent backward toward recliner, having him or her sit down when he or she feels the edge of the chair against the calves of the legs. Reconnect the ETT to the ventilator tubing.
3. Assist the parent in being comfortable by raising the footrest, position the infant in a flexed position with head and neck in a neutral position to avoid ETT movement (e.g., downward into the bronchi with head flexion or possible extubation with head extension) and/or obstructive apnea with head flexion or extension if the infant is on nasal continuous positive airway pressure.
4. Secure the ventilator tubing by draping it over the parent's shoulder. ***Do not tape the tubing to the blanket, parent clothing, etc.***
5. If using ISC temperature control (on the radiant warmer/incubator), turn to air control, set temperature at 33° C while the baby is receiving KC, and monitor the infant's skin temperature from the temperature gauge on the radiant warmer/incubator. (There is then no need to uncover or cold stress the infant to take a temperature.)
6. Maintain continuous electronic monitoring throughout KC; check both the infant's and/or parent's condition every 10 minutes during KC.
7. If the infant's condition remains stable, facilitate KC for a minimum of 1 hour.

Transfer After Kangaroo Care

1. Slowly place the recliner in an upright position, and assist parent to move forward to the front edge of the chair.
2. One staff handles the lines and another disconnects the ETT from the ventilator lines.
3. Assist the parent to stand, reconnect the ETT to the ventilator tubing, and let the infant stabilize.
4. In one movement, disconnect the ventilator tubing and place the infant in the radiant warmer/incubator.
5. Reconnect the ventilator tubing to the ETT, stabilize, and secure all lines inside the radiant warmer/incubator.
6. Document KC, length of session, and how the infant and parent tolerated KC.

Modified from Ludington-Hoe S, Ferreira C, Swinth J: Safe criteria and procedure for kangaroo care with intubated preterm infants, *J Obstet Gynecol Neonat Nurs* 32:586, 2003; Ludington-Hoe S, Morgan K, Abouelfrettoh A: A clinical guideline for implementation of kangaroo care with premature infants of 30 or more weeks' postmenstrual age, *Adv Neonatal Care* 8:S3, 2008.
ISC, Infant servocontrol.

frequency, increase or decrease in heart rate, and decrease in oxygen saturation.[211] These detrimental effects caused by handling were exhibited most frequently by neonates of younger gestational ages. Because sponge bathing of critically ill preterm infants clearly increases physiologic risk and provides no clear benefits, the procedure of routine bathing of these infants is unnecessary and not recommended.[212] Frequency of sponge bathing can be reduced to every 4 days without increasing skin flora colony counts or colonization with pathogens.[95] Waiting to bathe these infants until they are physiologically stable with introduction of the bath as a "recovery milestone" for parents to complete is a more developmentally and physiologically appropriate practice.[212] Parents may tub bathe the premature grower, and this may provide a soothing, relaxing, tension-relieving experience of multiple textures (i.e., water, water temperature, soap, washcloth). However, a recent study of the effects of tub bathing on preterm infants (done by nurses) found disruption of sleep and an increase in stress behaviors; the study recommended considering the effects of "routine" nursing procedures and modifying handling of the preterm to promote recovery, growth, and development and to decrease stress.[152]

Self-Consoling. Consoling hand-to-mouth behaviors are observed more frequently during caregiving (by nurses, rather than parents) and before and after feeding (especially in gavage-fed infants). **Hand-to-midline behaviors are encouraged by cradling the infant for feedings (for both bottle and gavage feedings if the infant tolerates it) with both arms in the midline.** If a premature infant needs an oxygen hood, using one large enough so that the infant's whole upper body will fit inside encourages hand-to-mouth quieting (Figure 13-3). VLBW preterm infants whose whole body was not inside the oxygen hood have been videotaped expending energy in persistent attempts (30 to 40 minutes) to self-console and reduce stress by trying to get their hands to their mouths.

Use arm restraints only when necessary, and immobilize the extremity in a physiologic position. Release and exercise the restrained extremity with each caregiving encounter. Avoid restraining both arms so that one is free for hand-to-mouth behaviors. If both must be restrained (e.g., the infant pulls out the orogastric tube), give the infant a pacifier.

Positioning. Preterm infants display motor development that is different from that of term infants.[197,238,256] A continuous assessment of muscle tone, response to positioning and handling, oral-motor function, and response to sensory stimuli provides data for individualizing intervention. The goal of intervention is to provide opportunities for normal development and organization of the sensory systems, detect early developmental problems, and educate parents about stimulation, handling, and positioning. Although some studies have shown that specific positioning for premature infants does not significantly affect development, others have shown that a developmental approach to care of VLBW infants greatly reduces the long-term effects of prematurity.[70,199] VLBW and full-term infants achieve the same fine and gross motor milestones although the developmental pathways of milestone achievement is different: early (in the first 8 months of life of the VLBW infant), fine motor control develops almost to the exclusion of gross motor development.

Preterm infants usually have less developed physiologic flexion in the limbs, trunk, and pelvis compared with term newborns (Table 13-5). Even at 40 weeks post-conceptual age, preterm infants have less flexion than their full-term counterparts have. For preterm infants, long periods of immobilization without a positioning device on a firm mattress with the influences of gravity result in a number of abnormal characteristics: (1) increased

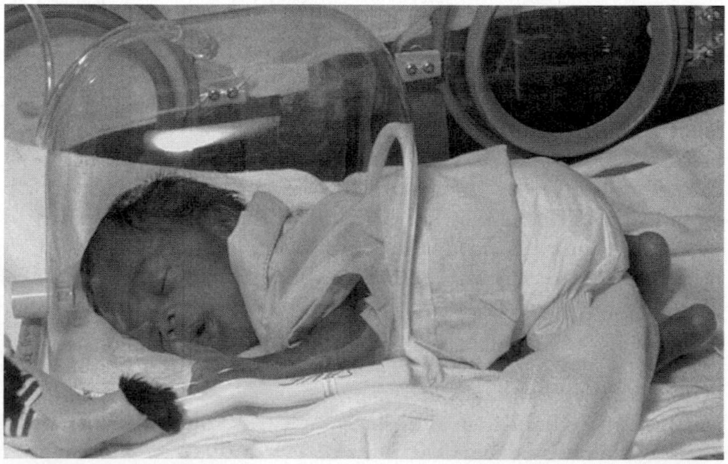

FIGURE 13-3 Preterm infant in oxygen hood that is large enough to accommodate upper body to facilitate hand-to-mouth behavior. Note sling that helps maintain flexion without frogleg position.

TABLE 13-5 DEVELOPMENT OF TONE*

GESTATIONAL AGE (wk)	DEVELOPMENT
28	Completely hypotonic and lacks all physiologic flexion
32	Hips and knees begin to show some flexion while arms remain extended
34	Flexor tone apparent in legs
36	Loose flexion of arms and legs evident and grasp reflex present
40	Develops tone in utero and develops flexed position in intrauterine space; after birth, reflex activity and central nervous system maturity help term infant unfold and extend; term infant holds all four limbs in flexed position

From Anderson J, Auster-Liebhaber J: *Phys Occup Ther Pediatr* 4(1): 1984; Dubowitz LM, Dubowitz V, Goldberg C: *J Pediatr* 77:1, 1970; Palisano R, Short M: *Phys Occup Ther Pediatr* 4(4):43, 1984.

*Muscle tone develops in caudocephalic and centripetal (distal to proximal) directions and interacts with simultaneous cephalocaudal development of movement to help affect posture. Although knowledge of normal development before term helps detect signs of abnormality, variability of ±2 weeks gestational age must be considered.[73,125]

neck extension with a right-sided head preference; (2) shoulder retraction and abduction (reduces forward rotation and ability to reach midline); (3) increased trunk extension with "arching" of the neck and back; (4) frogleg position: hips abducted and externally rotated; and (5) ankle and feet eversion (Figure 13-4).[125,197,256,273] These characteristics interfere with development of eye-hand coordination, head control in prone/sitting, crawling/walking, cognitive development, and equilibrium.[238,256] **Box 13-5 lists the reasons for proper positioning in the NICU.**

To prevent overstretching of the joints, facilitate development of flexor tone, and prevent deformities, the infant should be provided with a variety of positions.[256] Goals of proper positioning include (1) optimize alignment (e.g., neutral neck/trunk and foot positions), semiflexed, midline extremity posture, (2) support posture and movement within containment boundaries (avoid producing a barrier of immobilization), (3) modify positioning and handling to support behavioral state regulation of sleep-wake states, and (4) provide positions that encourage controlled, individual exposure to stimuli while monitoring for signs of behavioral stress from overstimulation and adjust stimuli accordingly.[256] A physical therapist can be helpful in facilitating these positions.

Side-lying is used to improve visual awareness of hands, encourage hands-to-midline

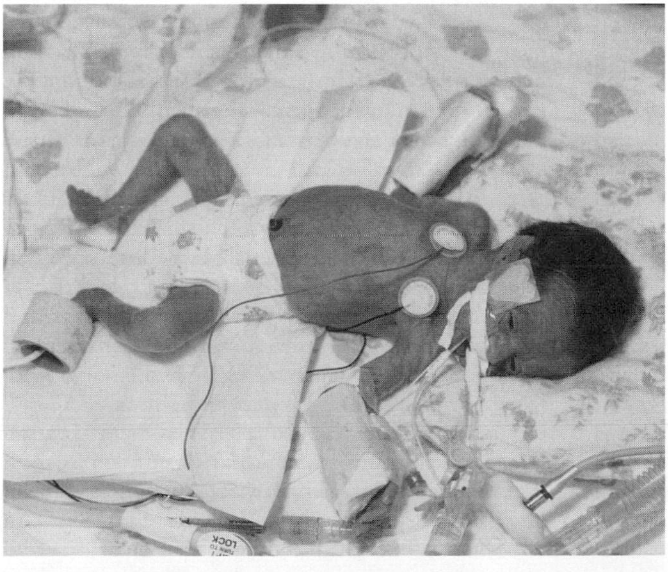

FIGURE 13-4 Premature infant hypotonic resting posture exhibiting the W configuration of arms, frogleg position of the legs, abducted hips, externally rotated ankles, everted feet, and asymmetric head position. This position promotes positional deformities and developmental gaps and delays. (From Hunter J: The neonatal intensive care unit. In Case-Smith J, editor: *Occupational therapy for children*, ed 4, St Louis, 2001, Mosby.)

BOX 13-5 REASONS FOR PROPER POSITIONING

1. Inhibits or shortens dystonic phase while infant remains in fetal position during postnatal period
2. Facilitates hand-to-midline and midline orientation[73,125]
3. Stimulates visual exploration of environment (through head to midline)
4. Facilitates development of head control (making feeding easier and helping respiratory problems)[73]
5. Helps balance flexors and extensors to facilitate symmetric posture[70,125,197,199,238]
6. Helps develop antigravity movement[125]
7. Enhances comfort and decreases stress[125]
8. Has an organizing effect that facilitates development of flexor tone[73,125,256]
9. Promotes normal and prevents abnormal development[70,73,125,238,256]
10. Helps enhance development of motor skills, reflexes, and postural tone*

From Pelletier-Sehnar JM, Palmeri A: High risk infants. In Pratt PN, Allen AS, editors: *Occupational therapy for children*, ed 2, St Louis, 1989, Mosby.
*References 70,125,199,238,256.

movement, and discourage the frogleg position. In this position, the infant can bring the hands to the mouth for sucking and self-comforting. Side-lying is best maintained with swaddling or commercial positioning devices rather than single blanket rolls (Figure 13-5). Position extremities so that the bottom arm is in a comfortable position and the upper shoulder and hip are slightly forward of the weight-bearing lower hip or shoulder, provide a small roll (e.g., folded cloth diaper or wash cloth or small bean-stuffed toy), and bundle for security but not so that the upper extremity compromises chest expansion.[125] Alternating sides reduces head molding and may prevent atelectasis of the dependent lung.[125,256] The head and trunk should be maintained in neutral alignment (e.g., the head and trunk are in the same vertical plane).[256]

To accommodate their ventilators, umbilical catheters, and other devices, acutely ill preterm infants may be positioned supine; the preterm's head should be in the midline. Positioning VLBW infants supine with their heads turned to either side causes mechanical obstruction of cerebral venous return and alters cerebral blood flow, which may contribute to the development of intraventricular hemorrhage (IVH).[210] **Supine positioning does not promote flexion and may be stressful to acutely ill infants.**[113,125] Earlier studies found an increase in apnea/bradycardia/periodic breathing in supine positioning,[113] although a recent study of 22 preterm infants with apnea and bradycardia found no significant difference in the incidence of clinically significant events between supine and prone positioning.[131] Placed supine, infants exhibit more startle behaviors, agitation, motor disorganization, calorie expenditure, and sleep disturbance from environmental stimuli.[125]

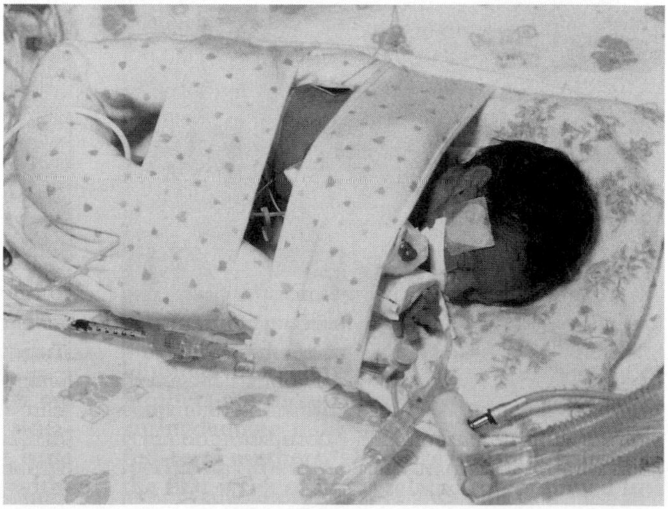

FIGURE 13-5 Small preterm infant in side-lying position supported in flexion and with a midline orientation of the extremities. (From Hunter J: The neonatal intensive care unit. In Case-Smith J, editor: *Occupational therapy for children*, ed 4, St Louis, 2001, Mosby.)

Prolonged supine positioning is associated with the hypertonic "arched" position (hyperextension of head, neck, and shoulder girdle) of many chronically ventilated infants (Figure 13-6); use of a gel or water pillow under the infant's head and neck (e.g., to the nipple level to prevent neck flexion; used as a mattress under the head or body of a VLBW infant) provides comfort and maintains neutral alignment.[125]

Supine positioning should promote as much flexion as possible. Use of a positioning device of foam with the middle cut out and sloping under the scapulae is another method of obtaining supine flexion. Use of hip support results in less lower extremity abduction and external rotation than in infants without such hip support.[125] Pillows filled with polystyrene beads (i.e., preterm bean bags) require skill for optimal positioning and close infant monitoring but are useful in providing positioning for very small premature infants (1000 to 1500 g).

Body containment increases the infant's feeling of security, promotes quieting and self-control, enhances physiologic stability, promotes energy conservation, reduces physiologic and behavioral stress, and enables stress to be better endured.[125,260] Without positional supports, many premature infants "travel" (no matter how many times they are returned) to the sides or bottom of their incubator. Parents and professionals are inclined to move the uncomfortable-looking infant back to the middle of a "boundary-less" world. Infants should be left where they feel safe and comfortable; if they become uncomfortable, they will let you know. Providing boundaries (e.g., blanket rolls, positioning devices) stops this migration and the expenditure of precious calories that could go to growth.

Small, acutely ill premature infants who are positioned supine often are extremely agitated, thrashing arms and legs, tachycardic, and expending precious energy and calories. Instead of needing medications, these infants often are calmed by providing a nest of blankets or a commercial nesting device (which simulates the boundaries and security of the uterus). This artificial womb must be closely surrounding the infant to promote flexion, security, and quiet rest (Figure 13-7). If agitation recurs, a limb (usually a leg) has extended outside the infant's secure boundary; flexing and returning it to the "womb" quiets the infant.[6,125]

Body containment maneuvers such as swaddling, holding onto a finger or hand, and crossing the infant's arms in the midline and holding them securely help with self-regulation during feeding, procedures, or other stressful manipulations.[57,125]

Because being wrapped in a blanket with extremities flexed simulates in utero position, swaddling (1) improves flexed posture and flexor muscle tone, (2) facilitates behavioral responses, and (3) improves the development of primitive reflexes.[125] Picking up the preterm infant from a supine position often produces startles, apnea, or head hyperextension. A better technique is to roll the infant prone, which flexes the head, and then flex the limbs onto the trunk and pick the infant up. If the infant has difficulty breathing in prone position, swaddle or contain the extremities before picking the infant up.

Prone positioning encourages the infant to work on using neck extension and promotes flexion of

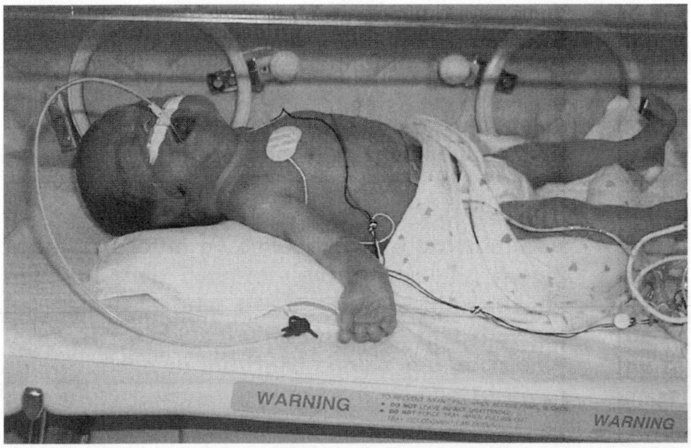

FIGURE 13-6 Supine positioning without positioning supports results in motor disorganization, agitation, arching posture, and burning of significant calories. (From Hunter J: The neonatal intensive care unit. In Case-Smith J, editor: *Occupational therapy for children*, ed 4, St Louis, 2001, Mosby.)

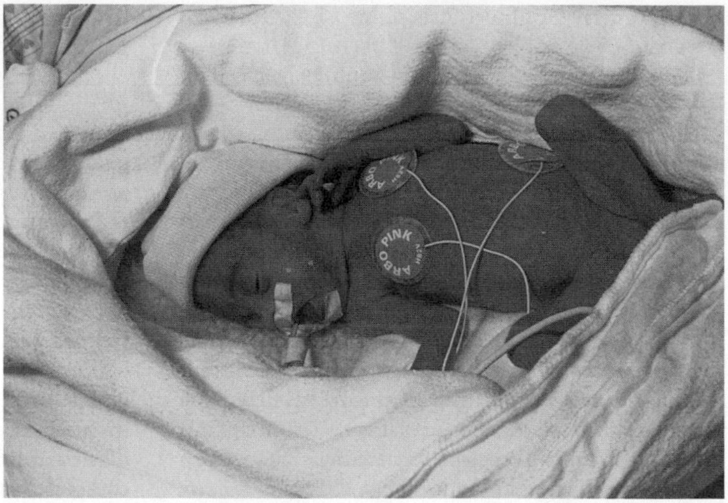

FIGURE 13-7 Very small premature infant resting quietly in a "nest" of pads and blankets.

the extremities. Position devices for prone include a small hip roll or sling to assist in maintaining flexion; use of gel/water pillows for head support; and secure lower boundary for foot bracing.[125] Use of a rolled cloth or gel pillow placed under the infant (from top of the head to the umbilicus) (1) provides elevation of the body to promote extremity flexion without placing excessive pressure on the knees and elbows, (2) enables the shoulders to round forward over the top of the roll, and (3) enables the legs to flex over the bottom edge of the roll.[125] **Prone (versus supine) positioning has numerous benefits and is the position of choice for many NICU infants (Box 13-6).** A recent study showed that sleeping in the prone position did not improve oxygenation in preterms 32 weeks post-menstrual age (PMA) or older for infants without respiratory problems.[129] The study concluded that preterms older than 32 weeks PMA, without respiratory difficulties, should be placed supine and monitoring continued to ensure adequate oxygen saturation.[129] Prone positioning of highly agitated, fretful narcotic-withdrawing neonates showed that they experienced less distress (i.e., lower withdrawal scores and lower caloric intake) than supine-lying infants.[164] Use of a sheepskin or lambskin helps to further facilitate flexion and prevents skin abrasion, especially on the knees.

Parents should be taught that when their baby is well enough to be weaned to an open crib, he or she will be physiologically and developmentally mature to tolerate supine sleep position in preparation for discharge.[20,151,154] **Many of the beneficial effects of prone positioning listed in Box 13-6 become detrimental in increasing the risk for sudden infant death syndrome (SIDS) (Table 13-6). In the American Academy of Pediatrics position paper on infant sleep, healthy infants should be placed *only* in the**

BOX 13-6 EFFECTS OF PRONE POSITIONING

1. Decreases heart rate variability[35]
2. Enhances respiratory control[166]
3. Improves oxygenation by 15% to 25%[21,29,176,279]
   a. Increased $TcPo_2$ values
   b. Increased Pao_2 values
   c. Decreased apnea, bradycardia, and periodic breathing[113]
4. Improves lung mechanics and lung volumes[129,279]
   a. Increased lung compliance
   b. Increased tidal volume
5. Decreases energy expenditure[104,167]
   a. Increased quiet sleep; higher arousal threshold[35,96]
   b. Decreased awake time; more sleep time[50]
   c. Decreased caloric expenditure (median difference supine vs. prone: +3.1 kcal/kg/day)
   d. Decreased heat loss[50]
   e. Less crying[35,50]
   f. Lower levels of activity[50]
6. Decreases gastric reflux in prone position with head of bed elevated 30 degrees

TABLE 13-6 SLEEP POSITION AS A RISK FACTOR FOR SUDDEN INFANT DEATH SYNDROME (SIDS): RESEARCH BASIS

SUPINE	PRONE
Preterm infants at 36-38 wk PCA[104] No significant difference in sleep organization based on body position. More awakenings in supine vs. prone position. Standard deviations of heart rate increase during quiet sleep in supine position; low frequency and high frequency of heart rate higher in supine vs. prone position in both active and quiet sleep states.	Prone position reduces spontaneous arousals from sleep in term infants.[121,130,207] First quiet sleep after feedings significantly longer, fewer number of awakenings, and decrease in overall heart rate variability in prone vs. supine.[104,121] Above characteristics of prone sleep constitute a higher arousal threshold, thus increased vulnerability to SIDS in prone position.[104,121,207] In preterm infants at 1 month corrected age, reduced heart rate variability during quiet sleep, no increase in total sleep, and a decrease in the number of sleep transitions.[19]
More sleep transitions, a lower arousal threshold and higher heart rate variability while sleeping supine contribute to decreased vulnerability to SIDS.	Sixty-two healthy, growing low-birth-weight infants (26-37 wk GA; 750-1600 g BW); sleeping position—a shift of EEG activity toward slower frequency, which may be related to mechanisms associated with a decrease in behavioral arousal in prone position.[121,237]
Full-term (n = 10) infants in prone/supine sleep positions given 0.4 mL water; instillation into the mouth resulted in airway protective responses of swallowing (95%) and arousal (54%).[126]	
Swallow rate rapid in supine position in response to small infusions of fluid, whereas respiratory rate remains largely unaffected. When supine, term infants can coordinate rapid swallowing while maintaining breathing.	A significant decrease in swallowing and breathing in active sleep in prone vs. supine position; airway protection is compromised in prone sleeping position during active sleep in healthy term infants exposed to minute pharyngeal fluid.
Full-term (n = 3240) ≥37 wk GA evaluated in the first 24 hrs of life for frequency/severity of spitting up incidents while asleep[259]: 96.6% did not spit up during sleep. 130 episodes of spitting up while sleeping supine (55% required no intervention; 37% brief bulb suction; 6% gentle stimulation; 2% wall suction). <4% spit up while sleeping supine, and none required significant intervention or experienced serious sequelae.	6 episodes of spitting up while infants side-lying (66.7% no intervention; 33.3% bulb suction).

BW, Birth weight; *GA*, gestational age; *EEG*, electroencephalogram; *PCA*, post-conceptual age.

supine position for sleep[16]; side-lying is no longer endorsed because the infant may spontaneously roll from side-lying to prone. Overheating sleeping infants; use of soft sleeping surfaces, stuffed toys, and positioning devices; and inappropriate sleep environments (e.g., waterbeds, pillows, bed railings) all should be avoided in healthy infants.[16] Use of a pacifier for sleep and sleeping in proximity (same room) as parents is also recommended.[16] Use of side-lying and prone positioning, as well as containment with soft bedding for physiologically compromised term and preterm infants, is safe and appropriate in a NICU setting.[154] Parents may question these practices; therefore their physiologic base and rationale should be explained.

Since the "Back to Sleep" campaign, the rate of SIDS has decreased by 40%,[16] it continues to decline by an additional 50%,[192] and infants who sleep supine are healthier than those who sleep prone.[124] In term infants, supine sleep position may delay some motor milestones by 1 month but does not delay walking. Increased amounts of time in supervised prone play ("tummy time") encourages earlier motor milestone attainment in supine sleepers[125] and helps prevent head molding.[256] A recent study of sleep positions in VLBW (<1500 g) infants, the group at highest risk for SIDS, found that they are more likely to sleep prone than larger LBW infants.[276] Reasons cited by mothers included (1) infant's preference and (2) advice from professionals (NICU doctors, nurses) who may remain uncomfortable recommending supine sleep in this population[44,151,253] despite American Academy of Pediatrics (AAP) recommendations[16] and the research that supports them.[129,151,276]

Head molding (i.e., bilateral flattening of the head and elongation of the face) is a significant problem in preterm infants; it results from flattening of the skull as the baby lies against the firm incubator mattress.[256] To parents, this head flattening is concerning, and they may find the infant less cute and desirable than a term infant with a rounded head. To prevent head molding, preterm infants are often placed on waterbeds, water pillows, air mattresses, or eggcrate-type mattresses, with variable results. Preterm infants (<32 weeks' gestation with birth weight <1500 g) who are turned every 3 hours, repositioned in one of six positions, and never placed in the same position twice in 8 hours had significantly rounder head shapes from 9 to 13 weeks of life compared with infants repositioned according to a standard NICU procedure.[115]

Kinesthetic. **A combination of vestibular and tactile stimulation increases quieting behaviors, decreases apneic and bradycardic episodes, entrains respirations, increases visual and auditory fixation, and increases brain growth.**[138,140] Waterbeds provide contingent stimuli, because they move in response to the infant's movement; oscillating waterbeds provide rhythmic motion. Kinesthetic stimulation is provided by rocking chairs, hammocks, baby swings, and baby carriers whose effects have not been investigated. Upright positioning in a car seat or infant seat encourages symmetry and spatial orientation. Soft rolls or foam padding maintains flexion; a rolled blanket in a horseshoe configuration around the infant's head and shoulders prevents lateral slouching. Carrying quiets the infant, provides sensory communication with the caregiver, changes the infant's environment, and provides visual, auditory, and tactile stimuli. A nasal cannula (see Chapter 23) and portable tank enable mobility for an infant receiving oxygen.

Rather than standardized protocols, tactile interventions must be individualized by assessing each infant's physiologic and behavioral responses before, during, and after touch (see Table 13-3). **While an infant is acutely ill, tactile intervention should include minimal handling, containment, and gentle touch (without stroking).** As the infant matures and becomes physiologically stable, stroking, rocking, and holding are integrated based on the individual infant's tolerance and preferences. In healthy preterm infants, a program of range-of-motion exercises with passive resistance is associated with an increase in weight gain and growth, bone mineral content and density, and muscle mass and a decreased risk for osteopenia.[10,153,278]

Co-bedding. Co-bedding, the practice of placing medically stable twins and higher-order multiples together in the same open warmer, incubator, or crib, was initiated after the observed stress response in separated siblings. **Postulated advantages of co-bedding are the following**[48]:

- **Improved stability of temperature, heart rate, and respirations (i.e., fewer episodes of apnea and bradycardia, better temperature regulation)**
- **Enhanced physiologic status: improved rates of growth (better weight gain) and development**
- **Co-regulation of sleep-wake cycles, soothing, and state regulation**
- **Decreased length of hospitalization and thus cost-effectiveness**
- **Improved parent-infant bonding and easier transition to home**
- **Improved staff-parent communication, individual care, and teaching of the family**

The major reluctance to co-bed is the potential risk for increased infection rates. To date, increased infection rates in co-bedded infants have not been reported. Infection concerns are addressed by good handwashing and color coding of equipment. Other safety concerns include proper identification for medication administration and medical emergencies and maintenance of temperature stability for all co-bedded infants.[9] Nesting and swaddling infants together and close monitoring of ambient temperature are necessary to achieve and maintain stable temperatures. Choosing medically stable infants (i.e., infants not requiring ventilator, continuous positive airway pressure, or oxygen hood therapy) and separating infants if one or more become unstable may prevent potential morbidity from co-bedding.

The practice of co-bedding has spread based on anecdotal information, because there is limited research (Table 13-7) to support or refute its use. Few differences between co-bedded and non–co-bedded infants have been demonstrated. Limitations on the research on co-bedding include small sample size, short follow-up periods, lack of

TABLE 13-7 CO-BEDDING MULTIPLES: RESEARCH BASIS

STUDY/DESIGN	OUTCOMES
11 sets of twins (<37 wk GA; without arterial lines/ventilators). VS recorded 12 hr before and 12 hr after co-bedding[272]	Safe—no adverse events Decreased apnea; may be caused by (1) change in sleep pattern (e.g., more frequent arousal by twin) or (2) more regular breathing pattern as a result of skin-to-skin contact between twins
Prospective, randomized repeated measure of 2 groups: n = 16 infants co-bedded in incubators; n = 21 infants in control group[48]	Safe—no infection/medication errors No significant clinical improvement in either infant or parental outcomes
Retrospective, comparative descriptive design with chart reviews and satisfaction surveys mailed to parents[221]	No negative clinical/developmental outcomes No significant differences in clinical/developmental outcomes between co-bedded and non–co-bedded All mothers reported positive experiences with NICU
Retrospective, descriptive design evaluating data on twins (23-35 wk GA) from co-bedded/non–co-bedded time periods in one NICU[143]	No association between co-bedding and incidence of infection (septicemia, NEC, pneumonia) At discharge, a significantly increased number of positive blood cultures in the non–co-bedded twins
Prospective randomized study of preterm twins (28-34 wk GA); n = 21 sets of co-bedded and n = 20 sets of non–co-bedded[51]	Significant increase in mean weight gain for co-bedded group No difference in number of apnea/bradycardia events between groups

GA, Gestational age; *NEC*, necrotizing enterocolitis; *NICU*, newborn intensive care unit; *VS*, vital signs.

randomization, and blinding of evaluators. Because parents continue care practices at home that they have witnessed and become accustomed to in the hospital, the possibility of continuing co-bedding at home (and the lack of evidence as to its safety) must be considered. Instituting co-bedding involves education of staff and parents about potential benefits/risks, the experimental nature of the practice, and the development of a clinical evaluation protocol to collect data on risks and benefits.[48,201] Both the National Association of Neonatal Nurses (NANN)[201] and the AAP[270] have concluded that neither the safety or benefit of co-bedding has been established by current research and that parents should be instructed to follow established safe sleeping practices[16] at home.

AUDITORY INTERVENTION

The NICU is a noisy environment that has no diurnal rhythm or predictability; it is as noisy at night as in the daytime (Table 13-8).[61,105,215,281] An infant in the NICU is exposed to an onslaught of noise 24 hours a day for days, weeks, or months. At follow-up, preterm infants exhibit a lower threshold for sound and a reduced responsiveness to auditory stimulation.[25] Neonatal illnesses, drug therapies, and possibly acoustic insult account for the increased risk (i.e., in up to 10% to 12% of low-birth-weight infants) for sensorineural hearing loss in NICU infants (regardless of gestational age).[15,106,109] An increased risk for sensorineural hearing loss in VLBW infants is related to more than 90 days of oxygen therapy, a maximum FIO_2 of 0.90, minimum plasma sodium less than 125 mEq/L, or maximum pH above 7.60[149] and use of ventilator therapy.[220] Moderate to severe conductive hearing loss also occurs in 42% of VLBW infants. "The danger of noise-induced hearing loss is greatest in preterm babies."[163]

The first goal in auditory intervention is to assess the current level of noise in the NICU[37,106,109] and decrease the noise decibel level wherever possible.[106,141,265,281] The noise environment of an individual infant depends on the ambient sounds in the nursery, the type of incubator and support equipment, and the baby's own behavior (i.e., quiet or crying). Noise measurement protocols must sample multiple noise sources and sites.[141,265] Some NICUs have installed decimeters that present a flashing or blinking light when the noise level exceeds a preset level (about 50 to 65 dB).[8] Sources of noise include heating, ventilation, and air conditioner flow units (noise levels may decrease by 2.5 to 10.5 dB when these units are turned off). **The greatest contributor to loud noise in the NICU is talking and conversation by the staff.**[8,106,109,215] Noise levels vary with location, time of day, and day of week within the NICU; therefore various locations or various times and days should be measured.[61,141,215,265]

Increased environmental noise levels are a stressor to all infants in the NICU—preterm infants, as well as ill term infants (e.g., infants with persistent pulmonary hypertension of the newborn [PPHN] or drug withdrawal) (Box 13-7). The sudden, high-pitched, shrill, dysrhythmic noise of equipment alarms alerts the care provider, but it also results in infants manifesting an extreme hypersensitivity to sound (as a learned conditioned response). CNS-injured preterms are particularly vulnerable to sound stress in the NICU, are less able to habituate to NICU noise, and respond with exaggerated and prolonged physiologic responses (e.g., alterations in respiratory rate, bradycardia, desaturations). **Noise is stressful not only to the infants but also to parents and care providers in the NICU.**[281] Three years after their NICU experience,

TABLE 13-8 NOISE LEVELS IN THE NICU

LEVEL (DB)	COMMENTS
48-69	Humidifiers and nebulizers
50-60	Normal speaking voice
50-73.5*†	Incubator (motor noise)
53	Median noise level on conventional ventilator
55-88	Bradycardia alarm
58-85‡	Noise in NICU (talking, equipment alarms, telephones, radio)
59	Median noise level on high-frequency oscillator
65-80†	Life support equipment (ventilator; intravenous pumps)
66-76	Sink on/off
67	Incubator alarm
70	Background noise mean level should not exceed
85§	Noise level at which hearing damage is possible for adult; (?) neonatal effects
90	Peak sound intensity in the NICU not to exceed
90§	Adult exposure for 8 hours requires protective device and hearing conservation program
92.8†	Opening incubator porthole
84-108	Placing a plastic bottle of formula on top of incubator
96-117†	Placing a glass bottle of formula on top of incubator
70-116†	Closing one or both cabinet doors
80-124†	Closing one or both portholes
120	Threshold for pain
130-140†	Banging incubator to stimulate apneic premature infant
160-165§	Recommendations for peak, single noise level not to exceed to prevent (adult) hearing loss; (?) neonatal effects

Data from Thomas KA, Uran A: How the NICU environment sounds to a preterm infant: update, *MCN Am J Matern Child Nurs* 32:250, 2007.

NICU, Neonatal intensive care unit.

*Modern incubators generate less than 60 dB; exceeds hourly recommendation of 50 dBA (see Table 13-9).

†Measures from inside the incubator.

‡Noise levels do not vary from morning to night.

§Occupational Safety and Health Administration (OSHA) standard. (No safety standards for neonates have been established.)

BOX 13-7 EFFECTS OF LOUD NOISE[8,43,103,106,134]

- Increase in stress behaviors:
  - State lability
  - Arousal state
  - Avoidance behaviors—more fussy, more startles, etc. (see the Critical Findings box on p. 291)
- Decrease in approach behaviors (see the Critical Findings box on p. 291)
- Cardiorespiratory changes:
  - Increased heart rate
  - Increased respiratory rate
  - Increased apnea or bradycardia
  - Increased hypoxemia (decreased pulse oximeter)
  - Increased peripheral and arterial vasoconstriction:
    - Increased systemic blood pressure
    - Increased intracranial pressure
  - Increased sensory neural hearing loss
  - Abnormal auditory development and processing
  - Prevents habituation
- Alters development of sleep-wake cycles:
  - Disturbs sleep; interrupts light sleep
  - Increases wakefulness and agitation
- Increased risk for intraventricular hemorrhage:
  - Increase in cerebral blood flow

mothers recall the noise level in the NICU as a stressor. NICU noise is stressful to care providers and has the potential to damage hearing; cause physiologic responses (e.g., increase blood pressure, alter immune response, increase stress hormone secretion, disturb sleep); cause fatigue, irritability, and "burnout"; interfere with communication with co-workers and parents; alter concentration; and increase errors.[264]

Although the AAP recommends that noise levels be below 45 dB,[56] most NICUs' noise levels range between 38 and 90 dB, with higher noise bursts (see Table 13-8).[37,47,61,141,265] To protect sleep, support stable vital signs, and improve speech intelligibility, recommended standards for noise criteria have been established. Recent noise studies in NICUs have found the following[37,47,61,141,265]:

- Noise levels are still louder than recommended.
- Environmental changes to reduce noise must be monitored because they may increase rather than decrease noise.
- Nurses perceived their own NICU as "pretty quiet" when, in fact, noise levels were above recommendations.
- Noise levels have not significantly decreased in the NICU.

Table 13-9 presents specific noise criteria and their rationale. Parents and care providers must be involved in planning, developing, and being educated about quieter NICUs.*

Strategies to minimize external auditory stimuli include quieting alarms with suction (and remembering to reset them); not taking a shift report over or allowing medical rounds near the infant's incubator; having noisy equipment repaired immediately; emptying sloshing water in ventilator or nebulizer tubing; maintaining cardiac monitors in a quiet state with alarms on (decreasing the sound of alarms by 50%); and purchasing quieter equipment (e.g., plastic instead of metal trash containers; quieter incubators).[47] Choosing heated humidifiers (48 dB) rather than nebulizers (69 dB) and keeping the containers full of water, rather than low, decrease noise from respiratory equipment. Nursery design changes[56,214,215] include smaller cubicles rather than one large room, soundproofing materials, lights for phones and alarm systems, and minimizing equipment noise. Placing a blanket on top of the incubator or using an incubator cover muffles the noise of equipment placement; gentle, considerate (to the infant) placement of equipment on or in the incubator muffles sound; and closing portholes and drawers gently decrease the structural noises of caregiving. Prohibiting placement of equipment (e.g., clipboards, stethoscopes, formula bottles) on top of the incubator prevents such noises.

Tapping (by parents or siblings) or banging (by medical, nursing, or ancillary personnel) on the incubator Plexiglas should *never* be permitted. This (along with a brisk startle reflex from the infant) is an opportunity to teach about the noise levels generated by such activity. Infants should be kept in incubators as long as necessary to maintain heat balance. **Older incubators do *not* protect the infant from noise. A well-managed NICU environment may be much quieter than the continuous noise of an incubator. Noise in modern incubators varies according to the model.** Sound sources within an incubator include its motor, infant sounds, equipment sounds inside the incubator, equipment sounds transmitted from outside the incubator, and ambient nursing noise (e.g., personnel, phones). **Modern incubator walls attenuate impulse noises from the NICU and may decrease the infant's noise exposure.** Inside modern

TABLE 13-9 RATIONALE FOR SPECIFIC NOISE CRITERIA[56]

NOISE CRITERION	RATIONALE
Hourly Leq (equivalent sound level) of 45 dB in infant room; 50 dB in staff work areas	Preserves sleep for healthy term infants most of the time
Hourly L_{10} of 50 dB in infant room; 55 dB in staff work areas (sound levels may exceed 55 dB only 10% of the time or a total of 6 min/hr)	Preserves sleep for infants; enables caregivers to speak at normal conversational levels and be clearly understood 12 feet away, approximately 90% of the time
L_{max} of 65 dB in infant room; not to exceed 70 dB in staff work areas (maximum decibel sound level ≤1 sec in duration—transient bursts of noise)	Minimizes rousing babies and causing startle responses

*References 37,47,109,127,141,214,215,254,265,281.

incubators, motor noise does not exceed 60 dB, but this level exceeds the more recent recommendation of 50 dB. However, impulse noises from the incubator (i.e., doors, latches) are louder on the inside of the incubator (see Table 13-8). Prolonged stays in an incubator not only expose the infant to repeated caregiving noises but also mean there will be a dearth of kinesthetic stimulation (e.g., carrying, holding, rocking, swinging, sitting upright in an infant seat) and socially relevant speech patterns. Both the internal noise generated by the incubator and how well the incubator attenuates external noise should be considered in incubator purchases.[37]

Conductive hearing loss is attributed to endotracheal intubation, poor eustachian tube function, increased otitis media, and chronic lung disease (CLD) in preterm infants. Noise levels in the NICU may interfere with development of other sensory systems and delay the development of hearing and language. Radios have been banned in most NICUs. **Day-night cycles (nap time, nighttime) when auditory stimulation is decreased should be established in the NICU.** Institution of a quiet time or rest period—through reduction of (1) noise from talking, equipment, telephones, and so on, (2) light by dimming overhead light, and (3) procedures to only emergency treatment—has resulted in enhanced infant sleep (34% to 85%), less crying (14% to 2.4%), and less parental and caregiver stress.[254] At discharge, NICU infants often will not sleep in a quiet room. Softly playing a radio facilitates sleep, and the infant gradually is weaned from it. Signs such as "Quiet… baby sleeping" or "Do not disturb, I'm asleep (talk to my nurse)" ensure undisturbed sleep *if* they are heeded.

The "in-turning" premature infant (see the Critical Findings box on p. 284) of less than 34 weeks' gestation probably receives enough auditory input from the NICU. Auditory enhancement at this stage is probably overstimulation. Just as high-frequency sounds arouse, low-frequency ones, such as the heartbeat, respiratory sounds, and vacuum cleaners, quiet and facilitate sleep.[71] One study showed less behavioral response and less salivary cortisol release by infants who were presented with a heartbeat sound or white noise (both at 85 dB) during and after heel stick.

Although music has been shown to soothe full-term babies, the use of music with preterm infants has not been well studied.[202] Presentation of in utero sounds and a female voice to agitated, intubated preterm infants has resulted in improved oxygen saturation and behavioral states. A meta-analysis of music therapy showed benefits to preterm infants including improved oxygen saturations, increased weight gain, decrease in hospitalization, an increase (over time) in tolerance for stimuli, reinforcement of nonnutritive sucking, and increase in the rate of feeding at 34 to 36 weeks in poor feeders.[252] A survey of staff attitudes about music therapy found that 68% would like music for preterms in the NICU and 86% agreed that music decreased stress and crying (79%), decreased pain (78%), improved sleep (79%), reduced parental stress (57%), and assisted staff in focusing or performing better (56%).[132] Recorded classical instrumental music was preferred.[262] However, caution is recommended in instituting music therapy until RCTs of substantial size evaluating short-term and long-term outcomes have been completed.[274]

Although the use of recordings of music or family voices has been advocated and widely practiced, some investigators have recommended that such recordings not be used. Among the reasons cited against their use are that their benefits and long-term consequences have not been established, their use places a nonresponsive machine between a caring person and the preterm infant, and recordings may replace exposure of the preterm to the contingent human voice.[106,109] However, if used with preterm infants, auditory stimuli should be (1) kept at a reasonable distance from the infant's ear (never use earphones), whether placed inside or outside the incubator, (2) played at levels below 55 dBA, (3) played for brief periods, and (4) used if the infant is soothed and discontinued if the infant becomes stressed, restless, or agitated.[106,274] However, because preterm infants cannot habituate to sound as well as term babies can, they may be unable to tolerate any added sound and may become exhausted by such stimuli.

The human voice is the most preferred sound. The preterm in an incubator may be isolated from important exposure to his or her mother's voice. Teach parents the neonate's preference for high-pitched voices speaking in typical speech patterns (not baby talk). The degree of attenuation of the higher frequency of mother's voice by the lower frequency of incubator noise, the incubator walls, and the ambient noise of the NICU has not been measured. Role model and teach parents to gently talk to the infant while touching and giving care.[106]

Teach parents to talk to their infant while presenting their faces in the infant's range of vision. Many explanations for the preference of mothers to cradle their babies on their left side have been postulated (i.e., hand dominance, importance of maternal heartbeat, left breast sensitivity, and advantage in monitoring the infant). A more recent hypothesis proposes that maternal affective signals (both auditory and visual) are given to the infant's free left ear and are processed by the more advanced right cerebral hemisphere. Watch for infant tolerance, and increase or decrease talk time to avoid overload. For older infants, imitate the infant's coos and babbles; this reinforces and encourages vocalizations.

For a neonate, hearing is more important than vision for attachment and bonding to the parents. Within seconds after birth, newborns are able to discriminate and prefer their mother's face. They have connected her familiar voice with her unfamiliar face. A high index of suspicion about hearing loss is warranted if caregivers do not observe normal responses to sound stimulation. All newborns—but especially those with a history of familial hearing loss; hyperbilirubinemia at exchange transfusion level; congenital viral infections; defects of the ear, nose, and throat; small preterm infants (<1500 g); those with bacterial sepsis or meningitis; respiratory distress; prolonged (>10-day) mechanical ventilation; low Apgar scores (0 to 3 at 5 minutes; 0 to 6 at 10 minutes); or physical stigmata associated with syndromes known to include hearing loss, as well as those receiving ototoxic drugs—are at increased risk for hearing loss.[12,15] **Because screening by these high-risk factors alone identifies only about 50% of newborns with significant hearing loss,[15] universal newborn hearing screening is the standard of care.[12,15]** Recent research has documented preliminary evidence that babies who have subsequently died of SIDS have asymmetry of hearing responses on their left side, which may suggest a relationship between inner ear function, respiratory control during sleep, and SIDS.[236]

VISUAL INTERVENTION

The NICU is lit with bright, cool-white fluorescent lights 24 hours a day. Light levels vary between and within various NICUs.[109] There is a trend toward decreasing NICU illumination.[109] Early studies showed light levels in the low range, from 34 to 100 lux at night and 184 to 1000 lux during the day; more recent studies report light levels ranging from low levels of 1 to 25 foot-candles (ftc) to high levels of 235 ftc.[249] However, the light levels in the LIGHT-ROP study were 399 and 447 lux, with and without goggles.[227] **The amount of light to which the preterm infant is exposed is influenced by (1) location in the NICU, (2) seasonal or climactic variations, (3) use of phototherapy, (4) ophthalmoscopic examinations (e.g., at birth and for retinopathy of prematurity [ROP] follow-up), and (5) infant-related factors (e.g., maturity and amount of eye opening, head position, or eye shielding).[91]** Ambient light levels in the NICU should be adjustable through a range of 10 to 600 lux (approximately 1 to 60 ftc) at every bedside.[13,56] Other light recommendations for newly built NICUs are outlined in Table 13-10.

Although decreased light levels and response to bright light have not been shown to reduce the incidence of ROP, ophthalmic sequelae of preterm birth are common. (See Chapter 23 for a discussion of ROP.) There are three broad categories

TABLE 13-10 LIGHT RECOMMENDATIONS IN THE NICU[13,56]

ILLUMINATION LEVEL	PURPOSE
High levels: 60-100 foot-candles (ftc)	Evaluate and assess skin color and perfusion.
Lower levels: 10-20 ftc	Safe and adequate because of concerns over retinal/ocular damage from continuous exposure to high levels (60-100 ftc).
Nighttime levels: 0-5 ftc	Diurnal variation in light levels.
Procedure light: 100-150 ftc	Available at every bedside to temporarily increase lighting for infant assessment/procedure without increasing light exposure to all other babies. Prevent light from reaching infant's eyes.
Support areas	For charting, medication preparation, etc., should provide adequate and separate light to accommodate sleeping babies and working health care providers. Lighting should be located to avoid any infant's direct line of sight to the fixture.
Daylight	One source visible from care areas for its psychologic benefit for staff and families.

NICU, Neonatal intensive care unit.

of ophthalmic sequelae: (1) decreased visual function; (2) strabismus; and (3) decreased eye size (arrested growth) and abnormal refractive state (increased myopia).[91] In addition, there is abundant animal, child, and adult research documenting negative biochemical and physical effects (e.g., change in endocrine function, increased hypocalcemia, cell transformations, immature gonadal development, chromosome breakage).[105] **Exposure to bright lights in the NICU is associated with the following[105]:**

- **Decreased oxygenation**
- **Increased incidence of retinopathy**
- **Poorer circadian rhythms**
- **Altered sleep patterns**
- **Alterations in state organization**
- **Skin changes (e.g., tanning, rashes)**
- **Alteration of nutrients in total parenteral nutrition (TPN) solution, formula, and breast milk**

Rapid increase in the intensity of ambient light causes a decrease in oxygen saturation in younger, immature preterm infants.

The first goal in visual intervention is to assess the current level of light and decrease it wherever possible.[281] A very immature preterm infant is accustomed to the muted light of the uterus (light filtered through the abdominal and uterine walls) and has fused eyelids (if the infant is less than 26 weeks gestational age). Draping blankets on top of the incubator or using a handmade or commercial incubator cover[109,146] decreases the light at the infant's level during rest but allows immediate maximal illumination when the cover is pulled back. Using adjustable lighting at each infant's bedside enables every infant to have more or less light, depending on the care and rest circumstances of the individual infant. Because infants are continuously monitored, not all infants need to be subjected to maximal illumination at all times.[105]

Cycled light, dimming the lights in day-night cycles, is associated with positive effects (Box 13-8). The Stanford cycled light trials consisted of a comparison of the development of circadian rhythms in two groups of preterm infants: (1) a dim group, with incubator or crib covered with a thick blanket except during feeding or other interventions; and (2) a cycled group, exposed to a regular light-dark cycle (e.g., a covered incubator/crib from 7 PM to 7 AM). At 36 weeks post-conceptual age, or 1 month and 3 months corrected age, there was a significant maturation in circadian rhythms of both temperature and sleep, but neither was benefited by cycled light. The researchers concluded that these circadian rhythms in preterm infants develop endogenously as a factor of post-conceptual age (e.g., maturation), independent of prematurity or environmental intervention.[191] Despite their findings, these researchers, citing sufficient data (see Box 13-8) and recommendations in the current AAP/ACOG Guidelines for Perinatal Care[13] to introduce regular day-night cycles, state that "there is no rationale for continuing a chaotic noncircadian environmental approach in the neonatal nursery for the care of the prematurely born infant."[191] A recent randomized controlled study showed that the circadian clock of the preterm infant is entrained by cycled light. Preterm infants exposed to low-level cycled light for 2 weeks before discharge showed night/day rest-activity patterns within the first week after discharge. Preterms exposed to low-level uncycled light were delayed in their development of day-night differences in activity and rest till 3 weeks after discharge.[228-230]

BOX 13-8 EFFECTS OF CYCLED LIGHT*

- Behavior:
  - Decreases movement or motor activity
  - Increases motor coordination
  - Increases sleep time
  - Decreases crying
  - More eye opening
- Cardiorespiratory changes:
  - Decreases heart rate
  - Decreases respiratory rate
- Feeding behavior:
  - Quicker progression to oral feedings
  - Feeds more efficiently and in less time
  - Increased weight gain and better growth
- Circadian rhythm development:
  - Melatonin level
  - Temperature
  - Heart rate
  - Rest and activity patterns
- Decreased cortisol levels
- Decreased incidence and severity of retinopathy of prematurity
- Decreased parental and/or care provider stress
- Decreased infant handling and noise levels

*References 36,191,213,229,230,254,292.

Visual attentiveness is correlated with birth weight and gestational age: the more mature the infant, the more the infant is able to fix and follow. An infant at 28 weeks' gestation fixes and follows but may become apneic, behaviorally disorganized, and stressed as a result. Visual stimulation is very tiring and taxing (increases the heart rate) for the immature infant: those of less than 34 weeks' gestation probably receive enough stimulation from the NICU environment. Premature visual stimulation also may interfere with auditory neurosensory development. When these infants reach the "coming-out stage" (see the Critical Findings box on p. 284), they may signal their readiness for visually enhancing activities.

Infants receiving phototherapy are deprived of visual sensory stimuli because of their protective eye pads. These should be removed during care and feeding and interaction with parents and professionals. Interesting visual stimuli include inanimate objects (e.g., toys, black-and-white faces and patterns, pictures of family members, artwork from siblings, mobiles) and animate objects (e.g., faces of parents, siblings, professionals) (Figure 13-8). Infants prefer the human face as a visual stimulus, especially the talking face, which stimulates both visual and auditory pathways. Parents often need to be encouraged that, rather than toys, their infant prefers to watch and listen to their faces and voices.

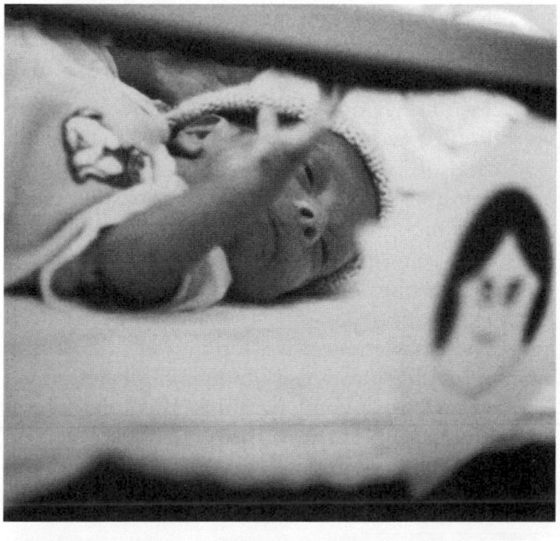

FIGURE 13-8 Premature infant fixing the gaze on a black-and-white face.

Teach parents the abilities of the infant and appropriate methods of visual stimulation:

- Place mobiles, pictures, and faces of high contrast (i.e., black and white) within the visual range of the newborn: 8 to 12 inches for term infants, a little closer for preterm infants.
- Quiet alert is the best state for visual encounters after feedings, if awake; swaddle the infant to quiet, or unwrap the infant to arouse; hold infant upright.
- Place the infant on the abdomen (called "Tummy Time") with objects of various sizes and shapes within visual range.
- Change toys and visual stimuli. Infants become bored with the same thing.
- When the preterm infant tolerates multiple stimuli, hold him or her in ***en face*** position (see Chapter 29) to feed, talk to, and rock. Whether the infant is nipple or gavage fed, alternate sides so the infant sees both sides of the care provider's face (especially important if the preterm infant exhibits the common preference for right-sided head turning).
- Place the infant at varied heights (in a baby carrier, crib, swing, infant seat, on the floor) so the infant sees the world from various angles.
- Place the infant so that he or she can bring the hands to midline and can see his or her hands and fingers and eventually reach for toys.

Infants who exhibit gaze aversion should not be "pursued" by the face of the parent or professional, because this only potentiates the time "spent away" with their gaze to protect themselves from overload. Gaze aversion, flat facial affect, and absence of a smile may cast doubt on the ability of these infants to see, because there is no eye "language" or caregiver feedback of preference, recognition, and delight. These infants do see, but they fix only fleetingly. **Minimizing the number of care providers is crucial for these babies so that they deal with as few caregiver cues, styles, and ways of being handled as possible. Most important, the caregiver must be sensitive and responsive to the infant's negative and positive cues.**

SMELL AND TASTE INTERVENTION

Newborns, including preterms, can detect, discriminate, respond (e.g., facial expression, change in respirations, apnea), learn, and remember olfactory stimuli.[241] The neonate's well-developed sense of smell is not stimulated in the NICU with pleasant odors. A high-risk infant is stimulated by the smell of forgotten alcohol, skin prep, or povidone-iodine (Betadine) pads inside the incubator and the unpleasant taste or smell of oral medications.[274] Because a premature infant cannot respond by crying or moving away, **the infant responds to noxious smells by a decrease in respiratory rate, transient apnea, or an increase in heart rate.** Removal of noxious odors from the incubator is as critical as removal of sharp instruments after a procedure. Even the smell of NICU detergent is detected, elicits a response that differs from the response to a pleasant odor, and decreases cerebral blood flow to the right hemisphere.[26]

Enhancing the olfactory environment includes having parents hold the infant or sit close if the infant cannot yet be held. The smell of the mother's breast milk is especially pleasant and elicits more suckling than the smell of formula.[30,241] Olfactory stimulation of sucking in preterm infants increases with increasing postnatal age.[30] Placing a drop of milk on the infant's lips with a cotton ball or gauze sponge helps the infant recognize the mother's smell[241] and associate that smell with food and feeding when the infant is able to nipple feed.[241]

Nonnutritive suckling (NNS) (during gavage and between feedings) is associated with better oxygenation; quieter, more restful behavior; increased readiness for nipple feedings because of a more alert state; fewer gavage feedings; acceleration of the sucking reflex; better weight gain; accelerated transition to full oral feedings; no alteration in breast feeding success; decreased tension; and increased insulin and gastrin secretion that may stimulate digestion and storage of nutrients.* Meta-analyses of NNS studies have found no consistency in these benefits but rather a decreased length of hospital stay, efficacy in pain relief, and no adverse effects (see Chapter 12).[219] Sucking on a pacifier satisfies the infant's sucking needs and may facilitate early learning that satiety and sucking are associated. However, nutritive and nonnutritive suckling are not alike (see Chapter 18); the fact that an infant vigorously sucks on a pacifier does not mean the infant will be able to suckle nutritively,[217] because the expressive and swallow phases have not been present in nonnutritive suckling and coordination of suck, swallow, and breathing has not been necessary. This is very confusing to most parents and many professionals and should be clarified for them.

High-risk infants often undergo prolonged periods during which a nil per os (NPO) status has been ordered, and during these times, their sensation of hunger is not relieved. Although pacifiers are soothing, these infants may learn that sucking and satiety are not related. NICU infants also experience many aversive stimuli around and within the mouth[287] (e.g., oral intubation, oral and endotracheal tube suction, intermittent gavage) that result in touch aversion of the mouth and a hypersensitive gag reflex. Feeding difficulties may result from the following:

- Severity of illness[179,235]
- Neurologic damage (e.g., IVH)[179]
- Structural abnormalities (e.g., cleft palate or submucous cleft, recessed chin)
- Prematurity: the infant is too neurologically immature and tires easily with "work" of feeding
- **Neural maturation (34 to 35 weeks' gestation) is the developmental guideline for initiation of oral feedings (Box 13-9); see also the Critical Findings box on p. 274),**[101,175,247] **although some infants are ready at an earlier age (30 to 34 weeks' gestation) (see the Critical Findings box on p. 284). Maturation of feeding skills occurs because of developmental changes in the CNS, coupled with experiential learning.*** So intimately interrelated are these indicators that maturity depends on experience and experience depends on maturity; therefore, the more opportunities to nipple feed, the more improved the preterm's feeding performance.[216] However, preterm infants may exhibit periods of apnea and tachypnea with bottle feeding, because consistent coordination of breathing with sucking and swallowing does not occur until 37 weeks' gestation (see the Critical Findings box on p. 275.
- Aversive feeder (acquired or developmental: sucking defect; psychologic: "hospitalitis," rumination)
- A combination of these types

The research basis for determining readiness for initiation of oral feedings is discussed in Chapter 18 and in the Critical Findings box on p. 284. An Early Feeding Skills (EFS) Assessment checklist has been developed to assess a preterm

*References 54,98,102,171,217,218,222,241.

*References 11,69,100,116,123,172,175,179,182,216,218,247.

BOX 13-9 STRATEGIES TO FACILITATE ORAL FEEDING

1. Minimize noxious stimuli to the mouth.
   a. Suction only as needed (not routinely).
   b. Consider indwelling gastric tube rather than intermittent gavage (e.g., an infant fed every 2 hours would have a gavage tube passed 12 times a day).
   c. Pass intermittent gavage tube down mouth through hole in pacifier nipple; if infant has hypersensitive gag, passing smaller tube down nose stimulates gag reflex less than passing tube down mouth.
   d. Perioral and intraoral stimulation techniques[31,98]:
      These techniques are only more aversive, rather than therapeutic, on babies with touch aversion at mouth area.
      When performing oral exercises, do so with care—do not stimulate aversion reflexes (e.g., gag reflex).
      Use of a new motorized pulsating pacifier results in faster emergence of NNS and increase in proportion of oral nutrition.[24]
2. Enhance pleasant stimuli to mouth (first experiences with suckling have lasting neurobehavioral effects).[92]
   a. Have infant smell or taste breast milk.
   b. Provide nonnutritive suckling[116] while tube feeding.
   c. Facilitate hand-to-mouth behaviors.
   d. Use nipple with proper flow rate.[169,179] If flow rate is too fast, increased flow stimulates anxiety and/or gag reflex and causes bradycardia—promotes incoordination. If flow rate is too slow, fatigue and frustration are increased and may result in inadequate consumption/growth failure.
   e. Perioral and intraoral stimulation—(?) facilitates development of normal sucking behaviors.[98]
   f. Use Lact-Aid nursing supplementer (see Chapter 18):
      Never frustrate infant with dry breast.
      Positive reinforcement for infant to nurse.
      Calorically and energy efficient method.
      Oral therapy—teaches infant proper nutritive suckle.
   g. For infants with difficulty in coordination of respiration with suck or swallow (prevents stress of apnea and hypoxia and enhances pleasure of feeding experience) (see Chapter 18)[267,268]:
      Assess feeding pattern (e.g., continuous or intermittent suck), pulse oximeter, muscle tone, breathing pattern, heart rate.[269]
      Remove nipple from mouth to enable infant to breathe.[145,266]
      Begin breast feeding before bottle feeding (see Chapter 18 Critical Findings: Readiness for Initiation of Oral Feedings: Research Basis on pp. 456-459).
      Use of orthodontic nipple results in physiologic stability and more effective feeding behavior in some infants.
3. Positioning: use proper position to facilitate swallow and improve suction—symmetric positioning with predominance of flexion.[179,269]
   a. Hold with feedings (even gavage) as much as possible.
   b. Consistent caregivers—parents, primary nurses, foster grandparents.
   c. Kangaroo care before feeding improves alertness; does not tire infant and should not be avoided before feeding.[55]
   d. Swaddle[179,269]:
      Decreases startles.
      Infant may become too warm and sleepy.
   e. Facilitate swallowing:
      Position with chin tucked.
      If breast feeding, turn infant's whole body toward mother so head and trunk are in alignment (infant is not trying to swallow with head turned to one side).
      Upright position with neck, shoulders, and back supported—slows gravitational flow of formula from nipple (as when infant is in semi-reclined position); restricted milk flow (e.g., milk flows only with active sucking, not with gravity) beneficial (e.g., more efficient; more volume obtained).
      Cuddling, semi-reclined position increases flow of formula by gravity—may be too fast, regardless of nipple chosen; results in increased gags, choking, and bradycardia.
      Prone with neck extended (slightly):
         Keeps tongue forward and airway unobstructed.
         Good for aversive feeder who chokes.
      Gentle, upward pressure under chin (chin support) or at base of tongue facilitates swallowing, because it mimics upward thrust of tongue with swallowing.
   f. Improve formation of suction:
      Semi-reclining (>45-degree angle) on lap of caregiver—frees both hands to work with infant on oral control.
      Cupping both cheeks (check support)[116] with fingers of free hand (i.e., hand not holding bottle) improves lip closure, suction formation, minimizes fluid loss, stabilizes the jaw, and organizes deglutition.[31,116,294]
      Gentle tugging at nipple (as if to take it out of mouth) may smooth and strengthen suck.
4. Timing
   a. Do not allow infant to cry to exhaustion before feeding—infant will be too tired to eat.
   b. Keep external stimuli to a minimum in immature preterm infants (<34 weeks) for optimal intake and weight gain.[179,244]
   c. If or when satiated, infant will not suck.
      Feed on demand/semidemand or when alert[58,173-175,179,266] (demand feeding reinforces sleep-wake cycle) and the development of self-regulation.[173,223]

NNS, Nonnutritive sucking; *VLBW*, very low birth weight.

Continued

BOX 13-9 STRATEGIES TO FACILITATE ORAL FEEDING—cont'd

If feeding on schedule, note whether infant gives cue of hunger: fussiness and crying, hand-to-mouth behaviors or rooting, hiccups. Infants as young as 32 to 33 weeks can provide cues so that feeding can be individualized.[172,175,179]

If feeding on schedule, space time and see whether infant exhibits cues of hunger (as above).

First, nipple what infant is able to feed; then tube feed (presence of an indwelling nasogastric tube may result in compromised respirations, oxygen desaturation, and bradycardia in the VLBW infant).[247]

d. Try to nipple feed for no longer than 20 to 30 minutes (infant becomes too tired and uses up energy and calories to feed instead of to grow).[179,235]

e. Infants of advanced age (around 6 months) may be unable to nipple if they have never had the opportunity. It may be more developmentally appropriate to cup feed or spoon feed infant because normal infants begin cup drinking between 6 and 8 months of age.

NNS, Nonnutritive sucking; *VLBW*, very low birth weight.

infant's readiness for oral feeding, oral feeding skill, and ability to maintain physiologic stability and tolerance of oral feeding.[269]

Preterm infants may not be at risk for chronic feeding problems if they are changed from non-oral methods (TPN and tube feeding) to oral methods by the end of the first month of life. Severe behavioral eating difficulties are associated with prematurity, low birth weight, CNS injury, distress during feeding in the first 6 months of life, and regular or frequent vomiting. Aversive feeding experiences may be the basis for early childhood eating difficulties.

Because criteria for discharge include full oral feedings with adequate weight gain,[13,179,188] transition to full oral feedings is being investigated. **Longer transition time to full oral feedings is significantly influenced by (1) apnea, (2) birth weight or gestational age, (3) younger age at first oral feeding, (4) BPD/CLD, (5) number of days being tube fed/receiving ventilatory therapy, and (6) desaturations of oxygen with feeding.*** Shorter transition time to complete oral feeding is associated with (1) greater weight and (2) older post-conceptual age at initiation of nipple feeding,[45,182] (3) use of oral stimulation (e.g., stroking, NNS),[98,173] and (4) a semi-demand or demand feeding protocol.[58,172,173,175] Post-conceptual age at first nippling indicates that neurodevelopmental maturation (e.g., state arousal, neuromotor skills, respiratory control) is a factor in transition time.[123,182,223,269]

A randomized study of early introduction of oral (bottle) feeding (e.g., within 48 hours of full tube feeding) found the following[247]:

- Transition time to all oral feedings was significantly shorter.
- Oral feeding was introduced 2.6 weeks earlier.
- Total oral feeding was achieved at earlier post-menstrual age (e.g., 54% of 33 weeks post-menstrual age infants versus 12.5% of control group).
- Weight gain and discharge weights were similar for both groups.
- Episodes of feeding-related bradycardia and desaturations were similar for both groups.
- Discharge was 10 days earlier for the earlier fed infants.

These researchers postulate that feeding opportunities in young infants provide them with practice and experiential opportunities to develop their oral motor skills and coordination of suck-swallow-breathe.[123,247]

For infants with BPD/CLD, the more days receiving positive pressure ventilation and supplemental oxygen, the older (in post-conceptual age) the infant when he or she is first fully nipple fed.[179] For these infants, transition time to full nipple feeding may be lengthened because of the increased work of breathing and the precedence of breathing (at an increased rate) over feeding.

The goals of intervention include (1) a safe feeding (i.e., diminished risk for aspiration), (2) a functional feeding (i.e., adequate caloric intake for optimal growth and with minimal energy expenditure),[287] and (3) a pleasant, social

*References 98,172,175,182,247,267.

interactive experience for the infant and parents or caregivers.[179,266,269] Box 13-9 outlines intervention strategies to facilitate oral feeding.

The use of individualized developmental care may assist VLBW and preterm infants with BPD/CLD in obtaining and maintaining an optimal condition for progression to oral feedings. **Use of skin-to-skin KC improves weight gain, supports and promotes breast feeding, and shortens length of stay (see Box 13-2). Because KC improves alertness and does not tire the infant, it can be used as a strategy to facilitate oral feeding (see Boxes 13-2 and 13-9).** The use of developmental care enables VLBW preterm infants to initiate the first oral feeding and have the last gavage feeding at an earlier age compared with VLBW infants not receiving developmental care. Preterm infants successfully completing oral feeding spent significantly more time in awake states than did preterm infants who were unsuccessful in their feeding.

Using developmental principles, health care providers are able to facilitate both the preterm infant and parents in effective feeding experiences. **A self-regulating preterm infant shows these signs of stability during feeding: (1) smooth, regular respirations (no or minimal increase in respiratory rate or effort); (2) consistent postural control—flexed, hands near face, maintains muscle tone, calm/organized behavior; (3) maintains optimal color; (4) quiet, alert state, focuses on feeding; and (5) coordinates suck-swallow-breathe.[244,269]** Coordination of feeding is facilitated by (1) imposing breaks (e.g., removing the nipple from the mouth; tipping the bottle so that the nipple is empty but remains in the infant's mouth), (2) limiting bolus size (the fewer the number of sucks, the smaller the bolus size) by limiting the number of successive sucks before the infant becomes stressed, and (3) slowing the flow rate (e.g., using low-flow-rate nipples,[169] upright positioning to decrease hydrostatic pressure and gravitational flow).[244]

Signs of stress during nipple feeding, their significance, and appropriate interventions are listed in the Critical Findings box on pp. 318-319. Even preterm infants who are near discharge still have oxygen desaturations when fed by their mothers; the incidence is decreased in infants receiving supplemental oxygen, beginning a feeding with a higher baseline oxygen saturation, and in those of an older post-conceptual age.[267,269] Parents must be taught how to interpret their infant's cues of stability and stress so that they can modify their behavior and learn to intervene to help their infant safely and successfully feed.[226,244,266] Skills parents need for effective feeding include (1) following the infant's lead about readiness to feed; preterms are able to root and open their mouths to the stimulus of a nipple, (2) assessing breathing cues, providing adequate rest (see the Critical Findings box on pp. 318-319) and not interrupting by "jiggling" or moving the nipple to stimulate sucking, and (3) recognizing that noisy swallowing and drooling indicate dysfunction[266] (see the Critical Findings box on pp. 318-319). Strategies that parents consider helpful in mastery of these skills are (1) being included in decision making about feeding and its success, (2) observing a nurse feed their baby, and (3) having a nurse spend time with them while they are feeding their baby to give them feedback, ideas, and tips about feeding.[226,266] For parents, learning to feed their infant is viewed as a significant symbol of parenting, as an opportunity to read and react to infant cues, and as a co-regulator of feeding.[179,226,266]

A feeding plan must be individualized for each infant and posted at the bedside (see Box 13-10 and the Case Study on p. 319). All care providers must adhere to the plan for consistency[179] of stimuli and to promote infant learning. Evidence-based approaches to nipple feeding (for NICU preterms and sick term infants) have been developed that integrate contingent, developmental principles with more nurse autonomy and multidisciplinary collaboration and support.[40,245]

CRYING OR SMILING INTERVENTION

Crying is the infant's innate care-eliciting behavior, a signal that he or she needs attention. The energy expenditure of a crying infant is increased by 7.5% compared with the resting state.[225] Immediate response decreases the infant's physiologic stress, increases the infant's trust in the environment, and enhances the sense of self and of control over the world.[157] The infant's need to escalate to "out-of-control" crying is decreased with immediate response, so that infants are easier to soothe. Consoling the crying infant also helps the infant change states so he or she is able to attend to and interact with the environment.

Term infants vocalize, cry, and look at their caregiver more than do preterm and ill infants.[75,105] Although preterm infants are more irritable than full-term infants, preterm infants cry

Critical Findings

STRESS DURING NIPPLE FEEDINGS

SIGN	SIGNIFICANCE	INTERVENTION
Color change Pallor, dusky, gray, central cyanosis—perioral/periorbital	Oxygen desaturation[168] Feeding too rapidly with brief, shallow breaths Low hematocrit level Breath-holding	Assess baseline color before feeding Periodic removal of nipple to facilitate deep breathing Monitor changes in color during feeding Use pulse oximeter during feeding to maintain saturation ≥92%[267,268]
Changes in state of alertness	Quiet alert state optimal for successful feeding[179,266] Increased infant focus on feeding Increased organization of oropharyngeal muscle movements Increasing drowsiness, falls asleep: Respiratory fatigue resulting from rapid feeding, desaturation, increased respiratory rate, and/or work of breathing Fatigue resulting from behavior/energy expenditure (e.g., crying; bathing) before feeding Fussiness/restlessness—resulting from oxygen desaturation (e.g., hypoxia) because of the work of breathing (WOB) and nippling; disorganized behavioral state	Offer preterm opportunity to suck on pacifier before feeding—encourages awake/alert behavior[268] Pulse oximeter monitoring during feeding—give and/or adjust oxygen to maintain saturations ≥92% during nippling efforts Unwrap if sleepy Periodic rest periods and pace energy expenditure with nipple feeding Swaddle/rock if fussy
Breathing	Increased respiratory effort resulting from work/exercise of feeding,[168,189,266,267] especially in the infant with CLD/BPD	
1. Respiratory fatigue: Falls asleep, ceases feeding before adequate volume obtained	WOB before feeding is increased further with effort of feeding Infants with poor endurance may be unable to feed or may demonstrate poor weight gain despite acceptable intake	Pulse oximeter monitoring with feeding to ensure adequate oxygenation; give oxygen PRN to keep saturation ≥92% Provide chin/cheek support (see Box 13-9) that decreases energy expenditure, enhances state organization and sucking activity
2. Tachypnea Respiratory rate >60/min	WOB increases with feeding; respiratory rate increased with work of feeding Increased incoordination of suck-swallow-breathe with feeding; predisposes to aspiration Increased risk for aspiration if gasping for breath	Brief and/or frequent breaks in feeding to enable deep breaths and reorganize breathing patterns[268]
3. Nasal flaring	Attempts to increase oxygen intake because of hypoxia or increased WOB	Pulse oximeter; supply adequate oxygen Brief breaks to reorganize breathing
Nasal blanching	Distress of breathing/hypoxia Incoordination of suck-swallow-breathe with possible aspiration if flaring/blanching occur	
4. Chin tugging/head bobbing/"catch up" breathing/grunting	Attempting to increase air entry because of "air hunger"/hypoxia/WOB/decreased tidal volume Incoordination of suck-swallow-breathe; increased risk for aspiration	As for signs 1 through 3
5. Crowing sounds—high-pitched stridorous noise on inspiration	Incoordination of opening/closing of vocal cords that increases the risk for aspiration into the trachea[294]	As for signs 1 through 3

Critical Findings—cont'd

SIGN	SIGNIFICANCE	INTERVENTION
Swallowing	Primary swallow dysfunction predisposes to aspiration,[266] swallowing may be evaluated by videofluoroscopy	
1. Drooling	Loss of bolus control because of: Inability of tongue to collect and hold fluid that is flowing too fast Rapid respiratory rate, excessive WOB that shortens time for swallowing to occur; so that only part of bolus is swallowed	Give fewer sucks in a row, followed by brief break so that bolus is smaller and easier to completely swallow[145]
2. Gulping	Use of prolonged sucking pattern or long sucking bursts (especially at the beginning of feeding) without deep breathing at the appropriate intervals Results in oxygen desaturation, bradycardia, apnea resulting from suppression of respiration Increases incoordination of suck-swallow-breathe and stimulates pharyngeal stretch receptors, resulting in vagally stimulated apnea	Give brief breaks to assist the infant in slowing down the feeding[145]
3. Gurgling sounds in the pharynx (breathing sounds are wet/noisy)[266]	Fluid collecting in the throat, pharynx, or supraglottic space above vocal cords Noisy respirations caused by breathing through fluid in hypopharynx because bolus is too large or flow is too fast	Brief break from feeding to enable extra swallow/dry swallow to clear fluid from throat
4. Swallowing (several times) in succession	Deliberate swallows in succession to clear bolus (that is too large/flow is too fast) from pharynx Breathing is delayed with successive swallowing and may result in apnea/bradycardia[170]	Break from feeding to clear throat and regain control of respiration
5. Coughing/choking/gagging/spitting up	Fluid has entered (or nearly entered) the airway[168] Changes in color, heart rate, respiratory rate suggest swallowing problems Occurrence toward end of feeding suggests gastroesophageal reflux; frequent or intense spitting up also may indicate reflux	Usually can be prevented by close attention and intervention to previous signs of feeding difficulty Breaks from feeding to clear airway, regain control of respiration and state organization Ability to cough enables infant to clear airway Inability to cough, color change, hypotonia, bradycardia, and apnea are symptoms of airway obstruction that may require suction and cardiopulmonary resuscitation Change nipple and/or bottle system

Modified from Shaker C: Nipple feeding preterm infants: an individualized, developmentally supportive approach, *Neonatal Netw* 18:15, 1999.
BPD, Bronchopulmonary dysplasia; *CLD*, chronic lung disease; *PRN*, as needed.

Case Study

Tommy was a 28-week preterm infant with severe RDS, prolonged ventilation, and now BPD. He is now 38 weeks post-conceptual age, receiving hood and nasal cannula oxygen and trying to learn to nipple feed. In the morning report, the night nurse says that Tommy "has bradycardia with tube passage so that 24 hours ago he had a cardiorespiratory arrest that required resuscitation. He also has bradycardia and tachypnea with bottle feeding."

Tommy's nurse evaluated his initial attempts to bottle feed (after waiting for him to demand) and wrote the care plan (Box 13-10) after feeding him 45 mL in 20 minutes without tachypnea, cyanosis, or bradycardia.

BPD, Bronchopulmonary dysplasia; *RDS*, respiratory distress syndrome.

BOX 13-10 TOMMY'S FEEDING PLAN

1. ***Sit upright.*** This decreases the flow of formula from the bottle and thus decreases:
   a. His gag reflex, which causes the bradycardia.
   b. His anxiety, which is caused by a bolus of formula in his mouth.
2. ***Use a blue nipple.*** This is the shortest nipple and decreases stimulation of his hypersensitive gag reflex, which causes his bradycardia. (All other nipples stimulated him to gag.)
3. ***Gently push up under his chin when he gets a mouthful of formula.*** This pushes his tongue upward against his palate, the same way the tongue moves during swallowing. (READER: Swallow and note your tongue motion.) He becomes frightened (i.e., eyes wide open and fearful; increased respiratory rate; arching and struggling) when he has a mouthful of formula, because he is used to sucking only on a dry pacifier and having nothing to swallow. His fear raises his heart rate, respiratory rate, and gag reflex, which causes bradycardia.
4. ***Talk to him.*** Softly and gently, tell him he can swallow and praise him when he does.
5. ***Nipple.*** Have him do this as much as possible (he will only get better with practice) and supplement feeding with the indwelling nasogastric tube (no more intermittent tube passage).

less throughout the day than do full-term infants. **NICU infants exhibit fewer care-eliciting behaviors (some preterm infants in one study never cried, vocalized, or looked at their caregiver).**[105] Preterm infants thus are less responsive to the caregivers (both parents and professionals), who receive less positive feedback from the infant and hence are less rewarded. In one study, those NICU infants who were able to cue the care provider (cry, look, vocalize) were consistently responded to 80% to 100% of the time.[105]

Intubated infants who cannot produce an audible cry signal their needs by agitation, heart rate changes, and changes in oxygenation. Preterm infants (<32 weeks' gestation) may recover better from agitation when left alone, because active consolation is overstimulating. How caregivers attempt to soothe a crying infant while giving NICU care includes (1) no response to cries (58.1% of the time), (2) response by talking (29.2% of the time), (3) response by social touching (5.5% of the time), and (4) response by talk and social touching (7.2% of the time).[105]

Parents and staff should use graduated interventions in quieting a crying infant by the following:

- Soothing with gentle, high-pitched talking (loud enough that the infant can hear it above his or her crying)
- Placing the palm of the hand across the infant's chest or holding arms on chest with the palm of the care provider's hand
- Swaddling with blankets to decrease self-upsetting startles
- Picking up infant, holding (upright is the most soothing position), and rocking
- Placing the infant skin-to-skin on the parent's chest
- Offering a pacifier

Most stimulation in the NICU is procedural. The lack of social stimulation in the NICU not only affects the infant but also teaches parents that their infant is too weak for, too fragile for, uninterested in, or incapable of social interaction. Again, social stimulation must be paced according to the stage of development and stability of the infant[77] **(see the Critical Findings box on p. 284).** Enhancing the infant's social environment includes presenting the smiling, moving, talking care provider's face to the alert infant; touching and stroking; and soothing and consoling the distressed infant.

In many busy NICUs, parents and a foster grandparent program provide this sensory integrated social experience. If the infant has been transported to a referral center, parents may live some distance away and be unable to visit daily. A chronically ill 4- to 5-month-old infant who begins to recognize the foster grandmother may smile, relax, and feed better for her and is often fussier and more irritable on her day off. A foster grandparent program benefits both infants and seniors—the infant receives love and socialization, and the senior "has a reason to get up in the morning."

If possible, parents should be encouraged to perform the "firsts" with their infant (e.g., first nipple feeding, first bath, first time out of the incubator). Because parents are not always present, they will miss some important milestones for their infant (e.g., extubation). Many NICUs have developed baby diaries (or calendars) in which the nurses, physicians, and foster grandparents write important information about the infant's day (as if the infant were the author). The text is accompanied by self-developing pictures with humorous captions (e.g., "Look at me. I've got my tube out!"). Staff are very creative in relating "what's been happening," so that the parents have not only a verbal report (that, over time, may be forgotten) but also a keepsake of NICU progress.

SUMMARY

Care of preterm infants began with a minimal handling policy. Research and knowledge of the unique anatomy and physiology of the neonate preceded the development of high-technology devices and high touch to manage both machines and newborns. Observation and research have documented the effect of the NICU environment on its vulnerable inhabitants. **Individualized developmental interventions in the NICU and beyond have resulted in decreased developmental delay, as well as medical benefits, improved parent competence and functioning, and cost savings (see Table 13-1).** Because individualized developmental care improves outcomes, several recommendations have been proposed: (1) third-party reimbursement may favor NICUs that are cost-effective; (2) NICUs choosing not to use developmental care should have clear reasons and consider randomized trials to disprove its effectiveness; and (3) the American Academy of Pediatrics should critically evaluate developmental care and make recommendations about its use.[187] Positive long-term effects and benefits of individualized developmental care continue to be documented at school age.[4,286] Individualized developmental care improves the lives of preterm infants and their families by preventing long-term complications and poor outcomes.[46]

The pursuit of "humane,"[133] relationship-based[4,5,127] developmental care continues with redesign of NICU environments,[56,127,214] including single-room care,[127,214] as well as changing the attitudes and care practices among health care providers. Creating an integrated, relationship-based, family-centered, developmental care philosophy requires the following:

- A commitment by individual care providers to alter practice for the benefit of neonates and families and to integrate family-centered developmental care into their individual practice[22,46,127]
- Relationship building with neonates, families, and colleagues[22,46,127]
- The use of effective change strategies[22] within the institution's organizational climate
- Implementing the guidelines of national professional organizations[13,14,56] to satisfy ethical, legal, and professional standards of care
- Changing health care providers' knowledge base, which requires multidisciplinary educational opportunities (e.g., orientation, in-service, continuing education, consultation) and written resource materials[2,22,46,127]

Two recent studies document the increased satisfaction of parents whose preterms were cared for with the NIDCAP model when compared with conventional, traditional care practices.[135,293]

Developmental care can no longer be considered "nice, but optional," especially with the evidence that not only brain function but also actual brain structure are positively affected by the early experiences of family-centered developmental care in the NICU.[3]

REFERENCES

1. Affonso D, Bosque E, Wahlberg V, et al: Reconciliation and healing for mothers through skin-to-skin contact provided in American tertiary level intensive care nursery, *Neonatal Netw* 12:25, 1993.
2. Als H: *Program guide: Newborn Individualized Developmental Care and Assessment Program (NIDCAP)—an education and training program for health care professionals,* ed 11, Boston, 2008, Children's Medical Center Corp.
3. Als H, Duffy F, McAnulty G, et al: Early experience alters brain function and structure, *Pediatrics* 113:846, 2004.
4. Als H, Gilkerson L: The role of relationship-based developmentally supportive newborn intensive care in strengthening outcome of preterm infants, *Semin Perinatol* 21:178, 1997.
5. Als H, Gilkerson L, Duffy F, et al: A three-center, randomized, controlled trial of individualized developmental care for very low birth weight preterm infants: medical, neurodevelopmental, parenting, and caregiving effects, *J Dev Behav Pediatr* 24:399, 2003.
6. Als H, Lawhon G, Brown E, et al: Toward a research instrument for the assessment of preterm infant's behavior (APIB). In Hiram E, Lester BM, Yogman MW, Fitzgerald HE, editors: *Dev Med Child Neurol,* vol 1, New York, NY, 1982, Springer.
7. Als H, Lawhon G, Duffy FH, et al: Individualized developmental care for VLBW preterm infants, *JAMA* 272:853, 1994.
8. Altimier L: Management of the NICU environment. In Kenner C, Lott J, editors: *Comprehensive neonatal nursing,* ed 3 Philadelphia, 2003, Saunders.
9. Altimier L, Lutes L: Co-bedding multiples, *Newborn Infant Nurs Rev* 1:205, 2001.
10. Aly H, Moustafa M, Hassanein S, et al: Physical activity combined with massage improves bone mineralization in premature infants: a randomized control trial, *J Perinatol* 24:305, 2004.

11. Amaizu N, Shulman R, Schanler R, et al: Maturation of oral feeding skills in preterm infants, *Acta Paediatr* 97:61, 2008.
12. American Academy of Pediatrics: Hearing assessment in infants and children: recommendations beyond neonatal screening, *Pediatrics* 111:436, 2003.
13. American Academy of Pediatrics: *American College of Obstetricians and Gynecologists (AAP/ACOG): Guidelines for perinatal care,* ed 6, Elk Grove Village, Ill, 2007, The Academy.
14. American Academy of Pediatrics: Committee on Hospital Care, and Institute for Family-Centered Care: family-centered care and the pediatrician's role, *Pediatrics* 120:683, 2007.
15. American Academy of Pediatrics: Joint Committee on Infant Hearing: Year 2007 Position Statement: Principles and guidelines for early hearing detection and intervention, *Pediatrics* 120:898, 2007.
16. American Academy of Pediatrics, Task Force on Sudden Infant Death Syndrome: The changing concept of sudden infant death syndrome: diagnostic coding shifts, controversies regarding sleep environment, and new variables to consider in reducing risk, *Pediatrics* 116:1245, 2005.
17. Anderson G, Chiu S, Dombrowski M, et al: Mother-newborn contact in a randomized trial of kangaroo (skin-to-skin) care, *J Obstet Gynecol Neonatal Nurs* 32:604, 2003.
18. Appleton S: "Handle with care": an investigation of the handling received by preterm infants in intensive care, *J Neonatal Nurs* 31:23, 1997.
19. Ariagno R, Mirmiran M, Adams M, et al: Effect of position on sleep, heart rate variability, and QT interval in preterm infants at 1 and 3 months' corrected age, *Pediatrics* 111:622, 2003.
20. Aris C, Stevens TP, LeMura C, et al: NICU nurses' knowledge and discharge teaching related to infant sleep position and risk of SIDS, *Adv Neonatal Care* 6:281, 2006.
21. Balaguer A, Escribano J, Roque M: Infant position in neonates receiving mechanical ventilation, *Cochrane Database Syst Rev* 4: CD003668 2006.
22. Ballweg D: Individualized care: actions for the individual staff member. In Kenner C, McGrath J, editors: *Developmental care of newborns and infants,* St Louis, 2004, Mosby.
23. Barker D: *Mothers, babies and health in later life,* ed 2, London, 1998, Churchill-Livingstone.
24. Barlow SM, Finan DF, Lee J, et al: Synthetic orocutaneous stimulation entrains preterm infants with feeding difficulties to suck, *J Perinatol* 28:541, 2008.
25. Barreto ED, Morris BH, Philbin MK, et al: Do former preterm infants remember and respond to neonatal intensive care unit noise? *Early Human Dev* 82:703, 2006.
26. Bartocci M, Winberg J, Papendieck G, et al: Cerebral hemodynamic response to unpleasant odors in the preterm newborn measured by near-infrared spectroscopy, *Pediatr Res* 50:324, 2001.
27. Bell SM, Ainsworth MD: Infant crying and maternal responsiveness, *Child Dev* 43:1171, 1972.
28. Bertelle V, Sevestre A, Laou-Hap K, et al: Sleep in the neonatal intensive care unit, *J Perinat Neonat Nurs* 21:140, 2007.
29. Bhat R, Leipala J, Singh N, et al: Effect of posture on oxygenation, lung volume, and respiratory mechanics in premature infants studied before discharge, *Pediatrics* 112:29, 2003.
30. Bingham PM, Churchill D, Ashikaga T: Breast milk odor via olfactometer for tube-fed, premature infants, *Behav Res Methods* 39:630, 2007.
31. Boiron M, DaNobrega L, Roux S, et al: Effects of oral stimulation and oral support on non-nutritive sucking and feeding performance in preterm infants, *Dev Med Child Neurol* 49:439, 2007.
32. Boukydis Z, Bigsby R, Lester B: Clinical use of the Neonatal Intensive Care Unit Network Neurobehavioral Scale (NNNS), *Pediatrics* 113:679, 2004.
33. Bowlby J: *Attachment*, New York, 1973, Basic Books.
34. Bowlby J: *Loss*, New York, 1980, Basic Books.
35. Brackbill Y, Douthitt T, West H: Neonatal posture: psychophysiological effects, *Neuropadiatrie* 4:145, 1973.
36. Brandon D, Holditch-Davis D, Belyea M: Preterm infants born at less than 31 weeks' gestation have improved growth in cycled light compared with continuous near darkness, *J Pediatr* 140:192, 2002.
37. Brandon DH, Ryan DJ, Barnes AH: Effect of environmental changes on noise in the NICU, *Neonatal Netw* 26:213, 2007.
38. Brazelton TB: *Neonatal behavioral assessment scale,* ed 2, Philadelphia, 1984, Spastics International Medical Publishers/Lippincott.
39. Brouwers E, van Baar A, Pop V: Maternal anxiety during pregnancy and subsequent infant development, *Infant Behav Devel* 24:95, 2001.
40. Brown VD, Gardner SL: *Nipple feeding the infant: Policy/Procedure/Protocol Packet NPDPA,* 2007 Nurse's Professional Development and Practice Association LLC. Available at www.npdpa.com.
41. Browne J: Considerations for touch and massage in the NICU, *Neonatal Netw* 19:61, 2000.
42. Browne J: Early relationship environments: physiology of skin-to-skin contact for parents and their preterm infants, *Clin Perinatol* 31:287, 2004.
43. Buehler DM, Als H, Duffy FH, et al: Effectiveness of individualized developmental care for low-risk preterm infants: behavioral and electrophysiologic evidence, *Pediatrics* 96:923, 1995.

44. Bullock L, Mickey K, Green J, et al: Are nurses acting as role models for the prevention of SIDS? *MCN Am J Matern Child Nurs* 29:172, 2004.
45. Bulock F, Woolridge M, Baum J: Development of coordination of sucking, swallowing, and breathing: ultrasound study of term and preterm infants, *Dev Med Child Neurol* 32:669, 1990.
46. Butler S, Als H: Individualized developmental care improves the lives of infants born preterm, *Acta Paediatr* 97(9):1173, 2008.
47. Byers JM, Waugh WR, Lowman LB: Sound level exposure of high-risk infants in different environmental conditions, *Neonatal Netw* 25:25, 2006.
48. Byers J, Yovaish W, Lowman L, et al: Co-bedding vs. single-bedding premature multiple-gestation infants in incubators, *J Obstet Gynecol Neonatal Nurs* 32:340, 2003.
49. Carfoot S, Williamson P, Dickson R: A systematic review of randomized controlled trials evaluating the effect of mother/baby skin-to-skin care on successful breast feeding, *Midwifery* 19:148, 2003.
50. Chang Y, Anderson G, Lin C: Effects of prone and supine positions on sleep state and stress responses in mechanically ventilated preterm infants during the first postnatal week, *J Adv Nurs* 40:161, 2002.
51. Chin SD, Hope L, Christos P: Randomized controlled trial evaluating the effects of cobedding on weight gain and physiologic regulation in preterm twins in the NICU, *Adv Neonatal Care* 6:142, 2006.
52. Christensson K, Cabrera T, Christensson E, et al: Separation distress call in the human neonate in the absence of maternal body contact, *Acta Paediatr* 84:468, 1995.
53. Christensson K, Siles C, Moreno L, et al: Temperature, metabolic adaptation and crying in healthy full-term newborns cared for skin-to-skin or in a cot, *Acta Paediatr* 81:488, 1992.
54. Collins C, Crowther C, Ryan P, et al: Effects of bottles, cups and dummies on breast feeding in preterm infants: a randomized controlled trial, *BMJ* 329:193, 2004.
55. Conde-Agudelo A, Diaz-Rossello J, Belzan J: Kangaroo mother care to reduce morbidity and mortality in LBW infants, *Cochrane Database Syst Rev* 2: CD002771 2003.
56. Consensus Committee on Recommendations: *Standards for newborn ICU design,* Feb 1, 2007. Accessed August 13, 2008, from www.nd.edu/nicudes/stan%2023.html.
57. Corff KE, Seideman R, Venkataraman PS, et al: Facilitated tucking: a nonpharmacologic comfort measure for pain in preterm neonates, *J Obstet Gynecol Neonatal Nurs* 24:143, 1995.
58. Crosson D, Pickler R: An integrated review of the literature on demand feedings for preterm infants, *Adv Neonatal Care* 4:216, 2004.
59. Danford DA, Miske S, Headley J, et al: Effects of routine care procedures on transcutaneous oxygen in neonates: a quantitative approach, *Arch Dis Child* 58:20, 1983.
60. Dangeman BC: The variability of Pao_2 in newborn infants in response to routine care, *Pediatr Res* 10:149, 1976.
61. Darcy A, Hancock LE, Ware EJ: A descriptive study of noise in the neonatal intensive care unit, *Adv Neonatal Care* 8:165, 2008.
62. DeCasper AJ, Fifer WP: Of human bonding: newborns prefer their mother's voices, *Science* 208:1175, 1980.
63. DeCasper AJ, Spence MJ: Prenatal maternal speech influences newborn's perception of speech sounds, *Infant Behav Dev* 9:133, 1986.
64. DeRoiste A, Bushnell I: Cardiorespiratory and transcutaneous oxygen monitoring of high-risk preterms receiving systematic stroking, *Int J Prenatal Perinatal Psychol Med* 12:89, 2000.
65. Diego MA, Field T, Hernandez-Reif M, et al: Preterm infant massage elicits consistent increases in vagal activity and gastric motility that are associated with greater weight gain, *Acta Paediatr* 96:1588, 2007.
66. Diego MA, Field T, Hernandez-Reif M: Temperature increases in preterm infants during massage therapy, *Infant Behav Dev* 31:149, 2008.
67. DiMenna L: Considerations for implementation of a neonatal kangaroo care protocol, *Neonatal Netw* 25:405, 2006.
68. Dobbing J, Sands J: Quantitative growth and development of the human brain, *Arch Dis Child* 48:757, 1973.
69. Dodrill P, Donovan T, Cleghorn G, et al: Attainment of early feeding milestones in preterm neonates, *J Perinatol* 28:549, 2008.
70. Downs JA, Edwards AD, McCormick DC, et al: Effect of intervention on development of hip posture in very preterm babies, *Arch Dis Child* 66:797, 1991.
71. Dreyfus-Brisac C: Organization of sleep in preterms: implications for caretaking. In Lewis M, Rosenblum LA, editors: *The effect of the infant on its caregiver,* New York, 1974, John Wiley & Sons.
72. Dreyfus-Brisac C: Ontogenesis of brain bioelectric activity and sleep organization in neonates and infants. In Faulkner F, Tanner JM, editors: *Human growth*, vol 3, New York, 1979, Plenum Publishing.
73. Dubowitz L, Dubowitz V, Mercuri E: The neurologic assessment of the preterm and full-term newborn infant, *Clinics in Developmental Medicine* 148, London, 1999, University Press.
74. Duxbury ML, Henly SJ, Broz LJ, et al: Caregiver disruptions and sleep of high-risk infants, *Heart Lung* 13:141, 1984.

75. Eckerman C, Hsu H, Molitor A, et al: Infant arousal in an *en face* exchange with a new partner: effects of prematurity and perinatal biological risk, *Dev Psychol* 35:282, 1999.
76. Eckerman C, Oehler J, Hannan T, et al: The development prior to term age of very prematurely born newborns' responsiveness in *en face* exchanges, *Infant Behav Dev* 18:283, 1995.
77. Eckerman C, Oehler J, Medvin M, et al: Premature newborns as social partners before term age, *Inf Behav Dev* 17:55, 1994.
78. Engler A, Ludington-Hoe S, Cusson R, et al: Kangaroo care: national survey of practice, knowledge, barriers, and perceptions, *MCN Am J Matern Child Nurs* 27:146, 2002.
79. Evans J: Comparison of two NICU patterns of caregiving over 24 hours for preterm infants, *Neonatal Netw* 13:87, 1994.
80. Evans J, McCartney E, Roth-Sautler C: Desaturation or bradycardic events following caregiving in the NICU, *Neonatal Intensive Care* 4:20, 2000.
81. Evans J, Vogelpohl D, Bourguignon C, et al: Pain behaviors in LBW infants accompanying some "nonpainful" caregiving procedures, *Neonatal Netw* 16:33, 1997.
82. Fantz RL, Fagan JF, Miranda SB: Early visual selectivity as a function of pattern variables, previous exposure, age from birth and conception and expected cognitive deficit. In Cohen L, Salaptic P, editors: *Infant perception,* vol 1, New York, 1975, Academic Press.
83. Feldman R: Mother-infant skin-to-skin contact (kangaroo care): theoretical, clinical, and empirical aspects, *Infants Young Child* 17:145, 2004.
84. Feldman R, Eidelman A: Mother-infant skin-to-skin contact (kangaroo care) accelerates autonomic and neurobehavioral maturation in premature infants, *Dev Med Child Neurol* 45:274, 2003.
85. Feldman R, Eidelman A, Sirota L, et al: Comparison of skin-to-skin (kangaroo) and traditional care: parenting outcomes and preterm infant development, *Pediatrics* 110:16, 2002.
86. Feldman R, Weller A, Eidelman A, et al: Testing a family intervention hypothesis: the contribution of mother-infant skin-to-skin contact (kangaroo care) to family interaction and touch, *J Fam Psychol* 17:94, 2003.
87. Feldman R, Weller A, Sirota L, et al: Skin-to-skin contact (kangaroo care) promotes self regulation in premature infants: sleep-wake cyclicity, arousal modulation, and sustained exploration, *Dev Psychol* 38:194, 2002.
88. Ferber S, Kuint J, Weller A, et al: Massage therapy by mothers and trained professionals enhances weight gain in preterm infants, *Early Hum Dev* 67:37, 2002.
89. Field T: Infant massage therapy. In Goldson E, editor: *Nurturing the premature infant,* New York, 1999, Oxford University Press.
90. Field T, Diego MA, Hernandez-Reif M, et al: Moderate versus light pressure massage therapy leads to greater weight gain in preterm infants, *Infant Behav Dev* 29:574, 2006.
91. Fielder A, Moseley M: Environmental light and the preterm infant, *Semin Perinatol* 24:291, 2000.
92. Fleisher BE, VandenBerg K, Constantinou J, et al: Individualized developmental care for very-low-birth-weight premature infants, *Clin Pediatr* 34:523, 1995.
93. Fohe K, Kropf S, Avenardius S: Skin-to-skin contact improves gas exchange in premature infants, *J Perinatol* 20:311, 2000.
94. Franck L, Bernal H, Gale G: Infant holding policies and practices in neonatal units, *Neonatal Netw* 21:13, 2002.
95. Franck L, Quinn D, Zahr L: Effect of less frequent bathing of preterm infants on skin flora and pathogen colonization, *J Obstet Gynecol Neonatal Nurs* 29:584, 2000.
96. Franco P, Pardou A, Hassid S, et al: Auditory arousal thresholds are higher when infants sleep in the prone position, *J Pediatr* 132:240, 1998.
97. Freedman DG: Ethnic differences in babies, *Hum Nat* 2:36, 1979.
98. Fucile S, Gisel E, Lau C: Oral stimulation accelerates the transition from tube to oral feeding in preterm infants, *J Pediatr* 141:230, 2002.
99. Gay C, Lee K, Lee S: Sleep patterns and fatigue in new mothers and fathers, *Biol Res Nurs* 5:311, 2004.
100. Gewolb IH, Vice FL: Maturational changes in rhythms, patterning, and coordination of respiration and swallow during feeding in preterm and term infants, *Dev Med Child Neurol* 48:589, 2006.
101. Goldson E: Non-nutritive sucking in the sick infant, *J Perinatol* 7:30, 1987.
102. Goltzbach S, Edgar D, Ariagno R: Biological rhythmicity in preterm infants prior to discharge from neonatal intensive care, *Pediatrics* 95:231, 1995.
103. Gorski PA, Davison MF, Brazelton TB: Stages of behavioral organization in the high risk neonate: theoretical and clinical considerations, *Semin Perinatol* 3:61, 1979.
104. Goto K, Mirmiran M, Adams M, et al: More awakenings and heart rate variability during supine sleep in preterm infants, *Pediatrics* 103:603, 1999.
105. Gottfried AW, Gaiter JL: *Infant stress under intensive care: environmental neonatology,* Baltimore, 1985, University Park Press.
106. Graven S: Sound and the developing infant in the NICU: conclusions and recommendations for care, *J Perinatol* 20:S88, 2000.

107. Hake-Brooks S, Anderson GC: Kangaroo care and breastfeeding of mother-preterm infant dyads 0–18 months: a randomized, controlled trial, *Neonatal Netw* 27:151, 2008.
108. Harrison L: Research utilization: handling preterm infants in the NICU, *Neonatal Netw* 16:65, 1997.
109. Harrison L, Lotas M, Jorgensen K: Environmental issues. In Kenner C, McGrath J, editors: *Developmental care of newborns and infants,* St Louis, 2004, Mosby.
110. Harrison L, Leeper J, Yoon M: Effects of early parent touch on preterm infants' arterial oxygen saturation and heart rate levels, *J Adv Nurs* 15:877, 1990.
111. Harrison L, Roane C, Weaver M: The relationship between physiological and behavioral measures of stress in preterm infants, *J Obstet Gynecol Neonatal Nurs* 33:236, 2004.
112. Harrison L, Williams A, Berbaum M, et al: Physiologic and behavioral effects of gentle human touch on preterm infants, *Res Nurs Health* 23:435, 2000.
113. Heimler R, Langlois J, Hodel D, et al: Effect of positioning on the breathing pattern of preterm infants, *Arch Dis Child* 67:312, 1992.
114. Hellerud B, Storm H: Skin conductance and behaviour during sensory stimulation of preterm and term infants, *Early Hum Dev* 70:35, 2002.
115. Hemingway M, Oliver S: Preterm infant positioning, *Neonatal Intensive Care* 13:18, 2000.
116. Hill A: The effects of nonnutritive sucking and oral support on the feeding efficiency of preterm infants, *Newborn Infant Nursing Reviews* 5:133, 2005.
117. Holditch-Davis D, Torres C, O'Hale A, et al: Standardized rest periods affect the incidence of apnea and rate of weight gain in convalescent preterm infants, *Neonatal Netw* 15:87, 1996.
118. Holsti L, Grunau RE, Oberlander TF, et al: Prior pain induces heightened motor responses during clustered care in preterm infants in the NICU, *Early Human Dev* 81:293, 2005.
119. Holsti L, Grunau RE, Whitfield MF, et al: Behavioral responses to pain are heightened after cluster care in preterm infants born between 30 and 32 weeks gestational age, *Clin J Pain* 22:757, 2006.
120. Holsti L, Weinberg J, Whitfield MF, et al: Relationship between adrenocorticotropic hormone and cortisol are related during clustered nursing care in preterm infants born at extremely low gestational age, *Early Hum Dev* 83:341, 2007.
121. Horne R, Franco P, Adamson T, et al: Effects of body position on sleep and arousal characteristics in infants, *Early Hum Dev* 69:25, 2002.
122. Horton J, Walderstrom U, Bowman E: Touch of LBW babies in NICU: observations over a 24 hour period, *J Neonatal Nurs* 4:24, 1998.
123. Howe TH, Sheu CF, Hinojosa J, et al: Multiple factors related to bottle-feeding performance in preterm infants, *Nurs Res* 56:307, 2007.
124. Hunt C, Leskko S, Vezina R, et al: Infant sleep position and associated health outcomes, *Arch Pediatr Adolesc Med* 157:469, 2003.
125. Hunter J: Positioning. In Kenner C, McGrath J, editors: *Developmental care of newborns and infants,* St Louis, 2004, Mosby.
126. Jeffery MA, Page M: Why the prone position is a risk factor for sudden infant death syndrome, *Pediatrics* 104:263, 1999.
127. Johnson B, Abraham M, Parrish R: Designing the neonatal intensive care unit for optimal family involvement, *Clin Perinatol* 31:353, 2004.
128. Johnston CC, Filion F, Campbell-Yeo M, et al: Kangaroo care diminishes pain from heel lance in very preterm neonates: a crossover trial, *BMC Pediatr* 8:13, 2008.
129. Kassim Z, Donaldson N, Khetriwal B, et al: Sleeping position, oxygen saturation and lung volume in convalescent, prematurely born infants, *Arch Dis Child Fetal Neonatal Ed* 82:F347, 2007.
130. Kato I, Franco P, Grosswasser J, et al: Incomplete arousal processes in infants who were victims of sudden infant death, *Am J Respir Crit Care Med* 168:1262, 2003.
131. Keene D, Wimmer J, Mathew O: Does supine positioning increase apnea, bradycardia and desaturation in preterm infants? *J Perinatol* 1:17, 2000.
132. Kemper K, Martin K, Block S, et al: Staff attitudes about music therapy for premature infants, *Pediatr Res* 85A:55, 2004.
133. Kennell J: The humane neonatal care initiative, *Acta Paediatr* 88:367, 1999.
134. Kent W, Tan A, Clarke M, et al: Excessive noise levels in the neonatal ICU: potential effects on auditory system development, *J Otolaryngol* 31:355, 2002.
135. Kleberg A, Hellstrom-Westas L, Widstrom AM: Mother's perception of Newborn Individualized Developmental Care and Assessment Program (NIDCAP®) as compared to conventional care, *Early Human Dev* 83:403, 2007.
136. Kleberg A, Westrup B, Stjernqvist K, et al: Indications of improved cognitive development at one year of age among infants born very prematurely who received care based on the Newborn Individualized Developmental Care and Assessment Program (NIDCAP®), *Early Hum Dev* 68:83, 2002.
137. Korja R, Maunu J, Kirjavainen J, et al, and the PIPARI study group: Mother-infant interaction is influenced by the amount of holding in preterm infants, *Early Hum Dev* 84:257, 2008.
138. Korner AF: The effect of the infants' state, level of arousal, sex and ontogenetic stage on the caregiver. In

Lewis M, Rosenblum LA, editors: *The effect of the infant on its caregiver,* New York, 1974, John Wiley & Sons.

139. Korones S: Disturbances and infant's rest. In Moore T, editor: *Iatrogenic problems in neonatal intensive care*, Report of the 69th Ross Conference on Pediatric Research, Columbus, Ohio, 1976, Ross Laboratories.
140. Kostandy RR, Ludington-Hoe SM, Cong X, et al: Kangaroo care (skin contact) reduces crying response to pain in preterm neonates: pilot results, *Pain Manag Nurs* 9:55, 2008.
141. Kreuger C, Wall S, Parker L, et al: Elevated sound levels within a busy NICU, *Neonatal Netw* 24:33, 2005.
142. Lahat S, Mimouni FB, Ashbel G, et al: Energy expenditure in growing preterm infants receiving massage therapy, *J Am Coll Nutr* 26:356, 2007.
143. LaMar K, Dowling DA: Incidence of infection for preterm twins cared for in cobedding in the neonatal intensive-care unit, *J Obstet Gynecol Neonatal Nurs* 35:193, 2006.
144. Langor V: Minimal handling protocol for the intensive care nursery, *Neonatal Netw* 9:23, 1990.
145. Law-Morstatt L, Judd D, Snyder P, et al: Pacing as a treatment for transitional sucking, *J Perinatol* 23:483, 2003.
146. Lee Y, Malakooti N, Lotas M: A comparison of the light-reduction capacity of commonly used incubator covers, *Neonatal Netw* 24:37, 2005.
147. Lehtonen L, Johnson M, Bakdash T, et al: Relation of sleep state to hypoxemic episodes in ventilated extremely-low-birth-weight infants, *J Pediatr* 141:363, 2002.
148. Leitch D: Mother-infant interaction: achieving synchrony, *Nurs Res* 48:55, 1999.
149. Leslie GI, Kalaw MB, Bowen JR, et al: Risk factors for sensorineural hearing loss in extremely premature infants, *J Pediatr Child Health* 31:312, 1995.
150. Lester BM, Tronick EZ: History and description of the Neonatal Intensive Care Unit Network Neurobehavioral Scale (NNNS), *Pediatrics* 113:634, 2004.
151. Levy J, Habib RH, Lipsten E, et al: Prone versus supine positioning in the well preterm infant: effects on work of breathing and breathing patterns, *Pediatr Pulmonol* 41:754, 2006.
152. Liaw JJ, Yang L, Yuh YS, et al: Effects of tub bathing procedures on preterm infants' behavior, *J Nurs Res* 14:297, 2006.
153. Litamanovitz I, Dolfin T, Friedland O, et al: Early physical activity intervention prevents decrease of bone strength in VLBW infants, *Pediatrics* 112:15, 2003.
154. Lockridge T, Taquino L: Infant sleep position protocols. In Kenner C, McGrath J, editors: *Developmental care of newborns and infants,* St Louis, 2004, Mosby.
155. Long J, Philip A, Lucey J: Excessive handling as a cause of hypoxemia, *Pediatrics* 65:203, 1980.
156. Ludington-Hoe S, Anderson G, Swinth J, et al: Randomized controlled trial of kangaroo care: cardiorespiratory and thermal effects on healthy preterm infants, *Neonatal Netw* 23:39, 2004.
157. Ludington-Hoe S, Cong X, Hashemi F: Infant crying: nature, physiologic consequences, and select interventions, *Neonatal Netw* 21:29, 2002.
158. Ludington-Hoe S, Ferreira C, Swinth J, et al: Safe criteria and procedure for kangaroo care with intubated preterm infants, *J Obstet Gynecol Neonatal Nurs* 32:579, 2003.
159. Ludington-Hoe SM, Hosseini R, Torowicz DL: Skin-to-skin contact (kangaroo care) analgesia for preterm infant heel stick, *AACN Clin Issues* 16:373, 2005.
160. Ludington-Hoe SM, Johnson MW, Morgan K, et al: Neurophysiologic assessment of neonatal sleep organization: preliminary results of a randomized, controlled trial of skin contact with preterm infants, *Pediatrics* 117:e909, 2006.
161. Ludington-Hoe SM, Morgan K, Abouelfettoh A: A clinical guideline for implementation of kangaroo care with premature infants of 30 or more weeks' postmenstrual age, *Adv Neonatal Care* 8:S3, 2008.
162. Ludington-Hoe SM, Thompson C, Swinth J, et al: Kangaroo care: research results and practice implications and guidelines, *Neonatal Netw* 13:19, 1994.
163. Lutes M, Graves C, Jorgensen K: The NICU experience and its relationship to sensory integration. In Kenner C, McGrath J, editors: *Developmental care of newborns and infants,* St Louis, 2004, Mosby.
164. Maichuk G, Zahorodny W, Marshall R: Use of positioning to reduce the severity of neonatal narcotic withdrawal syndrome, *J Perinatol* 19:510, 1999.
165. Maroney D: Recognizing the potential effect of stress and trauma on premature infants in the NICU: how are outcomes affected? *J Perinatol* 23:679, 2003.
166. Martin R, DiFiore JM, Korenke CB, et al: Vulnerability of respiratory control in healthy preterm infants placed supine, *J Pediatr* 127:609, 1995.
167. Masterson J, Zucker C, Schulze K, et al: Prone and supine positioning effects on energy expenditure and behavior of low birth weight neonates, *Pediatrics* 80:689, 1987.
168. Mathew O: Respiratory control during nipple feeding in preterm infants, *Pediatr Pulmonol* 5:220, 1988.
169. Mathew O, Belan M, Thoppil C: Sucking patterns of neonates during bottle feeding: comparison of different nipple units, *Am J Perinatol* 9:265, 1992.
170. Mathew O, Bhatia J: Sucking and breathing patterns during breast- and bottle-feeding in term newborns, *Am J Dis Child* 143:588, 1989.
171. McCain G: Promotion of preterm infant nipple feeding with nonnutritive sucking, *J Pediatr Nurs* 10:3, 1995.

172. McCain G: An evidence-based guideline for introducing oral feeding to healthy preterm infants, *Neonatal Netw* 22:45, 2003.
173. McCain G, Fuller EO, Gartside PS: Heart rate variability and feeding bradycardia in healthy preterm infants during transition from gavage to oral feeding, *Newborn Infant Nurs Rev* 5:124, 2005.
174. McCain G, Gartside P: Behavioral responses of preterm infants to a standard-care and semi-demand feeding protocol, *Newborn Infant Nurs Rev* 2:187, 2002.
175. McCain G, Gartside P, Greenberg J, et al: A feeding protocol for healthy preterm infants that shortens time to oral feeding, *J Pediatr* 139:374, 2001.
176. McEvoy C, Mendoza M, Bowling S, et al: Prone positioning decreases episodes of hypoxemia in ELBW infants (1000 grams or less) with chronic lung disease, *J Pediatr* 130:305, 1997.
177. McGehee L, Eckerman C: The preterm infant as a social partner: responsive but unreadable, *Infant Behav Dev* 6:461, 1983.
178. McGrath J, Block N: Efficacy and utilization of skin-to-skin care in the NICU, *Newborn Infant Nurs Rev* 2:17, 2002.
179. McGrath J, Braescu A: State of the science: feeding readiness in the preterm infant, *J Perinatal Neonatal Nurs* 18:353, 2004.
180. McGrath J, Thillet M, Van Cleave L: Parent delivered infant massage: are we truly ready for implementation? *Newborn Infant Nurs Rev* 7:39, 2007.
181. Meaney M: Maternal care, gene expression, and the transmission of individual differences in stress reactivity across generations, *Annu Rev Neurosci* 24:1161, 2001.
182. Medoff-Cooper B, Bilker W, Kaplan J: Suckling behavior as a function of gestational age: a cross-sectional study, *Infant Behav Dev* 24:83, 2001.
183. Mellien A: Incubators vs. mother's arms: body temperature conservation in VLBW premature infants, *J Obstet Gynecol Neonatal Nurs* 30:157, 2001.
184. Meltzoff AN, Moore MK: Imitation of facial and manual gestures by human neonates, *Science* 198(4312):74, 1977.
185. Mendes EW, Procianoy RS: Massage therapy reduces hospital stay and occurrence of late-onset sepsis in very preterm neonates, *J Perinatol* 28(12):815, 2008.
186. Mennella J, Jagnow C, Beauchamo G: Prenatal and postnatal flavor learning by human infants, *Pediatrics* 107:E88 (editorial) 2001.
187. Merenstein G: Individualized developmental care: an emerging new standard for neonatal intensive care units? *JAMA* 272:890, 1994.
188. Merritt T, Pillers D, Prows S: Early NICU discharge of very low birth weight infants: a critical review and analysis, *Semin Neonatol* 8:95, 2003.
189. Miller M, Kiatchoosakun P: Relationship between respiratory control and feeding in the developing infant, *Semin Neonatol* 9:221, 2004.
190. Miranda SB, Fantz RL: Visual abilities and pattern preference of preterm infants and full-term neonates, *J Exp Child Psychiatry* 10:189, 1970.
191. Mirmiran M, Ariagno R: Influence of light in the NICU on the development of circadian rhythms in preterm infants, *Semin Perinatol* 24:247, 2000.
192. Mitchell EA, Hutchison L, Stewart AW: The continuing decline in SIDS mortality, *Arch Dis Child* 92:625, 2007.
193. Modrcin-Talbott M, Harrison L, Groer M, et al: The biobehavioral effects of gentle human touch on preterm infants, *Nurs Sci Q* 16:60, 2003.
194. Moles A, Kieffer B, D'Amato F: Deficit in attachment behavior in mice lacking the mu-opioid receptor gene, *Science* 304:1983, 2004.
195. Reference deleted in proofs.
196. Montagu A: *Touching,* New York, 1971, Harper & Row.
197. Monterosso L, Kristjanson L, Cole J: Neuromotor development and the physiologic effects of positioning in very low birth weight infants, *J Obstet Gynecol Neonatal Nur* 31:138, 2002.
198. Moon C, Fifer W: Evidence of transnatal auditory learning, *J Perinatol* 20:S37, 2000.
199. Mouradian L, Als H: The influence of neonatal intensive care unit caregiving practices on motor functioning of preterm infants, *Am J Occup Ther* 48:527, 1994.
200. Nathaniels P: Fetal programming: how the quality of fetal life alters biology for a lifetime, *Pediatrics* 1:E126, 2000.
201. National Association of Neonatal Nurses: *Co-bedding of twins or higher order multiples,* Glenview, Ill, 2006, NANN.
202. Neal DO, Lindeke LL: Music as a nursing intervention for preterm infants in the NICU, *Neonatal Netw* 27:319, 2008.
203. Neu M: Kangaroo care: is it for everyone? *Neonatal Netw* 23:47, 2004.
204. Neu M, Browne J: Infant physiologic and behavioral organization during swaddled vs. unswaddled weighing, *J Perinatol* 17:193, 1997.
205. Norris S, Campbell LA, Brenkert S: Nursing procedures and alterations in transcutaneous oxygen tension in premature infants, *Nurs Res* 31:330, 1982.
206. Ohgi S, Fukuda M, Moriuchi H, et al: Comparison of kangaroo care and standard care: behavioral organization, development, and temperament in healthy, low-birth-weight infants through 1 year, *J Perinatol* 22:374, 2002.
207. Paluszynska D, Harris K, Thach B: Influence of sleep position experience on ability of prone-sleeping infants to escape from asphyxiating

microenvironments by changing head position, *Pediatrics* 114:1634, 2004.

208. Parker L, Anderson G: Kangaroo care for adoptive parents and their critically ill preterm infant, *MCN Am J Matern Child Nurs* 27:230, 2002.
209. Parmalee AH: Sleep states in premature infants, *Dev Med Child Neurol* 9:70, 1967.
210. Pellicer A, Gaya F, Madero R, et al: Noninvasive continuous monitoring of the effects of head position on brain hemodynamics in ventilated infants, *Pediatrics* 109:434, 2002.
211. Peters K: Selected physiologic and behavioral responses of the critically ill premature neonate to a routine nursing intervention, *Neonatal Netw* 15:74, 1996.
212. Peters K: Bathing premature infants: physiological and behavioral consequences, *Am J Crit Care* 7:90, 1998.
213. Peters K: Infant handling in the NICU: does developmental care make a difference? An evaluative review of the literature, *J Perinat Neonatal Nurs* 13:83, 1999.
214. Philbin M: Planning the acoustic environment of a neonatal intensive care unit, *Clin Perinatol* 31:331, 2004.
215. Philbin M, Gray L: Changing levels of quiet in an intensive care nursery, *J Perinatol* 22:455, 2002.
216. Pickler R, Best AM, Reyna B, et al: Prediction of feeding performance in preterm infants, *Newborn Infant Nurs Rev* 5:116, 2005.
217. Pickler R, Frankel H, Walsh K, et al: Effects of non-nutritive sucking on behavioral organization and feeding performance in preterm infants, *Nurs Res* 45:132, 1996.
218. Pickler R, Reyna B: Effects of non-nutritive sucking on nutritive sucking, breathing and behavior during bottle feedings of preterm infants, *Adv Neonatal Care* 4:226, 2004.
219. Pinelli J, Symington A: Non-nutritive sucking for promoting physiologic stability and nutrition in preterm infants, *Cochrane Database Syst Rev* 4:CD001071, 2005.
220. Polinski C: Hearing outcomes in the NICU graduate, *Newborn Infant Nurs Rev* 3:99, 2003.
221. Polizzi J, Byers JF, Kiehl E: Co-bedding versus traditional bedding of multiple-gestation infants in the NICU, *J Healthc Qual* 25:5, 2003.
222. Premji S, Paes B: Gastrointestinal function and growth in premature infants: is non-nutritive sucking vital? *J Perinatol* 1:46, 2000.
223. Pridham K, Kosorok MR, Greer F, et al: Comparison of caloric intake and weight outcomes of an ad lib feeding regimen for preterm infants in two nurseries, *J Adv Nurs* 35:751, 2001.
224. Provence S, Lipton RC: *Infants in institutions,* New York, 1962, International Universities Press.
225. Rao M, Blass E, Brignol M, et al: Effects of crying on energy metabolism in human neonates, *Pediatr Res* 33:309A, 1993.
226. Reyna BA, Pickler RH, Thompson A: A descriptive study of mothers' experiences feeding their preterm infants after discharge, *Adv Neonatal Care* 6:333, 2006.
227. Reynolds JD, Hardy RJ, Kennedy KA, et al: for the Light Reduction in ROP (LIGHT-ROP) Cooperative Group: Lack of efficacy of light reduction in preventing ROP, *N Engl J Med* 338:1572, 1998.
228. Rivkees S: Developing circadian rhythmicity in infants, *Pediatrics* 112:373, 2003.
229. Rivkees S: Emergence and influences of circadian rhythmicity in infants, *Clin Perinatol* 31:217, 2004.
230. Rivkees S, Mayes L, Jacobs H, et al: Rest-activity patterns of premature infants are regulated by cycled lighting, *Pediatrics* 113:833, 2004.
231. Roberts KL, Paynter C, McEwan B: A comparison of kangaroo mother care and conventional cuddling care, *Neonatal Netw* 19:31, 2000.
232. Rogers N, Szuba M, Staab J, et al: Neuroimmunologic aspects of sleep and sleep loss, *Semin Clin Neuropsychiatry* 6:295, 2001.
233. Rojas M, Kaplan M, Quevedo M, et al: Somatic growth of preterm infants during skin-to-skin care versus traditional holding: a randomized, controlled trial, *J Dev Behav Pediatr* 24:163, 2003.
234. Roller CG: Getting to know you: mother's experiences of kangaroo care, *J Obstet Gynecol Neonatal Nurs* 34:210, 2005.
235. Ross E, Browne J: Developmental progression of feeding skills: an approach to supporting feeding in preterm infants, *Semin Neonatol* 7:469, 2002.
236. Rubens DD, Vohr BR, Tucker R, et al: Newborn oto-acoustic emission hearing screening tests: preliminary evidence for a marker of susceptibility to SIDS, *Early Human Dev* 84:225, 2008.
237. Sahni R, Schulze KF, Kashyap S, et al: Sleeping position and electrocortical activity in low birthweight infants, *Arch Dis Child Fetal Neonatal Ed* 90:F311, 2005.
238. Samsom J, deGroot L: The influence of postural control on motility and hand function in a group of high risk preterm infants at 1 year of age, *Early Hum Dev* 60:101, 2000.
239. Sauls D: Effects of labor support on mothers, babies, and birth outcomes, *J Obstet Gynecol Neonatal Nurs* 31:733, 2002.
240. Scafidi F, Field T, Schanberg S, et al: Massage stimulates growth in preterm infants: a replication, *Infant Behav Dev* 13:167, 1990.
241. Schaal B, Hummel T, Soussignan R: Olfaction in the fetal and premature infant: functional status and clinical implications, *Clin Perinatol* 31:261, 2004.

242. Schanberg S, Field T: Maternal deprivation and supplemental stimulation. In Field T, McCabe P, Schneiderman N, editors: *Stress and coping across development,* Hillsdale, NJ, 1988, Erlbaum.
243. Shaker C: Nipple feeding premature infants: a different perspective, *Neonatal Netw* 8:9, 1990.
244. Shaker C: Nipple feeding preterm infants: an individualized, developmentally supportive approach, *Neonatal Netw* 18:15, 1999.
245. Shaker C, Woida A: An evidence-based approach to nipple feeding in a level III NICU: nurse autonomy, developmental care and teamwork, *Neonatal Netw* 26:77, 2007.
246. Shimada M, Takahashi K, Segawa M, et al: Emerging and entraining patterns of the sleep-wake rhythm in preterm and term infants, *Brain and Development* 21:468, 1999.
247. Simpson C, Schanler R, Lau C: Early introduction of oral feeding in preterm infants, *Pediatrics* 110:517, 2002.
248. Sizun J, Ansquer H, Browne J, et al: Developmental care decreases physiologic and behavioral pain expression in preterm neonates, *J Pain* 3:446, 2002.
249. Slevin M, Farrington N, Duffy G, et al: Altering the NICU and measuring infants' responses, *Acta Paediatr* 89:577, 2000.
250. Sontheimer D, Fischer C, Buch K: Kangaroo transport instead of incubator transport, *Pediatrics* 113:920, 2004.
251. Spitz R: Hospitalism, *Psychoanal Study Child* 1:53, 1945.
252. Standley J: A meta-analysis of the efficacy of music therapy for premature infants, *J Pediatr Nurs* 17:107, 2002.
253. Stastney P, Ichinose T, Thayer S, et al: Infant sleep position by nursery staff and mothers in newborn hospital nurseries, *Nurs Res* 53:122, 2004.
254. Strauch C, Brandt S, Edwards-Beckett J: Implementation of a quiet hour: effect on noise levels and infant sleep states, *Neonatal Netw* 12:31, 1993.
255. Sullivan R, Toubas P: Clinical usefulness of maternal odor in newborns: soothing and feeding preparatory responses, *Biol Neonat* 74:402, 1998.
256. Sweeney J, Guiterrez T: Motor development chronology: a dynamic process. In Kenner C, McGrath J, editors: *Developmental care of newborns and infants,* St Louis, 2004, Mosby.
257. Symanski M, Hayes M, Akilesh K: Patterns of premature newborns' sleep-wake states before and after nursing interventions on the night shift, *J Obstet Gynecol Neonatal Nurs* 31:305, 2002.
258. Symington A, Pinelli J: Developmental care for promoting development and preventing morbidity in preterm infants, *Cochrane Database Syst Rev* 2: CD001814, 2006.
259. Tablizo MA, Jacinto P, Parsley D, et al: Supine sleeping position does not cause clinical aspiration in neonates in hospital newborn nurseries, *Arch Pediatr Adolesc Med* 161:507, 2007.
260. Taquino L, Blackburn S: The effects of containment during suction and heelstick on physiological and behavioral responses of preterm infants, *Neonatal Netw* 13:55, 1994.
261. Thoman E: The breathing bear and the remarkable premature infant. In Goldson E, editor: *Nurturing the premature infant,* New York, 1999, Oxford University Press.
262. Thoman E: Temporal patterns of caregiving for preterm infants indicate individualized developmental care, *J Perinatol* 23:29, 2003.
263. Thomas K: Differential effects of breast-and-formula feeding on preterm infants' sleep-wake patterns, *J Obstet Gynecol Neonatal Nurs* 29:145, 2000.
264. Thomas K, Martin P: NICU sound environment and the potential problems for caregivers, *J Perinatol* 20:594, 2000.
265. Thomas KA, Uran A: How the NICU environment sounds to a preterm infant: update, *MCN Am J Matern Child Nurs* 32:250, 2007.
266. Thoyre S: Techniques for feeding preterm infants, *Am J Nurs* 103:69, 2003.
267. Thoyre S, Carlson J: Breathing problems during feeding for preterm infants nearing discharge, *Early Hum Dev* 72:25, 2003.
268. Thoyre S, Carlson J: Preterm infants' behavioral indicators of oxygen decline during bottle feeding, *J Advan Nurs* 43:631, 2003.
269. Thoyre SM, Shaker CS, Pridham KF: The Early Feeding Skills Assessment for preterm infants, *Neonatal Netw* 24:7, 2005.
270. Tomashek KM, Wallman C, and Committee on Fetus and Newborn, American Academy of Pediatrics: Cobedding twins and higher-order multiples in a hospital setting, *Pediatrics* 120:1359, 2007.
271. Torres C, Holditch-Davis D, O'Hale A, et al: Effect of standard rest periods on apnea and weight gain in preterm infants, *Neonatal Netw* 16:35, 1997.
272. Touch S, Epstein M, Pohl C, et al: The impact of cobedding on sleep patterns in preterm infants, *Clin Pediatrics* 41:425, 2002.
273. Tronick EZ, Scanlon KB, Scanlon JW: Protective apathy: a hypothesis about the behavioral organization and its relation to clinical and physiologic status of the preterm infant during the newborn period, *Clin Perinatol* 17:125, 1990.
274. Turnage-Carrier C: Caregiving and the environment. In Kenner C, McGrath J, editors: *Developmental care of newborns and infants,* St Louis, 2004, Mosby.
275. Van den Bergh B, Marcoen A: High antenatal maternal anxiety is related to ADHD symptoms, externalizing

problems, and anxiety in 8- and 9-year-olds, *Child Dev* 75:1085, 2004.

276. Vernacchio L, Corwin M, Lesko S, et al: Sleep position of low birth weight infants, *Pediatrics* 111:633, 2003.
277. Vickers A, Ohlsson A, Lacy J, et al: Massage for promoting growth and development of preterm and/or LBW infants, *Cochrane Database Syst Rev* 2: CD000390, 2004.
278. Vignochi C, Miura E: Effect of motor physiotherapy in bone mineralization of prematures: a randomized and controlled study, *J Perinatol* 28:624, 2008.
279. Wagaman MJ, Shutack JG, Moomjian AS, et al: Improved oxygenation and lung compliance with prone positioning of neonates, *J Pediatr* 94:787, 1979.
280. Walker C, Kudreikis K, Sherrard A, et al: Repeated neonatal pain influences maternal behavior, but not stress responsiveness in rat offspring, *Dev Brain Res* 140:253, 2003.
281. Walsh-Suyks M, Reitenbach A, Hudson-Barr D, et al: Reducing light and sound in the NICU: an evaluation of patient safety, staff satisfaction and costs, *J Perinatol* 21:230, 2001.
282. Weiss S, Wilson P: Origins of tactile vulnerability in high-risk infants, *Adv Neonatal Care* 6:25, 2006.
283. Weiss S, Wilson P, Hertenstein M, et al: The tactile context of a mother's caregiving: implications for attachment of LBW infants, *Infant Behav Dev* 23:91, 2000.
284. Weiss S, Wilson P, Morrison D: Maternal tactile stimulation and the neurodevelopment of LBW infants, *Infancy* 5:85, 2004.
285. Werner N, Conway A: Caregiver contacts experienced by premature infants in the neonatal intensive care unit, *Matern Child Nurs J* 19:21, 1990.
286. Westrup B, Boehm B, Lagercrantz HKS: Preschool outcome in children born very prematurely and cared for according to the Newborn Individualized Developmental Care and Assessment Program (NIDCAP), *Acta Paediatr* 93:498, 2004.
287. Westrup B, Kleberg A, von Eichwald W, et al: A randomized, controlled trial to evaluate the effects of the Newborn Individualized Developmental Care and Assessment Program in a Swedish setting, *Pediatrics* 105:66, 2000.
288. White R: Mother's arms: the past and future locus of neonatal care? *Clin Perinatol* 31:383, 2004.
289. White-Traut RC, Nelson MN, Silvestri JM, et al: Effect of auditory, tactile, visual, and vestibular intervention on length of stay, alertness, and feeding progression in preterm infants, *Dev Med Child Neurol* 44:91, 2002.
290. White-Traut RC, Nelson MN, Silvestri JM, et al: Developmental patterns of physiological response to a multisensory intervention in extremely premature and high-risk infants, *J Obstet Gynecol Neonatal Nurs* 33:266, 2004.
291. Whitfield M: Psychosocial effects of intensive care on infants and families after discharge, *Semin Perinatol* 8:185, 2003.
292. Whitman T, O'Callaghan M, Maxwell S: The effects of cycled vs. noncycled lighting on growth and development in preterm infants, *Infant Behav Dev* 18:87, 1995.
293. Wielenga JM, Smit BJ, Unk LK: How satisfied are parents supported by nurses with the NIDCAP® model of care for their preterm infant? *J Nurs Care Qual* 21:41, 2006.
294. Wolf L, Glass R: *Feeding and swallowing disorders in infancy: assessment and management,* Tucson, 1992, Therapy Skill Builders.
295. World Health Organization: *Report of consensus conference on kangaroo care for premature and low birth weight infants,* Trieste, Italy, 1996, WHO.

RESOURCES FOR PROFESSIONALS

Ludington-Hoe S, Morgan K, Abouelfrettoh A: A clinical guideline for implementation of kangaroo care with premature infants of 30 or more weeks' postmenstrual age, *Adv Neonatal Care* 8:S3, 2008.

National Association of Neonatal Nurses (NANN): Advanced competency in developmental care, Available at www.nann.org.

Noise measurement devices: Available at and www.talklight.com. and www.noisemetes.com.

Vida Health Communications: Promoting Preterm Infant Development Toolkit: Contains, *Focus on the Brain: Parts I and II* (DVD); *Focus on the Brain Professional Resources* (CD-ROM); *No Matter How Small* (DVD); 20 copies of *No Matter How Small,* home edition for NICU families, Available at www.vida-health.com.

RESOURCES FOR PARENTS

Dorner A: *Prematurely yours (video),* Boston, 1983, Polymorph Films.

Dorner A: *To have and not to hold: helping parents cope (video),* Boston, 1983, Polymorph Films.

Fern D, Graves C: *Developmental care guide for families with infants in the NICU,* Weymouth, Mass, 1996, Children's Medical Ventures. Website: www.childmed.com.

Flushman B, Gale G, Deverman S, et al: *My special start: a guide for parents in the neonatal intensive care unit,* Palo Alto, Calif, VORT.

Healy T: *Guiding your child through preterm development,* Alexandria, VA, 1988, Parent Care.

Hussey B: *Understanding my signals,* Palo Alto, Calif, 1988, VORT.

Institute for Family-Centered Care: *Newborn intensive care: changing practice, changing (video),* Bethesda, MD, 1996, The Institute.

Ludington-Hoe S, Golant S: *Kangaroo care: the best you can do to help your preterm infant,* New York, 1993, Bantam Books.

Rosenberg S: *Kangaroo care: a parent's touch (video),* Chicago, 1996, Prentice Women's Hospital.

VandenBerg K, Browne J, Perez L, et al: *Getting to know your baby: a developmental guide for community service providers and parents of NICU graduates,* Oakland, Calif, 2003, Special Start Training Program, Mills College, Department of Education. Website: www.specialstart.org.

Vergara E, Bigsby R: *Developmental and therapeutic interventions in the NICU,* Baltimore, 2004, Brooks Publishing.

14 FLUID AND ELECTROLYTE MANAGEMENT

JAMES E. JONES, RAY D. HAYES, ALISA L. STARBUCK, AND PETER J. PORCELLI

Advances in the management of specific neonatal disorders have contributed to a remarkable decline in morbidity and mortality in newborns. Fluid and electrolyte therapy, thermal regulation, and maintenance of oxygenation remain central features of modern, supportive neonatal intensive care. Thus infants requiring tertiary care (and most infants requiring intermediate level II or secondary care) will initially receive parenteral fluid and electrolytes. Fluid and nutrition data have been accumulated for full-term infants, but some crucial information is still missing regarding very-low-birth-weight (VLBW) infants (infants with birth weights <1500 g). For example, it is clear that the restrictive fluid policies of the 1950s aimed at reducing the observed postnatal diuresis were misguided efforts that caused hyperosmolality, hyperbilirubinemia, and hypoglycemia. On the other hand, the degree to which initial fluid, electrolyte, and glucose administration should be "liberalized" remains uncertain,[1,3,4] largely because patent ductus arteriosus, necrotizing enterocolitis, bronchopulmonary dysplasia (BPD), intraventricular hemorrhage (IVH), and hyperglycemia in VLBW infants are associated with larger volumes of fluid, electrolyte, and glucose administration.[1] At best, clinicians make approximations for therapy in many clinical situations, which is why good measures of fluid and electrolyte requirements are needed. In addition, the fluid requirements of VLBW infants may be modified by prenatal steroid administration to mothers and the use of artificial surfactant in infants.

This chapter discusses implementation of the following fundamental principles: (1) rapidly assessing the infant's initial condition; (2) developing a short-term, time-oriented management plan; (3) initiating therapy; and (4) monitoring the infant and modifying the plan based on clinical and biochemical data.

PHYSIOLOGY

Neonates show significant physiologic differences when compared (on a per-kilogram basis) with older children and adults: (1) their basic metabolic rate is greater, even double; (2) their fluid requirements are four to five times higher; (3) their sodium excretion is only 10% of that in older children and adults; and (4) their glomerular filtration rate is 5 to 10 times less than that of adults.[3] The subdivisions of total body mass (TBM) are illustrated in Figure 14-1. Total body water (TBW) as a percentage of TBM demonstrates a curvilinear decline with increasing gestational age (Figure 14-2). During the early fetal period, the fetus's TBW is 95% of total weight and decreases to 80% at 8 months gestation and then to 75% at term.[3] Intracellular fluid (ICF) and extracellular fluid (ECF) as percentages of TBM change in opposite directions as gestational age advances, whereas ECF decreases as ICF increases with growth.[2]

These physiologic and body composition phenomena result in a narrow margin of safety when calculating fluids and electrolytes for small infants,

Please note that the **PURPLE** type in each chapter is intended to make it easier to identify clinically applicable material.

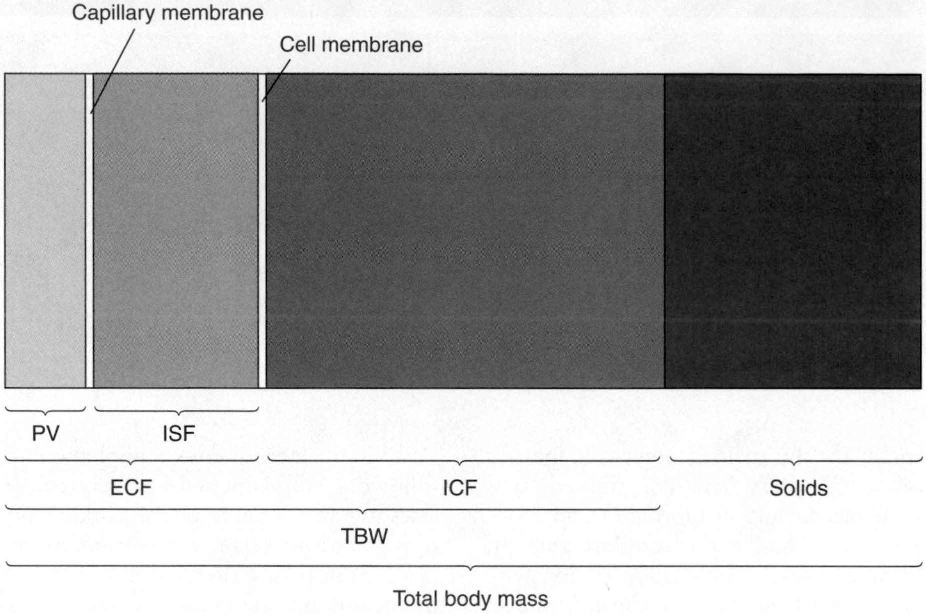

FIGURE 14-1 Major subdivisions of total body mass. *ECF,* Extracellular fluid; *ICF,* intracellular fluid; *ISF,* interstitial fluid; *PV,* plasma volume; *TBW,* total body water. (From Winters RW, editor: *The body fluids in pediatrics,* Boston, 1973, Little, Brown.)

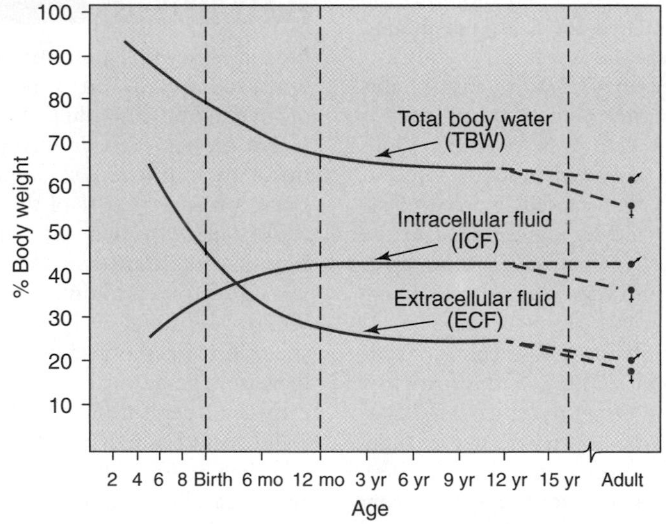

FIGURE 14-2 Effects of age on TBW, ICF, and ECF. Note curvilinear changes that are maximal during perinatal period. (From Winters RW, editor: The *body fluids in pediatrics,* Boston, 1973, Little, Brown.)

especially those less than 1250 g. Caregivers should independently calculate all requirements and compare calculations with standard guidelines. **Intravenous (IV) fluid should be administered by a special infusion pump that can regulate fluid with precision of at least 0.1 mL/hr. Intake should be measured hourly and all output measured. The balance of intake versus output should be assessed at least every 8 to 12 hours using a standard form (Figure 14-3).** Once clinical signs of fluid overload

Output

Closed drainage system∆ Chest tube #					Urine					Stools Last stool					Gastric Tube∆d			Blood out Balance forward		
Times	Site / Activity	cm H2O / Color	Pleurovac reading / Drainage in cc's		Type / Color	Specific gravity	pH / Glucose	Protein / Blood	Amt. / Cumul	Type	Hematest / Clinitest				Amt.	Color / Irrig.	Cumul. total	Reason	Amt. out	Cumul. total
0700																				
0800																				
0900																				
1000																				
1100																				
1200																				
1300																				
1400																				
1500																				
1600																				
1700																				
1800																				
1900																				
2000																				
2100																				
2200																				
2300																				
2400																				
0100																				
0200																				
0300																				
0400																				
0500																				
0600																				
24° Totals:																				

Chest tube activity
B - Bubbling
F - Fluctuating
D - Draining
C - Clamped
N - No movement

Chest tube color
BL - Bloody
S - Serosanguinous
Y - Yellow
W - White or milky
Other: ____________

Urine type
VD - Void
CATH - Catheterized
CR - CREDÉ

Urine color
A - Amber
Y - Yellow
BL - Bloody
Other: ____________

Stool type, size, and color
F - Formed
P - Pasty
LO - Loose
M - Mucus
MEC - Meconium
SDY - Seedy
SOF - Soft
W - Watery
LG - Large
MED - Medium
S - Small
T - Transitional
Y - Yellow
BR - Brown
BLK - Black
BL - Bloody
G - Green

Brenner Children's Hospital • Winston-Salem, N.C. **Neonatal day record**

FIGURE 14-3 Model intake and output sheet. (Courtesy Brenner Children's Hospital, Winston-Salem, North Carolina.)

Continued

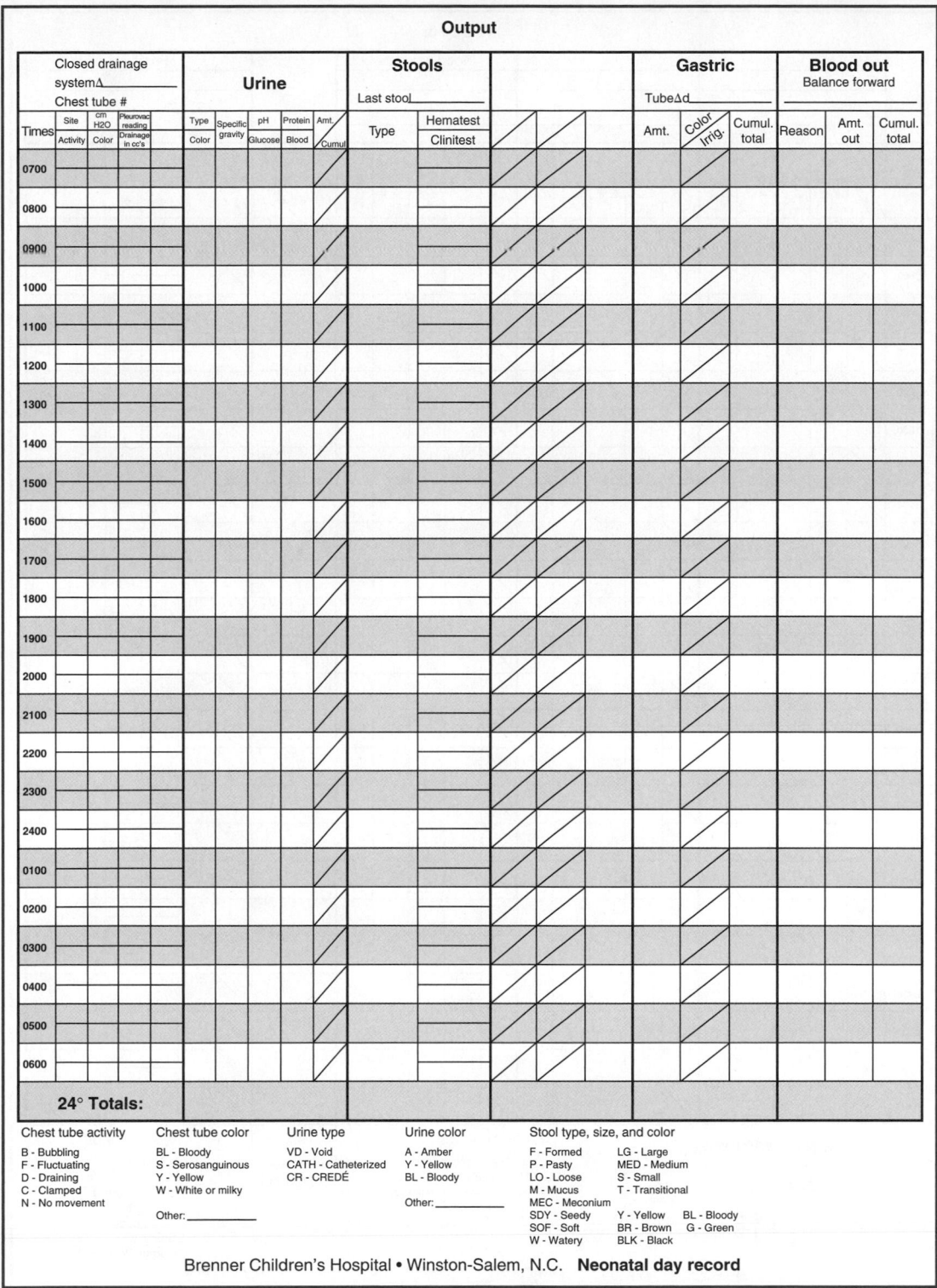

IV Intake

	#1 Bottle∆ / Line∆					#2 Bottle∆ / Line∆					Blood products						Feedings Tube size: / Tube∆:				
Time	Site check / Location	Rate per hour	Pump reading	Amount infused	Cumul. total	Site check / Location	Rate per hour	Pump reading	Amount infused	Cumul. total	Site check / Location	Rate per hour	Pump reading	Amount infused	Cumul. total	IV Intake hourly total	Type / Amt. ordered	Amount given	Emesis / Resid.	Set∆ / pH	Cumul.
0700																					
0800																					
0900																					
1000																					
1100																					
1200																					
1300																					
1400																					
1500																					*
1600																					
1700																					
1800																					
1900																					
2000																					
2100																					
2200																					
2300																					*
2400																					
0100																					
0200																					
0300																					
0400																					
0500																					
0600																					

24° Total

BRENNER CHILDREN'S HOSPITAL

Blood products

FFP - Fresh frozen plasma
PLTS - Platelets
PRBC's - CMV (-) Packed red blood cells

Type of feeding

N - Nipple
NG - Nasogastric
OG - Oral gastric
GT - Gastrostomy
TP - Transpyloric
Other:____________
* Cumul. IV/feedings

Brenner Children's Hospital • Winston-Salem, N.C. **Neonatal day record**

FIGURE 14-3 cont'd—Model intake and output sheet. (Courtesy Brenner Children's Hospital, Winston-Salem, North Carolina.)

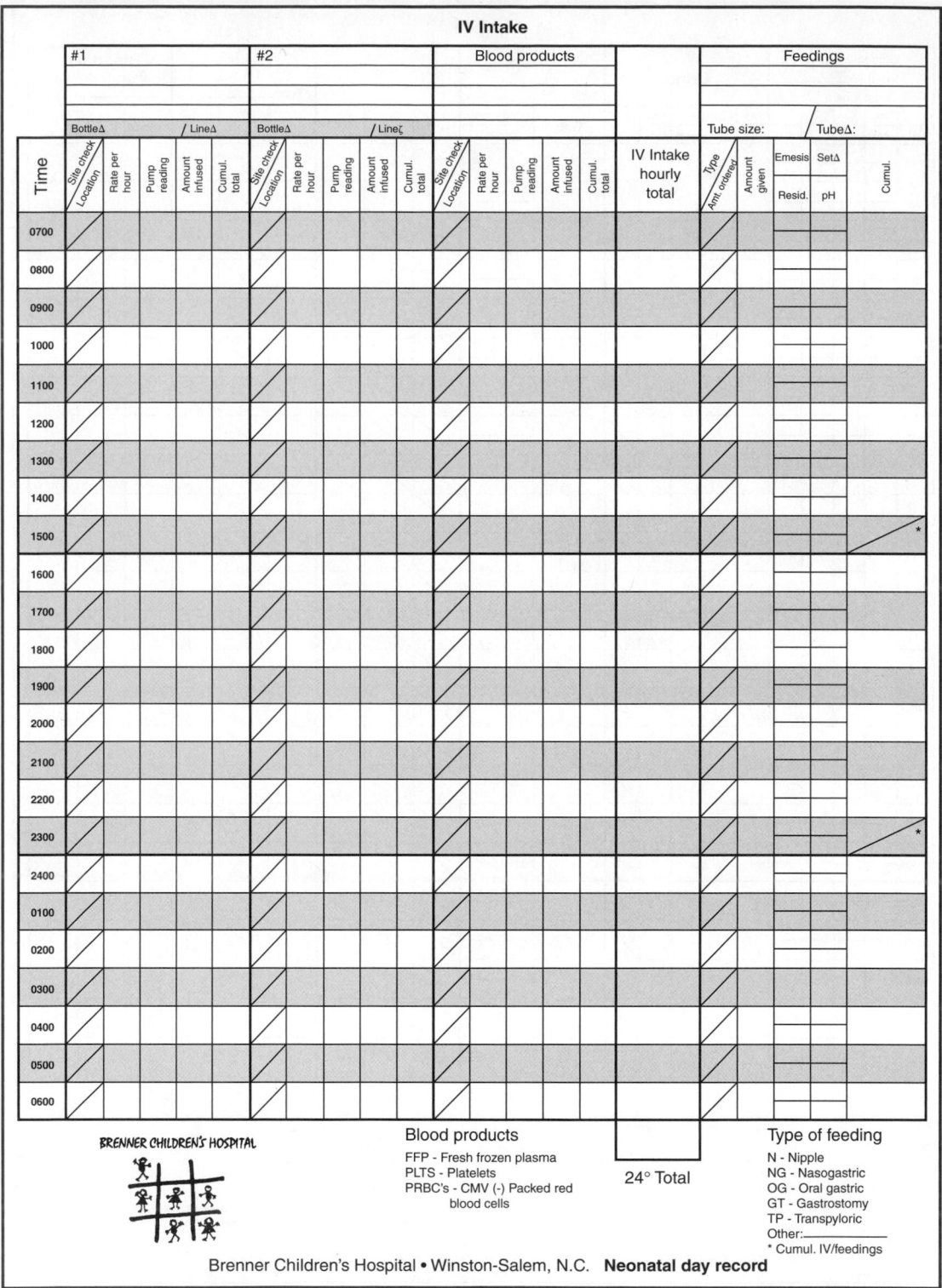

or deficit occur, it may be difficult to regain balance. Fluid balance should be managed prospectively with consistent procedures as a part of every initial care plan.

The effect of gestational age on body composition is striking (Figure 14-4). Because gestational age is a significant determinant of the percentage and distribution of TBW, accurate assessment is important. Changes in distribution and percent of body water will be influenced by intrauterine growth, maternal fluid balance, postnatal age, postnatal diet, daily water intake, and changing fluid and electrolyte absorption and excretion.

The initial (first 1 to 3 days) weight loss of both healthy term (up to 5% to 10% of TBM) and preterm (up to 10% to 15% of TBM) infants should be considered a normal physiologic loss of fluid from the interstitial fluid (ISF), rather than a pathophysiologic catabolism of body tissues. After birth, contraction of the ECF compartment occurs, followed by natriuresis, diuresis, and weight loss.[2,3] This weight loss is then regained over 7 to 10 days as muscle and fat. Preterm neonates often demonstrate relative oliguria during the first 24 to 48 hours. Neonates with respiratory distress syndrome (RDS) will have delayed postnatal contraction of the ECF compartment, further delaying diuresis. Onset of the diuresis after several days old usually coincides with the initial stages of recovery from RDS.[5]

Despite the period of natriuresis after birth, infants usually require no additional sodium during the first 24 to 48 hours of life. This strategy can promote decreased oxygen requirement and possibly decreased incidence of chronic lung disease.[2] It is normal to have an initial negative sodium balance, but later it is necessary to retain sodium and often additional sodium supplementation is required for appropriate growth.[5]

Reviewing the maternal history and the intrapartum course may be helpful to calculate the infant's fluid and electrolyte requirements. For example, if the mother received large amounts of electrolyte-free fluids in the intrapartum period, the neonate may be hyponatremic and have an expanded ECF space at birth. Because small-for-gestational-age (SGA) infants have reduced amounts of fat, body water (as a percentage of TBM) increases. Conversely, large-for-gestational-age (LGA) infants with an increased amount of body fat have a lower percentage of TBW.

ECF comprises both intravascular fluid (plasma) and ISF. The electrolyte composition of ISF and plasma is similar, but it is strikingly different from ICF (Figure 14-5). Sodium is the major cation

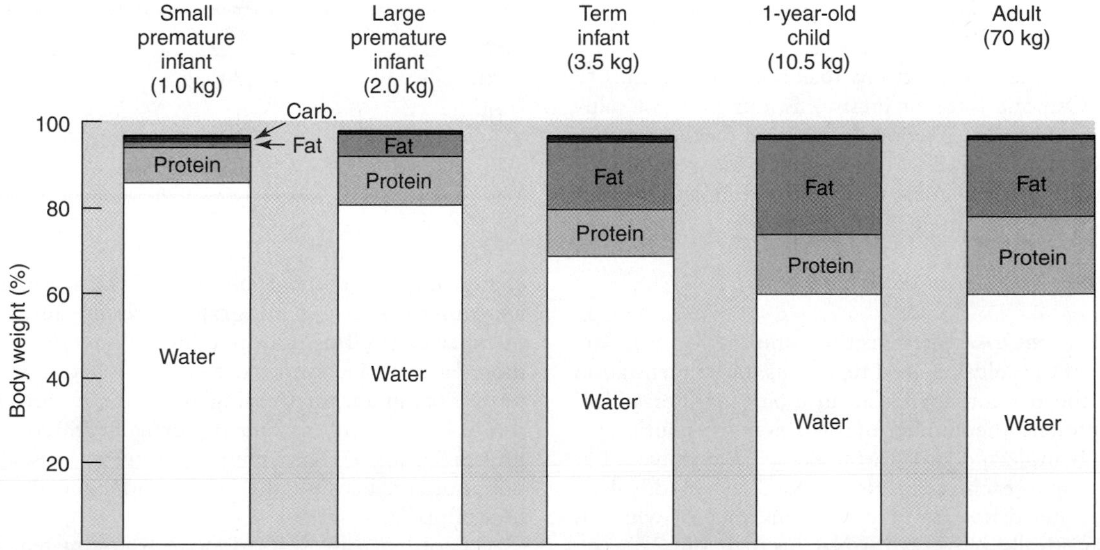

FIGURE 14-4 Effects of gestational age on body composition compared with older children and adults. (From Heird WC, Driscoll JM Jr, Schullinger JN, et al: Intravenous alimentation in pediatric patients, *J Pediatr* 80:351, 1972.)

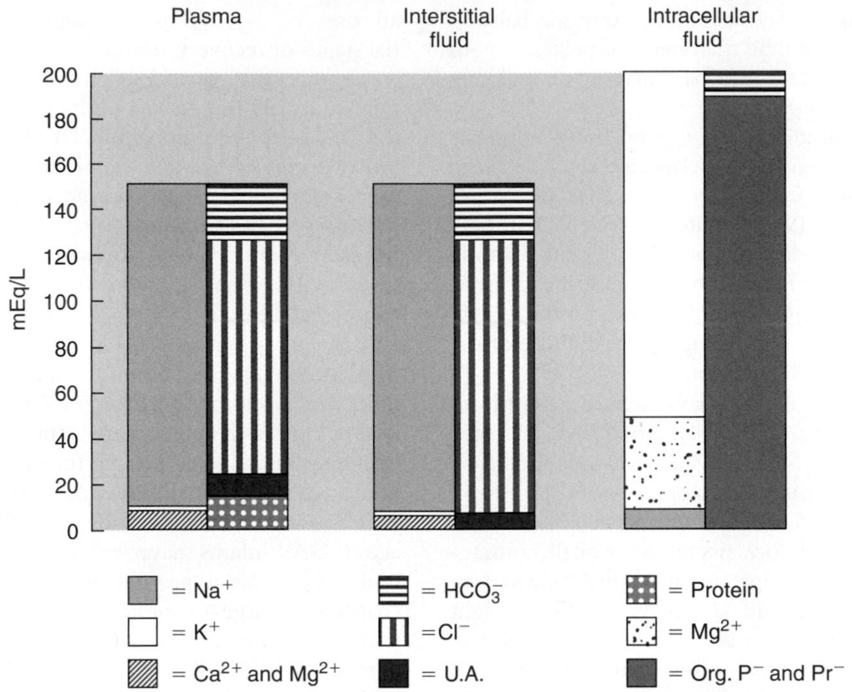

FIGURE 14-5 "Gamblegram" of plasma interstitial fluid and intracellular fluid. (From Winters RW, editor: *The body fluids in pediatrics.* Boston, 1973, Little, Brown.)

in ECF (both ISF and plasma) and is easily measured. Potassium, the major cation in ICF, on the other hand, cannot be measured readily because ICF is not easily accessible. Because 90% of the total body potassium is intracellular, low levels of plasma potassium are assumed to reflect low total body potassium.

Osmotic force or pressure is a property of solutions. Osmotic phenomena depend on the number (N) of particles in a solution regardless of size or charge and are measured in milliosmoles (mOsm) according to this equation:

$$mOsm = (mM) \times (N)$$

where ***mOsm*** represents the osmolality or osmolarity of the solution, ***mM*** represents the concentration of the measured particles in moles per liter and ***N*** represents the number of particles in the solution for each molecule after the substance is dissolved. For example, each molecule of NaCl when dissolved in water dissociates into two ions, each of which is osmotically active. N for NaCl is therefore 2.

Table 14-1 shows three examples. **Unfortunately, two physical chemistry terms are used interchangeably in clinical medicine: (1) osmolality (milliosmole per kilogram of *water*) and (2) osmolarity (milliosmole per liter of *solution*).** In most laboratories, osmotic forces are determined by the technique of freezing point depression, so osmolality is the correct term (normally 280 to 300 mOsm/kg water). The difference in terms is usually unimportant, because the total solid content per liter of plasma is small.

Osmolality can be satisfactorily estimated in many clinical settings by the following formula (Figure 14-6):

TABLE 14-1 EXAMPLES OF OSMOTIC FORCE

	mM	N	mOsm
NaCl	1	2	2
Glucose	1	1	1
$CaCl_2$	1	3	3

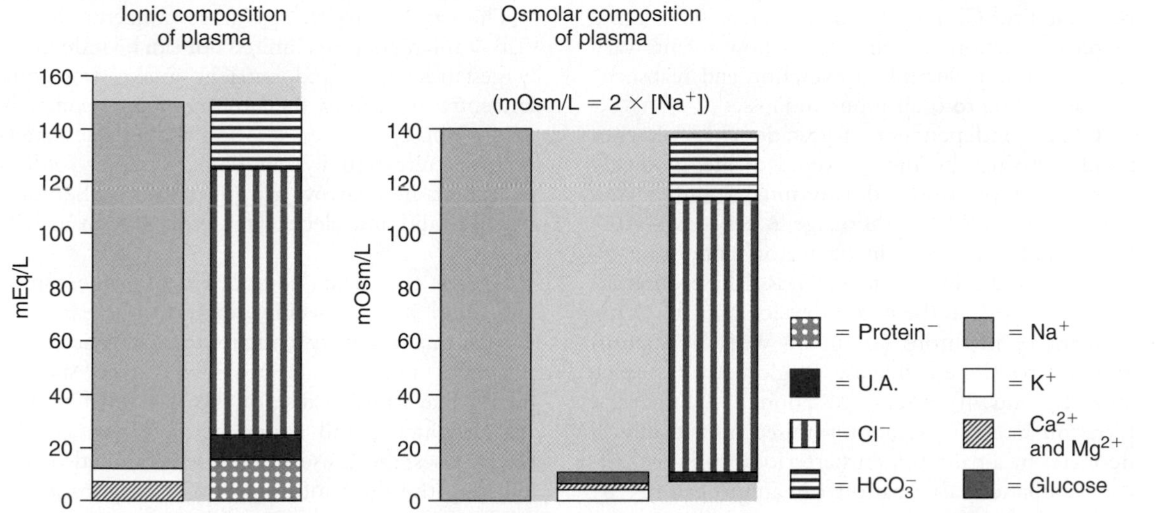

FIGURE 14-6 Ionic and osmolar composition of plasma. (From Winters RW, editor: *The body fluids in pediatrics*, Boston, 1973, Little, Brown.)

$$\text{Osmolality} = 2[\text{Na}^+] + \frac{\text{Glucose (mg/dL)}}{18} + \frac{\text{BUN (mg/dL)}}{2.8}$$

The coefficients 1/18 and 1/2.8 for the glucose and blood urea nitrogen (BUN) terms are present to convert milligrams per deciliter values to millimolar concentrations. For example, a patient with a serum sodium concentration of 135 mEq/L, a glucose of 72 mg/dL, and a BUN of 28 mg/dL has a calculated osmolality of:

$$2[\text{Na}^+] = 270$$

$$\frac{[\text{Glucose}]}{18} = 4$$

$$\frac{[\text{BUN}]}{2.8} = 10$$

$$\text{Osmolality} = 270 + 4 + 10 = 284 \text{ mOsm/L}$$

Osmotic forces are responsible for apparently low plasma electrolyte concentrations in some common clinical settings. For example, in hyperglycemia, the plasma sodium concentration reported by the laboratory is usually low but the total effective osmolality may be normal, as seen in this example:

$$\text{Glucose} = 720 \text{ mg/dL}$$

$$(\text{Na}^+) = 120 \text{ mEq/L}$$

$$\text{BUN} = 19 \text{ mg/dL}$$

$$\text{mOsm/L} = 280$$

$$(120 \times 2) + \frac{720}{18} + \frac{19}{2.8} = 287 \text{ mOsm/L}$$

An analogous situation exists for the less frequent condition, hyperlipidemia, in which low laboratory plasma sodium values are reported with a normal osmolality (Figure 14-7). Low laboratory values for plasma sodium occur because the increase in plasma solids (lipids) causes a lower plasma water content because of water displacement and hence a lower sodium concentration per liter of whole plasma. In this case, the plasma water and sodium concentration may be normal.

Osmotic forces largely determine shifts in the internal redistribution of water in hydration disturbances. Four pure disturbances of hydration exist: (1) too much electrolyte; (2) too little electrolyte; (3) too much water; and (4) too little water. Combinations of these disturbances often occur. Another example of changes in osmolality occurs in preterm infants who undergo insensible water loss because of skin immaturity, decreased body fat, and a large surface-to-volume ratio leading to increased evaporation. This water loss from the interstitial space results in a hyperosmolar extracellular compartment exhibited by hypernatremia and occasionally hyperkalemia and hyperglycemia.[2,3]

Neonatal renal "immaturity" affects fluid balance and electrolyte needs. Renal functions do not develop at the same rate. Neonatal glomerular filtration rate (GFR) is low in utero but increases rapidly within a few hours after delivery because renal blood flow increases as a result of the increasing mean arterial blood pressure and increasing glomerular permeability.[5] Glomerular filtration rate is a measure of renal function, which assesses how infants vary their fluid and electrolyte excretion and reabsorption according to their input and losses.

GFR is independent of gestational age. It rises rapidly during the first 6 weeks of life, gradually increasing more slowly during infancy, and reaches adult values by 12 months of age. A very-low-birth-weight (VLBW) infant in satisfactory condition at 6 weeks should have adequate GFR. These observations are based on the infant developing a full complement of nephrons (about 34 weeks' gestation) and the continued increase in glomerular surface area (beyond 40 weeks' gestation).[3,4] Glomerular filtration rate can be compromised in critically ill neonates by a patent ductus arteriosus and mechanical ventilation. Extubation can improve GFR by up to 15%.[5]

Renal tubular function is responsible for mineral and electrolyte excretion and reabsorption. Renal tubular function is influenced by gestational age.[5] Therefore urine sodium losses are a function of gestational age and sodium intake. Preterm infants with immature tubular function have a limited ability to excrete sodium. Urine sodium excretion increases slowly during the first 2 years of life. When increased amounts of sodium are provided to more mature infants, there will be a renal response resulting in elevated urine sodium as the renal system attempts to normalize serum sodium.

The capacity to change urine concentration in VLBW infants appears limited but can be influenced by gestational age and nutrient intake. Immature concentrating ability (maximum of approximately 600 mOsm/L) (Figure 14-8) coupled with an inability to excrete (rapidly) an acute water or sodium load results in a narrow margin of safety when prescribing fluid and electrolytes, especially in VLBW infants.[1,3,4]

Urea is the major component of urine osmolality (and hence specific gravity), whereas electrolytes quantitatively contribute less. When total parenteral nutrition is provided, urine specific gravity may rise because of the low renal threshold for glucose and amino acids. When specific gravity rises, the cause should be identified before adjusting the fluid infusion rate. A diagnostic test (Multistix 10 SC or Chemstrip) can screen for glucose and protein but not for amino acids, which must be detected by amino acid chromatography when necessary.

Neonatal urinary acidification is limited, and the threshold for bicarbonate excretion is reduced. Both physiologic and pathologic factors can contribute to alkaline urine. VLBW infants have a limited capacity for hydrogen ion excretion, whereas other infants may have acute illnesses such as bicarbonate-losing tubular necrosis or urinary tract infection.

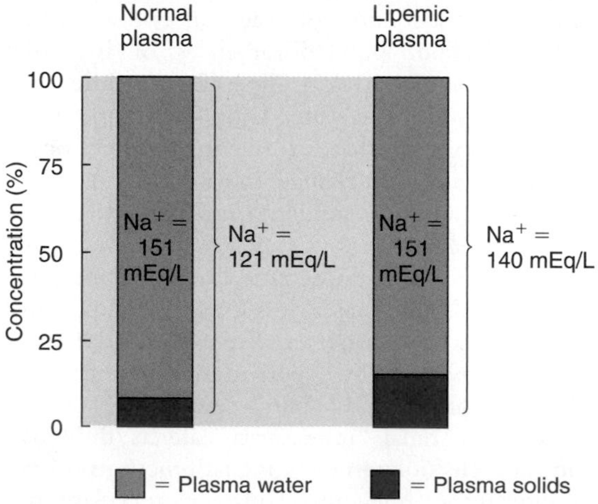

FIGURE 14-7 Effects of hyperlipidemia on plasma water and plasma sodium concentration. (From Winters RW, editor: *The body fluids in pediatrics*, Boston, 1973, Little, Brown.)

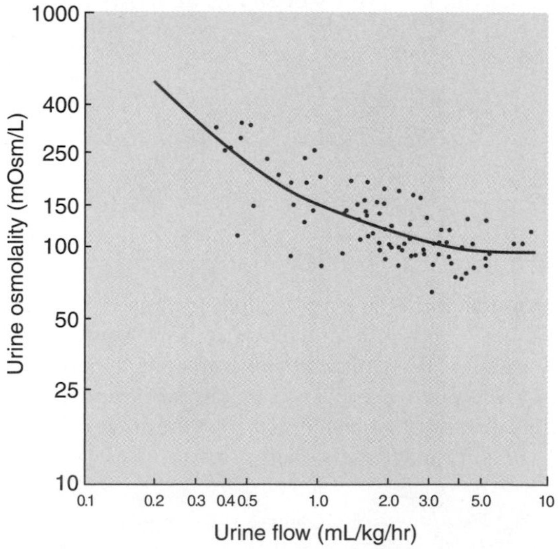

FIGURE 14-8 Normal urine flow rates. (From Jones MD, Gresham EL, Battaglia FC: Urinary flow rate and urea excretion rates in newborn infants, *Biol Neonate* 21:322, 1972.)

The roles of hormones including antidiuretic hormone, aldosterone, atrial natriuretic factor, and parathormone to regulate neonatal fluid and electrolyte balance are not well defined. Hormonal influences can be primary, such as in the syndrome of inappropriate secretion of antidiuretic hormone and in some cases of hypocalcemia. Secondary hormonal influences can be caused by certain drugs, such as the aldosterone antagonist ***spironolactone.***

Insensible water loss (IWL) occurs via pulmonary and cutaneous routes and is influenced by the factors listed in Table 14-2. However, IWL varies greatly depending on gestational age and birth weight (Table 14-3). The neonate's environment significantly affects fluid balance. Radiant warmer

TABLE 14-2 FACTORS THAT INFLUENCE INSENSIBLE WATER LOSS (IWL)

DECREASE IWL	INCREASE IWL
Heat shield or double-walled incubators	Inversely related to gestational age and weight
Plastic blankets	Respiratory distress
Clothes	Ambient temperature above thermoneutral
High relative humidity (ambient ventilator gas)	Fever
Emollient use	Radiant warmer
	Phototherapy
	Activity

TABLE 14-3 GUIDELINES FOR FLUID (mL/kg/day) AND SOLUTE PROVISION BY PATIENT WEIGHT AND DAYS OF AGE

WEIGHT (g)	RANGES OF WATER LOSS		DAY 1*	DAYS 2-3*	DAYS 4-7*
Less than 1250	IWL†	40-170			
	Urine	50-100			
	Stool	5-10			
	TOTAL	**95-280**	**120**	**140**	**150-175**
1250-1750	IWL†	20-50			
	Urine	50-100			
	Stool	5-10			
	TOTAL	**75-160**	**90**	**110**	**130-140**
More than 1750	IWL†	15-40			
	Urine	50-100			
	Stool	5-10			
	TOTAL	**70-150**	**80**	**90**	**100-200**

Increment for phototherapy: 20-30 mL/kg/day if patient is in open warmer and has radiant phototherapy. No adjustment if baby is in humidified environment and/or has fiberoptic phototherapy source.
Increment for radiant warmer: 20-30 mL/kg/day.
Maintenance solutes: Glucose: 7-12 g/kg/day (4-8 g/kg in VLBW infants)
Na: 1-4 mEq/kg/day (2-8 mEq/kg/day in VLBW infants)
K: 1-4 mEq/kg/day
Cl: 1-4 mEq/kg/day
Ca: 1 mEq/kg/day

*Adjustment based on a urine flow rate of 2 to 5 mL/kg/hr and a stable weight.
†May be reduced by 30% if the infant is on a ventilator.
IWL, Insensible water loss; *VLBW,* very-low-birth-weight.

usage decreases the neonate's radiant heat loss but can increase IWL by 50% to 200%, resulting in hypernatremic dehydration.[6] Incubators reduce radiant heat loss via their double-walled Plexiglas design.

Modern incubators provide sterile humidity (up to 80%) and are very effective in decreasing IWL by reducing evaporative heat loss. Internal incubator humidification was discontinued in the 1970s when it was associated with *Pseudomonas* infections.[7] Presumably, the nature of *Pseudomonas* promoted its stability and growth in the water humidification reservoirs. However, present humidification designs provide for direct heating of water in an external reservoir to a temperature that kills most organisms. The water is transformed into vapor, rather than mist, and carried in a gaseous state by the incubator's convective air flow, thus reducing the possibility of airborne bacterial transfer.[7]

Because added environmental humidity reduces transcutaneous evaporative water loss, a preterm infant nursed in humidity needs less fluid than if nursed without humidity to achieve the same water balance. A relative humidity of 80% can reduce water loss to one tenth of the water loss of preterm infants receiving care in 50% humidity.[6] This reduction in evaporative water loss has a significant impact on fluid requirements and electrolyte balance in premature infants. For infants with birth weight less than 1000 grams, the use of humidity results in lower fluid intake as well as fewer episodes of hypernatremia, hyperkalemia, and azotemia in the first 96 hours of life.[6] Despite these improvements, the optimal level and duration of humidification have yet to be determined.

ETIOLOGY

The causes of common electrolyte problems and common clinical syndromes are discussed in the "Treatment" section.

PREVENTION

Prevention of fluid and electrolyte imbalance in neonates begins with knowing how to calculate fluid and electrolyte requirements correctly. The estimated metabolic rate forms the reference base for all calculations. The metabolic rate (and hence oxygen consumption) normally increases steadily over the first weeks of life, so changes in water and electrolyte requirements should be anticipated.

If the daily caloric requirement is approximately 100 *cal/kg/day*, the physiologic basis of metabolic rate may be used to calculate needs; however, most institutions determine an infant's daily fluid need on a *mL/kg* basis, which is modified by factors that influence IWL and is usually adjusted depending on body weight, clinical composition, serum chemistry results, and urine volume and composition (Figure 14-9; see also Table 14-3).

Preterm infants usually have slightly lower metabolic rates than those of term infants. SGA infants may have higher metabolic rates than those of preterm infants of similar weight,[2] which may be because of their relatively large brain/body mass ratio. Both SGA and preterm infants, especially VLBW infants, should be expected to require more frequent assessment and modification of requirements.

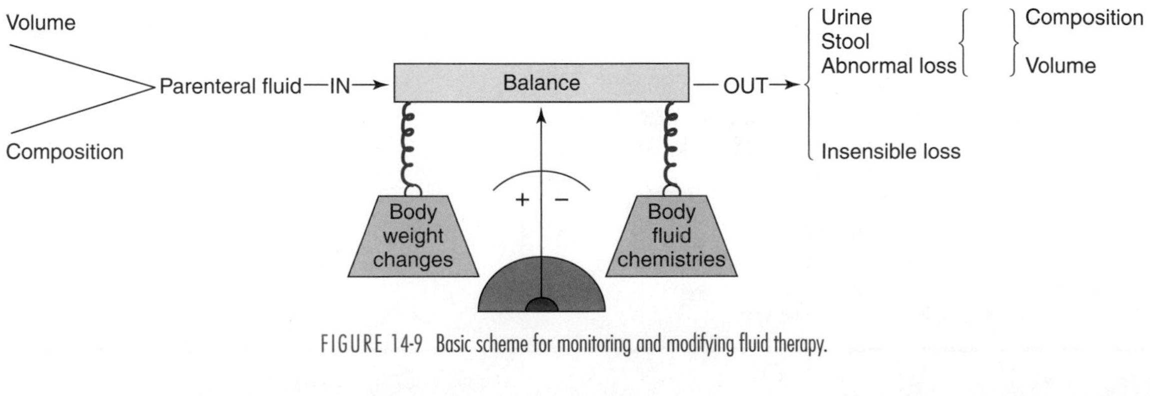

FIGURE 14-9 Basic scheme for monitoring and modifying fluid therapy.

Preterm infants, however, are subject to other problems that may diminish the influence of this metabolic rate when calculating fluid needs. SGA infants may require more water per kilogram than either preterm or term, appropriately grown infants (AGA infants). **Input should be recorded every hour, and output should be recorded as produced.** VLBW infants require frequent monitoring of fluid balance, so if output is unusually large, intake must be adjusted immediately. If fluid intake lags behind losses, critically ill infants may develop hypernatremia and may not tolerate "catching up." Continuous monitoring is necessary to ensure that fluid is administered in appropriate amounts. **Current infusion pumps can accurately infuse volumes of 0.1 mL/hr and must be used for the smallest, sickest infants.**

Requirements for fluid and electrolytes are divided into maintenance and deficit needs. ***Maintenance*** indicates the infant remains in a zero balance state and can be subdivided into (1) normal loss, which consists of water and electrolyte loss through stool, urine, and insensible (lung and skin) routes and (2) abnormal or increased losses, such as gastrointestinal/diarrhea, ostomy, and chest tube drainage.

All diapers should be preweighed using a gram scale and marked with dry/tare weight. After each stool or void, the diaper is reweighed; the difference equals the amount of loss. For example, if the dry weight is 20 g and the wet weight is 26 g, the difference is 6 g, or 6 mL of stool or urine. All losses should be calculated to the nearest milliliter.

The term ***deficit*** refers to previously incurred losses. These should be uncommon in the newborn but can occur when there are unrecognized losses such as "third space" or interstitial losses with necrotizing enterocolitis (NEC) (see below). In older neonates, deficits may occur with disorders that have an insidious or delayed onset, such as renal tubular dysfunction or nonvirilizing congenital adrenal hyperplasia.

Deficits are best estimated by body weight comparisons. Weight loss greater than 10% to 15% in 1 week should be considered excessive. VLBW infants are particularly difficult to maintain within 10% to 15% of birth weight during the first week of life.[6] Growth charts assist with calculations of weight loss and/or gain, and help consider the normal physiologic weight loss that occurs during the first several days after birth when calculating an infant's fluid needs.

The initial choice of parenteral solution depends on the weight and postnatal age of the infant (see Table 14-3). Also important is whether the infant is in an incubator with a heated humidified environment or under a radiant warmer without a plastic blanket or heat shield. **Uncovered VLBW infants under radiant warmers demonstrate IWL of up to 170 mL/kg/day,[5] and thus use of radiant warmers should be avoided if possible. Maintenance of water and glucose needs in larger infants on the first day of life can usually be met by a 10% glucose solution infused at 80 mL/kg/day, which provides an acceptable glucose infusion of about 5.5 mg/kg/min.** The infusion rate can be increased gradually to 100 to 120 mL/kg/day using principles of monitoring discussed below.

All sick infants require IV access for fluid administration.[5] The IV equipment should include (1) a needle or catheter, (2) connecting tubing, and (3) an infusion pump.

Electrolytes such as sodium and potassium are usually omitted the first day and then added as the salt of acetate, chloride, or phosphate in amounts of 1 to 4 mEq/kg/day. Mildly acidotic and VLBW infants may be given their sodium requirements as sodium acetate, which is metabolized to bicarbonate.[3] **Potassium should never be added to IV fluid until urine flow and renal function have been assessed.** The maintenance requirement for calcium is 0.5 to 1 mEq/kg/day (about 100 to 200 mg/kg/day) of calcium gluconate. This maintenance is most important in VLBW infants and those who are severely ill.

Factors that influence IWL must be identified early and maintenance needs adjusted appropriately to prevent problems with water and electrolyte balance. Management of VLBW infants presents special, complex problems, and further research is needed. The following observations may help:

- **Total fluid requirements** should start at 110 to 120 mL/kg/day at birth and often need to be increased by 20 to 40 mL/kg/day over days 2 to 4 of life, plateauing at 150 to 175 mL/kg/day.
- **Sodium requirements** (including medications) are 2 to 3 mEq/kg/day after 24 hours of age and may reach a maximum of 5 to 7 mEq/kg/day on days 5 and 6.
- **Cumulative weight loss plateaus at 11% to 15% of birth weight (95% confidence limits) by postnatal day 3 to 4.**
- **Maintaining normal serum glucose concentrations** (50 to 150 mg/dL) in VLBW infants

requires relatively less glucose (4 to 8 g/kg/day) than in term infants. The glucose concentration of the fluids administered may need to be changed, sometimes frequently, to maintain an appropriate serum glucose concentration. With the larger initial fluid requirements of very tiny babies, lower glucose concentrations, sometimes down to D_5W (5 mg% or 5 mg/dL) in IV fluids are often prescribed as the initial fluid. As anticipated, infants weighing less than 1000 g are the most difficult to manage without inducing either excessive weight loss, hypernatremia, or hyperglycemia.

VLBW infants, especially those stabilized under radiant warmers, may have greatly increased IWL with fluid requirements in the range of 175 to 200 mL/kg/day. By the end of the first week of life, as the epithelium cornifies, their daily requirements decrease to 120 to 150 mL/kg/day. When oral caloric intake is low (<50 kcal/kg/day), neonates will require significant administration of IV fluids, which should be provided as parenteral nutrition[6] containing glucose, amino acids, lipids, vitamins, and micronutrients (see Chapter 16).

DATA COLLECTION

Parenteral therapy should be based on the following principles: (1) assess the patient's clinical status for maintenance needs, factors that modify IWL, and confounding medical or surgical disorders; (2) calculate short-term (12 to 24 hours) fluid and electrolyte needs; (3) initiate therapy at the proper site and infusion rate; and (4) monitor and adjust the fluid infusion rate and content based on clinical and biochemical data.

History

Factors influencing IWL (see Table 14-2) include gestational age, birth weight, and postnatal age. It is important to know the fluids that the mother received during labor, since, for example, large volumes of hypotonic fluids administered to the mother may dilute the infant's serum electrolytes and expand the intravascular volume. When the patient's condition changes, it is important to detail the change to evaluate the potential effect of the new condition on fluid and electrolyte balance and requirements. Thus NEC may be associated with an acute need for additional volume expansion–type fluids because of "third space losses," whereas with acute renal failure, anuria should prompt clinical reassessment and usually indicates reducing daily fluid administration.

Signs and Symptoms

Weight, urine output (see the Data Collection box below), and **serum sodium concentration** (see the Data Collection box below) are the best overall clinical guides to assess whether therapy is adequate. **Weight is the most sensitive index of IWL and must be accurately determined at least every 24 hours.** Accurate daily weights in VLBW infants require special nursing efforts and often electronic bed scales.

Data Collection

CLINICAL EVALUATION OF FLUID AND ELECTROLYTE STATUS

- Serial weight (sometimes 2 to 3 times per day)
- Heart rate
- Blood pressure
- Skin perfusion
- Urine output
- Other drainage (ostomies, gastric, chest tubes)

Data Collection

LABORATORY EVALUATION OF FLUID AND ELECTROLYTE STATUS

Essential values are included in this box. Other measurements are routinely made but are less valuable in the rapid determination of fluid status and complications of imbalances.

- ***Sodium*** (most sensitive indicator of water loss in excess of electrolytes, as is insensible water loss)
- ***Potassium*** (may rise with decreased kidney perfusion and acidosis)
- ***Hematocrit*** (will rise with extracellular fluid contraction)
- ***BUN*** (relatively insensitive indicator of dehydration in neonate)
- ***Creatinine*** (will rise slowly with renal failure)
- ***Total CO_2*** (low level indicates acidosis, either because of bicarbonate loss or metabolic acidosis from poor tissue perfusion and anaerobic metabolism)

Urine output should be 2 to 5 mL/kg/hr with a specific gravity of 1.002 to 1.010 (60 to 300 mOsm). Blood pressure and peripheral perfusion may be used to reflect changes in vascular volume and cardiac output. Normal capillary refill is typically less than 3 seconds and is more reliable when tested on the forehead or sternum. However, its sensitivity and specificity have been questioned in older infants and should be interpreted with caution as a sign of adequate hydration. Blood pressure and heart rate should be evaluated in conjunction with capillary refill time.

Loss of skin turgor is a late and variable sign and usually is not helpful in assessing therapy, but vital signs (heart rate, respiratory rate, and temperature) provide useful signs about metabolic rate and stress. However, temperature may be affected by many external factors. Drainage volume and content from ostomies, chest tubes, nasogastric tubes, and other sites should be quantitated accurately. Fluid samples can be submitted for laboratory analysis to improve the accuracy of the replacement fluids. The amounts of drainage represent maintenance requirements that must be added to the calculation of baseline daily maintenance needs (abnormal + normal = total maintenance).

Laboratory Data

Tests for concentrations of electrolytes (Na^+, K^+, Cl^-, Ca^{2+}), red blood cells (hematocrit), glucose, BUN or creatinine, and acid-base status should be performed serially (see the Data Collection box on p. 344). Occasionally, serum osmolality and protein concentrations are helpful in assessing the neonate's condition. The anion gap may be calculated from the difference of the positive and negative ions, sodium, chloride, and bicarbonate: ($Na^+ - [Cl^- + HCO_3^-]$). A relatively low anion gap associated with the metabolic acidosis generally reflects bicarbonate loss in the urine, which can be normal in VLBW or abnormal in renal tubular acidosis.

Urine volume must be recorded with every void. Measuring urine osmolality and glucose and electrolyte concentrations helps clarify fluid and electrolyte balance when amounts of glucose, protein, or other solutes appear in the urine.

All drainage must be collected and measured, with the concentration of solutes determined (see the Data Collection box on p. 344). Accumulations over 4 to 6 hours are preferable to a single "spot" collection, which may be misleading. Occasionally, determining trace electrolyte elements, hematocrit, and protein content of urine or drainage can be crucial to management. However there are no "normal" values for urine electrolyte concentrations because they must be interpreted with respect to the infant's clinical diagnosis and the serum electrolyte concentrations.

TREATMENT

Techniques of IV Therapy

In modern neonatal intensive care, percutaneously placed central venous catheters have become an invaluable tool. Placement permits long-term administration of IV fluids, avoiding multiple painful procedures for peripheral IV placement and the need for surgical placement of a long-term central catheter. **This is particularly valuable for extremely-low-birth-weight (ELBW) infants for whom the time to establish full enteral feedings may be prolonged.** This technique is also helpful for long-term parenteral nutrition. Complications of long-term indwelling central catheters include infection, thrombosis, phlebitis, perforation, and infiltration. The risk for infection is directly related to the duration of the line's placement. Therefore these catheters should be discontinued as soon as enteral nutrition is adequately established. Thrombosis is more likely to occur when the flow rate of IV fluids is extremely low (<1 mL/hr). Infiltration usually occurs at the site of the catheter tip. This includes infiltration into the mediastinum, pleural space, or pericardium, depending on the location of the tip of the catheter (see Chapter 16).

Percutaneous insertion of Silastic catheters can be accomplished readily but requires clinical training and experience. Insertion sites include the saphenous, antecubital, axillary, basilic, cephalic, and external jugular veins. Advancing the catheter to a deep vein such as the superior or inferior vena cava is relatively simple but may be associated with thrombotic complications. The position of the catheter tip must be confirmed radiographically. Cannulation of the subclavian vein of VLBW infants requires insertion by a pediatric surgeon. Venesection or cutdown of peripheral or central vessels can be performed with appropriate training.

Peripheral venous access continues to be a valuable approach to IV therapy when short-term vascular access is needed. The advent of extremely small catheter and introducer sets (e.g., Quick Caths, Angiocaths) has permitted prolonged (5 to 7 days) use of a single peripheral infusion site. "Butterfly" infusion sets are rarely used for IV access.

A rubber band is an effective tourniquet for the extremity of a small infant. Attention must be paid to antiseptic technique when acquiring venous access. The skin should be cleaned with an antiseptic of 2% chlorhexidine and 70% isopropyl alcohol. Avoid shaving the head because parents may find this upsetting. Before puncturing the skin, prepare materials for placement. It is important to recognize the significant risk for infiltration and skin necrosis with a peripherally inserted IV line. The risk is greatest in the foot, less with the hand, and the least on the scalp. Calcium-containing solutions in parenteral nutrition present an additional risk, particularly for skin damage. Prevention of such extravasation injuries is paramount because few treatment options are available. Although the needle or catheter must be taped in place, the tape should allow for adequate visualization of the site. **The fluid administered should be recorded at least every hour, and the site should be observed for signs of infiltration. Syringe infusion pumps are used to administer IV fluids so that volumes as small as 0.1 mL/hr can be infused accurately.** The arm or leg can be positioned and stabilized on a padded board to prevent movement and minimize catheter displacement. The need for immobilization is less with catheters than with butterfly infusion sets. However, the board may need to be removed after several hours to visually ensure that no infiltration has occurred and to intermittently mobilize the limb. The most common complication of IV therapy is infiltration, with rates as high as 78%.[2] **If extravasation occurs, the infusion should be stopped immediately and the IV catheter removed. The affected extremity should then be elevated to limit swelling.**[6] Hyaluronidase is an enzyme that degrades hyaluronic acid, a constituent of the normal interstitial barrier, which increases the distribution and absorption of locally injected substances.[8] By facilitating more rapid absorption of potentially damaging fluid, tissue necrosis may be lessened. A plastic surgery consultation should be considered when tissues necrosis occurs.

Umbilical vessel catheterization should be limited to several days' duration until a central catheter can be placed (see Chapter 7).

Common Problems

In neonatal intensive care units (NICUs), virtually all patients initially receive IV fluid therapy. Therefore conventional rules of pediatric fluid therapy that estimate losses and project deficit replacement may not be appropriate. Weight, urine output and concentration, and the concentration of various solutes in serum and other body fluids are usually known. The correct diagnosis usually rests on clinical and laboratory measurements (not estimates), which are supported by the clinical setting. For example, one can compute the amount of sodium required to correct a deficit using the following formula:

$$\text{Necessary sodium} = (\text{Sodium desired} - \text{Sodium observed}) \times 0.6 \times \text{Weight (in kilograms)}$$

This calculation considers that the sodium will be given as a "dry salt." The total amount and the rate given are a matter of clinical judgment. In practice, often the clinician prescribes 50% of the calculated sodium deficit, remeasures serum sodium, and then modifies the IV solution. Attempts should be made to identify the etiology of the deficit while these conditions are being corrected, or it may recur.

Common Electrolyte Disorders

HYPOCALCEMIA (INFANTS WITH SERUM CALCIUM LESS THAN 7 mg/dL)

Hypocalcemia is a common finding in critically ill babies. Clinical findings may correlate poorly with biochemical data (total or ionized calcium). Jitteriness, irritability, and twitching are common initial, but nonspecific, signs. Both serum calcium and glucose should be measured. Hypocalcemia is strongly associated with infants of diabetic mothers and in infants with asphyxia, prematurity, and delayed nutrition. Risk for "early" hypocalcemia within 72 hours of birth is minimized by supplementing IV fluids with 35 or more mg/kg/day of elemental calcium[2] or initiating parenteral nutrition with 60 or more mg/kg/day for preterm infants.[2] Alternatively, early neonatal hypocalcemia may be prevented with oral calcium supplementation of 80 mg/kg/day of calcium gluconate.[2] (100 mg of calcium gluconate = 9.1 mg of elemental calcium.)

Attempts to rapidly correct hypocalcemia, using bolus infusions and slow infusions over 2 to 3 minutes, are not as successful and may induce dysrhythmias, compared with more gradual attempts to correct hypocalcemia. Either repeated slow infusions every 6 hours or a continuous infusion is best. Additional calcium should be given intravenously as 100 to 200 mg/kg/dose of calcium gluconate over 4 to 6 hours if seizures or biochemical abnormality persists. "Late" hypocalcemia, occurring at more than 7 days of age, usually has a specific cause such as malabsorption, hypomagnesemia, hypoparathyroidism, long-term diuretic therapy, or rickets and should be evaluated in detail.

Care should be taken when administering IV calcium: (1) the infant should receive cardiac monitoring to detect bradycardia; (2) calcium administration should be discontinued immediately if bradycardia occurs; and (3) the peripheral IV site should be checked for patency before and during administration because of the potential for skin necrosis, sloughing, and calcification caused by infiltrated calcium.

HYPERNATREMIA (INFANTS WITH SERUM SODIUM MORE THAN 150 mEq/L)

Clinical signs of hypernatremia are rare, except for late-occurring seizures. The most common causes of hypernatremia are (1) dehydration, usually caused by too little "free water" administration, (2) injudicious use of sodium-containing solution, such as sodium bicarbonate bolus infusion and sodium-containing medications, and (3) congenital or acquired reduction in antidiuretic hormone resulting in excess loss of "free water," diabetes insipidus. Intracranial bleeding correlates strongly with hypernatremia.[6] **Management should be directed toward prevention, and infants with hypernatremia should have serum sodium reduced slowly to prevent seizures.** Infants who experience hypernatremic dehydration often appear better hydrated than they are because hypernatremia shifts fluid into the intravascular space.

HYPONATREMIA (INFANTS WITH SERUM SODIUM LESS THAN 130 mEq/L)

Hyponatremia is usually asymptomatic because it develops chronically rather than as an acute imbalance; however, a late clinical sign is seizure. The most common causes include (1) excess hydration as a result of maternal or neonatal administration of electrolyte-free solutions, (2) renal loss of sodium in neonates receiving diuretic therapy, especially in VLBW infants, and (3) the syndrome of inappropriate antidiuretic hormone secretion (SIADH) that is suspected when decreased serum sodium and decreased urine output occur. This syndrome is associated with central nervous system (CNS) and lung pathologic conditions. Clinical criteria include (1) low serum sodium, (2) continued inappropriately high urine sodium loss, (3) urine osmolality greater than plasma, and (4) normal adrenal and renal function. Management is by water restriction until diuresis follows, and treatment is directed toward resolving the etiology.

HYPERKALEMIA (INFANTS WITH SERUM POTASSIUM MORE THAN 7 mEq/L)

Causes of hyperkalemia include (1) acidosis with or without tissue destruction, (2) renal failure (water overload may limit management), (3) adrenal insufficiency (relatively uncommon), and (4) iatrogenic secondary to inappropriate potassium administration. Table 14-4 outlines clinical signs and electrocardiogram (ECG) changes. **Management is directed toward resolving the causes and nonspecific treatment,** depending on the severity of the hyperkalemia and the associated clinical signs:

- Stop all potassium administration.
- Evaluate total and ionized calcium.
- If hypocalcemia is present, infuse 100 to 200 mg/kg of calcium gluconate to lower the cell membrane threshold. This is transient therapy but may be lifesaving.
- Infuse sodium bicarbonate 1 to 2 mEq/kg, slowly over 30 minutes or longer. This is also transient therapy designed to promote intracellular sodium and hydrogen exchange

TABLE 14-4 HYPERKALEMIA (INFANTS WITH MORE THAN 7 mEq/L SERUM POTASSIUM)

CLINICAL SIGNS	ELECTROCARDIOGRAM CHANGES
Muscular weakness	Short QT interval
Cardiac dysrhythmias	Widening QRS
Ileus	Sine wave QRS/T

for potassium. It is particularly useful when the hyperkalemia is associated with acidosis. However, if hyperkalemia is associated with acute renal failure, the relatively large volume of fluid required to deliver the sodium bicarbonate may be concerning.

- Administer 1 g/kg cation exchange resin (sodium polystyrene sulfonate [Kayexalate]) as an oral or rectal solution. Little experience has been reported in neonates, and technical problems of retention can be substantial. Furthermore, this may not be an option if the infant is nil per os (NPO) status or has an injured gastrointestinal tract. When this resin is used, sodium in the resin is exchanged for serum potassium, which may result in hypernatremia. Therefore careful attention must be paid to serum electrolyte concentrations.
- An insulin infusion given simultaneously with a dextrose infusion can help shift potassium to the intracellular space. There are several challenges to this form of therapy. First, the actual dose of insulin administered to the patient varies unpredictably since the insulin adsorbs to plastic IV tubing. Second, significant hypoglycemia and seizures may occur. Serum glucose concentration must be monitored frequently and the glucose infusion adjusted accordingly.
- Perform peritoneal dialysis. With neonatal hyperkalemic peritoneal dialysis, sodium bicarbonate frequently must be added to dialysate to prevent acidosis. Peritoneal dialysis is a complicated procedure in neonates, involving catheter placement and dialysis monitoring. It may be technically impossible in VLBW babies and difficult or impossible when there is injured bowel, as with necrotizing enterocolitis.

HYPOKALEMIA (INFANTS WITH SERUM POTASSIUM LESS THAN 3.5 mEq/L)

About 90% of the body's total potassium is intracellular. Management is directed toward the causes:

- Low serum potassium always implies significant intracellular depletion, most potassium is intracellular and can be low with normal serum potassium, and IV solutions usually should not exceed 40 mEq/L potassium.
- Diuretic-induced hypokalemia can be minimized by choosing a potassium-sparing diuretic such as spironolactone or providing supplemental potassium.

Clinical signs of hypokalemia are related to muscular weakness and cardiac dysrhythmias. Ileus may occur also. Electrocardiographic changes include decreased T waves and ST depression. The most common causes of hypokalemia are (1) increased gastrointestinal losses from an ostomy or nasogastric tube and (2) renal losses from diuretic therapy.

Common Clinical Syndromes

Acute renal failure is most often caused by (1) extrinsic factors such as perinatal asphyxia, shock, and heart failure, (2) intrinsic factors such as congenital or acquired lesions, and (3) obstructive uropathy, including urethral obstruction or extra-genitourinary mass. Oliguria or anuria usually occurs initially.

During initial oliguria, electrolyte-free glucose infusion should be limited to IWL and urine output. Frequently, this entails providing total fluids of 50 to 80 mL/kg/day. Recovery is usually associated with natriuresis (excessive urinary sodium loss) and osmotic diuresis. This may develop rapidly with sodium losses as high as 20 mEq/kg/day. **Body weight and fluid losses must be carefully and frequently measured, at least every 12 hours.**

Nonrenal losses, such as gastrointestinal drainage, must also be measured. Ideally, fluid and electrolyte therapy is directed toward maintaining the current weight or a weight loss of 1%/day until recovery is nearly complete. This may be accomplished initially by ordering replacement of IWL as a basal fluid order and replacing a percentage of additional fluid losses on a per-volume basis. The choice of fluid used for replacement depends on the electrolyte content of the fluid lost. Thus it may be helpful to measure urinary sodium and potassium loss concentrations and urine volume, recognizing that any "spot check" of these electrolytes will not fully reflect the loss over a 24-hour period.

Serial determination of serum electrolytes will help refine the fluid orders. As the patient recovers and renal function normalizes, transition to more standard fluids and electrolytes should occur. The renal ability of the patient to concentrate urine must be evaluated serially. If the patient remains in high-output renal failure and fluids are restricted, dehydration may occur. Dehydration will result in weight loss, increased serum electrolyte concentration, and hypernatremia with dilute urine. **Weight change during renal failure demands careful reevaluation of the fluid plan.**

Diuretics and Electrolytes

Diuretics represent one of the most common classes of drugs administered to sick neonates and infants. Electrolyte disturbances are the most common adverse effects of diuretic therapy and can lead to a variety of consequences. **Clinical indications for the use of diuretics in neonates and infants include RDS, BPD, congenital heart disease, and renal failure.** The classes of diuretics most commonly used in this age-group include loop diuretics, thiazides, and potassium-sparing diuretics. A discussion of the mechanism of action, diuretic efficacy, and common side effects follows.

LOOP DIURETICS

Loop diuretics bind to one of the chloride binding sites on the $Na^+/K^+/2Cl^-$ transporter, thus inhibiting reabsorption of sodium and chloride in the thick ascending limb of the loop of Henle. Water passively follows the movement of sodium and thus allows for diuresis.

Furosemide is the most widely studied diuretic in neonates and is consequently the prototype loop diuretic. It produces a 10-fold to 35-fold increase in sodium excretion and a 10-fold increase in urine flow. Therefore hyponatremia, hypochloremia, and hypovolemia are common with chronic use of furosemide. Hypokalemia is also of significant concern with chronic use of furosemide. The site of action of furosemide blocks tubular reabsorption of potassium. Potassium losses are also related to increased aldosterone production in the presence of sodium losses.[2]

In addition to potassium losses, furosemide also promotes urine calcium and magnesium excretion. The reabsorption of these cations is decreased because of furosemide's ability to eliminate the transepithelial potential difference. Chronic hypercalciuria leads to hypocalcemia and the possibility of renal calcifications and nephrocalcinosis. Compensatory mechanisms lead to increased parathyroid hormone secretion with associated bone resorption, bone demineralization, osteopenia, and possibly rickets.

Bumetanide is another loop diuretic commonly used in neonates and infants. It is 40 times more potent than furosemide. Side effects are the same as those seen with furosemide.

THIAZIDES

Hydrochlorothiazide and chlorothiazide are the most widely used thiazide diuretics in neonates and infants. Thiazides exert their effect by blocking the Na^+-Cl^- transporter at the distal convoluted tubule, collecting tubule, and early collecting duct. Because only a small portion of sodium reabsorption occurs in the distal tubule, thiazide diuretic efficacy is limited. However, chlorothiazide in combination with spironolactone has been shown to improve pulmonary mechanics in patients with BPD.[6]

Chronic use of thiazide diuretics leads to electrolyte disturbances, although usually they are less severe than with loop diuretics. Hyponatremia and hypokalemia are the most common side effects. Hypokalemia is the result of greater sodium-potassium exchange that occurs secondary to a higher concentration of sodium found in the distal tubule.

Whereas loop diuretics promote calcium loss, thiazide diuretics can increase serum calcium concentrations by increasing renal calcium reabsorption both proximally and distally.[6] This decrease in urinary calcium can be used to reverse loop diuretic–induced renal calcifications.

POTASSIUM-SPARING DIURETICS

Whereas loop and thiazide diuretics directly alter sodium reabsorption via direct inhibition of sodium transporters, potassium-sparing diuretics such as spironolactone competitively antagonize the aldosterone receptor. The primary binding site is the principal cell of the cortical collecting tubule. Aldosterone enhances sodium reabsorption in the collecting tubule and promotes potassium secretion. Therefore antagonizing aldosterone results in diminished sodium reabsorption with a consequent increase in serum concentrations of potassium and hydrogen. However, spironolactone inhibits the reabsorption of less than 2% of filtered sodium and is thus not an effective primary diuretic. The major use is to prevent urinary potassium loss induced by other diuretics.

Hyperkalemia is the primary electrolyte disturbance to monitor with the use of spironolactone. This side effect is usually not of great concern since spironolactone is frequently used in conjunction with other potassium-wasting diuretics. Spironolactone should be avoided in renal failure.

Major Surgery

Surgical trauma is superimposed on the normal metabolic responses of the neonate. The clinical impact is determined by the type and extent of surgery and gestational and postnatal age of the infant. In healthy term infants, negative balance of water, electrolytes, nitrogen, and calories with associated weight loss occurs during the first 3 to 5 days followed by transition to positive balance and weight gain by 7 to 10 days. Parallel transition times for preterm infants vary enormously. Deficits may exist as a result of delayed diagnosis, with external loss or internal loss. "Third space" losses can be significant, with peritoneal losses a notorious source of deficit underestimation.

Predicting the metabolic response to surgery is difficult, reflecting wide variation among individual patients, even patients with similar lesions. Uncontrollable and unmeasurable variables prevent a standardized postoperative physiologic response for neonates, especially those weighing less than 2 kg. Thermoregulation is a particular challenge for operative procedures. The patient is draped and shielded from radiant heat sources. Measuring and managing the patient's internal temperature with evaporative heat and water loss complicating the situation is difficult once the incision is made. Transport incubators, prewarmed operating rooms, radiant warmers, warming pads, and prewarmed solutions may help achieve thermoneutrality. Intraoperative fluid balance is rarely precise despite the clinicians's best efforts. Blood loss on sponges, drapes, and other objects should be measured, but IWL from open body cavities is difficult to estimate.

The principles of postoperative management are as follows:

- Monitor clinical and chemical variables frequently, every 4 to 6 hours; evaluate fluid balance, and measure drainage.
- Recognize that insensible water losses may include "third space losses." These include water lost into the lumen of the bowel or into the peritoneum secondary to peritonitis, resulting in the loss of both water and electrolytes from the intravascular compartment. At least a proportion of the fluids used to anticipate these losses should contain high sodium content similar to plasma, such as lactated Ringer's solution. Clinical judgment is used to estimate the third space losses since they cannot be measured. Serial evaluations of blood pressure, heart rate, urine output, and skin perfusion together may help determine if the volume prescribed is sufficient.
- Provide 30 to 40 kcal/kg/day as glucose.
- Provide parenteral nutrition early if significant enteral feedings (<50 kcal/kg) cannot be achieved by 3 to 5 days postoperative. Gastrointestinal motility returns rapidly in term infants compared with adults. Almost all VLBW infants require parenteral nutrition after surgery.

COMPLICATIONS

Excessive fluid administration (>180 mL/kg/day) has been associated with chronic lung disease and patent ductus arteriosus (PDA). Inadequate fluid administration has been associated with dehydration, decreased urine output, hypernatremia, poor tissue perfusion, and, potentially, tissue damage.

PARENT TEACHING

The need for and presence of an IV line in a newborn may be frightening for the parents. Clear, medically and physiologically sound explanations (in nonmedical jargon) of the need for fluid and electrolyte support for their infant help allay parents' fears (see the Parent Teaching box on p. 351). Scalp vein IVs are of particular concern (1) if the hair must be shaved and (2) because a common misconception is that the needle is positioned in the infant's brain. Explain to parents that scalp vein IVs are in the large veins of the head and not the brain and that an IV in the head stays in longer, thus decreasing the need for multiple vein punctures and allows the infant mobility of all four extremities. In answer to the question "Does it hurt?" a truthful answer is "Yes, when it is put in, but not after it is in the vein."

The concept of the use of central venous catheters should be presented to the parents early in the hospital course. The advantages are fewer painful procedures, increased mobility of the patient, and decreased risk for infiltrate. These should be clearly explained in lay language, as well as the potential complications such as infection, thrombosis, and the specific risk for the extravasation of fluid into body cavities, pleura, and pericardium. Well-illustrated

Parent Teaching

PARENT TEACHING ABOUT FLUID AND ELECTROLYTE MANAGEMENT

- Most babies cannot be feed immediately and will require intravenous (IV) fluids.
- Umbilical venous and arterial catheters must be removed in a few days.
- IV fluids will be given through percutaneous central venous catheters, peripheral IV lines, or surgically placed lines.
- Scalp IVs go only into subcutaneous veins, not into the brain.
- Placing the IV will hurt only during the procedure and will be painless afterward.
- Peripheral IVs are subject to infiltration, which may be serious if the fluid is hyperalimentation fluid or contains calcium.
- Central venous catheters (percutaneously or surgically placed) carry the risks of thrombosis, infection, or infiltration into body cavities such as the pleura or pericardium.
- IV fluids will be discontinued as soon as enteral nutrition is sufficiently advanced.

parent education materials often are very helpful when explaining these situations to parents.

Potential infiltration of peripheral IV sites should be addressed *prospectively* with parents. Erythema and edema are expected. Sloughing of the skin occasionally occurs in VLBW infants and is more common on the feet and hands than on the scalp.

Including parents in the care of their sick neonate requires an explanation about the importance of measuring intake and output. Inadvertent disposal of diapers and giving fluids that are not recorded should be prevented, and the importance of saving diapers for the infant's nurse should be emphasized. "A little spitting up" after feeding may seem insignificant if parents are not instructed in the importance of telling the nurse and saving it for evaluation.

REFERENCES

1. Aiken CG, Sherwood RA, Kenney IJ, et al: Mineral balance studies in sick preterm intravenously fed infants during the first week after birth: a guide to fluid therapy, *Acta Pediatr Scand Suppl* 355:1, 1989.
2. Bhatia J: Fluid and electrolyte management in the very low birth weight neonate, *J Perinatol* 26:S19, 2006.
3. Costarino AT Jr, Gruskay JA, Corcoran L, et al: Sodium restriction versus daily maintenance replacement in very low birth weight premature neonates: a randomized, blind, therapeutic trial, *J Pediatr* 120:99, 1992.
4. El-Dahr SS, Chevalier RL: Special needs of the newborn infant in fluid therapy, *Pediatr Clin North Am* 37:323, 1990.
5. Hartnoll G: Basic principles and practical steps in the management of fluid balance in the newborn, *Semin Neonatol* 8:307, 2003.
6. Modi N: Management of fluid balance in the very immature neonate, *Arch Dis Child Fetal Neonatal Ed* 89:F108, 2004.
7. Moffet HL, Allan D, Williams T: Survival and dissemination of bacteria in nebulizers and incubators, *Am J Dis Child* 114:13, 1967.
8. Thigpen JL: Peripheral intravenous extravasation: nursing procedure for initial treatment, *Neonatal Netw* 26:379, 2007.

SELECTED READINGS

Bauer K, Bovermann G, Roithmaier A, et al: Body composition, nutrition, and fluid balance during the first two weeks of life in preterm neonates weighing less than 1500 grams, *J Pediatr* 118:615, 1991.

Bell EF, Warburton D, Stonestreet BS, et al: Effect of fluid administration on the development of symptomatic patent ductus arteriosus and congestive heart failure in premature infants, *N Engl J Med* 302:598, 1980.

Chemtob S, Kaplan BS, Sherbotie JR, et al: Pharmacology of diuretics in the newborn, *Pediatr Clin North Am* 36:1231, 1989.

Chessex P, Reichman B, Verellen G, et al: Metabolic consequences of intrauterine growth retardation in very low birthweight infants, *Pediatr Res* 18:709, 1984.

Gaylord MS, Wright K, Lorch K, et al: Improved fluid management utilizing humidified incubators in extremely low birth weight infants, *J Perinatol* 21:438, 2001.

Greene HL, Hambidge KM, Schanler R, et al: Guidelines for the use of vitamins, trace elements, calcium, magnesium, and phosphorus in infants and children receiving total parenteral nutrition, *Am J Clin Nutr* 48:1324, 1988.

Hammarlund K, Sedin G, Strömberg B: Transepidermal water loss in newborn infants. VIII. Relation to gestational age and post-natal age in appropriate and small for gestational age infants, *Acta Paediatr Scand* 72:721, 1983.

Hay WW Jr: Intravenous nutrition of the very preterm neonate, *Acta Paediatr Suppl* 94:47, 2005.

Heimler R, Doumas BT, Jendrzejczak BM, et al: Relationship between nutrition, weight change, and fluid compartments in preterm infants during the first week of life, *J Pediatr* 122:110, 1993.

Kelly LK, Seri I: Renal developmental physiology: relevance to clinical care, *NeoReviews* 9:e150, 2008.

Peters O, Ryan S, Matthew L, et al: Randomised controlled trial of acetate in preterm neonates receiving parenteral nutrition, *Arch Dis Child Fetal Neonatal Ed* 77:F12, 1997.

Salle BL, David L, Chopard JP, et al: Prevention of early neonatal hypocalcemia in low birth weight infants with continuous calcium infusion: effect on serum calcium, phosphorus, magnesium, and circulating immunoreactive parathyroid hormone and calcitonin, *Pediatr Res* 11:1180, 1977.

Sann L, David L, Chayvialle JA, et al: Effect of early oral calcium supplementation on serum calcium and immunoreactive calcitonin concentration in preterm infants, *Arch Dis Child* 55:611, 1980.

Sherman TI, Greenspan JS, St Clair N, et al: Optimizing the neonatal thermal environment, *Neonatal Netw* 25:251, 2006.

15 GLUCOSE HOMEOSTASIS

JANE E. McGOWAN, PAUL J. ROZANCE, WEBRA PRICE-DOUGLAS, AND WILLIAM W. HAY, JR.

During intrauterine life, the fetus depends on the constant transfer of glucose across the placenta to meet its glucose requirements. After birth, neonates must maintain their own glucose homeostasis by producing and regulating their own glucose supply. This requires activation of a number of metabolic processes, including gluconeogenesis (synthesis of glucose from endogenous substrates) and glycogenolysis (release of glucose via breakdown of glycogen stores), as well as intact regulatory mechanisms for glucose metabolism and an adequate supply of metabolic substrates.

FETAL PHYSIOLOGY

Throughout gestation, maternal glucose provides the principal source of energy for the fetus via facilitated diffusion across the placenta. Fetal glucose uptake varies directly with maternal glucose concentration; fetal glucose concentration usually is about 70% of the maternal value. Changes in maternal metabolism, including increased caloric intake and decreased sensitivity of the maternal tissues to insulin, augment maternal glucose production and provide the additional glucose necessary to meet fetal energy demands. With normal maternal glucose concentrations and rates of glucose supply to the fetus, the fetus produces little, if any, glucose, although the enzymes for gluconeogenesis are present by the third month of gestation.[68] If fetal energy demands cannot be met, however, as is the case when maternal starvation is severe enough to produce maternal and fetal hypoglycemia, the fetus is capable of adapting by using alternate substrates, such as ketone bodies. In addition, data from animal models suggest that, under these conditions, there may be fetal glucose production.[54] Even in the basal state, the fetus relies on fuels such as lactate and amino acids to meet up to 25% to 30% of its energy demands, whereas lipids are used primarily for fat production.

Fetal glycogen synthesis begins as early as the ninth week of gestation, but the majority of fetal glycogen is produced in the third trimester. The major sites of glycogen deposition are skeletal muscle (>90% of body glycogen), liver (the only organ whose glycogen can be released for use by other organs), lung, and heart.[73] By 40 weeks' gestation, hepatic and skeletal muscle glycogen contents are several times adult levels. By contrast, lung and cardiac muscle glycogen stores decrease as the fetus approaches term, although these stores are still of physiologic significance. Survival in animals exposed to anoxia and in human infants after asphyxia, for example, is directly related to cardiac glycogen content. The decrease in lung glycogen, which begins at 34 to 36 weeks' gestation, may be related to ongoing developmental processes such as the synthesis of surfactant.

In addition to glycogen, the human fetus also stores energy as fat in adipose tissue. Most triglyceride synthesis occurs during the third trimester. By 40 weeks' gestation, the human fetus has a fat content of about 16%, making it the fattest of all terrestrial newborn mammals. The human placenta transports some free fatty acids, although the amount transported to the fetus is not sufficient to account for the amount of adipose tissue present; therefore the fetus also must synthesize triglycerides, using glycerol derived from glucose, as well as fatty acids transported across the placenta. As with glycogen, conditions in which fetal glucose supply is reduced will result in less adipose tissue accumulation.

Insulin is a major stimulus for fetal growth. Fetal pancreatic insulin content and glucose-stimulated insulin secretion increase to levels comparable to those found in neonates over the second half of gestation.[49] Fetal insulin secretion is augmented by

Please note that the PURPLE type in each chapter is intended to make it easier to identify clinically applicable material.

higher glucose concentrations; increased concentrations of amino acids add to this effect. Increased concentrations of insulin increase fetal glucose utilization and glucose oxidation rates without increasing total fetal oxygen consumption.[22,40] This implies that other substrates (e.g., amino acids) become available for nonoxidative metabolism when glucose and insulin are plentiful; such conditions promote tissue accretion and growth. Animal studies have demonstrated increased rates of amino acid utilization, incorporation of amino acids into protein synthesis, suppression of amino acid oxidation, and increased glucose uptake with increased insulin concentration and, conversely, decreased cell numbers and deoxyribonucleic acid (DNA) content with insulin deficiency, supporting insulin's role as a growth-promoting factor.

The fetuses of diabetic mothers who have very unstable plasma glucose concentrations during late gestation have an increased islet cell response to hyperglycemia compared with controls, releasing more insulin than normal fetuses at any given blood glucose concentration.[49] The higher insulin levels in turn lead to increased growth consisting primarily of adipose tissue, producing the macrosomia typically seen in infants of diabetic mothers (IDMs). In contrast, fetuses with intrauterine growth restriction (IUGR) have reduced numbers of pancreatic islet beta cells and produce less-than-normal amounts of insulin in response to glucose and amino acid stimulation. It is interesting to note that although correction of acute insulin deficiency promotes growth, exogenous insulin appears to have little effect on growth in human newborns or animal models with chronic insulin deficiency, suggesting that insulin infusion to promote growth in growth-restricted infants is unlikely to be beneficial and may lead to additional complications.

The related pancreatic hormone ***glucagon,*** which, like insulin, does not cross the placenta, has been detected as early as 15 weeks of gestation. In postnatal life, glucagon is a potent inducer of gluconeogenic enzymes, the opposite of insulin, which suppresses gluconeogenesis.[68] In fetal life, glucagon plays a much less important role in regulating glucose metabolism than insulin, reflecting the developmental insensitivity of fetal glucagon receptors. As a result, the insulin-to-glucagon effectiveness ratio in the fetus is high, which is important in preferentially maintaining glycogen synthesis and suppressing gluconeogenesis.

NEONATAL PHYSIOLOGY

At birth, the newborn infant is removed abruptly from its glucose supply and blood glucose concentration falls. Several hormonal and metabolic changes occur at birth that facilitate the adaptation necessary to maintain glucose homeostasis. Catecholamine levels increase markedly at birth, possibly as a response to the decrease in environmental temperature, as well as to the loss of the placenta, which may remove as much as 50% of circulating fetal epinephrine.[82] Glucagon concentrations and receptor sensitivity also increase, reversing the relatively high insulin/glucagon effectiveness ratio characteristic of fetal life.[76] The increased glucagon and norepinephrine concentrations activate hepatic glycogen phosphorylase, which induces glycogenolysis. Simultaneously, the decreasing glucose concentration and perinatal surge in fetal cortisol secretion stimulate hepatic glucose-6-phosphatase activity. Together these changes lead to an increase in hepatic glucose release.[18] Increased catecholamines also stimulate lipolysis, releasing fatty acids that can be metabolized to provide precursors for gluconeogenesis, as well as providing energy in the form of adenosine triphosphate (ATP) and cofactors such as nicotinamide adenine dinucleotide phosphate (NADPH) that enhance the activity of gluconeogenic enzymes. Catecholamine release also activates brown fat triglyceride turnover, producing heat necessary for postnatal thermoregulation. The normal postnatal decrease in insulin effect and increase in glucagon effects induce synthesis of phosphoenolpyruvate carboxykinase (PEPCK), which is considered the rate-limiting enzyme in hepatic gluconeogenesis. The concentrations of PEPCK and other gluconeogenic enzymes continue to increase over the first 2 weeks of life, regardless of gestational age. These changes act in concert to provide glucose to replace the supply previously received via the placenta.

Maintenance of glucose homeostasis depends on the balance between hepatic glucose output and glucose utilization by the brain and peripheral tissues. Hepatic glucose output is a function of rates of glycogenolysis and gluconeogenesis. Peripheral glucose utilization varies with the metabolic demands placed on the neonate. **Studies in normal human newborn infants using several different methods have determined that the steady-state glucose production/utilization rate in a term neonate**

is 4 to 6 mg/min/kg, approximately twice the weight-specific rate measured in adults.[21] As in the fetus, it appears that approximately half of this glucose is oxidized to CO_2 during normal metabolic processes, whereas the remainder is used in nonoxidative pathways, such as glycogen and fat synthesis. Perinatal glucose utilization increases (1) during hypoxia because of the inherent inefficiency of anaerobic glycolysis; (2) in the presence of hyperinsulinemia, which increases glucose uptake by insulin-sensitive tissues; (3) in newborns with respiratory distress because of increased muscle activity; and (4) during cold stress, which leads to increased sympathetic nervous system activity with subsequent release of norepinephrine, epinephrine, and thyroid hormone, which increase metabolic rate. If rates of glycogenolysis and gluconeogenesis do not match the rate of glucose utilization because of failure of the hormonal control mechanisms or variability of substrate supply, disturbances of glucose homeostasis occur. These disturbances are recognized clinically by the presence of hypoglycemia or hyperglycemia.

HYPOGLYCEMIA

Definition

The absolute blood or plasma glucose concentration that defines hypoglycemia as a pathologic condition remains difficult to establish and has not been determined. Further, there is no absolute correlation between blood or plasma glucose concentrations, clinical signs or symptoms, and either short-term or long-term sequelae. Instead, "reference" glucose concentrations generally reflect the lower limit of the normal range in a specific population of newborn infants, determined by statistical analysis of data collected in that population. Thus there is no consensus about threshold glucose concentrations below which diagnostic evaluation or treatment is mandated or that identify those infants likely to have adverse neurodevelopmental outcome.

Published definitions of hypoglycemia range from a blood glucose concentration of less than 20 mg/dL in preterm infants and less than 30 mg/dL in term infants to a plasma concentration of less than 45 mg/dL.[11-13] Some sources have even suggested raising the lower limit of normal to 50 to 70 mg/dL, although others have emphasized that such higher concentrations should be used primarily as target values during treatment for relatively severe and symptomatic hypoglycemia, rather than thresholds for instituting treatment.[11] Published reports fail to distinguish between threshold glucose concentrations below which physiologic responses may occur (and below which clinical monitoring may be indicated) and those below which pathological consequences are likely to develop (thus requiring aggressive treatment). In 1992, the majority of pediatricians in one survey in the United Kingdom defined a safe glucose concentration to be at least 2 mmol/L (36 mg/dL) in blood or 2.5 mmol/L (45 mg/dL) in plasma.[47,48] Figure 15-1 shows that 95% of normal term infants had a blood glucose concentration of more than 30 mg/dL in the first 24 hours of life and more than 45 mg/dL after 24 hours of life.[77] **A number of current references use 40 to 45 mg/dL as the lower limit of "normal" plasma glucose concentrations in the first 72 hours of life.***

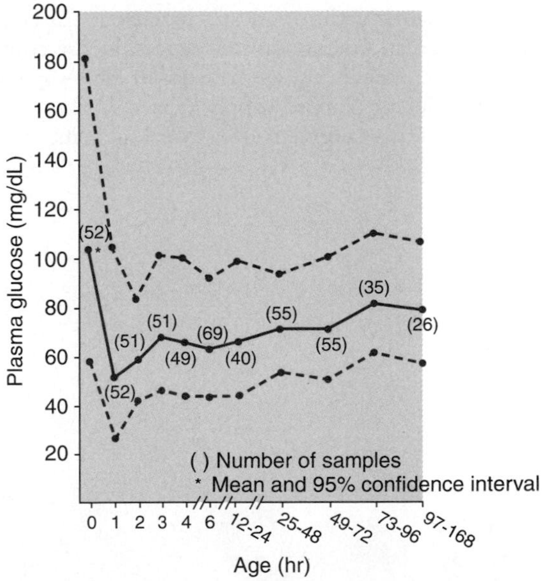

FIGURE 15-1 Plasma glucose concentrations during the first week of life in healthy appropriate-for-gestational-age term infants. (From Srinvasan G et al: Plasma glucose values in normal neonates: a new look, *J Pediatr* 109:114, 1986.)

*References 11,45,59,60,75,77,81.

Using these definitions of hypoglycemia, the overall incidence has been estimated at 1.3 to 4.4/1000 live births. Differences in incidence figures probably reflect variable inclusion of data from symptomatic versus asymptomatic infants. In preterm infants, the incidence of hypoglycemia is increased; estimates range from 1.5% to 5.5% (Figure 15-2). The incidence of hypoglycemia in term infants with IUGR may be as high as 25%, with an even higher rate seen in preterm small-for-gestational-age (SGA) infants.[56]

Hypoglycemia also may be defined clinically as the glucose concentration in a neonate that is associated with signs or symptoms that resolve when glucose is administered. This value is difficult to determine, however, because the symptoms of hypoglycemia are nonspecific and may not be noticed initially. **From a physiologic point of view, an infant may be said to be hypoglycemic when glucose supply is inadequate to meet demand.** Unfortunately, no method is available to establish this value in a given infant. Infants with increased demand or limited capability to alter glucose delivery (which is a function of both blood supply and glucose concentration) are at increased risk for impaired organ function at low blood glucose concentrations. Specifically, animal studies have shown that insufficient glucose supply may contribute to neuronal death, augment functional deficits, and increase the risk for long-term neurologic injury in the presence of concurrent cerebral hypoxia and/or ischemia. Clinical studies suggest this may be true also in newborn infants, although it is not clear whether the low glucose concentrations in cases of hypoxia and ischemia contributed directly to worse outcomes or were simply a marker for those infants with more significant metabolic compromise during hypoxia-ischemia who were therefore more likely to have worse outcomes.

Rather than defining hypoglycemia as an absolute blood glucose value, some investigators have suggested using specific glucose concentrations as an indicator that further investigation is needed to assess whether an infant's glucose homeostasis is compromised. Threshold values are based on evidence available in the literature (see further discussion in the "Treatment" section).[11] This approach **considers the overall metabolic and physiologic status of the infant when determining what constitutes an acceptable blood glucose concentration.** Some infants may undergo metabolic derangements at glucose concentrations above the "hypoglycemic" threshold, whereas others may be able to tolerate lower concentrations of blood glucose without developing metabolic stress. An infant with polycythemia, for example, may have a normal blood glucose concentration but decreased cerebral delivery of glucose because of reduced plasma flow.

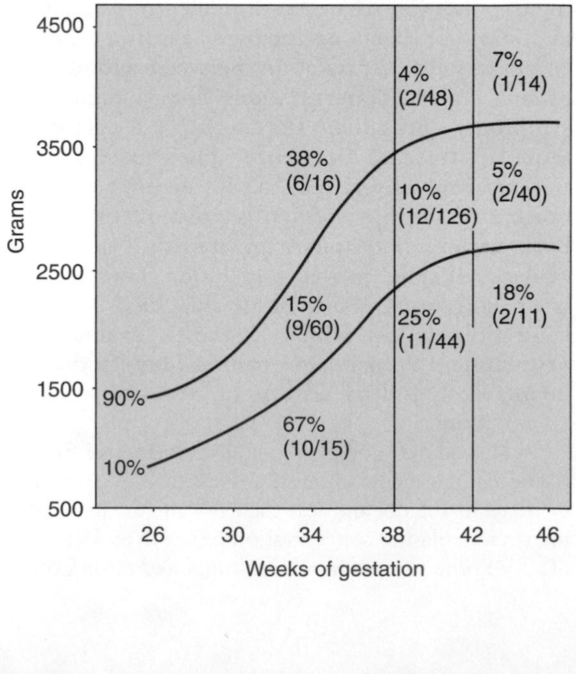

FIGURE 15-2 Incidence of neonatal hypoglycemia (blood glucose <30 mg/dL) by birth weight and gestational age. (From Lubchenco LO, Bard H: Incidence of hypoglycemia in newborn infants classified by birth weight and gestational age, *Pediatrics* 47:831, 1971.)

In contrast, breast-fed infants have normal substrate delivery to the brain even with "hypoglycemic" blood glucose values because they have increased plasma concentrations of ketone bodies compared with formula-fed infants.[37] Concentrations of ketones are lower in preterm and IUGR/SGA infants than in term infants who are feeding normally, suggesting that prematurity and IUGR are associated with less capacity to generate alternate brain energy substrates. This decreased capacity might increase the vulnerability of such infants to cerebral energy deficits when plasma glucose concentrations are decreased.[37,38]

In summary, **the definition of the blood glucose concentration at which intervention is indicated must be tailored to the clinical situation and the particular characteristics of a given infant.** Kalhan and Peter-Wohl recently suggested that further investigation and treatment should be instituted in the symptomatic infant at blood glucose concentrations of less than 45 mg/dL, whereas asymptomatic term infants with known risk factors should be treated if their blood glucose concentration is less than 36 mg/dL.[45] Several authors suggest that these thresholds for intervention should be higher in preterm infants and lower in breast-fed full-term infants.[11,36] However, it is important to recognize that there have been no systematic studies to demonstrate the risks or benefits of using any specific blood glucose concentration as a threshold for intervention in neonatal hypoglycemia. Given the apparently wide range of glucose values associated with normal neonatal outcomes, as well as the inherent inaccuracies in measuring glucose concentrations and the absence of a specific level below which injury inevitably occurs, any individual blood glucose measurement should be considered as representing the general status of the baby's glucose supply rather than as an absolute indicator of glucose sufficiency or insufficiency.

Hypoglycemic Neuronal Injury and Neuropathology

A schema of how hypoglycemia can contribute to neuronal injury is presented in Figure 15-3. Hypoglycemic brain damage in the newborn infant occurs predominantly in gray matter structures, although severe hypoglycemia in newborn infants may also be associated with white matter injury, particularly when the hypoglycemia occurs simultaneously with hypoxic-ischemic injury.[69,83] Pathologic studies of such severely hypoglycemic newborn infants have shown widespread neuronal injury in cerebral cortex, hippocampus, basal ganglia, thalamus, brainstem, and spinal cord. Late neuropathologic lesions associated with severe and prolonged low glucose concentrations include microcephaly associated with cortical atrophy and diffuse neuronal loss, as well as astrogliosis. Abnormalities may also be seen in white matter, whereas the cerebellum is generally spared.

Neuroimaging of Hypoglycemic Injury

Magnetic resonance imaging (MRI) performed 2 to 3 weeks after severe hypoglycemia demonstrates abnormal signals in the cortex, often most apparent in the occipital lobes.[2] More recent neuroradiologic investigations have shown a much wider variety in the pattern of injury involving both white matter and gray matter as a consequence of severe neonatal hypoglycemia.[9] Radiographically defined lesions after severe hypoglycemia in the newborn period can be transient and not associated with long-term neurologic consequences, indicating that follow-up MRI scans must be done to determine the permanency of the lesions.

HYPERGLYCEMIA

Definition

Hyperglycemia in newborns is usually defined, based on population data, as a blood glucose concentration of more than 125 mg/dL (>150 mg/dL plasma) in a term infant or more than 150 mg/dL in blood in a preterm infant. Unlike neonatal hypoglycemia, there are no reported "clinical" definitions of hyperglycemia (i.e., the appearance of physiologic disturbances associated with a specific high blood glucose concentration). The incidence of statistically defined neonatal hyperglycemia is difficult to determine; estimates range from 5.5% of all infants receiving intravenous (IV) infusions of $D_{10}W$ to as high as 40% in infants weighing less than 1000 g who are receiving IV dextrose infusions. Dweck and Cassady noted that 86% of infants with birth weights under 1100 g were hyperglycemic, and of these infants, 84% had one or more serum glucose concentrations greater than 300 mg/dL.[25]

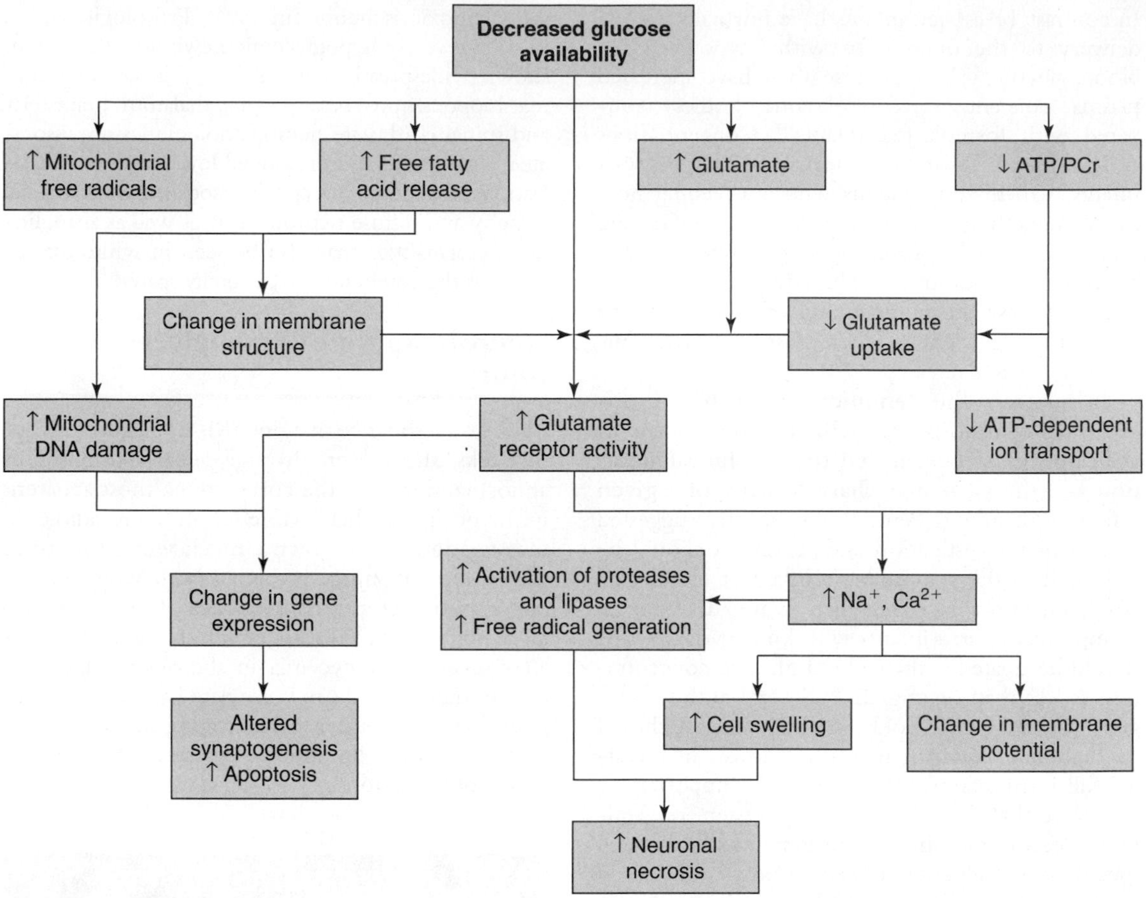

FIGURE 15-3 Proposed mechanism for the pathogenesis of hypoglycemic brain injury in the newborn. *ATP,* Adenosine 5′-triphosphate; *DNA,* deoxyribonucleic acid; *PCr,* phosphocreatine. (From McGowan JE: Role of glucose in cerebral function. In William W. Hay, Jr, editor, *Semin Neonat Nutr Metab,* 4:2-3, Columbus, Ohio, 1997, Ross Products.)

More recently, Blanco et al found that 88% of infants with birth weights less than 1000 g had at least one blood glucose concentration greater than 150 mg/dL in the first week of life.[8]

ETIOLOGY OF HYPOGLYCEMIA AND HYPERGLYCEMIA

Hypoglycemia

The causes of hypoglycemia can be grouped into several broad categories based on the mechanisms producing the hypoglycemia (Box 15-1; Table 15-1). These categories include inadequate substrate supply, abnormal endocrine regulation of glucose metabolism, and increased rate of glucose utilization. There also are several proposed causes for which mechanisms are not well defined.

INADEQUATE SUBSTRATE SUPPLY

If substrate availability is inadequate, hepatic glucose output will not meet metabolic demands. Most often this results from subnormal fat and glycogen stores that consequently do not provide sufficient energy to maintain glucose homeostasis until gluconeogenesis reaches adequate levels. Because most hepatic glycogen is accumulated during the

BOX 15-1

INDICATIONS FOR ROUTINE MONITORING OF BLOOD GLUCOSE FOR PREVENTION OF NEONATAL HYPOGLYCEMIA

Maternal Conditions

- Presence of diabetes or abnormal result of glucose tolerance test
- Preeclampsia and pregnancy-induced or essential hypertension
- Previous macrosomic infants
- Substance abuse
- Treatment with beta-agonist tocolytics
- Treatment with oral hypoglycemic agents
- Late antepartum to intrapartum administration of intravenous glucose

Neonatal Conditions

- Prematurity
- Intrauterine growth restriction
- Perinatal hypoxia-ischemia
- Sepsis
- Hypothermia
- Polycythemia-hyperviscosity
- Erythroblastosis fetalis
- Iatrogenic administration of insulin
- Congenital cardiac malformations
- Persistent hyperinsulinemia
- Endocrine disorders
- Inborn errors of metabolism

third trimester, infants born preterm have diminished glycogen stores. Infants with IUGR secondary to placental insufficiency also may be at risk for decreased glycogen accumulation, presumably because of diminished transfer of glycogen precursors (e.g., glucose, lactate) across the placenta. In these infants, relative hypoxemia caused by placental dysfunction may stimulate increased production of adrenaline and noradrenaline, leading to increased glycogen breakdown and further compromising substrate supply. Recent evidence from animal studies and human observations, however, suggesting that, because of increased glucose uptake mechanisms (e.g., increased expression of cell membrane glucose transporters) in response to glucose deficiency, muscle and hepatic glycogen stores may be normal or even increased in IUGR infants. Postnatally, catecholamine- and glucagon-stimulated glycogenolysis rapidly deplete glycogen supplies at a time when gluconeogenesis is still impaired because of low levels of PEPCK and other gluconeogenic enzymes, and hypoglycemia may result. After the first few postnatal days, preterm infants may still be at risk for hypoglycemia even though glycogen stores are adequate, because of low levels of hepatic microsomal glucose-6-phosphatase activity. Activity of this enzyme in preterm infants is low before birth and, in some infants, can remain low for several months after birth.[68,80,81] Because this enzyme catalyzes the dephosphorylation of glucose-6-phosphate to glucose and regulates the final step in hepatic glucose production, the decreased activity could contribute to diminished glucose production from both glycogenolysis and gluconeogenesis. Infants with low hepatic glucose-6-phosphatase activity may not be symptomatic with the initial episode of hypoglycemia but can become symptomatic if the hypoglycemia persists. Up to 18% of preterm infants have problems in maintaining normoglycemia at the time of discharge if a feeding is omitted or delayed.[41] Inadequate cortisol secretion in very preterm infants, particularly during periods of stress, also has been cited as a cause of limited activation of gluconeogenic enzymes. The underlying mechanisms are not clear but may be related to a lack of stimulation as a result of limited hypothalamic-pituitary axis activity.

ABNORMALITIES OF ENDOCRINE REGULATION

Hyperinsulinemia is the most common endocrinologic disturbance producing neonatal hypoglycemia and may be the most common cause of the infrequent cases of persistent hypoglycemia in infants. Excessive insulin secretion in the newborn increases glucose utilization by stimulating cellular glucose uptake in insulin-dependent tissues, including muscle and liver; however, brain glucose uptake does not appear to be significantly altered by increased insulin levels. At the same time, the high circulating insulin concentration promotes continued glycogen synthesis and inhibits both glycogenolysis and gluconeogenesis, impairing the infant's glucogenic response to the increased glucose demand and decreasing plasma

TABLE 15-1 NEONATAL HYPOGLYCEMIA: ETIOLOGY AND TIME COURSE

MECHANISM	CLINICAL SETTING	EXPECTED DURATION
Decreased substrate availability	Intrauterine growth restriction	Transient
	Prematurity	Transient
	Reduced glycogen stores	Transient
	Reduced fat stores	Transient
	Reduced ketogenesis	Transient
	Glycogen storage disease	Prolonged
	Inborn errors (e.g., fructose intolerance)	Prolonged
Endocrine disturbances		
Hyperinsulinemia	Infant of diabetic mother	Transient
	Persistent hyperinsulinism of infancy	Transient
	Congenital hyperinsulinism (HI)	Prolonged
	Recessive K_{ATP} HI	
	Focal K_{ATP} (focal adenomatosis) HI	
	Dominant K_{ATP} HI	
	Dominant glucokinase (GCK) HI	
	Dominant glutamate dehydrogenase (GDH) HI	
	Short-chain 3-hyroxyacyl-CoA dehydrogenase (SCHAD) HI	
	Beckwith-Wiedemann syndrome	Prolonged
	Erythroblastosis fetalis	Transient
	Exchange transfusion	Transient
	Islet cell dysplasias	Prolonged
	Maternal beta-agonist tocolytics	Transient
	Improperly placed umbilical artery catheter	Transient
	Inadvertent insulin administration	Transient
Other endocrine disorders	Immaturity of hepatic enzymes necessary for glucose production	Transient
	Reduced or failed counterregulation	Prolonged
	Hypopituitarism	Prolonged
	Hypothyroidism	Prolonged
	Adrenal insufficiency	Prolonged
Increased utilization	Increased brain weight to body weight and liver weight ratio with increased brain consumption of glucose	Prolonged
	Perinatal asphyxia	Transient
	Hypothermia	Transient
Miscellaneous/multiple mechanisms	Sepsis	Transient
	Congenital heart disease	Transient
	Central nervous system abnormalities	Prolonged

glucose concentration. Suppression of ketone body production from free fatty acids by high levels of insulin also might limit the availability of alternative fuels for cerebral metabolism, thereby contributing to the increased risk for adverse long-term outcomes in this patient population.

The most common clinical situation in which hyperinsulinemia occurs is in the infant of a diabetic mother (IDM). In utero, the fetus becomes hyperglycemic because of increased transfer of glucose across the placenta during episodes of maternal hyperglycemia. The fetal pancreatic beta cells are stimulated by the increased fetal glucose concentration to produce increased quantities of insulin. The pancreatic islet beta cells seem to become abnormally sensitive to increases in glucose concentration after repeated hyperglycemic stimuli. Before birth, the increase in cellular glucose uptake in response to the increased insulin secretion is matched by the increased availability of glucose from the mother. However, after delivery, the source of glucose is abruptly removed, whereas the hyperinsulinemia persists, producing hypoglycemia. The decrease in glucose concentration after birth is a result of insulin-stimulated peripheral glucose uptake, as well as inhibition of gluconeogenesis and glycogenolysis by the high insulin concentrations. Although some studies have reported other abnormalities in glucose metabolism in IDMs, Cowett et al found no difference in glucose kinetics in IDMs versus controls, perhaps because maternal diabetic control was well maintained during pregnancy in the group studied.[15] A large review of pregnancies in diabetic mothers found no association between the incidence of neonatal hypoglycemia and the number of episodes of maternal hyperglycemia (a reflection of the degree of control) late in pregnancy.[39] Recent studies have found that the incidence of neonatal hypoglycemia in IDMs correlates better with intrapartum, rather than antepartum, maternal glucose concentrations. The results of these studies emphasize that it is a sudden increase in glucose concentration that stimulates insulin secretion after a longer period in utero during which the fetal pancreatic beta cells have been sensitized to hypersecrete insulin as a result of repeated episodes of hyperglycemia.[16] The incidence of hypoglycemia in IDMs ranges from 15% to 75%; these infants are usually asymptomatic. A recent study has shown (1) that the complications typically associated with IDMs, including neonatal hypoglycemia, may be seen in women without overt gestational diabetes but who have glucose values on formal glucose tolerance testing at the upper end of the "normal" range, and (2) that the incidence correlates with increased glucose values. This suggests that there is a continuum of abnormal glucose tolerance during pregnancy that is associated with increased fetal insulin secretion, with gestational diabetes representing the most severe degree of disturbed glucose homeostasis.[64]

Other causes of islet cell hyperplasia and resultant hyperinsulinemia include (1) severe erythroblastosis fetalis,[3] possibly resulting from inactivation of insulin by glutathione released from hemolyzed red blood cells; (2) exchange transfusion,[70] in which insulin release is stimulated by the high dextrose content of commonly used blood preservative agents; and (3) in utero exposure to drugs such as beta-agonist tocolytics.[67] In utero exposure to valproate and postnatal exposure to indomethacin also may result in hypoglycemia, but the mechanisms responsible are not known.

Idiopathic hyperinsulinism (i.e., increased, persistent insulin secretion without a known predisposing factor) may occur as a result of altered regulation of insulin secretion in pancreatic beta cells.[33,42] Two general forms of persistent idiopathic hyperinsulinism are recognized: (1) prolonged neonatal hyperinsulinism; and (2) congenital (genetic) hyperinsulinism. Prolonged idiopathic neonatal hyperinsulinism appears to be common, although not well recognized or understood. Affected neonates usually have some evidence of stress before or during delivery, such as low birth weight (LBW) with IUGR (this disorder may affect 10% or more of IUGR/SGA infants), birth asphyxia, or maternal preeclampsia. Prolonged neonatal hyperinsulinism usually manifests in the first days after birth and often may be severe, requiring high dextrose infusion rates providing up to 15 or occasionally more mg per kg per minute of glucose. Prolonged neonatal hyperinsulinism also may last up to 4 weeks, does not respond well to glucocorticoids or frequent feedings, but can be treated with diazoxide at doses of 5 to 10 mg/kg/day.

Congenital (genetic) persistent hyperinsulinism is the most common form of persistent hypoglycemia in neonates and infants and also is the most difficult to diagnose and treat. The pancreatic abnormalities observed may be diffuse or focal, depending on the mutation present. Although the overall incidence of persistent hyperinsulinemic hypoglycemia (PHIHG) is low (approximately 1 in 50,000 births), the incidence of the inherited forms may be as high as 1 in 2500 infants in certain genetically homogeneous populations.[34] Depending on the degree of hyperinsulinemia in utero, these infants also may be macrosomic at birth. Most often, infants with PHIHG present with severe, recurrent hypoglycemia within the first few days of life. Recognizing such infants requires prolonged evaluation of an infant's capacity to maintain normal blood glucose concentrations between feedings after initial episodes of hypoglycemia are noted.

In recent years, at least five different genes have been associated with congenital hyperinsulinism. Mutations in several regions on the short arm of chromosome 11 have been found in approximately 50% of infants with PHIHG; these mutations are most often inherited in an autosomal recessive pattern. Infants who have this form of hyperinsulinism typically are large for gestational age (LGA), present with early neonatal hypoglycemia, and often require extremely high rates of IV glucose infusion (20 to 30 mg/kg/min). Affected infants have abnormalities of either the SUR1 or the Kir6.2 component of the K_{ATP} complex. Because the K_{ATP} complex, which is the site of diazoxide action, is disrupted by the mutations, these infants usually do not respond to diazoxide treatment. Octreotide (long-acting somatostatin) can be more helpful in the short term, but near-total (95% to 98%) pancreatectomy usually is necessary, along with continuous feedings and even insulin therapy.

Hyperinsulinism resulting from a focal pancreatic lesion (focal adenomatosis) may occur in 40% to 70% of hyperinsulinemic infants. In this disorder, a localized clone of beta cells expresses a paternally derived mutation in the gene for either SUR1 or Kir6.2 because of loss of heterozygosity for the maternal allele. The adenomas are small—3 to 5 mm in diameter. The clinical course of these infants is similar to that of infants with hyperinsulinism because of widespread mutations of the pancreatic K_{ATP} channel. Localization of the focal adenomatous region of the pancreas via catheterization of the pancreatic circulation and localized sampling of insulin production or via the more recently developed use of positron emission tomography (PET) with ^{18}F-fluoro-L-dopa may allow definition of the abnormal region of the pancreas, thereby guiding limited resection and avoiding more extensive, often near-total pancreatectomy.[42]

Several other mutations lead to genetic forms of PHIHG, including mutations in genes coding for glucokinase (GCK HI), an enzyme that regulates cellular metabolism and production of ATP, missense mutations of SUR1 leading to abnormal regulation of the K^+ channel, and mutations of glutamate dehydrogenase (GDH), which impair this enzyme's sensitivity to inhibition by guanine triphosphate. GDH is a key step in leucine-stimulated insulin secretion, and loss of GDH inhibition leads to excessive basal insulin secretion, as well as hypersensitivity to leucine stimulation. These different genetic disorders are much less common and have variable presentations, usually later in the neonatal period or even in early infancy.

In addition to hyperinsulinemia, global endocrine disturbances also can result in hypoglycemia.[44] These disturbances include a range of abnormalities of the hypothalamic-pituitary axis, the most severe being panhypopituitarism. Such infants frequently have growth hormone deficiency and hypothyroidism in addition to severe hypoglycemia. If pituitary dysfunction has resulted from a structural central nervous system (CNS) lesion, other neurologic problems, including abnormal muscle tone and neonatal seizures, may be present. Adrenal failure and hypoglycemia can occur as a result of adrenal hemorrhage, often in association with neonatal sepsis. Isolated endocrine defects, including primary hypothyroidism and cortisol deficiency, also may be associated with hypoglycemia.

Infants with Beckwith-Wiedemann syndrome also are macrosomic and hyperinsulinemic; in addition, they have other associated anomalies, including macroglossia, which may cause airway obstruction, and omphalocele. Asymptomatic hypoglycemia may occur in 30% to 50% of infants with Beckwith-Wiedemann syndrome and usually resolves in the first 3 days of life. However, up to 5% of affected infants may have persistent, frequently symptomatic hypoglycemia.[19] Although the specific mechanisms responsible for the syndrome and the associated hyperinsulinemia are not known, infants with Beckwith-Wiedemann syndrome have been found to have mutations in the short arm of chromosome 11, the same region in which mutations associated with other hyperinsulinemic syndromes have been identified (see below).

ENZYMATIC AND GENETIC DISORDERS[44]

Hormone Deficiencies. Hypoglycemia resulting from abnormal hormone production sometimes manifests in the neonatal period. Growth hormone and cortisol are counterregulatory hormones (i.e., they oppose the actions of insulin) and increase blood glucose concentrations by reducing glucose uptake in muscle tissue and stimulating lipolysis and gluconeogenesis during hypoglycemia. Although the counterregulatory effects of cortisol and growth hormone are less important than those of glucagon and catecholamines, hypoglycemia is a common complication of growth hormone and cortisol deficiency. Appropriate hormone replacement is the treatment of choice. It is of interest that several cases of panhypopituitarism and hyperinsulinemia have been reported in children.

Enzyme Deficiency Conditions. Hereditary disorders associated with deficiencies of specific enzymes that regulate substrate mobilization, interconversion, or utilization of carbohydrate, fat, or amino acids individually are rare disorders but collectively are frequently associated with hypoglycemia. These disorders are almost always inherited as autosomal recessive traits. Because of the interactions of fat, carbohydrate, and amino acid metabolism in the maintenance of normal fuel homeostasis, abnormalities in the metabolism of a single substrate can have primary and secondary effects on other metabolic pathways.

Defective Carbohydrate Metabolism

Glycogen Storage Diseases. In these inherited disorders, hypoglycemia results not from inadequate glycogen stores but, rather, from one of several enzyme deficiencies that prevent or limit glycogenolysis and release of glucose into the circulation. The glycogen storage diseases (I to VII) are inherited autosomal recessive defects, characterized by a deficient or abnormally functioning enzyme involved in the formation or degradation of glycogen in liver or muscle.

Fructose 1,6-Diphosphatase Deficiency. Hepatic fructose 1,6-diphosphatase deficiency results in a defect in gluconeogenesis. The initial signs and symptoms can be similar to those of glycogen storage disease type I (i.e., failure to thrive, hepatomegaly, lactic acidosis, and hypoglycemia).

Pyruvate Carboxylase and Phosphoenolpyruvate Carboxykinase Deficiencies. Pyruvate carboxylase and PEPCK are key gluconeogenic enzymes. Patients with pyruvate carboxylase deficiency are severely retarded and die early in infancy, and some have neuropathologic evidence of subacute necrotizing encephalopathy. Deficiency of hepatic phosphoenolpyruvate carboxykinase is a rare disorder; hypoglycemia is a common feature, although not clearly associated with defects of hepatic gluconeogenesis.

Galactose-1-Phosphate Uridylyl Transferase Deficiency (Classic Galactosemia). Infants with classic galactosemia are intolerant of products containing galactose. These infants present with hypoglycemia, failure to thrive, sepsis, diarrhea, and vomiting after meals containing galactose. Postprandial hypoglycemia seems to be caused by inhibition of phosphoglucomutase by galactose-1-phosphate, thereby resulting in sudden inhibition of glycogenolysis. Today, most infants with galactosemia are identified based on the results of routine neonatal screening.

Defective Amino Acid Metabolism. Several other inborn errors of metabolism, including propionic and methylmalonic acidemia and glutaric aciduria, may present with hypoglycemia in the first week of life.[66] Hypoglycemia and profound hypoalaninemia are observed in patients with classic maple syrup urine disease (branched-chain alpha-keto acid dehydrogenase deficiency) at times when their branched-chain amino acids and alpha-keto acids are markedly elevated.

Defective Fatty Acid Metabolism. A group of rare but severe metabolic disorders resulting in hypoglycemia and hypoketonemia are associated with abnormalities in fatty acid oxidation and ketone body formation.[44] During periods of fasting or intercurrent illness, free fatty acids (FFAs) are mobilized from adipose tissue. FFAs are utilized directly by body tissue (e.g., heart, skeletal muscle, gut, skin) or undergo beta-oxidation in the liver with the resultant production and release of ketone bodies, which can partly replace glucose in many tissues such as the brain, and acetyl coenzyme A (CoA) and reducing equivalents (NAD/NADH), which provide energy fuel for the gluconeogenesis process. Oxidation of FFA includes activation of fatty acids by acyl-CoA synthetase, carnitine-dependent transport into the mitochondrial matrix, and mitochondrial beta-oxidation of the fatty acids. Infants and children with disorders of fatty acid oxidation often present with profound hypoglycemia and altered level of consciousness, which may not improve despite normalization of the plasma glucose concentration.

Other markers of impaired fatty acid oxidation are absolute or relative hypoketonemia, marked increase in plasma FFA concentrations, hypotonia, hepatomegaly with microvesicular fat accumulation, elevated plasma activities of both liver and muscle enzymes, congestive heart failure, rhabdomyolysis, and, frequently, cerebral edema. Although the pathophysiology of the hypoglycemia in these children is not known, two mechanisms have been suggested: (1) decreased hepatic glucose production; or (2) more commonly understood, accelerated rates of glucose utilization, because glucose might serve as the primary substrate for all tissues in the absence of ketone body availability and defective FFA oxidation. These disorders should be considered in infants and children with severe hypoglycemia, decreased plasma concentrations of free and total carnitine, and relatively low plasma ketone body concentrations in combination with very high FFA concentrations.

INCREASED GLUCOSE UTILIZATION

Some term infants may have normal energy stores at birth and intact regulating mechanisms but may be stressed by one of several conditions so that the available supplies do not meet their energy requirements. An asphyxiated newborn is one common example. During and after asphyxia, when tissue oxygen supply is limited, the neonate relies largely on anaerobic metabolism for energy production. Because this process is relatively inefficient, more glucose is metabolized to produce the amount of energy necessary than would be used under aerobic conditions. As a result, glucose produced by lipolysis and glycogenolysis is rapidly consumed. Hypoxic-ischemic damage to the liver may further impair synthesis of gluconeogenic enzymes and thus delay the normal postnatal onset of gluconeogenesis. Elevated insulin concentrations also may be present, providing an additional cause for the hypoglycemia.[17] Other conditions in neonates that lead to a shift from aerobic to anaerobic metabolism, thus predisposing the infant to hypoglycemia, include hypotension, severe lung disease with hypoxemia and hypoventilation, and septic shock.

Hypothermia may result in hypoglycemia through rapid depletion of brown fat stores for nonshivering thermogenesis and secondary breakdown and exhaustion of glycogen stores. Hypothermia is most often seen in infants born at home, but milder degrees may occur in the delivery room. Hypoglycemia also has been observed in some infants with sepsis. A study done in several such infants found that they had an increased rate of glucose disappearance in response to an IV glucose infusion, suggesting an increased rate of glucose utilization.[51] Stimulation of glucose utilization may be a result of circulating endotoxins, which increase the rate of glycolysis.

Several other factors also contribute to the risk for hypoglycemia in infants with other identified risk factors. Preterm infants with respiratory distress syndrome (RDS), for example, have increased metabolic demands because of the increased work of breathing. Chronic hypoxia in IUGR fetuses stimulates catecholamine secretion, which can deplete glycogen stores. Infants with IUGR and hypoglycemia may have increased rates of glucose disappearance when receiving an IV glucose infusion, as well as reduced fat mobilization in response to hypoglycemia, when compared with normoglycemic SGA newborns. Because of the increased brain weight/liver weight and brain weight/body weight ratios in all newborns (12% in term newborns for the latter comparison versus 2% in adults), cerebral glucose requirements are markedly higher relative to the liver's capacity to respond than in the adult, even if glycogen stores are normal for size (Figure 15-4).[50] This is especially true in infants with asymmetric growth restriction. In addition, increased insulin sensitivity has been reported in SGA newborns within the first 48 hours of life.[4,72] These observations indicate that disturbances in glucose metabolism in addition to lower-than-normal energy stores may be present in some growth-restricted infants.

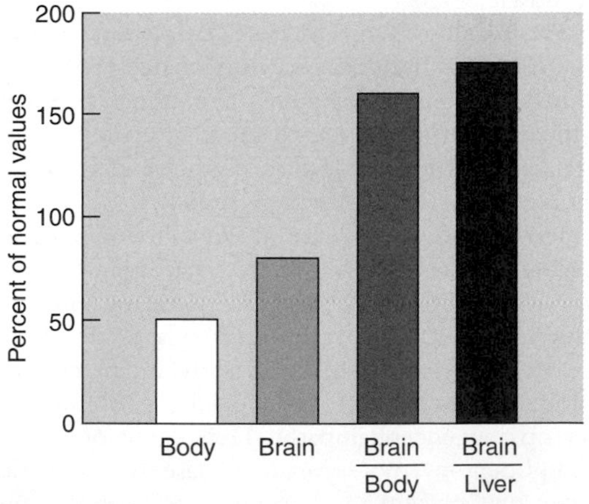

FIGURE 15-4 Differences in organ/body weight ratios in small-for-gestational-age infant compared with appropriate-for-gestational-age counterpart. (From Lafeber HN, Jones CT, Rolph TP: Some of the consequences on intrauterine growth retardation. In Visser HKA, editor: *Nutrition and metabolism of the fetus and infant,* Boston, 1979, Martinus Nijhoff.)

Hyperglycemia

Hyperglycemia is most common during the first week after birth (Box 15-2). Typically, a neonate with hyperglycemia is a LBW infant (<32 weeks' gestation and <1200 g birth weight), often one with IUGR, who cannot tolerate an IV glucose infusion at the usual rate of 4 to 8 mg/kg/min (i.e., $D_{10}W$ at 60 to 100 mL/kg/day). This relative glucose intolerance appears to be caused by general immaturity of the usual regulatory mechanisms, including absolute or decreased insulin release in response to glucose, insulin resistance (both peripheral, leading to decreased glucose utilization, and hepatic, leading to increased glucose production), and glucose intolerance caused by diminished basal glucose transport capacity.[25] These infants also have decreased insulin-sensitive tissue (e.g., skeletal muscle and fat) as a fraction of body weight. There also is some evidence of abnormal insulin processing by the pancreatic beta cells such that more immature forms of insulin (proinsulin and proinsulin split products) are released. Because these immature forms of insulin are much less active in stimulating the insulin receptor, they may contribute to a relative insulin resistance in these infants.[65] Some investigators also have reported that, unlike fetuses and adults, most preterm and some term infants fail to suppress endogenous glucose production despite the administration of an adequate exogenous supply (e.g., IV infusion)[14]; however, other investigators did not measure any glucose production in premature infants receiving IV glucose at a rate of more than 2 mg/kg/min.[86]

BOX 15-2 ETIOLOGIC FACTORS IN NEONATAL HYPERGLYCEMIA

- Iatrogenic (e.g., during intravenous glucose infusion)
- Decreased insulin production (e.g., with increased catecholamine production in very-low-birth-weight or intrauterine-growth-restricted infant; catecholamine infusion side effect)
- Decreased insulin sensitivity (e.g., with increased catecholamine production in very-low-birth-weight infant or transient diabetes mellitus; catecholamine infusion side effect)
- Sepsis
- Methylxanthine side effect
- Glucocorticoid side effect

Hyperglycemia also may be iatrogenic in an extremely-low-birth-weight (ELBW) infant (<750 g) who requires excess water to replace fluid lost through insensible water losses and who receives excess glucose along with the infused water because it is necessary to provide an isotonic IV solution. The risk for developing hyperglycemia is significantly increased with decreasing birth weight (up to 18 times greater in infants with birth weights <1000 g than among those weighing 1000 to 2000 g), as well as with an increasing rate of glucose infusion, even if the absolute infusion rate remains within the accepted range.

Delay in initiating enteral feedings may be an additional risk factor. The incidence of hyperglycemia is higher in LBW infants receiving all of their nutrition parenterally than in those who receive at least a part of their nutrition enterally, and prolonged intravenous nutrition may contribute to insulin resistance.[65] The rate at which the glucose concentration is increased in IV solutions, including intravenous nutrition, also may contribute; hyperglycemia is increasingly common at glucose infusion rates greater than 6 to 8 mg/kg/min. The presence of illness (e.g., sepsis), treatment with corticosteroids, and RDS that requires mechanical ventilation are associated with increased risk for developing hyperglycemia, most likely because of increased circulating catecholamine concentrations that lead to increased lipolysis and glycogenolysis and inhibit pancreatic insulin secretion and insulin action.

Several other etiologic factors must be considered in infants with hyperglycemia. Increased blood glucose concentrations have been reported in association with gram-negative sepsis.[43] Intravenous lipid infusions also may produce hyperglycemia if given rapidly at rates of more than 0.25 g/kg/hr; however, current practice is to administer lipids at a slower rate.[84] Methylxanthines are frequently used to treat apnea in preterm infants and may be a cause of hyperglycemia. This problem has been well documented after theophylline overdose but may occur also with appropriate administration. One study, for example, found that blood glucose concentrations in infants with therapeutic theophylline levels were higher than in untreated control subjects, with glucose concentrations in the hyperglycemic range in two treated infants.[78] Neonates undergoing surgical procedures also are at increased risk for hyperglycemia, probably because of a combination of the large quantities of glucose-containing fluids and blood products that may be administered during the procedure and the effects of stress-related hormones.

NEONATAL DIABETES

Although infants with IUGR are more commonly hypoglycemic, a few cases of what has been called ***transient neonatal diabetes mellitus (TNDM)*** have been reported, primarily in growth-restricted infants. In these cases, hyperglycemia is thought to be a result of partial insulin insensitivity, but increased levels of catecholamines and other stress-related hormones may play an important role. Recent studies have identified mutations in chromosome 6 in some infants with neonatal diabetes.[74] However, in transient diabetes mellitus, unlike true diabetes mellitus, ketosis does not develop. Most cases self-resolve or respond to decreasing the glucose administration rate; occasionally, insulin therapy may be necessary, but this should be reserved for infants with severe hyperglycemia (blood glucose concentration >300 mg/dL, despite decreasing IV glucose infusion rate) that is persistent and associated with clinically significant hyperosmolality and glucosuria. Permanent neonatal diabetes mellitus (PNDM) also occurs, although this is a rare disorder, with incidence estimated at 2 to 3/100,000 live births. Only about 25% of infants with PNDM have IUGR. Causes include mitochondrial diseases, pancreatic hypoplasia or aplasia, abnormal pancreatic glucokinase activity, and mutations of pancreatic K_{ATP} channel. Neonatal diabetes may be associated with other abnormalities including developmental delay, skeletal dysplasias, and intestinal atresia.

PREVENTION OF HYPOGLYCEMIA AND HYPERGLYCEMIA

Recognition of those infants at risk for disturbances in glucose homeostasis is the most important step in preventing both hypoglycemia and hyperglycemia. In infants with conditions predisposing to hypoglycemia, such as preterm infants, infants with IUGR, or IDMs, **early feeding and frequent monitoring of blood glucose concentrations may prevent a decrease in blood glucose concentration or allow early detection of decreased blood glucose levels. Maintenance of a neutral thermal environment is especially critical to minimize energy expenditure in those infants at risk for hypoglycemia.** Other conditions associated with hypoglycemia, such as asphyxia and hypothermia, may be avoided through appropriate obstetric and neonatal intervention.

Hyperglycemia occurs most often in preterm infants receiving high rates of IV glucose. In a very-low-birth-weight (VLBW) infant, hyperglycemia may be avoided by starting IV glucose infusions at rates of 2 to 3 mg/kg/min and checking blood glucose concentrations frequently (as often as every 3 to 4 hours) while the infant continues to receive IV glucose. However, hyperglycemia may be unavoidable in a very immature infant. There is some evidence that starting amino acid infusions shortly after birth in very preterm infants may limit the development of hyperglycemia, perhaps by increasing insulin production and secretion and also by promoting protein turnover and its attendant glucose (energy) requirements. Introduction of small-volume enteral feeds as soon as possible may also reduce the incidence or duration of hyperglycemia in VLBW infants.

DATA COLLECTION

History

The history of any neonate must include a detailed prenatal and family history. **Important maternal risk factors associated with neonatal hypoglycemia are listed in Box 15-1.** Other important data include a history of family members with atypical diabetes or other abnormalities of glucose homeostasis, family history of metabolic disease, and previous unexplained stillbirths.

The most important information to be obtained from the infant's history is gestational age, Apgar scores, and details of events in the delivery room, especially any findings that suggest the presence of significant perinatal compromise. **An infant with a history of any of the conditions listed in Box 15-1 or Table 15-1 should be considered at high risk for developing a problem with glucose homeostasis.**

Physical Examination

Careful measurement of birth weight and head circumference in combination with accurate gestational age assessment will establish whether the infant is preterm, LBW, SGA, or LGA and thus at increased risk for hypoglycemia. IDMs frequently have small heads relative to their general macrosomia and have been described as having "tomato facies" because of plethora and increased buccal fat. The physical findings associated with Beckwith-Wiedemann syndrome have already been described. The presence of midline facial defects, such as cleft lip or hypertelorism, may indicate the presence of a CNS malformation with associated pituitary dysfunction. Glycogen storage diseases should be considered in infants with hepatomegaly.

Signs and Symptoms

Signs of neonatal hypoglycemia are nonspecific and extremely variable (Box 15-3). They include general findings, such as abnormal cry, poor feeding, hypothermia, and diaphoresis; neurologic signs, including tremors and jitteriness, hypotonia, irritability, lethargy, and seizures; and cardiorespiratory disturbances, including cyanosis, pallor, tachypnea, periodic breathing, apnea, and cardiac arrest. These features also occur in preterm infants and in neonates with sepsis, intraventricular hemorrhage, asphyxia, hypocalcemia, congenital heart disease, and structural CNS lesions, among other causes. In the presence of any of the preceding signs, however, hypoglycemia always should be considered, because the diagnosis of insufficient brain energy supply can be made relatively easily and prompt treatment is essential.

BOX 15-3

CLINICAL SIGNS OF HYPOGLYCEMIA

- Mild to moderate changes in level of consciousness*
- Stupor or lethargy*
- Tremulousness*
- Irritability*
- Coma
- Seizures (depend on duration, repetitive occurrence, and severity of hypoglycemia)
- Respiratory depression or apnea, leading to cyanosis
- Hypotonia, limpness, inactivity
- High-pitched cry
- Poor feeding (after previously feeding well)
- Hypothermia

*Most frequent, and should be alleviated with correction of low glucose concentrations.

Hyperglycemia usually is asymptomatic and most often is diagnosed on routine screening of the infant at risk.

If a problem with glucose homeostasis is suspected, documentation of the aforementioned data, history (Box 15-1), physical examination, and signs and symptoms (Box 15-3) must reflect ongoing monitoring and measures taken. The use of risk assessments, guidelines, or protocols that consider the data just mentioned is encouraged (Figure 15-5).

Laboratory Data

When hypoglycemia is suspected, the plasma or blood glucose concentration must be determined promptly. **Ideally, this determination should be made with one of the laboratory enzymatic methods, such as the glucose oxidase or hexokinase method, but even bedside reagent test strip glucose analyzers (i.e., glucometers) can be used if the test is performed carefully with awareness of the more limited accuracy of these devices.** In the clinical setting, early and rapid determination of glucose concentrations in the high-risk or symptomatic neonate is essential.[29] Prompt detection of hypoglycemia permits early treatment and potentially helps avoid long-term neurologic sequelae.[12] Although laboratory measurements of glucose concentrations are the most effective methods for detecting hypoglycemia, results may not be available for up to 1 hour—far longer than appropriate for diagnosing hypoglycemia and thereby delaying the initiation of treatment. Rapid measurement methods available to the clinician at the bedside include several different systems using a handheld reflectance colorimeter, electrochemical detector, or ion-selective electrode methods (e.g., glucometer, i-STAT®). The sample of blood can be obtained from a warmed heel-stick or venipuncture specimen.

These methods can be useful in screening infants in whom abnormal glucose concentrations are suspected if the user is aware of their limitations. The accuracy of test strip results depends in part on the technique used. An adequate sample

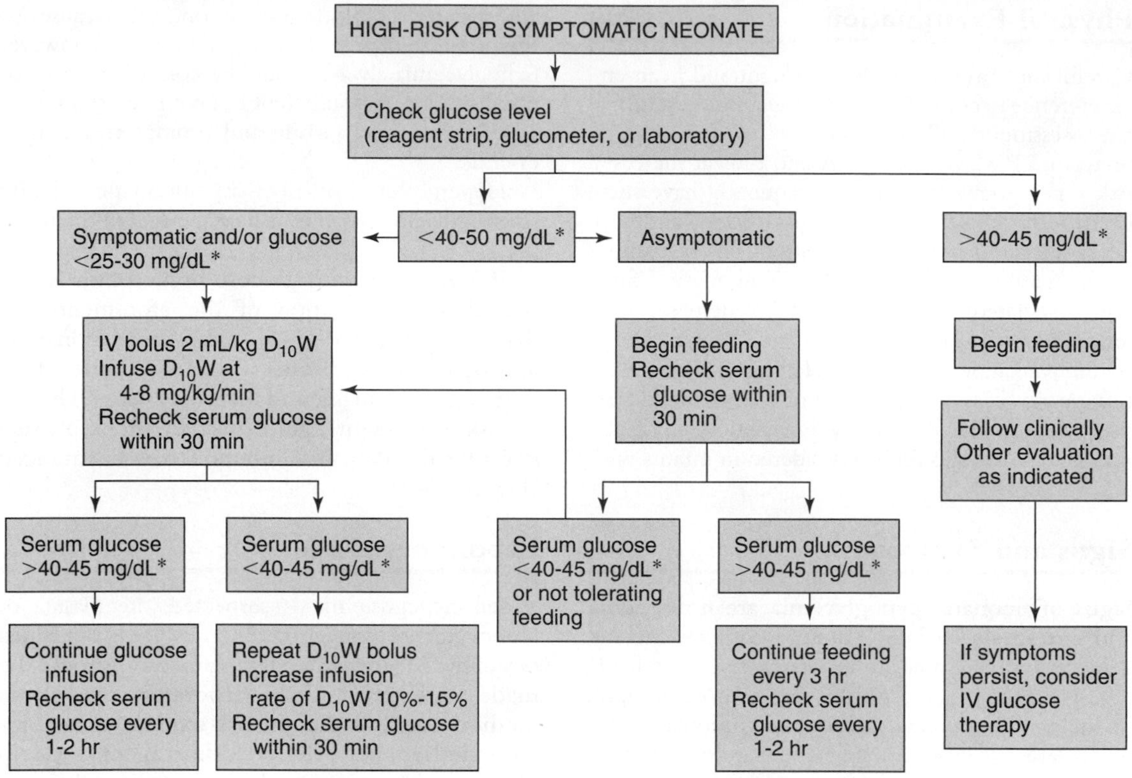

FIGURE 15-5 Decision tree for management of neonate with acute hypoglycemia. *IV*, Intravenous.

must be placed on the test strip pad, and the timing of reading the result is critical. Recently developed devices automatically read the result at the appropriate time, reducing one source of error. Hospital personnel should be trained and certified in the use of test strip methods and the bedside instruments used to quantify glucose concentration. **With proper technique, test strip results demonstrate a reasonable correlation with actual blood glucose concentrations, but the variation from the actual blood glucose value may be as much as 10 to 20 mg/dL.** A number of studies have compared the results obtained with specific commercial products with results obtained with laboratory methods.[1,32,58] Regardless of the test strip or instrument used, correlations with actual blood glucose concentrations are lowest at the lower glucose concentrations at which neonatal hypoglycemia must be accurately determined. **Several studies have shown that use of test strips alone may fail to detect from 11% to as many as 67% of infants with statistically defined hypoglycemia.[31,32,52] There also is a significant incidence of false-positive results.**

Because of the limitations of these methods, **whenever a diagnosis of hypoglycemia is suspected by test strip or glucometer results, the blood glucose concentration should be confirmed by a specimen sent to the chemistry laboratory for prompt (STAT) determination and reporting.** Although laboratory results are more accurate and reliable than screening methods, a long delay in processing the specimen can result in a falsely low level as the erythrocytes in the sample metabolize the glucose in the plasma. This problem can be avoided by transporting blood in a tube containing a glycolytic inhibitor. *Treatment of suspected hypoglycemia, however, should not be postponed until confirmation is obtained from the laboratory. Also, if hypoglycemia is suspected on the basis of clinical symptoms, initial*

treatment should be instituted even if the test strip result is "normal." If the actual value is abnormal, a delay in therapy could be harmful; if the actual value is within the normal range, therapy can be stopped without serious side effects.

Most cases of neonatal hypoglycemia have an identifiable cause (e.g., maternal diabetes or IUGR). In a term infant with no known risk factors for hypoglycemia, sepsis must be considered as the most likely cause of hypoglycemia and an appropriate evaluation should be performed. Of those infants without an identifiable cause, most have idiopathic hypoglycemia, which resolves spontaneously within 2 to 5 days, and no further evaluation is needed. However, in rare cases, hypoglycemia persists beyond the first week of life with no obvious cause detected, requiring a logical and rapid approach to diagnosis of the particular form of persistent hypoglycemia. The diagnostic evaluation of these infants should include (1) simultaneous determination of glucose and insulin concentrations, as well as alternate substrates, such as ketones and FFAs; (2) evaluation of pituitary function, including measurement of thyroid-stimulating hormone (TSH), thyroxine (T_4), adrenocorticotropic hormone (ACTH), cortisol, and growth hormone levels; and (3) appropriate studies to diagnose inborn errors of metabolism, such as lactate and pyruvate concentrations. Ideally, these studies should be obtained during an episode of hypoglycemia. Once hypoglycemia is identified in a neonate as persistent, a fasting study should be performed to measure plasma insulin concentration when plasma glucose concentration drops below 45 to 50 mg/dL. If this fasting study demonstrates hyperinsulinism, treatment should be immediately instituted (see "Treatment" section).

TREATMENT

Hypoglycemia

Early identification of an infant at risk for developing hypoglycemia and institution of prophylactic measures to prevent its occurrence constitute the best treatment for this disorder. The goals are to recognize at-risk infants, evaluate early and frequently for decreasing glucose concentrations, treat when indicated, and provide glucose and enteral feeding as needed to achieve and maintain glucose concentrations in the range that most normal infants develop via their own homeostatic mechanisms within 6 to 12 hours after birth.

A decision tree suggesting guidelines for management of infants with hypoglycemia is shown in Figure 15-5. Although most asymptomatic infants can be managed with frequent breast feeding/expressed breast milk or formula feedings, all symptomatic neonates should receive treatment with IV dextrose infusion to provide glucose at an initial rate of 4 to 6 mg/kg/min. In some circumstances, it may be useful to use a "minibolus" of 200 mg/kg dextrose (2 mL/kg of $D_{10}W$) plus the dextrose infusion regimen originally described by Lilien et al.[53] Advantages of the minibolus regimen include the following: (1) there is a lower incidence of hyperglycemia immediately after the bolus than was observed with use of boluses of solutions with higher dextrose concentrations; (2) the slower rate of administration decreases the insulin response to glucose infusion, thus lowering the risk for rebound hypoglycemia after the bolus; and (3) glucose concentration reaches the normal range more quickly than if continuous infusion is started without a preceding bolus (Figure 15-6). Rapid normalization of blood glucose may

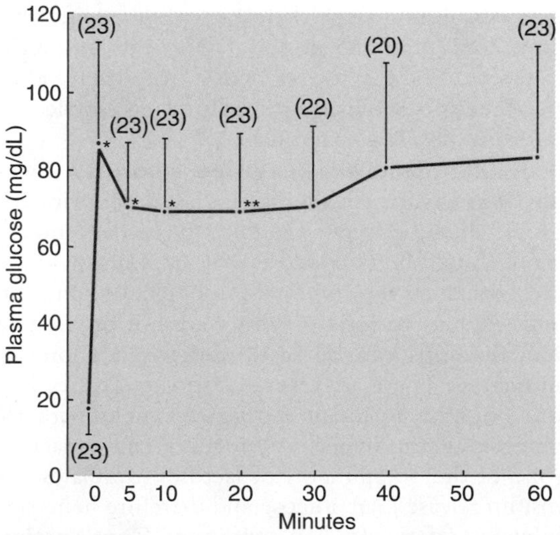

FIGURE 15-6 Plasma glucose response to glucose "minibolus" followed by continuous glucose infusion (8 mg/min/kg) as therapy for neonatal hypoglycemia. (From Lilien LD, Pildes RS, Srinivasan G, et al: Treatment of neonatal hypoglycemia with minibolus and intravenous glucose infusion, *J Pediatr* 97:295, 1980.)

be particularly beneficial in symptomatic infants, although no data confirm this assumption. The suggested infusion rates cover the range of hepatic glucose production in normal term newborns. In IDMs with asymptomatic hypoglycemia, the initial minibolus can be eliminated and the infusion rate should be kept at the minimum necessary to produce and maintain normal blood glucose concentrations to prevent an excessive insulin response. When glucose infusion rates are being calculated, it is important to remember that commercially prepared glucose solutions actually contain glucose in its hydrated form (molecular weight [MW] 198, versus MW 180 for anhydrous glucose), which lowers the actual glucose content of the solution by approximately 8%. Thus $D_{10}W$ contains approximately 9.2 g of glucose per deciliter.

Once the infant's glucose requirement has been determined, the glucose infusion should be maintained at that level until blood glucose concentrations are stable and in the desired range. The target blood glucose concentration during IV therapy should be above the "hypoglycemic threshold" defined for that particular infant; for example, if hypoglycemia is defined as 40 mg/dL, glucose concentrations should be maintained at or above 50 mg/dL.

Adjusting therapy to maintain a blood glucose concentration higher than the "diagnostic" threshold allows a margin of safety in the absence of any data establishing a correlation between specific glucose concentrations in this range and long-term outcome. There is no evidence that diagnosis or treatment thresholds for preterm infants should differ from those for term infants.

If the infant was being fed before IV therapy was instituted, feedings may be continued. However, the calculated minimum glucose requirement should be provided by the IV infusion alone rather than by the combination of glucose infusion and feedings. **In infants who were not previously fed, feedings can be instituted when clinically indicated.** There are several advantages to feeding a hypoglycemic infant during treatment with IV glucose. In the hyperinsulinemic infant, galactose (one of the components of lactose) stimulates less insulin release than glucose and therefore helps stabilize blood glucose concentrations. **Continuation of oral feedings also aids in the process of weaning the infant off IV glucose.** When feedings are well tolerated, the IV infusion generally can be slowly tapered if the glucose concentration and clinical status remain stable. Although enteral feeding has the theoretical risk for augmenting insulin secretion and subsequent hypoglycemia as a result of the food-stimulated release of gut peptides that may potentiate insulin release from the pancreas, there is no evidence that withholding feedings actually prevents this potential problem. **It probably is better to continue breast milk or formula feedings using smaller, more frequent amounts or continuous gastric infusion than to stop enteral feedings and maintain normoglycemia exclusively with IV glucose.** However, in rare cases, such as infants with severe, refractory hyperinsulinemic hypoglycemia, feedings may have to be stopped until glucose concentrations are stabilized.

ADJUNCTIVE THERAPY

See Table 15-2 for a summary of adjunct therapies for hypoglycemia.

Glucagon. Glucagon, 30 mcg/kg IV or intramuscular (IM), releases glycogen from hepatic stores when insulin concentrations are normal. However, IDMs and other infants with hyperinsulinemia may require much larger doses, up to 300 mcg/kg, to produce a response. Administration of glucagon may be useful diagnostically, because failure to respond to glucagon administration with an increase in serum glucose concentration suggests depletion of hepatic glycogen stores. Glucose infusion should be maintained after glucagon is administered, because there is a risk for increased insulin secretion in response to the glucagon-produced surge in glucose production. In addition, the rapid but transient increase in glucose concentration immediately after glucagon injection may produce a false sense that the hypoglycemia has resolved, even though the underlying cause still exists. Continuous infusions of glucagon have been used to treat refractory hypoglycemia[10]; however, this mode of administration has been associated with adverse side effects, including hyponatremia and thrombocytopenia.[6]

Other Agents. Glucocorticoids (hydrocortisone), somatostatin, and diazoxide have been used to treat hypoglycemia in refractory cases. Use of glucocorticoids to reduce peripheral glucose utilization and increase gluconeogenesis should be limited to those infants requiring more than 12 to 15 mg/kg/min

TABLE 15-2 ADJUNCT THERAPIES FOR HYPOGLYCEMIA

THERAPY	EFFECT	DOSAGE
Corticosteroids	Decrease peripheral glucose utilization Enhance gluconeogenesis	Hydrocortisone 5-15 mg/kg/day or Prednisone 2 mg/kg/day
Glucagon	Stimulates glycogenolysis Releases glycogen from hepatic stores when insulin concentrations are normal	30 mcg/kg IV or IM 300 mcg/kg if hyperinsulinism is present
Diazoxide	Inhibits insulin secretion	15 mg/kg/day
Somatostatin (long-acting: octreotide acetate)	Inhibits insulin and growth hormone release	5-10 mcg/kg every 6-8 hr
Pancreatectomy	Decreases insulin production/secretion	

From McGowan JE: Neonatal hypoglycemia, *Pediatr Rev*, 20:6-15, 1999.
IM, Intramuscular; *IV*, intravenous.

glucose infusion to maintain normal glucose concentrations. Somatostatin and diazoxide, which suppress insulin release, are most often used in infants with islet cell dysplasias who have persistent hypoglycemia after a partial pancreatectomy.

Miscellaneous. In infants with hypoglycemia caused by a specific medical problem, therapy should be directed toward alleviating the underlying illness. This includes administration of antibiotics to treat sepsis, partial exchange transfusion to reduce hyperviscosity, hormone replacement in cases of hypopituitarism, and dietary intervention for metabolic disorders. A trial of diazoxide should be initiated in infants who have been identified as having hyperinsulinism. If diazoxide is not effective at a maximum dose of 15 mg/kg per day divided into two doses per day, it should be stopped and octreotide should be tried. However, medical therapy alone fails to control hypoglycemia in 40% to 90% of infants with severe PHIHG.[20] If octreotide is not successful, surgical management is generally necessary. Before surgery, procedures should be performed to determine whether the pancreatic abnormalities are focal or diffuse. Focal disease generally is cured with partial pancreatectomy, whereas diffuse disease requires near-total pancreatectomy and then treatment of the exocrine and endocrine deficiencies that invariably result.[28]

Hyperglycemia

GLUCOSE

Most cases of hyperglycemia can be treated by reducing the neonate's IV glucose infusion rate. Many LBW infants will tolerate glucose infusions at rates of up to 4 mg/kg/min, although Zarif et al reported that more than 40% of infants weighing less than 1000 g had a blood glucose concentration higher than 125 mg/dL while receiving glucose at an average rate of 4.4 mg/kg/min.[85] In addition, a VLBW infant, with high fluid requirements resulting from large insensible water losses through the skin, may require a combination of water and glucose intake that could be administered only by using a hypotonic solution such as $D_{2.5}W$. The use of a low glucose concentration in the IV infusate necessitates the addition of sodium (e.g., $D_{2.5}W$ has approximately 130 mOsm/L, requiring the addition of sodium chloride to produce an isotonic solution with 280 mOsm/L), which may further complicate management of fluids and electrolytes. A VLBW infant needs adequate caloric intake (50 to 60 kcal/kg/day) to avoid a negative nitrogen balance and tissue catabolism. These needs often cannot be met without resultant hyperglycemia. If the glucose is only mildly elevated (e.g., concentrations of 150 to 250 mg/dL) and the infant has no evidence of adverse effects, reducing the rate of IV glucose administration is not necessary.

LIPID AND AMINO ACIDS

Intravenous lipid infusion rates can be decreased to help reduce hyperglycemia. This limits the contribution of free fatty acids produced by lipid metabolism that, upon oxidation, generate energy to drive gluconeogenesis (acetyl CoA and reducing equivalents, NAD/NADH). Decreasing lipid supply also limits the competition of fatty acids with glucose for oxidation, as well as the direct enhancement of gluconeogenic enzymes in the liver and thus the production of glucose. Limiting lipid supply also reduces the supply of glycerol, which is the primary support for gluconeogenesis in newborn infants.

Amino acid infusions should be started early to promote insulin secretion and enhance protein turnover with its obligatory energy (hence, glucose) requirements. Amino acids do not contribute measurably to enhancing gluconeogenesis, even though they provide more substrate.

INSULIN INFUSION

Because of the foregoing considerations, some authors have suggested the **use of a continuous insulin infusion in the infant who cannot tolerate infusion of glucose solutions with concentrations greater than 5 g/dL (e.g., D_5W).**[7,23] **Infusion of insulin at rates of 0.2 to 0.8 milliunit/kg/min (0.01 to 0.05 unit/kg/hr) for 12 to 24 hours may improve glucose tolerance.** However, insulin avidly binds to plastic IV tubing; thus the actual rate of insulin administration may be difficult to determine and may vary over time. Although various methods, such as priming the tubing with insulin-containing solution or albumin, have been proposed, these have not been shown to be consistently effective.

Hypoglycemia during administration of exogenous insulin can be avoided by starting with a low infusion rate (0.05 to 0.1 milliunit/kg/min) and increasing the rate by 10% to 20% every 60 to 90 minutes until the glucose concentration is less than 200 mg/dL. Blood glucose concentrations should be monitored every 15 to 20 minutes during initiation of the insulin infusion, and an IV glucose infusion should be maintained to avoid any abrupt changes in blood glucose concentration and to allow rapid correction of glucose concentration if it starts to fall below "normal" values. Use of insulin infusion has been reported to improve tolerance to glucose infusion, resulting in increased carbohydrate intake and weight gain. Most of the weight gain is fat, however, and there is risk for fatty infiltration in the liver and heart when insulin and glucose infusions are maintained for long periods. Such insulin treatment inhibits glucose production, but its effect on promoting glucose utilization is more modest, given the small amount of insulin-sensitive tissue per body weight. Acutely, insulin infusion has been noted to increase lactate production, with lactate concentrations up to threefold greater than baseline, and may be associated with metabolic acidosis. Administration of glucose and insulin at high rates also enhances CO_2 production, which might lead to hypercarbia in infants with respiratory disease. Also, episodes of hypoglycemia can occur even with careful monitoring during insulin infusion. **The use of insulin to treat hyperglycemia in neonates has recently been evaluated in a randomized prospective study, and it showed no obvious benefit and considerable morbidity.** The authors of this study and an editorial commentary concluded that **chronic insulin infusion cannot be recommended and must be used cautiously even in cases of acute hyperglycemia.**[5,46] This is especially true because there are no clinical studies that have demonstrated a cause-and-effect relationship between brief periods of neonatal hyperglycemia and adverse long-term outcomes.

MISCELLANEOUS

In addition to specific measures to lower the blood glucose concentration, close attention must be paid to fluid balance in the hyperglycemic infant, because, theoretically, hyperglycemia can induce an osmotic diuresis. However, this is rarely seen at blood glucose concentrations less than 400 mg/dL or when hyperglycemia occurs intermittently and for brief periods. Finally, as in hypoglycemia, efforts should be made to treat any underlying etiology, such as sepsis.

COMPLICATIONS

Hypoglycemia

The outcome for infants with neonatal hypoglycemia appears to be related to the duration, repetitive occurrence, and severity of the hypoglycemia, as well as the underlying etiology. Those with ***asymptomatic hypoglycemia*** usually have a normal neurodevelopmental outcome. Furthermore, although learning disabilities and abnormal electroencephalograms (EEGs) without seizure disorder occasionally have been reported in infants who had asymptomatic hypoglycemia, there is no evidence that treatment prevents such abnormal outcomes.[35] ***Symptomatic hypoglycemic*** infants (primarily those with severe, protracted, and recurrent neurologic abnormalities such as seizures and coma associated with plasma glucose concentrations <20 to 25 mg/dL for several hours or more) have a poorer prognosis, with abnormalities ranging from learning disabilities to cerebral palsy and persistent or recurrent seizure disorders, as well as mental retardation of varying degrees.[27] Prompt initiation of treatment is thought to be associated with a more positive outcome, although this has not been well documented.

In preterm infants, recent data indicate that hypoglycemia may adversely affect long-term outcome.[24,57] A follow-up study of more than 600 former preterm infants found significantly lower mental and motor indices in those with five or more documented episodes of moderate hypoglycemia (defined as a blood glucose concentration <45 mg/dL) during the neonatal period. This difference remained significant even when confounding factors such as intraventricular hemorrhage (IVH), need for ventilator support, and asphyxia were considered. However, differences in cognitive function were less apparent at school-age follow-up in the same cohort of patients. Hypoglycemic preterm infants who were also small for gestational age were found to have lower scores on psychometric tests at both 3 years and 5 years of age, with a greater effect seen in those infants with recurrent hypoglycemia. These results indicate that further long-term studies in preterm infants are needed.

The incidence of neurodevelopmental abnormalities in IDMs ranges from 0% to 35%; the lower figures are from more recent studies and may represent improvement in obstetric and neonatal care. Most of the long-term follow-up studies have not shown an association between the presence of neonatal hypoglycemia and later neurodevelopmental impairment.[39,71] Instead, outcome has been related to such factors as prematurity, presence of congenital anomalies, congenital iron deficiency, and degree of control of maternal disease. However, Stenninger et al found that IDMs who were hypoglycemic as newborns (glucose <27 mg/dL) had an increased frequency of deficits in attention, motor control, and perception at 8 years of age compared with both IDMs without hypoglycemia and normal newborn controls.[79] A number of other neonatal complications are associated with maternal diabetes, including polycythemia, which may add to disturbances of glucose homeostasis; hypocalcemia secondary to maternal hypoparathyroidism; dystocia secondary to macrosomia; and congenital anomalies. Infants of mothers with severe diabetic vasculopathy, in contrast to most IDMs, may have IUGR caused in part by decreased placental blood flow, with hypoglycemia resulting from inadequate glycogen and fat stores as occurs in all cases of IUGR rather than hyperinsulinemia alone.

Adverse neurologic outcomes have been reported in as many as 40% to 50% of infants with PHIHG, possibly because these infants cannot effectively generate ketone bodies, which could serve as an alternative source of energy for cerebral metabolism during periods of hypoglycemia.[61-63] In addition, infants with PHIHG who require a greater than 95% pancreatectomy often develop glucose intolerance or even frank diabetes mellitus later in life.[55] Hypoglycemia secondary to hypopituitarism is also associated with a poor outcome; often this results from other CNS or endocrine dysfunction, rather than from the hypoglycemia itself.

Hyperglycemia

Although there is no direct evidence, it has been postulated that hyperglycemia in the preterm infant can increase the risk for IVH by causing rapid changes in osmolarity with resultant rapid fluid shifts within the brain and germinal matrix. One study did report an increased mortality in hyperglycemic premature infants as compared with their normoglycemic counterparts, although hyperglycemia may have been a marker for those infants with more severe illness rather than a direct cause of the increased mortality. Increased morbidity may be seen in the form of greater difficulty with fluid and electrolyte management since use of dextrose-containing fluids must be limited, as well as problems establishing adequate nutrition. Several studies also suggest an association between hyperglycemia in ELBW infants and increased incidence of retinopathy of prematurity, but no cause-and-effect relationship has been demonstrated.[26,30]

Infants with TNDM usually recover spontaneously within the first week; persistent insulin resistance is extremely rare. However, those infants with chromosomal mutations have an increased incidence of adult-onset diabetes later in life.[74] No neurologic sequelae have been directly attributed to the presence of transient hyperglycemia in these neonates.

PARENT TEACHING

Parent teaching should begin before delivery, with emphasis placed on good nutrition and early and regular prenatal care. Teaching also should include information about those conditions that increase the risk for hypoglycemia (e.g., IUGR associated with maternal cigarette smoking and poor maternal nutrition). Regular prenatal care ensures the early detection of potentially serious problems, including preeclampsia, gestational diabetes, and abnormal fetal growth.

Prenatal teaching is especially important in the woman with known diabetes mellitus, because overall outcome (although not necessarily the incidence of hypoglycemia) is directly related to the degree of control before and during pregnancy. Breastfeeding information and encouragement to breast feed must be included in the prenatal education. In addition, the possibility of neonatal hypoglycemia and requirement for IV therapy can be discussed with the parents before delivery so that they will be aware that the infant may require a longer hospital stay even if delivered at term.

If IV therapy is selected to treat neonatal hypoglycemia, regardless of cause, a thorough explanation of the treatment plan must be given to the parents at the time therapy is instituted. Frequent progress reports should be provided to resolve unanswered (and often unasked) questions and relieve parental anxiety. Parents of children with islet cell dysplasias need to be aware of the clinical signs of hypoglycemia and emergency treatment measures that can be instituted, because recurrent hypoglycemia may occur in these cases. Parents of infants with inborn errors of metabolism also need counseling with regard to prognosis, as well as genetic counseling about risks for recurrence in future pregnancies.

Acknowledgments

Supported by NIH grants HD 20337 (JEM, PI), HD42815 (WWH, PI), DK52138 (WWH, PI), HD28794 (WWH, PI), HD07186 (WWH, PI), NIH U54RR025217 (WWH, Co-Director), and 2 L40 CA117814 (PJR, PI).

REFERENCES

1. Altimier L, Roberts W: One Touch II hospital system for neonates: correlation with serum glucose values, *Neonatal Netw* 15:15, 1996.
2. Barkovich AJ, Ali FA, Rowley HA, et al: Imaging patterns of neonatal hypoglycemia, *Am J Neuroradiol* 19:523, 1998.
3. Barrett CT, Oliver TK: Hypoglycemia and hyperinsulinism in infants with erythroblastosis fetalis, *N Engl J Med* 278:1260, 1968.
4. Bazaes RA, Salazar TE, Pittaluga E, et al: Glucose and lipid metabolism in small for gestational age infants at 48 hours of age, *Pediatrics* 111:804, 2003.
5. Beardsall K, Vanhaesebrouck S, Ogilvy-Stuart AL, et al: Early insulin therapy in very-low-birth-weight infants, *N Engl J Med* 359:1873, 2008.
6. Belik J, Musey J, Trussell RA: Continuous infusion of glucagon induces severe hyponatremia and thrombocytopenia in a premature neonate, *Pediatrics* 107:595, 2001.
7. Binder N, Raschko PK, Benda GI, et al: Insulin infusion with parenteral nutrition in extremely low birth weight infants with hyperglycemia, *J Pediatr* 114:273, 1989.
8. Blanco CL, Baillargeon JG, Morrison RL, et al: Hyperglycemia in extremely low birth weight infants in a predominantly Hispanic population and related morbidities, *J Perinatol* 26:737, 2006.
9. Burns CM, Utherford MA, Boardman JP, et al: Patterns of cerebral injury and neurodevelopmental outcomes after symptomatic neonatal hypoglycemia, *Pediatrics* 122:65, 2008.
10. Carter P, Lloyd D, Duffy P: Glucagon for hypoglycaemia in infants small for gestational age, *Arch Dis Child* 63:1264, 1988.
11. Cornblath M, Hawdon JM, Williams A, et al: Controversies regarding definition of neonatal hypoglycemia: suggested operational thresholds, *Pediatrics* 105:1141, 2000.
12. Cornblath M, Schwartz R: Hypoglycemia in the neonate, *J Pediatr Endocrinol* 6:113, 1993.
13. Cornblath M, Schwartz R, Aynsley-Green A, et al: Hypoglycemia in infancy: the need for rational definition, *Pediatrics* 85:834, 1990.
14. Cowett RM, Oh W, Schwartz R: Persistent glucose production during glucose infusion in the neonate, *J Clin Invest* 71:467, 1983.
15. Cowett RM, Susa JB, Gill DL, et al: Glucose kinetics in infants of diabetic mothers, *Am J Obstet Gynecol* 146:781, 1983.
16. Curet LB, Izquierdo LA, Gilson GJ, et al: Relative effects of antepartum and intrapartum maternal blood

glucose levels on incidence of neonatal hypoglycemia, *J Perinatol* 17:113, 1997.
17. Davis DJ, Creery WD, Radziuk J: Inappropriately high plasma insulin levels in suspected perinatal asphyxia, *Acta Paediatr Scand* 88:76, 2000.
18. Dawkins MJ: Biochemical aspects of developing function in newborn mammalian liver, *Br Med Bull* 22:27, 1966.
19. DeBaun MR, King AA, White N: Hypoglycemia in Beckwith-Weidemann syndrome, *Semin Perinatol* 24:164, 2000.
20. DeLonlay-Debeney P, Poggi-Travert F, Fournet J, et al: Clinical features of 52 neonates with hyperinsulinism, *N Engl J Med* 340:1169, 1999.
21. Denne SC, Kalhan SC: Glucose carbon recycling and oxidation in human newborns, *Am J Physiol* 251: e71: 1986.
22. DiGiacomo JE, Hay WW Jr: Effect of hypoinsulinemia and hyperglycemia on fetal glucose use, *Am J Physiol* 259:e506, 1990.
23. Ditzenberger GR, Collins SD, Binder N: Continuous insulin intravenous infusion therapy for VLBW infants, *J Perinatal Neonatal Nurs* 13:70, 1999.
24. Duvanel CB, Fawer CL, Cotting J, et al: Long-term effects of neonatal hypoglycemia on brain growth and psychomotor development in small-for-gestational age infants, *J Pediatr* 134:492, 1999.
25. Dweck HS, Cassady G: Glucose intolerance in infants of very low birth weight: incidence of hyperglycemia in infants of birth weights 1100 grams or less, *Pediatrics* 53:189, 1974.
26. Ertl T, Gyarmati J, Gaal V, et al: Relationship between hyperglycemia and retinopathy of prematurity in very low birth weight infants, *Biol Neonate* 89:56, 2006.
27. Fluge G: Neurological findings at follow-up in neonatal hypoglycaemia, *Acta Paediatr Scand* 64:629, 1975.
28. Fourtner SH, Stanley CA: Genetic and nongenetic forms of hyperinsulinism in neonates, *NeoReviews* 5:e370, 2004.
29. Gardner S, Hagedorn M: High risk neonatal care: level III nursery. In Gardner S, Hagedorn M, editors: *Legal aspects of maternal-child nursing practice,* Menlo Park, Calif, 1997, Addison-Wesley.
30. Garg R, Agthe AG, Donohue PK, et al: Hyperglycemia and retinopathy of prematurity in very low birth weight infants, *J Perinatol* 23:186, 2003.
31. Garland J, Alex C, Gleisberg D, et al: Clinical utility of a glucose reflectance meter for screening neonates for hypoglycemia, *J Perinatol* 16:250, 1996.
32. Giep TN, Hall RT, Harris K, et al: Evaluation of neonatal whole blood versus plasma glucose concentration by ion-selective electrode technology and comparison with two whole blood chromogen test strip methods, *J Perinatol* 16:244, 1996.
33. Glaser B: Hyperinsulinism of the newborn, *Semin Perinatol* 24:150, 2000.
34. Glaser B, Thornton P, Otonkoski T, et al: Genetics of neonatal hyperinsulinism, *Arch Dis Child Fetal Neonatal Ed* 82:F79, 2000.
35. Griffiths AD, Bryant GM: Assessment of effects of neonatal hypoglycaemia, *Arch Dis Child* 46:819, 1971.
36. Hawdon JM: Hypoglycaemia and the neonatal brain, *Eur J Pediatr* 158(suppl 1):9, 1999.
37. Hawdon JM, Ward Platt MP: Patterns of metabolic adaptation for preterm and term infants in the first neonatal week, *Arch Dis Child* 67:357, 1992.
38. Hawdon JM, Ward Platt MP: Metabolic adaptation in small for gestational age infants, *Arch Dis Child* 68:262, 1993.
39. Haworth JC, McRae KN, Dilling LA: Prognosis of infants of diabetic mothers in relation to neonatal hypoglycaemia, *Dev Med Child Neurol* 18:471, 1976.
40. Hay WW Jr, Meznarich HK, DiGiacomo JE, et al: Effects of insulin and glucose concentrations on glucose use in fetal sheep, *Pediatr Res* 23:381, 1988.
41. Humea R, Burchella A, Williams FLR, et al: Glucose homeostasis in the newborn, *Early Hum Dev* 81:95, 2005.
42. Hussain K: Diagnosis and management of hyperinsulinaemic hypoglycaemia of infancy, *Horm Res* 69:2, 2008.
43. James T III, Blessa M, Boggs TR Jr: Recurrent hyperglycemia associated with sepsis in a neonate, *Am J Dis Child* 133:645, 1979.
44. Kahler SG: Metabolic disorders associated with neonatal hypoglycemia, *NeoReviews* 5(9):e377, 2004.
45. Kalhan S, Peter-Wohl S: Hypoglycemia: what is it for the neonate? *Am J Perinatol* 17:11, 2000.
46. Kashyap S, Polin RA: Insulin infusions in very-low-birth-weight infants, *N Engl J Med* 359:1951, 2008.
47. Koh TH, Eyre JA, Aynsley-Green A: Neonatal hypoglycaemia: the controversy regarding definition, *Arch Dis Child* 63:1386, 1996.
48. Koh TH, Vong SK: Definition of neonatal hypoglycemia: is there a change? *J Pediatr Child Health* 32:302, 1996.
49. Ktorza A, Bihoreau M, Nurjhan N, et al: Insulin and glucagon during the perinatal period: secretion and metabolic effects on the liver, *Biol Neonate* 48:204, 1985.
50. Lafeber HN, Jones CT, Rolph TP: Some of the consequences of intrauterine growth retardation. In Visser KHA, editor: *Nutrition and metabolism of the fetus and infant,* Boston, 1979, Martinus Nijhoff.
51. Leake RD, Fiser RH, Oh W: Rapid glucose disappearance in infants with infection, *Clin Pediatr* 20:397, 1981.
52. Leonard M, Chessall M, Manning D: The use of a HemoCue blood glucose analyser in a neonatal unit, *Ann Clin Biochem* 34:287, 1997.
53. Lilien LD, Pildes RS, Srinivasan G, et al: Treatment of neonatal hypoglycemia with minibolus and intravenous glucose infusion, *J Pediatr* 97:295, 1980.

54. Limesand SW, Rozance PJ, Smith D, et al: Increased insulin sensitivity and maintenance of glucose utilization rates in fetal sheep with placental insufficiency and intrauterine growth restriction, *Am J Physiol Endocrinol Metab* 293:e1716, 2007.
55. Lovvorn HNIII, Nance ML, Ferry RJ Jr, et al: Congenital hyperinsulinism and the surgeon: lessons learned over 35 years, *J Pediatr* 34:786, 1999.
56. Lubchenco LO, Bard H: Incidence of hypoglycemia in newborn infants classified by birth weight and gestational age, *Pediatrics* 47:831, 1971.
57. Lucas A, Morley R, Cole TJ: Adverse neurodevelopmental outcome of moderate neonatal hypoglycaemia, *BMJ* 297:1304, 1988.
58. Maisels MJ, Lee C: Chemstrip glucose test strips: correlation with true glucose values less than 80 mg/dl, *Crit Care Med* 71:457, 1983.
59. McGowan JE: Neonatal hypoglycemia, *NeoReviews* 1:e6, 1999.
60. McGowan JE: Neonatal hypoglycemia: 50 years later, the questions remain the same, *NeoReviews* 5:e363, 2004.
61. Meissner T, Brune W, Mayatepek E: Persistent hyperinsulinaemic hypoglycaemia of infancy: therapy, clinical outcome and mutational analysis, *Eur J Pediatr* 156:754, 1997.
62. Meissner T, Wendel U, Burgard P, et al: Long-term follow-up of 114 patients with congenital hyperinsulinism, *Eur J Endocrinol* 149:43, 2003.
63. Menni F, de Lonlay P, Sevin C, et al: Neurologic outcomes of 90 neonates and infants with persistent hyperinsulinemic hypoglycemia, *Pediatrics* 107:476, 2001.
64. Metzger BE, Lowe LP, Dyer AR, et al: Hyperglycemia and adverse pregnancy outcomes. HAPO Study Cooperative Research Group, *N Engl J Med* 358:2008, 1991.
65. Mitanchez-Mokhtari D, Lahlou N, Kieffer F, et al: Both relative insulin resistance and defective islet beta-cell processing of proinsulin are responsible for transient hyperglycemia in extremely preterm infants, *Pediatrics* 113:537, 2004.
66. Ozand PT: Hypoglycemia in association with various organic and amino acid disorders, *Semin Perinatol* 24:172, 2000.
67. Procianoy RS, Pinheiro CEA: Neonatal hyperinsulinism after short-term maternal beta sympathomimetic therapy, *J Pediatr* 101:612, 1982.
68. Sadava D, Frykman P, Harris E, et al: Development of enzymes of glycolysis and gluconeogenesis in human fetal liver, *Biol Neonate* 62:165, 1992.
69. Salhab WA, Wyckoff MH, Laptook AR, et al: Initial hypoglycemia and neonatal brain injury in terms of infants with severe fetal acidemia, *Pediatrics* 114:361, 2004.
70. Schiff D, Aranda JV, Colle E, et al: Metabolic effects of exchange transfusion. II. Delayed hypoglycemia following exchange transfusion with citrated blood, *J Pediatr* 79:589, 1971.
71. Sells CJ, Robinson NM, Brown Z, et al: Long-term developmental follow-up of infants of diabetic mothers, *J Pediatr* 125:S9, 1994.
72. Setia S, Sridhar MG, Bhat V, et al: Insulin sensitivity and insulin secretion at birth in intrauterine growth retarded infants, *Pathology* 38:236, 2006.
73. Shelley HJ: Glycogen reserves and their changes at birth and in anoxia, *Br Med Bull* 17:137, 1961.
74. Shield JP: Neonatal diabetes: new insights into aetiology and implications, *Horm Res* 53(suppl 1):7, 2000.
75. Sinclair JC: Approaches to the definition of neonatal hypoglycemia, *Acta Paediatr Jpn* 39(suppl 1):S17, 1997.
76. Sperling MA, Ganguli S, Leslie N, et al: Fetal-perinatal catecholamine secretion: role in perinatal glucose homeostasis, *Am J Physiol* 247:e69: 1984.
77. Srinivasan G, Pildes RS, Caughy M, et al: Plasma glucose values in normal neonates: a new look, *J Pediatr* 109:114, 1986.
78. Srinivasan G, Singh J, Cattamanchi G, et al: Plasma glucose changes in preterm infants during oral theophylline therapy, *J Pediatr* 103:473, 1983.
79. Stenninger E, Flink R, Eriksson B, et al: Long-term neurological dysfunction and neonatal hypoglycaemia after diabetic pregnancy, *Arch Dis Child Fetal Neonatal Ed* 79:F174, 1998.
80. Sunehag A, Gustafsson J, Ewald U: Very immature infants (<30 weeks) respond to glucose infusion with incomplete suppression of glucose production, *Pediatr Res* 36:550, 1994.
81. Sunehag AL, Haymond MW: Glucose extremes in newborn infants, *Clin Perinatol* 29:245, 2002.
82. Tenenbaum D, Cowett RM: Mechanisms of beta sympathomimetic action on neonatal glucose homeostasis in the lamb, *J Pediatr* 107:588, 1985.
83. Vanucci RC, Vanucci SJ: Hypoglycemic brain injury, *Semin Neonatal* 6:147, 2001.
84. Vileisis RA, Cowett RM, Oh W: Glycemic response to lipid infusion in the premature neonate, *J Pediatr* 100:108, 1982.
85. Zarif MA, Pildes RS, Vidyasagar D: Insulin and growth-hormone responses in neonatal hyperglycemia, *Diabetes* 25:428, 1976.
86. Zarlengo KM, Battaglia FC, Fennessey PV, et al: Relationship between glucose use rate and glucose concentration in preterm infants, *Biol Neonate* 49:181, 1986.

SELECTED READINGS

Aynsley-Green A: Glucose: a fuel for thought, *J Paediatr Child Health* 27:21, 1991.

Chen Y-T, Burchall A: Glycogen storage diseases. In Scriver CR, Beaudet AL, Sly WS, et al, editors: *The metabolic and molecular bases of inherited disease,* ed 7, New York, 1995, McGraw-Hill.

Cornblath M, Schwartz R, editors: *Semin Perinatol* 24(2):2000 (entire issue is devoted to topics pertaining to glucose homeostasis in the newborn and infant).

Cowett RM: Neonatal glucose metabolism. In Cowett RM, editor: *Principles of perinatal-neonatal metabolism,* New York, 1991, Springer Verlag.

DiGiacomo JE, Hay WW Jr: Disorders of metabolic adaptation: abnormal glucose homeostasis. In Sinclair JC, Bracken MB, editors: *Effective care of the newborn infant,* Oxford, 1992, Oxford University Press.

Farrag HM, Cowett RM: Glucose homeostasis in the micropremie, *Clin Perinatol* 27:1, 2000.

Hay WW Jr: Reliability of blood glucose analysis. In Schwartz R, Cornblath M, editors: *Hypoglycemia in infancy: the need for a rational definition, Ciba Symposium Report,* 1990.

Kalhan SC, Raghavan CV: Metabolism of glucose and methods of investigation in the fetus and newborn. In Polin RA, Fox WW, editors: *Fetal and neonatal physiology,* ed 3, Philadelphia, 2003, Saunders.

Kalhan S, Saker F: Metabolic and endocrine disorders. Part I: Disorders of carbohydrate metabolism. In Fanaroff AA, Martin RJ, editors: *Neonatal-perinatal medicine: diseases of the fetus and newborn,* ed 6, St Louis, 1997, Mosby.

Kelly DP, Strauss AW: Inherited cardiomyopathies, *N Engl J Med* 330:13, 1994.

Meetze W, Bowsher R, Compton J, et al: Hyperglycemia in extremely-low-birth-weight infants, *Biol Neonate* 74:214, 1998.

Ogata ES: Carbohydrate metabolism in the fetus and neonate and altered glucoregulation, *Pediatr Clin North Am* 33:25, 1986.

Segal S, Berry GT: Disorders of galactose metabolism. In Scriver CR, Beaudet AL, Sly WS, et al: *The metabolic and molecular bases of inherited disease,* ed 7, New York, 1995, McGraw-Hill.

Siesjo BK: Hypoglycemia, brain metabolism, and brain damage, *Diabetes Metab Rev* 4:113, 1988.

Stanley CA, Hale DE: Genetic disorders of mitochondrial fatty acid oxidation, *Curr Opin Pediatr* 6:476, 1994.

Stokowski L: Metabolic disorders (glucose homeostasis). In Deacon J, O'Neil P, editors: *Core curriculum for neonatal intensive care nursing,* ed 3, Philadelphia, 2004, Saunders.

Widdowson EM, Spray CM: Chemical development in utero, *Arch Dis Child* 26:205, 1951.

Williams AF: Hypoglycaemia in the newborn: a review, *WHO Publications #5778,* 1997.

Ziegler EE, O'Donnell AM, Nelson SE, et al: Body composition of the reference fetus, *Growth* 40:329, 1976.

16 TOTAL PARENTERAL NUTRITION

HOWARD W. KILBRIDE, MARY KAY LEICK-RUDE, STEVEN L. OLSEN, AND JILL STIENS

Total parenteral nutrition (TPN) support for critically ill newborns was first reported four decades ago.[28] However, in the modern era of neonatal care, TPN continues to be a critical aspect of intensive newborn care. Availability of TPN has been one of the developments responsible for improved outcome of neonatal surgical patients.[77,81,84] Increased survival of extremely preterm infants has provided new challenges for neonatal parenteral nutrition.[21] Current evidence would suggest that early nutritional support is important to prevent postnatal growth restriction, which has been commonly recognized in these infants.[29]

This chapter discusses the nutritional needs of the high-risk newborn, specific indications for TPN, and guidelines for formulation and administration of intravenous (IV) nutritional solutions. It also provides an overview of mechanical, infectious, and metabolic complications, with emphasis on prevention and early identification.

PHYSIOLOGY

Fuel Stores

During periods of fasting, tissue stores of energy provide the major source of fuel for the body. Carbohydrate is stored in the liver and muscle as glycogen. Stable blood sugar levels are maintained by hormonal regulation of glycogen production (glycogenesis) and break down to glucose (glycogenolysis). Newborns, particularly those who are growth retarded or preterm, have low glycogen stores and often have insufficient regulatory mechanisms.[96]

The body's greatest energy stores are in the form of fat, which provides a calorie yield of 9 kcal/g when metabolized. In addition to normal deposits of adipose tissue, newborns (and hibernating adult animals) have unique stores called ***brown fat.*** These stores, which are anatomically located between the scapulae, in the axillae and mediastinum, and around the adrenal glands, protect the body from hypothermia through nonshivering thermogenesis[70] (see Chapter 6).

Protein makes up lean body mass. Although protein generally is not used as an energy source postnatally, in fetal life, amino acids are oxidized apparently for energy.[100] This may be true for brief periods postnatally, but extended periods of protein catabolism (breakdown of endogenous substrates), such as during times of starvation, may lead to body dysfunction, as noted later.

The Effects of Insufficient Nutrition

The last trimester of gestation is a time of rapid fetal growth, with active transplacental transport of most nutritional substrates. Preterm delivery interrupts the nutritional supply and abruptly results in a catabolic state, which, if prolonged, may alter growth potential. It is unclear whether it is possible or desirable to achieve in utero growth rates for the postnatal preterm infant, but reestablishment of an anabolic state and maintenance of micronutrient sufficiency are necessary.[100] During this period of neonatal life, the rapidly growing brain is responsible for much of the nutritional requirements. **Inadequate early nutrition may have irreversible effects on later neurodevelopmental outcome.**[62]

Postnatal growth retardation also is associated with neonatal medical complications, including apnea, ventilator dependence, and chronic lung disease.[21] Immune responses may be depressed with increased

Please note that the PURPLE type in each chapter is intended to make it easier to identify clinically applicable material.

susceptibility to infection (see Chapter 22). Protein malnutrition is most frequently seen in extreme preterms and may contribute to poor growth potential and long-term morbidity in these infants.[21,100,101] Poor postnatal growth for most extremely-low-birth-weight (ELBW) infants has emphasized the need for additional strategies to improve nutrition for this population.[25,26]

Nutritional Requirements of the Neonate

CALORIC

Caloric requirements for term or near-term infants are 105 to 120 kcal/kg/day. These estimates are based on enteral intake (see Chapter 17). Parenteral requirements are about 20% less, or approximately 85 to 100 kcal/kg/day. Requirements are greater for very-low-birth-weight (VLBW) infants, whether extremely preterm or small for gestational age (SGA), but optimal intakes have not yet been determined.[89]

Factors affecting caloric requirements include the infant's activity level, body temperature, and degree of stress. Nosocomial infections may also contribute to additional caloric needs.[102] Physical activity, which usually is infrequent in preterm infants, contributes less than 10% to the energy needs.[60] However, in pathologic states, such as with repetitious seizures or neonatal abstinence syndrome, increased activity may increase caloric needs. **An elevation of body temperature increases caloric expenditure by approximately 12% for each degree Celsius above 37.8° C (100° F).** Metabolic demands of surgery or severe cardiac or pulmonary distress may increase caloric requirements by 30% and chronic failure to thrive by 50% to 100%. In addition, postnatal dexamethasone therapy may slow weight and linear growth rates and potentially may affect brain growth.[21,68,94]

WATER

Water requirements vary with gestational and postnatal age (post-conceptual age) and environmental conditions (e.g., care in an incubator versus radiant heat warmer, use of phototherapy) (see Chapter 14).

MINERAL

Sodium requirements are minimal for the first days of life. After 1 week, the average requirement is 3 to 4 mEq/kg/day. Large renal losses (>5 mEq/kg/day) may occur in very immature infants (<28 weeks' gestation) in the first weeks of life. Potassium and chloride requirements are approximately 2 mEq/kg/day and 3 to 4 mEq/kg/day, respectively. Glucosuria with resulting osmotic diuresis may increase sodium and potassium urinary losses.[32]

Calcium is an important cofactor in hemostasis, enzyme function, muscle contraction, and cell membrane stability. In the newborn, 98% of calcium is stored in the bone. The initial calcium requirement is 1 mEq/kg/day to maintain calcium homeostasis and to avoid irritability and tetany associated with low serum ionized calcium levels. **In utero, the accretion rate is 4 to 5 mEq/kg/day, which the growing preterm infant should receive in addition to adequate phosphorus and vitamin D to avoid osteopenia, rickets, and bone fractures.**[109] Excess calcium intake may cause central nervous system (CNS) depression or signs of renal toxicity.

The phosphorus requirement for the growing preterm infant is 40 to 60 mg/kg/day (31 mg = 1 mmol). Bone contains 80% of the body's phosphorus. Low phosphorus intake causes increased renal calcium excretion and a depletion of bone calcium phosphate. Low phosphorus intake or chronic furosemide diuretic therapy also may lead to hypercalciuria and nephrolithiasis.[27] Because phosphorus is a major constituent of cellular energy function (adenosine triphosphate, 2,3-diphosphoglycerate, creatinine phosphate), severe depletion may result in muscle paralysis, respiratory failure, and interruption of important cellular functions, such as the hemoglobin-oxygen dissociation curve and leukocyte activity.

Magnesium is essential for intracellular enzyme systems. The requirement is 0.25 to 0.5 mEq/kg/day.[4] Magnesium deficiency states mimic hypocalcemia, manifesting as irritability, tremulousness, tetany, and cardiac dysrhythmias. Magnesium excess may manifest as lethargy, hypotonia, and delayed stooling.

CARBOHYDRATE

During fetal life, glucose is the primary source of energy.[100] At birth, the preterm infant has only a small supply of glycogen, the storage form of glucose (equivalent to about 200 kcal of energy). Glucose is particularly important for the CNS, because other substrates are not available. Initially, a glucose infusion rate (GIR) of 6 mg/kg/min is sufficient to meet metabolic needs of the newborn infant. Requirements are greater for infants who are stressed (e.g., from sepsis or hypothermia) or hyperinsulinemic (e.g., infants of diabetic mothers or infants with Beckwith-Wiedemann syndrome). **With long-term parenteral nutrition, at least 50% of total caloric requirement should be provided as carbohydrate (GIR 8 to 10 mg/kg/min), generally as dextrose (calculated as 3.4 kcal/kg of hydrated carbohydrate). To avoid metabolic consequences of excessive glucose loads, a GIR of more than 12 mg/kg/min (18 g/kg/day of glucose) should be avoided.**

PROTEIN

The quantity of daily nitrogen required by a term newborn infant, based on estimates from breast milk intake, is approximately 325 mg/kg/day (approximately 2 g/kg/day of protein).[5,35] Requirements for preterm infants are much higher, as indicated by in utero accretion rates during the latter half of pregnancy. At 28 weeks' gestation, the fetus requires 350 mg/kg/day of nitrogen. This figure declines to 150 mg/kg/day by term gestation. **When the estimated accretion rate is added to the obligatory postnatal nitrogen excretion, the requirement for a 28-weeks' gestation preterm may be calculated to be approximately 495 mg/kg/day (3.1 g/kg/day of protein). If one assumes parenterally administered amino acids are converted to body proteins at 75% efficiency, the estimated parenteral amino acid requirement would be as high as 3.7 g/kg/day.**[31,40,101]

In fetal life, protein is actively transported from mother's circulation across the placenta in quantities greater than needed for accretion, with the excess being oxidized for energy.[99] Clinicians have found that increasing protein intake postnatally at all energy intake levels above 40 kcal/kg/day results in increased protein accretion. **Current evidence indicates that protein intake up to 4 g/kg/day is safe with no clinically significant increase in azotemia, acidosis, or hyperaminoacidemia.**[79] Further investigations are needed to determine safe upper limits for maximum protein administration beyond that level.

Studies have shown that administration of amino acids shortly after birth decreases protein catabolism, which is extremely important particularly for VLBW infants.[31,99] Based on the current evidence, providing VLBW infants with 3 g/kg/day of protein on the first day of life is safe.[25] **Many units have created a "stock" or "starter TPN (protein-containing) solution" to achieve the goal of providing 2 to 3 g/kg/day of protein immediately after admission to the neonatal intensive care unit (NICU) to promote anabolism.** Although current studies overwhelmingly support the early use of parenteral protein nutrition, further investigation is needed to document the effect of this supplementation on long-term growth and development.

The quality of the amino acid mixture infused is important for efficacy and safety.[1] **Although there is no formulation specifically for preterm infants, pediatric solutions provide greater quantities of essential amino acids and result in plasma amino acid levels similar to that of postprandial breastfed infants.** An essential amino acid is one that cannot be synthesized in adequate quantity to meet the requirements for normal growth and development. The differentiation between essential and nonessential amino acids is not clear in newborn infants, because the ability to synthesize some amino acids may vary with the clinical situation or stage of maturity. Lysine and threonine are essential in their entirety. There is a high requirement for branched-chain amino acids (e.g., leucine, isoleucine, valine) in the growing newborn. These are metabolized primarily in skeletal muscle.[41]

Methionine is an essential sulfur-containing amino acid that is metabolized to cysteine and taurine. **For preterm infants of less than 32 weeks' gestation, cystathionase activity is insufficient for cysteine synthesis.**[108] **Some investigators have found cysteine supplementation results in greater nitrogen retention, and for this reason it is recommended for short-term supplementation for high-risk preterms, although the effects of prolonged use have not been fully investigated.**[92] **Cysteine is not stable in amino acid solutions, so cysteine hydrochloride supplements must be added separately to the parenteral nutrition.** Taurine is a nonprotein amino sulfonic acid that is converted from cysteine by cysteine sulfonic acid decarboxylase. Taurine concentrations are low in infants who have received nonsupplemented TPN infusions. Taurine deficiency may have a detrimental effect on the developing nervous system. **It is a general practice to add taurine to TPN for VLBW infants because this may prevent cholestasis in some newborns by more effectively conjugating bile salts and creating soluble end-products.**[42,93,107]

Tyrosine is another amino acid that appears to be essential in the newborn period. It is present in small amounts in most amino acid solutions, although one manufacturer uses a soluble form, *N*-acetyl-L-tyrosine, which infants slowly metabolize to tyrosine.[82] Tyrosine is a by-product of phenylalanine metabolism, so supplementation has an effect on the phenylalanine requirement. Histidine is considered to be an essential amino acid for newborns, with the lowest levels evident in preterm infants. Arginine may be essential only for the newborn with reduced arginine synthetase activity. This amino acid is thought to facilitate clearance of nitrogenous waste products by "priming the urea cycle." Use of amino acid infusate with insufficient arginine has been associated with hyperammonemia.[39] Glutamine also has been considered a conditionally essential amino acid; however, in a randomized trial, no benefit was shown for parenteral glutamine in relation to days to enteral feedings, incidence of necrotizing enterocolitis (NEC), or growth rates.[78]

Nonessential amino acids make up the largest percentage of the amino acid pool in the fetal body. The desired quantities of these amino acids for parenteral solutions are not known. It is thought they should be provided in a balanced formulation. Pediatric solutions differ from adult solutions by providing glutamic acid and aspartic acid with lower glycine concentrations.[1,104]

FAT

Long-chain fatty acids are essential in the newborn for brain development and appear to be important for gene expression and other molecular mechanisms.[106] Essential fatty acids (EFAs) include linoleic and linolenic, and in the newborn, arachidonic acid.[4] Biochemical evidence of EFA deficiency may be seen in less than 1 week in VLBW infants receiving a deficient diet, and the administration of parenteral glucose and amino acids may accelerate these abnormalities.[100] EFA deficiency results in an imbalance in fatty acid production with an overproduction of nonessential fatty acids. **Clinical manifestations appearing at variable times after biochemical changes of EFA deficiency include scaly dermatitis, poor hair growth, thrombocytopenia, failure to thrive, poor wound healing, and increased susceptibility to bacterial infection.** Clinical manifestations of EFA deficiency can be avoided if 3% to 4% of caloric intake is supplied as linoleic acid (approximately 0.5 g/kg/day of intravenous [IV] lipid).[33]

In addition to preventing EFA deficiency, lipid emulsion is a concentrated source of nonprotein calories, which promotes nitrogen retention. Preterm infants appear to have limited capability to oxidize fatty acids. This limitation may be related to deficiency of carnitine, which, in the form of acylcarnitine, promotes transfer of fatty acids into mitochondria, where oxidative metabolism occurs. However, a systematic review of randomized studies found no benefit for carnitine supplementation on weight gain, lipid utilization, or ketogenesis, so routine supplementation is not recommended.[15]

VITAMINS

The biologic role of vitamins, signs and symptoms of deficiency states, and recommended oral requirements are available in Chapter 17. Although there is not a multivitamin formulation specifically for preterm infants, the American Society for Clinical Nutrition (ASCN) has suggested that preterm infants receive 40% to 65% of the daily recommended vitamin doses for term infants and children.[89] These guidelines may result in excessive intakes of some water-soluble vitamins, particularly pyridoxine and riboflavin. Although preterm infants have limited stores of lipid-soluble vitamins because of low body fat, potential toxicity from excess administration is a concern. Vitamin A is a lipid-soluble vitamin important for tissue growth, protein synthesis, and epithelial differentiation. Vitamin A may be administered more effectively in lipid emulsion rather than dextrose amino acid solutions.[4,24] However, vitamin A supplementation has been proven to be effective in lowering chronic lung disease rates only when given by intramuscular (IM) injections three times per week.[105]

Vitamin E is a lipid-soluble biologic antioxidant that is deficient in preterm infants. However, daily parenteral intake of 2 to 3 mg/kg has been associated with serum levels generally in the recommended range of 1 to 2 mg/dL. Pharmacologic doses have been tried unsuccessfully for prevention of bronchopulmonary dysplasia and retinopathy of prematurity, and IV high-dose vitamin E may increase risk for sepsis.[14] Therefore aiming for tocopherol levels greater than 3.5 mg/dL is not recommended. Vitamin K production by intestinal flora is impaired by insufficient enteral feedings and use of broad-spectrum antibiotics in infants on long-term TPN. Vitamin K is provided at the recommended dosage through parenteral pediatric multivitamin solutions.[4]

TRACE MINERALS

Although trace minerals are relatively scarce (<0.01% of the weight of the human body by definition), they play an important role in normal growth and development.[111] Deficiencies of both zinc and copper have been identified in infants on long-term TPN not supplemented with trace minerals. Postsurgical infants with ongoing gastrointestinal losses may have negative zinc balance even if given usual zinc replacement in TPN.[88]

Manifestations of deficiency and recommendations for intake are provided in Chapter 17. Parenteral recommendations are lower than enteral, which are based on physiologic requirements. For infants not receiving frequent blood transfusions, iron therapy may be necessary by 2 months of age. Infants receiving erythropoietin therapy need additional iron supplementation, given either enterally or parenterally.[66]

INDICATIONS

Parenteral nutrition, including protein supplementation and carbohydrate at basal levels, should begin on the first day of life for preterm infants not being fed, as well as for other newborns who are not likely to tolerate enteral feedings within a few days. A preterm infant has limited nutritional stores and quickly develops negative protein balance without early supplementation. TPN continues to be a critical aspect of long-term management for neonatal surgical patients.[84] **When parenteral nutrition solutions are administered through a peripheral vein, caloric intake is limited because the fluid osmolarity should not exceed 900 mOsm/L, which results in relatively limited concentrations of carbohydrate (<12.5% dextrose) and amino acids (<3%). Some recommend even more conservative limits on osmolarity for peripheral lines (500 mOsm/L).**[44] When used with lipid emulsions, peripheral parenteral nutrition (PPN) allows caloric intake of about 70 to 80 kcal/kg/day and protein intake of 2.5 to 3.0 g/kg/day. This level of nutritional intake prevents catabolism and, in some cases, results in moderate growth. PPN usually is adequate for term newborns with transient bowel disease (such as may be seen after the repair of a small omphalocele) or for larger preterm infants whose enteral feedings are delayed for a few days. PPN is used commonly to supplement nutrition in newborns who are receiving partial enteral feedings. When caloric needs can be met by PPN, this route is preferred to the central route, because the catheter insertion risks are avoided and generally the risk for infection is less.

If parenteral nutritional duration is longer than 1 week, administration of TPN solution through a central line is recommended. The placement of a central line for parenteral nutrition allows a higher carbohydrate load to be used, giving more calories with less fluid. In preterm infants at risk for a patent ductus arteriosus and pulmonary edema, diminishing fluid intake and improving nutritional status may be important aspects of management. **Specific indications for TPN by a central catheter include the following:**

- ELBW infants (<1000 g birth weight) and others who do not tolerate a significant volume of enteral feeding within the first week of age or who cannot receive adequate caloric intake by PPN
- Infants who have had gastrointestinal surgery and will have a significant delay in enteral nutrition, such as those with a gastroschisis, bowel resection after NEC, or meconium peritonitis
- Infants with chronic gastrointestinal dysfunction, such as intractable diarrhea

DATA COLLECTION

Monitoring Growth

Weight loss or insufficient weight gain is the initial effect of inadequate caloric intake. Linear growth, although less affected, is diminished after long periods of poor nutrition. Because of "brain-sparing," head circumference growth is the least affected. Measurements should be obtained in a standardized fashion and recorded weekly.

Fetal weight gain in utero at each week of gestation is currently used as the standard to assess adequacy of postnatal growth. In the midtrimester (24 to 27 weeks' gestation), expected weight gain is 1.5% of body weight.[100] Charts are available to monitor postnatal growth rates based on data from a large preterm population, although for long-term monitoring, use of growth curves from normal populations may be more appropriate, as available from the Centers for Disease Control and Prevention (CDC) (*www.cdc.gov/growthcharts/*).[34]

Minimum monitoring of growth should consist of the following:

- Weigh daily, or more frequently in ELBW infants with rapidly changing extracellular fluid status. Maintenance of a thermostable environment with minimal handling of ELBW infants can be achieved through the use of in-bed scales. Strict attention to consistency of technique during the weighing process is essential to obtain accurate, reliable measurements.[103] Monitoring weight gain on a weekly basis in grams per kilogram of weight gained daily (g/kg/day) may help in reducing postnatal growth restriction and positively impact long-term neurodevelopmental outcome. An ideal rate of weight gain for ELBW infants appears to be 18 to 21 g/kg/day.[30]
- Measure length weekly.
- Head circumference measured weekly.

Biochemical Monitoring

In addition to anthropometric measurements, biochemical parameters may be monitored to assess nutritional adequacy. Periodic assessment of calcium, phosphorus, and alkaline phosphatase levels is important to detect metabolic disturbances associated with osteopenia.[109] Tests for protein malnutrition include serum total protein, albumin, transferrin, retinol-binding protein, and transthyretin (prealbumin), the latter two suggested primarily for preterm infants.[5,35] Routine clinical use of these measurements awaits greater definition of normal variation and independent effects of systemic illness and medications.

Biochemical monitoring of the infant's physiologic status is necessary to avoid complications of TPN. Usefulness of the laboratory data should be balanced with the economic costs and risks from iatrogenic blood losses for the infant (Table 16-1).

When serum electrolyte levels are abnormal, urinary electrolyte levels may be useful to clarify sodium and potassium requirements (e.g., if body sodium is depleted, low urine concentration would be expected).

TABLE 16-1 METABOLIC MONITORING FOR INFANTS RECEIVING PARENTERAL NUTRITION

	FREQUENCY	
VARIABLE	ACUTE	STABLE
Electrolytes, BUN	Daily	2×/wk
Calcium, phosphorus	Weekly	Biweekly
Alkaline phosphatase	—	Biweekly
Serum glucose screen	q 8 hr	Daily
Urine glucose	q 8 hr	Daily
Hemoglobin/hematocrit	Daily	Weekly
Liver function:		
Bilirubin	2×/wk	PRN
Transaminase	Weekly	Biweekly
Triglyceride*	—	Weekly

BUN, Blood urea nitrogen; *PRN,* as needed.
*When on lipid emulsion.

TREATMENT

Vascular Access

UMBILICAL ARTERY CATHETERS AND UMBILICAL VEIN CATHETERS

Umbilical artery catheters (UACs) and umbilical vein catheters (UVCs) are commonly placed in sick newborns to provide vascular access for IV fluids, blood samplings, and blood pressure monitoring. Because of the risks for thromboembolic and infection complications, these lines generally are removed by 1 week of age.[22,36]

PERIPHERAL AND MIDLINE CATHETERS

If continued venous access is necessary after this time, a peripheral, midline, or peripherally inserted central catheter (PICC) can be placed. The type of line used is determined by the anticipated length of time needed and the osmolarity of the substances to be infused.[44] Peripheral IVs are indicated for short-term IV access. A midline catheter, which is threaded to the proximal portion of an extremity or neck, can provide longer intravenous access than a peripheral IV when prolonged peripheral strength TPN is indicated. Midline catheters appear to be associated with lower rates of phlebitis than short peripheral catheters and with lower rates of infection and cost than central lines.[59]

PERIPHERALLY INSERTED CENTRAL CATHETERS

A PICC line can provide maximal nutritional intake when long-term parenteral access is necessary.[2] Percutaneous placement of a 20- to 26-gauge (1.9- to 2.6-Fr) Silastic (silicone) or polyurethane catheter can be performed routinely in even the smallest of neonatal patients by trained nurses and physicians.[72,76] The catheter usually is placed in the antecubital or axillary veins in the arms; however, leg, scalp, or external jugular veins may be used to achieve central access. Veins that may be needed for percutaneous central line placement should not be sites for routine venipuncture (see Chapter 7).

Percutaneous line placement involves stabilization of the vein, maximum barrier precautions (sterile gloves, gown, large drape, masks), and antiseptic preparation of the skin with 2% chlorhexidine or povidone-iodine and alcohol product.[16,54,87] Fully equipped prepackaged kits are available for this procedure from a number of manufacturers. Most kits include an 18- or 19-gauge insertion needle that is used to puncture and tunnel through the subcutaneous tissue before entering the vein. Once the needle is within the vein, the catheter, which has been flushed with heparinized saline solution, is passed through the needle into the vein and advanced to a premeasured distance, which is the estimated location of the superior vena cava.[44] (If the basilic vein is used, turn the infant's head to face the insertion site to minimize the risk for the catheter entering neck vessels.) The catheter tip position should be documented radiographically. If the catheter is placed in the saphenous vein, obtain a lateral roentgenogram if the anteroposterior film suggests possible vertebral vessel cannulation rather than inferior vena cava placement.[67] Remove the needle carefully from the skin and discard it. A Steri-Strip should be placed over the catheter insertion site to maintain its position before the dressing is completed. The addition of heparin to IV fluids is commonly used by practitioners to prevent occlusion of vascular catheters. However, there is no indisputable evidence for this practice.[86]

The length of tubing outside the infant's body should be measured and recorded. Excess may be carefully curled at the site of insertion and covered with a sterile, transparent dressing. If an arm board was used for stabilization, it may be removed. Arm restraints should not be necessary.

BROVIAC® CATHETER

Large-bore Silastic catheters (Broviac®) are placed surgically in infants in whom the percutaneous method is not successful and long-term access is anticipated. Generally, the catheters are placed in the internal or external jugular veins or common facial vein by cutdown and threaded to a central venous site. The distal end is tunneled subcutaneously and exited through the anterior chest wall. The catheter must be secured and dressed sterilely.

OTHER VASCULAR ACCESS OPTIONS

Other sites that may be used for TPN infusion on a short-term basis include subclavian, jugular, and femoral veins. Some centers use a UVC for short-term parenteral nutrition when another site is not feasible.

Composition of Infusate

CARBOHYDRATE

The prime source of calories for the neonate usually is dextrose. Peripherally, 10% to 12% solution is used. When central access is obtained, a 15% to 30% dextrose concentration may be used. The glucose load is increased if either the infusion rate or glucose concentration of the infusate is increased. Too rapid an increase in glucose load may exceed an infant's carbohydrate tolerance and result in hyperglycemia. A rapid decrease in the infusion rate or the glucose concentration of the infusate may result in hypoglycemia.

When calculating caloric intake, use the following:

$$1 \text{ g dextrose} = 3.4 \text{ kcal}$$

or

$$100 \text{ mL/kg of } D_{10}W = 34 \text{ kcal/kg}$$

or

$$100 \text{ mL/kg of } D_{30}W = 102 \text{ kcal/kg}$$

The glucose infusion rate (GIR) can be calculated:

$$\text{GIR (mg/kg/min)}$$

$$= \frac{\text{g glucose/day} \times 1000}{1440 \text{ (min/day)}} / \text{weight (kg)}$$

Generally, a newborn of 28 weeks' gestation or more (>1000 g body weight) initially tolerates a GIR of about 6 mg/kg/min. Daily increases in dextrose concentration or fluid volume to increase carbohydrate administration by 2.0 mg/kg/min usually are tolerated. ELBW infants may be carbohydrate intolerant, and initial GIR should be lower (4 or 5 mg/kg/min) for these infants. An insulin infusion may be considered for ELBW infants experiencing persistent hyperglycemia with physiologic glucose infusion rates.[32]

Blood glucose determinations and screening for glucosuria should be performed several times each day when glucose delivery is initiated or altered.

LIPIDS

Lipid emulsion at a rate of 0.5 to 1 g/day/100 kcal is sufficient to prevent EFA deficiency; however, additional lipids should be provided to supplement nonprotein caloric intake and support growth.[100] Lipids should never make up more than 50% of total caloric intake. Fat emulsions should be given cautiously, beginning with 0.5 to 1 g/kg/day and advanced 0.5 g/kg every 1 to 2 days as tolerated to 3 g/kg/day maximum. Fat emulsions are available as either 10% or 20%, but the 20% concentration is universally used for VLBW infants, because its lower phospholipid concentration results in lower plasma levels of triglyceride and cholesterol and less fluid administration (Table 16-2).[80]

Emulsified fat particles are similar in size and metabolic rate to naturally occurring chylomicrons. Most are cleared through passage in the adipose and muscle tissue. The capillary endothelial lipoprotein lipase hydrolyzes triglycerides and phospholipids, generating free fatty acids (FFAs), glycerol, and other glycerides. Most of the FFAs diffuse into the adipose tissue for re-esterification and storage. A small portion circulates to be used by other tissues for fuel or for conversion by the liver into very-low-density lipoprotein. **Extremely preterm and SGA infants with decreased adipose tissue have prolonged clearance of fat emulsion. In general, because complications of lipids are related to delay in clearance, lipids should be infused over a 24-hour period to provide the lowest hourly rate.[80]** The rate-limiting step for lipid clearance is the metabolism by lipoprotein lipase. The use of heparin stimulates the release of this enzyme and may enhance clearance of IV lipids. Carbohydrate also must be administered with fat to facilitate fatty acid oxidation and to promote FFA clearance.

TABLE 16-2 COMPOSITION OF FAT EMULSIONS

COMPOSITION	INTRALIPID (CLINITEC) 20%	LIPOSYN II (ABBOTT) 20%
FATTY ACID DISTRIBUTION (%)		
Linoleic acid	50	54.5
Oleic acid	26	22.4
Palmitic acid	10	10.5
Linolenic acid	9	8.3
Stearic acid	3.5	4.2
COMPONENTS (%)		
Soybean oil	20	20
Safflower oil	—	—
Egg phospholipids	1.2	1.2
Glycerin	2.25	2.5
Caloric contents (kcal/dL)	200	200
Osmolarity (mOsm/L)	260	292

AMINO ACID SOLUTION

The compositions of two crystalline amino acid solutions available for neonatal parenteral use are presented in Table 16-3. The maximum concentration of the amino acid solution generally is 2% for peripheral use and 3% for central use. Each solution supplies an excess of nonessential amino acids, although more recently available solutions have sought to balance the nonessential amino acid profile.

Cysteine, which is an essential amino acid in preterm infants, is not stable for long periods in solution. This amino acid is commercially available to be added immediately before the solution is administered. TrophAmine and Aminosyn-PF include taurine, which is not available in other solutions.

A minimum quantity of energy substrates must be provided for effective utilization of parenteral protein. For ELBW infants, approximately 40 kcal/kg/day of carbohydrates or fat and 1.5 g/kg/day of protein are necessary for resting metabolic needs to prevent catabolism. However, urinary protein losses are greatest for preterm infants,

TABLE 16-3 CONCENTRATIONS (mg/dL) OF AMINO ACIDS ADJUSTED TO 3% SOLUTION

	SOLUTIONS	
AMINO ACID	AMINOSYN-PF (ABBOTT)	TROPHAMINE (KENDALL McGAW)
ESSENTIAL		
L-Leucine	356	420
L-Phenylalanine	129	144
L-Methionine	54	102
L-Lysine	204	246
L-Isoleucine	228	246
L-Valine	194	234
L-Histidine	94	144
L-Threonine	154	126
L-Tryptophan	54	60
NONESSENTIAL		
L-Alanine	210	162
L-Arginine	369	360
L-Proline	244	204
L-Tyrosine	19	69
L-Cysteine	*	<10*
L-Serine	149	114
L-Glycine	116	108
L-Glutamine	—	—
L-Taurine	21	7.5

*Cysteine hydrochloride supplement may be added.

so additional supplementation is needed to prevent protein deficits. For each gram of protein provided above the basal amount, approximately 10 kcal of nonprotein energy is needed.[25,31,100]

ELECTROLYTES

Sodium and potassium may be supplied with chloride, acetate, or phosphate anions. The daily chloride requirement is approximately 3 mEq/kg/day and should be balanced with acetate to avoid alkalosis or acidosis (acetate is converted to bicarbonate). Amino acid preparations also supply anions that must be recognized to calculate a balanced anion solution. For example, TrophAmine supplies 1 mEq of acetate per gram of protein. On the other hand, cysteine addition to the TPN solution reduces the pH, necessitating buffering with acetate.

MINERALS

Phosphorus may be provided as sodium or potassium phosphate. Calcium may be provided as 10% calcium gluconate (9.7 mg of elemental calcium/100 mg of salt). Both calcium gluconate and potassium phosphate have relatively high levels of aluminum and should be used judiciously for chronic TPN in infants with renal dysfunction (see discussion of aluminum toxicity in the "Trace Elements" section).[43] When preparing a solution with both calcium and phosphate, care must be taken to avoid calcium phosphate precipitation, which may limit the intake of these important minerals. Magnesium is supplied as magnesium sulfate.

If one is using a potassium phosphate solution at pH 7.4, 4.4 mEq of potassium supplies 93 mg of elemental phosphorus (3 mM). When a solution of sodium phosphate is used at pH 7.4, 4.0 mEq of sodium is given with each 93 mg of elemental phosphorus.

CALCIUM

- **Because of increased risk for precipitation, calcium chloride generally should not be used (but may be considered for an infant at risk for aluminum toxicity).**
- **An elevation in ambient temperature, increased storage time, rise in pH, and decrease in protein or glucose concentration may increase the likelihood of precipitation. The addition of cysteine, which lowers solution pH, may enhance calcium and phosphate solubility.[104]**
- **When one is preparing the solution, calcium and phosphate salts should be added separately, but not in sequence, during the last stages of solution mixing. The solubility of the added calcium should be calculated from the volume at the time the calcium is added, not the final volume.**
- **The use of a physiologic ratio of calcium to phosphorus (1.8:1) in the TPN solution allows increased concentration of these minerals.[73,91]**

VITAMINS

A preparation approximating the American Medical Association's recommended formulation of IV vitamins is available (MVI-Ped). **The daily recommended dose is one vial for infants weighing more than 3 kg, 65% vial for infants 1 to 3 kg, and 30% vial for infants less than 1 kg.[4]**

TRACE ELEMENTS

Zinc is supplied as zinc sulfate. Serum zinc levels usually approximate the maternal levels at birth and decline over the first week of life. **By the second week of life, neonates not receiving dietary zinc should have supplementation.** It may be necessary to initiate zinc intake earlier in neonates with intestinal loss, such as after gastrointestinal surgery.

Copper is supplied as cupric sulfate. Approximately two thirds of stored copper is accumulated during the last trimester. Therefore a preterm infant may need early supplementation but a term infant has adequate hepatic stores for at least several weeks. Because copper is excreted through the biliary system, this mineral should be removed from parenteral fluids for infants with cholestasis.[111]

Manganese, chromium, and selenium salts should be provided for long-term parenteral nutrition. Manganese supplementation should not be provided to infants with cholestasis. The chromium dose may be reduced or discontinued in an infant with impaired renal function. A commercially available trace element solution is available that provides zinc, copper, manganese, and chromium.

Traces of aluminum are incorporated into parenteral solutions during processing.[53] Although aluminum is not known to have a physiologic role in the body, high aluminum levels have been associated with bone disease, encephalopathy, anemia, and hepatic cholestasis and may contribute to neurodevelopmental damage in preterm infants on chronic parenteral nutrition.[12] **Infants with disturbance of renal clearance are at greatest risk for aluminum loading.** The U.S. Food and Drug Administration requires manufacturers to report the aluminum content of parenteral products.[43]

Definitions of safe and potentially toxic levels of contamination are available.[6] **Clinicians should attempt to reduce aluminum intake and should monitor levels for infants at highest risk.**[3]

Table 16-4 outlines a suggested composition for a TPN solution (guideline only). Even in the most knowledgeable hands, accurate calculation and ordering of parenteral nutrition for preterm or ill infants is a complex task. Online TPN ordering programs are available in many units to assist the clinician with this task. Use of such programs has been shown to decrease order entry errors.[58] The Case Study on p. 388 illustrates considerations in writing orders for TPN solutions.

TABLE 16-4 SUGGESTED COMPOSITION FOR INTRAVENOUS NUTRITION REGIMEN

COMPONENT	DAILY AMOUNT
CALORIES	
Dextrose 3.4 kcal/g	10-15 g/kg
Lipids 2.0 kcal/mL (20%) solution	1-3 g/kg
Protein (6.25 g protein = 1 g N_2)	3.5-4 g/kg
ELECTROLYTES	
Sodium	3 mEq/kg
Potassium	2-3 mEq/kg
Chloride	3-4 mEq/kg
Acetate	3 mEq/kg
Phosphate	2 mM/kg
Calcium	3 mEq/kg
Magnesium	0.3 mEq (20 mg)/kg
VITAMINS	
MVI-Ped	1 vial*
Vitamin A	0.7 mg
Thiamine (B_1)	1.2 mg
Riboflavin (B_2)	1.4 mg
Niacin	17 mg
Pyridoxine (B_6)	1 mg
Ascorbic acid (C)	80 mg
Ergocalciferol (D)	10 mcg
Vitamin E	7 mg
Pantothenic acid	5 mg
Cyanocobalamin	1 mcg
Folate	140 mcg
Vitamin K	200 mcg
TRACE ELEMENTS	
Zinc (zinc sulfate)†	300 mcg/kg
Copper (cupric sulfate)†	20 mcg/kg
Manganese sulfate†	5 mcg/kg
Chromium chloride†	0.2 mcg/kg
Selenium	2 mcg/kg

*MVI Pediatric (Astra Pharmaceuticals), reduced amount provided for very-low-birth-weight infants (see text).
†As Multitrace-4 Neonatal (American Regent Laboratories, Inc.).

Preparing the Solution

Solutions should be prepared in the hospital pharmacy under a laminar flow hood in a work area isolated from traffic and contaminated supplies.

Case Study

The following case example illustrates considerations in writing orders for total parenteral nutrition (TPN).

History

A male infant born at 26 weeks' gestation at 900 g is now 10 days old and unable to be fed because he has developed necrotizing enterocolitis (NEC). Because there will be a prolonged delay in enteral alimentation, a central vein catheter is placed for TPN. He is currently receiving $D_{10}W$ at 140 mL/kg with maintenance electrolytes. His current weight is 850 g. Serum electrolytes and blood glucose are normal. The approach to calculating TPN requirements is as follows.

Caloric Requirement

Because the patient has already had a significant postpartum period without adequate nutrition, achieving caloric intake necessary for growth is a very important part of his care. The infant will probably require 100 kcal/kg or more for tissue repair and growth. We will begin with approximately 60 to 70 kcal/kg (the birth weight is used until weight gain is established) and advance the intake daily to reach this level.

Carbohydrate

Initially, a dextrose load just above what has been previously tolerated should be used. Thus the patient may receive $D_{12.5}W$ at approximately 140 mL/kg/day; the volume could vary depending on the infant's fluid requirements.

This represents:

$$12.5 \text{ g glucose/dL} \times 140 \text{ mL/kg} = 17.5 \text{ g glucose/kg}$$
$$17.5 \text{ g glucose/kg} \times 3.4 \text{ kcal/g glucose} = 60 \text{ kcal/kg}$$

Fat

Lipid emulsion should be added to increase the caloric intake, starting with 1.0 g/kg/day.

$$5 \text{ mL/kg } 20\% \text{ lipid emulsion } (1.0 \text{ g}) \times 2 \text{ kcal/mL} = 10 \text{ kcal/kg/day}$$

Thus the total non-nitrogen calories on the first day of TPN are 70 (60 + 10).

Protein

Provision of protein nutrition is critical to this preterm infant for growth and to repair damaged tissues. The initial amino acid replacement is 2.5 to 3 g/kg/day.

Electrolytes

The patient should receive maintenance sodium ion (approximately 3 mEq/kg) and potassium ion (2 to 3 mEq/kg) unless there are excessive renal or gastrointestinal losses.

Anions

Balancing anions is the next consideration. The 3 g/kg of amino acids, if given as TrophAmine, adds approximately 3 mEq/kg of acetate to the solution (1 mEq acetate/1 g amino acids). If 3 mEq/kg of potassium is provided as potassium chloride, the solution has balanced anions. Giving 3 mEq/kg of sodium as sodium phosphate provides approximately 2.2 mM/kg of elemental phosphorus:

$$(3 \text{ mM } PO_4/4 \text{ mEq } Na^+) = (3 \text{ mEq } Na^+/\text{kg}) = 2.25 \text{ mM } PO_4$$

Minerals, Vitamins, and Trace Elements

Calcium, magnesium, phosphorus, vitamins, and trace elements should be ordered at this point. Calcium initially should be started at 2 to 3 mEq/kg/day but may be increased as tolerated with growth to 4 to 5 mEq/kg/day.

Use of an online TPN ordering program may assist the clinician by automating many of these calculations.[58]

TPN Orders

Thus the TPN orders would be written for this patient as follows:

125 g Dextrose ($D_{12.5}W$) with the Following per Liter to Run 5.3 mL/hr	***Quantity Provided per kg/day (in 140 mL):***
20 g amino acids	2.8 g AA
20 mEq potassium as potassium chloride	2.8 mEq K^+
	2.8 mEq Cl^-
20 mEq sodium as sodium phosphate	2.8 mEq Na^+
15 mM phosphate*	2.1 mM Phos
20 mEq calcium	2.8 mEq Ca^{2+}
2 mEq magnesium	0.3 mEq
21.7 mL MVI-Ped	3 mL/day
1.3 mL trace element solution†	0.18 mL

Run 20% lipid emulsion at 0.14 mL/hr for 24 hr (approximately 0.5 g/kg of lipids/day).

*3 mM of sodium phosphate = 4 mEq sodium; if potassium phosphate is used, 3 mM of potassium phosphate = 4.4 mEq potassium.

†Commercially available trace element solution (Multitrace[4]—Neonatal, includes zinc, copper, manganese, and chromium).

Progression

On subsequent days, the dextrose concentration and lipids would be advanced slowly to increase the caloric intake to requirement as tolerated. The quantity of protein would also be increased to about 4 g/kg/day.

There should be quality control checks to monitor for sterility breaks in equipment, personnel, environment, and solutions.

Because many additives potentially can be insoluble in combination, a mixing sequence should be established that separates the most incompatible ingredients. Storage increases the risk for microbial contamination; therefore, TPN solutions should be prepared on the day they are needed.[64] However, to be able to provide an amino acid infusion to preterm infants immediately after admission, some units maintain a "stock" amino acid solution (10% dextrose with 3 g of amino acids per 100 mL).[97]

Administering the Total Parenteral Nutrition Solution

Proper administration of the TPN solution is as important as its preparation in preventing complications. The label on the solution always should be checked to correctly identify the patient, using at least two identifiers, and to verify current formulation order.

Standardized procedures must be established to avoid infectious complications from solution contamination. Solutions on the nursing units may be returned to the pharmacy for additives before hanging, but no additives should be placed in the solution once it is hanging. **The bag or bottle of TPN solution should be changed every 24 hours, and the tubing administration sets should be changed at least every 72 hours. Lipid emulsions and tubing should be changed every 24 hours.[16,54,63] Polyvinyl chloride (PVC) tubing and IV bags containing phthalates should be avoided to reduce potential toxicity from plasticizers.[45,71]**

Exposure of TPN to light generates peroxides, which induce vasoconstriction and oxidant stress associated with bronchopulmonary dysplasia (BPD). Photoprotection of bags, syringes, and tubing used to deliver TPN and lipids may reduce the oxidant effect on the lungs and mesenteric blood flow. Light shielding also appears to diminish oxidative stress and alterations of lipid metabolism, resulting in lower levels of triglyceride and better substrate delivery. Amber-colored tubing may be used for this purpose.[18,49,50]

Changes in TPN infusion rates result in changes in glucose delivery to the newborn and may lead to hypoglycemia or hyperglycemia if the glucose homeostatic mechanisms do not adjust fast enough. Reactive hypoglycemia may occur if the glucose load is abruptly discontinued.[9] **Parenteral nutrition solutions must infuse at a constant rate via an infusion pump. Infusion rates should not be increased or decreased. If the parenteral nutrition infusion is suddenly discontinued because of a clotted catheter or accidental removal, an appropriate solution with dextrose should be infused via a peripheral vein and blood glucose should be monitored.**

Use of parenteral nutrition may increase an infant's risk for hyperglycemia during surgery. Because rapid fluid infusions may be necessary during operative procedures, the TPN solution should be discontinued and replaced with a physiologic infusate during the perioperative period. After surgery, TPN should be as when the patient is euglycemic, with recent evidence of early postoperative protein tolerance and improved protein balance.[81]

Tapering of the TPN solution occurs as the infant begins to tolerate enteral feedings. When the patient is taking approximately two thirds of the necessary calories enterally, the central line may be removed.

Administering Fat Solution

Rapid infusion of the fat emulsion may exceed its clearance rate from the body and accentuate complications; therefore fat emulsions should not be infused faster than 0.15 g/kg/hr.[4,80] Lipids generally are given through a Y-site connection to bypass the filter in the TPN line or may be given through a separate venous site. However, some hospitals use a combined dextrose, amino acid, and lipid solution known as ***three-in-one*** or ***total nutrient admixture (TNA).***[83,89] A 1.2-micron filter is used with this solution to remove certain drug precipitates (Ca/PO_4), air, and *Candida,* but it is not effective in removing bacteria. The decision to use TNA should be approached with caution in infants. Lipid emulsions increase the pH of the TPN solution, limiting the amount of calcium and phosphorus that can be delivered because of the risk for precipitation. Precipitates are particularly difficult to detect in TNA, which is a milky solution. High concentration of calcium and low pH of the solution also can disrupt TNA, causing it to "crack," leading to separation of oil from the rest of the solution. One must store the admixture emulsion at an ambient temperature below 28° C to prevent coalescence.[56]

When administering lipids to ill infants receiving other infusions, care must be taken to ensure that medications are compatible with lipids or medications must be provided by a separate intravenous route to prevent precipitation.

COMPLICATIONS

Mechanical Complications

Pneumothorax, hemothorax, hydrothorax, air embolism, thromboembolism, catheter misplacement, cardiac perforation, and tamponade are all recognized complications of Broviac®, subclavian, or jugular catheter insertions. Potential mechanical complications of percutaneous central lines include catheter occlusion, accidental dislodgement, erythematous tracking, phlebitis, thrombosis, superior vena cava syndrome, catheter migration, and catheter entrapment or breakage.[69,72,74,75] A pleural or pericardial effusion may be blood or chyle or may be a signal that the catheter has eroded into the pleural or pericardial space. The effusion may be the infusate. **Therefore chest roentgenogram examination is necessary to document correct catheter placement before a hypertonic solution is instilled.**

The preceding complications may occur at any time while the catheter is present. Documentation of catheter position should be repeated if there is any history of pulling or tension on the catheter or any apparent change in its external position or change in the clinical condition associated with the preceding complications.

Any signs of catheter malfunction require troubleshooting and assessment for potential interventions to salvage the line. Some clinicians will flush a partially occluded line with a thrombolytic agent, such as recombinant tissue plasminogen activator (rt-PA).[48] The risk of this practice must be weighed against the benefits of maintaining the central line. In most cases, if the catheter is a temporary line, it may be better to remove it and place a new line in another site.

Infectious Complications

Infections associated with the central line may occur from contamination of the solution, tubing connections, or hubs. Although organisms may contaminate the solution during preparation, usually **colonization occurs with entry into the line or bag. Intermittent administration of medications, removal of blood samples through the line, or multiple tubing changes provide opportunity for organisms to contaminate the solution.**

Rigid criteria for sterile preparation of the solutions are mandatory (see "Preparing the Solution" section).

An in-line 0.22-μm membrane filter, which is incorporated into the IV tubing, is capable of trapping bacteria and fungi (although not endotoxin) and should help minimize the risk for septicemia from a contaminated IV bag. In addition, filters lessen the risk for an air embolism. An in-line filter setup is available that decreases the number of connections.

Nothing should be added to the TPN solution after it leaves the pharmacy.

AVOIDING LINE COLONIZATION

- When changing IV fluids, one should avoid bleed-back into the catheter.
- Line setups should be designed to minimize the number of ports and connections.[52]
- Generally, medications should not be given into injection ports in the IV tubing but, rather, should be given into a dedicated heparin-locked Y-site entry port. Stopcocks are not recommended.
- The source of an infection is usually contamination with an organism that has colonized the hub or surrounding skin. Scrupulous attention to hand hygiene and disinfection of catheter tubing, hubs, ports, and connections by vigorous rubbing with 70% alcohol before tubing changes or entry are critical infection prevention strategies.[51,52,72]

Dressings are not routinely changed on PICC lines. If the dressing becomes nonocclusive or moistened, the site should be cleaned according to hospital protocol and redressed with a sterile transparent dressing.[87] This should be performed using sterile gloves. The exposed catheter should be remeasured to ensure that it was not inadvertently moved during this process. **Dressings are changed routinely on Broviac®, subclavian, jugular, and femoral catheters.** Dressing changes are recommended at least weekly or more frequently if drainage is noted or the dressing is no longer occlusive.

EVALUATING INFANTS FOR INFECTIOUS DISEASE COMPLICATIONS

Central line–associated bacteremia represents an important source of nosocomial infections in the intensive care nursery. The prevalence of this complication varies by unit, based on patient demographics, including birth weight, gestational age, diagnoses (proportion of surgery and medicine), and care practices.

Bacteremia must be considered in a newborn with a central line in place who presents with signs of sepsis (e.g., temperature instability, lethargy, poor skin perfusion, increased cardiopulmonary distress, apnea). Some neonatal infections may be treated successfully with the line in place. However, if the infant remains systemically ill, even if the blood culture result is negative, the central line should be removed.[13]

Altered immune function by lipid deposition in macrophages and the reticuloendothelial system must be considered in infants with sepsis. *Malassezia furfur* is a lipophilic, opportunistic fungal organism that may cause sepsis in infants receiving long-term lipid infusions.[90] This organism may contaminate the line and appear as a white film. This organism often will not grow in routine blood culture media. Specific culture techniques are necessary when *Malassezia* is suspected.[20]

Guidelines for management of an infant with a central line in place with suspected sepsis are as follows:

- The infant should be evaluated for potential sources of infection, including a general physical examination looking for non–TPN-related sources and inspection of peripheral and central venous sites for erythema.
- Laboratory assessment should include (1) complete blood cell count with platelet count and (2) aerobic blood cultures. Other cultures, including urine, tracheal aspirate, and cerebrospinal fluid, may be indicated, based on clinical findings. A blood fungal culture should be considered if the infant has had preceding antibiotic treatment or signs of fungal infection.[10,11,46]
- A chest x-ray evaluation should be performed if the infant demonstrates signs of respiratory distress or there is a need to reassess catheter position.
- Consider decreasing or discontinuing lipid infusion until the infection has been treated for 24 to 48 hours.[7]
- If the infant is critically ill, the central line should be removed immediately. If the infant is stable, treatment may be considered through the line.
- A positive blood culture generally is considered to indicate bacteremia or sepsis in a newborn with a central line in place. However, the coagulase-negative *Staphylococcus,* an opportunistic organism that is a common cause of catheter-related sepsis, also is normal skin flora and frequently contaminates blood cultures. Use of ancillary diagnostic tools, such as the C-reactive protein levels and complete blood counts, are helpful to distinguish false-positive results from true infections. Some clinicians also recommend obtaining two cultures (two peripheral, or one peripheral and one from the line) before starting antibiotics. If both yield positive results, catheter-related sepsis is confirmed.[65]
- If bacteremia is documented but the sepsis signs are improved, the catheter may remain in place while being used for antibiotic treatment. One should be sure that the antibiotics are compatible with the TPN solution (to avoid stopping the TPN during the antibiotic infusion). A follow-up blood culture and close clinical monitoring are necessary to document that the infection has been treated adequately.

If a central line is pulled because of sepsis, a new central line should not be placed for 48 to 72 hours.

Metabolic Complications

GLUCOSE METABOLISM

Hyperglycemia may occur with increased carbohydrate load, especially in ELBW infants who may have inadequate endogenous insulin production or decreased sensitivity to insulin. Elevated blood sugar may lead to hyperosmolality and osmotic diuresis, resulting in dehydration. Manifestations include polyuria, glucosuria, and excessive weight loss. Serum sodium is not a reliable measure of serum osmolality if there is hyperglycemia. Direct measurement or estimate by use of the following formula is necessary:

$$\text{Serum osmolality} = (1.86)\ Na^{+} + (BUN/2.8) + (Glucose/18)$$

Transient glucose intolerance may be seen with stress. If hyperglycemia occurs without apparent change in glucose infusion, the possibility of sepsis, pain, hypoxemia, intraventricular hemorrhage (especially if the infant is <34 weeks' gestation), or inadvertent increase in carbohydrate administration (mistake in preparation or rate of infusion) should be considered. Glucose intolerance also may be accentuated during infusions of lipid emulsion, especially in an ELBW infant. Discontinuation of the lipid infusion without alteration of the carbohydrate load will often eliminate hyperglycemia in this situation. Some ELBW infants remain hyperglycemic even on reduced carbohydrate intakes. These infants may benefit from a continuous insulin infusion to attain adequate caloric intake. Treatment varies, but the usual infant dose is 1 unit/kg/min.[32] Routine use of insulin to promote growth in the preterm infant is not advised because of side effects.[8]

Hypoglycemia may result from an abrupt interruption of glucose infusion or excessive exogenous insulin administration. Manifestations of hypoglycemia include apnea, lethargy, jitteriness, and seizures. If these signs occur immediately after an interruption of the TPN infusion, an IV glucose infusion must be initiated at once, followed by close monitoring of the blood glucose to allow appropriate glucose administration. The glucose concentration of the infusate may usually be safely decreased by 5 g/dL every 12 hours. Blood glucose values should be monitored hourly until stable after each change.

AMINO ACID METABOLISM

Hyperammonemia may be seen in preterm infants given excessive protein loads. Hyperammonemia will occur also in an infant with a congenital metabolic disturbance, such as a urea cycle defect, when challenged with an amino acid load. **Hyperammonemia may be manifested as somnolence, lethargy, seizures, and coma.** Biochemical screening is necessary to identify this complication before symptoms appear.

Azotemia may occur before hyperammonemia, but blood urea nitrogen (BUN) elevation in the first week of life of a preterm infant is usually associated with dehydration and has not been a reliable marker of protein excess.[25] Therefore, although daily monitoring is common in the first week, rising BUN is not an indication by itself to decrease the protein load.

CHOLESTASIS

Infants receiving TPN for more than 2 weeks frequently develop cholestatic jaundice (direct bilirubin >2 mg/dL).[19,95,98] The risk appears greatest for the least mature infants and those receiving the longest period of TPN without enteral feeding. The cause appears to be multifactorial, including lack of bile flow stimulation, delayed enteral feedings, malnutrition, or inflammation after localized or generalized infection and may be influenced by the amino acid composition of the TPN.[110] Serum amino transferases often are normal early in the clinical course. Serum albumin and prealbumin levels usually remain normal. An abnormality in hepatic synthetic function or early rise in isoenzyme levels should lead the clinician to investigate other forms of liver disease. **The differential of cholestatic jaundice includes the following:**

- **Bacterial sepsis**
- **Congenital viral infection**
- **Postpartum acquisition of cytomegalovirus**
- **Neonatal hepatitis**
- **Bile duct obstruction, such as biliary atresia or choledochal cyst**
- **Galactosemia**
- **Cystic fibrosis**
- **Alpha$_1$-antitrypsin deficiency**

Management of cholestatic jaundice should include (when possible) the following:

- Increase enteral feedings as tolerated and decrease proportionately the parenteral nutrition
- Eliminate copper and manganese from trace minerals in TPN
- Protect solutions from light by covering the bag and IV tubing to reduce levels of light-induced toxic peroxides[49,55]
- Trial of an agent that induces bile flow[17,61]
- For infants with short bowel syndrome, control intestinal bacterial overgrowth[47]
- Consider an alternative type of fat emulsion (Omegaven®)[38,57]

LIPID METABOLISM

High-risk infants, including preterm and SGA low-birth-weight infants, may demonstrate intolerance to fat emulsion infusions. Hyperlipidemia may result, causing elevation of triglyceride, FFA, and lipoprotein levels. In extreme cases, lactescence may be visible in serum on a spun blood specimen (increased plasma turbidity). For screening, a triglyceride level should be checked after initiation of therapy and then weekly and doses adjusted based on results. Steroid therapy may elevate the triglyceride level.[85] Transient hyperglycemia may result from lipid infusion. This complication is usually dose related and rarely requires treatment.[23]

Competitive displacement of bilirubin by FFA theoretically may increase the risk for kernicterus in preterm infants with hyperbilirubinemia. However, studies of preterm infants have indicated lipid infusions may be used in jaundiced infants but attention to the infusion rate and monitoring of FFAs are necessary.[80]

PARENT TEACHING

In-Hospital Total Parenteral Nutrition

Clinicians caring for an ill newborn must be attentive to the involvement and emotional state of the parents. There remain a number of concerns for child abuse, foster placement, and relinquishment among infants who have been cared for in the NICU compared with healthy term newborns, especially when care has been prolonged and complex.

Clinical conditions or policies that promote separation of parents from their infant increase the risk for bonding problems. When a newborn infant cannot be fed orally, an important, normal part of the infant's care is no longer available for the parents. The placement of a central line may be frightening to parents and result in less handling and caregiving. **Infants requiring continuous care, including TPN, should have primary nursing (one regular nurse), and the parents should have regular and consistent communication with a primary physician. Care providers should attempt to keep the parents involved in other parts of the infant's care, because the parents are unable to feed the infant. Parents should be fully informed about the purpose and appropriate care of the infant's central line so they will feel comfortable handling their infant with the line in place.**

A neonatal service that uses TPN has the best results if it includes an experienced "nutrition team," comprising a neonatologist, surgeon, nutrition support nurse, pharmacist, dietitian, and social worker, with each member playing a vital role to make TPN a safe and effective therapy.

Home Total Parenteral Nutrition

Home parenteral nutrition has been used in infants with congenital intestinal anomalies or after massive bowel resection for NEC. TPN is initiated in the hospital. If growing and otherwise well, the infant may be a candidate for TPN at home. Issues to be addressed include ability and willingness of parents to care for the infant at home, available financial support, adequate home setting, pharmacy support services, and additional skilled nursing care needed. The infant should have a more permanent central line placed as early in the discharge process as possible. Parent teaching should begin early, including verbal and written instruction and hands-on practice and return demonstrations (see the Parent Teaching box below.)

Administration of TPN at home is different from hospital administration of TPN and is typically managed by a pediatric gastroenterology service in conjunction with a home infusion therapy or pharmacy service. Infants often go home on a cyclic TPN regimen (12 hr/day). An ambulatory pump improves the mobility and flexibility of the parent and infant and allows a more normal life.

Compliance and success with home TPN are greatly increased when the parents understand the need for and the appropriate way to administer TPN and how to troubleshoot and care for the catheter.[37]

Parent Teaching

HOME ADMINISTRATION OF PARENTERAL NUTRITION

- Strict handwashing and aseptic handling of tubing connections and hubs
- Use of infusion pump
- Monitoring of site for signs of infection, phlebitis, or leaking
- Troubleshooting for occlusion, leaking, extravasation
- Evaluation for signs of systemic infection
- Emergency response to broken or dislodged catheter, loss of electrical power
- Developmental care: oral stimulation, holding, appropriate play activities
- Dressing care and changes
- Monitoring for signs and symptoms of hypoglycemia
- Securing or taping of line to avoid dislodgement with positioning and handling

REFERENCES

1. Adamkin DD, Radmacher P, Rosen P: Comparison of a neonatal versus general-purpose amino acid formulation in preterm neonates, *J Perinatol* 15:108, 1995.
2. Ainsworth SB, Clerihew L, McGuire W: Percutaneous central venous catheters versus peripheral cannulae for delivery of parenteral nutrition in neonates, *Cochrane Database Syst Rev* 2:CD004219, 2004. Accessed August 24, 2009, from www.nichd.nih.gov.
3. American Academy of Pediatrics, Committee on Nutrition: Aluminum toxicity in infants and children, *Pediatrics* 97:413, 1996.
4. American Academy of Pediatrics, Committee on Nutrition: Parenteral nutrition. In Kleinman RE, editor: *Pediatric nutrition handbook,* ed 6, Elk Grove Village, Ill, 2008, The Academy.
5. American Academy of Pediatrics, Committee on Nutrition: Protein. In Kleinman RE, editor: *Pediatric nutrition handbook,* ed 6, Elk Grove Village, Ill, 2008, The Academy.
6. ASCN/ASPEN Working Group on Standards for Aluminum Content of Parenteral Nutrition Solutions: *JPEN J Parenter Enteral Nutr* 15:194, 1991.
7. Avila-Figueroa C, Goldmann DA, Richardson DC, et al: Intravenous lipid emulsions are the major determinant of coagulase-negative staphylococcal bacteremia in very low birth weight newborns, *Pediatr Infect Dis J* 17:10, 1998.
8. Beardsall K, Vanhaesebrouck S, Ogilvy-Stuart AL, et al: Early insulin therapy in very-low-birth-weight infants, *N Engl J Med* 359:1873, 2008.
9. Bendorf K, Friesen CA, Roberts CC: Glucose response to discontinuation of parenteral nutrition in patients less than 3 years of age, *JPEN J Parenter Enteral Nutr* 20:120, 1996.
10. Benjamin DK Jr, Miller W, Garges H, et al: Bacteremia, central catheters, and neonates: when to pull the line, *Pediatrics* 107:1272, 2001.
11. Benjamin DK Jr, Ross K, McKinney RE Jr, et al: When to suspect fungal infection in neonates: a clinical comparison of *Candida albicans* and *Candida parapsilosis fungemia* with coagulase-negative staphylococcal bacteremia, *Pediatrics* 106:712, 2000.
12. Bishop NJ, Morley R, Day JP, et al: Aluminum neurotoxicity in preterm infants receiving intravenous-feeding solutions, *N Engl J Med* 336:1557, 1997.
13. Borghesi A, Stronati M: Strategies for the prevention of hospital-acquired infections in the neonatal intensive care unit, *J Hosp Infect* 68:293, 2008.
14. Brion LP, Bell EF, Raghuveer TS: Vitamin E supplementation for prevention of morbidity and mortality in preterm infants, *Cochrane Database Syst Rev* 3: CD003665, 2003.
15. Cairns PA, Stalker DJ: Carnitine supplementation of parenterally fed neonates, *Cochrane Database Syst Rev* 4: CD000950, 2004.
16. Centers for Disease Control and Prevention: Guidelines for the prevention of intravascular catheter-related infections, *MMWR Recomm Rep* 51(RR-10):1, 2002.
17. Chen CY, Tsao PN, Chen HL, et al: Ursodeoxycholic acid (UDCA) therapy in very-low-birth-weight infants with parenteral nutrition associated cholestasis, *J Pediatr* 145:317, 2004.
18. Chessex P, Harrison A, Khashu M, et al: In preterm neonates, is the risk of developing bronchopulmonary dysplasia influenced by the failure to protect total parenteral nutrition from exposure to ambient light? *J Pediatr* 151:213, 2007.
19. Christensen RD, Henry E, Wiedmeier SE, et al: Identifying patients, on the first day of life, at high-risk of developing parenteral nutrition-associated liver disease, *J Perinatol* 27:284, 2007.
20. Chryssanthou E, Broberger U, Petrini B: *Malassezia pachydermatis* fungaemia in a neonatal intensive care unit, *Acta Paediatr* 90:323, 2001.
21. Clark RH, Thomas P, Peabody J: Extrauterine growth restriction remains a serious problem in prematurely born neonates, *Pediatrics* 111:986, 2003.
22. Coleman MM, Spear ML, Finkelstein M, et al: Short-term use of umbilical artery catheters may not be associated with increased risk for thrombosis, *Pediatrics* 113:770, 2004.
23. Cooke RJ, Yeh YY, Gibson D, et al: Soybean oil emulsion administration during parenteral nutrition in the preterm infant: effect of essential fatty acid, lipid, and glucose metabolism, *J Pediatr* 111:767, 1987.
24. Dahl GB, Svensson L, Kinnander NJ, et al: Stability of vitamins in soybean oil fat emulsion under conditions simulating intravenous feeding of neonates and children, *JPEN J Parenter Enteral Nutr* 18:234, 1994.
25. Denne SC, Poindexter BB: Evidence supporting early nutritional support with parenteral amino acid infusion, *Semin Perinatol* 31:56, 2007.
26. Dinerstein A, Nieto RM, Solana CL, et al: Early and aggressive nutritional strategy (parenteral and enteral) decreases postnatal growth failure in very low birth weight infants, *J Perinatol* 26:436, 2006.
27. Downing GJ, Egelhoff JC, Daily DK, et al: Kidney function in very low birth weight infants with furosemide-related renal calcifications at ages 1 to 2 years, *J Pediatr* 120:599, 1992.
28. Dudrick SJ: Early developments and clinical applications of total parenteral nutrition, *J Parenter Entera Nutr* 27:291, 2003.
29. Ehrenkranz RA: Early, aggressive nutritional management for very low birth weight infants: what is the evidence? *Semin Perinatol* 31:48, 2007.

30. Ehrenkranz RA, Dusick AM, Vohr BR, et al: Growth in the neonatal intensive care unit influences neurodevelopmental and growth outcomes of extremely low birth weight infants, *Pediatrics* 117:1253, 2006.
31. Embleton ND: Optimal protein and energy intakes in preterm infants, *Early Hum Dev* 83:831, 2007.
32. Farrag HM, Cowett RM: Glucose homeostasis in the micropremie, *Clin Perinatol* 27:1, 2000.
33. Farrell PM, Gutcher GR, Palta M, et al: Essential fatty acid deficiency in premature infants, *Am J Clin Nutr* 48:220, 1988.
34. Fenton TR: A new growth chart for preterm babies: Babson and Benda's chart updated with recent data and a new format, *BMC Pediatr* 3:13, 2003.
35. Fomon SJ: Requirements and recommended dietary intake of protein during infancy, *Pediatr Res* 30:391, 1991.
36. Furdon SA, Horgan MJ, Bradshaw WT, et al: Nurses' guide to early detection of umbilical arterial catheter complications in infants, *Adv Neonatal Care* 6:242, 2006.
37. Grant J: Recognition, prevention, and treatment of home total parenteral nutrition central venous access complications, *JPEN J Parenter Enteral Nutr* 26(suppl 5):S21, 2002.
38. Gura KM, Duggan CP, Collier SB, et al: Reversal of parenteral nutrition-associated liver disease in two infants with short bowel syndrome using parenteral fish oil: implications for future management, *Pediatrics* 118:e197, 2006.
39. Hanning RM, Zlotkin SH: Amino acid and protein needs of the neonate: effects of excess and deficiency, *Semin Perinatol* 13:131, 1989.
40. Heird WC: Amino acid and energy needs of pediatric patients receiving parenteral nutrition, *Pediatr Clin North Am* 42:765, 1995.
41. Heird WC: Amino acids in pediatrics and neonatal nutrition, *Curr Opin Clin Nutr Metab Care* 1:73, 1998.
42. Howard D, Thompson DF: Taurine: an essential amino acid to prevent cholestasis in neonates? *Ann Pharmacother* 26:1390, 1992.
43. Hubbard W: Aluminum in large and small volume parenterals used in total parenteral nutrition, *Fed Reg* 63:176, 1998.
44. Infusion Nurses Society: Infusion nursing standards of practice, *J Infus Nurs* 29(suppl 1):S1, 2006.
45. Jaeger RJ, Weiss AL, Brown K: Infusion of di-2-ethylhexylphthalate for neonates: a review of potential health risk, *J Infus Nurs* 28:54, 2005.
46. Karlowicz MG, Hashimoto LN, Kelly RE, et al: Should central venous catheters be removed as soon as candidemia is detected in neonates? *Pediatrics* 106:e63: 2000.
47. Kaufman SS: Prevention of parenteral nutrition-associated liver disease in children, *Pediatr Transplant* 6:37, 2002.
48. Kerner JA, Garcia-Carenga MG, Fisher AA, et al: Treatment of catheter occlusion in pediatric patients, *JPEN J Parenter Enteral Nutr* 30:S73, 2006.
49. Khashu M, Harrison A, Lalari V, et al: Photoprotection of parenteral nutrition enhances advancement of minimal enteral nutrition in preterm infants, *Semin Perinatol* 30:139, 2006.
50. Khashu M, Harrison A, Lalari V, et al: Impact of shielding parenteral nutrition from light on routine monitoring of blood glucose and triglyceride in preterm neonates, *Arch Dis Child Fetal Neonatal Ed* 94(2):F111, 2009.
51. Kilbride HW, Powers R, Wirtschafter DD, et al: Evaluation and development of potential better practices to prevent neonatal nosocomial bacteremia, *Pediatrics* 111:e504, 2003.
52. Kilbride HW, Wirtschafter DD, Powers RJ, et al: Implementation of evidence-based potentially better practices to decrease nosocomial infections, *Pediatrics* 111:e519, 2003.
53. Klein GL: Aluminum in parenteral solutions revisited-again, *Am J Clin Nutr* 61:449, 1995.
54. Kline AM: Pediatric catheter-related bloodstream infections: latest strategies to decrease risk, *AACN Clin Issues* 16:185, 2005.
55. Laborie S, Lavoie JC, Pineault M, et al: Protecting solutions of parental nutrition from peroxidation, *JPEN J Parenter Enteral Nutr* 23:104, 1999.
56. Lee MD, Yoon JF, Kim SI, et al: Stability of total admixtures in reference to ambient temperatures, *Nutrition* 19:886, 2003.
57. Lee S, Gura KM, Kim S, et al: Current clinical applications of omega-6 and omega-3 fatty acids, *Nutr Clin Pract* 21:323, 2006.
58. Lehmann CU, Conner KG, Cox JM: Preventing provider errors: online total parenteral nutrition calculator, *Pediatrics* 113:748, 2004.
59. Leick-Rude MK, Haney B: Midline catheter use in the intensive care nursery, *Neonatal Netw* 25:189, 2006.
60. Leitch CA, Denne SC: Energy expenditure in the extremely low-birth weight infant, *Clin Perinatol* 27:181, 2000.
61. Levine A, Maayan A, Shamir R, et al: Parenteral nutrition-associated cholestasis in preterm neonates: evaluation of ursodeoxycholic acid treatment, *J Pediatr Endocrinol Metab* 12:549, 1999.
62. Lucas A, Morley R, Cole TJ: Randomised trial of early diet in preterm babies and later intelligence quotient, *BMJ* 317:1481, 1998.
63. Matlow AG, Kitai I, Kirpalani H, et al: A randomized trial of 72- versus 24-hour intravenous tubing set changes in newborns receiving lipid therapy, *Infect Control Hosp Epidemiol* 20:487, 1999.
64. McKinnon BT: FDA safety alert: hazards of precipitation associated with parenteral nutrition, *Nutr Clin Pract* 11:59, 1996.

65. Mermel LA, Farr BM, Sherertz RJ, et al: Guidelines for the management of intravascular catheter-related infections, *Infect Control Hosp Epidemiol* 22:222, 2001.
66. Meyer MP, Haworth C, Meyer JH, et al: A comparison of oral and intravenous iron supplementation in preterm infants receiving recombinant erythropoietin, *J Pediatr* 129:258, 1996.
67. Mitsufuji N, Matsuo K, Kakita S, et al: Extravascular collection of fluid around the vertebra resulting from malpositioning of a peripherally inserted central venous catheter in extremely low birth weight infants, *J Perinatal Med* 30:341, 2002.
68. Murphy BP, Inder TE, Huppi PS, et al: Impaired cerebral cortical gray matter growth after treatment with dexamethasone for neonatal chronic lung disease, *Pediatrics* 107:217, 2001.
69. Nadroo AM, Lin J, Green RS, et al: Death as a complication of peripherally inserted central catheters in neonates, *J Pediatr* 138:599, 2001.
70. Nedergaard J, Cannon B: Brown adipose tissue: development and function. In Polin RA, Fox WW, Abman S, editors: *Fetal and neonatal physiology*, ed 3, Philadelphia, 2003, Saunders.
71. Pak VM, Nailon RE, McCauley LA: Controversy: neonatal exposure to plasticizers in the NICU, *MCN Am J Matern Child Nurs* 32:244, 2007.
72. Paulson PR, Miller KM: Neonatal peripherally inserted central catheters: recommendations for prevention of insertion and postinsertion complications, *Neonatal Netw* 27:245, 2008.
73. Pelegano JF, Rowe JC, Carey DE, et al: Simultaneous infusion of calcium and phosphorus in parenteral nutrition for premature infants: use of physiologic calcium/phosphorus ratio, *J Pediatr* 114:115, 1989.
74. Pettit J: Assessment of infants with peripherally inserted central catheters: Part 1. Detecting the most frequently occurring complications, *Adv Neonatal Care* 2:304, 2002.
75. Pettit J: Assessment of infants with peripherally inserted central catheters: Part 2. Detecting less frequently occurring complications, *Adv Neonatal Care* 3:14, 2003.
76. Pettit J: Technological advances for PICC placement and management, *Adv Neonatal Care* 7:122, 2007.
77. Pierro A, Eaton S: Metabolism and nutrition in the surgical neonate, *Semin Pediatr Surg* 17:276, 2008.
78. Poindexter BB, Ehrenkranz RA, Stoll BJ, et al: Parenteral glutamine supplementation does not reduce the risk of mortality or late-onset sepsis in extremely low birth weight infants, *Pediatrics* 113:1209, 2004.
79. Premji S, Fenton T, Sauve R: Does amount of protein in formula matter for low-birthweight infants? *JPEN J Parenter Enteral Nutr* 30:507, 2006.
80. Putet G: Lipid metabolism of the micropremie, *Clin Perinatol* 27:57, 2000.
81. Reynolds RM, Bas KD, Thureen PJ: Achieving positive protein balance in the immediate postoperative period in neonates undergoing abdominal surgery, *J Pediatr* 152:63, 2008.
82. Roberts SA, Ball RO, Moore AM, et al: The effect of graded intake of glycly-L-tyrosine on phenylalanine and tyrosine metabolism in parenterally fed neonates with an estimation of tyrosine requirement, *Pediatr Res* 49:111, 2001.
83. Rollins CJ: Total nutrient admixtures: stability issues and their impact on nursing practice, *J IV Nurs* 20:299, 1997.
84. Rowe MI, Rowe SA: The last fifty years of neonatal surgical management, *Am J Surg* 180:345, 2000.
85. Sentipal-Walerius J, Dollberg S, Mimouni F, et al: Effect of pulsed dexamethasone therapy on tolerance of intravenously administered lipids in extremely low birth weight infants, *J Pediatr* 134:229, 1999.
86. Shah PS, Kalyn A, Satodia P, et al: A randomized, controlled trial of heparin versus placebo infusion to prolong the usability of peripherally placed percutaneous central venous catheters (PCVCs) in neonates: the HIP (Heparin Infusion for PCVC) study, *Pediatrics* 119:e284, 2007.
87. Sharpe EL: Tiny patients, tiny dressings: a guide to the neonatal PICC dressing change, *Adv Neonatal Care* 8:150, 2008.
88. Shulman RJ: Zinc and copper balance studies in infants receiving total parenteral nutrition, *Am J Clin Nutr* 49:879, 1989.
89. Shulman RJ, Phillips S: Parenteral nutrition in infants and children, *J Pediatr Gastroenterol Nutr* 36:587, 2003.
90. Sizun J, Karangwa A, Giroux JD, et al: *Malassezia furfur*-related colonization and infection of central venous catheters: a prospective study in a pediatric intensive care unit, *Intensive Care Med* 20:496, 1994.
91. So K-W, Ng P-C: Treatment and prevention of neonatal osteopenia, *Curr Paediatr* 15:106, 2005.
92. Sogheir LM, Brion LP: Cysteine, cystine or N-acetylcysteine supplementation in parenterally fed neonates, *Cochrane Database Syst Rev* 4: CD004869, 2006.
93. Spencer AU, Yu S, Tracy TF, et al: Parenteral nutrition–associated cholestasis in neonates: multivariate analysis of the potential protective effect of taurine, *JPEN J Parenter Enteral Nutr* 29:337, 2005.
94. Stark AR, Carlo WA, Tyson JE, et al: Adverse effects of early dexamethasone in extremely-low-birth-weight infants: National Institute of Child Health and Human Development Neonatal Research Network, *N Engl J Med* 344:95, 2001.
95. Steinbach M, Clark RH, Kelleher AS, et al, for the Pediatrix Amino-Acid Study Group: Demographic

and nutritional factors associated with prolonged cholestatic jaundice in the premature infant, *J Perinatol* 28:129, 2008.

96. Sunehag A, Gustafsson J, Ewald U: Very immature infants (<30 wk) respond to glucose infusion with incomplete suppression of glucose production, *Pediatr Res* 36:550, 1994.
97. Te Braake FWJ, Van Den Akker CHP, Wattimena DJL, et al: Amino acid administration to premature infants directly after birth, *J Pediatr* 147:457, 2005.
98. Teitelbaum DH, Tracy T: Parenteral nutrition-associated cholestasis, *Semin Pediatr Surg* 10:72, 2001.
99. Thureen PJ, Anderson AH, Baron KA, et al: Protein balance in the first week of life in ventilated neonates receiving parenteral nutrition, *Am J Clin Nutr* 68:1128, 1998.
100. Thureen PJ, Hay WW Jr: Intravenous nutrition and postnatal growth of the micropremie, *Clin Perinatol* 27:197, 2000.
101. Thureen P, Heird WC: Protein and energy requirements of the preterm/low birthweight (LBW) infant, *Pediatr Res* 95R:57:2005
102. Torine IJ, Denne SC, Wright-Coltart S, et al: Effect of late-onset sepsis on energy expenditure in extremely premature infants, *Pediatr Res* 61:600, 2007.
103. Torrence CR, Horns KM, East C: Accuracy and precision of neonatal electronic incubator scales, *Neonatal Netw* 14:35, 1995.
104. Trissel LA, editor: *Handbook on injectable drugs,* ed 12, Bethesda, Md, 2003, American Society of Health-System Pharmacists.
105. Tyson JE, Wright LL, Oh W, et al: Vitamin A supplementation for extremely-low-birth-weight infants, *N Engl J Med* 340:1962, 1999.
106. Uauy R, Hoffman DR: Essential fat requirements of preterm infants, *Am J Clin Nutr* 71(suppl):S245, 2000.
107. Verner A, Craig S, McGuire W: Effect of taurine supplementation on growth and development in preterm or low birth weight infants, *Cochrane Database Syst Rev* 4: CD006072, 2007.
108. Viña J, Vento M, Garcia-Sala F, et al: L-Cysteine and glutathione metabolism are impaired in premature infants due to cystathionase deficiency, *Am J Clin Nutr* 61:1067, 1995.
109. Williford AL, Pare LM, Carlson GT: Bone mineral metabolism in the neonate: calcium, phosphorus, magnesium, and alkaline phosphate, *Neonatal Netw* 27:57, 2008.
110. Wright K, Ernst KD, Gaylord MS, et al: Increased incidence of parenteral nutrition-associated cholestasis with Aminosyn PF compared to TrophAmine, *J Perinatol* 23:444, 2003.
111. Zlotkin SH, Atkinson S, Lockitch G: Trace elements in nutrition for premature infants, *Clin Perinatol* 22:223, 1995.

17 ENTERAL NUTRITION

MARIANNE SOLLOSY ANDERSON, LINDA LEE WOOD, JACQUELINE A. KELLER, AND WILLIAM W. HAY, JR.

Advances in perinatal care have decreased morbidity and mortality for many infants,[80] but the provision of adequate and optimal nutrition to support term and preterm infants in the neonatal intensive care unit continues to be a difficult, though important, challenge. Recent research in neonatal nutrition has provided some evidence-based guidance for clinicians, resulting in the adoption of earlier, more substantial parenteral and enteral strategies for nutrition of newborn infants, particularly those born very preterm. Other research has emphasized the importance of early enteral feeding for the best support of gastrointestinal development, somatic growth, metabolic homeostasis, prevention of infection, and future health. Together, such research has demonstrated that immediate parenteral support and early enteral feedings are fundamental and not optional in neonatal management.

This chapter provides an overview of the physiology of fetal and neonatal nutrition and growth, gastrointestinal anatomic and functional development, and the fundamentals of neonatal nutritional requirements. More specific detail about the assessment and monitoring of growth, feeding strategies and techniques, and the possible complications of enterally feeding at-risk infants is included. The ongoing nutritional needs of infants recovering from complications of preterm birth and other disorders also are presented, as well as the elements of providing for those needs after hospital discharge.

PHYSIOLOGY

Fetal Growth

Fetal growth is regulated by complex genetic, nutritional, endocrine, environmental, and epigenetic factors.[15,42,117] Genetic potential alone has a relatively minor impact.[64,65] Maternal factors such as prepregnancy weight and weight gain during pregnancy directly correlate with fetal size.[1,13,62,114] The quality of the maternal diet (protein, energy, vitamins, minerals) also directly affects fetal growth.[94] In general, however, a large maternal reserve of nutrients is available to the fetus, and in most circumstances, changes in maternal diet do not limit fetal growth.

The growth and function of the placenta strongly determine fetal growth by providing oxygen and essential nutrients.[21,57,58,97] Critical fetal anabolic hormones, such as the insulin-like growth factors (IGF)–I/II and insulin, are regulated by circulating concentrations of nutrients and are themselves regulators of fetal nutrient uptake and metabolism. Apancreatic infants, who have no circulating insulin, are among the most severely growth restricted of all newborns (Figure 17-1); infants of diabetic mothers, who respond to increased maternal-fetal glucose delivery with increased insulin secretion, are among the largest (Figure 17-2). Thyroid hormone also contributes to fetal growth by regulation of oxidative metabolism. Infants with other endocrine deficiencies, such as those resulting from anencephaly, panhypopituitarism, or hypothyroidism, are near normal in age-specific size at birth, indicating a complex interplay between the fundamentally required supply of nutrients to the fetus and the supporting roles of the fetal endocrine milieu that regulates intrauterine growth.

Gastrointestinal Development

Enteral feeding continues to support gastrointestinal development that begins in early fetal life. The fetal gut is anatomically complete by 20 to 22 weeks after conception; functional development of the gastrointestinal system begins in utero and continues into infancy (Table 17-1). In utero, the fetal intestine is exposed to nutrients and growth factors from the mother, placenta, amniotic fluid, and the fetal tissues. The fetal gut is in communication with the external amniotic fluid

Please note that the **PURPLE** type in each chapter is intended to make it easier to identify clinically applicable material.

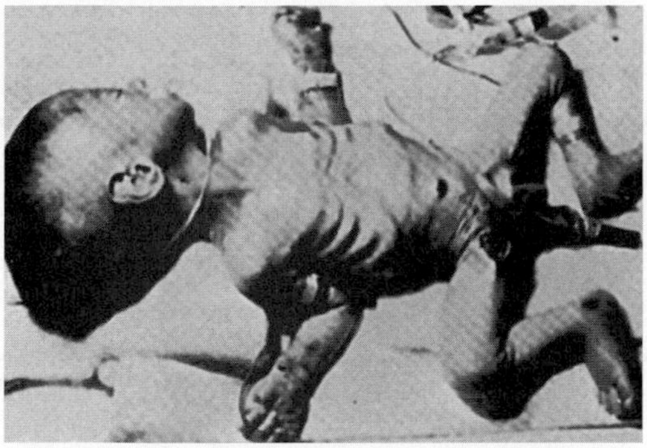

FIGURE 17-1 Term newborn (birth weight 1280 g) with pancreatic agenesis confirmed at autopsy. Plasma insulin was absent. Note marked deficiency of adipose tissue and muscle development. (From Hill D: Effect of insulin on fetal growth, *Semin Perinatol* 2:319, 1978.)

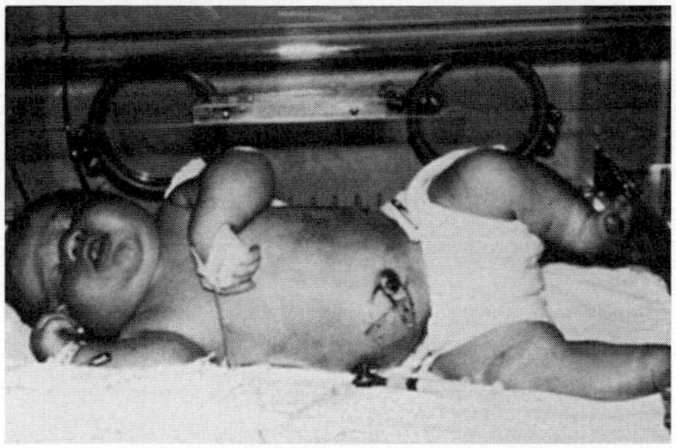

FIGURE 17-2 Characteristic large-for-gestational-age infant of diabetic mother. (Courtesy Newborn Service, University of Colorado Hospital, Denver, Colo [WW Hay, Jr].)

TABLE 17-1 DEVELOPMENT OF THE HUMAN GASTROINTESTINAL TRACT: FIRST APPEARANCE OF DEVELOPMENTAL MARKERS

DEVELOPMENTAL MARKER	WEEKS OF GESTATION
Gastrulation	3
Gut tube formed, early differentiation of foregut, midgut, and hindgut	4
Gut lumen in continuity with amniotic cavity	7
Growth of intestines into umbilical cord	7
Intestinal villus formation	9
Intestines into abdominal cavity	10
Δ glucosidase, dipeptidase, lactase enzymes	10
Glucose transporters	10
Liver lobules, bile metabolism	11
Swallowing	11
Parietal cells, pancreatic islets, bile secretion	12
Stomach fundus, body, pylorus, greater and lesser curvature	14
Gastric glands	14
Intestinal crypts, elongation of intestinal villi	14
Intestinal lymph nodes	14
Differentiation of pancreatic endocrine and exocrine tissue	14
Active transport of amino acids	14
Sucking movements	19
Superficial esophageal glands	20

Data from Lebenthal E: The impact of development of the gut on infant nutrition, *Pediatric Ann* 16:211, 1987; Montgomery RK, Mulberg AE, Grand RJ: Development of the human gastrointestinal tract: twenty years of progress, *Gastroenterology* 116:702, 1999.

Continued

TABLE 17-1 DEVELOPMENT OF THE HUMAN GASTROINTESTINAL TRACT: FIRST APPEARANCE OF DEVELOPMENTAL MARKERS—cont'd

DEVELOPMENTAL MARKER	WEEKS OF GESTATION
Gastric motility and secretion	20
Fatty acid absorption	24
Coordination of suck and swallow	33-36

Data from Lebenthal E: The impact of development of the gut on infant nutrition, *Pediatric Ann* 16:211, 1987; Montgomery RK, Mulberg AE, Grand RJ: Development of the human gastrointestinal tract: twenty years of progress, *Gastroenterology* 116:702, 1999.

environment by 7 weeks post-conception, and early development and functional priming are supplied by growth factors, enzymes, immunoglobulins, and hormones present in that fluid.[87] Fetal swallowing can be observed as early as 11 weeks' gestation.[29] The components of the amniotic fluid, including carbohydrates and amino acids, change during development, as does the volume of amniotic fluid ingested, varying from a few milliliters per day to more than 450 mL per day, or 20% of fetal weight, late in gestation.[10] Amniotic fluid contains growth factors that promote gut cell differentiation. Such growth factors and nutrients in the amniotic fluid stimulate production of enteric hormones that act locally to promote further gut development. The timing of the appearance of gastrointestinal hormones, polypeptides, neurotransmitters, and digestive enzymes in the fetus is variable, but most are present in the gastrointestinal tract by the end of the first trimester of pregnancy. Nutrient transport systems are in place by 14 weeks for amino acids, 18 weeks for glucose, and 24 weeks for fatty acids.

After birth, the gastrointestinal system must further adapt for enteral digestion, absorption, mucosal growth and differentiation, and peristalsis. Some gastrointestinal functions are "switched on" at birth (e.g., decrease in intestinal permeability, increase in mucosal lactase activity), regardless of the length of gestation. Others, however, are intrinsically "programmed" to occur at a certain post-conceptual age (e.g., the onset of peristalsis at 28 to 30 weeks and the coordination of suck, swallow, and breathing at 33 to 36 weeks). Environmental influences, including colonization of the gut by bacteria and the introduction of nutrients into the gut, also affect postnatal gastrointestinal and immunologic development.[2,18,77]

Infants born before term have both anatomic and functional limits to the digestion and tolerance of enteral feedings. Neurologic maturation is important not only for coordination of sucking, swallowing, and breathing during feeding but also for gastrointestinal motility. Peristalsis in the esophagus is immature and bidirectional in the preterm infant, with forward movement of food to the stomach developing only near term.[56] Abnormal esophageal peristalsis and transient relaxations of the lower esophageal sphincter muscle likely contribute to the common problem of gastroesophageal reflux seen in preterm infants. Enteral feeding promotes the ongoing maturation and development of the gastrointestinal system in both the term and preterm infant.[17] Once enteral feedings are established, gastric emptying rate seems to be similar in term and preterm infants.[89,113]

Intestinal motor activity in the preterm infant is immature and disorganized compared with that in term infants, with term infants having distinct fasting phases of gastrointestinal quiescence, nonmigrating motor activity, and migrating motor complexes. After feeding, term infants show a dramatic increase in the intensity of motor activity that is not observed in preterm infants. A measure of gastrointestinal motility is provided by the passage of stool within 24 hours of birth in more than 95% of full-term infants; however, the more preterm the infant, the greater the delay in passing the first stool. Coordinated, mature gastrointestinal motility and peristalsis with feeding develop in the preterm infant between 33 weeks and term.

Protein digestion and absorption are remarkably efficient in the preterm infant despite the fact that enterokinase, a rate-limiting enzyme in the activation of pancreatic proteases, has only 20% of activity found in the term newborn and 10% of adult activity. In the newborn, protein digestion is aided by the activity of brush border and cytosolic peptidases. Carbohydrate absorption is limited by a relative deficiency of lactase, which splits lactose into glucose and galactose. Lactase in the infant of less than 34 weeks' gestation is present at only about 30% of the activity found in the normal term infant, although lactose intolerance is rare in these infants, particularly when they are fed human milk. Preterm infants malabsorb 10% to 30% of dietary fat because of a small bile acid pool size and relative lack of pancreatic lipase.[78] Some compensation is provided by lingual and gastric lipases, as well as the lipase present in human milk. Despite relative deficiencies in many enzymes important in nutrient processing, the preterm infant usually can digest and absorb complex nutrient mixtures such as human milk quite effectively.

Postnatal Growth of Preterm Infants

After birth, usual nutritional regimens, even when provided more aggressively, fail to produce growth rates in preterm infants that mimic normal rates of intrauterine growth, the accepted goal of nutrition for the preterm infant.[27,32,96] A variety of complications contribute to this growth failure, but the primary problem is that most preterm infants are fed less protein and calories immediately after birth than are needed to support normal fetal rates of protein accretion and body growth. In addition, the preterm infant is exposed to environmental factors that increase energy expenditure, including low relative humidity and radiant and convective heat losses, as well as energy-consuming demands of breathing, resistance to gravity, and the processes of digestion, absorption, and synthesis of nutrients into body structure. Stress-induced hormones that are catabolic in sick infants, particularly corticosteroids and catecholamines, limit the production and action of anabolic growth factors, particularly insulin and IGFs, further preventing normal rates of growth and weight gain at rates comparable to those of healthier infants of the same gestational age. Overall, however, even in sick or physiologically unstable infants, the principal factor causing postnatal growth failure is delayed and inadequate intake of protein and energy.[32]

After birth, all infants lose excess extracellular salt and water. Term infants usually lose 5% to 8% of birth weight by the third day of life. In extremely-low-birth-weight (ELBW, <1000 g birth weight) preterm infants, normal diuresis and fluid management strategies to limit fluid overload over the first 10 to 14 days of life usually produce a net loss of body weight. Such infants may lose 8% to 15% of birth weight. Further weight loss and failure to gain weight are exacerbated by inadequate nutritional support, particularly of protein and energy. Deficits accumulated daily during early neonatal life may take weeks to months to replenish. Accurate measurement of body length can be helpful in the early newborn period. More recent methodologies to assess the neonate include (1) dual x-ray absorptiometry (DXA), and (2) air displacement plethysmography, which partitions new tissue accrual into water, fat, and lean body mass components, thus helping define needs for additional specific nutrients (protein, lipids, carbohydrates) for body growth (even during the early postnatal period of fluctuating water weight). Early provision of both adequate calories and protein to sustain optimal nutrition is difficult without the addition of parenteral nutrition for preterm infants and sick infants of all gestational ages (see Chapter 16).

Assessment of Growth and Nutritional Status

The generally accepted goal of postnatal nutrition for preterm infants is to achieve and maintain the normal rate of intrauterine growth (Figure 17-3). Unfortunately, there is no clear standard for normal fetal growth. Many growth curves have been developed from anthropometric measurements taken at birth in populations of infants born at different gestational ages.[3,32] Because preterm birth is not a normal outcome, cross-sectional anthropometric measurements obtained at birth do not accurately describe normal growth parameters for any given gestational age. Growth curves based on serial ultrasound measurements of fetuses who were born at term in healthy condition and with normal measurements provide continuous, rather than cross-sectional, data that correlate better with the expected fetal growth rate of a particular fetus or newborn (Figure 17-4).[16,36] **For the average, appropriately grown, preterm infant, expected weight gain is approximately 15 to 20 g/kg/day.**

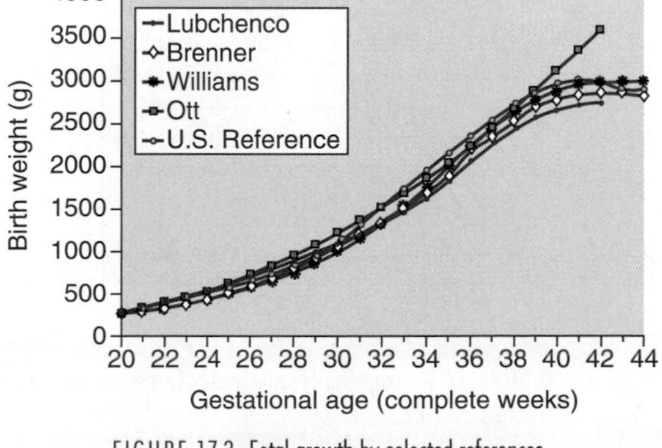

FIGURE 17-3 Fetal growth by selected references.

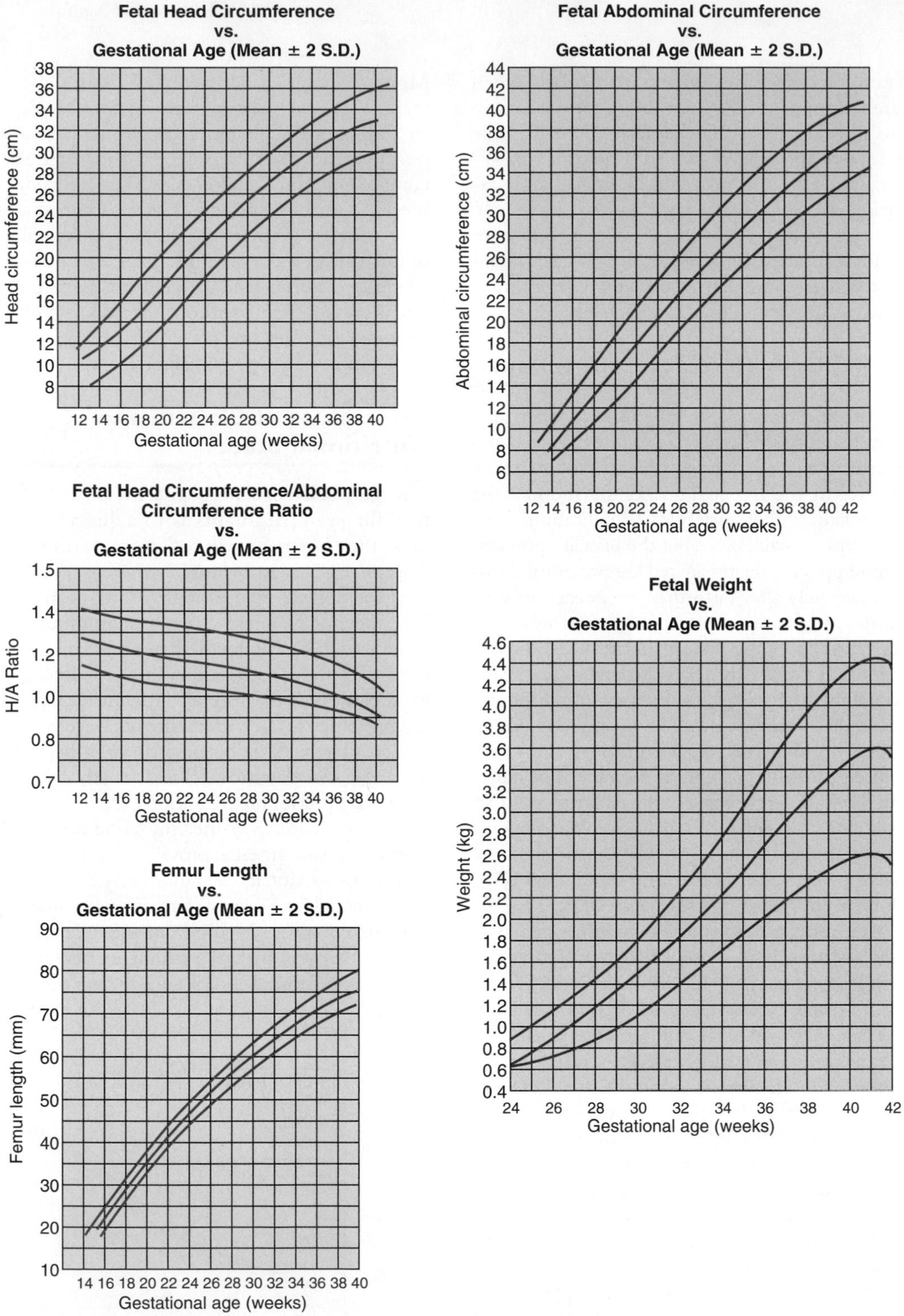

FIGURE 17-4 Composite of serial fetal body measurements by ultrasound examination. *H/A,* Head/abdominal circumference; *S.D.,* standard deviation.

We lack good methods to assess nutritional adequacy over time in very small infants. Rates of change in anthropometric measurements provide some retrospective information, but they do not tell us what an infant needs to maintain a normal growth rate (Box 17-1; Figure 17-5). Too often, growth charts simply document the failure to provide adequate nutrition during the previous days to weeks. Indirect calorimetry offers some advantage, but instruments that are clinically practical and sufficiently accurate to quantify nutrient metabolism in tiny infants are not yet available. Similarly, application of stable isotope methodology to measure utilization and oxidation rates of individual nutrients remains confined to large medical centers with expensive and sophisticated mass spectrometry facilities. Evaluation of an individual infant's immediate nutrient requirements and responses to the administration of different mixtures and amounts of nutrients remains an elusive but still necessary goal.

NUTRITIONAL REQUIREMENTS

Nutritional requirements should be considered in general categories: energy (or calories), protein, carbohydrate, fats, minerals and solutes, and vitamins. Water requirements and limits also must be considered when designing nutrition support strategies. The source, complexity, and constituents of these nutrients are important, as well as the route of administration. Box 17-2 on p. 405 lists commonly used nutritional conversion factors and formulas. See Chapter 16 for parenteral nutrition and Chapter 18 for breast feeding.

BOX 17-1 GROWTH MONITORING

1. ***Weight*** is subject to large variations based on fluctuations in fluid balance (e.g., presence or absence of edema, congestive heart failure, renal failure) and attached equipment (e.g., intravenous lines and boards, endotracheal tubes). Infant weight should be measured daily as follows:
   a. Use the same scale and weigh infant naked or using supportive weighing method as possible. Supportive weighing, or swaddled weights, help ensure an infant's physiologic and behavioral stability during the weighing procedure.[61] Remove "attached" equipment if possible, or weigh similar items separately and subtract from total weight. Swaddled weights are equal to the naked weight after the weight of the diaper and blanket are subtracted. Unswaddled weights still can be used to improve accuracy for very small infants or if swaddling puts the infant at risk or interferes with the infant's care needs. In-bed scales are useful for extremely-low-birth-weight infants or infants who become unstable with handling. An electronic scale that averages several measurements reduces movement artifact and may be useful for active infants.
   b. Reference standards for the weights of nursery equipment (e.g., diapers, intravenous boards, tubing, endotracheal tubes) should be available for nursery use.
   c. Weigh the infant at the same time daily, preferably before a feeding.
   d. Record the infant's weight, the time of weight measurement, and the scale used on the chart. Energy (calories) and fluid intake should be recorded on the same chart. This information combined with biochemical parameters (e.g., serum electrolytes, hemoglobin, albumin) and the physical examination provides the best overview of the infant's nutritional status. Daily weight should be plotted on the appropriate preterm or term growth chart. Weekly review of the infant's weight change provides useful information on trends in overall growth or weight loss that may be overlooked in the daily charting.
2. ***Crown-heel length and head circumference*** are measured and recorded on admission and at least weekly thereafter. Accurate length measurements are difficult to obtain without special equipment such as a length board, but accuracy can be improved by repeated measurements and use of the tonic-neck reflex to straighten the hip and knee. Increase in head circumference is used as an indicator of brain growth.
   a. To measure the crown-heel length, place the infant supine on a firm surface with the knees extended and the ankles flexed 90 degrees. Measure the length from the top of the head (crown) to the bottom of the heel.
   b. Head circumference is obtained using a paper or soft tape measure. Record the largest measurement obtained with the tape placed over the frontal, parietal, and occipital prominences.
3. ***The ponderal index*** (or weight-length index; see Figure 17-5) is used to assess "quality" of growth. The index is calculated as the weight in grams multiplied by 100, divided by the cube of the length in centimeters. True organ growth and tissue accretion are accompanied by increases in both weight and length and can be evaluated partly using the ponderal index.
4. ***Biochemical monitoring*** of the growing infant may include periodic measurement of serum electrolytes, calcium, phosphorus, alkaline phosphatase, total protein, albumin, and hemoglobin. These data can be used to help prevent specific deficiencies in the diet, such as hyponatremia in preterm infants with excessive renal solute losses or hypophosphatemia with increased alkaline phosphatase as seen in rickets and osteopenia.

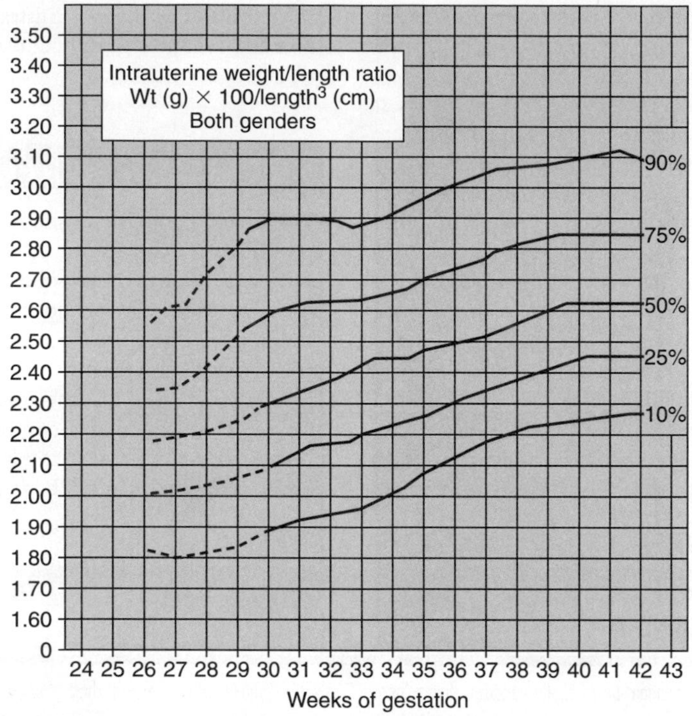

FIGURE 17-5 Ponderal index. (From Lubchenco L, Hansman C, Boyd E: Intrauterine growth in length and head circumference as estimated from live birth at gestational ages from 26 to 42 weeks. Reproduced with permission from *Pediatrics* 37:403, 1966, copyright by the American Academy of Pediatrics.)

Energy

Negative energy balance is frequent in preterm infants because they have limited energy stores, high energy expenditures, and low intake. Energy requirements are determined by an infant's total energy expenditure, energy excretion, and energy stored in new tissue as growth. Total energy expenditure can be subdivided into contributions of basal metabolic rate, activity, thermoregulation, and the energy costs of digestion and metabolism. Energy excretion is composed of fecal and urinary losses, as well as heat lost by radiation and evaporation. Nursing infants in thermoneutral, humidified incubators, starting at admission to the NICU, can substantially decrease energy expenditure in preterm infants. Estimates of energy requirements for growing preterm infants are shown in Table 17-2 on p. 406. The large range of these estimates reflects the variability of infant activity and environmental conditions. Therefore it is essential to adjust nutrient delivery to individual requirements. For example, if an infant is particularly active and showing poor growth, nutrient delivery should be adjusted upward accordingly.

Caloric requirements for the healthy term infant average 110 kcal/kg/day, much lower than the energy requirements of preterm infants. Increased energy requirements can be anticipated during sepsis, acute and chronic respiratory illness, and recovery from surgery (Figure 17-6). Daily caloric intake should be calculated for each infant growing or recovering from illness in the neonatal intensive care unit. A useful approach for calculating caloric intake is shown in Box 17-3 on p. 407.

Protein

Protein accretion is critical for normal growth. The amount and type of protein necessary for optimal growth in preterm infants have been difficult to establish. Metabolic balance studies support a need for higher protein intakes in the growing preterm infant than in the term infant. Throughout the normal period of breast feeding, the concentration of protein in human milk decreases; however, the preterm infant's need for protein continues to be much

BOX 17-2 COMMONLY USED CONVERSION FACTORS AND FORMULAS

Energy
- 1 kcal = 4.184 kJ

Gross energy (kcal/g)
- Protein = 5.65
- Carbohydrate = 3.95
- Fat = 9.25

Metabolizable energy (kcal/g)
- Protein = 4
- Carbohydrate = 4
- Fat = 9

Protein
- Total protein (g/dL) = total nitrogen (g/dL) × 6.25

Vitamins
- 1 International unit vitamin A = 0.3 retinol equivalent
  - = 0.3 mcg retinol
  - = 1.8 mcg beta-carotene
- 400 International units vitamin D = 10 mcg vitamin D
- 1 International unit vitamin E = 1 mg DL-α-tocopherol

Minerals
- 1 mEq Na = 1 mmol Na = 23 mg Na
- 1 mEq K = 1 mmol K = 39 mg K
- 1 mEq Cl = 1 mmol Cl = 35 mg Cl
- 2 mEq Ca = 1 mmol Ca = 40 mg Ca
- 1 mmol P = 31 mg P

Osmolarity (mOsm/L) = Osmolality (mOsm/kg H_2O) × kg H_2O/L solution

Renal solute load (mOsm/dL) = [Protein (g/dL)] × 4 + [Na + K + Cl (mEq/dL)]

Potential renal solute load (mOsm/dL) = [Protein (g/dL)] × 5.7 + [Na + K + Cl (mEq/dL)] + [P (mg/dL)/31]

higher than the term infant. Mature human milk provides adequate protein to meet the recommended goals of 2 to 2.5 g/kg/day for term infants, but it is inadequate to meet the goals of 3.5 to 4 g/kg/day for preterm infants.[74] In one study, preterm infants receiving both protein and energy supplementation during enteral feedings (to as much as 3.6 g/kg/day protein and 149 kcal/kg/day energy) had increased gains only in length and head circumference in relation to increased protein intake. In the same study, extra energy increased primarily weight and triceps skinfold thickness, demonstrating the need for protein to grow bone, brain, and lean body mass, whereas excess energy leads primarily to increased fat deposition (Figure 17-7).[59,60] These benefits unique to protein and energy have since been supported by a Cochrane Review of the literature.[68]

Although infants with growth failure may be at higher neurodevelopmental risk,[40] it has been difficult to establish long-term benefits to developmental outcome with particular feeding strategies. Studies of preterm infants maintained on diets fortified with protein and energy have shown improved neurodevelopmental test scores in early life. Neurodevelopmental outcome appears to be even better when human milk is supplemented with protein and energy.[75,76] More recent studies have shown such benefits extended into adolescence when previously preterm infants had increased brain size, caudate nucleus volume, and intelligence quotient (IQ) in direct relation to their protein and energy intake during their postnatal period.[51,54]

Human milk from an infant's own mother is unique and the preferred source of protein for that newborn. Human milk contains whey-predominant protein (whey:casein ratio of 70-80: 30-20), whereas cow's milk has a whey:casein ratio of 18:82. Whey protein is particularly rich in essential and conditionally essential amino acids. Milk expressed from mothers of preterm infants is somewhat higher in protein than milk from mothers of term infants. Nonetheless, fortification of preterm maternal milk with protein (as well as calcium, phosphorus, sodium, potassium, and lipid) usually is necessary to promote growth rates approximating those of normal human fetuses, particularly in the very-low-birth-weight (VLBW) preterm infant.[99] Given the multiple benefits of mother's milk feeding for preterm infants, including provision of antimicrobial factors and improved feeding tolerance, mother's milk feeding with protein and energy supplementation, (e.g., with Enfamil® Human Milk Fortifier produced by Mead Johnson Nutritionals or Similac® Human Milk Fortifier produced by Abbott Nutrition) is highly recommended (see Table 17-3 on p. 408). A human milk–based fortifier, ProlactPlus HMF™ (Prolacta Bioscience, Monrovia, Calif.), is also available.

An average protein intake of 3.5 g/kg/day is recommended for most preterm infants born before 30 weeks' gestation. Protein requirements are higher (4.0 g/kg/day) in ELBW infants (i.e., <27 weeks' gestation and <1000 g). Growth should be monitored and supplementation provided expectantly. Term infants in general do not require protein or energy supplementation unless their dietary fluid is restricted because of illness (e.g., congestive heart failure).

TABLE 17-2 ESTIMATED DAILY ENERGY REQUIREMENT (kcal/kg) FOR PRETERM INFANTS

		EUROPEAN SOCIETY OF GASTROENTEROLOGY AND NUTRITION	
FACTOR	AMERICAN ACADEMY OF PEDIATRICS	AVERAGE	RANGE
Energy expenditure			
Resting metabolic rate	50	52.5	45-60
Activity	15	7.5	5-10
Cold stress	10	7.5	5-10
Energy cost of digestion	8	17.5	10-25
Energy stored	25	25	20-30
Energy excreted	12	20	10-30
Total requirements	120	130	95-165

Modified from American Academy of Pediatrics, Committee on Nutrition: Nutrition needs of low-birthweight infants, *Pediatrics* 112:622, 1988; Committee on Nutrition of the Preterm Infant, European Society of Pediatric Gastroenterology and Nutrition: *Nutrition and feeding of the preterm infant,* Oxford, UK, 1987, Blackwell.

	Normal Requirements		Likely Changes in Requirements with Illness						
	Well Term	Well Preterm	RDS	CLD	CHD Cyanotic	CHD CHF	Sepsis	NEC/SBS	IUGR
Free water (mL/kg)	100 to 120	120 to 140	↓	↓	Ø	↓	↑	↑	↑
Energy (kcal/kg)	100	120	↑	↑↑	↑	↑↑	↑↑	↑↑	↑
Carbohydrate (g/kg)	10	12 to 14	↑	↓	↑	↑	↑	↑	↑
Protein (g/kg)	1.5 to 2.2	3.0 to 4.0	Ø	↑	↑	↑	↑↑	↑	↑
Fat (g/kg)	3.3 to 6	4 to 7	Ø	↑	↑	↑	Ø	↑↑*	↑
Calcium (mg/kg)	45 to 60	120 to 230	Ø	↑↑•♦	↑◊	↑•◊	Ø	↑*	↑
Iron (mg/kg)	1	2 to 4	Ø	↑♦	↑	Ø	Ø	↑	↑
Vitamin A (IU/kg)	333	700 to 1500	↑◊	↑◊	Ø	Ø	Ø	Ø	Ø

Ø No change.

* Particularly with loss of the terminal ileum.

• Particularly with calciuric diuretics such as furosemide.

◊ Particularly if postoperative.

♦ In <1500-g preterm infants.

FIGURE 17-6 Daily nutritional requirements and changes with illness. *CHD,* Congenital heart disease; *CHF,* congestive heart failure; *CLD,* chronic lung disease; *IUGR,* intrauterine growth restriction; *NEC,* necrotizing enterocolitis; *RDS,* respiratory distress syndrome; *SBS,* short bowel syndrome. (Modified from Thureen P, Hay WW Jr: Conditions requiring special nutritional management. In Tsang RC, Lucas A, Uauy R, et al, editors: *Nutritional needs of the preterm infant,* Baltimore, 1993, Williams & Wilkins.)

The amino acid profile in the newborn diet is as important as the amount of protein provided. Growth rate of lean body mass is determined directly by the intake of the essential amino acids. Conditionally, or developmentally, essential amino acids (those that are uniquely required in larger amounts at certain developmental stages and cannot be synthesized at sufficient rates for requirements [e.g., cysteine, taurine, histidine, arginine, lysine]) also are important to the infant, especially if preterm. Normal growth,

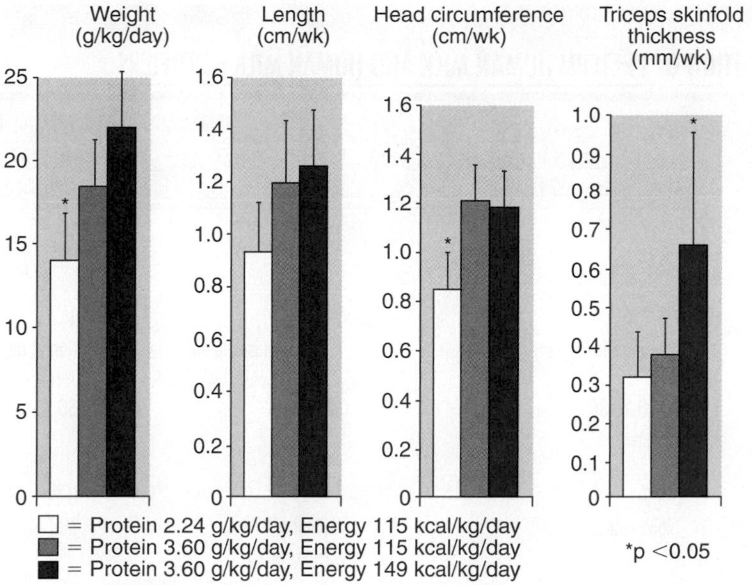

FIGURE 17-7 Growth rates with varying protein and energy intakes. (From Kashyap S, Schulze KF, Forsyth M, et al: Growth nutrient retention and metabolic response in low-birth-weight infants fed varying intakes of protein and energy, *J Pediatr* 113:713, 1988; Kennaugh JM, Hay WW, Jr: Nutrition of the fetus and newborn, *West J Med* 147:435, 1987.)

BOX 17-3 CALCULATING DAILY CALORIC INTAKE (kcal/kg/day)

Conversion Factors

20 kcal/oz = 0.67 kcal/mL
24 kcal/oz = 0.80 kcal/mL
1 kcal = 1 calorie
1 oz = 30 mL

Calculation

1. Add total daily feeding intake (in mL)
2. Divide total intake (mL) by the infant's weight (kg)
   This equals enteral intake in mL/kg/day
3. Multiply mL/kg/day intake by kcal per ounce of feeding
4. Multiply by 1 oz/30 mL

This equals enteral intake in kcal/kg/day.

energy metabolism, and immune function depend on appropriate availability of these amino acids. Particularly in the rapidly growing infant, growth requirements may not be met by the relatively limited intake of essential amino acids common with most current nutritional regimens or by the limited biosynthesis of conditionally essential amino acids.

Fat

Human neonates are unique among neonatal mammals in having a relatively high white fat content of 16% to 18% of body weight at term. The term infant also has stores of brown fat, which is necessary for neonatal thermogenesis. In utero fat deposition occurs predominantly during the last 12 to 14 weeks of gestation. Thus infants born preterm are deficient in fat stores, both for use as energy and for thermogenesis. Dietary fats are important to sustain growth, provide essential fatty acids, and promote the absorption of fat-soluble vitamins. Newborn infants absorb fat less efficiently than older children. Preterm infants demonstrate even greater deficiencies in fat digestion and metabolism. Pancreatic lipase and bile acids are less available for fat digestion and absorption. Lingual and gastric lipases, present in newborn secretions, compensate for deficient pancreatic lipase, as does mammary gland lipase if the infant is receiving breast milk. Current recommendations for dietary fat consist of provision of 40% to 52% of total calories (4.4 to

TABLE 17-3 **COMPOSITION OF PRETERM HUMAN MILK AND HUMAN MILK FORTIFIERS**

		HUMAN MILK FORTIFIERS (per 4 PACKETS)	
	MATURE PRETERM HUMAN MILK (28 DAYS, APPROXIMATE per 100 mL*)	ENFAMIL® HUMAN MILK FORTIFIER†	SIMILAC® HUMAN MILK FORTIFIER‡
Energy (kcal)	67-75	14	14
PROTEIN			
Amount (g)	1.3-1.8	1.1	1
Source	Human milk	Milk protein isolate and whey protein isolate hydrolysate	Nonfat milk and whey protein concentrate
Whey:casein ratio	70-80:20-30	60:40	60:40
FAT			
Amount (g)	3-3.9	1	0.36
Source	Triglycerides	MCT oil (70%) Soy oil (30%)	MCT oil
CARBOHYDRATE			
Amount (g)	6-11	<0.4	1.8
Source	Lactose and glucose	Mineral salts and corn syrup solids	Corn syrup solids
MINERALS			
Calcium (mg)	25	90	117
Phosphorus (mg)	13	50	67
Sodium (mEq))	0.9 ± 0.2	0.7	0.7
Potassium (mEq)	1.2 ± 0.3	0.7	1.6
Chloride (mEq)	1.5 ± 0.2	0.4	1.1
Iron (mg)	0.2	1.44	0.35
Zinc (mg)	0.3	0.72	1
Magnesium (mg)	3	1	7
OTHER CHARACTERISTICS			
Potential renal solute load (mOsm/100 mL)	12.6	9.7	11.2
Osmolality (mOsm/kg water)	290	+35 (above human milk when mixed)	+90 (above human milk when mixed)

This table lists the major constituents; refer to product inserts for a complete listing of vitamins, minerals, and trace elements.
MCT, Medium-chain triglyceride.
*Data from Klein CJ, editor: Nutrient requirements for preterm infant formulas, *J Nutr* 132:1395S, 2002.
†Mead Johnson Nutritionals, Evansville, Indiana.
‡Ross Products Division, Abbott Nutrition, Columbus, Ohio.

5.7 g/100 kcal). Long-chain polyunsaturated fatty acids (LC-PUFAs) are essential for normal growth and development, particularly of the retina and brain. LC-PUFA supplementation, therefore, has been a topic of much discussion and research in recent years. Of particular interest are the n-3 and n-6 essential fatty acids, alpha-linolenic acid (ALA) and linoleic acid (LA), and their metabolites, docosahexaenoic acid (DHA) and arachidonic acid (ARA), respectively.[52] Both term and preterm human milk contain considerable quantities of linolenic acid. The preterm infant can synthesize DHA from its precursor linolenic acid, but whether the synthesized amount is sufficient remains uncertain. Human milk also contains preformed LC-PUFAs. In an effort to make formula more like the gold-standard human milk, manufacturers in the United States have added DHA and ARA to both term and preterm infant formulas.

LC-PUFA supplementation is thought to be safe for both term and preterm infants.[34,37,53,67] The evidence for long-term benefit, however, particularly for term infants, is mixed.[39,107] The inconsistent conclusions among studies have been recently reviewed.[48] For preterm infants, in whom PUFAs are particularly important for growth and brain and visual development and who have not had the opportunity for late gestation accumulation of fats, there may be benefit and little risk with supplementation.[39,66,102] Areas of ongoing research include (1) maternal supplementation of n-3 long-chain polyunsaturated fats to promote fetal growth and improve the length of gestation, (2) exploration of the effects of LC-PUFAs on preventing necrotizing enterocolitis, and (3) the relationship of neonatal fat composition to the development of atherosclerosis in later life.

Medium-chain triglycerides (MCTs) do not require bile salts for absorption and can be directly absorbed into the portal venous circulation. This offers theoretical advantages for the preterm infant, although there is little evidence that inclusion of MCTs improves growth of the healthy preterm infant. MCTs do improve fat absorption and energy intake in infants with hepatic dysfunction or short bowel syndromes.

Some fats (e.g., essential fatty acids) are essential for normal infant growth. All fatty acids provide a concentrated source of energy. The polyunsaturated n-3 fatty acids are important components of cell membranes, particularly significant for the developing nervous system. There is no place for "fat restriction" in the nutritional support of preterm or term infants within the guidelines just mentioned.

Carbohydrates

Carbohydrate reserves begin to accumulate as glycogen in the developing fetus as early as the start of the second trimester. Most of this glycogen (as much as 90% of total body glycogen in term infants) serves local cellular needs in different organs, whereas hepatic glycogen specifically provides glucose for other glucose-dependent tissues, primarily the brain. Immediately after birth, with cessation of glucose supply from the placenta, the neonate must use stored glycogen for energy. The newborn can exhaust the supply of stored glucose from the liver within 12 hours of birth under severely stressful conditions (e.g., hypoxia, hypotension, increased catecholamine and glucagon release) if food or IV glucose is not provided. The normal glucose utilization rate in the term newborn is 4 to 6 mg/kg/min. The brain accounts for most of the glucose use, especially in preterm and asymmetrically growth-restricted infants, who have a larger-than-normal brain:body-weight ratio.

The predominant carbohydrate in human milk is lactose, a disaccharide composed of glucose and galactose. Glucose has a central role in energy metabolism. Galactose provides 50% of the calories derived from lactose; its major metabolic role is in energy storage, because the newborn liver readily incorporates galactose from the portal circulation into hepatic glycogen.

Provision of 40% to 50% of total caloric intake as carbohydrate (12 to 14 g/kg/day) prevents accumulation of ketone bodies and other adverse metabolic effects (e.g., hypoglycemia) in the newborn. This amount of carbohydrate generally is supplied as lactose in human milk or commercial formulas. If there are signs of lactose intolerance, such as frequent loose stools, abdominal distention or apparent cramping, or positive stool reducing substances (Clinitest), then a portion of the carbohydrate may be given as sucrose or glucose polymers. Glucose polymers have the added advantage of keeping formula osmolality low. Lactose-free infant formulas are commercially available (Table 17-4). Use of such non-lactose products should be reserved for those rare infants with clinically proven lactose intolerance.

Vitamins

Vitamins are organic substances that are present in trace amounts in natural food sources and are essential to normal metabolism. Lack of vitamins in the diet produces well-recognized deficiency states in

TABLE 17-4 COMPARATIVE NUTRITIONAL COMPOSITION OF TERM INFANT FEEDINGS per 100 kcal

		COW'S MILK–BASED				SOY PROTEIN–BASED	
				LACTOSE FREE			
	MATURE HUMAN MILK (28 DAYS)*	ENFAMIL® LIPIL® WITH IRON†	SIMILAC® ADVANCE® WITH IRON‡	ENFAMIL® LACTOFREE® LIPIL®†	SIMILAC® SENSITIVE® WITH IRON‡	ENFAMIL® ProSobee® LIPIL®†	SIMILAC® ISOMIL® ADVANCE®‡
Nutrient density (kcal/oz)	20	20	20	20	20	20	20
Energy (kcal)	98-110	100	100	100	100	100	100
PROTEIN							
Amount (g)	1.8	2.1	2.07	2.1	2.14	2.5	2.45
% Total calories	7	8.5	8	8.5	9	10	10
Source	Human milk	Reduced minerals; whey and nonfat milk	Nonfat milk and whey protein concentrate	Milk protein isolate	Milk protein isolate	Soy protein isolate	Soy protein isolate and L-Methionine
FAT							
Amount (g)	4.3-4.9	5.3	5.4	5.3	5.4	5.3	5.46
% Total calories	50	48	49	48	49	48	49
Source	Triglycerides	Palm olein Soy oil Coconut oil High oleic vegetable oil Single cell oil products (DHA and ARA)	High oleic safflower oil Soy oil Coconut oil Single cell oil products (DHA and ARA)	Palm olein Soy oil Coconut oil High oleic vegetable oil Single cell oil products (DHA and ARA)	High oleic safflower oil Soy oil Coconut oil	Palm olein Soy oil Coconut oil High oleic vegetable oil Single cell oil products (DHA and ARA)	High oleic safflower oil Soy oil Coconut oil Single cell oil products (DHA and ARA)
Linoleic acid (mg)	440-1500	860	1000	860	1000	860	1000

CARBOHYDRATE							
Amount (g)	10-11	10.9	10.8	10.9	10.7	10.6	10.3
% Total calories	40-44	44	43	44	43	42	41
Source	Lactose and glucose	Lactose	Lactose	Corn syrup solids	Corn maltodextrin and sucrose	Corn syrup solids	Corn syrup and sucrose
MINERALS							
Calcium (mg)	39-45	78	78	82	84	105 (5.2)	105 (5.2)
Phosphorus (mg)	18-24	43	42	46	56	69	75
Ca:P ratio	1.9-2.1	1.8	1.8	1.5	1.5	1.5	1.4
Sodium (mg [mEq])	18-26 [0.8-1.1]	27 [1.2]	24 [1]	30 [1.3]	30 [1.3]	36 [1.6]	44 [1.9]
Potassium (mg [mEq])	60-80 [1.5-2]	108 [2.8]	105 [2.7]	110 [2.8]	107 [2.7]	120 [3.1]	108 [2.8]
Chloride (mg [mEq])	55-63 [1.6-1.8]	63 [1.8]	65 [1.8]	67 [1.9]	65 [1.8]	80 [2.3]	62 [1.8]
Iron (mg)	0.05-0.75	1.8	1.8	1.8	1.8	1.8	1.8
Zinc (mg)	0.2-0.3	1	0.75	1	0.75	1.2	0.75
Magnesium (mg)	4.5-5	8	6	8	6	11	7.5
VITAMINS							
Vitamin A (international units)	110-320	300	300	300	300	300	300
Vitamin D (international units)	3-3.2	60	60	60	60	60	60

This table lists the major constituents; refer to product inserts for a complete listing of vitamins, minerals, and trace elements.

ARA, Arachidonic acid; *DHA,* docosahexaenoic acid.

*Data from Klein CJ, editor: Nutrient requirements for preterm infant formulas, *J Nutr* 132:1395S, 2002; and Tsang RC, Uauy R, Koletzko B, et al, editors: *Nutrition of the preterm infant: scientific basis and practical guidelines,* ed 2, Cincinnati, 2005, Digital Educational Publishing.

†Mead Johnson Nutritionals, Evansville, Ind.

‡Abbott Nutrition, Columbus, Ohio

Continued

TABLE 17-4 COMPARATIVE NUTRITIONAL COMPOSITION OF TERM INFANT FEEDINGS per 100 kcal—cont'd

		COW'S MILK–BASED				SOY PROTEIN–BASED	
				LACTOSE FREE			
	MATURE HUMAN MILK (28 DAYS)*	ENFAMIL® LIPIL® WITH IRON†	SIMILAC® ADVANCE® WITH IRON‡	ENFAMIL® LACTOFREE® LIPIL®†	SIMILAC® SENSITIVE® WITH IRON‡	ENFAMIL® ProSobee® LIPIL®†	SIMILAC® ISOMIL® ADVANCE®‡
VITAMINS—cont'd							
Vitamin E (international units)	0.3-0.6	2	1.5	2	3	2	1.5
Vitamin K (mcg)	0.3	8	8	8	8	8	11
Vitamin C—ascorbic acid (mg)	5.6-6	12	9	12	9	12	9
Vitamin B_1—thiamine (mcg)	29-31	80	100	80	100	80	60
Vitamin B_2—riboflavin (mcg)	49-51	140	150	140	150	90	90
Vitamin B_6 (mcg)	10-46	60	60	60	60	60	60
Folic acid (mcg)	2.5-18	16	15	16	15	16	15
OTHER CHARACTERISTICS							
Potential renal solute load (mOsm)	14	19.4	18.7	20	19.9	23.9	22.8
Osmolality (mOsm/kg water)	290-305	300	300	200	200	200	200

This table lists the major constituents; refer to product inserts for a complete listing of vitamins, minerals, and trace elements.

ARA, Arachidonic acid; *DHA,* docosahexaenoic acid.

*Data from Klein CJ, editor: Nutrient requirements for preterm infant formulas, *J Nutr* 132:1395S, 2002; and Tsang RC, Uauy R, Koletzko B, et al, editors: *Nutrition of the preterm infant: scientific basis and practical guidelines,* ed 2, Cincinnati, 2005, Digital Educational Publishing.

†Mead Johnson Nutritionals, Evansville, Ind.

‡Abbott Nutrition, Columbus, Ohio

adults. The biologic roles of many vitamins are not completely understood in preterm infants, and recognition of clinical deficiency states often is difficult.[98] Certain vitamins have received close attention in neonatology, in particular vitamin C for its role in enhancing iron absorption from the gastrointestinal tract, vitamin K for prevention of hemorrhagic disease of the newborn,[4] vitamin D for the prevention of rickets,[103,116] and vitamins A and E as antioxidants.[49] Vitamin A supplementation has been shown in some studies to decrease chronic lung disease in ELBW infants.[112]

Because vitamins have a central role in many metabolic processes, signs of vitamin deficiency can be nonspecific, such as lethargy, irritability, and poor growth. Table 17-5 is a summary of the recommended vitamin intake for enterally fed infants. For comparison, the average vitamin content of term human milk and commercial infant formulas is included in Table 17-4.[110] Routine supplementation of vitamins above the recommended doses is not advised because of possible toxicity and lack of clearly demonstrated benefits. For example, although supplementing vitamin D at 1000 international units/day has not been shown to result in full repletion,[25] there is no evidence that supplementation above the recommended dose prevents osteopenia in preterm infants.

Minerals and Trace Elements

The content of minerals in human milk is the gold standard for mineral requirements in term infants. Mineral requirements for the preterm infant have been estimated from in utero accretion rates. Preterm infants are relatively lacking in some important minerals (e.g., iron, calcium, zinc), because their accumulation occurs mostly in the third trimester. Published recommendations for selected daily intakes in healthy, enterally fed preterm infants are shown in Tables 17-5 and 17-6 and discussed in detail in Reference 63. Supplementation with calcium and phosphorus to achieve the recommended intakes (a Ca:P ratio of 1.7:1, by weight) has been shown to decrease the incidence of metabolic bone disease in preterm infants. Mineral supplementation of human milk or use of an enriched preterm formula (as shown in Table 17-7 on pp. 416-417) usually is necessary to achieve the recommended mineral requirements.

TABLE 17-5 RECOMMENDED ENTERAL MINERAL AND VITAMIN INTAKE FOR INFANTS

	TERM (per 100 kcal)	PRETERM (per 100 kcal)
MINERALS		
Calcium (mg)	50-140	123-185
Phosphorus (mg)	20-70	82-109
Ca:P ratio by weight	1-2:1	1.7-2:1
Sodium		
mg	25-50	39-63
mEq	1.1-2.2	1.7-2.7
Potassium		
mg	60-160	60-160
mEq	1.5-4.1	1.5-4.1
Chloride		
mg	50-160	60-160
mEq	1.4-4.6	1.7-4.6
Iron (mg)	0.2-1.65	1.7-3
Zinc (mg)	0.4-1	1.1-1.5
Magnesium (mg)	4-17	6.8-17
VITAMINS		
Vitamin A (mcg RE)	61-152	204-380
(international units)	203-506	679-1265
Vitamin D (international units)	40-100	75-270
Vitamin E (international units)	0.5-?	2-8
Vitamin K (mcg RE)	1-25	4-25
Vitamin C—ascorbic acid (mg)	6-15	8.3-37
Vitamin B_1—thiamine (mg)	30-200	30-250
Vitamin B_2—riboflavin (mg)	80-300	80-620
Vitamin B_6—pyridoxine (mg)	30-130	30-250
Folate (mcg)	11-40	30-45

Data from Klein CJ, editor: Nutrient requirements for preterm infant formulas, *J Nutr* 132:1395S, 2002; Reidel BD, Greene HL: Vitamins. In Hay WW Jr, editor: *Neonatal nutrition and metabolism,* St Louis, 1991, Mosby.
RE, Retinol equivalents.

COMPOSITION OF ENTERAL FEEDINGS

Human Milk

The ideal enteral diet for almost all term newborn infants is human milk,[5] providing sufficient energy, protein, fat, carbohydrate, micronutrients, and water

TABLE 17-6 MINERALS AND TRACE ELEMENTS IN NEONATAL NUTRITION

MINERAL OR ELEMENT	BIOLOGIC ROLE	DEFICIENCY STATE	RECOMMENDED INTAKE FOR GROWING PRETERM INFANTS
Sodium	Growth and tissue accretion, body fluid equilibrium, cellular energy, electrical charge balance	Poor growth, fluid imbalance, neurologic dysfunction, lethargy, seizures	3-5 mEq/kg/day
Potassium	Growth and tissue accretion, acid-base balance, cellular energy, electrical charge balance	Myocardial damage, dysrhythmia, hypotonia, muscle weakness	2-3 mEq/kg/day
Chloride	Growth and tissue accretion, cellular energy, electrical charge balance	Failure to thrive, muscle weakness, vomiting	3-5 mEq/kg/day
Calcium	Bone and tooth formation, fat absorption, nerve conduction, muscle contraction	Bone demineralization, tetany, dysrhythmias, seizures	200 mg/kg/day
Phosphorus	Bone and tooth formation, energy transfer compounds	Bone demineralization, weakness	100-140 mg/kg/day
Magnesium	Metalloenzymes, cellular electrical charge balance	Neurologic dysfunction, anorexia, diarrhea, renal disease	5-10 mg/kg/day
Iron	Hemoglobin formation, metalloenzymes	Anemia, apathy	2 mg/kg/day after 1 month of age
Zinc	Metalloenzymes, DNA-RNA synthesis, wound healing, host defenses	Growth restriction, dermatitis, alopecia, diarrhea, delayed wound healing	1.2-1.5 mg/kg/day
Copper	Metalloenzymes, protein metabolism	Neurologic dysfunction, anemia, neutropenia, bone demineralization	100-200 mcg/kg/day
Manganese	Metalloenzymes, carbohydrate metabolism, antioxidants, hemostasis	Neurologic dysfunction, defects in lipid metabolism, reduced coagulants, growth restriction in animals	10-20 mcg/kg/day
Chromium	Carbohydrates metabolism, component of nucleic acids	Impaired glucose tolerance, impaired growth	2-4 mcg/kg/day
Selenium	Metalloenzymes, antioxidants	Cardiomyopathy	1.5-3 mcg/kg/day
Iodine	Thyroid hormone synthesis	Hypothyroidism	1 mcg/kg/day
Molybdenum	Metalloenzymes	Neurologic and visual dysfunction, growth restriction in animals	2-3 mcg/kg/day

Data from Forbes SB: *Pediatric nutrition handbook,* Elk Grove Village, Ill, 1985, American Academy of Pediatrics; Tsang R, editor: *Vitamin and mineral requirements of preterm infants,* New York, 1985, Marcel Dekker.
DNA, Deoxyribonucleic acid; *RNA,* ribonucleic acid.

for normal growth. Contraindications to the use of human milk are found in Box 17-4. The development of a beneficial gastrointestinal flora, characterized by a large prevalence of bifidobacteria and lactobacilli, is strongly supported by human milk feedings.[47,71,79,93] In addition, human milk, unlike formulas, provides a variety of antimicrobial factors that protect against infection, such as secretory immunoglobulins (IgA), leukocytes, complement, lactoferrin, and lysozyme.[88] Human milk also contains

BOX 17-4 CONTRAINDICATIONS TO THE USE OF HUMAN MILK

- Maternal miliary tuberculosis
- Galactosemia
- Maternal drug abuse
- Some maternal medications
- Maternal human immunodeficiency virus infection

hormones and growth factors such as epidermal and nerve growth factors, insulin-like growth factors (IGF) I/II, erythropoietin, prolactin, calcitonin, steroids, thyrotropin-releasing hormone (TRH), and thyroxine. These milk hormones and trophic factors play active roles in organ maturation, growth, and health. Several essential and conditionally essential amino acids are present in high concentrations in human milk. The protein and fat components of human milk are readily digestible, and human milk contains large numbers of enzymes that aid in nutrient digestion and processing (e.g., lipase). Exclusive human milk feeding of infants at high risk may reduce the risk for developing atopic disease or milk protein allergy in infancy.[45,70] There also are obvious psychologic benefits to a mother who provides her own milk for her sick infant (see Chapter 18).

Human milk is the recommended basis of nutrition for the preterm infant.[5] The preterm infant will not grow at the normal rate of fetal growth on human milk alone, however, because of the special nutritional requirements addressed previously. Recommended daily requirements for energy, protein, calcium, sodium, phosphorus, magnesium, iron, zinc, and several vitamins necessary to meet the normal rate of in utero growth usually will not be achieved in the growing "healthy" preterm infant who is fed with unsupplemented human milk. The preterm infant with respiratory distress, infection, excessive heat losses, or increased activity has even greater nutritional needs. Nonetheless, milk from mothers of preterm infants has more protein and sodium than milk obtained at term and occasionally provides for adequate growth in larger and healthier preterm infants. The nutritional composition of term human milk is compared with commercial term infant formulas in Table 17-4. The nutrient content of "mature" preterm human milk is compared with fortified preterm human milk and preterm formulas in Table 17-7. Use of commercially available supplements to human milk that provide additional energy, protein, vitamins, and minerals is recommended.[98] Nutrient composition of these fortifiers is shown in Table 17-3.

Formulas

Cow's milk–derived formulas have been designed to mimic human milk to provide biologically available protein mixtures with appropriate protein:energy ratios for normal growth. In general, formulas designed for term infants contain 20 kcal/oz and are adequate to meet the needs of term infants with an intact gastrointestinal tract and "normal" fluid requirements. A whey and casein mixture approximating that of human milk is preferred. Preterm formulas contain whey:casein ratios of 60:40 and have higher protein contents than those of term formulas. Preterm formulas also contain less lactose as a carbohydrate source and substitute corn syrup solids and lactose to provide approximately 42% to 44% of the calories derived from carbohydrate. Preterm formulas provide some of the fat in the form of medium-chain triglycerides because of the ease with which they are absorbed. Calcium and phosphorus content is increased, with a Ca:P ratio of 1.8 to 2:1, which provides for improved bone mineralization. Other minerals and vitamins also are present in higher concentrations in preterm formulas to reflect the special nutritional needs of the VLBW infant. Preterm formulas are available in 20 and 24 kcal/oz preparations, with similar osmolalities and renal solute loads.

Soy protein formulas should be reserved for term infants with galactosemia, severe lactose intolerance, hereditary lactase deficiency, vegan families, or those who have IgE-mediated cow's milk protein allergy. **Soy-derived formulas should not be used for preterm infants because of the poorer quality of protein, lower digestibility and bioavailability, and lower calcium and zinc accretion rates seen with these formulas.**[9] In addition, there are concerns for all infants about the concentrations of phytates, aluminum, and phytoestrogens that these formulas contain.[35,86,111] If necessary, a protein hydrolysate formula should be used for preterm infants with protein intolerance. For term infants, formulas derived from protein hydrolysates should be reserved for infants who are allergic to cow's milk proteins and are not breast fed or do not tolerate soy-derived formulas. Soy formulas have no role in

TABLE 17-7 COMPARATIVE NUTRITIONAL COMPOSITION OF PRETERM INFANT FEEDINGS (per 100 kcal)

	MATURE PRETERM HUMAN MILK (UNFORTIFIED)*	PREMATURE INFANT FORMULAS		POST-DISCHARGE FORMULAS	
		ENFAMIL® PREMATURE LIPIL®†	SIMILAC® SPECIAL CARE® WITH IRON‡	ENFACARE® LIPIL®†	SIMILAC NEOSURE®‡
NUTRIENT DENSITY (kcal/oz)	19-21	20 or 24	20 or 24	22	22
ENERGY (kcal)	100	100	100	100	100
PROTEIN					
Amount (g)	2.2 ± 0.2	3	2.71	2.8	2.8
% Total calories	8	12	11	11	11
Source	Human milk	Whey protein concentrate and nonfat milk	Nonfat milk and whey protein concentrate	Nonfat milk and whey protein concentrate	Nonfat milk and whey protein concentrate
FAT					
Amount (g)	5.4 ± 0.9	5.1	5.43	5.3	5.5
% Total calories	44-52	46	49	47	50
Source	Triglycerides	MCT oil Soy oil High oleic vegetable oil Single cell oil products (DHA and ARA)	MCT oil Soy oil Coconut oil Single cell oil products (DHA and ARA)	High oleic oil Soy oil MCT oil Coconut oil Single cell oil products (DHA and ARA)	Soy oil Coconut oil MCT oil Single cell oil products (DHA and ARA)
Oil ratio (approximate)	99	40:30:27:2:1	50:30:18.3:0.25:0.4	34:29:20:14:2.2:0.8	44.7:29:24.9:0.15:0.4
Linoleic acid (mg)	440-1500	810	700	950	750
CARBOHYDRATE					
Amount (g)	10 ± 0.6	11	10.3	10.4	10.1
% Total calories	40-44	44	41	42	40
Source	Lactose and glucose	Corn syrup solids and lactose	Corn syrup solids and lactose	Lactose and corn syrup solids	Corn syrup solids and lactose
MINERALS					
Calcium (mg)	37-44	165	180	120	105
Phosphorus (mg)	19-21	83	100	66	62
Ca:P ratio	1.9-2.2:1	2:1	1.8:1	1.8:1	1.7:1

Sodium mg (mEq)	30-37 (1.3-1.6)	58 (2.5)	43 (1.9)	35 (1.5)	33 (1.4)
Potassium mg (mEq)	78-85 (2-2.2)	98 (2.5)	129 (3.3)	105 (2.7)	142 (3.6)
Chloride mg (mEq)	63-82 (1.8-2.3)	90 (2.5)	81 (2.3)	78 (2.2)	75 (2.1)
Iron (mg)	0.2	1.8	1.8	1.8	1.8
Zinc (mg)	0.5	1.5	1.5	1.25	1.2
Magnesium (mg)	4.4-4.9	9	12	8	9
VITAMINS					
Vitamin A					
(mcg RE)	104-125	375	375	135	138
(international units)	(345-416)	(1250)	(1250)	(450)	(460)
Vitamin D (international units)	3-3.2	240	150	80	70
Vitamin E (international units)	1.9	6.3	4	4	3.6
Vitamin K (mcg)	0.3	8	12	8	11
Vitamin C—ascorbic acid (mg)	5-6.25	20	37	16	15
Vitamin B_1—thiamine (mcg)	200	200	250	200	220
Vitamin B_2—riboflavin (mcg)	270-310	300	620	200	150
Vitamin B_6 (mcg)	18-20	150	250	100	100
Folic acid (mcg)	12	40	37	26	25
OTHER CHARACTERISTICS					
Potential renal solute load (mOsm)	18.7	27.4	27.8	24.5	25.2
Osmolality (mOsm/kg water)	290	240	235	250	250

This table lists the major constituents; refer to product inserts for a complete listing of vitamins, minerals, and trace elements.

ARA, Arachidonic acid; *DHA,* docosahexaenoic acid; *MCT,* medium-chain triglycerides.

*Data from Klein CJ, editor: Nutrient requirements for preterm infant formulas, *J Nutr* 132:1395S, 2002; and Tsang RC, Uauy R, Koletzko B, et al, editors: *Nutrition of the preterm infant: scientific basis and practical guidelines,* ed 2, Cincinnati, 2005, Digital Educational Publishing.

†Mead Johnson Nutritionals, Evansville, Ind.

‡Abbott Nutrition, Columbus, Ohio.

the prevention of atopic disease. In contrast, extensively hydrosylated formulas may delay or prevent atopic dermatitis in infants at high risk.[45] In general, families with a strong history of cow's milk protein allergy should be encouraged to breast feed.

Elemental formulas are used in infants with malabsorption, abnormal gastrointestinal tracts, or severe protein allergy. The protein source in these formulas is derived from free amino acids, and 52% of the fat is from MCT oil. Use of elemental formulas generally is indicated in the infant with severe liver disease and fat malabsorption, with short bowel syndrome (e.g., after necrotizing enterocolitis [NEC] with surgical resection), or with dysmotility syndromes (e.g., in gastroschisis). Occasionally, elemental formulas are useful after a severe episode of infectious gastroenteritis with mucosal injury and resulting protein or lactose intolerance. A lactose-free formula also may be used in this setting. It is not necessary to use an elemental formula in the routine care of VLBW infants. A variety of other modified formulas are available for infants with special nutritional needs.

In some circumstances, infants require fluid restriction (e.g., because of pulmonary edema, congestive heart failure, or renal failure) while on full enteral feedings. **Caloric delivery and nutritional support can be maintained by increasing the caloric density of feedings when feeding volumes cannot be tolerated or fluid intake must be limited.** This can be done by adding human milk fortifiers, glucose polymers, vegetable oil, Microlipid (a lipid emulsion, Sherwood Medical), or MCT oil to the milk or formula as tolerated to achieve acceptable concentrations and intakes of these nutrients. Liquid formula concentrates also are used to increase the caloric density of infant feedings. **Powdered infant formulas should not be used for feeding or fortification in hospitalized newborns in an intensive care unit,** unless no alternative is available, because of information linking *Enterobacter sakazakii* infections in neonates to the use of powdered infant formulas (Food and Drug Administration [FDA] recommendation 4-11-02). Caloric densities of greater than 24 kcal/oz can be achieved with fortification, although infants tolerate these supplements in a highly individual fashion and should be monitored for signs of feeding intolerance (e.g., abdominal distention, increased stooling, presence of fat or sugar in the stool). Consider the distribution of calories to maintain a balance of protein, fat, and carbohydrate, about 10%, 45%, and 45%, respectively. Increasing caloric density of feedings also necessitates less water delivery to the infant and generally leads to an increase in formula osmolality as well. Therefore careful monitoring of feeding tolerance, electrolytes, and fluid balance (renal function) is necessary on a high–caloric density feeding regimen.

FEEDING TECHNIQUES

Gavage Feeding

Gavage feedings are indicated in infants requiring endotracheal intubation or those with an immature, weak, or absent suck, swallow, or gag reflex (Box 17-5). Most infants tolerate intermittent feedings delivered slowly over 30 to 60 minutes. ***Continuous feedings*** may be helpful for infants

BOX 17-5 GAVAGE FEEDING GUIDELINES

Equipment

1. Breast milk/formula in syringe (4-hour amount, or unit protocol, maximum)
2. Tape, optional transparent dressing
3. Lubricant, optional
4. Stethoscope
5. For intermittent feeding: infant feeding set with syringe, medicine cup, 4-Fr to 8-Fr gavage tube
6. For indwelling feeding tubes: infant less than 1 kg, 4-Fr tube; greater than 1 kg, 5-Fr to 6-Fr tube (tube size may also depend on placement [i.e., oral versus nasal], amount of feeding, and rate of delivery of feeding).[61] Short-term feeding tube (generally made of polyvinyl chloride [PVC]) should be changed every 24 to 72 hours.
   Long-term feeding tube (made of polyurethane) should be changed every 4 weeks.
   Note: Always follow manufacturer's recommendations.
7. Syringe pump and extension tubing as needed

BOX 17-5 GAVAGE FEEDING GUIDELINES—cont'd

Feeding Tube Insertion

1. Wash hands and assemble equipment in a clean area.
2. Measure for tube placement by placing tip of feeding tube at the tip of nose, draw to base of ear, then to halfway between the xiphoid process and the umbilicus.
3. Mark tube with indelible ink pen to indicate the distance from the tip of the tube to the corner of the mouth or edge of the naris.
4. Insert tube (swaddling the infant may help with tolerance of this procedure).
   NEVER FORCE THE TUBE.
   Oral placement (usually for infants less than 1 kg, those on nasal continuous positive airway pressure (NCPAP) or ventilator, those with high oxygen need, or those with excoriated nares): insert tip into the oropharynx, gently pushing tube in a downward arc into the esophagus until reaching the premeasured mark.
   Nasal placement (generally preferred for infants greater than 1 kg with mature or strong gag reflex and infants who are breast feeding or nippling): moisten tip with water or lubricant. Insert tip gently into one nostril and advance slowly as above.
5. Gastric tube tip placement is verified by abdominal radiograph or pH measurement of the aspirate. The tube landmark should be checked with every caregiving procedure to determine that it is still visible and at the correct location.
6. Soft Silastic tubes are generally used for transpyloric feedings and require the use of a stylet for insertion. The tube must be inspected visually and by flushing with water before insertion to ensure that it has not been perforated by the stylet. The stylet is removed after insertion and is stored in package by the bedside. Tip placement usually is verified by radiographic imaging.

Securing Feeding Tube

1. Intermittent feeding tubes can be taped to the cheek.
2. Indwelling tubes must be taped securely to the face, leaving the landmark visible. For tubes placed nasally, a narrow piece of tape may be placed along the tubing on the upper lip, with a transparent dressing applied over the tube on the cheek.

Feeding

1. Aspirate entire stomach contents to assess quantity, as well as color and appearance.
2. To prevent loss of electrolytes, slowly return aspirate to the stomach. Exceptions to this include aspirates that are bloody or "coffee ground," green or bright yellow, or fecal appearing or contain large amounts of mucus. Do not refeed, and discuss feeding plan with physician or practitioner. Also report aspirates of undigested formula if amount is more than one half of the feeding or occurs more than once or if there is a change in abdominal assessment. Reducing the feeding by the amount of the refed aspirate is recommended for one or two feedings.
3. Instill human milk or formula via intermittent gavage feeding:
   Detach syringe from feeding tube and remove plunger; reattach syringe to feeding tube. Pour the predetermined amount of milk into the syringe. Flow may begin spontaneously or require a gentle nudge from the plunger. Allow feeding to run in slowly by gravity. Never push a feeding. The higher the syringe is held, the faster the feeding will flow (about 8 inches is ideal). For most infants, a feeding should run in over 30 minutes. Gavage sets may be rinsed carefully and used for up to 24 hours unless labeled "single use only" or manufacturer's directions indicate otherwise.
4. Intermittent gavage feeding via indwelling feeding tube:
   Check aspirate and feed as above. When feeding is complete, instill 1 to 2 mL sterile water to clear tubing of residual food and cap or close off the tube by attaching syringe with plunger.
5. Continuous drip feedings via indwelling feeding tube:
   Check feeding tube placement and feeding residuals every 2 to 4 hours using stopcock, which is placed between the feeding tube and the extension tubing. Check ink landmark on feeding tube hourly to ensure proper placement of the tube. Prepare up to 4 hours of breast milk or formula (or amount according to institutional studies of bacterial growth). Fill syringe with predetermined feeding amount plus enough to prime the extension tubing. Place syringe into syringe pump and program to deliver feeding at desired rate. To help prevent loss of milk fat by settling, place syringe in an upward vertical position and use mini-bore tubing.

Care, Assessment, and Documentation

1. Assess infant's tolerance of feeding tube placement. If gagging occurs, attempt to insert tube down one side of the oropharynx rather than down the middle. If the infant becomes apneic, bradycardic, or cyanotic during feeding tube placement, pause to allow recovery or remove the tube and allow infant to rest before trying again. If these symptoms occur during the feeding, stop the feeding by lowering the syringe or stopping the pump. If recovery occurs quickly, resume feeding slowly and observe. If distress continues or recurs, stop feeding and inform the physician or practitioner.
2. Change short-term (PVC) feeding tube every 24 to 72 hours (or manufacturer's recommendations).
3. Change long-term nasal feeding tube (polyurethane) to opposite nostril weekly. Discard and replace tube after 4 weeks (or manufacturers' recommendations).
4. Document all details of the feeding and the infant's tolerance, proper placement of the indwelling feeding tube, and when feeding tube or equipment is to be changed.

recovering from necrotizing enterocolitis (NEC) or infants with short bowel syndrome, congenital heart disease, or intolerance of bolus feedings. There is some evidence that these infants have better absorption of nutrients and therefore improved growth. The caregiver should monitor the number and consistency of stools or stoma output. **Stools should be tested for occult blood or reducing substances** (to detect undigested or partially digested carbohydrate [e.g., with Clinitest]) when feeding intolerance or malabsorption is suspected. If short bowel syndrome is present, transition from continuous to bolus feedings should proceed slowly and cautiously by infusing feedings over gradually shorter periods of time, with increasing intervals between feedings until bolus feedings every 3 to 4 hours are tolerated. Prolonged oral or nasal gastric tube feedings cause adverse oral stimulation and promote gastroesophageal reflux and problems of oral aversion. Some neonates require gastrostomy tube placement after certain surgical procedures (see Chapter 28).

For most infants, intragastric feedings are preferred to transpyloric feedings. Routine use of transpyloric feedings has increased mortality without proven benefits.[83,84] Even when indicated because of severe reflux and aspiration, transpyloric feedings have additional complications, including intestinal perforations requiring surgery. Use of transpyloric feeding should be restricted to short-term use in those infants who cannot tolerate gastric feedings because of excessive reflux with aspiration, pneumonia, and apnea.

PRECAUTIONS

Aspiration is a serious problem in an infant of any gestational age who does not have a neurologically mature swallow, gag, or cough reflex (<34 to 36 weeks). Tachypneic infants with labored respirations or with an endotracheal tube also are at increased risk for aspiration. Gavage tube position must be checked carefully using bedside testing of pH[90] or abdominal radiograph, if necessary; feedings should run in slowly; infants should not be overfed. Gavage feedings should never be pushed.

Oral Feeding

Development of appropriate neuromuscular coordination is necessary to successfully initiate oral feedings. Criteria for initiating oral feeding must be individualized. Coordination of suck, swallow, and breathing emerges at about 34 weeks' gestation, regardless of postnatal age. Respiratory illness leads to energy depletion. **Oral feeding usually is not possible unless the respiratory rate is less than 60 breaths/min.** Neonates with craniofacial malformation (e.g., cleft lip or palate, choanal stenosis or atresia, mandibular hypoplasia) are at increased risk for aspiration. Use of different nipple shapes and sizes and sitting the infant in the upright position facilitate safe oral feeding. Gastrostomy tube placement may be necessary if oral feedings are not adequately established (see Chapter 28).

The ability to suck on a pacifier, fingers, or a gavage tube does not ensure the infant's ability to perform nutritive sucking. **A preterm infant without a gag reflex is at risk for aspiration with nipple feedings. An infant who is successful at oral feeding should exhibit an active suck, coordinated swallow, minimal fluid loss around the nipple, and completion of feeding within 15 to 30 minutes.**[105] The preterm infant hospitalized in the neonatal intensive care unit (NICU) usually has been exposed to many unpleasant oral sensations, such as endotracheal tubes, suction catheters, gavage tubes, and facial tape. These infants often become "disorganized feeders" and develop oral aversion.

The first few feedings in the preterm infant often last only a few minutes. Coordination of sucking with breathing is the first lesson for the preterm infant. Stress behaviors (e.g., increase or decrease in respiratory or heart rate, decreased oxygen saturation, color change, gagging, choking, emesis, fatigue, irritability, or a "panicked look") should result in a rest period or cessation of the feeding. Provider "pacing" is important until the infant learns to self-pace feedings (see Chapter 13).

An infant receiving supplemental oxygen should be monitored by pulse oximetry to determine oxygen requirements during oral feedings. Softer nipples may be used for infants with weak suck and swallow capacity. Strategies to facilitate oral feedings include a relaxed caregiver, a quiet environment with subdued light, and a snugly wrapped infant (see Chapter 13).

Extremely preterm infants appear to benefit from a minimal enteral nutrition regimen (often called ***trophic feedings,*** since the purpose is to develop gut growth and development but not body growth). Such feedings should begin slowly at approximately 20 mL/kg/day, about every 4 hours, and then increase after 3 to 5 days as tolerated to once every 2 to 3 hours and finally to full enteral feeding volumes and full nipple (or breast) feedings. **Even for the very preterm infant, scheduling oral feedings for parent visits enables them to actively participate in their infant's care.** Too rapid a change to oral feeding results in weight loss, primarily because the infant tires with feeding and is unable to take in a sufficient amount of food. Diligent attention is warranted, and nipple feedings often have to be limited and gavage feedings continued to prevent dehydration and malnutrition.

FEEDING INTOLERANCE AND COMPLICATIONS

Assessment for signs of feeding intolerance is imperative because, although some feeding complications are mild and respond to nursing interventions, others are more serious and require medical intervention. **Feeding intolerance frequently is the first sign of illness (e.g., hypoxia, dyspnea, congestive heart failure, sepsis, NEC).** At first, such signs often are subtle, so the caregiver should be constantly aware of any change in the infant's overall condition and feeding tolerance.

Residuals

The feeding tube is aspirated every 2 to 4 hours before a feeding to determine whether gastric emptying is adequate. Incompletely digested aspirates of less than 50% of the previous feeding, 2 to 4 mL/kg, or a 1-hour volume if on continuous feedings may be normal and generally should be refed to the infant (Figure 17-8). Increasing residuals can indicate feeding intolerance, and the infant should be evaluated for intestinal obstruction or NEC. If such serious disorders are not discovered, feedings can be started again with decreased feeding volumes and/or slower rates of instillation, as well as slower rates of feeding advancement. Medications such as metoclopramide or erythromycin have been used to accelerate bowel motility and improve feeding tolerance, but few data from clinical trials are available to confirm these outcomes.[55] **The presence of bile or blood in the gastric aspirate warrants further investigation and possibility of NEC.**

Emesis

Infants with emesis should always be evaluated for intestinal obstruction or diseases that produce ileus,

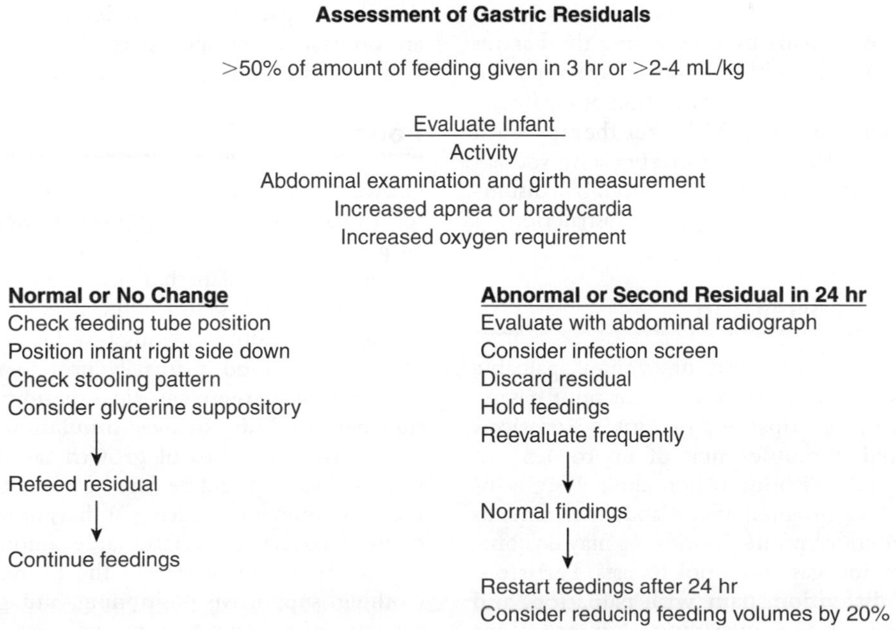

Assessment of Gastric Residuals
>50% of amount of feeding given in 3 hr or >2-4 mL/kg
Evaluate Infant
Activity
Abdominal examination and girth measurement
Increased apnea or bradycardia
Increased oxygen requirement
Normal or No Change
Check feeding tube position
Position infant right side down
Check stooling pattern
Consider glycerine suppository
Refeed residual
Continue feedings
Abnormal or Second Residual in 24 hr
Evaluate with abdominal radiograph
Consider infection screen
Discard residual
Hold feedings
Reevaluate frequently
Normal findings
Restart feedings after 24 hr
Consider reducing feeding volumes by 20%

FIGURE 17-8 Assessment of gastric residuals.

such as NEC and sepsis. With persistent emesis of increasing amounts, feedings should be held and the infant evaluated for sepsis, NEC, obstruction (including Hirschsprung's disease and, in infants of diabetic mothers, microcolon), metabolic disorders, or increased intracranial pressure. Emesis also results from an overdistended stomach, gastroesophageal reflux, poorly positioned feeding tube, gastric irritation from enterally administered medications, drug withdrawal, or overstimulation in a very small infant. Interventions include allowing the feeding to flow more slowly by use of a smaller gavage tube, instilling the feeding over a longer period, decreasing feeding volumes, prone positioning, giving medications at the end of the feeding, or modifying a stressful environment (see Chapter 13). Litmus testing or abdominal radiographs should be used to assess feeding tube position.

GASTROESOPHAGEAL REFLUX

Gastroesophageal reflux should be suspected in an infant with irritability, emesis, apnea and bradycardia, respiratory deterioration, refusal to eat, or otherwise unexplained blood in the stools. **The use of histamine-2 (H-2) receptor blocker therapy for gastroesophageal reflux or feeding intolerance in infants is not supported by good evidence. H-2 blockers have been implicated in neonatal sepsis for being permissive to pathologic organisms** by eliminating the barrier function of gastric acid.[43] Studies have reported decreased NEC with the acidification of feedings[92] and the **association of H-2 blocker therapy with an increased risk for necrotizing enterocolitis.**[46] Postoperative emesis and abdominal distention may indicate a stricture, partial obstruction, or inflammatory abscess.

Abdominal Distention

Abdominal distention with or without palpable or visible loops of bowel is a sign of poor gastric motility, ileus, constipation, or "gas." **Variations in abdominal circumference of up to 1.5 cm can occur and, without other clinical signs of illness, may be normal.** If the abdomen remains soft and nontender, prone positioning may be comforting, allowing gas and stool to pass. **Persistent abdominal distention, pain with palpation, and discoloration of the overlying skin are signs of pathology (e.g., anatomic obstruction or infection) and require investigation.** An abdominal x-ray examination is indicated in these patients. **Abdominal girth is measured every 4 to 8 hours to document increased distention.** Place paper or cloth tape around the abdomen at a consistent point marked on the abdomen.

Diarrhea

Diarrhea, or frequent water-loss stools, signifies intolerance of the caloric density of feedings, transient lactase deficiency, highly osmotic medications, or other pathology, including, rarely, allergy. **Stool culture for bacterial or viral pathogens and stool Clinitest should be performed if the infant also appears ill or if there is blood in the stool.** In lactose malabsorption, short-term use of a non–lactose-containing formula or hydrolysate formula should result in return to normal stools.

Apnea and/or Bradycardia

Apnea and/or bradycardia frequently occurs during or after feeding. These signs are vagally mediated by the passage or presence of a feeding tube, gastric distention, or gastroesophageal reflux or occur with abdominal distention and compromise of lung volumes or airway obstruction. **Interventions to decrease vagal stimulation include changing to an orogastric gavage tube, decreasing feeding volume, and feeding more slowly.**

Poor Growth

Growth is an essential requirement for the preterm infant. When normal growth does not occur, all possible factors should be considered, but most commonly, the infant has not been fed sufficient amounts of food. If this is the case and the infant is not sick in some obvious way, he or she should be fed more food, primarily protein and energy. **Factors that increase caloric expenditure, such as thermal instability or overstimulation, should be considered as causes of growth failure.** Preterm infants always should be cared for in a thermoneutral environment, wearing a hat or other form of head covering (because large amounts of heat are lost from the surface of the head). Additional clothing, supportive positioning, and grouping of care and stimulation to conserve energy often help improve growth.

Danger Signs

Bile in the gastric aspirate is generally a sign of significant ileus or obstruction. The presence of blood in the stools or gastric aspirate, a tense or tender abdomen, and abdominal wall erythema are more ominous signs of feeding intolerance and may indicate frank NEC (see the Critical Findings box below. The presence of these signs and symptoms warrants a careful physical examination and usually further investigation including x-ray examinations. Feedings should be postponed while these signs and symptoms are being investigated. Other useful studies include a complete blood count with differential to evaluate extent of blood loss, presence of thrombocytopenia (a marker of necrotic bowel), and change in white blood cell count as evidence of infection. Although feeding of human milk may help protect against developing NEC and 5% to 10% of cases of NEC occur in infants who have never been fed enterally, NEC can occur in any infant. **Abnormal abdominal distention or bilious or bloody gastric aspirates should be investigated carefully regardless of feeding status.**

THE PRETERM INFANT

Much progress has made in providing nutritional support for ELBW (<1000 g) and VLBW (<1500 g) preterm infants. The nutritional requirements of these very small infants are marked, unique, incompletely understood, and frequently inadequately provided for, despite improvement in both the quality and quantity of nutrients in currently used intravenous (IV) and enteral nutrient regimens (Box 17-6). Also, many of these infants are growth restricted at birth. Thus their nutritional needs for normal rates of metabolism and growth are very likely to differ from those of normal-growth infants.[24] **Table 17-8 shows enteral intake recommendations for stable, growing preterm infants.** Whether additional nutritional supplementation should be provided for some or all of these infants to support "catch-up" growth and the best "recipe" for that supplementation are currently controversial.[38,69,101,108,109]

In spite of increasingly aggressive in-hospital nutritional management, the majority of prematurely born infants remain growth restricted and are small for post-conceptual age at the time of discharge.[32,33] In fact, the fraction of these infants who are small for gestational age at discharge is several-fold greater than the fraction at birth (Figure 17-9).[32] **There is increasingly strong evidence that early nutritional support of preterm and growth-restricted infants can have lasting consequences for neurodevelopmental outcome.**[11,30] Many previous studies in humans and animals have documented that prolonged postnatal undernutrition and malnutrition add far greater insult than does prenatal undernutrition alone.[73] Such observations have important

Critical Findings

DANGER SIGNS REQUIRING IMMEDIATE ATTENTION

1. Bile in the gastric aspirate
2. Presence of blood in the stools or gastric aspirate
3. Tense or tender abdomen
4. Abdominal wall erythema
5. Unexplained anemia, thrombocytopenia, and neutropenia

BOX 17-6 SPECIAL NUTRITIONAL CONDITIONS IN EXTREMELY-LOW-BIRTH-WEIGHT INFANTS

1. Minimal energy reserves (both carbohydrates and fat)
2. Intrinsically higher metabolic rate (greater relative mass of more metabolically active organs: brain, heart, liver)
3. Higher protein turnover rate (especially when growing)
4. Higher glucose needs for energy and brain metabolism
5. Higher lipid needs to match the in utero rate of fat deposition
6. Excessive evaporative rates (immature skin)
7. Occasionally very high urinary water and solute losses (depending on intake and renal maturation)
8. Low rates of gastrointestinal peristalsis
9. Limited production of gut digestive enzymes and growth factors
10. Higher incidence of stressful events (hypoxemia, respiratory distress, sepsis)
11. Metabolic effects of medications used frequently (steroids, antibiotics, sedatives, catecholamines)
12. Abnormal neurologic outcome if not fed adequately

Modified from Thureen P, Hay WW Jr: Conditions requiring special nutritional management. In Tsang RC, Lucas A, Uauy R, et al, editors: *Nutritional needs of the preterm infant*, Baltimore, 1993, Williams & Wilkins.

TABLE 17-8 ENTERAL INTAKE RECOMMENDATIONS FOR STABLE, GROWING PRETERM INFANTS*

		CONSENSUS RECOMMENDATIONS BY THE AUTHORS OF THIS CHAPTER			
		INFANT WEIGHT <1000 g	INFANT WEIGHT >1000 g	AAPCON†	ESPGAN-CON‡
Water	mL	125-167	125-167	—	115-154
Energy	kcal	100	100	100	100
Protein	g	3-3.16	2.5-3	2.9-3.3	2.25-3.1
Carbohydrate	g			9-13	7-14
Lactose	g	3.16-9.5	3.16-9.8	—	—
Oligomers	g	0-7	0-7	—	—
Fat	g			4.5-6.0	3.6-7
Linoleic acid	g	0.44-1.7	0.44-1.7	0.4	0.5-1.4
Linolenic acid	g	0.11-0.44	0.11-0.44	—	>0.055
18:2/C18:3		>5	>5	—	5-15
Vitamin A—lung disease	International units	583-1250 1250-2333	583-1250 1250-2333	75-225 —	270-450 —
Vitamin D	International units	125-333§	125-333§	270	800-1600/day
Vitamin E	International units	5-10	5-10	>1.1	0.6-10
Supplement (human milk)		2.9	2.9	—	—
Vitamin K	mcg	6.66-8.33	6.66-8.33	4	4-15
Ascorbate	mg	15-20	15-20	35	7-40
Thiamine	mcg	150-200	150-200	>40	20-250
Riboflavin	mcg	200-300	200-300	>60	60-600
Pyridoxine	mcg	125-175	125-175	>35	35-250
Niacin	mg	3-4	3-4	>0.25	0.8-5.0
Pantothenate	mg	1-1.5	1-1.5	>0.30	>0.3
Biotin	mcg	3-5	3-5	>1.5	>1.5
Folate	mcg	21-42	21-42	33	>60
Vitamin B_{12}	mcg	0.25	0.25	>0.15	>0.15
Sodium	mg	38-58	38-58	48-67	23-53
Potassium	mg	65-100	65-100	66-98	90-152
Chloride	mg	59-89	59-89	—	57-89
Calcium	mg	100-192	100-192	175	70-140
Phosphorus	mg	50-117	50-117	91.5	50-87
Magnesium	mg	6.6-12.5	6.6-12.5	—	6-12
Iron	mg	1.67	1.67	1.7-2.5	1.5

*120 kcal/kg/day was used where conversion was made from per kg recommendations.
†American Academy of Pediatrics, Committee on Nutrition.
‡European Society of Paediatric Gastroenterology and Nutrition, Committee on Nutrition of the Preterm Infant.
§Aim = 400 international units/day.

TABLE 17-8 ENTERAL INTAKE RECOMMENDATIONS FOR STABLE, GROWING PRETERM INFANTS—cont'd

		CONSENSUS RECOMMENDATIONS BY THE AUTHORS OF THIS CHAPTER			
		INFANT WEIGHT <1000 g	INFANT WEIGHT >1000 g	AAPCON†	ESPGAN-CON‡
Zinc	mcg	833	833	>500	550-1100
Copper	mcg	100-125	100-125	90	90-120
Selenium	mcg	1.08-2.5	1.08-2.5	—	—
Chromium	mcg	0.083-0.42	0.083-0.42	—	—
Manganese	mcg	6.3	6.3	>5	1.5-7.5
Molybdenum	mcg	0.25	0.25	—	—
Iodine	mcg	25-50	25-50	5	10-45
Taurine	mg	3.75-7.5	3.75-7.5	—	—
Carnitine	mg	Approximately 2.4	Approximately 2.4	—	>1.2
Inositol	mg	27-67.5	27-67.5	—	—
Choline	mg	12-23.4	12-23.4	—	—

*120 kcal/kg/day was used where conversion was made from per kg recommendations.
†American Academy of Pediatrics, Committee on Nutrition.
‡European Society of Paediatric Gastroenterology and Nutrition, Committee on Nutrition of the Preterm Infant.
§Aim = 400 international units/day.

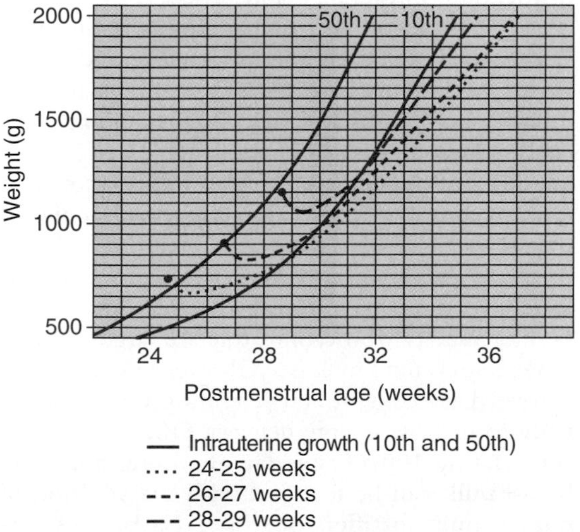

FIGURE 17-9 Average body weight versus postmenstrual age in weeks for infants with gestational ages 24 to 25 weeks *(dotted line)*, 26 to 27 weeks *(short dashes)*, and 28 to 29 weeks *(long dashes)*. The reference intrauterine growth curves were plotted using the smoothed 10th and 50th percentiles birth weight data reported by Alexander et al.[3] (From Ehrenkranz RA, Younes N, Lemons JA, et al: Longitudinal growth of hospitalized very low birth weight infants. Reproduced with permission from *Pediatrics* 104:287, 1999, © American Academy of Pediatrics.)

implications. First, we cannot now think of "early" nutrition of these small infants simply in terms of providing immediate nutrient needs just for metabolic maintenance (e.g., glucose to prevent hypoglycemia); we also must consider that early nutrition has biologic effects that have lasting or lifelong significance. Second, we can no longer regard nutritional practices in preterm infants as simply a matter of personal choice. The major impact of sufficient early nutritional support on long-term outcome should be a stimulus to new research that defines consistent approaches to the nutrition of preterm infants to optimize their future health and development.[20,23]

Concerns about the safety of enteral feeding of preterm infants have frequently delayed the initiation of feedings, but evidence is accumulating to suggest **early initiation of low-volume enteral feedings ("minimal enteral nutrition"), especially with human milk, improves gastrointestinal development, motility, and function in the preterm infant and protects against NEC and systemic infection.**[7,31,81] Enteral feedings are associated with surges in gut hormone production that mediate trophic effects on gastrointestinal growth and mucosal maturation. Absorption of nutrients is improved with increased amount and length of villous absorptive surface. Provision of only small quantities of milk into the neonatal gastrointestinal tract promotes the production of locally acting gut hormones, such as gastrin, enteroglucagon, and motilin, which are thought to be very important for normal intestinal maturation.[85] Feeding tolerance is improved and full enteral feedings are achieved earlier in these infants.[82,85] **Minimal enteral feedings also have been shown to improve nutritional outcome (weight gain, bone mineralization) in preterm infants.**[100] The potential advantages of minimal enteral feeding are listed in Box 17-7. Failure to provide any enteral nutrition for prolonged periods to the newborn infant should be avoided unless small-volume feeding is specifically contraindicated.

During the acute phase of a preterm infant's illness, aggressive nutrition should be provided by the parenteral route (see Chapter 16), but studies have shown that **minimal enteral feedings can safely be started by day of life 2 or 3, even in very small or ill infants. Feedings from 6 to 20 mL/kg/day divided into every 2- to 24-hour slow bolus feeds are given without advancement for several days.** The transition to nutritive enteral feedings then can proceed slowly as described below, with continuous assessment of feeding tolerance to avoid complications such as NEC. Mother's colostrum/milk is the preferred initial feeding choice, but, if necessary, donor human milk or full-strength formula may be used as an alternative for minimal enteral feeding.

BOX 17-7 ADVANTAGES OF MINIMAL ENTERAL FEEDING

- No increase in incidence of necrotizing enterocolitis
- Decreased sepsis[82]
- Decreased permeability of mucosa to foreign antigens
- Increased intestinal peptides and hormones[85]
- Increased mucosal thickness and villi
- Maturation of intestinal motor activity[81]
- Improved feeding tolerance[82]
- Improved bone mineralization[118]
- Earlier achievement of full enteral feedings[82]
- Improved weight gain[82]
- Shorter hospital stay[82]
- Reduced requirement for supplemental oxygen[82]

Although most infants benefit from early enteral feeding, those who are asphyxiated, hypotensive, severely hypoxemic, or symptomatic with patent ductus arteriosus or those with evidence of NEC should not be fed enterally. These infants should be managed with aggressive full parenteral nutrition.

Few controlled trials support any given feeding strategy, although rapid advances to large feeding volumes are poorly tolerated by most preterm infants.[8] There is some evidence of calorie loss from expressed human milk and increased bacterial contamination during continuous gavage feeding.[12,28] **Benefits of continuous feedings include decreased energy expenditure and improved growth in the preterm infant.**[44] **Similar growth usually is achieved whether infants are fed intermittently or continuously.**[95,104,106] However, infants fed by continuous tube feeding take longer to achieve full enteral feeds.[95] Studies indicate that an intermittent "slow" infusion (e.g., 3 hours of volume given over 1 hour out of three) improves gastric emptying and duodenal motility.[6,26] The following guidelines reflect just one approach to enteral feedings; caution and flexibility must be used in following any feeding schedule. **In general, the smaller the infant, the greater attention must be paid to feeding tolerance, although large infants certainly can develop serious feeding intolerance and NEC.**

After a period of gut priming, usually 5 to 7 days, with minimal enteral feedings, advancement to full nutritive enteral feedings for the infant who weighs less than 2000 g should proceed in increments not greater than 15 to 20 mL/kg/day. Full feedings of human milk or formula (approximately 160 mL/kg/day) are achieved over 7 to 10 days. In most cases, breast milk should be fed to the infant in the order in which it is collected, with the colostrum given first. An alternative for infants who cannot tolerate large volumes of feedings is hind milk (see Chapter 18), which has increased fat content and may be given preferentially to increase energy delivery. **Once the infant is tolerating 100 mL/kg/day of enteral nutrition, breast milk can be fortified with the addition of human milk fortifiers** (see Table 17-3). Thus progression to full enteral feedings of fortified human milk or 24 kcal/oz preterm infant formula occurs over a minimum of 2 weeks. During this time, parenteral nutritional support is tapered to maintain from birth at least 3.5 g/kg/day protein, 30% to 54% of total calories from fat, and 40% to 60% of total calories from carbohydrate. **In general, infants weighing less than 1200 g are fed every 2 hours and those weighing more are fed every 3 hours if bolus feedings are tolerated without emesis or residuals.** Firm experimental support for any feeding guidelines for preterm infants is sorely lacking, however. The suggested approach is both arbitrary and conservative. Individualization of feeding strategy is necessary for either more sick and physiologically unstable infants or more well and stable infants.

Late-Preterm Infant

The late-preterm infant, born at 34 to 37 weeks' gestation, represents the fastest growing preterm population, now accounting for more than 70% of all preterm births. Although generally these babies are larger and healthier than less mature newborns, NICU admission is frequently for feeding issues. The infant has intact, functional digestive and absorptive functions, but motility and intestinal colonization may be delayed. Of particular clinical importance is the immaturity of oromotor tone, function, and neural integration. As mentioned, the suck-swallow-breathing reflex develops between 33 and 36 weeks' gestation. **Infants born during this period may initially seem to feed well but cannot maintain successful feeding the first week of life.** Poor feeding is much more frequent in this group of babies, potentially contributing to problems of hypoglycemia and hyperbilirubinemia. **The ideal food for these infants is not well studied, but it is reasonable to fortify mother's milk or use preterm formulas and provide supplemental vitamins and minerals until the infant is taking full enteral feedings appropriate for a term infant.**

THE INTRAUTERINE GROWTH-RESTRICTED INFANT

Nutritional support for the small-for-gestational-age infant requires separate consideration, because decreased size-for-dates occurs with various pathologic conditions or no pathology at all. Small size at birth is related to any number of diseases or abnormalities, both intrinsic and extrinsic to the fetus and newborn. Early events in gestation, including chromosomal and genetic abnormalities or early infection, lead to symmetric growth restriction. In contrast, asymmetric growth restriction occurs in response to late placental insufficiency or other insults that restrict nutrient supply to the fetus. Many completely healthy and normal infants are constitutionally small. Complicating these issues is the fact that preterm infants often are growth restricted at birth (i.e., whatever led to growth restriction also contributed to processes that caused or promoted preterm birth). **Such infants require more individualized management, because they may not tolerate advancing enteral feedings and do not necessarily respond to increased nutrient intake with appropriate rates of growth.**[11,115] Furthermore, overfeeding a growth-restricted infant has been considered a cause of adult diseases such as obesity, insulin resistance, diabetes, and cardiovascular disease.[72]

In general, growth-restricted infants are likely to have increased energy needs and low stores of energy, nutrients, and minerals.[24,91] Hypoglycemia,[50] hyperglycemia, increased need for heat production, and increased risk for gastrointestinal ischemia and NEC are more likely in the early postnatal period in these infants than in their normally grown peers. These problems require anticipatory nutritional monitoring and management. Early parenteral glucose, protein, and energy supplementation is necessary while cautious enteral feedings are started.

CHANGES IN NUTRITIONAL REQUIREMENTS WITH ILLNESS

Studies in adult patients have shown dramatic changes in nutritional requirements depending on type of illness, degree of illness, surgery, and premorbid nutritional status. Although these changes are not well studied in neonates, preliminary data and clinical experience indicate similar changes should be expected in ill infants. In fact, these patients have even greater nutritional needs because of requirements for growth and development. The overriding observation from all studies, however, is that ELBW and VLBW preterm infants are underfed during the early postnatal period and that this undernutrition, combined with additional stresses from various diseases, increases the risk for long-term adverse neurologic sequelae. The value of achieving a specific body composition and growth rate is less certain.

There remains a critical need for determining the right quality, as well as quantity, of nutrients for these infants. **The effects of common disease states on the nutrient requirements in preterm and term infants are shown in Figure 17-6.**

Acute and chronic respiratory diseases are the most common illnesses in neonates. **Acute respiratory problems, such as respiratory distress syndrome, pneumonia, and aspiration, all increase the infant's metabolic needs for energy and protein. Energy requirements are met by increasing carbohydrate and fat delivery.** However, the metabolism of excessive carbohydrate feeding (>12.5 mg/kg/min) may be detrimental to pulmonary status by increasing oxygen consumption and carbon dioxide production, increasing respiratory work, and adding to respiratory failure. Lipid is a good alternative source of concentrated energy because its metabolism has a lower respiratory quotient and produces less carbon dioxide. Lipids provide dense calories for volume and prevent essential fatty acid deficiency. Protein wasting and catabolism with illness increase the infant's requirement for exogenous support. Adequate provision of amino acids, especially branched-chain amino acids, prevents catabolism of body protein stores, including respiratory and diaphragmatic muscle protein, and may improve minute ventilation by decreasing carbon dioxide production.

Infants with chronic lung disease and bronchopulmonary dysplasia present difficult nutritional problems. Poor nutrition is associated with abnormal lung development, increased toxic effects of oxygen, decreased surfactant production, and increased risk for infection. Although energy and metabolic demands are increased in these patients, many routine management strategies make the disease process worse. Excessive fluid volumes increase pulmonary edema and contribute to lung injury. **Increased work of breathing limits intake.** Steroid therapy and chronic disease have negative effects on protein balance. Diuretic use can waste calcium and potassium. Decreasing the proportion of energy provided by carbohydrates has been shown in older infants with chronic respiratory disease to decrease lipogenesis and therefore carbon dioxide production. Vitamin supplementation should be provided at the estimated advisable intake.

Congenital heart disease, especially when accompanied by cyanosis or congestive heart failure, significantly impairs nutritional status and growth. These infants have ***increased basal metabolic needs*** and experience the additional catabolic stress of early surgery. Nutritional management also is complicated by underlying hypoxemia, diuretic therapy, respiratory distress, malabsorption, and delicate fluid balance. Mineral derangement is common postoperatively with diuretic therapy and suboptimal intake. Iron supplementation is necessary to provide for increased erythropoiesis with chronic hypoxemia.

Good nutritional status can decrease the risk for infection and sepsis, as well as improve recovery in neonates. Normal immune response depends on adequate protein energy, micronutrients, and trace elements. Although not well studied in this population, it appears that the metabolic requirements of septic infants, especially for energy and amino acids, are much greater than the requirements of otherwise similar, but uninfected, infants.

The infant with NEC or short bowel syndrome is at additional risk for malnutrition because of malabsorption and increased nutrient losses. During the acute illness, these patients must receive adequate parenteral nutrition. Recovery needs to be supported by gradual increases in enteral nutrition and slowly decreasing parenteral supplementation. Of particular concern are excessive water losses with electrolyte imbalance and malabsorption of fats and fat-soluble vitamins.

Any infant recovering from asphyxia or shock should probably not receive enteral feedings for 24 to 72 hours to allow recovery of the bowel from the ischemic injury and decrease the risk for NEC.

Neonates who have undergone surgery are at increased risk for nutritional deficiencies resulting from the stresses of illness and surgery and possible abnormal nutrient and water losses. In these infants, enteral feedings are preferred because they are safe and more economical, preserve the integrity of the intestinal mucosa, and promote continued development of the gastrointestinal tract. **After an operative procedure, the infant is often nil per os (NPO) status for 3 to 14 days until the return of intestinal motility and function** (e.g., stooling, lack of abdominal distention, decreased gastric aspirates, absence of bilious aspirates). The method of feeding chosen, rapidity of feeding advancement, formula composition, and type of feeding depend on the infant's general medical condition, gastrointestinal function, and type of surgery. The choice of formula for the postsurgical neonate depends on bowel integrity. An infant recovering from mild NEC may be started on human milk or regular formula. With serious or surgically treated NEC, human milk is preferred but an elemental or hydrolysate formula may be used.

Oral feedings should be started postoperatively in the term infant if he or she is awake, hungry, and able to suck, swallow, and gag and has normal intestinal motility and no respiratory distress. Preterm infants usually need gavage feeding. Daily and weekly growth should be monitored and assessed relative to caloric intake. Inadequate growth may be treated with increased volumes, increased caloric density, or a less stressful method of feeding (e.g., a combination of nipple and gavage feedings).

DEVELOPMENTAL SUPPORT

The importance of developmentally supportive feeding cannot be overlooked when discussing infant nutrition. Prematurity resulting in delayed introduction of feeding skills, surgical interventions for congenital or genetic abnormalities sometimes necessitating alternative feeding methods such as gastrostomy tube feedings, and prolonged interruption of normal feeding patterns are all examples of the impact that hospitalization can have on patients and their families.[22]

Being aware of the impact that prolonged hospitalization can have on feeding is the first step in being able to provide support and guidance to families of fragile infants. By using a team approach, the family can help support their infant in attaining and strengthening feeding skills in preparation for discharge and hopefully prevent or minimize long-term feeding difficulties that often are associated with an extended hospital stay, such as loss of feeding skills and feeding aversion issues.[14,61]

A ***supportive feeding team*** should include the parents, physicians, nurse practitioners, lactation specialists, nutritionists, occupational and physical therapists, developmental specialists, and nursing staff educated in the developmental support of infants with specialized feeding needs. This support should start as soon as an infant is admitted and continue beyond discharge to promote the best possible outcome with regard to feeding ability.

FAMILY SUPPORT

Parents of the NICU patient may feel overwhelmed by their infant's illness, appearance, and uncertain future. Loss of control of the infant's care and unclear parental roles make bonding difficult and add to feelings of helplessness, frustration, and isolation. It is imperative that the **health care team and especially the bedside nurse be supportive of the parents as caregivers. This support can begin with education about early feeding** practices in the nursery and anticipated infant growth and development. Feeding is an excellent way to involve parents in their infant's care. **Parents should be involved in discussions of feeding practices and food choices. During gavage feedings, parents should be encouraged to hold their infant and support the pacifier to encourage nonnutritive sucking.** Frequent communication about the ups and downs of feeding the sick newborn, as well as weekly progress updates on growth charts, is helpful.

A mother's ability to provide breast milk remains the one aspect of care that she alone can do for her infant. Preterm birth and prolonged illness, as well as the inability to breast feed the infant directly, are major barriers to successful breast feeding. Lactation support in the NICU increases mothers' success at maintaining lactation through discharge from the NICU. Guidelines for expression and collection of human breast milk, gavage feeding of human milk, and identification of oral feeding readiness all are essential elements of lactation support and success (see Chapter 18).

FEEDING THE PREMATURELY BORN INFANT AFTER HOSPITAL DISCHARGE

Many preterm infants are still preterm when they are discharged from the NICU, and most are small for their corrected gestational age (i.e., they are growth restricted) despite attempts to improve in-hospital nutrition.[32] These infants require continued attention to nutritional support after hospital discharge. **Infants who are discharged on breast milk feedings can be supplemented with powder formula fortification of mother's milk or a 24 kcal/oz formula if growth is suboptimal.** Vitamins and minerals should be supplemented for all breast-feeding infants. **Demand feeding should**

be initiated before discharge to document adequate growth on the chosen feeding regimen.

Efforts to wean formula-fed infants to 20 kcal/oz formula before discharge may be counterproductive. Transitional or post-discharge formulas have been used for such infants. These products are intermediate between preterm and term formulas in their energy, protein, calcium, phosphorus, vitamin, and mineral contents. **Providing preterm infants with a formula containing higher protein and energy contents after discharge until a corrected age of 12 months has resulted in improved growth.**[19,41] See Table 17-7 for post-discharge formula nutritional composition.

Infants with significant chronic lung disease who require supplemental oxygen at home are particularly likely to need 24 kcal/oz formula after discharge to maintain adequate growth at home. Oxygen supplementation itself also improves growth in these infants when normal oxygen saturation is maintained. The ideal composition of feedings in "recovering" preterm infants has yet to be determined; however, efforts to continue feeding with a 22- or 24-kcal/oz infant formula with a higher protein and mineral content for several months after hospital discharge are supported by studies showing long-term improvement in growth and neurodevelopmental outcome, even for preterm infants who do not have significant chronic illnesses.

REFERENCES

1. Abrams B, Selvin S: Maternal weight gain pattern and birth weight, *Obstet Gynecol* 86:163, 1995.
2. al Tawil Y, Berseth CL: Gestational and postnatal maturation of duodenal motor responses to intragastric feeding, *J Pediatr* 129(3):374, 1996.
3. Alexander G, Himes JH, Kaufman RB, et al: A United States national reference for fetal growth, *Obstet Gynecol* 87:2, 163, 1996.
4. American Academy of Pediatrics: Committee on Fetus and Newborn: Controversies concerning vitamin K and the newborn, *Pediatrics* 112:191, 2003.
5. American Academy of Pediatrics, Section on Breastfeeding: Breastfeeding and the use of human milk, *Pediatrics* 115:496, 2005.
6. Baker JH, Berseth CL: Duodenal motor responses in preterm infants fed formula with varying concentrations and rates of infusion, *Pediatr Res* 42:618, 1997.
7. Berseth CL: Minimal enteral feedings, *Clin Perinatol* 22:195, 1995.
8. Berseth CL, Bisquera JA, Paje VU: Prolonging small feeding volumes early in life decreases the incidence of necrotizing enterocolitis in very low birth weight infants, *Pediatrics* 111:529, 2003.
9. Bhatia J, Greer F, and the Committee on Nutrition: Use of soy protein-based formulas in infant feeding, *Pediatrics* 121(5):1062, 2008.
10. Bloomfield FH, Harding JE: Fetal nutrition. In Thureen PJ, Hay WW Jr, editors: *Neonatal nutrition and metabolism,* ed 2 New York, 2006, Cambridge University Press.
11. Brandt I, Sticker EJ, Lentze MJ: Catch-up growth of head circumference of very low birth weight, small for gestational age preterm infants and mental development to adulthood, *J Pediatr* 142:463, 2003.
12. Brennan-Behan M, Carlson G, Meier P, et al: Calorie loss from expressed mother's milk during continuous gavage infusion, *Neonatal Netw* 13:27, 1994.
13. Brown JM, Murtaugh MA, Jacobs DR Jr, et al: Variation in newborn size according to prepregnancy weight change by trimester, *Am J Clin Nutr* 76:205, 2002.
14. Browne J, Gabrielski L, Paul D: *Guidelines for oral feeding,* Denver, 1998, Center for Family & Infant Interaction.
15. Burdge GC, Hanson MA, Slater-Jeffries JL, et al: Epigenetic regulation of transcription: a mechanism for inducing variations in phenotype (fetal programming) by differences in nutrition during early life? *Br J Nutr* 97(6):1036, 2007.
16. Burkhardt T, Schaffer L, Zimmermann R, et al: Newborn weight charts underestimate the incidence of low birthweight in preterm infants, *Am J Obstet Gynecol* 199(2):139.e6, 2008.
17. Burrin DG, Stoll B: Key nutrients and growth factors for the neonatal gastrointestinal tract, *Clin Perinatol* 29:65, 2002.
18. Caicedo RA, Schanler RJ, Li N, et al: The developing ecosystem: implications for the neonate, *Pediatr Res* 58(4):625, 2005.
19. Carver JD, Wu PYK, Hall RT, et al: Growth of preterm infants fed nutrient-enriched or term formula after hospital discharge, *Pediatrics* 107(4):683, 2001.
20. Clark R, Thomas P, Peabody J: Extrauterine growth restriction remains a serious problem in prematurely born neonates, *Pediatrics* 111:986, 2003.
21. Cleal JK, Lewis RM: The mechanisms and regulation of placental amino acid transport to the human foetus, *J Neuroendocrinology* 20:419, 2008.
22. Comrie JD, Helm JM: Common feeding problems in the intensive care nursery: maturation, organization, evaluation and management strategies, *Semin Speech Lang* 18:239, 1997.
23. Cooke R, Ainsworth S, Fenton A: Postnatal growth retardation: a universal problem in preterm infants, *Arch Dis Child Fetal Neonatal Ed* 89:F428, 2004.

24. Davies PSW, Clough H, Bishop NJ, et al: Total energy expenditure in small for gestational age infants, *Arch Dis Child Fetal Neonatal Ed* 74:F208, 1996.
25. Delvin EE, Salle Bl, Claris O, et al: Oral vitamin A, E, and D supplementation of pre-term newborns either breast-fed or formula-fed: a 3-month longitudinal study, *J Pediatr Gastroenterol Nutr* 40(1):43, 2005.
26. De Ville K, Knapp E, Al-Tawil Y, et al: Slow infusion feedings enhance duodenal motor responses and gastric emptying in preterm infants, *Am J Clin Nutr* 68:103, 1998.
27. Dinnerstein A, Nieto RM, Solana CL, et al: Early and aggressive nutrition strategy (parenteral and enteral) decreases postnatal growth failure in very low birth weight infants, *J Perinatol* 26:436, 2006.
28. Dodd V, Freman R: A field study of bacterial growth in continuous feedings in a NICU, *Neonatal Netw* 9:17, 1991.
29. Dumont RC, Rudolph CD: Development of gastrointestinal motility in the infant and child, *Gastroenterol Clin North Am* 23:655, 1994.
30. Dusick AM, Poindexter BB, Ehrenkranz RA, et al: Growth failure in the preterm infant: can we catch up? *Semin Perinatol* 27:302, 2003.
31. Ehrenkranz RA: Early, aggressive nutritional management for very low birth weight infants: what is the evidence? *Semin Perinatol* 31:48, 2007.
32. Ehrenkranz RA, Younes N, Lemons JA, et al: Longitudinal growth of hospitalized very low birth weight infants, *Pediatrics* 104:280, 1999.
33. Embleton NE, Pang N, Cooke RJ: Postnatal malnutrition and growth retardation: an inevitable consequence of current recommendations in preterm infants? *Pediatrics* 107:270, 2001.
34. Eritsland J: Safety considerations of polyunsaturated fatty acids, *Am J Clin Nutr* 71:197, 2000.
35. ESPGHAN Committee on Nutrition, Agostino C, Axelsson I, Goulet O, et al: Soy protein infant formulae and follow-on formulae: a commentary by the ESPGHAN Committee on Nutrition, *J Pediatr Gastroenterol Nutr* 42:352, 2006.
36. Fenton TR: A new growth chart for preterm babies: Babson and Benda's chart updated with recent data and a new format, *BMC Pediatrics* 3:13, 2003.
37. Fewtrell MS, Abbott RA, Kennedy K, et al: Randomised, double-blind trial of long-chain polyunsaturated fatty acid supplementation with fish oil and borage oil in preterm infants, *J Pediatr* 144:471, 2004.
38. Fewtrell MS, Morley R, Abbott RA, et al: Catch-up growth in small-for-gestational-age term infants: a randomized trial, *Am J Clin Nutr* 74:516, 2001.
39. Fewtrell MS, Morley R, Abbott RA, et al: Double-blind, randomized trial of long-chain polyunsaturated fatty acid supplementation in formula fed to preterm infants, *Pediatrics* 110:73, 2002.
40. Franz AR, Pohlandt F, Bode H, et al: Intrauterine, early neonatal, and postdischarge growth and neurodevelopmental outcome at 5.4 years in extremely preterm infants after intensive neonatal nutritional support, *Pediatrics* 123(1):e101, 2009.
41. Gibson AT, Carney S, Cavazzoni E, et al: Neonatal and post-natal growth, *Horm Res* 53(Suppl 1):42, 2000.
42. Gicquel C, El-Osta A, LeBouc Y: Epigenetic regulation and fetal programming, *Best Pract Res Clin Endocrinol Metab* 22(1):1, 2008.
43. Graham III PL, Begg MD, Larson E, et al: Risk factors for late onset gram-negative sepsis in low birth weight infants hospitalized in the neonatal intensive care unit, *Pediatr Infect Dis J* 25:113, 2006.
44. Grant J, Denne SC: Effect of intermittent versus continuous enteral feeding on energy expenditure in premature infants, *J Pediatr* 118:928, 1991.
45. Greer FR, Sicherer SH, Burks AW, et al: Effects of early nutritional interventions on the development of atopic disease in infants and children: the role of maternal dietary restriction, breastfeeding, timing of introduction of complementary foods, and hydrolyzed formulas, *Pediatrics* 121(1):183, 2008.
46. Guillet R, Stoll BJ, Cotton CM, et al: Association of H2-blocker therapy and higher incidence of necrotizing enterocolitis in very low birth weight infants, *Pediatrics* 117(2):e137, 2006.
47. Harmsen HJ, Wildeboer-Veloo AC, Raangs GC, et al: Analysis of intestinal flora development in breast-fed and formula-fed infants by using molecular identification and detection methods, *J Pediatr Gastroenterol Nutr* 30:61, 2000.
48. Heird WC, Lapillonne A: The role of essential fatty acids in development, *Annu Rev Nutr* 25:549, 2005.
49. Henriksen C, Helland IB, Ronnestad A, et al: Fat-soluble vitamins in breast-fed preterm and term infants, *Eur J Clin Nutr* 60(6):756, 2006.
50. Holtrop PC: The frequency of hypoglycemia in full-term large and small for gestational age newborns, *Am J Perinatol* 10:150, 1993.
51. Huppi PS: Nutrition for the brain, *Pediatr Res* 63(3):229, 2008.
52. Innis SM: Perinatal biochemistry and physiology of long-chain polyunsaturated fatty acids, *J Pediatr* 143:S1, 2003.
53. Innis SM, Adamkin DH, Hall RT, et al: Docosahexaenoic acid and arachidonic acid enhance growth with no adverse effects in preterm infants fed formula, *J Pediatrics* 140:547, 2002.
54. Isaacs EB, Gadian DG, Sabatini S, et al: The effects of early human diet on caudate volumes and IQ, *Pediatr Res* 63(3):308, 2008.
55. Jadcherla SR, Berseth CL: Effect of erythromycin on gastroduodenal contractile activity in developing neonates, *J Pediatr Gastroenterol Nutr* 34(1):16, 2002.

56. Jadcherla SR, Duong HG, Hoffmann RG, et al: Esophageal body and upper esophageal sphincter motor responses to esophageal provocation during maturation in preterm newborns, *J Pediatr* 143:31, 2003.
57. Jansson T, Cetin I, Powell TL, et al: Placental transport and metabolism in fetal overgrowth: a workshop report, *Placenta* 27(1):109, 2006.
58. Jansson T, Powell TL: IFPA 2005 Award in Placentology Lecture. Human placental transport in altered fetal growth: does the placenta function as a nutrient sensor?—a review, *Placenta* 27(Suppl A):S91, 2006.
59. Kashyap S, Forsyth M, Zucker C, et al: Effects of varying protein and energy intakes on growth and metabolic response in low birth weight infants, *J Pediatr* 108:995, 1986.
60. Kashyap S, Schulze KF, Forsyth M, et al: Growth, nutrient retention, and metabolic response in low birth weight infants fed varying intakes of protein and energy, *J Pediatr* 113:713, 1988.
61. Kenner C, Lott JW: Newborn and infant neurodevelopmental development. In *Comprehensive neonatal nursing: a physiological perspective*, ed 3, Philadelphia, 2003, Saunders, p 258.
62. Kirchengast S, Harlmann B: Maternal prepregnancy weight status and pregnancy weight gain as major determinants for newborn weight and size, *Annals of Human Biol* 25(1):17, 1998.
63. Klein CJ: Nutrient requirements for preterm infant formulas, *J Nutr* 132:1395S, 2002.
64. Knight B, Shields BM, Hill A, et al: The impact of maternal glycemia and obesity on early postnatal growth in a nondiabetic Caucasian population, *Diabetes Care* 30(4):777, 2007.
65. Knight B, Shields BM, Turner M, et al: Evidence of genetic regulation of fetal longitudinal growth, *Early Hum Dev* 81(10):823, 2005.
66. Koletzko B, Agostoni C, Carlson SE, et al: Long chain polyunsaturated fatty acids (LC-PUFA) and perinatal development, *Acta Paediatr* 90:460, 2001.
67. Koletzko B, Sauerwald U, Keicher U, et al: Fatty acid profiles, antioxidant status, and growth of preterm infants fed diets without or with long-chain polyunsaturated fatty acids, *Eur J Nutr* 42(5):243, 2003.
68. Kuschel CA, Harding JE: Protein supplementation of human milk for promoting growth in preterm infants (review), *Cochrane Database Syst Rev* 2:CD000433, 2000.
69. Latal-Hajnal B, Von Siebenthal K, Kovari H, et al: Postnatal growth in VLBW infants: significant association with neurodevelopment outcome, *J Pediatr* 143:163, 2003.
70. Laubereau B, Brockow I, Zirngibl A, et al: Effect of breast-feeding on the development of atopic dermatitis during the first 3 years of life: results from the GINI-birth cohort study, *J Pediatr* 144:602, 2004.
71. Liepke C, Adermann K, Raida M, et al: Human milk provides peptides highly stimulating to the growth of bifidobacter, *Eur J Biochem* 269:712, 2002.
72. Lucas A: Programming by early nutrition: an experimental approach, *J Nutr* 128(Suppl 2):410S, 1998.
73. Lucas A, Cole TJ: Randomised trial of early diet in preterm babies and later intelligence quotient, *BMJ* 317:1481, 1998.
74. Lucas A, Hudson G: Preterm milk as a source of protein for low birth weight infants, *Arch Dis Child* 59:831, 1984.
75. Lucas A, Morley R, Cole TJ, et al: Early diet in preterm babies and developmental status at 18 months, *Lancet* 335:1477, 1990.
76. Lucas A, Morley R, Cole TJ, et al: Breast milk and subsequent intelligence quotient in children born preterm, *Lancet* 339:261, 1992.
77. Mackie RI, Sghir A, Gaskins HR: Developmental microbial ecology of the neonatal gastrointestinal tract, *Am J Clin Nutr* 69(Suppl):1035S, 1999.
78. Manson WG, Weaver LT: Fat digestion in the neonate, *Arch Dis Child Fetal Neonatal Ed* 76:F206, 1997.
79. Martin R, Langa S, Reviriego C, et al: Human milk is the source of lactic acid bacteria for the infant gut, *J Pediatr* 143:754, 2003.
80. Mathews MS, MacDorman MF: Infant mortality statistics from the 2005 period linked birth/infant death data set, *National Vital Statistics Reports* 57(2):1, 2008.
81. McClure RJ, Newell SJ: Randomised controlled trial of trophic feeding and gut motility, *Arch Dis Child Fetal Neonatal Ed* 80:F54, 1999.
82. McClure RJ, Newell SJ: Randomised controlled study of clinical outcome following trophic feeding, *Arch Dis Child Fetal Neonatal Ed* 82:F29, 2000.
83. McGuire W, McEwan P: Transpyloric versus gastric tube feeding for preterm infants, *Cochrane Database Syst Rev* 3:2002 CD003487.
84. McGuire W, McEwan P: Systematic review of transpyloric versus gastric feeding for preterm infants (review), *Arch Dis Child Fetal Neonatal Ed* 89:F245, 2004.
85. Meetze WH, Valentine C, McGuigan JE, et al: Gastrointestinal priming prior to full enteral nutrition in very low birth weight infants, *J Pediatr Gastroenterol Nutr* 15:163, 1992.
86. Miniello VL, Moro GE, Tarantino M, et al: Soy-based formulas and phyto-oestrogens: a safety profile, *Acta Pediatr Suppl* 441:93, 2003.
87. Montgomery RK, Mulberg AE, Grand RJ: Development of the human gastrointestinal tract: twenty years of progress, *Gastroenterology* 116:702, 1999.
88. Newburg DS, Walker WA: Protection of the neonate by the innate immune system of developing gut and of human milk, *Pediatr Res* 61(1):2, 2006.

89. Newell SJ, Chapman S, Booth IW: Ultrasonic assessment of gastric emptying in the preterm infant, *Arch Dis Child* 60(1 Spec No):32, 1993.
90. Nyqvist KH, Sorell A, Ewald U: Litmus tests for verification of feeding tube location in infants: evaluation of their clinical use, *J Clin Nurs* 14:486, 2005.
91. Olivares M, Llaguno S, Marin V, et al: Iron status in low-birth-weight infants, small and appropriate for gestational age: a follow up study, *Acta Paediatr* 81:824, 1992.
92. Ortiz JE, Sottile FD, Siegel P, et al: Gastric colonization as a consequence of stress ulcer prophylaxis: a prospective, randomized trial, *Pharmacotherapy* 18:486, 1998.
93. Penders J, Thijs C, Vink C, et al: Factors influencing the composition of the intestinal microbia in early infancy, *Pediatriacs* 118(2):511, 2006.
94. Phillips C, Johnson NE: The impact of quality of diet and other factors on birth weight of infants, *Am J Clin Nutr* 30:215, 1977.
95. Premji S, Chessell L: Continuous nasogastric milk feeding versus intermittent bolus milk feeding for premature infants less than 1500 grams, *Cochrane Database Syst Rev* 1: CD001819, 2001.
96. Radmacher PG, Looney SW, Rafail ST, et al: Prediction of extrauterine growth retardation (EUGR) in VLBW infants, *J Perinatol* 23:392, 2003.
97. Regnault TR, Friedman JE, Wilkening RB, et al: Fetoplacental transport and utilization of amino acids in IUGR: a review, *Placenta* 26(Suppl A):S52, 2005.
98. Reidel BD, Greene HL: Vitamins. In Hay WW Jr, editors: *Neonatal nutrition and metabolism,* St Louis, 1991, Mosby.
99. Reis BB, Hall RT, Schanler RJ, et al: Enhanced growth of preterm infants fed a new powdered human milk fortifier: a randomized, controlled trial, *Pediatrics* 106:581, 2000.
100. Rigo J, Pieltain C, Salle B, et al: Enteral calcium, phosphate, and vitamin D requirements and bone mineralization in preterm infants, *Acta Pediatr* 96(7):969, 2007.
101. Robertson C: Catch-up growth among very-low-birth-weight preterm infants: a historical perspective, *J Pediatr* 143:145, 2003.
102. Rodriquez A, Raederstorff D, Sarda P, et al: Preterm infant formula supplementation with alpha linolenic acid and docosahexanoic acid, *Eur J Clin Nutr* 57:727, 2003.
103. Salle BL, Delvin EE, Lapillonne A, et al: Perinatal metabolism of vitamin D, *Am J Clin Nutr* 71(Suppl 5):1317S, 2000.
104. Schanler RJ, Schulman RJ, Lau C, et al: Feeding strategies for premature infants: randomized trial of gastrointestinal priming and tube-feeding, *Pediatrics* 103:434, 1999.
105. Shaker CS: Nipple feeding premature infants: a different perspective, *Neonatal Netw* 8:9, 1990.
106. Silvestre MA, Morbach CA, Brans YW, et al: A prospective randomized trial comparing continuous versus intermittent feeding methods in very low birth weight neonates, *J Pediatr* 128:748, 1996.
107. Simmer K: Long chain polyunsaturated fatty acid supplementation in infants born at term, *Cochrane Database Syst Rev* 4:CD000376, 2001.
108. Singhai A, Cole T, Fewtrell M, et al: Is slower early growth beneficial for long-term cardiovascular health? *Circulation* 109:1108, 2004.
109. Singhai A, Fewtrell M, Cole T, et al: Low nutrient intake and early growth for later insulin resistance in adolescents born preterm, *Lancet* 361:1089, 2003.
110. Tsang RC, Uauy R, Koletzko B, et al: *Nutrition of the preterm infant: scientific basis and practical guidelines*, ed 2 Cincinnati, 2005, Digital Educational Publishing.
111. Turck D: Soy protein for infant feeding: what do we know? *Curr Opin Clin Nutr Metab Care* 10:360, 2007.
112. Tyson JE, Wright LL, Oh W, et al: Vitamin A supplementation for extremely-low-birth-weight infants, *N Engl J Med* 340:1962, 1999.
113. Van Den Driessche M, Peeters K, Marien P, et al: Gastric emptying in formula-fed and breast-fed infants measured with the 13C-octanoic acid breath test, *J Ped Gastroenterol Nutr* 29(1):46, 1999.
114. Villar J, Cogswell M, Kestler E, et al: Effect of fat and fat-free mass deposition during pregnancy on birth weight, *Am J Obstet Gynecol* 167(5):1344, 1992.
115. Vohr BR, McKinley LT: The challenge pays off: early enhanced nutritional intake for VLBW small-for-gestation neonates improves long-term outcome, *J Pediatr* 142:459, 2003.
116. Wagner CL, Greer FR, and the AAP Section on Nutrition Breastfeeding and the Committee on Nutrition: Prevention of rickets and vitamin D deficiency in the infant, child, and adolescent, *Pediatrics* 122(5):1142, 2008.
117. Waterland RA: Epigenetic mechanisms and gastrointestinal development, *J Pediatr* 149(Suppl 5):S137, 2006.
118. Weiler HA, Fitzpatrick-Wong SC, Schellenberg JM: Minimal enteral feeding within 3 d of birth in prematurely born infants with birth weight < or = 1200g improves bone mass by term age, *Am J Clin Nutr* 83(1):155, 2006.

18 BREAST FEEDING THE NEONATE WITH SPECIAL NEEDS

SANDRA L. GARDNER AND RUTH A. LAWRENCE

Human milk has been recognized as the gold standard for infant nutrition for centuries. Published studies from 1918 on have confirmed that problems develop when human milk is replaced with artificial formulas made from the milk of other species. Milk of other species that is fed to human infants has been known to contribute to increased infant mortality. Over the years, increasing research has confirmed the presence of the anti-infective properties of human milk, which protect against infections of the gastrointestinal tract, the upper and lower respiratory tracts, and the urinary tract, as well as against otitis media, bacteremia, bacterial meningitis, botulism, and necrotizing enterocolitis (NEC), leading to lower infant mortality.[3,8,108] In numerous studies, human milk also has been shown to have a protective effect against sudden infant death syndrome (SIDS), type 1 and type 2 diabetes, obesity, Crohn's disease, ulcerative colitis, lymphoma, childhood leukemia, allergic diseases, asthma, chronic digestive disorders, heart disease, and hypertension.[3,108] Breast feeding also enhances cognitive and visual development and neurodevelopment.[116,149] A recent study showed less of a pain response in full-term infants undergoing heel lance when they were breast fed before, during, and after the procedure (see Chapter 12). **In preterm infants, human milk provides both short-term and long-term advantages (Table 18-1) in a dose-dependent relationship—the more breast milk the preterm receives, the more benefits received.**

Because of a lack of experience and knowledge about breast feeding, a new mother who is discharged early (24 to 48 hours) from the hospital may find it challenging to initiate breast feeding for her healthy newborn infant. The mother of a newborn with special needs, such as a preterm infant, a sick term newborn, or an infant with a congenital anomaly, may have even more difficulty in establishing breast feeding because of the stress of separation and concerns about the infant's well-being. The tremendous benefits of providing human milk for all infants, but especially the premature, outweigh any apparent difficulties.[144]

Healthy People 2010,[209] the health policy statement for the United States, states the following goal about breast feeding: 75% of women breast feeding in the early postpartum period, at least 50% still breast feeding their infant at 6 months, and 25% breast feeding their infant at 1 year of age. A report published by the Institute of Medicine from the Subcommittee on Nutritional Status During Pregnancy and Lactation,[91] the American Academy of Pediatrics (AAP) Section on Breast Feeding,[8] and the U.S. Surgeon General's *Blueprint for Action on Breast Feeding*[207] state that (1) all infants in the United States should be breast fed, (2) "human milk is uniquely superior for infant feeding,"[91] (3) "infants should be exclusively breast fed for 5 to 6 months,"[8] and (4) "breast feeding is the ideal method of feeding and nurturing infants."[207] The policy statement by the AAP provides additional recommendations for high-risk infants, including preterm infants. They state that the "hospitals and physicians should recommend human milk for premature and other high-risk infants either by direct breast feeding or using the mother's own expressed milk." The statement continues by recognizing that maternal

Please note that the PURPLE type in each chapter is intended to make it easier to identify clinically applicable material.

TABLE 18-1 ADVANTAGES OF BREAST FEEDING AND HUMAN MILK INTAKE FOR PRETERM INFANTS[77]

BENEFIT	COMMENT
Protection from NEC[30,172,185]	Formula-fed infants developed NEC 6 to 10 times more often than infants receiving only human milk. Infants ≥30 weeks' gestation: incidence of NEC 20 times more in formula-fed than in human milk–fed infants. Lower incidence of intestinal perforations and less severity of NEC with human milk intake before NEC. Dose-dependent relationship between human milk intake and reduced risk for NEC/death after 2 weeks of life in ELBW preterms.[142]
Protection from infection or sepsis[142]	Lowered infection and severity of infections in hospitalized ELBW, VLBW, or LBW infants fed human milk,[59,90,185] resulting in shortened LOS. Decreased protection if formula feeding added to human milk feedings. Increased rehospitalization: sevenfold for formula-fed compared with 0-1 for infants who are breast fed (both partially and completely).
Increased feeding tolerance[133]	Whey protein in human milk is more digested, which results in more rapid gastric emptying and less gastric residual.[22] Fat globules in human milk provide optimal absorption.[13] It is possible to achieve complete enteral feedings by 6 weeks of age in VLBW infants fed own mother's milk (compared with VLBW infants fed donor milk or formula).[115] Formula-fed infants: increased vomiting, gastric residuals, and longer time to achieve complete enteral feedings.[115] Early enteral feeding with human milk is as well tolerated in preterms treated with indomethacin for PDA as in matched controls.[19]
Earlier attainment of full enteral feedings,[194] which is associated with a significant reduction in late-onset sepsis among extremely premature infants[177]	Preterms ≤1250 grams receiving at least 50% human milk attained earlier full enteral feeding.
Decreased risk for later allergy	Lower incidence of allergic symptoms (especially eczema) at 18 months in human milk–fed preterm infants.[114]
Improved retinal function[38,89,159]	Better retinal function, depending on omega-3 fatty acid concentration (found in human milk, but not previously in formula) in enteral feedings. Less ROP and less severe ROP in human milk–fed compared with formula-fed infants.[89] In ELBW infants fed human milk, there was no decreased risk for severe ROP.[75]
Improved neurocognitive development[21,38,51,78,196,214]	Long-term advantages: higher intelligence quotients at 30 months[215] and 7 to 8 years of age[84]; better development at 18 to 22 months of age[116,149,214]; and better behavioral scores (orientation/engagement, motor regulation, and total scores).[214] Faster brainstem maturation—resulting in better control of breathing.[10] No or small effect on neurodevelopmental outcomes.[60] Early supplementation of human milk with DHA/ARA for VLBW associated with better recognition memory and problem-solving skills at 6 months.[78]
Suppression of oxidative stress	Oxidative DNA damage in VLBW infants is suppressed at 14 and 28 days of age by measuring urinary 8-0 HdG excretion.[190]
Reduced heart disease in later life	Lower cardiorespiratory levels and LDL to HDL ratios in adolescents born premature who were fed human milk.

Modified from Meier P, Brown L: Breast feeding for mothers and low birth weight infants. *Nurs Clin North Am* 31:351, 1996.

ARA, Arachidonic acid; *DHA*, docosahexaenoic acid; *DNA*, deoxyribonucleic acid; *ELBW*, extremely-low-birth-weight; *HDL*, high-density lipoprotein; *LBW*, low-birth-weight; *LDL*, low-density lipoprotein; *LOS*, length-of-stay; *HdG*, hydroxy-deoxy-guanosine; *NEC*, necrotizing enterocolitis; *PDA*, patent ductus arteriosus; *ROP*, retinopathy of prematurity; *VLBW*, very-low-birth-weight.

support and education, mother-infant skin-to-skin contact, and direct breast feeding as early as possible are keys to success. State-by-state breast feeding data on the percentage and length of breast feeding are available from the Centers for Disease Control and Prevention (CDC) at *www.cdc.gov* and have been published by Ryan.[181] In 2008, the CDC reported that 77% of mothers in the United States were discharged from the hospital breast feeding their newborns—the highest rate in more than a decade.

The goal of this chapter is to give the health care provider the skill and knowledge to support the breast feeding dyad, especially when it involves the neonate with special needs.

PHYSIOLOGY OF BREAST FEEDING

Nutritional Value of Breast Milk

The components of breast milk vary with the (1) stage of lactation, (2) time of day, (3) sampling time during a feeding, and (4) extremes of maternal nutrition. In addition, there is variation among individuals.[97,108]

Colostrum is produced immediately at delivery and within 5 days gradually changes to transitional milk with increased lactose and finally mature milk by 2 weeks with an increasing concentration of fat. Colostrum contains higher ash content and higher concentrations of sodium, potassium, chloride, protein, fat-soluble vitamins, and minerals than does mature milk. Colostrum has a lower fat content, especially of lauric and myristic acids, than does mature milk. This milk is yellowish, thick, and rich in antibodies, has specific gravity between 1.040 and 1.060, and contains 67 kcal/dL. Multiparas and women who have previously breast fed have more colostrum during the first few days than do women who have not.

Transitional milk is produced between 7 and 10 days postpartum, remains high in protein and lower in fat, and has a dramatic increase in water content compared with colostrum. Among mothers, the high variability of transitional milk accounts for 67 to 75 kcal/dL.

Mature milk is produced after 10 days postpartum and contains 75 kcal/dL. By the second week of life, maternal milk production averages about 30 mL/hr (i.e., 750 to 800 mL/day). During a feeding, the relative content of protein and the absolute content of fat increase. Morning feedings have a higher fat content than do afternoon and evening feedings. Foremilk is lower in fat than hindmilk. Severely malnourished mothers have been shown to produce less milk, and water-soluble vitamins may be affected by deficient diets, as may occur in strict vegetarians.

Human Milk Versus Cow's Milk

Cow's milk differs significantly from human milk. Cow's milk has 18 parts whey to 82 parts casein, whereas human milk has 60 parts whey to 40 parts casein. Casein is composed of proteins with ester-bound phosphate, high proline content, and low solubility at a pH of 4 to 5. Casein forms curd by combining with calcium caseinate and calcium phosphate. The cysteine and taurine content is low in cow's milk but high in human milk, whereas the methionine content is high in cow's milk and low in human milk (the human infant lacks the enzyme to digest methionine). Human milk also has lower levels of aromatic amino acids, phenylalanine, and tyrosine. Human milk contains 6.8 g/dL of lactose, and cow's milk contains 4.9 g/dL of lactose. Sodium, phosphorus, calcium, magnesium, citrate, and total ash content are higher in cow's milk, but potassium and the calcium:phosphorus ratio are higher in human milk. Formula attempts to mimic human milk but still lacks cholesterol, omega-3 fatty acids, enzymes, antibodies, lactoferrin, and other protective anti-infective properties.

Human milk contains more iron than unsupplemented cow's milk but less iron than supplemented cow's milk. Only 10% of iron is absorbed from formula, whereas about 80% is absorbed from human milk. Iron in formula encourages the growth of *Escherichia coli* and inactivates lactoferrin. Cow's milk has a mean pH of 6.8, osmolality of 350 mOsm, and 221 mOsm renal osmolar load. Human milk has a mean pH of 7.1, osmolality of 286 mOsm, and 79 mOsm renal osmolar load.

Cow's milk forms indigestible curds much more easily and thus delays gastric emptying. The newborn cannot handle certain proteins well because cow's milk lacks specific enzymes necessary for metabolism. These enzymes are readily available in human milk. **However, 95% of human milk protein is nutritionally available to term infants, whereas the gastrointestinal immaturity of the preterm infant enables four to six times higher daily losses of human milk protein if human milk is pasteurized or has cow milk–based fortifier**

added. Some human milk proteins are immunoglobulins, which have a protective effect on the gut and are preserved by antiproteases from being digested (i.e., are found in stool). In very-low-birth-weight (VLBW) infants, the antiproteases persist so that there are more immunoglobulins and lactoferrin in the stool early on (i.e., six and four times more IgA and lactoferrin, respectively). This is a function of the milk of mothers who deliver prematurely, not a deficiency of VLBW gut. **Iron is more bioavailable in human milk, and iron absorption from human milk is more efficient,** but cow's milk has a higher concentration of zinc and contains more fluorine than does human milk. Human milk, however, contains a ligand specific to zinc absorption, and thus more zinc actually is absorbed and used. Human milk has been used as a therapy for zinc deficiency (see Chapter 17 for other human milk components).

Preterm Versus Term Breast Milk

Significant evidence exists that there are many differences in the breast milk that a mother produces when she has a preterm infant compared with breast milk produced for a term infant: (1) preterm breast milk has increased protein content; (2) the types of protein, predominantly whey, have a more physiologic balance of amino acids and contain many anti-infective properties; (3) the lipid content in preterm breast milk is more specific for the preterm neonate (i.e., an increased supply of medium-chain to intermediate-chain fatty acids); (4) lactose, the major carbohydrate in breast milk, has increased absorption in preterm infants; and (5) IgA concentrations are higher (see Chapter 17 for a comparison of preterm and term breast milk).

The Immunologic Value of Breast Milk

Because human milk protects neonates through its many anti-infective properties, breast-fed infants have decreased morbidity compared with bottle-fed infants.[70,154] **The immunologic benefits of human milk depend on dose, duration, and exclusivity.**[74] The main defense factors in human milk are (1) antimicrobial agents, (2) anti-inflammatory factors, and (3) immunomodulators and leukocytes. In addition to providing protective agents, the components in human milk also modulate the development of the newborn's own immune functions.[70] Bioactive factors in human milk and their functions are listed in Table 18-2. Because the highest concentration of some of these factors is found in colostrum,[70,175] this early milk should be pumped, preserved, and fed to a neonate with special needs. **Pumped milk should be labeled chronologically so that it is fed to preterm infants in the same sequence in which it was collected. In this fashion, the preterm infant**

TABLE 18-2 BIOACTIVE FACTORS IN HUMAN MILK

COMPONENT	FUNCTION
ANTIBODIES	
Secretory IgA (sIgA)	Attaches to mucosal epithelium of digestive tract, thus preventing attachment of pathogens,[102,176] sIgA against enteric, respiratory, and viral pathogens, as well as specific pathogens to which the mother has been exposed; highest concentration in colostrum peaks during first 3 to 4 days postpartum, present in mature milk through first year of life[27,184]; antiallergic properties: inhibits absorption of macro-molecular antigens from neonatal small intestine.
MAJOR NUTRIENTS	
Protein	
sIgA: IgM, IgG	Immune protection.
Lactoferrin	Binds iron, thwarts growth of pathogens (e.g., bactericidal, antiviral), modulates cytokine function and is anti-inflammatory; highest levels in colostrum; present in mature milk through first year of life.[102] May attenuate iron-induced oxidation products in preterms.[170]

Modified from Hamosh B: Bioactive factors in human milk, *Pediatr Clin North Am* 48:69, 2001.

Continued

TABLE 18-2 **BIOACTIVE FACTORS IN HUMAN MILK—cont'd**

COMPONENT	FUNCTION
MAJOR NUTRIENTS—cont'd	
Protein—cont'd	
Lysozyme	Destroys pathogens (e.g., gram-positive and few gram-negative bacteria) by cell wall lysis; human milk contains 300 times the concentration in cow's milk; concentration increases with prolonged lactation.[176]
Casein	Inhibits microbial adhesion to mucous membranes of respiratory and gastrointestinal tracts. Promotes growth of *Lactobacillus bifidus*, the normal intestinal flora for breast-fed infants, and inhibits pathogens[112]; by 1 month of age, *Bifidobacterium* level in infants fed human milk is 10 times that of formula-fed infants.
Fibronectin	Enhances antimicrobial activity of macrophages[176]; assists in repair of intestinal tissue damage by immune reactions.
Carbohydrate	
Oligosaccharides	Bind to microorganisms (microbial ligands), thus preventing pathogens from attaching to respiratory mucosal surfaces.[184]
Glycoconjugates mucin; lactadherin	Microbial and viral ligands.[70] Provide receptor site binding for organisms so that the organism is made less harmful or passes from the body in the stool.[176]
Fat	
Free fatty acids (FFAs)	Disrupt and destroy lipid-enveloped virus, bacteria, and protozoa.[70]
MINOR NUTRIENTS	
Nucleotides	Enhance T-cell maturation, antibody response to vaccines, intestinal maturation, repair after diarrhea and natural killer cell activity; promote growth of *Lactobacillus bifidus*.
VITAMINS	
A, C, E, D	Anti-inflammatory: scavenges oxygen radicals. Vitamin D content of breast milk is 25 international units/L or less. For prevention of rickets and vitamin D deficiency, all breast-fed infants should be given supplemental vitamin D (e.g., 400 international units/day) beginning within the first few days of life.[9]
ENZYMES	
Bile salt–dependent lipase	Production of FFA with antibacterial/protozoan activity.
Catalase	Anti-inflammatory: degrades H_2O_2.
Glutathione peroxidase	Anti-inflammatory: prevents lipid peroxidation.
Platelet-activating factor (PAF) acetyl hydrolase	Degrades PAF, a potent cause of ulceration; protects against necrotizing enterocolitis.[172]
GROWTH FACTORS	
Epithelial growth factors	Enhances maturation of gut epithelial barrier; limiting penetration by foreign antigens, thus decreasing immune stimulation.[176]
Transforming growth factors	Alpha: promotes epithelial cell growth. Beta: suppresses lymphocyte function: anti-inflammatory.
HORMONES	
Prolactin	Enhances B- and T-lymphocyte development; affects differentiation of intestinal lymphoid tissue.
Cortisol, thyroxine, insulin	Promotes maturation of neonatal intestine and development of intestinal host-defense mechanisms.
Erythropoietin	Influences erythropoiesis, gut maturation, apoptosis, neurodevelopment, and immunity.[187]

Modified from Hamosh B: Bioactive factors in human milk, *Pediatr Clin North Am* 48:69, 2001.

TABLE 18-2 **BIOACTIVE FACTORS IN HUMAN MILK—cont'd**

COMPONENT	FUNCTION
CELLS	
B-lymphocytes	Synthesize IgA and other antibodies targeted against specific pathogens.
Macrophages	90% of cells in breast milk; phagocytize microorganisms and kill bacteria in neonatal intestine; produce lysozyme, lactoferrin, and complement.
Neutrophils	Phagocytize bacteria in neonatal gastrointestinal tract.
T-lymphocytes	Phagocytosis against organisms in gastrointestinal tract; mobilize other host defenses; antigens introduced into maternal respiratory and/or gastrointestinal systems stimulate development of antibodies in breast milk; incorporation into neonatal tissue bestows short-term adoptive immunity.[109]
Cytokines	Modulate functions and maturation of immune system.
Proinflammatory: interleukin 1b, 6, 8, 12; interferon-gamma; tumor necrosis factor-alpha	Enhances inflammation.
Anti-inflammatory: interleukin 10; tumor growth factor-beta	Suppresses function of macrophages, natural killer and T-cells.

receives the high concentration of protective qualities that have been shown to protect the gastrointestinal and respiratory systems. Banked human milk can be used if the mother is unable or unwilling to provide sufficient quantities of breast milk. Human milk banks in the United States have rigorous guidelines for donations and adhere to strict quality controls.[8]

The normal microflora found in the neonatal gastrointestinal tract is the first line of defense against many pathogenic bacteria. After birth, the first exposure of the neonatal gut is to the maternal vaginal flora, and colonization continues with development of an environment of flora by 1 week of age. **With breast feeding or provision of breast milk, the dominant flora are bifidobacteria, which seem to suppress other organisms.** When infants are provided formula, the growth of bifidobacteria is very slow and at the end of the first week, there is only one-tenth the concentration compared with that in infants fed breast milk. Breast milk has been shown to be effective in reducing the colonization with *Klebsiella, Enterobacter,* and *Citrobacter.*[50] Reduction of anti-infective activity occurs with the addition of formula but not breast milk fortifier to the diet.[71,109,186] Yet in one study, when infection and NEC were combined, preterm infants fed fortified breast milk had more infectious events than did a partial-supplement group. Continued surveillance in the use of fortifiers is recommended.[186]

Normal Lactation

Breast development during pregnancy is stimulated by luteal and placental hormones—lactogen, prolactin, and chorionic gonadotropin.[154] Production of breast milk depends on both mammogenesis and lactogenesis. Mammogenesis is the growth and development of the glandular tissue of the breast and the differentiation of secretory epithelial cells or lactocytes during pregnancy.[72] **Estrogen stimulates growth of the milk collection (ductal) system, whereas progesterone stimulates growth of the milk production system.** These hormones, however, inhibit the initiation of breast milk production in significant quantity. With the birth of the infant, the hormones of pregnancy decline abruptly when the placenta is delivered, permitting the initiation of milk secretion. There is some speculation that mammogenesis and lactogenesis I may be truncated with the birth of preterm infants, especially the VLBW premature infant. In addition, cesarean section delivery may affect lactogenesis II as it affects the hormone balance stimulated by labor. Breast growth varies greatly during pregnancy, and it is unclear how much breast tissue is necessary to support full lactation. Many factors other than breast size affect milk production, such as stress and fatigue, both of which are increased when a preterm infant is born.

If a woman aborts as early as 16 weeks, her breasts secrete colostrum; therefore mothers are prepared to breast feed any viable infant.[108]

Estrogen and progesterone function as inhibitors to actual milk production because they inhibit the breast receptors for prolactin. Therefore stimulation of the breast before delivery does not create milk but may induce uterine contractions because oxytocin is released. Once the infant and placenta are delivered, stimulation of the nipple becomes effective in producing milk.

Stimulating the nipple by the infant's sucking action causes an increase in the prolactin released in the bloodstream and induces the synthesis and release of oxytocin, which is initiated by nipple stimulation and other sensory pathways (Figure 18-1). The amount of prolactin is directly related to the quantity and quality of nipple stimulation; because prolactin stimulates the synthesis and secretion of milk, the surges in prolactin levels are related to the quantity of milk. **A decrease in the quality of stimulation causes a decrease in prolactin surges and thus a decrease in milk production.** Recent studies show that overweight/obese mothers have a diminished prolactin response to infant suckling (e.g., less milk production) in the first postpartum week.[171] These mothers may benefit from earlier lactation counseling and support that will enable them to continue breast feeding.[171,193]

Adequate prolactin secretion controls the maintenance of milk supply. The sooner the

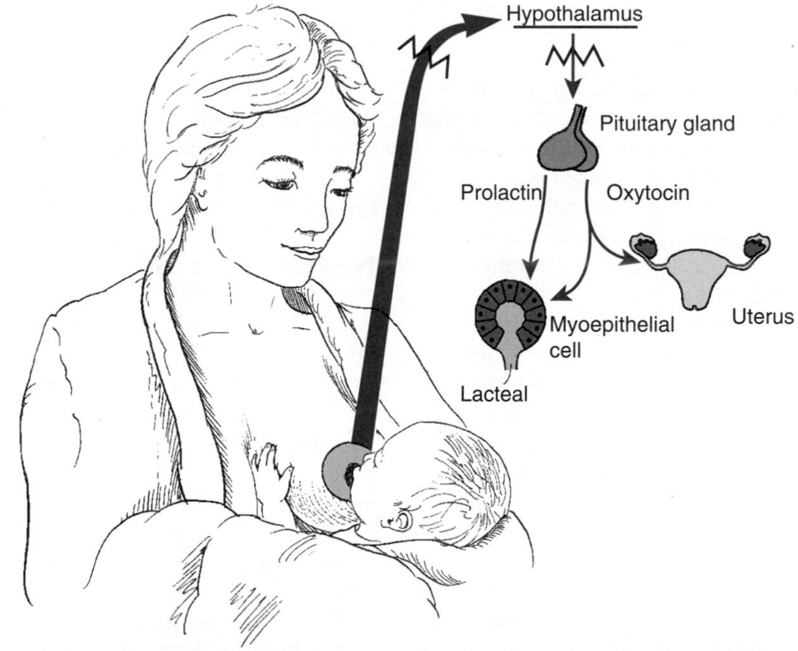

FIGURE 18-1 Ejection reflex arc, or letdown reflex. Infant suckling stimulates mechanoreceptors in the mother's nipple and areola that send the stimuli along the nerve pathways to the hypothalamus. Stimulation of the posterior pituitary releases oxytocin that (1) stimulates myoepithelial cells of the breast to contract and eject milk and (2) stimulates the uterus to contract. Stimulation of the anterior pituitary releases prolactin, which is responsible for milk production in mammary alveoli. (Modified from Lawrence RA, Lawrence RM: *Breast feeding: a guide for the medical profession*, ed 5, St Louis, 1999, Mosby.)

infant nurses, the sooner the milk comes in and becomes established. Initially, production of milk is on a more consistent basis because the basal level of prolactin is very high immediately after birth. Maintenance of milk depends on adequate stimulation of the breast and removal of milk on a regular and frequent basis. Initially, a newborn needs to nurse for a longer time to stimulate milk production and letdown. As the infant grows, sucking becomes more efficient, with the infant stimulating sequential letdowns early in the nursing period, thereby shortening the length of nursing. Establishing a generous milk supply is critical in long-term maintenance. Research has demonstrated that for mothers who are separated from their infants, pumping both breasts simultaneously stimulates a higher prolactin surge with increased milk supply than pumping one breast at a time.[79,94,152]

PSYCHOLOGIC VALUES OF BREAST FEEDING

The short-term advantage of breast feeding is early mother-infant contact. The en face position of breast feeding enhances this contact. During the first 1 to 2 hours after birth, the infant's suckling and touching of the mother's areola increases maternal attentiveness to the baby's needs for at least the first week of life. Because several studies show that maternal analgesia alters the infant's initial breast-feeding behavior, the mother's behavior may also be altered. Early contact—whether by breast feeding or another physical means—sometimes must be delayed or modified in a sick neonate. **Prolactin and oxytocin affect the initiation of maternal behavior and are involved in stress management in humans.** Oxytocin has been shown to reduce depression and anxiety in lactating mothers when compared with nonlactating mothers.[210] Feldman and Eidelman[51] found that providing breast milk functions to initiate a more optimal bonding process between mothers and their premature infants by operating on physiologic, behavioral, and representational (mood) systems. **Maternal depression as measured by the Beck Depression Inventory was reduced significantly when mothers provided more than 75% of breast milk nutrition for their preterm infant.**[51]

The long-term psychologic effect for the mother of unrestricted nursing appears to be a more even mood cycle as a result of elevated prolactin, oxytocin, and endorphin levels,[210] **which enhance coping mechanisms associated with caring for a new family member by diminishing maternal stress responses to physical, intrapersonal, or interpersonal stress.**[65] **Providing her own milk, including pumping and gavaging breast milk and eventual feeding at the breast, enhances maternal attachment and maternal behaviors**[65,96,204] **and enables the mother to contribute to her infant's care (see Chapter 29).** Proximity of mother and infant, as well as the infant's initial experience at the breast, contributes to maternal and infant regulation and the establishment of innate behaviors and emotional and social ties between mother and infant.[204] **Kavanaugh et al described rewards to the mother from breast feeding as follows**[96]**:**

- **Knowing that she is providing the healthiest nutrition**
- **Enhancing closeness between her and her preterm infant**
- **Perceiving her preterm infant's contentment and tranquility during breast feeding**
- **Convenience for the mother**
- **Giving her a tangible claim to her preterm infant**

All referring physicians and nursing personnel who admit infants to the neonatal intensive care unit (NICU) should encourage, support, and assist mothers who wish to breast feed their infants. Use of kangaroo care (see Chapter 13) in the NICU facilitates early initiation of breast feeding and increases maternal confidence, competence, and breast-feeding duration. If the infant is able to take oral nourishment, he or she can be breast fed at 1000 to 1200 g and about 28 weeks gestational age (see Chapter 13, Box 13-9, "Strategies to Facilitate Oral Feeding").

Neurobehavioral Development in Premature Infants

The positive impact of breast feeding on neurobehavioral and cognitive development in infants has been posited for several decades. **Two theories have been proposed to explain improved neurobehavioral development, nutritional content of breast milk that improves neurologic growth, and the effect of breast feeding on mother-infant relationship that indirectly supports cognitive development.** Evidence continues to mount demonstrating positive effects of human milk in the preterm infant. Breast feeding increases maternal responsiveness and higher levels of synchrony observed between mothers and preterm infants, hence leading to higher cognitive outcomes. A study of 86 preterm infants with mean gestation age at birth of 30 weeks and average birth weight of 1300 g found that amount of breast milk provided made a significant impact on the neurodevelopment of the infant when assessed at 37 weeks and 6 months of corrected age. **The preterm infants who received more than 75% of their nutrition from breast milk demonstrated a more mature neurodevelopmental profile at 37 weeks corrected for gestational age (CGA) and higher mental and psychomotor skills at 6 months corrected age.**[51] One hundred and nineteen VLBW infants with mean birth weight of 1056 g and mean gestational age of 28 weeks were followed for 20 months corrected age. Infants were fed both fortified breast milk for the first 4 weeks of life with premature formula as needed. Twenty-nine received formula only, 25 received less than 25 mL/kg/day, 16 received 25 to 49 mL/kg/day, and only 28 received more than 50 mL/kg/day. At 20 months, there was no difference in neurodevelopmental behavior and amount of human milk fed. The authors concluded that provision of breast milk did not increase poor outcomes and recognize that limitation of the amount of breast milk available may have decreased the ability to detect difference in outcome. They also recognized that other variables should be studied including longer duration and increased amount of breast milk provided, assessment of maternal-infant interactions, and kangaroo care techniques.[60]

FACILITATING SUCCESSFUL BREAST FEEDING

Although breast feeding is a normal, natural function, it is not a reflex but, rather, a highly complex interaction and interdependence between mother and infant. To be successful, the breast-feeding dyad must synchronize their behavior and physiology and receive support from their environment. Delayed breast feeding may be as successful as immediate feeding when (1) problems are prevented, (2) the mother receives support and encouragement in maintaining her milk supply, and (3) everyone is patient and knowledgeable about teaching the infant to suckle. **Initiating breast feeding as early as possible is important to prevent problems.** Thorough evaluation of the effectiveness of the nursing couple is important in achieving adequate nutrition and breast-feeding success. Knowledgeable health care providers and licensed, certified lactation consultants, where available, can perform these evaluations.[40,164] Development of an evidence-based and mother-friendly breast-feeding service has been shown to dramatically improve the volume of mother's milk that is available and to prolong the duration of milk provision for preterm infants.[140]

Sucking

Sucking is a primitive reflex appearing as early as 15 to 16 weeks' gestation. Although isolated components of feeding behaviors (e.g., root, suck, swallow, gag) are all present early in gestation, they are not effectively coordinated for bottle feedings before 32 to 34 weeks gestational age (see the Critical Findings box on p. 275). The infant can coordinate suck and swallow while breast feeding as early as 28 weeks' gestation. Two distinct types of sucking, nonnutritive and nutritive, develop in the human infant.

Nonnutritive Sucking

Nonnutritive sucking is sucking activity in which no fluid or nutrition is delivered to the infant. Characterized by short bursts of rapid motion, pauses, and few swallows, nonnutritive sucking has a stabilizing effect on physiologic responses (i.e., better oxygenation; quieter, more restful behavior; decreased tension; increased insulin and gastrin secretion that may stimulate digestion and storage of nutrients; and improved readiness for oral feedings) (see Chapter 13). Because there is no bolus of fluid to swallow, nonnutritive sucking results in an alternation of inspiration and expiration without the regular apneic periods of nutritive sucking.

Nutritive Sucking

Nutritive sucking, used by an infant when fluid or nutrition is available, is characterized by an organized, rhythmic pattern that is about half the rate of nonnutritive sucking (i.e., one per second). During nutritive sucking, each milk expression is followed by a reflexive swallow and an occasional brief pause. In a term neonate, rates of sucking range from 40 to 100/min. Nutritive sucking provides the neonate with positive reinforcement, which encourages a steady level of behavior. A variety of factors affect nutritive sucking, including maternal anesthesia and/or analgesia, length of labor, type of delivery, gestational age, birth weight, age (in hours), severity of illness, infant state, type of fluid, disorders of the central nervous system, and individual variations.* Although nutritive sucking is associated with faster heart rate (when bottle feeding), little information is available describing energy requirements of nutritive sucking. The findings of one study suggest that, during bottle feeding, preterm infants expend significantly less energy to suck the same volume than do full-term infants.[92] **Bottle feeding requires more energy than breast feeding in all infants.**[92]

Two patterns of nutritive sucking have been identified: continuous sucking and intermittent sucking.[124] ***Continuous sucking*** occurs at the beginning of bottle feeding, when the suck is strong and continuous for at least 30 seconds.[121,124] ***Intermittent sucking,*** an alteration of sucking bursts with periods of pause/no sucking,[121,124] occurs first during breast feeding, followed by continuous sucking (with breast milk letdown).[123,138] Breathing and oxygenation are affected more during continuous than during intermittent sucking,[205] even in full-term infants who can exhibit apnea and bradycardia with feeding.[120]

An increasing level of organization of nutritive sucking occurs with increasing gestational age, maturity, and experience.† Preterm sucking patterns exhibit more sucking-to-breathing ratio (2:1 to 4:1) than well-coordinated sucking breathing ratios (e.g., 1:1) of full-term newborns.[162] By 32 to 34 weeks post-conceptual age (PCA), there is a change in sucking bursts (i.e., increase in number of sucks, number of suck bursts and pressure; decrease in time between sucking bursts). This developmental maturation enables nutritive sucking to take less time and is less tiring.

Nutritive sucking requires coordination between suck, swallow, and breathing. During coordinated sucking bursts, suck/swallow/breathing occur in a 1:1:1 sequential pattern. The lack of a suck, swallow, and breathing ratio of 1:1:1 contributes to a preterm infant's apnea with feeding, a reflexive protection of the airway.[123,164,205] Although suck/swallow is achieved by 32 weeks' gestation,[132] respiration may still not be well coordinated so the preterm infant may develop apneic episodes with bottle feeding.[164,205] With increasing PCA and neuromuscular maturity, *consistent* coordination of suck-swallow-breathe (with bottle feeding) occurs by 35 to 37 weeks PCA.[57]

A recent randomized study of early introduction of oral (bottle) feeding (e.g., within 48 hours of full tube feedings) found the following[192]:

- Transition time to all oral feedings was significantly shorter.
- Oral feeding was introduced 2.6 weeks earlier.
- Total oral feeding was achieved at earlier postmenstrual age (PMA) (e.g., 54% of 33-week-PMA infants versus 12.5% of control group infants).
- Weight gain and discharge weights were similar in both groups.
- Episodes of feeding-related bradycardia and desaturations were similar for both groups.
- The early feeding group was discharged 10 days earlier than the control group.

In this study and others, researchers postulate that **feeding opportunities in young infants provide them with practice and experiential opportunities to develop their oral motor skills and coordination of suck-swallow-breathe.**[56,125,192]

Human nutritive suckling is composed of five separate yet interrelated processes: rooting, orienting, suction, expression, and swallowing (Figure 18-2).[26] ***Rooting,*** the tactile stimulating of the infant's face and lips, elicits the head to turn toward the stimulus. Stimulation of the center of the lower lip enables the infant to root by coming forward extending the tongue, drawing in the nipple and areola, and latching on, rather than turning the head to one side. ***Orienting, or latching on,*** occurs when the tongue draws the nipple and areola into an elongated teat and compresses it against the hard palate.[73]

Suction, the application of negative pressure in the infant's mouth, holds the nipple and areola in place.[73] At the beginning of breast feeding, a strong suction stretches and shapes the nipple, but only moderate suction is necessary to maintain adequate grasp of the nipple. During the feeding, occasional bursts of suckling enable milk to be expressed. ***Expression*** of milk occurs when the peristaltic motion of the tongue[73] stimulates the release of oxytocin, which stimulates myoepithelial cells surrounding the milk ducts (Figure 18-3) to contract, and milk is ejected from the ducts. The lips should be flanged out to

*References 57,63,105,123,128,130,131,158,162,169,192.
†References 57,63,105,125,128,130,131,158,162,164,192.

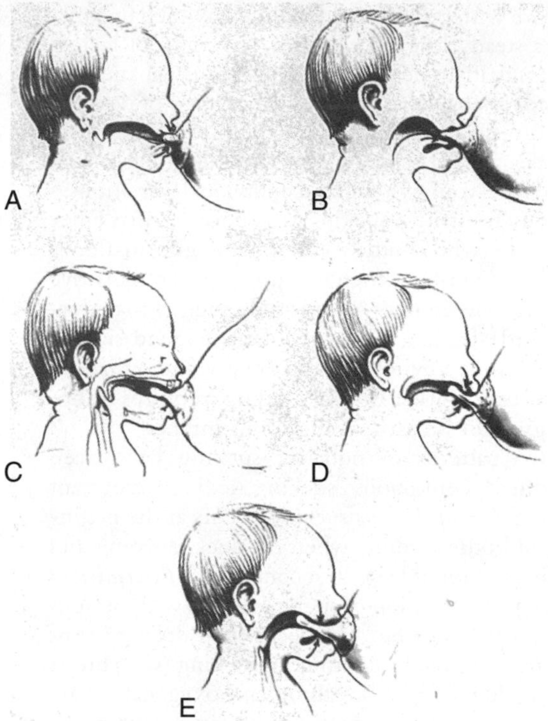

FIGURE 18-2 Normal suckling. **A**, Infant grasps breast (note *arrows* showing jaw action). **B**, Tongue moves forward to draw nipple in. **C**, Nipple and areola move toward palate as glottis still permits breathing. **D**, Tongue moves along nipple, pressing it against hard palate, creating pressure. **E**, Ductules under areola are milked, and flow begins because of peristaltic movement of tongue. Glottis closes and swallow follows. (From Lawrence RA, Lawrence RM: *Breast feeding: a guide for the medical profession*, ed 6, St Louis, 2005, Mosby.)

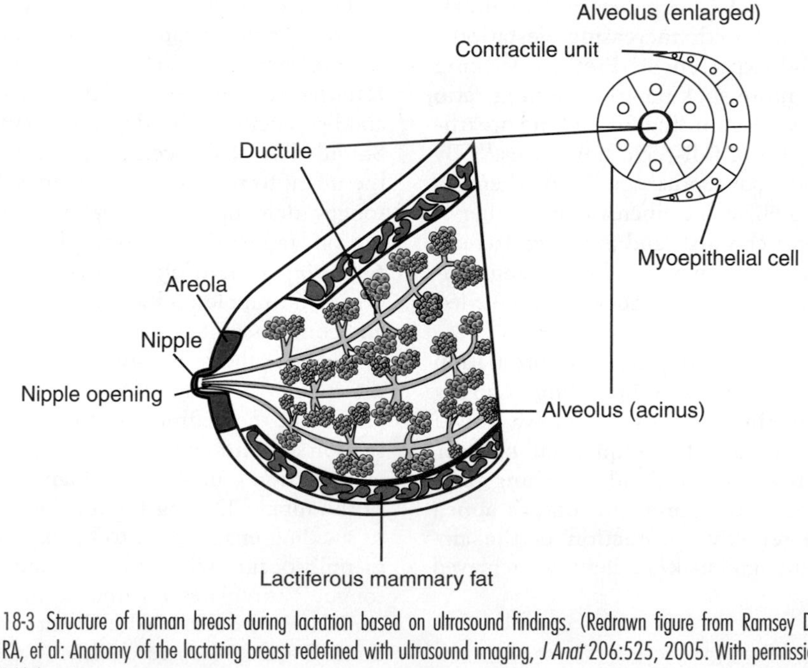

FIGURE 18-3 Structure of human breast during lactation based on ultrasound findings. (Redrawn figure from Ramsey DT, Kent JC, Hartmann RA, et al: Anatomy of the lactating breast redefined with ultrasound imaging, *J Anat* 206:525, 2005. With permission of Wiley-Blackwell Publishing.)

create a seal as peristaltic motion of the tongue stimulates milk ejection. After maximal compression of the nipple with peristaltic motion, milk is expressed from the lactiferous sinuses.

Swallowing milk occurs as the peristaltic motion of the tongue triggers peristaltic motion of the posterior pharynx (reflexive swallowing)[73] and propulsion down the esophagus (which also shows peristalsis). These peristaltic motions coordinate suck and swallow so breast-feeding infants do not choke, unless letdown reflex is excessive. Swallowing milk also reflexively initiates the expression cycle of jaw and tongue movements. Therefore nutritive suckling is primarily expression and swallowing of milk. During nursing, just enough suction to keep the nipple in proper position is used, even during the expressive phase of suckling. **Breast feeding is an infant-regulated system; milk flow depends on the active suckling by the infant. When an infant pauses to regain physiologic stability, the flow of milk from the breast ceases.**

Ultrasonographic studies of full-term infants' breast feeding note (1) an elongation to twice the resting size of the maternal nipple, (2) formation of a passive seal by the neonate's oral cavity, and (3) milk ejection coinciding with the downstroke of the tongue and jaw, creating negative pressure by oral cavity enlargement. Ultrasonographic studies of full-term infants bottle feeding note (1) less elasticity and less elongation of artificial nipples (compared with human nipple), (2) similar mechanism used to suckle artificial nipples as used to breast feed, which is quickly replaced by the thrusting motion to close the holes and control the flow, and (3) milk expression dependent on a vacuum phenomenon by oral cavity enlargement rather than by nipple compression.[73] Artificial nipples have also been shown to vary in their rate of milk flow.[117,119,121] Nipple hole size, rather than the type of nipple,[117,122] has been found to be the major determinant in the variability in milk flow.[119] With an artificial nipple, fluid flows into the posterior oropharynx by gravity (Figure 18-4). Artificial nipples and bottles are gravity-regulated systems requiring the infant to actively inhibit milk flow to permit swallowing and breathing. In an attempt to regulate milk flow and prevent choking or gagging, infants may clench their jaws or obstruct the nipples' holes with their tongues in a thrusting motion. Orthodontic nipples result in physiologic stability and more effective feeding behavior in some infants.[45]

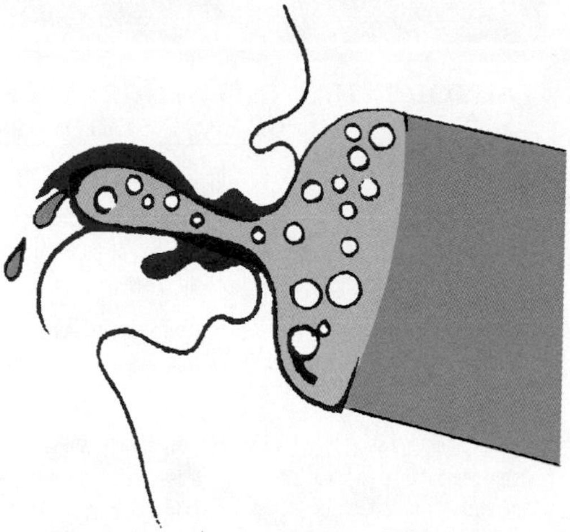

FIGURE 18-4 Artificial nipple. (From Lawrence RA, Lawrence RM: *Breastfeeding: a guide for the medical professional*, ed 6, St Louis, 2005, Mosby.)

PREVENTION OF BREAST-FEEDING PROBLEMS

Problems with breast feeding may be with the mother or with the neonate or may arise from a combination of problems in the dyad. Lack of information about common problems in the early weeks of breast feeding is a common reason for breast-feeding failure.[198] In descriptive studies addressing breast-feeding problems, mothers have frequently identified concerns related to sore nipples, breast discomfort, and inadequate milk supply.[29,42] Breast-feeding problems should be prevented. To solve a breast-feeding problem, the mother must be observed feeding the infant.

Maternal Problems

INADEQUATE MILK SUPPLY

Inadequate milk supply, a major problem for both mother and infant, is the most commonly cited reason for discontinuation of breast feeding in the NICU and after discharge.[29,82,95,136] Predictors of maternal perception of inadequate milk supply at 8 to 12 weeks postpartum (after preterm birth) include inadequate milk supply at 6 weeks postpartum, unemployment, and infant

Critical Findings

FACTORS THAT INFLUENCE THE MOTHER'S MILK SUPPLY AND SUCCESSFUL BREAST FEEDING OF THE PRETERM INFANT

ENHANCES	REDUCES	COMMENTS
Early initiation of pumping, preferably with a double-pumping setup and breast massage[94]	Immediate separation at birth, delayed initiation of pumping or feeding at the breast	Initiate within 2 to 3 hours of birth, if possible[58]; pumping both breasts simultaneously is associated with higher prolactin levels, milk yield, fat concentration, and maternal preference.[79,94,203]
Frequent milk expression with complete breast emptying at each session	Failure to express frequently or incomplete emptying of the breasts	5 to 8 expressions/day (every 3 to 4 hr): duration of pumping >100 min/day (about 15 to 20 minutes with double-pump setup); longest non-pumping interval <6 hours.[58,203]
Rest, relaxation, and stress management (see Chapters 29 and 30)	Fatigue, anxiety, stress (i.e., maternal illness, return to work, more commitments in and outside the home)	Inverse relationship between maternal anxiety scores and milk volume for mothers of preterm infants; uninterrupted sleep of at least 6 hours.[109,210]
Adequate nutrition	Inadequate nutrition	At least 60% of recommended daily allowances produces milk of adequate quantity and quality to promote infant growth.[31]
Medications		
Metoclopramide, oxytocin, reserpine, phenothiazines	Bromocriptine, antihistamine, oral contraceptives (especially estrogen and progesterone combination)	Knowledge of maternal medication use enables effective counseling.
Herb		
Fenugreek		Two or three capsules two or three times per day; maternal diarrhea; lowers blood glucose; may increase asthma symptoms; maple syrup smell to sweat, urine, milk; colic.[67]
Positive feedback to mother regarding infant growth; infant's condition improving	Worsening infant's condition	Mothers report feeling rewarded by infant's growth while receiving expressed mother's milk by gavage.[136]
Skin-to-skin contact (kangaroo care); co-bedding of multiples; simultaneous feeding and caregiving schedules (see Chapter 13)	Parental separation	Maternal reinforcement of lactation, maternal behaviors, confidence, and attachment; ensures maternal exposure to pathogens in neonatal intensive care unit (NICU) so that her immune system is stimulated to produce environmentally specific antibodies that are passed in maternal milk and protect the preterm.
Educational information (e.g., video, brochure) readily available for both mothers and fathers[195,201] of preterm infants	No verbal or written information for parents; conflicting opinions about breast feeding	Decision about type of pump, frequency; written instructions on collection and storage per NICU protocol; information about maternal rest, fluid intake, and nutrition. Positive effects of breast feeding, advantages of human milk to preterm infant; how to interpret infant cues and behaviors.[157,201,203]

Modified from Schanler R, Hurst N: Human milk for the hospitalized preterm infant, *Semin Perinatol* 18:476, 1994.

hospital discharge after postpartum day 42.[82] Initially, some neonates with special needs are unable to breast feed. In this common situation, the most compelling breast-feeding issue is establishing an adequate milk supply without the neonate's assistance[81] (see the Critical Findings box above and on p. 447). Preterm mothers are three times more likely to produce an inadequate milk supply at 6 weeks than are full-term mothers.[81] Because low milk volume in the first week of life is related to continued low production,[81] developing a very early program

Critical Findings—cont'd

ENHANCES	REDUCES	COMMENTS
Knowledgeable professional care providers (e.g., primary nurses, lactation specialists, physicians) who educate, support, and assist through consistent, practical advice	Nonsupportive care providers and/or inconsistent advice and information	Prevention of maternal problems (e.g., inadequate supply, sore nipples, engorgement) through self-education and professional interaction and education enhances success and prevents discontinuation of breast feeding.
Initiation of breast feeding before bottle feeding	Initiation of bottle feeding before breast feeding	Early breast feeding is less stressful than early bottle feeding[24,57,134-136,138,219] because of difference in the patterns of sucking and breathing; during bottle feedings, preterm infants alternate short bursts of sucking with breathing and do not breathe within sucking bursts; during breast feeding, breathing is integrated within sucking bursts.[135] Test weighing (i.e., weighing before and after breast feeding, with differences in weight representing milk intake [1 g = 1 mL) using electronic scales is a reliable method of documenting milk intake in preterm infants.[203] For specific problems, maximizing milk intake may be assisted by lactational support devices and/or breast pump stimulation of the opposite breast during infant feeding.[109,136] For multiples: Introduce simultaneous feeding as soon as possible, encourage maternal independence with position suggestions, comfort measures, experimenting, and verbalizing what mother needs or wants.[157] Need for privacy, taking babies out of NICU, rooming-in with father to assist with care and feeding.[157] Lactational support devices and/or breast pump stimulation of the opposite breast during infant feeding.[185]

of education and support for the mother will help her establish an early milk supply and prevent low milk volume.

Initiating, establishing, and maintaining a milk supply must be accomplished mechanically when the infant is unable to breast feed. Because milk production depends on adequate and frequent expression, maternal education is the key to establishing an adequate supply (see the Critical Findings box above and on p. 446). Mothers should be encouraged to provide their milk for their compromised infants and should be educated about the benefits of human milk feedings for their fragile infant so that they are able to make an informed choice and decision.* The mother who wants to or is willing to breast feed should be instructed about initiating and maintaining a milk supply until the infant can breast feed. In general, instruction includes information about pumping, which is individualized to the mother's situation. Milk production through pumping should be encouraged early and regularly to (1) collect colostrum, rich in anti-infective properties, (2) ease initial engorgement associated with lack of regular stimulation and maintain continued stimulus to produce milk, (3) provide quality nutrition for the neonate, and (4) alleviate concerns about available volume once the infant begins breast feeding. The early postpartum period in the hospital is the optimal time to teach pumping methods, while support and encouragement are readily available.

*References 113,137,140,144,175,198.

BREAST DISCOMFORT

Maternal problems include engorgement, painful nipples, and cracked nipples.[173] A primipara is at high risk for developing engorgement. Frequent emptying of the breast is the best prevention.

Engorgement occurring in the early postpartum period is characterized by general breast swelling, usually in both breasts in a well, afebrile woman. A little engorgement is normal. Areolar engorgement blocks the nipple and makes grasping the areola difficult for the infant. **Gentle breast massage and manual expression of a small amount of milk soften the areola so the infant is able to "latch on."** When the body of the breasts and the areolae become excessively engorged and painful, **the goal of management is to make the mother comfortable so that nursing may continue. Supporting the breasts is crucial, and the mother should wear a well-fitting but adjustable brassiere 24 hours a day.**[109] **Applying cold packs between nursing decreases pain and swelling. Pain relievers also may be prescribed. Applying heat (packs or a warm shower) and expressing some milk before feeding help initiate milk flow. A nursing infant, manual expression, or an effective pump helps initiate and maintain milk flow.** Breast massage before and during breast pumping/feeding also facilitates milk flow.

Prenatal stimulation of the nipple by pulling or rolling (to toughen it for breast feeding) is not recommended because of the possibility of initiating uterine contractions and premature labor.[109]

Breast feeding should not be painful. When it is, the problem is most often an incorrect latch. Sore nipples are another major discomfort and concern for the new mother. The initial grasp of the nipple by the infant or with pumping can be uncomfortable. **Poor positioning of the infant, however, can cause painful and eventually cracked nipples. Prevention and treatment involve educating the mother about careful positioning of the infant facing the mother, looking directly at the breast, and tummy-to-tummy with her (Figure 18-5). Changing the infant's position on the nipple at different feedings is helpful.**

Positioning the infant correctly at the breast assists in the prevention of sore nipples.[25] **There are three common positions that can be used with breast feeding: the cradle hold (see Figure 18-5), the football hold (Figure 18-6), and lying down.** Initially, the cradle or football hold allows the most control for the mother and infant to learn breast feeding. Breast feeding in the lying-down position becomes easier once latch-on techniques are developed.

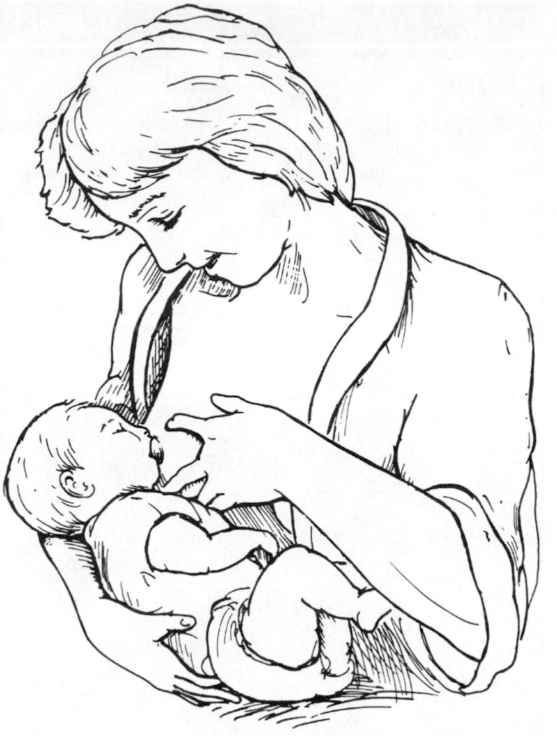

FIGURE 18-5 Proper positioning for breast feeding infant tummy-to-tummy facing the mother.

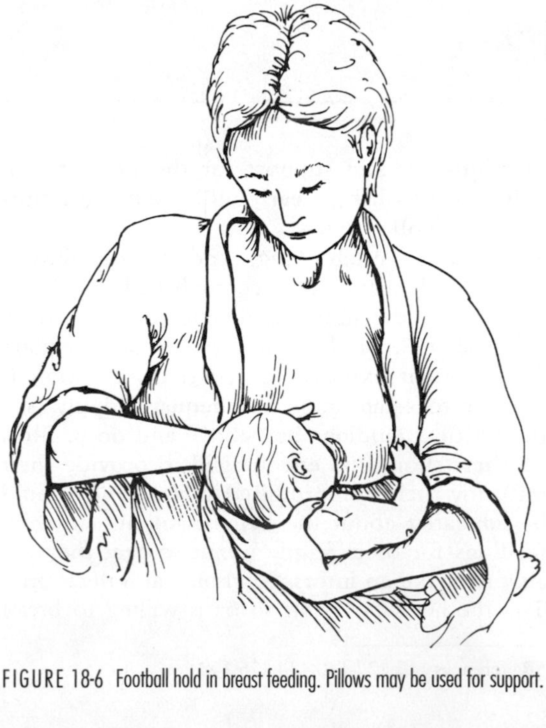

FIGURE 18-6 Football hold in breast feeding. Pillows may be used for support.

Nipple care involves keeping nipples clean and dry. Clear water (no soap or alcohol) is all that is necessary to keep the nipples clean. Drying nipples well, not using plastic nursing pads, and exposing nipples to air and dry heat (sunlight, light bulb sauna, or a low setting on a hair dryer) are comforting. **Using ointments may be helpful, especially in dry climates. If used, a small amount (i.e., one drop) should be gently massaged into the nipple after the feeding. Purified lanolin (if there is no allergy to wool), A&D ointment, or vitamin E may be used to treat, but will not prevent, sore nipples.** A recent randomized clinical trial (RCT) found that use of breast shells and lanolin cream to treat sore nipples promoted healing and prevented infections.[28] Another recent RCT comparing the use of hydrogel dressings with lanolin ointment in the prevention and treatment of sore nipples found a greater reduction in pain, no infections, and earlier discontinuation of therapy in the hydrogel dressing group.[44]

Severe and/or persistent nipple pain may be caused by bacterial or yeast infection, which should be promptly treated. Yeast infection of the breast (Table 18-3) manifests as a burning sensation in the nipples, stabbing pain throughout the breast, and edema/shiny skin or flaking

TABLE 18-3 PERINATAL COMPLICATIONS AND BREAST FEEDING

COMPLICATIONS	BREAST FEED YES	BREAST FEED NO	COMMENTS
MATERNAL COMPLICATIONS			
Cesarean section	X		Regional anesthesia enables contact and feeding in recovery room. Pain medication is best given after feeding so levels peak before next feeding.
Pregnancy-induced hypertension	X		Preterm or small-for-gestational-age infants may be delivered, making delayed breast feeding and pumping necessary. Maternal drugs may affect infant (see Table 18-4).
Venous thrombosis and pulmonary embolism	X		Depending on mother's ability; radioactive materials may be used for diagnosis, and pulmonary embolism anticoagulants may be used for therapy (see Table 18-4).
BACTERIAL INFECTIONS			
Urinary tract	X		Choice of antibiotics is important (see Table 18-4).
Mastitis	X		Continued emptying of breast (i.e., nursing baby or breast pump), bedrest, antibiotic therapy that is safe for infant, application of heat and cold, and use of analgesics are therapeutic.
Sexually transmitted diseases	X		No contraindication once mother is treated appropriately.
Tuberculosis	X	X	Culture-positive mothers must be separated from their infants regardless of mode of feeding; may pump and provide breast milk because tubercle bacillus is not passed through milk but through respiratory contact.[109]
	X		After therapy, when it is safe for mother to contact infant, then it is safe to breast feed directly.
Diarrhea	X		Proper handwashing should be done and breast feeding continued.
VIRAL INFECTIONS			
Cytomegalovirus (CMV)	X		Both virus and protective antibodies occur in breast milk; the relative incidence and severity of CMV infection acquired from breast milk in low-birth-weight (LBW) infants is low.[145] For preterm infants with lower concentration of transplacental antibodies: freeze milk (which decreases viral titer) for 3 to 7 days before feeding (for the first few weeks) until antibodies received via milk increase.[104,109]

Data from American Academy of Pediatrics: *Report of the committee on infectious disease*, ed 27, Elk Grove Village, Ill, 2006, The Academy; Lawrence RA, Lawrence RM: *Breast feeding: a guide for the medical profession*, ed 6, St Louis, 2005, Mosby.

Continued

TABLE 18-3 PERINATAL COMPLICATIONS AND BREAST FEEDING—cont'd

COMPLICATIONS	BREAST FEED YES	BREAST FEED NO	COMMENTS
VIRAL INFECTIONS—cont'd			
Enterovirus	X		Maternal antibodies in breast milk protect infants from enteroviral infections, especially if the infant was breast fed for >2 weeks.[183]
Rubella	X		Isolate infected infant from other infants and susceptible personnel. Mother is not contagious postpartum and need not be isolated from infant. Rooming-in may be considered.
Rubella immunization	X		There is no known adverse effect on infant.
Herpes simplex virus (HSV)	X	X	May breast feed if there is no active lesion on breast. Strict handwashing, as well as covering of genital lesions, is necessary. Rooming-in supports breast feeding while isolating infant from others in nursery.
Varicella (chickenpox)	X	X	If mother has chickenpox within 6 days of delivery, isolate mother and do not allow her to breast feed until she is no longer contagious. Infant should be separated regardless of mode of feeding.
Measles (rubeola)	X	X	If infant has measles, may isolate mother and infant together and allow breast feeding. Mothers with postpartum measles have breast fed, and neonates have acquired mild disease. Secretory antibodies are probably present in milk in 45 hours. Mother exposed before delivery without active disease should be isolated from infant, because 50% of infants contract disease.
Hepatitis	X		Hepatitis A: may breast feed as soon as mother receives gamma globulin.
	X		Hepatitis B antigen has been found in breast milk, but transmission by this route is not well documented. Both infants of chronic HBsAg carriers and those with acute hepatitis should receive high-titer hepatitis B immunoglobulin and hepatitis vaccine, and breast feeding is permitted.
	X		Hepatitis C virus (HCV) infection rate is 4% in both breast-fed and bottle-fed infants; breast feeding permitted: HCV-positive women do not increase the infection risk to their infants.
Human immunodeficiency virus (HIV), acquired immunodeficiency syndrome (AIDS)		X	Breast feeding is absolutely contraindicated in mothers who are HIV positive and living in developed countries where safe alternatives are available.[7,108,109] The risk for HIV transmission with exclusive breast feeding has recently been studied in the developing world. Exclusive breast feeding decreases the risks of HIV transmission (14.1% at 6 weeks and 19.5% at 6 months of age) and mortality (6.1% at 3 months of age) when compared with infants who received solids in addition to breast feeding.[37]
Human T-cell leukemia virus type I (HTLV-I)		X	Infected lymphocytes found in breast milk; unknown if able to cause disease. Current U.S. position: breast feeding contraindicated.[109]
West Nile virus	X		Transmission through human milk occurs but is rare.[83]
PARASITIC INFECTIONS			
Toxoplasmosis	X		No transmission of toxoplasmosis has been demonstrated in humans. Antibodies are present in breast milk.
FUNGAL INFECTIONS			
Candida albicans infection of the nipple/breast	X		Antifungal topical medication (nystatin) for the mother and simultaneous oral nystatin for the infant. Persistent yeast infections are treated with oral fluconazole (see Table 18-4).
OTHER INFECTIONS			
Trichomoniasis		X	Metronidazole is contraindicated for infant; milk may be pumped and discarded until therapy is completed. Mother's dose can be modified so she can pump and discard milk for 24 to 48 hours.

Data from American Academy of Pediatrics: *Report of the committee on infectious disease*, ed 27, Elk Grove Village, Ill, 2006, The Academy; Lawrence RA, Lawrence RM: *Breast feeding: a guide for the medical profession*, ed 6, St Louis, 2005, Mosby.

TABLE 18-3 PERINATAL COMPLICATIONS AND BREAST FEEDING—cont'd

COMPLICATIONS	BREAST FEED YES	BREAST FEED NO	COMMENTS
OTHER MATERNAL COMPLICATIONS			
Anemia	X		Severe maternal anemia, but not mild to moderate anemia, adversely affects the iron status of breast milk. Maternal nutritional status significantly influences fetal iron status but not breast milk iron content.[101]
Diabetes	X		Lactation is antidiabetogenic. Lactosuria must be differentiated from glycosuria.
Thyroid disease	X	X	Radioisotopes and thiouracil are found in breast milk and may adversely affect infant. Mother who is taking propylthiouracil can breast feed. Neither hypothyroidism nor hyperthyroidism is contraindication alone.
Cystic fibrosis	X	X	May cause nutritional drain on mother. Milk composition is normal. The Cystic Fibrosis Association has guidelines for lactation.
Smoking	X	X	Nicotine interferes with letdown and is excreted in milk. Of mothers who smoke, breast-fed infants are healthier than bottle-fed infants.
Opiate withdrawal	X		One small study. See "Methadone" in the "Other Substances" section in Table 18-4.
NEONATAL COMPLICATIONS			
Medical			
Diarrhea	X	X	Maintain breast feeding in infectious diarrhea unless milk is source of infection. Congenital lactase deficiency is rare but requires lactose-free formula.
Respiratory disease	X	X	Breast milk by gavage may be used if infant's condition permits.
Galactosemia		X	Galactose (lactose)-free diet is required.
Inborn errors of metabolism (e.g., phenylketonuria)	X	X	Combination of breast milk and special formula may sometimes be used. Careful monitoring of blood and urine levels of the amino acid is required.
Acrodermatitis enteropathica	X		Low plasma zinc levels are corrected by human milk and zinc sulfate supplementation.
Down syndrome	X		Hypotonia and poor suck reflex contribute to poor letdown and inadequate supply. Proper positioning, manual expression to begin feeding, and supporting the breast so infant does not lose nipple are helpful. Support from another mother with an infant with Down syndrome is helpful.
Hypothyroidism	X		Enough T_3 may be ingested to avoid serious symptoms.
Hyperbilirubinemia	X		May have slightly higher bilirubin than bottle-fed infant. There is no evidence that supplements are beneficial (see Chapter 21).
Breast milk jaundice	X	X	Uncommon occurrence; diagnosis of exclusion; if all other causes are excluded, a temporary cessation of breast milk may be indicated (see Chapter 21).
Cystic fibrosis	X		Increased losses of and lower electrolyte content of breast milk may cause electrolyte imbalance, which is less likely than with formulas.
Surgical			
Cleft lip and/or palate	X		Associated lesions, size, and position of defect influence successful feeding. Positioning and stabilizing breast in infant's mouth may help seal defect. Consult plastic surgeon.
Gastrostomy	X		If gastrostomy feedings are used, expressed breast milk is appropriate.

Continued

TABLE 18-3 PERINATAL COMPLICATIONS AND BREAST FEEDING—cont'd

COMPLICATIONS	BREAST FEED YES	BREAST FEED NO	COMMENTS
Surgical—cont'd			
Partial obstruction (meconium plug, ileus, Hirschsprung's disease)	X		If oral feedings are indicated, breast milk is feeding of choice because of digestibility and mild cathartic effect.
Necrotizing enterocolitis	X		Breast feeding may be partially protective and may be used when feeding resumes.
Gastrointestinal bleeding	X		Most common cause is maternal bleeding from nipple. Perform Apt test to differentiate fetal from adult hemoglobin.
Central nervous system	X		Weak suck and uncoordinated suck and swallow may be problems; however, infants with malformations may breast feed more effectively than bottle feed.

Data from American Academy of Pediatrics: *Report of the committee on infectious disease*, ed 27, Elk Grove Village, Ill, 2006, The Academy; Lawrence RA, Lawrence RM: *Breast feeding: a guide for the medical profession*, ed 6, St Louis, 2005, Mosby.

skin on the nipple/areola.[150] A recent study showed that a significant risk factor for yeast infections of the breast and oral thrush in the baby was use of bottles in the early postpartum period.[150] In this study,[150] yeast infection was associated with cessation of breast feeding (in 65% of infected mothers) by 9 weeks postpartum because of pain with feeding.[55]

Another recognized cause of nipple pain is Raynaud's phenomenon of the nipple, which is often misdiagnosed and mistreated as a yeast infection.[11] Twenty percent of childbearing-age women may have Raynaud's, and symptoms are exacerbated by cold temperatures.[11] Raynaud's phenomenon of the breast, associated with a history of breast surgery, is characterized by extreme or severe nipple pain with breast feeding; nipple blanching, cyanosis or erythema; and accompanying throbbing pain, burning, and paresthesia. Treatment includes (1) preventing and/or decreasing exposure to cold and emotional stress, (2) avoiding vasoconstrictive drugs (e.g., nicotine), (3) using nifedipine for its vasodilator effects[11] (see Table 18-4), and (4) including fish oil and evening primrose oil in the mother's diet.[108] If the mother does not have Raynaud's of fingers or toes, it is unlikely she has it of the breast.

In the past, nipple shields were not recommended because they are awkward for the mother, confusing for the infant, and decrease milk production by 50%. More recently, supervised temporary use of silicone nipple shields has been found to be a useful tool in treatment of sore nipples and latch-on problems and as a bridging technique to direct breast feeding.[198] A recent study showed that for preterm infants, use of a nipple shield increased breast milk intake and promoted longer duration of breast feeding.[139] Breast pumping after use of nipple shields is necessary to express residual milk, maintain adequate milk supply, and obtain milk for supplemental feeding.[198] Nipple shields are helpful also if the mother's nipple is too large for her infant's mouth.

Flat or inverted nipples may be difficult for the infant to grasp and result in maternal engorgement, decreased milk supply, infant frustration, and suboptimal infant breast feeding behavior[42] (Figure 18-7). Inverted nipples may be treated by using a breast pump to draw out the nipple before attempting to latch the baby onto the nipple.

Neonatal Problems

Ideally, no term or preterm infant who will be breast fed should ever be fed with an artificial nipple, but this is not always possible, especially for a sick premature infant who requires prolonged hospitalization. However, teaching a premature infant to suck often starts long before nutrition is obtained from a nipple. When a premature infant is gavage fed, giving a pacifier

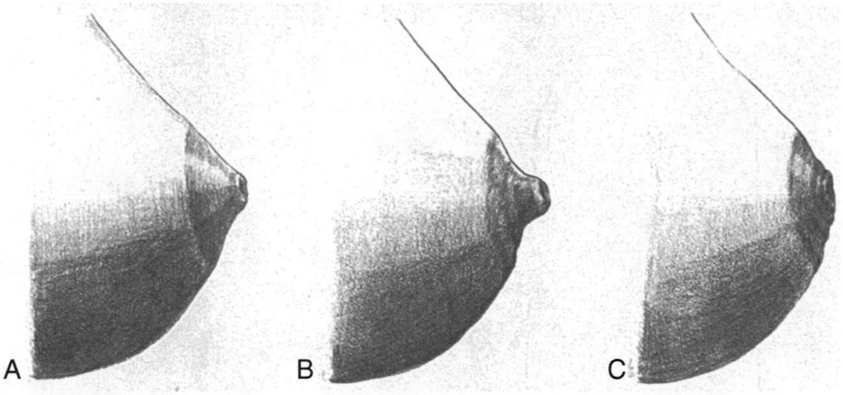

FIGURE 18-7 Inverted nipples. **A,** Normal and inverted nipples may look similar when nipple is not stimulated. **B,** Normal nipple protrudes when stimulated. **C,** Inverted nipple retracts when stimulated. (Courtesy Jimmy Lynne Scholl Avery.)

teaches the infant to equate satiety with sucking. Using a pacifier provides nonnutritive sucking that calms and soothes the preterm infant and also provides the opportunity to develop sucking skill. A recent RCT in preterm infants showed no influence of pacifier use on any breast-feeding outcome (e.g., breast feeding at discharge or several months later).[36] These findings agree with an RCT of reducing pacifier use in term infants that showed no effect on early weaning.[100] When the mother is present for gavage feeding, the infant can be given the breast instead of an artificial nipple. If it is necessary to avoid swallowing any fluid, the breast can be prepumped. Placing the infant in direct skin-to-skin contact with the mother's breast enables nuzzling and licking behaviors and teaches that relief from hunger and the breast-feeding position are associated. Because increased stimulation creates an increased milk supply, it is possible to breast feed multiple infants. In the early weeks, it will be difficult and time consuming, but eventually it can become faster and more convenient than bottle feeding. Two infants can be fed at the same time, in the cradle position or in the football hold position (Figure 18-8). A study of breast-feeding twins found that mothers preferred simultaneous feeding using the football hold (possibly because of the bias of the observers because not all mothers of twins agreed).[157] Infants should change breasts with each feeding, because one may have a stronger suck than the other and each breast should receive an equal amount of stimulation.

Understanding the mechanisms of suckling is essential to preventing, assessing, and intervening in neonatal suckling problems. Infants are born ready to suckle the breast. Nipple confusion describes the difficulty of infants who have been fed with artificial nipples before learning to breast feed. The infant who has learned to feed from a bottle nipple often sucks incorrectly at the breast, preventing milk flow.

The infant's confusion creates frustration and crying, which may inhibit milk letdown. The best means for preventing nipple confusion is to enable the infant to learn breast feeding *before* bottle feeding is established[153] (see the Critical Findings box on pp. 446-447).

Assessment of the problem includes evaluating the method of feeding and possibly using alternative nutritional methods (gavage feedings) until the cause is determined. If the infant is bottle fed, choking may be a result of a soft nipple, a fast flow that the infant cannot control, or a nipple that is too long for the infant's (particularly the preterm infant's) mouth. If the mother is breast feeding and the ejection is strong, the first rush of milk could cause choking, which may be prevented by manual expression of a small amount (several spurts) of milk before offering the nipple to the infant. Collins et al[36] studied the effect of bottles, cups, and dummies (pacifiers) on breast feeding in preterm infants using an RCT. Included in the study were 319 preterm neonates born at 23 to 34 weeks' gestation, with 303 included in the final analysis. The primary outcome measure was

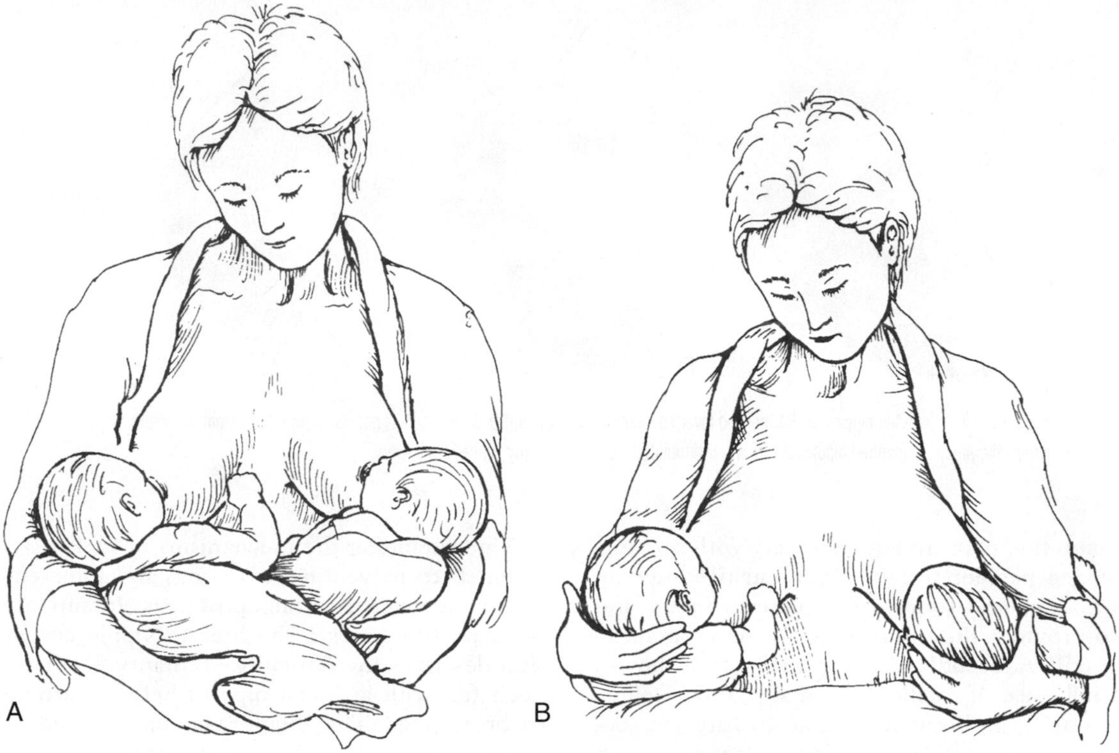

FIGURE 18-8 Breast feeding twins. **A**, Cradle position. **B**, Football hold position.

continuation of any breast feeding on discharge home from the NICU. **The results demonstrated that there were no significant differences with the use of a dummy (pacifier).** However, infants randomized to cup feeds were more likely to be fully breast fed on discharge home but had a longer length of stay in the hospital (cup = 59 days; bottle = 48 days). Cup feeding did not have a difference in the incidence of any breast feeding at discharge. **On the other hand, Howard et al[85] found in a cohort of 750 healthy newborns that early use of a pacifier did decrease success and duration of breast feeding through 1 year.** A recent analysis of four studies found that cup feeding cannot be recommended over bottle feeding as a supplemental method for breast feeding because (1) there is no significant benefit in maintaining breast feeding beyond hospital discharge and (2) there is an unacceptable consequence: longer length of stay with cup feeding.[54] **Furthermore, the National Association of Neonatal Nurses (NANN) states that, despite growing use of cup (and finger feeding), there is no research to support physiologic soundness, risks and safety, efficacy, or possible benefits, especially when used with premature and low-birth-weight infants.[151]**

Some suckling problems result from the sequelae of perinatal events (e.g., low Apgar score, preterm low-birth-weight (LBW), small-for-gestational-age (SGA), large-for-gestational-age (LGA), late-preterm infants, infant of a diabetic mother (IDM), and multiple births) or of physical disorders (e.g., hyperbilirubinemia, hypoglycemia, cardiorespiratory conditions, sepsis, neuromotor/developmental problems, and structural abnormalities of the oral cavity)[18,108,153] and represent developmental delays. **These suckling difficulties require diagnostic evaluation of the underlying cause and appropriate intervention.[18,108,153]**

Late-preterm infants (e.g., 34⁰⁄₇ to 36⁶⁄₇ weeks of gestation) (see Chapter 5) are often poor feeders because of their developmental

immaturity in coordination of suck-swallow-breathe and because they are awake less frequently, give fewer if any cues of readiness to feed, and are easily fatigued and fall asleep before a feeding is completed.[62] All of these problems contribute to poor stimulation of the breast, incomplete breast emptying, and inadequate milk production. While in the hospital, lactation assistance should focus on strategies to initiate and maintain maternal milk supply and provide adequate fluids and calories for the late-preterm infant.[62] **Hallmarks of breast feeding the late-preterm infant include proper positioning; use of breast pump, nursing supplementer (see Figure 18-9), or breast shield; waking every 2 to 3 hours to feed (for 8 to 12 breast feedings a day); use of skin-to-skin care; pre– and post–breast-feeding weights; and use of alternative methods of enteral nutrition.**[2,62] Collaboratively creating a feeding plan with parents that they understand and are able to carry out at home is essential before discharge.[2,15,47]

Some mothers may not establish or may have difficulty maintaining an adequate milk supply, yet infants with problems require an easily obtainable milk supply. **The Lact-Aid Nursing Trainer system (Figure 18-9) addresses a variety of breast feeding problems, including suckling defects.**[17] Expressed breast milk (EBM) or formula is contained in a presterilized, disposable bag suspended between the mother's breasts by a cord, and the liquid is delivered by a thin, flexible tube attached to the bag. The end of the tube is placed against the mother's nipple to enable the infant to suckle the tube and nipple at the same time. **This device provides the correct rate of flow and volume of liquid that elicits the reflexes of swallowing and expression. The Lact-Aid trainer provides oral therapy and nutritional supplementation for the infant and the mammary stimulus necessary to enhance the mother's lactation.**[108] **It is effective in managing low milk production in the mother that has resulted from separation, delayed breast feeding, poor technique, or other correctable problems, and the device gives nutritional and oral therapy to an infant who is slow in gaining weight or has a suckling dysfunction.**

CAUTION: **To prevent the spread of serious infections, the Lact-Aid trainer should never be borrowed, rented, or loaned from another mother.**

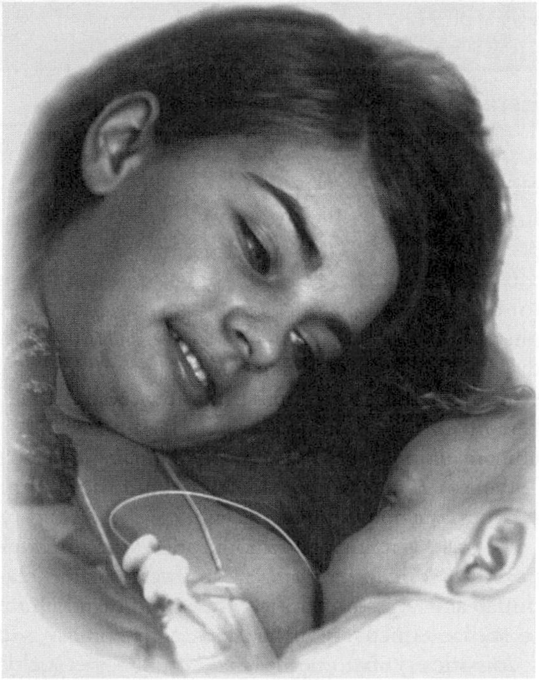

FIGURE 18-9 Lact-Aid Nursing Trainer. (Courtesy Lact-Aid International, Inc.)

Problems with the letdown reflex may originate with the mother, the neonate, or both. The mother's emotional state may interfere with letdown—a tense mother will not have a letdown reflex. Often, especially in breast feeding a premature infant, this is because of fear of failure or a lack of privacy. Knowledge of the mechanisms of lactation can help the mother avoid a fear of failing. **Give the mother as much privacy and the least stressful environment possible when she is pumping her breasts and breast feeding. If a mother experiences a weak or delayed letdown, she should massage the colostrum or milk down to the nipple before putting the infant to the breast.** Infants with a poor suck, such as preterm infants or infants with Down syndrome or a neurologic deficit, understimulate the breast and do not trigger the letdown reflex. **Use of the Lact-Aid trainer provides oral therapy, improves these infants' suckling ability, and facilitates a successful nursing relationship. The breast also can be stimulated with a good pump between feedings to increase the milk supply.**

DATA COLLECTION AND INTERVENTION

Establishment of Breast Feeding

AVAILABLE FEEDING AND SUCKLING NEONATE

Infants who have been admitted to a NICU often present a dilemma to care providers as to the most favorable time to begin putting the infant to the breast. The infant's current physical status, plus considerations of nutrition and energy expenditure, helps determine such decisions. In a national survey, criteria used to determine readiness for oral feedings included the following: (1) 75% used gestational age (e.g., 34 weeks by 60%) or weight (e.g., 1500 g by 50%); and (2) infant behavioral cues (e.g., sucking behaviors)[191] (see the Critical Findings box below and on pp. 457-459). **Few empirical data support the contention that either weight or gestational age affects the ability of a preterm infant to suckle effectively as the suck and swallow will automatically be coordinated by the peristaltic motion at the breast.** In the same survey, a majority (85% to 93%) responded that bottle feeding is started first, before breast feeding.[191] **Professional caregivers believe and teach parents that breast feeding is too stressful and requires more energy and exertion than bottle feeding.**[217] Contrary to physiologic evidence, progression of nutritional support for the preterm has proceeded from intravenous (IV) fluids → total parenteral nutrition → gavage (continuous → intermittent) → bottle feeding (at 1500 to 1800 g or 34 to 35 weeks post-conceptual age) → breast feeding (after bottle feeding without distress). **Problems arising from this approach include the following*:**

- **Delay in initial oral feedings**
- **Establishment of a sucking method that may not easily transfer to breast feeding**
- **Initiation of breast feeding when discharge is imminent so the mother receives little, if any, breast-feeding assistance and support**
- **Each additional week of hospitalization reduces the likelihood of the infant transitioning to direct breast feeding by 14%**

*References 57,68,136,166,192,197,198,217.

Critical Findings

READINESS FOR INITIATION OF ORAL FEEDINGS: RESEARCH BASIS

BREAST FEEDING	CRITERIA	BOTTLE FEEDING
Preterm		*Preterm*
28-32 weeks: Better able to coordinate suck, swallow, and breathing.[134,135,138]	←*Gestational/ post-conceptual age*→	34 to 35 weeks: PCA is a developmental guideline—based on belief that sucking pattern is similar to that of full-terms*; infants may be ready at an earlier age (i.e., 28-34 weeks).[132] Coordination of respirations with sucking and swallowing is consistently achieved by infants >37 weeks PCA.[128,162]
<1500 g: Better able to coordinate suck, swallow, and breathing.[134-136,138]	←*Weight*→	1500 to 1800 g: Traditional criteria without research basis.
Full-Term	←*Mechanics of Sucking*→	*Full-Term*
Ultrasound study shows human nipple elongates to twice its resting length; neonatal cheeks act as a passive seal for the oral cavity. Sucking pressures of −50 to −155 mm Hg.[165]		Higher maximum pressure and number of sucks or bursts; greater suck widths and greater intake/suck. Able to alter sucking to accommodate nutrient composition, nipple, and hole size to minimize energy expenditure[123] and autoregulate milk flow by controlling pressure generated during sucking.[123] Regulates sucking pressure by coordination of various oral motor structures so that intraoral pressure is controlled to enable milk flow in a manageable fashion.

AC, Before feeding; *BPD*, bronchopulmonary dysplasia; *CA*, corrected age; *PC*, after feeding; *PCA*, post-conceptual age; *PMA*, post-menstrual age; *VLBW*, very-low-birth-weight.
*References 56,105,125,128,132,162.

Critical Findings—cont'd

BREAST FEEDING	CRITERIA	BOTTLE FEEDING
Preterm		***Preterm***
Sucking pressures of −2.5 to −15 mm Hg.[165]		Burst width (interburst and intersuck width) similar to that of full-term infant.[92,130,131] At the beginning of a feeding, preterms generate weaker sucking pressure within the oral cavity that changes over time to pressures and duration in the same range as for term infants, because of neural maturation and sucking experience.
Full-Term	***←Energy Expenditure→***	***Full-Term***
50% of feeding obtained in first 2 min; 80% to 90% by 4 min; last 5 min, minimal obtained from each breast.[165]		86% of feeding obtained in first 4 min of sucking.[105] Generate larger negative pressure with sucks with higher energy expenditure.[92] Able to alter sucking to accommodate nutrient composition, nipple and hole size to minimize energy expenditure[123] and autoregulate milk flow by controlling pressure generated during sucking.[123]
Preterm		***Preterm***
After 34 weeks: 70% to 80% of feeding ingested in first 6 min, then intake sluggish, rest periods increase; and sucking and nourishment decrease. At 36 to 37 weeks: Sucking standards are similar to those in mature neonate.[158] The younger the gestational age, the higher the variability.[158] Longer duration of breast than bottle feeding.[134,138] No differences in duration of breast versus bottle feeding.		40% of total volume ingested in first min, less energy to suck same volume as full-term infant.[92] Infants born 26 to 29 weeks gestational age benefit from restricted milk flow (i.e., milk is obtained only with active sucking; no milk flows to infant by gravity or high-low nipples during rest periods). At initiation of oral feeding (with restricted milk flow), an intake of 1.5 mL/min and a proficiency of 30% (e.g., intake of 9 mL in first 5 min; intake of 30 mL in 20 min) are indicative of earlier attainment of full oral feeding.[105] Consumes an average of 2.6 mL/min of feeding.[162]
At 35 weeks CA: Small volume of milk intake in same duration of feeding; fed less efficiently and with fewer suck bursts.[57]		At 35 weeks CA: Greater volume of milk intake in same duration of feeding with more sucking bursts; fewer single sucks, better nipple seal.[57]
Preterm	***←Temperature→***	
Skin temperature higher (than when bottle feeding) because of bodily contact with mother.[35,134,138] No temperature change before feeding (ac) or after feeding (pc).		

Continued

Critical Findings—cont'd

BREAST FEEDING	CRITERIA	BOTTLE FEEDING
Preterm Less weight gain after breast feeding compared with bottle feeding.[68]	***←Weight Gain→***	***Preterm*** No difference in weight gain between experimental self-demand feeding protocol and control group (standard care).[125]
	←Heart Rate→	Preterm Bradycardia occurred with bottle feeding but not breast feeding; bradycardia possibly related to faster milk flow and interference with breathing[134,138]; apnea and bradycardia with bottle feeding in otherwise healthy preterms.[128]
	←Coordination of Suck, Swallow, and Breathing→	Full-Term Suck, swallow, breathe in a 1:1:1 pattern.[128] Alteration of breathing pattern—prolongation of expiration and shortening of inspiration.[124,138] No difference in sucking frequency or pressure when bottle feeding expressed milk or formula. Differences in sucking and/or breathing patterns attributed to nutrient delivery rather than nutrient composition.[122]
Preterm Different patterns of sucking bursts and better coordination, breathing is integrated within sucking bursts.[135]	***←Coordination of Suck, Swallow, and Breathing→***	***Preterm*** Initial feedings at 32 to 34 weeks are characterized by periods of apneic suckle alternating with respirations; as PMA increases, the percentage of apneic swallows decreases and suck-swallow-breathing is more synchronized.[63,212] High-flow nipples result in apnea[123,189] or bradycardia.[117-119,121] Do not breathe within sucking bursts but in alternate short bursts of sucking with breathing.[138] Consistently achieved by infants 37 weeks PCA. Use of orthodontic nipples results in physiologic stability and effective feeding behavior in some preterms.[45] At 34 weeks PCA, sucking pattern primarily expression component; with maturation, experience, endurance, and strength gains, there is a shift to more frequent use of term sucking pattern.[192] Not necessary to wait for full-term sucking pattern for successful oral feeding.[56,192]
Full-Term No desaturation with feeding.[69] 18% of pc saturations <90%.	***←Oxygen Saturation→***	***Full-Term*** No desaturation with feeding.[124] 29% of pc saturations <90%. More oxygen desaturations (<90%) than breast feeding.[122]
Preterm No difference in oxygenation with breast versus bottle feeding;[134,138] no pc decline of oxygenation; oxygenation more stable than with bottle feeding—fewer desaturations.[45] Desaturations (<90%) in 21% of breast feedings.[35] With BPD, saturation higher than with bottle feeding.[35]		***Preterm*** Decreased oxygenation during initial sustained sucking, but oxygenation increased as sucking pattern modulated.[178] 32 to 36 weeks: Range of 94% to 97% with feeding, with sucking decreased saturation from 2.5% to 16% (range 80% to 100%).[132] Fluctuations and sharper decrease in saturation with bottle feedings versus breast feeding[35,134,138,178]; 10 min pc saturation 50% below baseline.[35] Desaturations (>90%) in 38% of bottle feeding.[35] Desaturation in VLBW infants at discharge: average of 10.8 events during feeding; 20% of feeding time with saturations less than 90% Behavioral cues of desaturation are unreliable; changes in breathing and sucking pauses to regulate breathing pattern and increase oxygenation may occur.

AC, Before feeding; *BPD*, bronchopulmonary dysplasia; *CA*, corrected age; *PC*, after feeding; *PCA*, post-conceptual age; *PMA*, post-menstrual age; *VLBW*, very-low-birth-weight.
*References 56,105,125,128,132,162.

Critical Findings—cont'd

BREAST FEEDING	CRITERIA	BOTTLE FEEDING
	←*Hypercapnia*→ (*elevated* Pco_2)	**Preterm** 34 to 35 weeks: Increased Pco_2 depresses sucking and swallowing so that respirations may supersede feeding in preterms with increased respiratory drive (e.g., BPD).
Preterm 32 weeks: Increased feeding in active/alert and quiet/alert.	←*Behavioral Cues*→ ←Quiet, alert→ state before and during feedings associated with more successful feeding behaviors.[125,128,129] Offer pacifier for nonnutritive suck (NNS) ac to promote awake behavior at beginning of feeding.[162,164] ←NNS pattern of sucking develops before nutritive pattern; mature NNS pattern not reliable cue for readiness to orally feed.[105,162] ←Cues include[8,128,192]→ Oral behaviors—sucking on pacifier, fingers, feeding tube. Rooting reflex, hand-to-mouth behaviors, mouthing movements. Presence of gag reflex. ←*Behavioral State*→ Changes—arousal from sleep, quiet alert state ac.[129] Exhibits stability in autonomic, motoric, and behavioral states. Able to self-regulate, interact, and tolerate outside stimuli.[128] ←Crying→ fussing and demanding to feed—a late sign.	**Full-Term and Preterm** Motor behavior: Change in arm posture (flexion) with feeding.

An ***Early Feeding Skills (EFS) Assessment*** checklist has been developed to assess both oral feeding readiness and oral feeding skills in preterm infants.[206] To individualize interventions, an infant's developmental stage regarding specific feeding skills (e.g., the ability to remain engaged in feeding; to organize oral-motor functioning; to coordinate swallowing and breathing; to maintain physiologic stability) is profiled. Content validity, as well as intrarater and interrater reliability have been established. The EFS is being tested for predictive, concurrent, and construct validity.[206]

Use of a breast-feeding protocol[200] without use of bottle feeding (either before breast feeding or to supplement breast feeding) is associated with the longest duration of breast feeding.[16] An RCT of this protocol in which nasogastric (NG) supplementation was compared with bottle feeding for a transition to feeding at the breast found that NG supplementation was associated with feeding from the breast at discharge, 3 days, 3 months, and 6 months compared with preterm infants supplemented with bottle feeding.[99] In this same study, earlier age at initiation of breast feeding also was associated with successful and longer duration of breast feeding.[99] Other protocols for transitioning from gavage to breast have been proposed but not tested in an NICU population.[156] After discharge from the NICU, mothers wean their preterm infants from the breast because of (1) infant resistance to latching on, (2) weak suck, (3) refusing the breast, and (4) difficulty with latch-on.[80] If the sucking pattern learned with bottle feeding impedes breast feeding, health care providers should promote early, exclusive breast feeding to prolong the duration of preterm breast feeding after discharge.[16,24,99,164]

Maturation of feeding skills depends on developmental changes in the infant's central nervous system coupled with experiential learning.* Studies show that preterm infants are able to breast feed far earlier (<1500 g or 28 to 36 weeks' gestation) than they can bottle feed.[134-136,138,198] A comparison of studies of breast feeding and bottle feeding shows less oxygen desaturation, warmer skin temperature, no bradycardia, and better coordination of sucking and breathing with breast feeding when compared with bottle feeding (see the Critical Findings box on pp. 456-459). According to these research data, the ability of the preterm infant to breast feed without alterations in homeostasis occurs *before* the ability to safely bottle feed. Oxygenation is more stable with breast feeding, because the type of sucking pattern (e.g., intermittent) and the flow of milk at the beginning of breast feeding may be easier for the VLBW infant to control and regulate.[118,189] In VLBW infants, breathing is compromised (e.g., desaturations, increase in heart and respiratory rates) more during continuous sucking than during intermittent sucking.[189]

When an NG tube is in place, a VLBW infant has even poorer oxygenation, shallower breathing, and inability to increase tidal volume.[189] The postfeeding period enables recovery of oxygen saturation and end-tidal CO_2 to the prefeeding levels.[189]

Health care providers and parents should closely observe VLBW infants during the continuous sucking period (e.g., the first minute of bottle feeding,[205] with letdown during breast feeding) for apnea, oxygen desaturation, and heart rate changes. Recommendations for continuous sucking periods include (1) not allowing breathing pauses of more than 10 seconds, (2) monitoring oxygen saturation and heart rate for continuous sucking of more than 30 seconds, and (3) interrupting sucking by withdrawing the nipple for breathing pauses and desaturations.[107,189] Desaturations especially in the first minute of bottle feeding, during the continuous sucking period, still occur in VLBW infants nearing discharge.[205]

Skin-to-skin (kangaroo) care provides a safe, effective alternative method of caring for premature infants (see Chapter 13). Use of kangaroo care has been shown to improve lactation for mothers of preterm infants.[30,57,198] During skin-to-skin contact, the infant may initiate nonnutritive suckling at the breast. Nonnutritive time at the breast is used to accustom both mother and baby to each other and the pleasant sensory stimuli at the breast. Nonnutritive suckling at the breast improves maternal letdown, enhances attachment and bonding, and shortens transition time to and lengthens the duration of breast feeding.[164,198] As the preterm matures, nonnutritive suckling is replaced by hunger cues, latching on, and effective nutritive suckling. Both appropriate-for-gestational-age (AGA) and SGA infants (700 to 2450 g) benefit from early (sometimes starting at birth) and sustained breast feeding as follows (see Chapter 13):

- More mothers breast feed and are more confident.
- More frequent feedings are given.
- More milk is produced.
- Infants breast feed longer (e.g., at 1 month after discharge, breast feeding rates increased from 11% to 50%).
- There is less bradycardia than with gavage or bottle feeding.
- There is better weight gain and earlier discharge.

*References 24,56,128,158,162,164,192,198,200.

Both maternal and neonatal responses to breast feeding should be monitored.[164,198] **Adequate milk volume is available when the milk ejection (letdown) reflex occurs. Breast massage may assist in bringing down the milk, thus making it easier for the infant to obtain. Letdown may be felt by the mother or observed as a change in the rhythm of infant suckling and audible swallowing. After letdown is established, the infant expends little energy in suckling.** He or she only needs to coordinate swallowing and breathing with an occasional burst of sucking. **The nurse should be available during the initial breast feeding to provide support to the mother, to ensure that the infant exhibits no signs of distress (e.g., color changes, bradycardia, oxygen desaturation, drop in temperature), and to provide guidance for the mother if the infant chokes with letdown.** The nurse also needs to reinforce to the mother that the infant's sucking pattern will be a pattern of bursts and pauses. The pauses are present in all infants and provide rest periods for the infant.

The infant's respiratory status should be reviewed. Infants requiring supplemental oxygen can breast feed. If the infant requires 35% oxygen or less, oxygen may be delivered through a nasal cannula to ensure adequate, consistent oxygenation. This will eliminate another source of concern for the mother: having to worry about juggling the blow-by oxygen line. If the infant has not been placed on a nasal cannula previously, the nurse should initiate the cannula and then assess oxygenation using a pulse oximeter before the feeding begins. The infant's temperature status requires review. Attention should be directed toward preventing hypothermia with infants who require significant thermal support. The infant should be swaddled, and a hat should be placed on his or her head to prevent heat loss.

Duration of breast feeding should be based on cues of satiety, such as sucking cessation or falling asleep, or cues of physiologic instability or fatigue. Frequency of breast feeding can be progressed, as can frequency of bottle feeding: from one breast feeding per day to one per shift to every other breast feeding. If the mother is available with this progression, bottle feeding may be deferred until breast feeding is well established, or bottle feeding may be avoided altogether. When the infant is taking all nutrition orally, the mother can be encouraged to breast feed as often as possible and institute an ad lib schedule.[137,198] **If the mother is available, the infant should breast feed as often as necessary and supplementation should not be provided. However, if the breast milk supply is insufficient, using a Lact-Aid Nursing Trainer provides nutritional supplementation and mammary stimulation to increase maternal milk supply. Total intake should be estimated to ensure adequate calories. If the infant weighs less than 1500 g, it may be necessary to augment calories, protein, and calcium with human milk fortifiers (fortifiers made from human milk are preferred to cow milk fortifiers)** (see Chapter 17).[103]

Families and staff often fear that the infant will not get enough during a breast feeding. This concern is especially predominant when infants have been hospitalized for prematurity and fluids and calories have been scrutinized closely. Health professionals should be sensitive to such concerns and refrain from employing methods such as weighing infants before and after feedings or using gavage tubes to attempt to determine the exact amount of breast milk ingested during the feeding. **With today's electronic NICU scales, however, test weighing (before and after feeding) (see the Critical Findings box on pp. 446-447) is accurate, if necessary.**[68,198] In one study, test weighing was not shown to increase maternal competence or confidence in breast feeding during and for 4 weeks after hospitalization.[68] Another study showed that in-home test weighing after discharge was helpful in reassuring mothers of VLBW infants that the infants were receiving adequate intake while nursing.[88] **However, health professionals should focus on cues that can be used during and after hospitalization by both caregivers and the family.**[68] **These cues include the infant's satisfaction after the feeding (asleep or fussy), the frequency of feedings, voiding pattern (minimum of six to eight wet diapers per day, weighing diapers, and checking specific gravity), and palpation of the mother's breasts before and after feeding. Trends in weight gain also can demonstrate the success of the mother-infant dyad in breast feeding.**

A small infant may have difficulty taking a large nipple into the mouth. The mother should shape her nipple by compressing behind the areola to allow more of the nipple to be placed in the infant's mouth. The thumb and index finger or the first two fingers should be parallel to

the infant's nose and chin. The breast must be soft enough to be compressed in this manner. The mother should hold the infant close for the comfort of both, with the infant's entire body, not just the head, turned toward the mother's body (see Figure 18-5).

A nipple shield allows the infant to get a nipple in the mouth but increases the amount of sucking necessary to obtain milk and decreases the amount of stimulation received at the nipple. Supervised temporary use of silicone nipple shields has been found to be a successful bridging technique for the infant to transfer to direct breast feeding (after only a few sessions of shield use).[173] Use of a nipple shield should be followed by breast pumping to express residual milk, maintain adequate milk supply, and obtain milk to freeze for supplemental feeding.

Because nonnutritive suckling does not stimulate prolactin secretion and milk production, infants should not be placed on an empty breast to feed. Without positive reinforcement (i.e., milk) for their efforts, infants soon learn that the breast does not give milk, become frustrated, and refuse to feed. The Lact-Aid trainer may be used to initiate proper suckle and supplement intake in a small premature infant who is able to nurse (see "Prevention" section on p. 455).

Supplementing breast feedings with bottle-fed formula is inefficient in terms of energy and calories, because the infant expends energy, and thus calories, to feed twice. More energy-efficient and calorically efficient methods of initiating breast feeding include offering smaller, more frequent feedings, supplementing by gavage feeding, and using a lactation supplementing device. Breast milk fortifiers (see Chapter 17) should be used when the mother's milk is not adequate for the infant's requirements. Breast milk substitutes should be used when the mother does not provide sufficient volume.

UNAVAILABILITY OF A FEEDING OR SUCKLING NEONATE

If premature birth or neonatal or maternal illness delays the onset of breast feeding, the mother experiences a decrease in her milk production. Depending on how long breast feeding has been delayed, mammary involution and the return of menstrual hormonal cycles may inhibit breast feeding. A preterm infant or one who is ill may be weak and tire easily, and thus adequate lactation is not established.

If a neonate is unable to feed at the breast, breast milk must be produced through artificial stimulation of the breast. The mother should establish a regular routine of breast massage[94,198] and pumping soon after the infant's birth. A comfortable chair with armrests or a pillow often helps, and the mother should be assured of privacy during breast feeding and breast pumping. It is often necessary for the care provider to help the mother start and to encourage her routine. Each breast should be pumped every 2 to 4 hours, preferably with a double pumping system to enhance milk supply.[79,94] Mothers should increase pumping time up to 15 to 20 minutes as the milk comes in, with the suction pressure increased as tolerated. At the beginning of pumping, mothers should awaken to pump at night to establish a good milk supply. Sleep and rest are necessary for good milk supply; however, the mother should not sleep when breasts are engorged because this will decrease the supply. Mothers should be advised that if their infant were with them, they would be feeding every 2 to 4 hours around the clock and therefore should develop that pattern to establish an adequate supply.

CAUTION: Mothers should be counseled about the potential risks of using breast shells or breast pump kits that have been used by other women. Breast shells, breast pump kits, and lactation aids are intimate-care items and are meant for use with one mother and one baby. Breast pump attachments and collection devices must be appropriately cleaned.[39]

Induction Aids. Various induction aids using tactile and mechanical principles are available to assist the mother in lactating and relactating. Knowledge of the different systems and their advantages and disadvantages enables the health care provider to help the mother choose the most helpful aid.

Breast massage (gentle, tactile stimulus usually in a circular motion using increasing pressure) before breast feeding or pumping may help unplug breast ducts and enable milk to flow more easily.

Breast massage during pumping provides the important tactile stimulation that is missing without the infant's nursing and facilitates prolactin release and milk yield.[108]

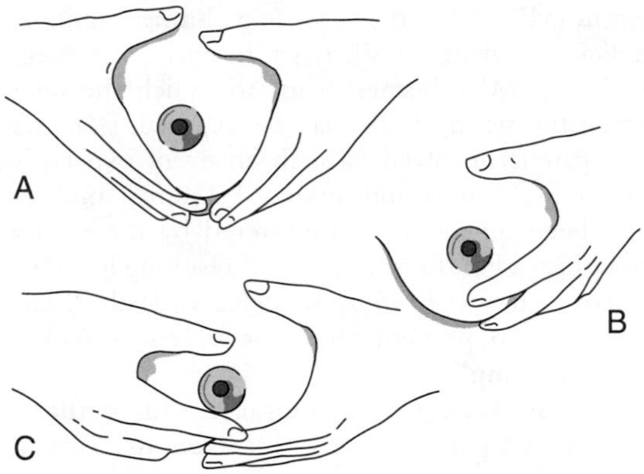

FIGURE 18-10 Breast massage. **A,** Place hands with palms toward chest at breast. Encircle breast with fingers and thumbs. **B** and **C,** Applying pressure, move hands forward, overlapping as they near nipple. Stop posterior to areola. Continue for 1 to 2 minutes or until milk is on nipple. Repeat on opposite breast. (From Lawrence RA, Lawrence RM: *Breastfeeding: a guide for the medical professional*, ed 6, St Louis, 2005, Mosby.)

Hand Expression. **Once the breast milk supply has been established, hand expression (Figure 18-10) is the simplest and most cost-effective way to collect milk; however, prolactin secretion and milk yields are less than with a pulsatile breast pump.**[220] Some mothers find hand expression aesthetically unsatisfactory, and they should use other methods.

Mechanical Devices. **Breast pumps work by application of negative pressure (e.g., −50 to −155 mm Hg) and compression in a suck-release pattern (e.g., rate of 40 to 50 suck-release cycles/min) by fitting the nipple cup (or flange) over the maternal nipple and areola.**[20] Nonautomated pumps are regulated by the number of times the mother manually exerts and releases pressure. Three types of nonautomated pumps are available: (1) bicycle horn pumps, which should never be used; (2) cylinder pumps; and (3) trigger or handle pumps.[20] Nonautomated pumps are best for occasional use. **Automated pumps (either fully or partially) exert more negative pressure, permit the greatest number of cycles per minute, and are the pumps of choice for establishing and maintaining lactation for a preterm or sick infant.**[20,198] A randomized trial comparing a novel manual breast pump (with compressive action on the areola) with a standard electric pump, used by mothers of preterm infants, found that the manual pump produced greater milk flow, resulted in greater total milk volume, was preferred by most mothers, and was more cost effective.[52] Automated pumps are available in the NICU and for home rental use. Health insurance (both public and private) may reimburse for pump rental.

Serum prolactin levels and increased milk yield more closely parallel those with natural infant suckling when an intermittent, pulsative pump is used.[220] **Just as nursing twins simultaneously results in a greater prolactin response, pumping both breasts simultaneously is more convenient and provides higher prolactin release (and higher milk yield) and saves time.**[79,220]

To increase milk supply when the infant is not nursing, the pump should be used frequently (see the Critical Findings box on pp. 446-447). Because the breast pump is not as efficient as the suckling infant,[20] **before initiating pumping, the mother may find that tactile stimulation and breast massage help increase the milk supply.** Looking at the infant's picture or listening to a tape recording of the infant's cry stimulates her milk production with a pump.

Beginning on the low or normal pump setting and carefully breaking the suction at the breast with a finger help prevent sore nipples. Painful engorgement is relieved by pumping each breast just enough to obtain relief. Nipple or areolar engorgement must be relieved so that the infant is able to grasp and suckle the nipple.

Lactoengineering. **To increase caloric density of EBM to improve growth/weight gain in VLBW infants, the pumping process can be altered to increase lipid content. Because the lipid content of hindmilk (e.g., milk expressed after letdown or later in the pumping session) is two to three times higher than the lipid content of foremilk, selectively feeding hindmilk to VLBW infants has been shown to increase growth and weight gain.**[184,211] **For VLBW infants with a consistent weight gain of less than 15 g/kg/day, hindmilk feedings may be initiated until a consistent weight gain of more than 30 g/kg/day is achieved.**[211]

To express hindmilk, breast pumping is interrupted an average of 2 to 5 minutes after milk ejection has begun. This milk is collected and

labeled "foremilk." Pumping is resumed until about 2 minutes after milk flow has ceased. This milk is placed in a separate container labeled "hindmilk." Another method of lactoengineering is to individualize the milk fractionation procedure by use of a "creamatocrit" that accurately estimates lipid and caloric content of EBM.[64,141] A small sample (<1.0 mL) of pumped breast milk is aliquoted into two capillary tubes that are sealed and centrifuged for 5 minutes. The lipid and cream layer rises to the top of the tubes and can be quantitated as a percentage of breast milk volume using a hematocrit reader and converted to estimates of lipid concentration and caloric density using published regression equations.[141] A recent study showed that mothers are able to cost-effectively and accurately perform creamatocrit assays; the mothers enjoyed the responsibility and increased involvement in their infant's care.[64] It is interesting to note that low-income mothers with fewer years of formal education and skilled rather than professional occupations were the most accurate in their performance of creamatocrits.

COMPLICATIONS OF BREAST FEEDING

Many complications other than prematurity may pose difficulties with breast feeding. **Information on perinatal complications and breast feeding is shown in Table 18-3.**[8,108] Because of the significant benefits of breast milk, infants with special needs should be encouraged and mothers should be assisted in breast feeding. Many principles used with the preterm and other variations of feeding styles and techniques may help facilitate these infants and their mothers in enjoying a successful breast-feeding experience.

Consultation with or referral to a certified licensed lactation consultant or specialist also may be helpful.[164] Many NICUs have such an expert on their staff.

Misappropriation of Breast Milk

Misappropriation of breast milk (giving the wrong expressed breast milk to the wrong infant) does occur. As a distillate of human blood, human milk may contain infectious bacteria (e.g., *Klebsiella, Staphylococcus,* methicillin-resistant *Staphylococcus aureus* [MRSA]) and viruses (e.g., human immunodeficiency virus [HIV], hepatitis virus, cytomegalovirus [CMV], herpes virus) to which the infant given the wrong milk may be exposed. Both staff and parents involved in such an event experience psychologic stress and anxiety.[46] Human milk has also been mistakenly administered by the intravenous instead of the enteral route, resulting in a range of consequences from no sequelae to death.[182] **Unit practices to prevent these occurrences include the following**[46,182]**:**

- **Use tubing for enteral feedings that is incompatible with intravenous tubing/connections.**
- **Check milk containers for two identifiers.**
- **Two nurses verify milk for administration; both nurses sign that verification has occurred.**
- **Two nurses verify and sign (that milk has been verified) at transfer and at discharge.**
- **Use commercial bar-coded devices.**

Drugs in Breast Milk

Table 18-4 provides information about specific drugs excreted in breast milk.[6,108] Protein binding, degree of ionization, molecular weight, and solubility of drugs influence the passage of drugs into milk. Protein-bound drugs and drugs of large molecular weight (>200) are less likely to pass into milk. Conversely, lipid-soluble drugs pass more easily into the milk. Because breast milk is slightly acidic when compared with plasma, weakly alkaline compounds are present in equal or greater amounts in breast milk compared with plasma. Weakly acidic compounds have a higher concentration in plasma than in breast milk.

Several factors influence the drug effect on the infant. **Most drugs appear in milk, but drug levels usually do not exceed 1% to 2% of the ingested dose and do not depend on the milk volume.**[108] The clinical dose of a drug to the infant can be calculated by the following formula[67]:

D-infant = Drug concentration in milk (at C-max, or C-av) × Volume of milk ingested

Drug transfers through breast milk may be minimized by feeding the infant before taking oral medications.[14] Many variables, such as gastric emptying, pH, and effects of intestinal enzymes, affect

Text continued on p. 470

TABLE 18-4 DRUGS EXCRETED IN BREAST MILK

DRUGS	BREAST MILK	CONSIDERATIONS IN INFANT
ANALGESICS		
Heroin, codeine, meperidine, fentanyl, morphine, pentazocine, dextropropoxyphene	Appears in variable amounts. FDA warning[208] about mothers who rapidly metabolize codeine (because of a genetic predisposition), resulting in increased morphine levels in their breast milk and morphine overdose to breast-feeding infants. Mothers who rapidly metabolize codeine will become so sleepy that they are unable to care for themselves or their infant. Rapid metabolizers of codeine include (1) 1% to 10% in whites, (2) 3% in blacks, (3) 1% in Asians and Hispanics, (4) 16% to 28% in North Africans, Ethiopians, and Saudi Arabians, and (5) those positive for *CYP2D6* genotype with genetic testing.	Symptoms of depression and floppiness have been associated with these drugs. Sleepiness, difficulty breast feeding, limpness, hypotonia, and respiratory distress. Severe, life-threatening events (respiratory arrest) caused by morphine overdose have occurred.
Aspirin	Safe on a single-dose schedule, although it passes into milk in low concentration.	In a deliberate overdose, metabolic acidosis resulted from an accumulation in the infant; use cautiously because of the risk for Reye's syndrome.
Acetaminophen	Appears in small amounts.	Well tolerated.
Ibuprofen	Appears in small amounts.	Well tolerated.
Sumatriptan succinate	Appears in small amounts.	Well tolerated.
ANTIBIOTICS AND SULFA DRUGS		
Sulfa drugs	Appear in breast milk and may interfere with bilirubin binding in neonate; infants with G6PD deficiency may develop hemolysis.	Should not be used for breast-feeding mother in the first month if infant is jaundiced or if infant has G6PD deficiency.
Chloramphenicol	Appears in breast milk.	Contraindicated in nursing mother because infant may accumulate drug and develop "gray baby syndrome."
Penicillins (ampicillin, amoxicillin)	Small amounts in breast milk.	Disruption of gastrointestinal (GI) flora, allergic sensitization/reactions. Observe for thrush, diarrhea, and rash. Breast milk assists recolonization of normal gut flora.
Tetracycline	Appears in breast milk at 50% of serum level.	Infants may develop stained and mottled teeth when therapy exceeds 10 days; should be given only for life-threatening maternal infections. Discontinue breast feeding during treatment.
ANTIFUNGALS		
Metronidazole/tinidazole	Appears in breast milk in levels equal to serum levels.	Side effects include decreased appetite, vomiting, blood dyscrasia, and animal evidence of tumorigenesis. Mother's dose can be modified (e.g., 2 g single-dose therapy) so she can pump and discard milk for 24 hours.
Antimalarial (chloroquine)	Very small amounts appear in breast milk.	Observe for GI symptoms (vomiting, diarrhea); hypotension.
Cephalosporins (cephalexin, cephalothin)	Very small amounts appear in breast milk.	Rash and sensitization are possible. Also may affect bacterial flora—diarrhea, thrush.

Modified from American Academy of Pediatrics, Committee on Drugs: The transfer of drugs and other chemicals into human breast milk, *Pediatrics* 108:776, 2001; Hale T: *Medications and mother's milk*, ed 13, Amarillo, Tex, 2008, Hale Publishing; Lawrence RA, Lawrence RM: *Breast feeding: a guide for the medical profession*, ed 6, St Louis, 2005, Mosby.

3′,5′-AMP, 3′,5′-Adenosine monophosphate; *FDA*, Food and Drug Administration; *G6PD*, glucose-6-phosphate dehydrogenase; *SIDS*, sudden infant death syndrome; T_3, triiodothyronine; T_4, thyroxine; *TSH*, thyroid-stimulating hormone.

*Drug of abuse; contraindicated during breast feeding—hazardous to both mother and infant.

†Only Food and Drug Administration–approved drug for opiate withdrawal.[5]

Continued

TABLE 18-4 DRUGS EXCRETED IN BREAST MILK—cont'd

DRUGS	BREAST MILK	CONSIDERATIONS IN INFANT
ANTIFUNGALS—cont'd		
Fluconazole (Diflucan)	Excreted into breast milk in small amounts (1% of the maternal dose; <5% of the therapeutic pediatric dose).	Considered safe for nursing infants.
Fluoroquinolones (levofloxacin, norfloxacin, ofloxacin, ciprofloxacin)	Varying levels in breast milk—use with caution.	Pseudomembranous colitis—observe for GI symptoms (vomiting, diarrhea). Tooth discoloration; phototoxicity. Arthropathy in animals.
ANTICHOLINERGICS		
Atropine, scopolamine, synthetic quaternary ammonium derivatives	Atropine appears, but quaternary ammonium derivatives do not appear in breast milk.	The neonate of nursing mother receiving atropine should be observed for tachycardia, constipation, and urinary retention.
Cimetidine	Appears in higher concentration than in serum.	No reported effects, although may suppress gastric activity, inhibit drug metabolism, and produce central nervous system stimulation. Use with caution until more information about anti-androgenic effects.
ANTICOAGULANTS		
Heparin and warfarin (Coumadin)	Do not appear in breast milk.	
ANTITHYROIDAL AGENTS		
Iodide	Passes into milk.	May affect thyroid activity and cause goiters. Not contraindicated during breast feeding.
Thiouracil	Higher concentration in maternal milk than in blood.	Neonatal problems include suppression of thyroid activity and agranulocytosis. If breast fed, infant should be given thyroid supplement, and thyroid function should be followed.
Propylthiouracil	Appears in small amounts (<0.3% of maternal dose).	No reported effects on infant. Follow with T_3, T_4, and TSH.
ANTICONVULSANTS		
Phenobarbital, phenytoin, carbamazepine (Tegretol), and valproic acid (Depakene)	All appear in small amounts.	Sedation is possible, but rarely are clinical symptoms significant enough to cause adverse effects. Accumulation may occur because of long half-life of valproic acid.
Lamotrigine	Mean milk-to-plasma ratio 41.3% with a non-significant trend toward higher levels in breast milk 4 hours after maternal dose.[155]	Infant plasma concentrations were 18.3% of maternal plasma concentrations; with a theoretical infant dose of 0.51mg/kg/day and a relative infant dose of 9.2%.[155] Mild thrombocytosis was the only adverse event noted.
CARDIOVASCULAR DRUGS		
Digoxin	Appears in small amounts.	Appears to be safe.
Reserpine	Appears in breast milk.	Symptoms include diarrhea, lethargy, nasal stuffiness, bradycardia, and respiratory difficulties; contraindicated in breast feeding.

Modified from American Academy of Pediatrics, Committee on Drugs: The transfer of drugs and other chemicals into human breast milk, *Pediatrics* 108:776, 2001; Hale T: *Medications and mother's milk*, ed 13, Amarillo, Tex, 2008, Hale Publishing; Lawrence RA, Lawrence RM: *Breast feeding: a guide for the medical profession*, ed 6, St Louis, 2005, Mosby.

3′,5′-AMP, 3′,5′-Adenosine monophosphate; *FDA*, Food and Drug Administration; *G6PD*, glucose-6-phosphate dehydrogenase; *SIDS*, sudden infant death syndrome; T_3, triiodothyronine; T_4, thyroxine; *TSH*, thyroid-stimulating hormone.

*Drug of abuse; contraindicated during breast feeding—hazardous to both mother and infant.

†Only Food and Drug Administration–approved drug for opiate withdrawal.[5]

TABLE 18-4 **DRUGS EXCRETED IN BREAST MILK—cont'd**

DRUGS	BREAST MILK	CONSIDERATIONS IN INFANT
CARDIOVASCULAR DRUGS—cont'd		
Propranolol, metoprolol, labetalol	Appear in breast milk in varying degrees; safest beta blockers with breast feeding.	Observe for beta blockade—respiratory depression, bradycardia, or hypoglycemia.
Verapamil, diltiazem	Appear in varying amounts in breast milk.	Appear to be safe.
Nifedipine	90% of the dose unavailable for transfer to breast milk because of binding to plasma proteins.[11] One to 3 hours after maternal dosing, low levels (<1 to 10.3 mcg/L) appear in breast milk.[67]	Appears to be safe.
CATHARTICS		
Aloin, cascara sagrada, and anthraquinone preparations	Appear in breast milk.	Colic and diarrhea are possible side effects.
CONTRACEPTIVES		
Birth control pills (combined; progestin only; minipill)	Appear in breast milk with peak levels 2 hours after intake.	Combined: may alter the quality and quantity of milk—suppress lactation, shorter breast feeding, and slower weight gain. Progestin only or minipill: no alteration of milk volume or infant weight gain. Unknown long-term risk for cancer—no evidence in past 30 years.[108]
Medroxyprogesterone (Depo-Provera)	Increased prolactin levels before/after sucking.	No adverse effects—3-month injection (increased protein and quantity of milk); 6-month injection (increased quantity but decrease in protein, fat, calcium).[108]
Birth control implant (IMPLANON)	Small amount of hormone passes into breast milk. Best to delay implant till 4 weeks postpartum.	Small number of children studied for 3 years after breast feeding—no effects on growth and development.
Barrier methods (diaphragm, condoms, foams, cervical cap)	No chemicals to be excreted into breast milk.	No effects on infant.
DIAGNOSTIC RADIOACTIVE COMPOUNDS		
^{67}Ga, ^{125}I, and ^{64}Cu	Appear for 24 to 48 hours.	Check half-life of specific compound. Pump and discard; then resume breast feeding.
DIURETICS		
Hydrochlorothiazide	May suppress lactation.	Inadequate milk; no significant risks are present; compatible with breast feeding.
IMMUNOSUPPRESSANT		
Azathioprine	One small study (n = 10 mothers; 31 breast milk samples) found small levels (1.2 and 7.6 ng/mL) of 6-mercaptopurine (6-MP) in breast milk samples at 3 and 6 hours after azathioprine ingestion.	Potential risks of bone marrow suppression, increased risk for infections and pancreatitis. No signs of clinical immunosuppression in the small study.

Continued

TABLE 18-4 DRUGS EXCRETED IN BREAST MILK—cont'd

DRUGS	BREAST MILK	CONSIDERATIONS IN INFANT
PSYCHOTHERAPEUTIC AGENTS		
Lithium	Appears in breast milk; infant serum level is 10% to 50% of mother's level.	Contraindicated in pregnancy; controversial during lactation. Cyanosis, hypotonia, electrocardiogram changes. Evaluate lithium levels. Inhibits cyclic 3′,5′-AMP, a substance significant to brain growth.
	A recent small study (n = 10 mother/baby pairs) found the average breast milk concentration of lithium to be 0.35 mEq/liter with an infant trough concentration of 0.16 mEq/liter.[213]	Carefully selected mothers may breast feed a healthy infant while taking lithium: (1) maternal mood stable, (2) simple medication regimen and/or monotherapy with lithium, and (3) a pediatrician collaborating to monitor the infant.[213]
Olanzapine	Small amount (1.02%). Avoid breast feeding during peak levels within 5 hours after dose.[61]	No adverse effects.
Phenothiazines	Appear in small amounts.	Evaluate each drug separately; observe for sedation.
Diazepam (Valium)	Appears in breast milk and may accumulate in infant because it is detoxified in liver.	Poor feeding, weight loss, hypoventilation, and drowsiness may be seen. Low incidence of toxicity and adverse events.
Tricyclic antidepressants (amitriptyline, nortriptyline, desipramine)	Appear in minimal amounts (<1%)	Careful considerations to select the safest for the infant. Nortriptyline may be the preferred choice.
Selective serotonin reuptake inhibitors (SSRIs) (fluoxetine, sertraline, paroxetine, citalopram, escitalopram)[127]	Appear in varying amounts. Fluoxetine—high levels, highly lipid bound. Produces the highest proportion (22%) of infant levels that are elevated above 10% of the average maternal level.[23] Citalopram produces elevated levels in 17% of infants.[23]	Sertraline is the drug of choice after birth because plasma levels are low (<2 ng/mL).[43,146,216] May alter short-term and/or long-term central nervous system development and function. Slower growth curve or weight gain with fluoxetine.[32] Most infants may continue breast feeding when mother is treated with 20 to 40 mg daily.[48] Citalopram—minimize maternal dose to decrease elevated infant levels.[216] Paroxetine levels are also low.[216] Escitalopram—somnolence and sedation in young infants.
STIMULANTS		
Amphetamines (methamphetamine*)	Amphetamine concentration 3 to 7 times higher in breast milk than in maternal plasma on the 10th and 42nd days of life.[199]	Stimulation of the infant—poor sleeping patterns and irritability. Infant death and SIDS-like syndrome reported with methamphetamine intake of mother.[12] Small amounts of amphetamine in infant's urine.[199]
Caffeine	Appears in small amounts (<1%) but may accumulate in infant.	Symptoms include jitteriness, wakefulness, and irritability. May alter iron concentration in milk and iron deficiency anemia at 1 month of age.
Theophylline	Appears in moderate amounts.	Irritability, jitteriness, and wakefulness may be seen in infant.
Cocaine*	Appears in breast milk.	Cocaine intoxication: neurotoxicity (e.g., irritability, hyperactive reflexes, tremulousness, and mood lability) and seizures have been reported (see Chapter 11).[33,34]

Modified from American Academy of Pediatrics, Committee on Drugs: The transfer of drugs and other chemicals into human breast milk, *Pediatrics* 108:776, 2001; Hale T: *Medications and mother's milk*, ed 13, Amarillo, Tex, 2008, Hale Publishing; Lawrence RA, Lawrence RM: *Breast feeding: a guide for the medical profession*, ed 6, St Louis, 2005, Mosby.

3′,5′-AMP, 3′,5′-Adenosine monophosphate; *FDA*, Food and Drug Administration; *G6PD*, glucose-6-phosphate dehydrogenase; *SIDS*, sudden infant death syndrome; T_3, triiodothyronine; T_4, thyroxine; *TSH*, thyroid-stimulating hormone.

*Drug of abuse; contraindicated during breast feeding—hazardous to both mother and infant.

†Only Food and Drug Administration–approved drug for opiate withdrawal.[5]

TABLE 18-4 **DRUGS EXCRETED IN BREAST MILK—cont'd**

DRUGS	BREAST MILK	CONSIDERATIONS IN INFANT
OTHER SUBSTANCES		
Methadone†	Appears in breast milk, concentration low (range 21.0 to 46.2 ng/mL).[93] Peak methadone levels occur in 4 hours after oral administration; the maximum amount secreted into breast milk is ≈2.2% g of the mother's dose.[109] Milk-to-plasma ratios range from 0.05 to 1.89.[126]	Management depends on maternal dosage—under 20 mg/24 hours probably safe.[5] Observe for sedation, withdrawal. Recent studies find that breast milk intake is associated with less neonatal abstinence syndrome (NAS) and less use of pharmacologic treatment, regardless of type of drugs and gestation.[1,93]
Ethanol (alcohol)	Quick equilibration between serum and breast milk levels.	Large quantities associated with lethargy, drowsiness, and affected motor development. The deficit in motor development was not replicated in a study of 18-month-olds exposed to moderate alcohol use during breast feeding.[111] May inhibit milk letdown reflex and suppress lactation. Avoid nursing within 2 to 3 hours of alcohol intake.
Marijuana*	May reach high concentrations.	May decrease prolactin levels, milk supply, and motor development. Exposure to secondary smoke. Avoid breast feeding for several hours after use.[108]
Nicotine	Appears in breast milk in proportion to number of cigarettes smoked and/or time from last cigarette.	Irritability; failure to thrive may result because of suppression of lactation. Effects of secondary smoke: increased incidence of upper respiratory infections, otitis media, bronchitis, pneumonia, and SIDS. Avoid smoking in the same room with the infant.
	Smoking reduces the transport of iodine into breast milk. Mothers should receive iodine supplement.[106]	Infants whose mothers smoke are at increased risk for iodine deficiency–induced brain damage if the mother does not receive iodine supplementation.[106]
Herbal tea mixtures (containing anise, fennel, licorice, galega) used to stimulate lactation (i.e., mother's milk tea)	Essential oils found in anise and fennel appear in breast milk.	Difficulty feeding; growth failure, hypotonia; lethargy; vomiting; weak cry; poor suck; decreased reaction to painful stimuli.[179]
Fenugreek	Appears in breast milk; milk has a maple syrup smell.	Urine may have a maple syrup smell.
Ginseng	No data on amount in breast milk.	May cause neonatal androgen effect and hirsutism.
Comfrey	No data on amount in breast milk; caution use in any form.	Associated with veno-occlusive disease and hepatotoxicity and is carcinogenic. Contraindicated in breast feeding.
Silicone breast implants	Silicon in cow's milk has been shown to be 10 times higher and even higher in commercial infant formulas than in mothers with silicone implants.[188] Breast-feeding mothers with silicone implants are similar to mothers without implants with respect to levels of silicon in their blood and breast milk.[188]	No adverse effects.
RESPIRATORY DRUGS		
Inhalants (steroids—budesonide)	Lower levels of budesonide (mean ratio of 0.46) in milk that in maternal plasma.[49]	Negligible systemic exposure to inhaled corticosteroids:[49] Mean infant dose 0.3% of daily maternal dose; average infant plasma concentration 1/600th of maternal plasma concentration.

absorption. Finally, the chronologic and gestational ages of the infant affect the maturity of the systems involved in excretion and detoxification (see Chapter 10).

PARENT TEACHING

Parent teaching has been discussed throughout this chapter because it is essential to a successful breast-feeding experience for both mother and infant (see the Parent Teaching box below).

Before a premature or sick infant is actually nursed at the breast, the colostrum and breast milk may have to be pumped and fed to the infant. If the mother's production is adequate, no supplementation is necessary. Before collecting the mother's milk, perform the following:

- Screen the mother (by history) for disease.
- Screen the mother (by history) for drugs that she has taken.
- Instruct the mother in sterile technique.

Proper collection and storage must be discussed with each family so that stored milk does not cause infections. Breast pumps can be a potential source of contamination, and therefore instructions on proper cleaning are paramount. D'Amico et al[39] describe a process used for review and updating procedures to decrease this risk in an NICU. A written handout of pumping, storing, and thawing practices is helpful. Often the mother pumps and collects the milk, and the father transports it to the NICU (see Chapter 29). In addition, fathers assist with pumping, assume more daily domestic duties, and provide moral support to pumping mothers.[195] Methods of treatment and storage are listed in Box 18-1. Rewarming techniques include (1) placing frozen milk in a room-temperature water bath, in a hot-water bath, in a microwave oven, or under cold running water and then tepid water or (2) using commercially available devices. Slow room-temperature rewarming is a concern because of bacterial overgrowth, especially if thawing is prolonged. Most nurseries use room-temperature water bath rewarming to avoid exposure to the high temperatures of the

Parent Teaching

KEY POINTS FOR SUCCESSFUL BREAST FEEDING

- Breast milk is the best milk for preterm or sick neonates. Teach parents the benefits and advantages of breast milk for their infant(s).
- Teach parents how to interpret their infant's cues/behaviors of self-regulation and stress (see Chapter 13), hunger, and satiety.
- Teach parents proper collection/storage/transport of pumped breast milk; proper care and cleaning of breast pump supplies to prevent infection.
- Teach mothers self-care: need for rest, diet, and fluid intake for lactation.
- Provide anticipatory guidance about pumping and a dwindling milk supply (see Figure 18-11).
- Teach parents realistic expectations for the first feeding at the breast and that breast feeding is a learned behavior for both mother and preterm or sick infant.
- Provide positive feedback, support, and encouragement to mother for pumping and with feeding at the breast.
- Teach parents the importance of their involvement in their infant's care, especially in skin-to-skin (kangaroo) care and its benefits for both mother and preterm infant.

BOX 18-1 TREATMENT AND STORAGE OF BREAST MILK

Treatment

1. Heat: Significant loss of lysozyme, lactoferrin, immunoglobulins, lactoperoxidase, lymphocyte function, complement, phagocytosis, and macromolecules may occur. Fat content altered (≈13%) by milk sterilization.[8,53] Pasteurization does not alter fat content or fatty acid composition, but fat absorption by small preterm infants may be reduced from inactivation of bile salt lipase.[102]
2. Lyophilization: Effects are similar to those of heat treatment.
3. Freezing: Limited information; cells are not viable, but there is no effect on IgA content. Fat content is altered by freezing and thawing.

Storage

1. Use sterile glass or polypropylene containers (amount for one feeding/bag).
2. Label with name, date, and time of collection.
3. Store in refrigerator for 24 hours (at 0° to 4° Centigrade [32° to 39.2° Fahrenheit]) or for longer periods (−18° Centigrade [0° Fahrenheit]).

hot-water bath and the microwave. Microwaving is contraindicated—*never* use microwave heating of breast milk because of the destruction of anti-infective properties (e.g., lysozyme and secretory IgA), resulting in an overgrowth of bacteria.[2,8,167] Fresh breast milk is preferable for feedings because it has the greatest amount of immunologic properties. If the mother visits the infant at feeding time, she may pump her breasts and the breast milk can be immediately fed to the infant, if the infant cannot be put to breast.

Human milk banks that collect, store, and distribute milk to infants other than those of the donating mother exist around the world. This support is not available to some NICUs; others intentionally choose not to store donor milk. The reservations about storing donor milk generally involve questions concerning adequate nutrition and immunologic benefit versus harm to a high-risk infant. A randomized controlled trial comparing donor milk to mother's own milk and preterm infant formula for extremely preterm infants found no short-term advantages of donor milk over preterm formula and slower weight gain (caloric value of donor breast milk was less than 20 cal/kg/oz).[168,185] Adequate screening of human milk donors (for CMV, HIV, and other viruses) is essential, as is informed consent. Because of the possibility of milk-borne pathogens (e.g., HIV, hepatitis C virus), all donor milk must be pasteurized.[108] Many nurseries do not give human milk other than the mother's. Milk banks ship human milk when necessary. For milk bank locations, contact the Human Milk Banking Association of North America, Inc. (HMBANA), 1500 Sunday Drive, Suite 102, Raleigh, NC 27607. Phone: (919) 787-5181. Website: *www.hmbana.org*.

A mother may be so concerned about the welfare of her infant that she spends most of her time at the hospital and receives inadequate rest, which is a common cause of milk production problems. The care plan includes encouraging, educating, and suggesting to the mother that she go home and rest, which may require someone to assist with the care of the newborn's siblings. The stress of having a sick infant and the time spent at the hospital may mean that the mother does not receive adequate nutrition.

It is necessary to add about 600 kcal to the nonpregnant diet and to replace elements, such as calcium, minerals, and fat-soluble vitamins, used in producing milk. The recommended dietary increases are even greater than those during pregnancy.[218] Adequate fluid intake (six to eight glasses of water, skim milk, or other non-caffeine liquids) should be consumed every day. Certain components of breast milk (e.g., quantity, protein and calcium content) do not vary with the mother's diet, whereas others (e.g., fatty and amino acids, lysine, methionine, water-soluble vitamins) vary with maternal intake.

A mother's diet does not have much effect on the quality of the breast milk (unless malnutrition intervenes)[91] but affects the mother's overall health. She should be reminded to eat a balanced diet. Vegetarian diets should be supplemented with about 4 mg of cyanocobalamin (vitamin B_{12}) per day to prevent neurologic impairment in the breast-fed infant.[31]

Anticipatory guidance is essential for mothers who are breast feeding preterm infants. Mothers must be informed in the beginning that their milk supply may dwindle, even though they closely adhere to the pumping schedule. This is normal, because no pump stimulates the breast as efficiently and physiologically as the suckling infant. When the pumping regimen begins, explaining and drawing the mother a picture (Figure 18-11) of what is commonly experienced helps alleviate guilt caused by a dwindling

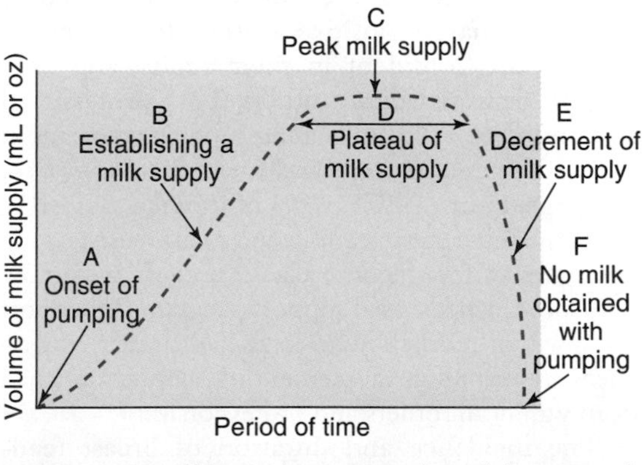

FIGURE 18-11 Establishing and maintaining milk supply by pumping. **A**, Pumping begins. **B**, Milk supply is established and increases. **C**, Peak or maximum volume of milk is established and plateaus. **D**, Gradually, supply begins to dwindle and may totally cease. ***E*** and ***F***, The volume of milk and time period for decline in supply to begin and end in no milk production is an individual process. Some women begin and end this cycle in days or weeks; others are able to pump for months. Even if the supply dwindles to no milk, nutritive SUCKLING of the infant with a Lact-Aid Nursing Trainer in place (see Figure 18-9) will reestablish the supply.

milk supply. A rather sparse supply of milk does not mean she cannot nurse the infant, because the milk supply builds in response to the infant's nutritive suckle. The parent should be taught that there is no correlation between the amount of breast milk expressed and the amount of milk a mother actually lets down when the infant is at the breast.

Breast-feeding problems may be particularly detrimental to the mother's perception of breast feeding success. **Disappointment with the breast feeding experience may result from unrealistic expectations about breast feeding the preterm infant. Establishing realistic parental expectations for the first time the infant breast feeds decreases disappointment from unattainable goals.** Breast feeding, like parenting, is not instinctual but, rather, is a learned behavior for both the mother and the infant. No one, including the health care provider, should expect immediate latch-on and vigorous sucking. **The first several attempts at breast feeding may consist only of direct skin contact, nuzzling, and licking behaviors by the infant and cuddling and positioning by the mother. Any actual sucking is an "extra" reward but should not be anticipated.**

Emotional support during breast feeding of a normal or sick infant facilitates a successful experience for both the mother and the infant.[41,66,144,160] Mothers are more successful with breast feeding when they have a positive attitude toward breast feeding, are confident in their ability, and have support from significant others (both professional and lay).[41,160,198] Breast-feeding support programs in the NICU result in improved breast-feeding rates at discharge. In one NICU, 73% of mothers of VLBW infants initiated breast feeding, and even breast-feeding outcomes of low-income black mothers were 63% with an evidence-based support program.[140] Support groups with mothers who have had similar experiences are helpful in supplementing support obtained from significant others and professionals.

The incidence and duration of breast feeding preterm or sick newborns vary among NICUs[143,163,198] and among countries. In the United States in 1995, only 32% to 38% of mothers of low-birth-weight infants initiated breast feeding compared with 62% of all mothers.[180] During the same period, 75% of mothers of hospitalized newborns in Switzerland succeeded in breast feeding their infants: 50% exclusively and 25% partially breast fed.[87] **There is an inverse relationship between gestational age and duration of breast feeding, with most mothers (>50%) abandoning breast feeding before their infants are discharged from the hospital.[98,136,143]** In a German cohort study, the average duration of breast milk feedings in VLBW infants was one third of that of a matched group of term infants.[98] Early cessation of breast milk feeding (e.g., during initial hospitalization) in VLBW infants was associated with the mother's smoking and low level of parental education. In the same study, prolonged breast milk feeding was associated with multiple pregnancies, infants of less than 29 weeks' gestation, maternal age greater than 35 years, and spontaneous pregnancy.[98] Another recent study found that white mothers born in the United States were less likely to breast feed preterm and term infants than black mothers born in the United States and mothers of any other ethnic/racial group in the state of Massachusetts.[143]

Hill et al[80] reported that 54% of preterm infants were receiving breast milk or breast feeding at discharge and only 51% at 4 weeks after discharge. A descriptive study of nutritional intake in the first 6 months of life in 31 mothers of LBW preterms found that whereas 70% of the infants were receiving breast milk at 40 weeks PCA, only 26% were still fed some breast milk at 6 months PCA.[221] The BEST (Breast Milk Early Saves Trouble) Program (initiated to improve use of breast milk in the first week of life in preterms <2000 g) resulted in 50% (versus 33%) of preterms receiving EBM, 82% (versus 74%) of babies receiving some breast milk, and 33% (versus 2%) of preterms receiving banked breast milk; trends of more mothers breast feeding and more discharged home breast feeding also occurred.[148] Another study of the transition from bottle/breast feeding to exclusive breast feeding for preterms of 30 to 35 weeks' gestational age (GA) in the first 4 weeks after hospital discharge found the following[219]:

- Sixty percent received exclusive breast milk in the first week.
- In weeks 2 to 4, 56% to 59% received breast milk exclusively.
- The number of feedings directly at the breast was initially low and increased over the first 4 weeks (e.g., 60% were fed directly at the breast less than 50% of the time in the first week; by the fourth week, 23% were exclusively breast fed and another 27% were primarily breast fed).
- Fifty percent of these infants were primarily breast fed by 1 month after discharge.

Establishing an adequate milk supply was a key factor in successful transition from primarily bottle feeding at discharge (e.g., 60% of the infants were discharged when direct breast feeding was less than 50% of the time) to primarily breast feeding at home.[219] The most common reason cited by mothers for discontinuation of breast feeding (both in the hospital and after discharge) is inadequate milk supply (or "not getting enough").[29,42,95,136,219] Early initiation and establishment of adequate feeding at the breast before discharge encourages both mothers and professionals that exclusive breast feeding is successful. **However, the early post-discharge period may be significantly stressful for mothers, because the breast-feeding pattern of a preterm infant may predispose to underconsumption (i.e., inability to compensate for inadequate intake in one feeding by increasing the number or intake of subsequent feedings), result in behaviors indicative of inadequate intake, and require nutritional supplementation.[95]**

Education and training about the many facets of breast feeding are essential for medical and nursing staff.* **Staff attitudes and behaviors are important to breast-feeding families and affect the breast-feeding experience.[147,161,174,202,203]** A multidimensional approach to such education includes providing the staff with manuals, guides, and other educational materials, as well as scheduling routine classes, in-service training, and workshops. **Moreover, professionals with clinical expertise should be identified; these resource personnel can increase the staff's competency in counseling and assisting breast-feeding families.**

Evidence-based protocols addressing breast feeding can outline a consistent approach for staff, as well as provide resource material that addresses successful strategies for handling common problems. Protocols can also reduce the amount of incorrect information that is disseminated. A number of protocols for managing breast-feeding issues have been developed by the Academy of Breastfeeding Medicine and are available from their website (see "Resource Materials for Professionals" on pp. 480-481).

Providing a breast-feeding program for preterm infants that is grounded in evidence-based practices demonstrates strong success. Meier et al[140] evaluated the effectiveness of such a program for mothers and their VLBW infants. The program provides assistance to low-income mothers who are a group known to have low breast-feeding rates. The program followed VLBW infants during a 24-month period. Of the 207 eligible, 151 initiated milk expression (72.9%); other data included mean birth weight of 1010 g, mean gestational age of 27.8 weeks, and 61-day average length of stay. **Results demonstrated a high level of lactation initiation that approximates the national health objective in *Healthy People 2010* of 75%, and provision of 61.3% nutrition from own mother's milk (OMM) over the duration of hospitalization.** In addition, at the time of discharge, 33.8% were receiving OMM exclusively, 35.8% were receiving both OMM and formula, and 30.5% were receiving formula exclusively. The exclusive breast-feeding rates are impressive and are similar to the data for overall exclusive breast feeding. **The authors speculate that the high rates of lactation initiation were the result of two primary interventions of the program. The first was the "clarity of the message that mothers received about the importance of OMM from health care providers and their immediate access to electric breast pump rental and professional assistance to get started."[140]** Estimates of breast-feeding initiation rates in previous reports have ranged from 48% to 73% in infants born preterm and at low birth weight.[58]

A recent study of lactation counseling for mothers (some who intended to breast feed and others who intended to formula feed) of VLBW preterms showed that more mothers decided to pump breast milk, mainly because of the health benefits for their infant.[193] In mothers who intended to formula feed, there was an 85% milk expression rate; in mothers intending to breast feed, the rate was 100%. Both black and Hispanic mothers pumped at 95% and 93% rate, respectively. All mothers believed that pumping was worth the effort and appreciated the help they received; none felt more stress or anxiety. Reasons given by the mothers for ceasing to pump included (1) low milk supply, (2) returning to school or work, and (3) inability to pump as often as needed. Success in breast feeding infants who were in the NICU depends on family support, timely breast-feeding information, and a supportive NICU environment.[110]

Breast milk is the best milk, especially for a sick or premature infant. By understanding normal lactation, the health care provider can support the breast-feeding dyad when breast feeding is delayed or disrupted.

*References 8,76,147,161,174,202,203.

REFERENCES

1. Abdel-Latif ME, Pinner J, Clews S, et al: Effects of breast milk on the severity and outcome of neonatal abstinence syndrome among infants of drug-dependent mothers, *Pediatrics* 117:e1163, 2006.
2. Academy of Breastfeeding Medicine: *Protocol #10: Breastfeeding the near-term infant (35-37 weeks' gestation),* 2004. Accessed September 6, 2009, from www.bfmed.org.
3. Agency for Healthcare Research and Quality: *Breastfeeding and maternal and infant health outcomes in developed countries,* Rockville, MD, 2007, The Agency. Accessed September 6, 2009 from www.ahrq.gov/clinic/tp/brfouttp.htm.
4. Reference deleted in proofs.
5. American Academy of Pediatrics: Committee on Drugs: Neonatal drug withdrawal, *Pediatrics* 101:1079, 1998
6. American Academy of Pediatrics: Committee on Drugs: The transfer of drugs and other chemicals into human breast milk, *Pediatrics* 108:776, 2001.
7. American Academy of Pediatrics: Committee on Pediatric AIDS: Human milk, breast feeding, and transmission of human immunodeficiency virus type 1 in the United States, *Pediatrics* 112:1196, 2003.
8. American Academy of Pediatrics, Section on Breast Feeding: Breast feeding and the use of human milk, *Pediatrics* 115:496, 2005.
9. American Academy of Pediatrics, Wagner CL, Greer FR, and the Section on Breastfeeding Medicine: Prevention of rickets and vitamin D deficiency in infants, children, and adolescents, *Pediatrics*; 122:1142 2008.
10. Amin S, Merle KS, Orlando MS, et al: Brainstem maturation in premature infants as a function of enteral feeding type, *Pediatrics* 106:318, 2000.
11. Anderson J, Held N, Wright K: Raynaud's phenomenon of the nipple: a treatable cause of painful breast feeding, *Pediatrics* 113:e360, 2004.
12. Ariagno R, Karch SB, Middleberg R, et al: Methamphetamine ingestion by a breast-feeding mother and her infant's death: People v Henderson, *JAMA* 275(3):183, 1995.
13. Armand M, Hamosh M, Mehta NR, et al: Effect of human milk or formula on gastric function and fat digestion in the premature infant, *Pediatr Res* 40:429, 1996.
14. Association of Women's Health, Obstetric and Neonatal Nurses (AWHONN): *Evidence-based clinical practice guideline: breast feeding support—prenatal care through the first year,* Washington, DC, 2000, The Association.
15. Association of Women's Health, Obstetric and Neonatal Nurses (AWHONN): *Near-term Infant Round Table Discussion,* Washington, DC, 2005, The Association.
16. Auer C, Steichen J, Fargo J: The relationship between first oral feeding (breast versus bottle), and pre- and post-discharge breast feeding in an NICU population, *Pediatr Res* 55:385A, 2004.
17. Auerbach K, Avery JL: Relactation and the premature infant: report from a survey, *Res Hum Nurtur (monograph 3)* 1979.
18. Ballard J, Auer C, Khoury J: Ankyloglossia: assessment, incidence and effect of frenuloplasty on the breast feeding dyad, *Pediatrics* 110:e63, 2002.
19. Bellander M, Ley D, Polberger S, et al: Tolerance to early feedings is not compromised by indomethacin in preterm infants with patent ductus arteriosus, *Acta Paediatr* 92:1074, 2003.
20. Biancuzzo M: *Breast feeding the newborn: clinical strategies for nurses,* ed 2, St Louis, 2003, Mosby.
21. Bier JA, Oliver T, Ferguson A, et al: Human milk improves cognitive and motor development of premature infants during infancy, *J Hum Lact* 18:361, 2002.
22. Billeaud C, Guillet J, Sandler B: Gastric emptying in infants with or without gastro-esophageal reflux according to the type of milk, *Eur J Clin Nutr* 44:577, 1990.
23. Birnbaum CS, Cohen LS, Bailey JW, et al: Serum concentrations of antidepressants and benzodiazepines in nursing infants: a case series, *Pediatrics* 104:e11, 1999.
24. Blackwell M, Eichenwald EC, McAlmon K, et al: Interneonatal intensive care unit variation in growth rates and feeding practices in healthy moderately premature infants, *J Perinatol* 25:478, 2005.
25. Blair A, Cadwell K, Turner-Maffei C, et al: The relationship between positioning, the breast feeding dynamics of latching process and pain in breast feeding mothers with sore nipples, *Breastfeeding Rev* 11:5, 2003.
26. Bosma JF, editor: *Oral sensation and perception,* Department of Health, Education and Welfare Pub No (NIH) 73-546. Bethesda, MD, 1973, Department of Health, Education and Welfare.
27. Brandtzaeg P: The secretory immunoglobulin system: regulation and biologic significance—focusing on human mammary glands. In Davis M, Isaacs C, Hanson L, et al, editors: *Integrating population outcomes, biologic mechanisms and research methods in the study of human milk and lactation,* New York, 2002, Plenum.
28. Brent N, Rudy SJ, Redd B, et al: Sore nipples in breast-feeding women: a clinical trial of wound dressings vs. conventional care, *Arch Pediatr Adolesc Med* 152:1077, 1998.
29. Callen J, Pinelli J, Atkinson S, et al: Qualitative analysis of barriers to breastfeeding in very-low-birthweight infants in the hospital and postdischarge, *Adv Neonatal Care* 5:93, 2005.
30. Carfoot S, Williamson P, Dickson R: A systematic review of randomized controlled trials evaluating the effect of mother/baby skin-to-skin care on successful breast feeding, *Midwifery* 19:148, 2003.

31. Center for Disease Control and Prevention: Maternal deficiency of B_{12} linked to neurologic impairment, *MMWR Morb Mortal Wkly Rep* 52:61, 2003.
32. Chambers CD, Anderson PO, Thomas RG, et al: Weight gain in infants breast fed by mothers who take fluoxetine, *Pediatrics* 104:1120, 1999.
33. Chaney NE, Franke J, Wadlington WB: Cocaine convulsions in a breast feeding baby, *J Pediatr* 112:134, 1988.
34. Chasnoff IJ, Lewis DE, Squires L: Cocaine intoxication in a breast feeding infant, *Pediatrics* 80:836, 1987.
35. Chen C, Wang T, Chang H, et al: The effect of breast- and bottle-feeding on oxygen saturation and body temperature in preterm infants, *J Hum Lact* 16:21, 2000.
36. Collins C, Crowther C, Ryan P, et al: Effects of bottles, cups, and dummies on breast feeding in preterm infants: a randomized control trial, *BMJ* 329:193, 2004.
37. Coovadia HM, Rollins NC, Bland RM, et al: Mother-to-child transmission of HIV-1 infection during exclusive breastfeeding in the first 6 months of life: an intervention cohort study, *Lancet* 369:1107, 2007.
38. Crawford M, Golfetto I, Ghebremeskel K, et al: The potential role for arachidonic and docosahexaenoic acids in protection against some central nervous system injuries in preterm infants, *Lipids* 38:303, 2003.
39. D'Amico C, DiNardo C, Krystofiak S: Preventing contamination of breast pump kit attachments in the NICU, *J Perinat Neonat Nurs* 17:150, 2003.
40. Dann MH: The lactation consult: problem solving, teaching, and support for the breastfeeding family, *J Pediatr Health Care* 19:12, 2005.
41. Dennis C, Hodnett E, Gallop R, et al: A randomized controlled trial evaluating the effect of peer support on breast feeding duration among primiparous women, *Can Med Assoc J* 166:21, 2002.
42. Dewey K, Nommsen-Rivers L, Heinig J, et al: Risk factors for suboptimal infant breast feeding behavior, delayed onset of lactation, and excess neonatal weight loss, *Pediatrics* 112:607, 2003.
43. Dodd S, Stocky A, Buist A, et al: Sertraline in paired blood plasma and breast-milk samples from nursing mothers, *Hum Psychopharmacol* 15:161, 2000.
44. Dodd V, Chalmers C: Comparing the use of hydrogel dressings to lanolin ointment with lactating mothers, *J Obstet Gynecol Neonatal Nurs* 32:486, 2003.
45. Dowling D: Physiological responses of preterm infants to breast-feeding and bottle-feeding with the orthodontic nipple, *Nurs Res* 48:78, 1999.
46. Drenckpohl D, Bowers L, Cooper H: Use of the six sigma methodology to reduce incidence of breast milk administration errors in the NICU, *Neonatal Netw* 26:161, 2007.
47. Engle WA, Tomashek KM, Wallman C, and the Committee on Fetus and Newborn: "Late-preterm" infants: a population at risk, *Pediatrics* 120:1390, 2007.
48. Epperson C, Jatlow P, Czarkowski K, et al: Maternal fluoxetine treatment in the postpartum period: effects on platelet serotonin and plasma drug levels in breast feeding mother-infant pairs, *Pediatrics* 112:e425, 2003.
49. Falt A, Bengtsson T, Kennedy BM, et al: Exposure of infants to budesonide through breast milk of asthmatic mothers, *J Allergy Clin Immunol* 120:798, 2007.
50. Fanaro S, Chierici R, Gueririni P, et al: Intestinal microflora in early infancy: composition and development, *Acta Paediatr Suppl* 441:48, 2003.
51. Feldman R, Eidelman A: Direct and indirect effects of breast milk on the neurobehavioral and cognitive development of premature infants, *Dev Psychobiol* 43:109, 2003.
52. Fewtrell MS, Lucas P, Collier S, et al: Randomized trial comparing the efficacy of a novel manual breast pump with a standard electric breast pump in mothers who delivered preterm infants, *Pediatrics* 107:1291, 2001.
53. Fidler N, Sauerwald TU, Koletzko B, et al: Effects of human milk pasteurization and sterilization on available fat content and fatty acid composition, *J Pediatr Gastroenterol Nutr* 27:317, 1998.
54. Flint A, New K, Davies MW: Cup feeding versus other forms of supplemental enteral feeding for newborn infants unable to fully breastfeed, *Cochrane Database Syst Rev* 2:CD005092, 2007.
55. Foxman B, D'Arcy H, Gillespie B, et al: Lactation mastitis: occurrence and medical management among 946 breast feeding women in the United States, *Am J Epidemiol* 155:103, 2002.
56. Fucile S, Gisel E, Lau C: Oral stimulation accelerates the transition from tube to oral feeding in preterm infants, *J Pediatr* 141:230, 2002.
57. Furman L, Minich N: Efficiency of breast-feeding as compared with bottle-feeding in very low birth weight (VLBW, less than 1.5 kg) infants, *J Perinatol* 24:706, 2004.
58. Furman L, Minich N, Hack M: Correlates of lactation in mothers of very low birth weight infants, *Pediatrics* 109:e57, 2002.
59. Furman L, Taylor G, Minich N, et al: The effect of maternal milk on neonatal morbidity of very low-birth-weight infants, *Arch Pediatr Adolesc Med* 157:66, 2003.
60. Furman L, Wilson-Costello D, Friedman H, et al: The effect of neonatal maternal milk feedings on the neurodevelopmental outcome of very low birth weight infants, *J Dev Behav Pediatr* 25:247, 2004.
61. Gardiner S, Kristensen J, Begg E, et al: Transfer of olanzapine into breast milk, calculation of infant drug dose, and effect on breast-fed infants, *Am J Psychiatry* 160:1428, 2003.

62. Gardner SL: Late-preterm ("near-term") newborns: a neonatal nursing challenge, *Nurse Currents* 1:1, 2007. Available at www.abbottnutritionlearning-center.com.
63. Gewolb IH, Vice FL: Maturational changes in the rhythms, patterning, and coordination of respiration and swallow during feeding in preterm and term infants, *Dev Med Child Neurol* 48:589, 2006.
64. Griffin TL, Meyer PP, Bradford LP, et al: Mothers' performing creamatocrit measures in the NICU: accuracy, reactions and cost, *J Obstet Gynecol Neonatal Nurs* 29:249, 2000.
65. Groer M, Davis M, Hemphill J: Postpartum stress: current concepts and the possible protective role of breast feeding, *J Obstet Gynecol Neonatal Nurs* 31:411, 2002.
66. Guise J, Palda V, Westhoff C, et al: The effectiveness of primary care–based interventions to promote breast feeding: systematic evidence review and meta-analysis for the U.S. Preventive Services Task Force, *Ann Fam Med* 1:70, 2003.
67. Hale T: *Medications and mother's milk*, ed 13, Amarillo, Tex, 2008, Hale Publishing.
68. Hall W, Shearer K, Mogan J, et al: Weighing preterm infants before and after breast feeding: does it increase maternal confidence and competence? *MCN Am J Matern Child Nurs* 27:318, 2002.
69. Hammerman C, Kaplan M: Oxygen saturation during and after feeding in healthy term infants, *Biol Neonate* 67:94, 1995.
70. Hamosh M: Bioactive factors in human milk, *Pediatr Clin North Am* 48:69, 2001.
71. Hansel L: *Immunobiology of human milk: how breast feeding protects the infant*, Amarillo, Tex, 2004, Pharmasoft.
72. Hartman P, Cregan M, Ramsay D, et al: Physiology of lactation in preterm mothers: initiation and maintenance, *Pediatr Ann* 32:351, 2003.
73. Hayashi Y, Haashi E, Nana T: Ultrasonographic analysis of sucking behavior of newborn infants: the driving force of sucking pressure, *Early Hum Dev* 49:33, 1997.
74. Heinig M: Host benefits of breast feeding for the infant: effect of breast feeding duration and exclusivity, *Pediatr Clin North Am* 48:105, 2001.
75. Heller CD, O'Shea M, Yau Q, et al: Human milk intake and retinopathy of prematurity in extremely low birth weight infants, *Pediatrics* 120:1, 2007.
76. Hellings P, Howe C: Breast feeding knowledge and practice of pediatric nurse practitioners, *J Pediatr Health Care* 18:8, 2004.
77. Henderson G, Anthony MY, McGuire W: Formula milk versus maternal breast milk for feeding preterm or low birth weight infants, *Cochrane Database Syst Rev* 4:CD002972, 2007.
78. Henriksen C, Haughholt K, Lindgren M, et al: Improved cognitive development among preterm infants attributable to early supplementation of human milk with docosahexaenoic acid and arachidonic acid, *Pediatrics* 121:1137, 2008.
79. Hill P, Aldag J, Chatterton R: Initiation and frequency of pumping and milk production in mothers of non-nursing preterm infants, *J Hum Lact* 17:9, 2001.
80. Hill P, Ledbetter R, Kavanaugh K: Breast feeding pattern of low birth weight infants after hospital discharge, *J Obstet Gynecol Neonatal Nurs* 26:190, 1997.
81. Hill PD, Aldag JC, Chatterton RT, et al: Comparison of milk output between mothers of preterm and term infants: the first 6 weeks after birth, *J Human Lactation* 21:22, 2005.
82. Hill PD, Aldag JC, Zinamen M, et al: Predictors of preterm infant feeding methods and perceived insufficient milk supply at week 12 postpartum, *J Human Lactation* 23:32, 2007.
83. Hinckley AF, O'Leary DR, Hayes EB: Transmission of West Nile virus through human breast milk seems to be rare, *Pediatrics* 119:e666, 2007.
84. Horwood L, Darlaw B, Mogridge N: Breast milk feeding and cognitive ability at 7-8 years, *Arch Dis Child Fetal Neonatal Ed* 84:F23, 2001.
85. Howard C, Howard F, Lanphear B, et al: Randomized clinical trial of pacifier use and bottle-feeding or cup-feeding and their effect on breastfeeding, *Pediatrics* 111:511, 2003.
86. Reference deleted in proofs.
87. Hunkeler B, Aebi C, Minder C, et al: Incidence and duration of breast-feeding of ill newborns, *J Pediatr Gastroenterol Nutr* 18:37, 1994.
88. Hurst N, Meier P, Engstrom J, et al: Mothers performing in-home measurement of milk intake during breast feeding of their preterm infants: maternal reactions and feeding outcomes, *J Hum Lact* 20:178, 2004.
89. Hylander M, Strobino D, Pezzullo J, et al: Association of human milk feedings with a reduction in retinopathy of prematurity among very low birthweight infants, *J Perinatol* 21:356, 2001.
90. Hylander MA, Strobino DM, Dhanireddy R, et al: Human milk feedings and infection among VLBW infants, *Pediatrics* 102:630, 1998.
91. Institute of Medicine: *Committee on Nutritional Status During Pregnancy and Lactation: Nutrition during pregnancy and lactation: an implementation guide*, Washington, DC, 1992, National Academy Press.
92. Jain L, Sivieri E, Abbasi S, et al: Energetics and mechanics of nutritive sucking in the preterm and term neonate, *J Pediatr* 111:894, 1987.
93. Jansson LM, Choo R, Velez ML, et al: Methadone maintenance and breastfeeding in the neonatal period, *Pediatrics* 121:106, 2008.
94. Jones E, Dimmock P, Spencer S: A randomized controlled trial to compare methods of milk expression after preterm delivery, *Arch Dis Child Fetal Neonatal Ed* 85:F91, 2001.

95. Kavanaugh K, Mead L, Meier P, et al: Getting enough: mothers' concerns about breast feeding a preterm infant after discharge, *J Obstet Gynecol Neonatal Nurs* 24:23, 1995.
96. Kavanaugh K, Meier P, Zimmerman B, et al: The rewards outweigh the efforts: breast feeding outcomes of mothers of preterm infants, *J Hum Lact* 13:15, 1997.
97. Kent JC, Mitoulas LR, Cregan MD, et al: Volume and frequency of breastfeedings and fat content of breast milk throughout the day, *Pediatrics* 117:e387, 2006.
98. Killersreiter B, Grimmer I, Buhrer C, et al: Early cessation of breast milk feeding in very low birthweight infants, *Early Hum Dev* 60:193, 2001.
99. Kliethermes PA, Cross ML, Lanese MG, et al: Transitioning preterm infants with nasogastric tube supplementation: increased likelihood of breast feeding, *J Obstet Gynecol Neonatal Nurs* 28:264, 1999.
100. Kramer M, Burr R, Digenesis S, et al: Pacifier use, early weaning, and cry/fuss behavior: a randomized controlled trial, *JAMA* 286:322, 2001.
101. Kumar A, Rai AK, Basu S, et al: Cord blood and breast milk iron status in maternal anemia, *Pediatrics* 121:e673, 2008.
102. Kunz C, Rodriquez-Palmero M, Koletzko B, et al: Nutritional and biochemical properties of human milk. I. General aspects, proteins and carbohydrates, *Clin Perinatol* 26:307, 1999.
103. Kuschel C, Harding J: Multicomponent fortified human milk for promoting growth in preterm infants, *Cochrane Database Syst Rev* 1:CD000343, 2004.
104. Landers S: Maximizing the benefits of human milk feeding for the preterm infant, *Pediatr Ann* 32:298, 2003.
105. Lau C, Alagugurusamy R, Schanler R, et al: Characterization of the developmental stages of sucking in preterm infants during bottle feeding, *Acta Paediatr* 89:846, 2000.
106. Laurberg P, Nohr S, Pedersen K, et al: Iodine nutrition in breast-fed infants is impaired by maternal smoking, *J Clin Endocrinol Metab* 89:181, 2004.
107. Law-Morstatt L, Judd D, Snyder P, et al: Pacing as a treatment technique for transitional sucking patterns, *J Perinatol* 23:483, 2003.
108. Lawrence RA, Lawrence RM: *Breast feeding: a guide for the medical profession*, ed 6, St Louis, 2005, Mosby.
109. Lawrence RM, Lawrence RA: Given the benefits of breastfeeding, what contraindications exist?, *Pediatr Clin North Am* 48:235, 2001.
110. Lessen R, Crivelli-Kovach A: Prediction of initiation and duration of breast-feeding for neonates admitted to the neonatal intensive care unit, *J Perinat Neonatal Nurs* 21:256, 2007.
111. Little RE, Northstone K, Golding J, and the ALSPAC Study Team: Alcohol, breast feeding, and development at 18 months, *Pediatrics* 109:e72, 2002.
112. Lonnerdal B: Nutritional and physiologic significance of human milk proteins, *Am J Clin Nutr* 77:1537S, 2003.
113. Lu M, Lange L, Slusser W, et al: Provider encouragement of breast feeding: evidence from a national survey, *Obstet Gynecol* 97:290, 2001.
114. Lucas A, Brooke OG, Cole TJ, et al: Early diet of preterm infants and development of allergic or atopic diseases: randomized prospective study, *BMJ* 300:837, 1990.
115. Lucas A, Cole T: Breast milk and neonatal necrotizing enterocolitis, *Lancet* 336:1519, 1990.
116. Lucas A, Morley R, Cole TJ, et al: A randomised multicentre study of human milk versus formula and later development in preterm infants, *Arch Dis Child Fetal Neonatal Ed* 70:F141, 1994.
117. Mathew O: Nipple units for newborn infants: a functional comparison, *Pediatrics* 81:688, 1988.
118. Mathew O: Respiratory control during nipple feeding in preterm infants, *Pediatr Pulmonol* 5:220, 1988.
119. Mathew O: Determinants of milk flow through nipples, *Am J Dis Child* 144:222, 1990.
120. Mathew O: Breathing patterns of preterm infants during bottle feeding: role of milk flow, *J Pediatr* 199:960, 1991.
121. Mathew O: Science of bottle feeding, *J Pediatr* 119:511, 1991.
122. Mathew O, Belan M, Thoppil C: Sucking patterns of neonates during bottle feeding: comparison of different nipple units, *Am J Perinatol* 9:265, 1992.
123. Mathew O, Bhatia J: Sucking and breathing patterns during breast- and bottle-feeding in term neonates, *Am J Dis Child* 143:588, 1989.
124. Mathew OP, Clark ML, Pronske ML, et al: Breathing pattern and ventilation during oral feeding in term newborn infants, *J Pediatr* 106:810, 1985.
125. McCain G: An evidence-based guideline for introducing oral feeding to healthy preterm infants, *Neonatal Netw* 22:45, 2003.
126. McCarthy J, Posey B: Methadone levels in human milk, *J Hum Lact* 16:115, 2000.
127. McCoy D, Holmberg S: Antidepressant medications during breast feeding: safety and efficacy for mother and infant, *Am J Nurse Pract* 5:9, 2001.
128. McGrath J, Braescu A: State of the science: feeding readiness in the preterm infant, *J Perinat Neonatal Nurs* 18:353, 2004.
129. McGrath J, Medoff-Cooper B: Alertness and feeding competence in extremely early born preterm infants, *Newborn Infant Nurs Rev* 2:174, 2002.
130. Medoff-Cooper B, Bilker W, Kaplan J: Suckling behavior as a function of gestational age: a cross sectional study, *Infant Behav Dev* 24:83, 2001.

131. Medoff-Cooper B, McGrath J, Shults J: Feeding patterns of full-term and preterm infants at forty weeks postconceptional age, *J Dev Behav Pediatr* 23:231, 2002.
132. Medoff-Cooper B, Verklan T, Carlson S: The development of sucking patterns and physiologic correlates in very-low-birth-weight infants, *Nurs Res* 42:100, 1993.
133. Mehall J, Kite C, Saltzman D, et al: Prospective study of the incidence and complications of bacterial contamination of enteral feeding in neonates, *J Pediatr Surg* 37:1177, 2002.
134. Meier P: Bottle and breast feeding: effects on transcutaneous pressure and temperature in preterm infants, *Nurs Res* 37:36, 1988.
135. Meier P: Suck-breathe patterning during bottle and breast feeding for preterm infants. In David T, editor: *Major controversies in infant nutrition*, London, 1996, Royal Society of Medicine Press.
136. Meier P: Breast feeding in the special care nursery: prematures and infants with medical problems, *Pediatr Clin North Am* 48:425, 2001.
137. Meier P: Supporting lactation in mothers with very low birth weight infants, *Pediatr Ann* 32:317, 2003.
138. Meier P, Anderson GC: Responses of small preterm infants to bottle and breast feeding, *Matern Child Nurs J* 12:97, 1987.
139. Meier P, Brown L, Hurst N, et al: Nipple shields for preterm infants: effect on milk intake and duration of breast feeding, *J Hum Lact* 16:106, 2000.
140. Meier P, Engstrom J, Mingolelli S, et al: The Rush Mothers' Milk Club: breast feeding interventions for mothers with very-low-birth-weight infants, *J Obstet Gynecol Neonatal Nurs* 33:164, 2004.
141. Meier P, Engstrom J, Murtaugh M, et al: Mothers' milk feedings in the NICU: accuracy of the creamatocrit technique, *J Perinatol* 22:646, 2002.
142. Meinzen-Derr J, Poindexter B, Wrage L, et al: Role of human milk in extremely low birth weight infants' risk of necrotizing enterocolitis or death, *J Perinatol* 29(1):57, 2009.
143. Merewood A, Brooks D, Bauchner H, et al: Maternal birthplace and breastfeeding initiation among term and preterm infants: a statewide assessment for Massachusetts, *Pediatrics* 118:e1048, 2006.
144. Miracle D, Meier P, Bennett P: Making my baby healthy: changing the decision from formula to human milk feedings for very low birthweight infants, *Adv Exp Med Biol* 554:317, 2004.
145. Miron D, Brosilow S, Felszer K, et al: Incidence and clinical manifestations of breast milk-acquired cytomegalovirus infection in low birth weight infants, *J Perinatol* 25:299, 2005.
146. Misri S, Kostaras X: Benefits and risks to mother and infant of drug treatment for postnatal depression, *Drug Saf* 25:903, 2002.
147. Mitra A, Khoury A, Carothers C, et al: The Loving Support Breastfeeding Campaign: awareness and practices of health care providers in Mississippi, *J Obstet Gynecol Neonatal Nurs* 32:753, 2003.
148. Montgomery D, Schmutz N, Baer VL, et al: Effects of instituting the "BEST Program" (Breast Milk Early Saves Trouble) in a level III NICU, *J Hum Lact* 24:248, 2008.
149. Morley R, Fewtrell M, Abbott R, et al: Neurodevelopment in children born small for gestational age: a randomized trial of nutrient-enriched versus standard formula and comparison with a reference breast fed group, *Pediatrics* 113:515, 2004.
150. Morrill J, Heinig J, Pappagianis D, et al: Risk factors for mammary candidosis among lactating women, *J Obstet Gynecol Neonatal Nurs* 34:37, 2005.
151. National Association of Neonatal Nurses (NANN): *Position Statement #3017: Cup and finger feeding of breast milk*, Glenview, Ill, 2003, The Association.
152. Neifert M: Prevention of breast feeding tragedies, *Pediatr Clin North Am* 48:273, 2001.
153. Neifert M, Lawrence R: Nipple confusion: toward a more formal definition, *J Pediatr* 126:5125, 1995.
154. Neville M: Anatomy and physiology of lactation, *Pediatr Clin North Am* 48:13, 2001.
155. Newport DJ, Pennell PB, Calamaras MR, et al: Lamotrigine in breast milk and nursing infants: determination of exposure, *Pediatrics* 122:e223, 2008.
156. Nye C: Transitioning premature infants from gavage to breast, *Neonatal Netw* 27:7, 2008.
157. Nyqvist K: Breast-feeding in preterm twins: development of feeding behavior and milk intake during hospital stay and related caregiving practices, *J Pediatr Nurs* 17:246, 2002.
158. Nyqvist N, Farnstrand C, Edebol E, et al: Early oral behavior in preterm infants during breast feeding: an electromyographic study, *Acta Paediatr* 90:658, 2001.
159. O'Connor D, Hall R, Adamkin D, et al: Growth and development in preterm infants fed long-chain polyunsaturated fatty acids: a prospective, randomized controlled trial, *Pediatrics* 108:359, 2001.
160. Philipp B, Merewood A, Malone K, et al: Effect of NICU-based peer counselors on breast feeding duration among premature infants, *Pediatr Res* 55:36A, 2004.
161. Philipp B, Merewood A, O'Brien S: Physicians and breast feeding promotion in the US: a call for action, *Pediatrics* 107:584, 2001.
162. Pickler R, Reyna B: Effects of non-nutritive sucking, breathing, and behavior during bottle feedings of preterm infants, *Adv Neonatal Care* 4:226, 2004.
163. Powers H, Clark R, Bloom B, et al: Site variation in rates of breast milk feedings in neonates discharged from intensive care units, *Acad Breastfeed Med News Views* 7:37, 2001.

164. Premji S, McNeil D, Scotland J: Regional neonatal oral feeding protocol: changing ethos of feeding preterm infants, *J Perinat Neonatal Nurs* 18:371, 2004.
165. Prieto CR, Cardenas H, Salvatierra AM, et al: Sucking pressure and its relationship to milk transfer during breastfeeding in humans, *J Reprod Fertility* 108:69, 1996.
166. Pugh L, Milligan R, Frick K, et al: Breast feeding duration, costs, and benefits of a support program for low-income breast feeding women, *Birth* 29:95, 2002.
167. Quan R, Yang C, Rubenstein S, et al: Effects of microwave radiation on anti-infective factors in human milk, *Pediatrics* 89:667, 1992.
168. Quigley MA, Henderson G, Anthony MY, et al: Formula milk versus donor breast milk for feeding preterm or low birth weight infants, *Cochrane Database Syst Rev* 4:CD002971, 2007.
169. Radzyminski S: The effect of ultra low dose epidural analgesia on newborn breast feeding behaviors, *J Obstet Gynecol Neonatal Nurs* 32:322, 2003.
170. Raghuveer T, McGuire E, Martin S, et al: Lactoferrin in the preterm infants' diet attenuates iron-induced oxidation products, *Pediatr Res* 52:964, 2002.
171. Rasmussen K, Kjolhede C: Prepregnant overweight and obesity diminish the prolactin response to suckling in the first week postpartum, *Pediatrics* 113:e465, 2004.
172. Reber K, Nankervis C: Necrotizing enterocolitis: preventive strategies, *Clin Perinatol* 31:157, 2004.
173. Riordan J: *Breast feeding and human lactation*, ed 3, Boston, 2005, Jones & Bartlett.
174. Riordan J, Gill-Hopple K: Breast feeding care in multicultural populations, *J Obstet Gynecol Neonatal Nurs* 30:216, 2001.
175. Rodriguez N, Miracle D, Meier P: Sharing the science on human milk feedings with mothers of VLBW infants, *J Obstet Gynecol Neonatal Nurs* 34:109, 2005.
176. Rodriguez-Palmero M, Koletzko B, Kunz C, et al: Nutritional and biochemical properties of human milk. II. Lipids, micronutrients and bioactive factors, *Clin Perinatol* 26:335, 1999.
177. Ronnestad A, Abrahamsen TG, Medbo S, et al: Late-onset septicemia in a Norwegian national cohort of extremely preterm infants receiving very early full human milk feeding, *Pediatrics* 115:e269, 2005.
178. Rosen C, Glaze D, Frost J: Hypoxemia associated with feeding in the preterm and full term neonate, *Am J Dis Child* 138:623, 1984.
179. Rosti L, Nardini A, Bettinelli ME, et al: Toxic effects of herbal tea mixture in two newborns, *Acta Paediatr* 83:683, 1994.
180. Ryan A: The resurgence of breast feeding in the United States, *Pediatrics* 99:e12, 1997.
181. Ryan AS, Wenjun Z, Acosta A: Breast feeding continues to increase into the new millennium, *Pediatrics* 110:1103, 2002.
182. Ryan CA, Mohammed I, Murphy B: Normal neurologic and development outcome after an accidental intravenous infusion of expressed breast milk in a neonate, *Pediatrics* 117:236, 2006.
183. Sadeharju K, Knip M, Virtanen SM, et al: Maternal antibodies in breast milk protect the child from enterovirus infections, *Pediatrics* 119:941, 2007.
184. Schanler R: The use of human milk for premature infants, *Pediatr Clin North Am* 48:207, 2001.
185. Schanler R, Lau C, Hurst N, et al: Randomized trial of donor human milk versus preterm formula as substitutes for mothers' own milk in the feeding of extremely premature infants, *Pediatrics* 116:400, 2005.
186. Schanler R, Shulman R, Lau C: Feeding strategies for premature infants: beneficial outcomes of feeding fortified human milk versus preterm formula, *Pediatrics* 103:1150, 1999.
187. Semba R, Juul S: Erythropoietin in human milk: physiology and role in infant health, *J Hum Lact* 18:252, 2002.
188. Semple JL, Lugowski SJ, Baines CJ, et al: Breast milk contamination and silicone implants: preliminary results using silicon as a proxy measurement for silicone, *Plast Reconstr Surg* 102:528, 1998.
189. Shiao S-Y: Comparison of continuous versus intermittent sucking in VLBW infants, *J Obstet Gynecol Neonatal Nurs* 26:313, 1997.
190. Shoji H, Shimizu T, Shinohara K, et al: Suppressive effects of breast milk on oxidative DNA damage in very low birthweight infants, *Arch Dis Child Fetal Neonatal Ed* 89:F136, 2004.
191. Sidell E, Froman R: A national survey of neonatal intensive care units: criteria used to determine readiness for oral feedings, *J Obstet Gynecol Neonatal Nurs* 23:783, 1994.
192. Simpson C, Schanler R, Lau C: Early introduction of oral feeding in preterm infants, *Pediatrics* 110:517, 2002.
193. Sisk PM, Lovelady CA, Dillard RG, et al: Lactation counseling for mothers of very low birth weight infants: effect on maternal anxiety and infant intake of human milk, *Pediatrics* 117:e67, 2006.
194. Sisk PM, Lovelady CA, Gruber KJ, et al: Human milk consumption and full enteral feeding among infants who weigh ≤1250 grams, *Pediatrics* 121:e1528, 2008.
195. Smith JR, Jamerson PA, Bernaix LW, et al: Fathers' perceptions of supportive behaviors for the provision of breast milk to premature infants, *Adv Neonatal Care* 6:341, 2006.
196. Smith M, Durkin M, Hinton V, et al: Influence of breast feeding on cognitive outcomes at ages 6–8 years: followup of very low birth weight infants, *Am J Epidemiol* 158:1075, 2003.
197. Smith M, Durkin M, Hinton V, et al: Initiation of breast feeding among mothers of very low birth weight infants, *Pediatrics* 111:1337, 2003.

198. Spatz D: Ten steps for promoting and protecting breast feeding for vulnerable infants, *J Perinat Neonatal Nurs* 18:385, 2004.
199. Steiner E, Villen T, Hallberg M, et al: Amphetamine secretion in breast milk, *Eur J Clin Pharmacol* 27:123, 1984.
200. Stine M: Breast feeding and the premature newborn: a protocol without bottles, *J Hum Lact* 6:167, 1990.
201. Sweet L, Darbyshire P: Fathers and breast feeding very-low-birthweight preterm babies, *Midwifery*, Epub ahead of print: January 10, 2008.
202. Taveras E, Li R, Grummer-Strawn L, et al: Mothers' and clinicians' perspectives on breast feeding counseling during routine visits, *Pediatrics* 113:e405, 2004.
203. Taveras E, Li R, Grummer-Strawn L, et al: Opinions and practices of clinicians associated with continuation of exclusive breast feeding, *Pediatrics* 113:e283, 2004.
204. Thoyre S: Mothers' ideas about their role in feeding their high-risk infants, *J Obstet Gynecol Neonatal Nurs* 29:613, 2000.
205. Thoyre S, Carlson J: Occurrence of oxygen desaturation events during preterm infant bottle feeding nearing discharge, *Early Hum Dev* 72:25, 2003.
206. Thoyre S, Shaker C, Pridham K: The Early Feeding Skills Assessment for preterm infants, *Neonatal Netw* 24:7, 2005.
207. U.S. Department of Health and Human Services: *HHS blueprint for action on breast feeding*, Washington, DC, 2000, U.S. Department of Health and Human Services, Office of Women's Health.
208. U.S. Food and Drug Administration (FDA), Center for Drug Evaluation and Research, FDA Public Health Advisory: *Use of codeine by some breastfeeding mothers may lead to life-threatening side effects in nursing babies*, August 17, 2007. Accessed September 6, 2009, from www.fda.gov/Cder/drug/advisory/codeine.htm.
209. U.S. Public Health Service: *Healthy People 2010*, Washington, DC, 1999, U.S. Department of Health and Human Services, U.S. Government Printing Office.
210. Uvnas-Moberg K, Johansson B, Lupoli B, et al: Oxytocin facilitates behavioral, metabolic and physiological adaptations during lactation, *Appl Anim Behav Sci* 72:225, 2001.
211. Valentine C, Hurst N, Schanler R: Hind milk improves weight gain in LBW infants fed human milk, *J Pediatr Gastroenterol Nutr* 18:474, 1994.
212. Vice FL, Gewolb IH: Respiratory patterns and strategies during feeding in preterm infants, *Dev Med Child Neurol* 50:467, 2008.
213. Viguera AC, Newport DJ, Ritchie J, et al: Lithium in breast milk and nursing infants: clinical implications, *Am J Psychiatry* 164:342, 2007.
214. Vohr BR, Poindexter BB, Dusick AM, et al: Beneficial effects of breast milk in the neonatal intensive care unit on the development outcome of extremely low birth weight infants at 18 months of age, *Pediatrics* 118:e115, 2006.
215. Vohr BR, Poindexter BB, Dusick AM, et al: Persistent beneficial effects of breast milk ingested in the neonatal intensive care unit on outcomes of extremely low birth weight infants at 30 months of age, *Pediatrics* 120:e953, 2007.
216. Weissman A, Levy B, Hartz A, et al: Pooled analysis of antidepressant levels in lactating mothers, breast milk and nursing infants, *Am J Psychiatry* 161:1066, 2004.
217. Wight N: Management of common breast feeding issues, *Pediatr Clin North Am* 48:321, 2001.
218. Wilson P, Pugh L: Promoting nutrition in breast feeding women, *J Obstet Gynecol Neonatal Nurs* 34:120, 2005.
219. Wooldridge J, Hall W: Posthospitalization breast feeding patterns of moderately preterm infants, *J Perinat Neonatal Nurs* 17:50, 2003.
220. Zinamen MJ, Hughes V, Queenan J, et al: Acute prolactin and oxytocin responses and milk yield to infant suckling and artificial methods of expression in lactating women, *Pediatrics* 89:437, 1992.
221. Zukowsky K: Breastfed low-birth-weight premature infants: a description of nutritional intake in the first 6 months of life, *Newborn Infant Nurs Rev* 7:161, 2007.

RESOURCE MATERIALS FOR PROFESSIONALS

Academy of Breastfeeding Medicine: *Clinical protocols for managing common medical problems affecting breast feeding success*. Available at www.bfmed.org.

Altman D: *Clinics in human lactation: history and assessment—it's all in the details*, Amarillo, Tex, 2008, Hale Publications.

Association of Women's Health: *Obstetrical and Neonatal Nurses: Evidence-based clinical practice guideline: breastfeeding support—prenatal care through the first year*, Washington, DC, 2000, The Association.

Breastfeeding and herbal supplements, Available at www.e-lactancia.org.

Brown VD: *Clinical practice tool: breastfeeding clinical practice algorithms*, Nurse's Professional Development and Practice Association, LLC 2008, Available at www.npdpa.com.

Buescher ES, Hatcher SW: *Breastfeeding and disease*, Amarillo, Tex, 2008, Hale Publications.

California Perinatal Quality Care Collaborative (CPQCC): *Quality Improvement Tool Kits: Nutritional support of the VLBW infant. Parts I and II.* Available at www.cpqcc.org.

Drugs in lactation. Website: www.neonatal.ttuhsc.edu/lact.

Gardner SL, Brown VD: *Policy/Procedure/Protocol Packet: Nipple feeding the infant,* Nurse's Professional Development and Practice Association, LLC, 2008. Available at www.npdpa.com.

Hale T, Wight N, Martin J, et al: *Best medicine: human milk in the NICU,* Amarillo, Tex, 2008, Hale Publications.

Neonatal Product Group, Overland Park, Kan: *The Penguin Nutritional Warmer (commercial device that warms breast milk to body temperature).* Available at www.neonatalproductgroup.com.

Robbins S, Beker L: *Infant feedings: guidelines for preparation of formula and breast milk in health care facilities,* Chicago, Ill, 2004, American Dietetic Association.

Schanler R, Dooley S, Gartner L, et al: *Breastfeeding handbook for physicians,* Chicago, 2005, American Academy of Pediatrics and The American College of Obstetricians and Gynecologists.

The Lactation Center at the University of Rochester Medical Center: (585) 275-0088.

RESOURCE MATERIALS FOR PARENTS

American Academy of Pediatrics: *New mother's guide to breast feeding,* New York, 2002, Bantam Books.

Bergman N: *Kangaroo mother care: restoring the original paradigm for infant care and breast feeding (video),* Cape Town, South Africa. 2000. Website: www.kangaroomothercare.com.

Eiger M, Olds S: *The complete book of breast feeding,* ed 3, New York, 1999, Workman Publishing.

Fogarty K, O'Hara M: *The real deal on breast feeding (video),* 2004. Playgroup Productions at www.realdealvideos.com.

Harrison H: *The premature baby book,* New York, 1983, St Martin's Press.

Huggins K: *The nursing mother's companion,* ed 4, Boston, 1999, Harvard Common Press.

Lact-Aid International: PO Box 1066, Athens, TN 37303; 1-866-866-1239. Available at www.lact-aid.com.

LaLeche League International: *The breastfeeding answer book,* ed 3, Schaumburg, Ill, 2003, The League.

LaLeche League International: *The womanly art of breastfeeding,* ed 7, Schaumburg, Ill, 2004, The League.

Lauwers J, Swisher A: *Counseling the nursing mother,* ed 4, Boston, 2005, Jones & Bartlett.

Meier P: *Breast feeding multiple babies,* Columbus, Ohio, 2003, Ross Products Division Abbott Laboratories (Available in English and Spanish.)

Meier P: *Breastfeeding your premature baby,* Columbus, Ohio, 2003, Ross Products Division Abbott Laboratories. (Available in English and Spanish.)

Meier P: *Expressing milk for your premature baby; breast feeding your premature baby with a nipple shield; troubleshooting milk volume problems in the NICU; choosing a correctly fitting breast shield,* McHenry, Ill, 2003, Medela, Inc.

Morton J: *A premie needs his mother: first steps to breast feeding your premature baby (video),* Palo Alto, Calif, 2001, DLD Productions. Website: www.breastmilksolutions.com/index.html.

National Breastfeeding, Awareness Campaign: *Breast feeding support,* Website: www.4woman.gov/breastfeeding. Breast feeding helpline: 1-800-994-9662.

Newman J, Pitman T: *The ultimate breast feeding book of answers: the most comprehensive problem solution guide to breastfeeding from the foremost expert in North America,* Roseville, Calif, 2000, Prima Lifestyles.

Pryor G: *Nursing mother, working mother,* Boston, 1997, Harvard Commons Press.

Renfrew M, Fischer C, Arms S: *Breast feeding, getting breast feeding right for you,* Berkeley, Calif, 2000, Celestial Arts.

Website: www.breastfeeding.com.

World Health Organization, *Relactation: a review of experience and recommendations for practice,* Geneva, Switzerland, 1998, The Organization.

19 SKIN AND SKIN CARE

CAROLYN HOUSKA LUND AND DAVID J. DURAND

The skin is a large organ in premature and term infants, making up at least 13% of body weight in contrast to 3% of body weight in adults.[65] Skin functions include thermoregulation, barrier against toxins and infections, water and electrolyte excretion, fat storage and insulation, and tactile sensation.

Like many other organs, the skin of a premature infant is immature. The combination of immaturity with the need for intensive care monitoring and procedures places premature infants at risk for skin trauma and loss of skin integrity. **Skin trauma and skin immaturity have serious consequences for infants in the neonatal intensive care unit (NICU), including problems in thermoregulation, fluid and electrolyte balance, diversion of calories for tissue repair, discomfort, potential toxicity from absorbed substances, and increased risk for infection.**

This chapter reviews the physiology of term and premature infants' skin, the differences in structure and function related to skin immaturity, and the prevention and treatment strategies to promote optimal skin integrity for infants in the NICU.

PHYSIOLOGY

There are three layers to the skin: the epidermis, the dermis, and the subcutaneous layer (Figure 19-1). The epidermis comprises the stratum corneum (a nonliving layer) and the basal layer. The stratum corneum is formed of lipids and protein in "brick and mortar" configuration. The basal layer replaces the stratum corneum with cells called ***keratinocytes.*** Approximately every 26 days, keratinocytes migrate from the basal layer to the exfoliated layers of the stratum corneum. In addition to keratinocytes, melanocytes also are found in the basal layer.

The dermis, a woven layer of collagen and elastin fibers, is 2 to 4 mm thick at birth. It contains nerves, blood vessels, and hair follicles. Sensations of heat, touch, pressure, and pain originate in the dermal layer. Sebaceous glands and sweat glands are located in the dermis, as well as in the subcutaneous layer of the skin. Sweat glands become mature in term infants during the first week of life, whereas maturation in premature infants occurs between 21 and 33 days and perhaps even longer in extremely premature infants.

The subcutaneous layer is composed of fatty connective tissue, with fat deposition occurring primarily during the last trimester of pregnancy. This layer provides heat insulation and functions as a calorie reservoir.

The skin of a normal term infant is covered with ***vernix caseosa,*** a "cheesy" substance composed of water (80%), lipids, and proteins,[113] sebum from sebaceous glands, broken-off lanugo, and desquamated cells from the amnion. Vernix production begins at the end of the second trimester, accumulates on fetal skin in a cephalocaudal manner,[53] and protects the fetus against maceration from the amniotic fluid and chafing caused by crowding in utero. Vernix detaches from fetal skin as the levels of pulmonary surfactant rise, resulting in a progressive increase in the turbidity of the amniotic fluid.[55,91] **Leaving residual vernix intact may be beneficial after delivery, because the presence of vernix produces earlier acidification of the skin and may act to facilitate colonization by the normal bacterial flora.**[113,120]

The skin of premature infants is thinner than that of term infants and may appear transparent or even

Please note that the **PURPLE** type in each chapter is intended to make it easier to identify clinically applicable material.

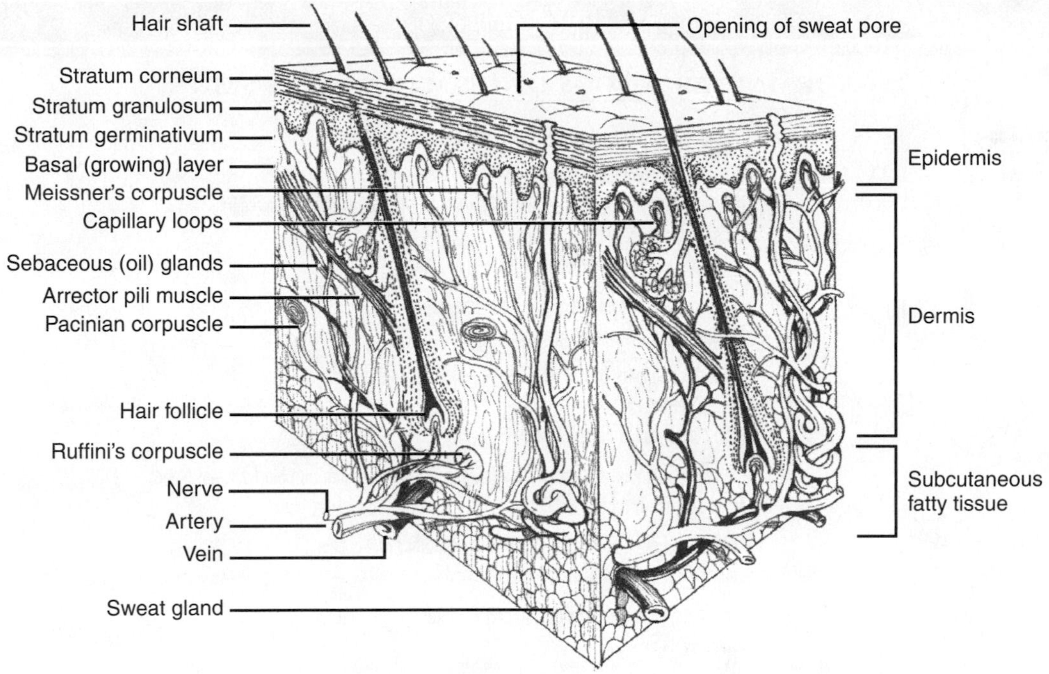

FIGURE 19-1 Cross section of skin layers and anatomic structures. (From *Principles of infant skin care,* Skillman, NJ, 1994, Johnson & Johnson.)

gelatinous in extremely immature infants. **There is usually a ruddy, red appearance caused by the underdeveloped stratum corneum, making skin color a poor tool for assessing the oxygenation status of very immature infants.** There are fewer wrinkles on skin surfaces than in term infants, and the skin is covered by ***lanugo*** to varying degrees, depending on maturity; these fine hairs cover the upper back, arms, and forehead. The subcutaneous layer in premature infants is often edematous because of an excess of cutaneous water and sodium (see Chapter 14).

ETIOLOGY

Term Newborn Skin Variations

Although the basic skin structures are the same in all term newborns without dermatologic disease, cutaneous variations may be seen on physical examination. These variations (see the Critical Findings box on p. 484) are not considered pathologic, but it is useful for clinicians to know them, because many parents ask the significance of physical variations as they examine their newborn.

Physiologic and Anatomic Differences in Premature Skin

Developmental differences in skin physiology and anatomy exist between full-term and premature infants when compared with older children and adults. This section discusses these differences and identifies the implications for care.

UNDERDEVELOPMENT OF THE STRATUM CORNEUM

The stratum corneum, the nonliving layer of the epidermis that is responsible for controlling evaporative heat loss and ***transepidermal water loss (TEWL),*** contains 10 to 20 layers in adults and term infants. **Term infants have been shown to have lower transepidermal water loss than adults, with the lowest levels seen on the first day of life.**[123] **Premature infants have fewer**

Critical Findings

NORMAL VARIATIONS OF TERM NEWBORN SKIN

Linea nigra	Line of increased pigmentation from umbilicus to genitalia
Mongolian spots	Irregular, blue-gray, bruiselike spots Usually seen over sacrum and buttocks, may extend over back and shoulders Caused by pigmented cells in dermis Most common in infants with darker pigmentation
Lanugo	Fine, downy hair over back, shoulders, and face Shed at 32 to 36 weeks' gestation
Milia	White, pinhead-size bumps over chin, cheeks, nose, and forehead Tiny epidermal cysts If on palate, called *Epstein's pearls*
Miliaria	Caused by retention of sweat from edema in stratum corneum that blocks sweat glands Most common is rubra (prickly pear), but there are also clear versions
Harlequin sign	Color of half of body turns deep red while the other half is pale Caused by immature autoregulation of blood flow
Vernix caseosa	Gray-white, cheesy substance that protects fetal skin in utero Gradually diminishes near term
Cutis marmorata	Mottling caused by vasomotor immaturity
Erythema toxicum neonatorum	Small, firm white or yellow pustules with erythematous margin Most often seen on trunk, arms, and perineal area Benign condition seen in 30% to 70% of newborns
Acne neonatorum	Acne-like rash seen in newborns at several weeks of age Caused by stimulation of sebaceous glands by maternal hormones More common in males Instruct caregivers not to use creams, lotion, or ointments because they can worsen the rash
Transient neonatal pustular melanosis	Resembles miliaria but present at birth Most frequently found on face, palms of hands, soles of feet Not infectious or contagious
Café au lait spots	Irregularly shaped oval lesions If large size (>4 × >6 cm), or if >6 in number, associated with neurofibromatosis

layers of stratum corneum, depending on their gestational age. At less than 30 weeks' gestation, they may have only two or three layers (Figure 19-2); and extremely premature infants of less than 24 weeks' gestation may have virtually no stratum corneum.[56,92] Another function of the stratum corneum—protection against toxins and infectious agents such as bacteria and viruses—is minimal in premature infants, leaving them vulnerable to transcutaneously transmitted infections and toxicity from topically applied substances.

The transition from the aquatic, intrauterine environment to the atmospheric, external environment has been thought to result in accelerated maturation of the stratum corneum and more mature function after the first 10 to 14 days of life.[41,52] However, other authors cite a slower process in **premature infants less than 27 weeks' gestation, with**

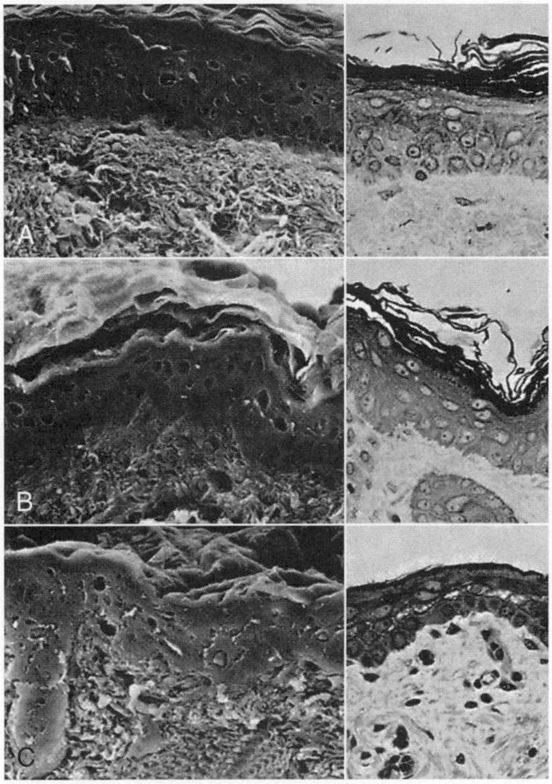

FIGURE 19-2 Photomicrograph of the stratum corneum in an adult **(A)**, a term newborn **(B)**, and a premature infant of 28 weeks' gestation **(C)**. Note fewer layers of stratum corneum in the premature infant. (From Holbrook KA: A histological comparison of infant and adult skin. In Maibach HI, Boisits EK, editors: *Neonatal skin: structure and function*, New York, 1982, Marcel Dekker.)

rates of TEWL nearly double adult levels even at 28 days of life.[106] Premature infants of 23 to 25 weeks' gestation have losses 10 times higher than term infants initially, and they continue to have elevated heat and water loss resulting from immature barrier function for a longer period.[1] The maturation process can take as long as 8 weeks in an infant of 23 weeks' gestation.[63]

DERMAL INSTABILITY

The dermis is made of collagen and elastin fibers in a gel matrix, providing mechanical strength, protection, and elasticity to the skin. The dermis of the term newborn is thinner than the adult dermis and has a higher water content.[56,73] Collagen deposition in the dermis increases with advancing gestational age, preventing fluid from accumulating in this layer. Premature infants have a tendency to become edematous, because they have less collagen and fewer elastin fibers in the dermis.

Both term and premature infants may be prone to necrotic injury from excessive edema because of alteration in blood flow and perfusion to the epidermis. Edematous infants need protection from pressure and ischemic injury, including routine turning and the use of surfaces to minimize pressure points such as water beds and gelled mattresses or pads.

DIMINISHED COHESION BETWEEN EPIDERMIS AND DERMIS

Numerous fibrils connect the epidermis to the dermis at the dermo-epidermal junction. These fibrils are more widely spaced and fewer in number in the premature infant[56] (Figure 19-3) but become stronger with advancing gestational and postnatal age. Genetically abnormal fibrils at this junction are found in certain types of the genetic disorder *epidermolysis bullosa,* a blistering skin condition that occurs with even minimal trauma. Premature infants also are prone to blistering from injury, although this decreases as they mature. **This diminished cohesion places premature infants at risk for injury from adhesive removal as well. Particularly if extremely aggressive adhesives are used, there may be a stronger bond of the adhesive to the epidermis than of the epidermis to the dermis, and epidermal stripping may result during adhesive removal.**

SKIN pH

The ability of the skin surface to form and maintain an acid surface is a function of various chemical and biologic processes. Acid skin surfaces with a pH less than 5 have been documented extensively in adults and children.[13] This ***acid mantle*** has protective qualities against some pathogens and other microorganisms. Because microbial colonization begins with delivery, the acid skin surface helps keep a state of equilibrium; if the pH shifts from acidic to neutral, there may be an increase in total numbers of bacteria and a shift in species. TEWL also may increase when skin pH rises.[122]

Term newborns are born with a relatively alkaline skin surface, measuring a mean pH of 6.34. Within 4 days, the pH declines to a mean of 4.95.[13] Skin pH measurements have been reported in premature infants of varying gestational ages, and

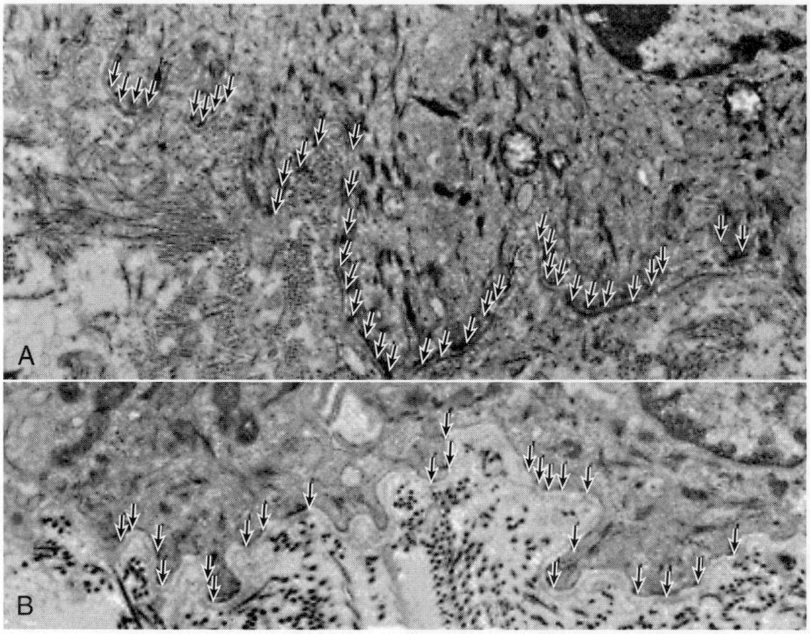

FIGURE 19-3 **A** and **B**, *Arrows* indicate fibrils called *hemidesmosomes*, which anchor the epidermis to the dermis. **B**, They are fewer in number and more widely spaced in the premature infant. (From Holbrook KA: A histological comparison of infant and adult skin. In Maibach HI, Boisits EK, editors: *Neonatal skin: structure and function*, New York, 1982, Marcel Dekker.)

the pH was above 6 on the first day, decreasing to 5.5 during the first week, and gradually declining to 5 during the first month.[43] **Bathing and other skin care practices alter skin pH; it may take an hour or longer to regenerate the acid mantle after bathing with an alkaline soap.** Skin that is occluded by wearing diapers has been shown to have a pH of 6, which is known to be a risk factor in the development of diaper dermatitis.[121]

NUTRITIONAL DEFICIENCIES

Fat and zinc accumulate in the fetus during the last trimester of pregnancy. Because these nutritional components are necessary for maintaining an intact, healthy skin surface, premature infants born before the last trimester may develop skin problems caused by deficiencies in either of these nutrients. Problems also may be seen in infants who are unable to receive adequate enteral nutrition unless appropriate parenteral supplements are employed.

Essential fatty acid (EFA) deficiency can be seen in premature and postmature infants because of decreased fat stores (see Chapter 17). In this condition, there is a superficial scaling and occasionally desquamation and irritation in the neck, groin, or perianal area. There may be decreased serum levels of EFAs, thrombocytopenia, and impaired platelet aggregation because EFAs are needed to promote platelet function.[44]

Providing adequate EFA prevents skin manifestations of EFA deficiency. In infants who are receiving small amounts of enteral nutrients or none at all, administration of intravenous (IV) lipid solutions at a total dose of 0.5 g/kg/day can prevent EFA deficiency (see Chapter 16). Once EFA deficiency occurs, IV lipids can reverse the process in 1 to 2 weeks. Dietary replacement takes longer and is effective only if gastrointestinal function is good. Topical therapy with sunflower seed oil, which is rich in linoleic acid, promotes transdermal absorption of EFA and raises serum levels but is variable in the rate of absorption. In a study of topical application, researchers found that safflower oil failed to yield improvements in patients with EFA deficiency.[57]

Zinc, an essential trace mineral, is a cofactor in many areas of metabolism, including lymphocyte transformation and metabolism of protein, nucleic acids, and mucopolysaccharides of skin and

Critical Findings

CLINICAL FEATURES OF ZINC DEFICIENCY

- Erythematous, scaly skin
- Excoriations of the groin and perianal areas, neck folds, circumoral area, and at sites of trauma, such as areas of adhesive removal
- Lethargy
- Poor growth
- Alopecia
- Diarrhea

subcutaneous tissues and is necessary for normal wound healing.[35] Two thirds of the transfer of zinc from mother to fetus occurs in the last 10 weeks of pregnancy. ***Zinc deficiency*** occurs when there are abnormal losses of zinc in stool or urine; when there are low or absent stores, as in premature birth; or during increased demands, such as during rapid growth, stress, or tissue healing. Thus premature infants and infants with pathologic conditions of the intestine (including chronic diarrhea, short bowel syndrome, intestinal diversions such as ileostomy, or intestinal resection) are at increased risk for zinc deficiency. In addition, **any infant receiving total parenteral nutrition should receive trace minerals to prevent zinc deficiency (see Chapter 16).**

Symptoms of zinc deficiency are listed in the Critical Findings box above. Serum zinc levels of less than 68 mcg/mL accompanied by a low alkaline phosphatase and clinical symptoms are diagnostic of zinc deficiency. Prevention of zinc deficiency for term infants receiving total parenteral nutrition includes zinc supplementation with 100 to 200 mcg/kg/day; premature infants require higher levels of supplementation (400 mcg/kg/day).[127] Premature infants have also been reported to develop zinc deficiency while fed breast milk; they may require an oral zinc sulfate supplement.[126]

PREVENTION

During daily skin care practices such as bathing, moisturizing, antimicrobial skin disinfection, and adhesive removal, the skin of newborns is at risk for trauma or disruption of normal barrier function. This is particularly true of newborns in the NICU, who may have been born prematurely or may be critically ill or require surgery.

This section reviews basic skin care practices in terms of impact on skin integrity, preventing potential toxicity, and reducing exposure to potentially sensitizing chemical. Recommendations for preventing trauma, protecting immature barrier function, and promoting skin integrity supported by scientific evidence are presented. These recommendations also are integrated into an ***evidence-based skin care guideline*** for health professionals.[7]

Bathing

Among the purposes of bathing the newborn are overall hygiene, aesthetics, and protection of health care workers by removing blood and body fluids. Bathing, however, is not an innocuous procedure. During the immediate postbirth period, bathing can result in hypothermia, increased oxygen consumption, and respiratory distress. **To prevent hypothermia, increased oxygen consumption, and respiratory distress, the first bath should be delayed until the infant's temperature has been stabilized in the normal range for 2 to 4 hours[95] or at 1 hour if radiant heat is provided during the bath.**[116] With appropriate attention to the environment, there is no difference in heat loss when the bath is performed at the bedside in the mother's room or in the nursery.[87] **Bathing also has been shown to destabilize vital signs and temperature in premature infants.**[96]

Bathing with antiseptic soaps and cleansers is still practiced in some nurseries. Studies have shown that although hexachlorophene reduced the number of *Staphylococcus aureus* strains present on the skin, toxicity was reported, especially in premature infants, associated with absorption through the skin; it should not be used.[3,67,104] Both povidone-iodine and chlorhexidine are sometimes used for the initial bath in newborn nurseries, although the effect on bacterial colonization is transient.[32] **Chlorhexidine has proved effective in reducing colonization for up to 4 hours[32] but also can be absorbed.**[31] Although toxicity from chlorhexidine has not been identified, many nurseries do not use it for routine bathing because of the potential risk. Antimicrobial soap is not recommended by the American Academy of Pediatrics and the American College of Obstetricians and Gynecologists[4] because of the harshness of the soap and the potentially negative effect it may have on normal skin colonization.

Soaps made with lye and animal fats are alkaline, with a pH above 7.0. Cleansing bars and liquids made with synthetic detergents are formulated to a more neutral pH of 5.5 to 7.0. **All soaps and cleansers are at least mildly irritating and drying to skin surfaces**[114,115] **and disrupt the skin surface pH.**[48] In addition, the degree to which the skin is irritated also depends on the length of contact and the frequency of bathing.

The recommendations are **(1) to select cleansers that have a neutral pH and minimal dyes and perfumes to reduce risk for potential sensitization to these products, and (2) to bathe the infant no more than every other day.**[7] The effects of bathing on skin parameters in small premature infants have not been studied to date. To reduce alterations in skin pH, dryness, and irritation in **premature infants less than 32 weeks, cleanse with warm-water baths during the first week, using soft cotton cloths, cotton balls, or the caregiver's hands.** It has been shown that **skin colonization with bacteria does not increase with bathing as infrequently as every 4 days.**[98] Less frequent bathing may offer other advantages for premature infants, who have demonstrated physiologic and behavioral disruptions during sponge baths.[96] Immersion bathing, even of stable infants on ventilators or nasal continuous positive airway pressure (NCPAP), may be soothing and less stressful.[2]

Immersion bathing places the infant's entire body, except the head and neck, into warm water (38° C [100.4° F]), deep enough to cover the shoulders. A recent study of immersion versus sponge bathing in 102 newborns for their first and subsequent baths showed that the **immersion-bathed infants had significantly less temperature drop and appeared more content** and their mothers reported more pleasure with the bath; there was no difference in cord healing scores with either immersion or sponge bathing.[19] Immersion bathing is also beneficial from a developmental perspective.[2,5] Stable premature infants after umbilical catheters are removed and term infants with umbilical clamps in place can be bathed safely in this way.[7] **Bathing is an excellent time to educate parents (1) about how to physically care for their baby and (2) about their baby's neurobehavioral status and social characteristics.**[64]

Emollients

The skin surface of term newborns is drier than that of adults but becomes gradually better hydrated as the eccrine sweat glands mature during the first year of life.[90,103] Maintaining the hydration of the stratum corneum is necessary for an intact skin surface and normal barrier function. Skin that is dry, scaly, or cracking not only is uncomfortable but also can be a portal of entry for microorganisms. **Products used to counteract dryness are called *moisturizers, emollients, or lubricants.*** Common emollients include mineral oils, petrolatum, and lanolin and its derivatives. Emollients are sometimes divided into oil-in-water or water-in-oil emulsions.

Emollient use to prevent dermatitis and improve skin integrity has been studied in several randomized, controlled trials in premature infants. In one report,[68] premature infants of 29 to 36 weeks' gestation were treated with **Eucerin cream daily** and had less dermatitis as measured by a visual grading scale but no differences in direct measurements of TEWL with an evaporimeter. In a later study, premature infants of both shorter gestation and younger postnatal age were treated with **Aquaphor ointment,** a water-miscible oil-in-water preparation that contains neither dyes nor perfumes. In this study, there was improvement in both TEWL and visual scale dermatitis. **No increases in skin surface temperatures or thermal burns were seen, even when the emollient was applied to infants under radiant heaters or phototherapy lights.** In addition, cutaneous cultures revealed **no increase in bacterial or fungal colonization on skin treated with emollients.** It was noted that fewer treated infants had positive blood or cerebrospinal fluid culture results compared with control subjects, although the study was not large enough to prove this effect.[93]

A large, randomized controlled trial of 1191 infants with birth weights of 501 to 1000 g was conducted to determine whether twice-daily application of Aquaphor ointment would reduce combined outcome measures of mortality and sepsis. Although skin integrity appeared improved with routine emollient use, no effect was seen in the outcomes of sepsis plus mortality. Of note, an increase in coagulase-negative *Staphylococcus epidermidis* bloodstream infections was seen in infants with birth weights below 750 g, although the mechanism and relationship to emollient use are not clearly understood.[40] Although a small case-control study had previously associated petrolatum-based emollients with a higher incidence of fungal infections,[22] this was not seen in the larger trial. The effects of emollients on TEWL or fluid balance were not studied in this trial.

The benefits of emollient use must be carefully weighed against the risk for infection. In general, emollients can be safely used to treat skin with excessive dryness, cracking, or fissures on an "as-needed" basis. They also may be effective in reducing TEWL and evaporative heat loss, although other methods, such as using a high-humidity environment or transparent adhesive dressings, also are available for this purpose. Avoiding products with perfumes or dyes is prudent, because these can be absorbed and are potential contact irritants.[26] **Small tubes or jars for single-patient use are recommended to prevent contamination with microorganisms.**

Skin Disinfectants

Decontamination of skin before invasive procedures such as venipuncture and placement of umbilical catheters and chest tubes is common practice in neonatal intensive care nurseries. However, there are **anecdotal reports of skin injury, including blistering, burns, and sloughing, from disinfectants including isopropyl alcohol, povidone-iodine, and alcohol-containing chlorhexidine use in premature infants.**[51,101,105] There have been case reports of high iodine levels, iodine goiter, and hypothyroidism associated with povidone-iodine use in premature infants.[27,60,97] Several prospective studies of routine povidone-iodine use in intensive care nurseries[70,94,107] and one study of presurgical skin preparation of infants younger than 3 months[89] found **alterations in iodine levels and thyroid effects from povidone-iodine exposure as a result of absorption through the skin.** Although one study did not find alterations in thyroid function from iodine absorption in neonates,[49] the study period (10 days) may be too short to see this effect.

Another important aspect of skin disinfection is how effectively disinfectant solutions reduce colonization and infection rates. During skin preparation before blood culture sampling in children and adults, **lower rates of microbial colonization were seen with povidone-iodine compared with isopropyl alcohol.**[30] A larger study of blood culture sampling in adults found **fewer contaminated cultures when chlorhexidine had been used compared with cultures from povidone-iodine–cleansed subjects.**[88]

Two studies in premature infants compared skin and peripheral intravenous catheter colonization with bacteria after skin preparation with either chlorhexidine or povidone-iodine. Malathi et al[82] found the rate of colonization was no different between disinfectants but the technique of application was important: the authors recommended **longer periods of cleansing (>30 seconds) or two consecutive cleansings for maximum reduction of colonization.** Garland et al[45] reported that **chlorhexidine reduced catheter colonization:** 4.3% with chlorhexidine compared with 9.3% with povidone-iodine.

A meta-analysis of eight studies involving 4143 central catheters in adult patients found that using chlorhexidine gluconate–containing disinfectants for insertion and routine site care reduced the risk for catheter-related bloodstream infections by 49%[28] and has led to recommendations to replace povidone-iodine with chlorhexidine disinfectants.[25] A comparison of isopropyl alcohol, povidone-iodine, and 2% chlorhexidine aqueous solution for disinfection of 668 central venous catheters in adults during insertion and routine dressing changes showed chlorhexidine to be significantly more effective in reducing catheter-related infections.[81] Similar studies have not been conducted in the NICU population. In a sequential study **in a single NICU, the rate of positive blood cultures and number of true infections were unchanged when the unit switched from povidone-iodine to chlorhexidine gluconate for skin disinfection.**[71] Of note, the typical dwell time for central catheters in many of the studies is 7 to 10 days, whereas peripherally inserted central catheters in neonates are often in 3 weeks or longer.

Chlorhexidine gluconate (CHG) is currently available in the United States as a 2% aqueous CHG skin preparation in 4-ounce bottles, as a tincture of 2% CHG in 70% isopropyl alcohol (ChloraPrep) in single-use packaging, and as a wipe containing 0.5% CHG in 70% isopropyl alcohol. **The tincture has been approved for infants older than 2 months, although many neonatal units use the tincture "off label"** because of the convenience and decreased risk for contamination of bottled products. However, **the combination of two disinfectants (CHG and isopropyl alcohol) has a significant potential for skin injury in very-low-birth-weight (VLBW) infants and cannot be recommended for them.** All CHG products should not come in contact with the eyes or ears, per manufacturer's recommendations, because of reports of damage to these structures. However, careful use before scalp intravenous or central line insertion is acceptable if splashing or using excessive amounts of CHG is avoided. **CHG is applied in two consecutive wipings or for a 30-second scrubbing period and then is removed with sterile water or saline solution when the procedure is completed.**

Many nurseries have chosen to continue the use of povidone-iodine disinfectants because of the lack of single-use CHG products that do not contain isopropyl alcohol. **Povidone-iodine** is available in a 10% aqueous solution in a variety of single-use applications. It is also **applied in two consecutive wipings or for a 30-second scrubbing period and then is allowed to dry for at least 30 seconds before the procedure. Any solution should be completely removed after the procedure, using sterile water or saline solution to prevent any further absorption. Disinfection with isopropyl alcohol is questionable in the NICU, because it is less effective than either povidone-iodine or chlorhexidine and can be irritating and drying to skin surfaces.**

The risks and benefits of routine skin antisepsis in infants is a subject that clearly deserves further investigation. Although there are insufficient comparative data on the costs, risks, and benefits of skin antisepsis regimens to mandate standard practice, **the use of alcohol pledgets alone provides the least-effective antimicrobial activity. Povidone-iodine and isopropyl alcohol carry significant risks of percutaneous toxicity.** The potential for subclinical toxicities must be considered with all products used on small newborns; therefore when several topical therapeutic options are available, the one with the least potential for toxicity should be chosen. **In addition, disinfectants should be removed completely from the skin with water or saline to prevent further absorption and contact.**

The routine use of antimicrobial sprays, creams, or powders for umbilical cord care has not been shown to be more effective in preventing infection compared with dry cord care.[128] The use of antibiotic ointments and antiseptics can prolong the time to cord separation, and it seems to have no beneficial effect on the frequency of infection.[6,62,128] A study of 1811 newborns randomized to receive either routine isopropyl alcohol with each diaper change or natural drying found no umbilical infections in either group, and time to cord separation was reduced from 9.8 days in the alcohol-treated group to 8.16 days in the natural-drying group.[38] Another study randomized 766 newborns to receive either triple dye applied to the umbilical cord immediately after delivery, followed by twice-daily applications of isopropyl alcohol, or "dry care" without any treatment. Infants in the dry-care group were more likely to be colonized with bacteria than those in the treatment group, and one infant in the dry-care group developed omphalitis on the third day of life. The days to cord separation were not reported.[61]

Recommendations for umbilical cord care to prevent contamination include the following[7]**:**
- **Washing hands before handling the cord**
- **If the cord becomes soiled with urine or stool, cleansing with water and drying with absorbent gauze**
- **Keeping the diaper folded down and away from the umbilical stump**

The development of omphalitis is not necessarily related to cord disinfection, because it occurs also in infants who have received topical disinfectants. However, **vigilant attention to the signs and symptoms is necessary by health professionals, and parents need guidance about how to manage the umbilical cord and when to consult their health care provider.**[37]

Adhesive Application and Removal

One of the most common practices in the NICU is the application and removal of adhesives that secure endotracheal tubes, IV devices, and monitoring probes and electrodes. A research utilization project involving 2820 premature and term newborns found that **adhesives were the primary cause of skin breakdown among NICU patients.**[78] Changes in TEWL and skin barrier function are seen in adults after ten consecutive removals of adhesive tape[72] and after one removal of adhesive tape in premature infants.[52] Types of damage from adhesive removal include epidermal stripping, tearing, maceration, tension blisters, chemical irritation, sensitization, and folliculitis.[54]

Solvents are sometimes used to prevent discomfort and skin disruption from adhesive removal. They contain hydrocarbon derivatives or petroleum distillates that have potential or proven toxicities. **Toxicity is a major concern, especially**

in premature infants with their underdeveloped stratum corneum, increased skin permeability, larger surface-area to body-weight ratio, and immature hepatic and renal function. A case report of toxic epidermal necrosis in a premature infant resulted from the use of a solvent.[59] **Mineral oil or petrolatum products may be helpful in removing adhesives but cannot be used if the site must be used again for reapplication of adhesives,** such as with the retaping of an endotracheal tube. **Removing adhesives with water-soaked cotton balls sometimes helps, and gently pulling the adhesive parallel to the skin surface rather than straight up at a 90-degree angle** may facilitate removal with less skin trauma.[80]

Skin bonding agents promote adherence. Unfortunately, they may create a stronger bond between adhesive and epidermis than the fragile cohesion of the epidermis to the dermis; when the adhesive is removed, epidermal stripping may result. Plastic polymers have been studied and are reported to reduce skin trauma.[42] An alcohol-free skin protectant is available that is less irritating to skin surfaces in adults than are comparable products containing alcohol.[51] This product has been approved for infants older than 30 days to treat mild diaper dermatitis and to prevent skin injury from adhesive removal.[112] A single study from England reports positive effects when using this skin protectant to tape intravenous lines in newborns.[58]

Pectin-based skin barriers such as Hollihesive™ and DuoDERM™ are used between skin and adhesive and mold well to curved surfaces while maintaining adherence in moist areas. Studies initially described less visible trauma to skin with pectin barriers.[36,76,86] However, a controlled trial of pectin barrier (Hollihesive), plastic tape (Transpore), and hydrophilic gelled adhesive found that significant skin disruption, as measured by TEWL and visual inspection, occurred after removal of both the pectin barrier and plastic tape.[77] Because the adhesives were left in place 24 hours before removal in this study, a time effect of peak adhesive aggressiveness may have been reached. Significant changes were measured after a single adhesive application and removal in all three weight groups studied (<1000 g; 1001 to 1500 g; and >1500 g), indicating that **even larger premature infants are at risk for skin injury from tape removal.** Despite this finding, pectin barriers and similar hydrocolloid adhesive products continue to be used in the NICU because they mold well to curved surfaces and adhere even with moisture.

Prevention of skin trauma from adhesive removal includes minimizing tape use when possible by using smaller pieces, backing the adhesive with cotton, and delaying tape removal until adherence is reduced. Pectin barriers and hydrocolloid adhesives may prove helpful, because they mold and adhere well to body contours and often attach better in moist conditions. As with tape, **removal of pectin barriers and hydrocolloid should be delayed, if possible, until the adherence lessens.** The use of soft gauze wraps to secure probes and hydrogel electrocardiogram electrodes and hydrogel tapes are helpful. **Adhesives should be removed slowly and carefully with warm water and cotton balls.** Mineral oil or an emollient may facilitate adhesive removal if reapplication of adhesives at the site of removal is not necessary. **Silicone-based adhesive products have been shown to improve adherence to wounds and reduce discomfort when removal is necessary**[39,50] and may prove beneficial if developed for a wider range of adhesive products for neonates.

DATA COLLECTION

History

The gestational age and postnatal age of neonates in the NICU are both important considerations for determining appropriate skin care practices. Premature infants of lower gestational ages have underdeveloped skin layers and function. With advancing postnatal age and maturation, skin integrity and skin barrier function are improved.

Reviewing the maternal history for any dermatologic diseases is also important. Many of the most severe skin diseases, such as forms of congenital ichthyosis or epidermolysis bullosa, are inherited disorders. A positive family history will alert the clinician to the potential for developing these rare disorders.

Signs and Symptoms

A thorough daily examination of all skin surfaces reveals the state of skin integrity for neonates

in the NICU. Early signs such as skin abrasions or small excoriations may call for either diagnostic or treatment procedures. **A scoring tool, such as the Neonatal Skin Condition Score (NSCS)** (see the Critical Findings box below), used in the Association of Women's Health, Obstetric and Neonatal Nurses (AWHONN)/National Association of Neonatal Nurses (NANN) research-based practice project,[75,78] **has been extensively used in both premature and full-term infants, with validity and reliability established.**[79] **This scoring system can be integrated into skin care protocols to identify neonates with excessive dryness, erythema, or skin breakdown.**[7] Risk factors for skin injury in individual patients are listed in the Critical Findings box below. In the first week of life in extremely-low-birth-weight (ELBW) infants (<30 weeks, <1000 g), there may be problems with thermoregulation (see Chapter 6) and dehydration (see Chapter 14) because of the large evaporative heat losses and transepidermal water losses through the immature stratum corneum.

Critical Findings

THE NEONATAL SKIN CONDITION SCORE

Dryness

1 = Normal, no sign of dry skin
2 = Dry skin, visible scaling
3 = Very dry skin, cracking/fissures

Erythema

1 = No evidence of erythema
2 = Visible erythema <50% body surface
3 = Visible erythema >50% body surface

Breakdown

1 = None evident
2 = Small localized areas
3 = Extensive

NOTE: Perfect score = 3; worst score = 9

From Lund C, Osborne J, Kuller J, et al: Neonatal skin care: clinical outcomes of the AWHONN/NANN evidence-based clinical practice guideline, *J Obstet Gynecol Neonatal Nurs* 30:41, 2001.

Laboratory Data

With the many skin excoriations in both small and large neonates that result from traumatic events such as adhesive removal or pressure necrosis, infection through this portal of entry in the skin is a potential. **In VLBW infants, it may be useful to obtain a skin culture, Gram stain, or potassium hydroxide (KOH) preparation**[11,12] for early detection of microorganisms that can lead to systemic illness in these immunocompromised patients. A ***skin surface culture*** is helpful if the skin breakdown cannot be traced to a traumatic injury, because the origin of the breakdown often is linked to infection, especially with fungal infections[102] or staphylococcal scalded skin syndrome. A more comprehensive workup for infection may be indicated if there is evidence of clinical deterioration in infants with extensive skin breakdown (see Chapter 22).

TREATMENT

Skin Excoriations

Skin excoriations are cleansed with warmed sterile water or half-normal saline solution; a 20- or 30-mL syringe with a Teflon IV catheter attached can be used to gently débride the excoriation. This technique is effective in flushing out debris and dead tissue from an infected or "dirty" wound, allowing a better surface for healing. **Moistening the tissue every 4 to 6 hours aids the healing process,** because drying of tissue actually impedes the migration of cells. Once the wound surface is clear, other dressings or ointments can be used.

Critical Findings

RISK FACTORS FOR SKIN INJURY

- Gestational age <32 weeks
- Edema
- Use of paralytic agents and vasopressors
- Multiple tubes and lines
- Numerous monitors
- Surgical wounds
- Ostomies
- Technologies that limit movement: high-frequency ventilation; extracorporeal membrane oxygenator

Ointments are sometimes used because of their antibacterial or antifungal properties and also because covering the wound with a semi-occlusive layer promotes healing by facilitating the migration of epithelial cells across the surface. Only if extensive bacterial colonization is suspected, Polysporin, Bacitracin, or Bactroban ointment is used sparingly every 8 to 12 hours. Many dermatologists do not recommend the use of Neosporin because of the potential for developing later sensitization to this ointment, although sensitization to Bacitracin is being reported with increasing frequency.[85] Overuse of antimicrobial ointments can be a problem in promoting more resistant strains of bacteria. If **fungal infection is suspected, Nystatin ointment is used, and it can be applied also to surrounding intact skin to prevent extension of the infection.** In general, ointments are preferable to creams for this use because of better adherence and healing properties.

Transparent adhesive dressings are made from a polyurethane film backed with adhesive that is impermeable to water and bacteria but allows airflow. A rim of intact skin must be around the wound to attach the dressing. Uses include wound care, dressings for IV devices including central venous lines and percutaneous silicone catheters, and prevention of friction injuries to areas such as the knees or sacrum.

When used for wound care, transparent adhesive dressing promotes "moist healing" that allows the rapid migration of epithelial cells across the site. These dressings should be used only on "clean" (uninfected) wounds because bacteria and fungi can proliferate under the dressing. When the dressing is placed over a clean wound, often a serous or milky exudate composed of leukocytes forms, which actually aids in the prevention of infection. **The dressings can be left in place for days at a time or until they become loose. Removing and reattaching the dressings on a daily basis is not recommended because the adhesive can injure the intact skin around the wound and further impede healing.**

Another use of transparent adhesive dressings in the NICU is the prevention of excessive TEWL in premature infants.[16,21,66,83,117] TEWL, as measured by an evaporimeter, can be reduced by as much as 50% by the creation of this "second skin." In one study,[83] a nonadherent transparent dressing (not commercially available) was used and the skin under the dressing not only had a lower TEWL while covered but also actually had lower TEWL when removed, suggesting that perhaps a faster maturation of the skin barrier function had occurred. Cultures were obtained both on covered and uncovered skin and showed no increase in either bacterial or fungal colonization under the dressings. Unfortunately, nonadherent dressings are not commercially available and transparent adhesive dressings can cause a significant amount of skin trauma when removed. Alternative ways to reduce TEWL in VLBW infants can be used, including double-walled incubators and heated humidity (see Chapter 6).

Other types of dressings used in wound management include hydrogels (dressings and gel) and hydrocolloid dressings (DuoDERM), both of which promote moist healing.[10,109] ***Hydrogel dressings*** can be used after irrigation of the wound and in conjunction with either antibacterial or antifungal ointment if the wound is infected. These dressings must be **changed every 8 to 12 hours, because they can dry out.** No adhesive attaches these dressings. It is best to avoid placing hydrogel dressings on intact skin surfaces, because they can macerate the skin and actually reduce barrier function. **Hydrocolloid dressings are used over uninfected wounds and can be left in place for 5 to 7 days while healing takes place.** Another wound treatment is **amorphous hydrogel applied directly onto the wound from a tube.** Amorphous hydrogels such as DuoDERM Gel and IntraSITE consist of 80% to 90% water to make it soothing to skin while keeping the wound moist, a cellulose polymer to extract and trap fluid, and propylene glycol to rehydrate tissues.[108-110]

Surgical wounds that open or dehisce are infrequent but require expert wound management. Nutrition is often a part of the process in getting these wounds to heal, as is the prevention of infection.[46] Often the surgeon or an enterostomal therapist will design the appropriate wound management program for these situations.

Intravenous Extravasations

Prevention of tissue injury from IV extravasations includes taping IV devices with transparent dressings or plastic tape so that the insertion site is clearly visible and observing the site with appropriate documentation every hour. If the IV device is placed in a limb, the tape that secures it to the rigid board should be placed loosely over a bony prominence, such as the elbow or knee, and not on skin in proximity to the insertion site. This allows extravasated fluid and medications to expand over a larger surface and not remain in a small, constricted area, which can result in greater tissue injury. It may be wise to avoid poorly perfused extremities in favor of scalp veins, except the forehead. Using central venous lines such as percutaneous catheters to infuse highly irritating solutions and medications is also recommended. Many nurseries limit the glucose concentrations in peripheral lines to 12.5% and the amino acid concentrations to 2%; calcium and potassium concentrations also are more dilute than those used in central lines.

If IV fluid has extravasated into surrounding tissue, the IV device should be removed and the extremity elevated. Use of moisture, heat, or cold is not recommended, because the tissue is vulnerable at this point to further injury.[17] **Hyaluronidase (Amphadase, Vitrase, Hylenex) can be extremely helpful if administered within an hour of extravasation** (see Chapter 10). This medication is an enzyme that causes a breakdown of interstitial barrier and allows the diffusion of the extravasated fluid over a larger area to prevent tissue necrosis.[69,100,124] **The dose of hyaluronidase is 15 to 20 units diluted to 1 mL,** although in one study using an animal model, 150 units was used without harmful effects.[69] **It is administered in five injections, inserted subcutaneously around the periphery of the extravasation site (Figures 19-4 and 19-5), and ideally is administered within 1 to 2 hours of the extravasation. Extravasations that may benefit from administration of hyaluronidase include any with evidence of blanching, discoloration, or blistering or those involving hypertonic or calcium-containing solutions, even if the site appears relatively undisturbed.** Calcium-containing solutions may cause deep tissue injury even when epidermal tissues are not involved. In addition to hyaluronidase administration, creating multiple puncture holes over the area of swelling and gently squeezing or letting the extravasated fluid leak out can facilitate the removal of the infiltrate and prevent skin sloughs.[29] **Saline washout is another technique described to facilitate the removal of extravasated irritants from tissues surrounding an IV site.**[24,33,47]

Hyaluronidase is not recommended in the extravasation of vasoconstrictive medications such as dopamine, because the vasoconstriction could extend with its use. Phentolamine (Regitine) is used in this case, because it directly counteracts the action of dopamine. The **method of delivery is the same as for hyaluronidase, with the total dose (0.5 mg) diluted to 1 mL, injected in five sites subcutaneously around the periphery of the extravasation.**[125]

When tissue injury occurs after extravasation, treating the wound with techniques using moist healing principles facilitates healing without scarring. There has been success using a generous application of amorphous hydrogel and placing the extremity in a plastic bag, the so-called "bag/boot" method.[111] In most cases, **skin grafts can be avoided by the use of appropriate wound healing techniques.** In all cases of tissue injury, open wounds should be considered a portal of entry for infection and topical or systemic treatment should be considered.

Diaper Dermatitis

Diaper dermatitis, which has a multitude of causes in infants, affects the perineum, groin, thighs, buttocks,

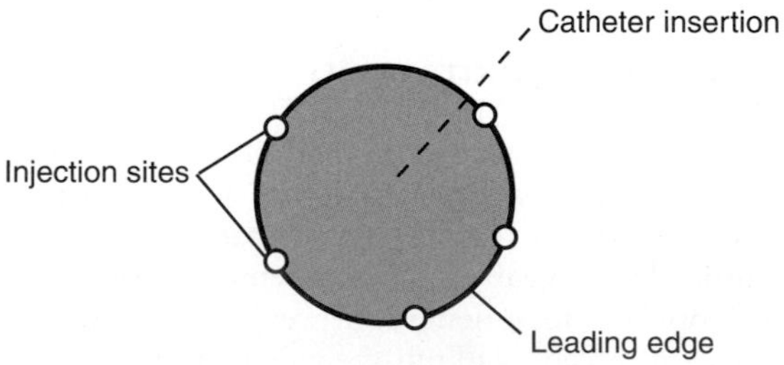

FIGURE 19-4 Technique for administration of hyaluronidase and/or phentolamine. A total volume of 1 mL is administered at five sites subcutaneously (0.2 mL each) around the periphery of the intravenous extravasation.

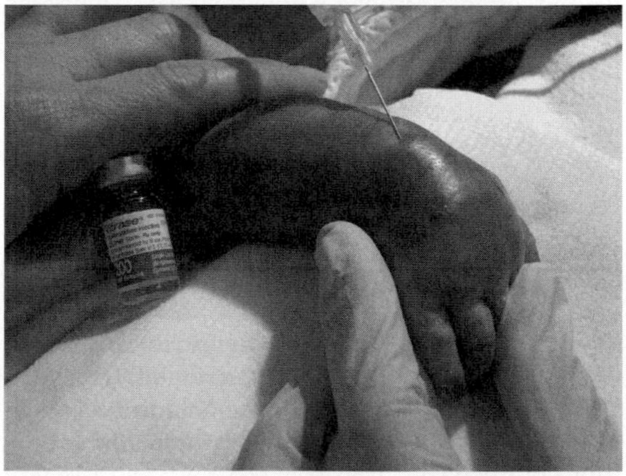

FIGURE 19-5 Hyaluronidase (Vitrase) being administered to extravasation in hand using 27-gauge needle.

and anal region. The underlying skin condition of the infant contributes to the degree of diaper dermatitis that occurs.

Another factor that influences the **development of diaper dermatitis is the degree of wetness of the skin; skin that is moist and macerated becomes more permeable and susceptible to injury.**[14,15,118] In addition, skin that is moisture-laden becomes more heavily colonized with microorganisms. Skin pH also has an effect; when the skin is exposed to urine, the **pH can rise from acid to alkaline ranges and tissues become more vulnerable to injury and penetration by microorganisms.**[8,118] The alkaline pH also can activate enzymes found in stool, protease, and lipase, which break down protein and fat, the building blocks of the stratum corneum.[20] This is the primary mechanism for direct contact dermatitis from exposure to stool, the most common form of diaper dermatitis.

Strategies for preventing diaper dermatitis include maintaining a skin surface that is dry and has a normal (acidic) skin pH. Frequent diaper changes are recommended, especially in the newborn period.

There is insufficient evidence to support that any specific type of diaper plays a central role in the prevention of diaper dermatitis.[9] However, superabsorbent gelled diapers with breathable covers have been shown to keep skin surfaces dryer by "wicking" the moisture away from the skin and separating urine from feces.[23,34] Use of powders is discouraged because of the risk for inhalation of particles into the respiratory tract. **After skin injury from diaper dermatitis has occurred, protecting injured skin to prevent re-injury is the primary goal of treatment.** Topical treatment for diaper dermatitis involves ointments and creams containing a variety of ingredients. Most contain zinc oxide or petrolatum and are generally similar in composition.[119] **Generous application of protective skin barriers that contain zinc oxide can prevent further injury while allowing skin to heal.** Once skin excoriations occur, keeping skin open to air may not be effective because the already impaired tissue may be reinjured with fecal contact and dryness is counterproductive to healing. **It is not necessary or desirable to completely remove skin barrier products with diaper changes, because this may disrupt healing tissue.** Instead, remove as much waste material as possible and reapply the barrier generously to the affected areas with each diaper change. Another class of barrier products is semipermeable barrier film, designed to repel moisture and protect the skin from irritants[119]; one of these products is approved for use in infants older than 30 days.[112]

If *Candida albicans* is involved in the diaper dermatitis, it is necessary to use an antifungal ointment or cream. Antifungal preparations include Mycostatin, miconazole, clotrimazole, and ketoconazole in ointment or cream forms; ointments are preferable to coat the skin and repel moisture. If the dermatitis is both fungal and a contact irritant dermatitis, it may be necessary to layer the ointment with the antifungal preparation. In this case, Mycostatin powder is used, followed by an application of alcohol-free skin protectant to seal the powder onto the skin surface, followed by a generous application of a skin barrier cream such as zinc oxide or pectin paste.

Occasionally infants may experience extremely severe diaper dermatitis from intestinal malabsorption syndromes or constant dribbling of stool, as in the case of infants who have problems with rectal enervation, such as those with myelomeningocele, bladder exstrophy, or after a "pull-through" procedure for Hirschsprung's disease. In the case of malabsorption, the stool may have a pH that is higher than normal because of rapid transit through the small intestine and there may be significant amounts of undigested carbohydrates and stool enzymes, as well as increased stool frequency. Severe diaper dermatitis in this case can be a symptom of a more severe nutritional deficiency, or even dehydration, and needs thorough medical evaluation. Stools in these infants should be regularly tested for pH, carbohydrates, and occult blood, and their number and total volume should be measured.

While optimal nutritional therapy is being addressed with special diets or parenteral nutrition, skin protection from injury should be initiated. **Products such as pectin paste without alcohol (e.g., Ilex, a non-alcohol pectin paste)** may provide a sturdier barrier for these infants than zinc oxide preparations. **The skin should be thoroughly cleansed before a very thick application of the pectin paste.** Then it is necessary to apply a greasy ointment over this, because the pectin-based paste may adhere to the diaper. **When the infant has a stool, it is not necessary to completely remove the barrier paste;** the stool can be wiped away as much as possible before reapplying the thick paste barrier. The skin will heal under this protective covering as long as it is protected from re-injury.[74]

If fungal infection is a component of the dermatitis, antifungal therapy must be instituted in addition to the protective barriers. In this case, Mycostatin powder attached with alcohol-free skin protectant is the first layer; then the barrier cream is applied as described previously.

COMPLICATIONS

Improper handling of newborn skin (and injudicious use of products) can cause damage, prevent healing, and interfere with normal maturation processes. **Compromised skin integrity can lead to infection, pain and discomfort, and diversion of calories for tissue repair. Other dangers include toxicity from topically applied substances** that are readily absorbed by small infants with a large surface-area to body-weight ratio, as well as immature renal and hepatic function that cannot detoxify chemicals readily.

Injury from infiltrated IV solutions can injure skin and occasionally cause deep tissue necrosis with both muscle and nerve damage. Factors that increase the risk for injury from IV extravasations include length of time between extravasation and treatment; hypertonic solutions, such as those with high calcium, potassium, amino acid, or glucose solutions; medications such as nafcillin that are irritating to veins; and the use of mechanical pumps for infusions. There may be an added risk for injury in patients with poor perfusion to extremities and in limbs that have been secured with restricting adhesives that obstruct venous return.

If the epidermis has been injured, it can easily become a portal of entry for infection. Thus a contact irritant diaper dermatitis can progress to a fungal or staphylococcal infection. *Staphylococcus aureus* can cause pustule formation at hair follicles and is a rare complication of diaper dermatitis. The mechanism for fungal diaper dermatitis is still debated. Some researchers believe that *Candida albicans* infection is a secondary invasion to skin that has been previously injured, whereas others see this organism as a primary cause of skin disruption.[99]

***Candida albicans* diaper dermatitis causes an intense inflammation that is bright red and sharply demarginated in the inguinal folds, buttocks, thighs, abdomen, and genitalia, often with satellite lesions that extend the rash over the trunk (Figure 19-6).** *Candida albicans* can be harbored in the gastrointestinal tract, necessitating oral therapy if lesions are found in the mouth.

PARENT TEACHING

It is the responsibility of professionals to teach parents informally during caregiving procedures such as bathing, cord care, and diaper changes and to prepare written materials about appropriate

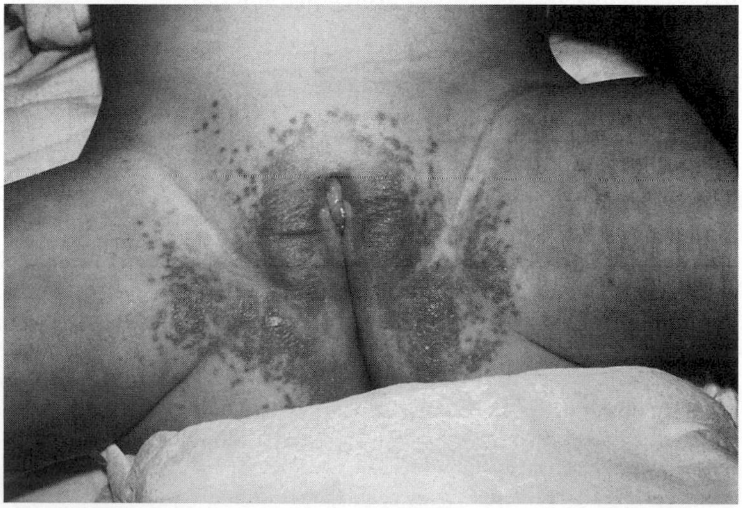

FIGURE 19-6 Diaper dermatitis caused by a *Candida albicans* infection. Red pustular satellite lesions extend into the periphery.

skin care practices for their infant after discharge from the NICU (see the Parent Teaching box below). Parents will need education about the normal mechanisms of cord healing, including the range of appearance in umbilical cords, because some cords can appear very moist and soggy. The cord can be cleansed with water if it becomes soiled with urine or stool.[7] Inform parents that minimal use of skin care products is optimal and may reduce the incidence of contact sensitization to chemicals.[18,26,84] It is also extremely useful to educate parents about the mechanisms that are involved in diaper dermatitis so that prevention is stressed and appropriate interventions are selected depending on the underlying cause.

Developmental differences in the anatomy and physiology of neonatal skin affect skin integrity for term and premature infants in the NICU. Prevention is the primary focus of care, and decisions about the best way to provide basic skin care and hygiene based on current research are essential for care providers, both professionals and parents.

Parent Teaching

APPROPRIATE SKIN CARE PRACTICES

- Baby needs to be bathed only two or three times per week. Sponge bath with water between tub bathings.
- Use on the skin only products that have as few additives and as little fragrance as possible; minimal skin care products reduce the incidence of contact sensitization of the skin by added chemicals.
- Do not use powder because of inhalation into baby's lungs.
- Prevent diaper rash by frequently changing wet and soiled diapers, cleansing diaper area, and using diapers that "wick" moisture away from the skin. If baby's skin becomes red and irritated with one brand of disposable diaper, try another brand.
- Treat diaper rash by using protective skin barriers (e.g., zinc oxide) with each diaper change to prevent further injury and allow skin to heal. Clean waste from skin barrier but do not clean off the skin barrier because this may disrupt skin healing.
- Diaper rash caused by a yeast infection requires antifungal medication.
- Umbilical cord dries and falls off within 7 to 10 days. Turn diaper back away from the cord till it falls off; as the cord separates, a small amount of blood stain may be on the diaper. Keep cord area clean, and rinse with water if it becomes soiled with urine or stool. Call the health care provider immediately if the cord develops an area of red, warm-to-touch skin at the base, a foul odor, or drainage from the base of the cord.

REFERENCES

1. Agren J, Sjors G, Sedin G: Transepidermal water loss in infants born at 24 and 25 weeks of gestation, *Acta Paediatr* 87:1185, 1998.
2. Als H, Lawhon G, Brown E, et al: Individualized behavioral and environmental care for the very low birth weight preterm infant at high risk for bronchopulmonary dysplasia: neonatal intensive care unit and developmental outcome, *Pediatrics* 78:1123, 1986.
3. American Academy of Pediatrics: *Red Book: report of the committee on infectious diseases,* ed 27, Elk Grove Village, Ill, 2006, The Academy.
4. American Academy of Pediatrics and The American College of Obstetricians and Gynecologists: *Guidelines for perinatal care,* ed 6, Elk Grove Village, Ill, 2007, The Academy.
5. Anderson GM, Lane A, Chang H: Axillary temperature in transitional newborn infants before and after tub bath, *Appl Nurs Res* 8:123, 1995.
6. Arad I, Eyal F, Fainmesser P: Umbilical cord care: a study of bacitracin ointment vs. triple dye, *Arch Dis Child* 56:887, 1981.
7. Association of Women's Health, Obstetric and Neonatal Nurses: *Evidence-based clinical practice guideline: neonatal skin care,* ed 2, Washington, DC, 2007, The Association.
8. Atherton DJ: A review of the pathophysiology, prevention and treatment of irritant diaper dermatitis, *Curr Med Res Opin* 20:645, 2004.
9. Baer EL, Davies MW, Easterbrook KJ: Disposable nappies for preventing napkin dermatitis in infants, *Cochrane Database Syst Rev* 3: CD004262, 2006.
10. Baharestani MM: An overview of neonatal and pediatric wound care knowledge and considerations, *Ostomy Wound Manage* 53:34, 2007.
11. Baley J, Kliegman RM, Boxerbaum B, et al: Fungal colonization in the very low birth weight infant, *Pediatrics* 78:225, 1986.
12. Baley J, Silverman R: Systemic candidiasis: cutaneous manifestations in low birth weight infants, *Pediatrics* 82:211, 1988.
13. Behrendt H, Green M: *Patterns of skin pH from birth through adolescence,* Springfield, Ill, 1971, Charles C Thomas.
14. Berg R: Etiologic factors in diaper dermatitis: a model for development of improved diapers, *Pediatrician* 14:27, 1987.
15. Berg R, Buckingham K, Stewart R: Etiologic factors in diaper dermatitis: the role of urine, *Pediatr Dermatol* 3:102, 1986.

16. Bhandari V, Brodsky N, Porat R: Improved outcome of extremely low birth weight infants with Tegaderm application to skin, *J Perinatol* 25:276, 2005.
17. Brown A, Hoelzer D, Piercy S: Skin necrosis from extravasation of intravenous fluids in children, *Plast Reconstr Surg* 64:145, 1979.
18. Bruckner A, Weston W, Morelli J: Does sensitization to contact allergens begin in infancy? *Pediatrics* e3:105, 2000.
19. Bryanton J, Walsh D, Barrett M, et al: Tub bathing versus traditional sponge bathing for the newborn, *J Obstet Gynecol Neonatal Nurs* 33:704, 2004.
20. Buckingham K, Berg R: Etiologic factors in diaper dermatitis: the role of feces, *Pediatr Dermatol* 3:107, 1986.
21. Bustamante S, Steslow J: Use of a transparent adhesive dressing in very low birth weight infants, *J Perinatol* 9:165, 1989.
22. Campbell J, Zaccaria E, Baker C: Systemic candidiasis in extremely low birth weight infants receiving topical petrolatum ointment for care: a case control study, *Pediatrics* 105:1041, 2000.
23. Campbell R, Seymour JL, Stone LC, et al: Clinical studies with disposable diapers containing absorbent gelling materials: evaluation on infant skin condition, *J Am Acad Dermatol* 17:978, 1987.
24. Casanova D, Bardot J, Magalon G: Emergency treatment of accidental infusion leakage in the newborn: report of 14 cases, *British J Plastic Surgery* 54:396, 2001.
25. Centers for Disease Control and Prevention: Guidelines for the prevention of intravascular catheter related infections, *MMWR* 51:1, 2002.
26. Cetta F, Lambert G, Ros S: Newborn chemical exposure from over-the-counter skin care products, *Clin Pediatr* 30:286, 1991.
27. Chabrolle J, Rossier A: Goiter and hypothyroidism in the newborn after cutaneous absorption of iodine, *Arch Dis Child* 53:495, 1978.
28. Chaiyakunapruk N, Veenstra DL, Lipsky BA, et al: Chlorhexidine compared with povidone-iodine solution for vascular catheter-site care: a meta-analysis, *Ann Intern Med* 136:792, 2002.
29. Chandavasu O, Garrow E, Valsa V, et al: A new method for the prevention of skin sloughs and necrosis secondary to intravenous infiltration, *Am J Perinatol* 3:4, 1986.
30. Choudhuri J, McQueen R, Inoue S, et al: Efficacy of skin sterilization for a venipuncture with the use of commercially available alcohol or iodine pads, *Am J Infect Control* 18:82, 1990.
31. Cowen J, Ellis S, McAinsh J: Absorption of chlorhexidine from the intact skin of newborn infants, *Arch Dis Child* 54:379, 1979.
32. Davies J, Babb J, Ayliffe A: The effect on the skin flora of bathing with antiseptic solutions, *J Antimicrob Chemother* 3:473, 1977.
33. Davies J, Gault D, Buchdahl R: Preventing the scars of neonatal intensive care, *Arch Dis Child Fetal Neonatal Ed* 70:F50, 1994.
34. Davis J, Leyden J, Grove G, et al: Comparison of disposable diapers with fluff absorbent and fluff plus absorbent polymers: effects on skin hydration, skin pH, and diaper dermatitis, *Pediatr Dermatol* 6:102, 1989.
35. Dixon A: Think zinc, *Neonatal Netw* 5:29, 1987.
36. Dollison E, Beckstrand J: Adhesive tape vs. pectin-based barrier use in preterm infants, *Neonatal Netw* 14:35, 1995.
37. Donlon CR, Furdon SA: Assessment of the umbilical cord outside of the delivery room, Part 2, *Adv Neonatal Care* 2:187, 2002.
38. Dore S, Buchan D, Coulas S, et al: Alcohol versus natural drying for newborn cord care, *J Obstet Gynecol Neonatal Nurs* 27:621, 1998.
39. Dykes PJ, Heggie R, Hill SA: Effects of adhesive dressings on the stratum corneum of the skin, *J Wound Care* 10:7, 2001.
40. Edwards W, Conner J, Soll R: The effect of prophylactic ointment therapy on nosocomial sepsis rates and skin integrity in infants of birth weights 501–1000 grams, *Pediatrics* 113:1195, 2004.
41. Evans N, Rutter N: Development of the epidermis in the newborn, *Biol Neonate* 49:74, 1986.
42. Evans N, Rutter N: Reduction of skin damage from transcutaneous oxygen electrodes using a spray on dressing, *Arch Dis Child* 61:881, 1986.
43. Fox C, Nelson D, Wareham J: The timing of skin acidification in very low birth weight infants, *J Perinatol* 18:272, 1998.
44. Friedman Z: Essential fatty acids revisited, *Am J Dis Child* 134:397, 1980.
45. Garland J, Buck R, Maloney P: Comparison of 10% povidone-iodine and 0.5% chlorhexidine gluconate for the prevention of peripheral intravenous catheter colonization in neonates: a prospective trial, *Pediatr Infect Dis J* 14:510, 1995.
46. Garvin G: Wound healing in pediatrics, *Nurs Clin North Am* 25:181, 1990.
47. Gault D: Extravasation injuries, *British J Plastic Surgery* 46:91, 1993.
48. Gfatter R, Hackl P, Braun F: Effects of soap and detergents on skin surface pH, stratum corneum hydration and fat content in infants, *Dermatology* 195:258, 1997.
49. Gordon C, Rowitch D, Mitchell M, et al: Topical iodine and neonatal hypothyroidism, *Arch Pediatr Adolesc Med* 149:1336, 1995.
50. Gotschall CS, Morrison M, Eichelberger M: Prospective, randomized study of the efficacy of Mepitel on children with partial-thickness scalds, *J Burn Care Rehabil* 19:279, 1998.

51. Grove G, Leydon J: *Comparison of the skin protectant properties of various film-forming products,* Broomall, Pa, 1993, Skin Study Center, KLG.
52. Harpin V, Rutter N: Barrier properties of the newborn infant's skin, *J Pediatr* 102:419, 1983.
53. Haubrich K: Role of vernix caseosa in the neonate: potential application in the adult population, *AACN Clin Issues* 14:457, 2003.
54. Hoath S, Narendran V: Adhesives and emollients in the preterm infant, *Semin Neonatol* 5:112, 2000.
55. Hoath S, Pickins WL: The biology and role of vernix. In Hoath S, Maibach H, editors: *Neonatal skin: structure and function,* ed 2 New York, 2003, Marcel Dekker.
56. Holbrook KA: A histological comparison of infant and adult skin. In Maibach HI, Boisits EK, editors: *Neonatal skin: structure and function,* New York, 1982, Marcel Dekker.
57. Hunt C, Engel RR, Modler S, et al: Essential fatty acid deficiency in neonates: inability to reverse deficiency by topical applications of EFA-rich oil, *J Pediatr* 92:603, 1978.
58. Irving V: Reducing the risk of epidermal stripping in the neonatal population: an evaluation of an alcohol free barrier film, *J Neonatal Nurs* 7:5, 2001.
59. Ittman P, Bozynski ME: Toxic epidermal necrolysis in a newborn infant after exposure to adhesive remover, *J Perinatol* 13:476, 1993.
60. Jackson H, Sutherland R: Effect of povidone-iodine on neonatal thyroid function, *Lancet* 2:992, 1981.
61. Janssen PA, Selwood BL, Dobson SR, et al: To dye or not to dye: a randomized, clinical trial of a triple dye/alcohol regime versus dry cord care, *Pediatrics* 111:15, 2003.
62. Johnson J, Malachowshi N, Vosti K, et al: A sequential study of various modes of skin and umbilical care and the incidence of staphylococcal colonization and infection in the neonate, *Pediatrics* 58:354, 1976.
63. Kalia Y, Nonato L, Lund C, et al: Development of the skin barrier function in premature infants, *J Invest Dermatol* 111:320, 1998.
64. Karl D: The interactive newborn bath: using infant behavior to connect parents and newborns, *Am J Matern Child Nurs* 24:280, 1999.
65. Klaus MH, Fanaroff AA: *Yearbook of perinatal/neonatal medicine,* Chicago, 1987, Year Book.
66. Knauth A, Gordin M, McNelis W, et al: Semipermeable polyurethane membrane as an artificial skin for the premature neonate, *Pediatrics* 83:945, 1989.
67. Kopelman AE: Cutaneous absorption of hexachlorophene in low-birth-weight infants, *J Pediatr* 82:972, 1973.
68. Lane A, Drost S: Effects of repeated application of emollient cream to premature neonates' skin, *Pediatrics* 92:415, 1993.
69. Laurie S, Wilson K, Kernahan D, et al: Intravenous extravasation injuries: the effectiveness of hyaluronidase in their treatment, *Ann Plast Surg* 13:191, 1984.
70. Linder N, Davidovich N, Reichman B, et al: Topical iodine-containing antiseptics and subclinical hypothyroidism in preterm infants, *J Pediatr* 131:434, 1997.
71. Linder N, Prince S, Barzilai A, et al: Disinfection with 10% povidone-iodine versus 0.5% chlorhexidine gluconate in 70% isopropanol in the neonatal intensive care unit, *Acta Paediatr* 93:205, 2004.
72. Lo J, Oriba H, Maibach H, et al: Transepidermal potassium, ion, and water flux across delipidized and cellophane tape-stripped skin, *Dermatologica* 180:66, 1990.
73. Loomis C, Koss TM, Chu D, et al: Fetal skin development. In Eichenfield L, Frieden I, Esterly N, editors: *Neonatal dermatology,* ed 2 Philadelphia, 2008, Saunders.
74. Lund C: Prevention and management of infant skin breakdown, *Nurs Clin North Am* 34:907, 1999.
75. Lund C, Kuller J, Lane A, et al: Neonatal skin care: evaluation of the AWHONN/NANN research-based practice project on knowledge and skin care practices, *J Obstet Gynecol Neonatal Nurs* 30:30, 2001.
76. Lund C, Kuller JM, Tobin C, et al: Evaluation of a pectin-based barrier under tape to protect neonatal skin, *J Obstet Gynecol Neonatal Nurs* 15:39, 1986.
77. Lund C, Nonato L, Kuller J, et al: Disruption of barrier function in neonatal skin associated with adhesive removal, *J Pediatr* 131:367, 1997.
78. Lund C, Osborne J, Kuller J, et al: Neonatal skin care: clinical outcomes of the AWHONN/NANN evidence-based clinical practice guideline, *J Obstet Gynecol Neonatal Nurs* 30:41, 2001.
79. Lund CH, Osborne JW: Validity and reliability of the neonatal skin condition score, *J Obstet Gynecol Neonatal Nursing* 33:320, 2004.
80. Lund CH, Tucker J: Skin adhesion. In Hoath S, Maibach H, editors: *Neonatal skin: structure and function,* ed 2 New York, 2003, Marcel Dekker.
81. Maki D, Ringer M, Alvarado C: Prospective randomized trial of povidone-iodine, alcohol, and chlorhexidine for prevention of infection associated with central venous and arterial catheters, *Lancet* 338:339, 1991.
82. Malathi I, Millar MR, Leeming JP, et al: Skin disinfection in preterm infants, *Arch Dis Child* 69:312, 1993.
83. Mancini A, Sookdeo-Drost S, Madison K, et al: Semipermeable dressings improve epidermal barrier function in premature infants, *Pediatr Res* 36:306, 1994.

84. Manzini B, Ferdani G, Simonetti V, et al: Contact sensitization in children, *Pediatr Dermatol* 15:12, 1998.
85. Marks J, Belsito D, DeLeo V, et al: North American Contact Dermatitis Group: standard tray patch test results, *Am J Contact Derm* 6:160, 1995.
86. McLean S, Kirchoff KT, Kriynovich K, et al: Three methods of securing endotracheal tubes in neonates: a comparison, *Neonatal Netw* 11:17, 1992.
87. Medves JM, O'Brien B: The effect of bather and location of first bath on maintaining thermal stability in newborns, *J Obstet Gynecol Neonatal Nurs* 33:175, 2004.
88. Mimoz O, Karim A, Mercat A, et al: Chlorhexidine compared with povidone-iodine as skin preparation before blood culture, *Ann Intern Med* 131:834, 1999.
89. Mitchell I, Pollock JC, Jamieson MP, et al: Transcutaneous iodine absorption in infants undergoing cardiac operation, *Ann Thorac Surg* 52:1138, 1991.
90. Mize M, Vila-Coro A, Prager T: The relationship between postnatal skin maturation and electrical skin impedance, *Arch Dermatol* 125:647, 1989.
91. Moraille R, Pickens W, Visscher M, et al: A novel role for vernix caseosa as a skin cleanser, *Biol Neonate* 87:8, 2005.
92. Nonato L: *Evolution of skin barrier function in neonates*, Unpublished doctoral dissertation, UMI Publication No. AAT9827176, Berkeley, 1998, University of California.
93. Nopper A, Horii K, Sookdeo-Drost S, et al: Topical ointment therapy benefits premature infants, *J Pediatr* 128:660, 1996.
94. Parravicini E, Fontana C, Paterlini G, et al: Iodine, thyroid function, and very low birth weight infants, *Pediatrics* 98:730, 1996.
95. Penny-MacGillivray T: A newborn's first bath: when? *J Obstet Gynecol Neonatal Nurs* 25:481, 1996.
96. Peters K: Bathing premature infants: physiological and behavioral consequences, *Am J Crit Care* 7:90, 1998.
97. Pyati SP, Ramamurthy RS, Krauss MT, et al: Absorption of iodine in the neonate following topical use of povidone-iodine, *J Pediatr* 91:825, 1977.
98. Quinn D, Newton N, Piecuch R: Effect of less frequent bathing on premature infant skin, *J Obstet Gynecol Neonatal Nurs* 34:741, 2005.
99. Rasmussen J: Classification of diaper dermatitis: an overview, *Pediatrician* 14:6, 1987.
100. Raszka W, Kueser T, Smith F, et al: The use of hyaluronidase in the treatment of intravenous extravasation injuries, *J Perinatol* 10:146-149, 1990.
101. Reynolds PR, Banerjee S, Meek JH: Alcohol burns in extremely low birthweight infants: still occurring, *Arch Dis Child Fetal Neonatal Ed* 90:F10, 2005.
102. Rowen JL, Atkins JT, Levy ML, et al: Invasive fungal dermatitis in the < or = 1000-gram neonate, *Pediatrics* 95:682, 1995.
103. Saijo S, Tagami H: Dry skin of newborn infants: functional analysis of the stratum corneum, *Pediatr Dermatol* 8:155, 1991.
104. Sarkany I, Arnold L: The effect of single and repeated applications of hexachlorophene on the bacterial flora of the skin of the newborn, *Br J Dermatol* 82:261, 1970.
105. Schick JB, Milstein JM: Burn hazard of isopropyl alcohol in the neonate, *Pediatrics* 68:587, 1981.
106. Sedin G, Hammarund K, Nilsson GE, et al: Measurements of transepidermal water loss in newborn infants, *Clin Perinatol* 12:79, 1985.
107. Smerdely P, Lim A, Boyages SC, et al: Topical iodine-containing antiseptics and neonatal hypothyroidism in very-low-birth weight infants, *Lancet* 16:661, 1989.
108. Sprung P, Hou Z, Ladin D: Hydrogels and hydrocolloids: an objective product comparison, *Ostomy Wound Manage* 44:36, 1998.
109. Taquino L: Promoting wound healing in the neonatal setting: process vs. protocol, *J Perinat Neonatal Nurs* 14:104, 2000.
110. Thomas S, Hay P: Fluid handling properties of hydrogel dressings, *Ostomy Wound Manage* 41:54, 1995.
111. Thomas S, Rowe HN, Keats J, et al: The management of extravasation injury in neonates, World Wide Wounds, *Elect J Wound Heal Manage*. www.smtl.co.uk. Accessed September 9, 2009, 1997.
112. 3M Health Care: *3M Cavilon No Sting Barrier Film (brochure)*, St Paul, Minn, 2001, 3M Company.
113. Tollin M, Bersson G, Kai-Larsen Y, et al: Vernix caseosa as a multi-component defense system based on polypeptides, lipids and their interactions, *Cell Mol Life Sci* 62:2390, 2005.
114. Tupker RA, Pinnagoda J, Coenraads PJ, et al: Evaluation of detergent-induced irritant skin reactions by visual scoring and transepidermal water loss measurement, *Dermatol Clin* 8:33, 1990.
115. Tupker RA, Pinnagoda J, Nater JP: The transient and cumulative effect of sodium lauryl sulphate on the epidermal barrier assessed by transepidermal water loss: inter-individual variation, *Acta Derm Venereol* 70:1, 1990.
116. Varda K, Behnke R: The effect of timing of initial bath on newborn's temperature, *J Obstet Gynecol Neonatal Nurs* 29:27, 2000.
117. Vernon H, Lane AT, Wischerath LJ, et al: Semipermeable dressing and transepidermal water loss in premature infants, *Pediatrics* 86:357, 1990.
118. Visscher MO: Recent advances in diaper dermatitis: etiology and treatment, *Pediatric Health* 3:81, 2009.
119. Visscher MO: Update on the use of topical agents in neonates, *Newborn Infant Nurs Rev* 9:31, 2009.
120. Visscher M, Narendran V, Pickens W, et al: Vernix caseosa in neonatal adaptation, *J Perinatol* 25:440, 2005.

121. Visscher MO, Chatterjee R, Munson KA, et al: Changes in diapered and nondiapered infant skin over the first month of life, *Pediatr Dermatol* 17:45, 2000.
122. Wilhelm K, Maibach H: Factors predisposing to cutaneous irritation, *Dermatol Clin* 8:17, 1990.
123. Yosipovitch G, Maayan-Metzger A, Merlob PP, et al: Skin barrier properties in different body areas in neonates, *Pediatrics* 106:105, 2000.
124. Zenk K: Management of intravenous extravasations, *Infusion* 5:77, 1981.
125. Zenk K, Sills J: Management of dopamine-induced perivascular blanching and extravasation in LBW infants, *J Perinatol* 6:82, 1986.
126. Zimmerman A: Acrodermatitis in breast-fed premature infants: evidence for a defect in mammary gland zinc secretion, *Pediatrics* 69:176, 1982.
127. Zlotkin S, Buchanan B: Meeting zinc and copper intake requirements in the parenterally fed preterm and full-term infant, *J Pediatr* 103:441, 1983.
128. Zupan J, Garner P, Omari AA: Topical umbilical cord care at birth, *Cochrane Database Syst Rev* 3: CD001057, 2004.

20 NEWBORN HEMATOLOGY

MARILYN MANCO-JOHNSON, DONNA J. RODDEN, AND TARU HAYS

RED BLOOD CELLS

Physiology

Red blood cells transport and deliver oxygen to vital organs and body tissues. Red blood corpuscles are simple cells composed of membrane encasing hemoglobin with an energy system to fuel the cells. Hemoglobin is the protein in red cells that carries oxygen, binding and releasing it based on concentration differences. Ex utero, red cells absorb oxygen by diffusion in the lungs, where the oxygen tension of the alveolar air is higher than that of the capillary blood, and release it from the systemic capillaries, where the oxygen tension is now higher than that of surrounding tissues. In utero, oxygen diffuses to the fetus from the placental venous circulation. Fetal red cells contain a unique hemoglobin (fetal hemoglobin) in which the two beta chains of adult hemoglobin (called ***hemoglobin A_1***) are replaced by two gamma chains. ***Fetal hemoglobin*** (called ***hemoglobin F***) has a higher affinity for oxygen than does adult hemoglobin, allowing fetal red cells to compete successfully for available oxygen. Normal fetal red cells are characterized by an increased mean corpuscular hemoglobin (MCH), mean corpuscular volume (MCV), hemoglobin, and hematocrit. After birth, with the transition to air breathing and a higher blood oxygen tension, the hypoxic stimulus driving fetal red cell production in the bone marrow is removed. The plasma concentration of erythropoietin, the hormone that stimulates bone marrow production of red blood cells, falls. The number of circulating reticulocytes, which are young red blood cells in the circulation, decreases. Subsequently, the hemoglobin and hematocrit diminish until a new equilibrium is reached. Postnatal changes in red cell production include an increase in the ratio of hemoglobin A to hemoglobin F and an increase in levels of the red cell enzyme 2,3-diphosphoglycerate (2,3-DPG). 2,3-DPG promotes the release of oxygen to tissues by decreasing hemoglobin affinity to oxygen within tissues. Oxygen delivery in the neonate is enhanced by increases in the concentrations of hemoglobin A and red cell concentration of 2,3-DPG.

The production of hematopoietic cells is first seen within the yolk sac in the 14-day embryo and disappears by the eleventh week of gestation.[15] Hematopoiesis in other tissues results from colonization by stem cells derived from the yolk sac.[7] By the fifth to sixth week, embryonic erythropoietic activity is present in the liver. The liver becomes the primary source of red cell production by 8 to 9 weeks.[10] Between the eighth and twelfth weeks, the spleen and lymph nodes are involved in erythropoiesis.[13] Other tissues and organs involved in erythropoiesis include the kidney, thymus, and connective tissue. Erythropoiesis is found in the bone marrow at 10 to 11 weeks. This activity increases rapidly until the twenty-fourth week, when bone marrow erythropoiesis replaces liver erythropoiesis. There is no evidence of erythropoietin production before the tenth week.[49] After the tenth week of gestation, erythropoietin production rises and appears to stimulate red cell production in the bone marrow during the third trimester.[14] Initially, production of erythropoietin is in the fetal liver, and by the last trimester, production is in the kidneys. The level of erythropoietin gradually rises to significant levels after the thirty-fourth

Please note that the **PURPLE** type in each chapter is intended to make it easier to identify clinically applicable material.

week of gestation.[13] Elevated erythropoietin levels can be found when the fetus is hypoxic.[10]

In more than 90% of healthy term infants, the hematocrit range is 48% to 60% and the hemoglobin range is 16 to 20 g/dL.[13] Changes in the blood count at the time of birth are shown in Table 20-1.[11,13] Normally after a term birth, hemoglobin concentrations fall from a mean of 17 g/dL to approximately 11 g/dL by 2 to 3 months of age. This nadir in red blood cell values is called ***physiologic anemia of the newborn*** and is a normal process in the adaptation to extrauterine life.

Several factors should be considered in the interpretation of hematocrit values in the newborn, including age of the infant (both in hours and in days), site of blood collection, and method of analysis. **Hematocrit changes significantly during the first 24 hours of life; it peaks at 2 hours of age and then progressively drops, with decreases determined at 6 and 24 hours of age.**[42] The method used to determine hematocrit can significantly affect the value. Capillary hematocrit measurements are highly subject to variations in blood flow; **hematocrit results generally are highest in capillary blood, intermediate in venous blood, and lowest in arterial samples.**[24,32,45] **Prewarming the site minimizes the artifactual increase in the hematocrit.** When obtaining blood counts, note that in both term and preterm infants, the hematocrit obtained from a capillary puncture (commonly termed ***heel stick***) can differ as much as 20% from the hematocrit of blood drawn from a central vein.

Adult red cells circulate for an average of 120 days. **Normal neonatal red blood cells have a circulating half-life reduction of 20% to 25% compared with the red blood cells of older children or adults. Survival of red cells of premature infants is reduced by approximately 50%.**

TABLE 20-1 CHANGES IN ERYTHROPOIESIS AROUND THE TIME OF TERM BIRTH

	IN UTERO	POSTDELIVERY
Oxygen saturation (%)	45*	95
Erythropoietin levels	High	Undetectable
Red cell production	Rapid	<10% (by day 7)
Reticulocyte count (%)	3-7	0-1 (by day 7)
Hemoglobin (g/dL)	16.8	18.4
Hematocrit (%)	53	58
MCV (fL)	107	98 (by day 7)
MCHC (g/dL)	31.7	33 (by day 7)

MCHC, Mean corpuscular hemoglobin concentration; *MCV*, mean corpuscular volume.
*Mean values represented.

Pathophysiology of Anemia

Anemia is a deficiency in the concentration of red cells and hemoglobin in the blood and results in tissue hypoxia and acidosis. Anemia is defined by a hemoglobin or hematocrit value that is greater than two standard deviations below the mean for post-conceptual and postnatal age.

Determination of the cause of anemia is important to direct treatment. Anemia in the newborn results from one or more of the following basic mechanisms:

- Blood loss (acute or chronic)
- Decreased red cell production
- Shortened red cell survival

BLOOD LOSS

Acute blood loss and chronic blood loss are the most common causes of anemia in the neonate. Blood loss can occur in utero, perinatally, or postnatally. Some degree of fetomaternal blood mixing occurs in 50% of all pregnancies.[11] Blood loss usually is insignificant; however, in 1% of pregnancies, blood loss is greater than 40 mL.[11] The blood volume of the fetus is approximately 90 mL/kg. Large blood loss can cause profound asphyxia and death; determination of profound drop in hemoglobin and hematocrit may lag by hours when blood volume is equilibrated. Anemia caused by chronic blood loss is better tolerated, because the neonate is able to compensate for the gradual loss in red cell mass. There is a large differential for blood loss in the neonate (Box 20-1).

Fetomaternal transfusion is a common cause of occult blood loss in the fetus. **The Kleihauer-Betke acid elution test is the method used to confirm the presence of fetal blood cells in the maternal circulation.**[48] Fetal cells retain red staining of hemoglobin after fixing, whereas adult cells (also called ***ghost cells***) are very pale because hemoglobin has been eluted. The volume of fetal blood in the maternal circulation is estimated by counting fetal red cells on the maternal blood smear under light microscopy. Ten fetal cells per 30 fields viewed under high power are equal to 1 mL of fetal blood.

Twin-to-twin transfusion is another cause of occult blood loss and is seen in 15% to 30% of all monochorionic twins with abnormalities of placental blood vessels.[43] The anemic twin is on the arterial side of the placental vascular malformation. The clinical significance of twin-to-twin transfusion depends on the duration of blood transfer. With chronic transfusion, a 20% weight discordance similar to that observed with placental insufficiency can be found.[34] Intracranial bleeding associated with prematurity, later birth order of a multiple-gestation delivery, rapid delivery, breech delivery, and massive cephalhematoma can cause anemia. Other forms of neonatal hemorrhage include umbilical, retroperitoneal, adrenal, renal, and gastrointestinal (GI) bleeding, as well as ruptured liver or spleen.

Swallowed maternal blood may be confused with GI bleeding. **The Apt test is used to distinguish swallowed maternal blood from neonatal blood** and is based on alkali resistance of fetal hemoglobin.[2] A 1% solution of sodium hydroxide is added to 5 mL of diluted blood. Fetal hemoglobin remains pink, but adult hemoglobin becomes yellow.

Iatrogenic blood loss results from blood sampling with inadequate replacement. A survey performed in the intensive care nursery of the University of California at San Francisco found that an average of 38.9 mL of blood was removed for laboratory tests during the first week of life.[39] For premature infants, whose blood volume can be as little as 50 mL, anemia is commonly caused by blood draws. **The majority of red cell transfusions given in nurseries are directly related to frequent blood sampling.**[32]

DECREASED RED CELL PRODUCTION

Anemia caused by decreased production of red cells tends to develop slowly, allowing time for physiologic compensation. Affected infants may have few signs of anemia other than pallor. The reticulocyte count will be low and inappropriate for the degree of anemia.

Worldwide, iron deficiency is the leading cause of anemia in infancy and childhood.

BOX 20-1 CAUSES OF BLOOD LOSS IN THE NEONATE

1. Hemorrhage before birth
   a. Fetomaternal
      - Traumatic amniocentesis or periumbilical blood sampling
      - Spontaneous
      - Chronic gastrointestinal bleeding
      - Blunt trauma to the maternal abdomen
      - Postexternal positioning
   b. Twin-to-twin
   c. External
      - Abruptio placentae
      - Placenta previa
2. Hemorrhage during birth
   a. Placental malformation
      - Chorangioma
      - Chorangiocarcinoma
   b. Hematoma of the cord or placenta
   c. Rupture of a normal umbilical cord
      - Precipitous delivery
      - Entanglement
   d. Rupture of an abnormal umbilical cord
      - Varices
      - Aneurysm
   e. Rupture of anomalous vessels
      - Aberrant vessel
      - Velamentous insertion of the cord
      - Communicating vessels in the multilobular placenta
   f. Incision of placenta during cesarean section
3. Internal fetal or neonatal hemorrhage
   a. Intracranial
   b. Giant cephalohematoma, caput succedaneum
   c. Pulmonary
   d. Retroperitoneum
   e. Subcapsular liver or spleen
   f. Renal or adrenal
4. External neonatal hemorrhage
   a. Delayed clamping of the umbilical cord
   b. Gastrointestinal
   c. Iatrogenic from blood sampling

Modified from Luchtman-Jones L, Schwartz A, Wilson D: Hematologic problems in the fetus and neonate. In Fanaroff A, editor: *Neonatal-perinatal medicine: diseases of the fetus and infant,* vol 2, St Louis, 1997, Mosby.

Iron-deficiency anemia can occur at any time when growth exceeds the ability of the stores and dietary intake to supply sufficient iron for erythropoiesis. Iron storage at birth is directly related to body weight. **Typically, infants are born with iron stores sufficient to support new red blood cell (RBC) production until they double their birth weight.**[33] Infants who are fed exclusively breast milk or iron-enriched formula and cereal are less likely to develop iron-deficiency anemia.

Premature infants have iron stores adequate for less than 3 months postnatally because of low birth weight, faster rate of growth, and iatrogenic blood losses. **Iron supplementation is necessary early in preterm infants to prevent anemia (Table 20-2).**

Iron deficiency causes a hypochromic, microcytic anemia. The peripheral smear shows small, pale red cells with a large variety of shapes and sizes resulting in an increased relative distribution of width (RDW). The platelet count is increased and may be greater than 1,000,000/mcL. Mild forms of iron deficiency may be confused with other causes of anemia, including infection and thalassemia. A therapeutic trial of iron can be used to diagnose iron deficiency.

Anemia of prematurity is common in infants born at less than 35 weeks' gestation. This is a normocytic, normochromic anemia appearing between 2 and 6 weeks characterized by a low reticulocyte count and an inadequate response to erythropoietin.[40] **If hemoglobin levels drop below 10 g/dL, the infant may display decreased activity, poor growth, tachypnea, and tachycardia.** Randomized placebo-controlled studies demonstrate that preterm infants can respond to erythropoietin with decreased amount of blood transfused if they are also supplemented with iron.[31] Because preterm infants currently receive fewer red cell transfusions compared with the past two decades, they are at increased risk for iron deficiency. Although the **Academy of Pediatrics recommends 2 to 4 mg/kg/day elemental iron for preterm infants and 4 to 6 mg/kg/day for preterm infants receiving concomitant erythropoietin,** higher doses for prevention of iron deficiency may be associated with improved outcomes.[22]

TABLE 20-2 RECOMMENDED IRON SUPPLEMENTATION FOR THE NEONATE

GROUP	DOSE (mg/kg/day)	INITIATION, DURATION
Full term	1	4 mo to 3 yr
Preterm, low birth weight	2 1	2 mo to 1 yr, then 1 yr to 3 yr
Very low birth weight	4 1	2 mo to 1 yr, then 1 yr to 3 yr

Hypothyroidism, deficiency of transcobalamin II, and inborn errors of cobalamin utilization cause macrocytic anemia because of decreased and ineffective bone marrow production.

Constitutional pure red cell aplasia is also known as ***Diamond-Blackfan anemia.***[25] Diamond-Blackfan anemia is caused by more than 200 unique mutations in ribosomal protein genes.[6] This normocytic or macrocytic anemia manifests at birth in 10% and by 1 month in 25% of affected infants. Signs and symptoms include pallor, anemia, and reticulocytopenia. In red cell aplasia, the platelet count may be moderately elevated and the leukocyte count may be slightly decreased. Bone marrow examination is normocellular with few erythroid precursors. Thirty percent of affected infants demonstrate congenital anomalies, primarily of the head, face, eyes, and thumbs. The syndrome can have autosomal dominant or recessive inheritance. As infants grow older, characteristics of fetal erythropoiesis persist, including elevations in fetal hemoglobin, *i* antigen, and red cell adenosine deaminase (ADA), as well as fetal patterns of red cell enzymes. Of affected infants, 70% respond to corticosteroid therapy, particularly if treatment is initiated early in infancy. Infants who do not respond to steroids require long-term red cell transfusion therapy and are at risk for subsequent iron overload. In Diamond-Blackfan anemia, the erythrocyte progenitors do not respond to erythropoietin but often respond to stem cell factor and, to a lesser degree, interleukin-3.

Fanconi's anemia is a congenital syndrome of progressive bone marrow failure with autosomal recessive inheritance.[1] At birth, infants may be recognized by one or more of the associated congenital defects, which include microcephaly, short stature, absent or abnormal thumb, and other cutaneous, musculoskeletal, and urogenital abnormalities. Thrombocytopenia and an elevated MCV usually are the first hematologic abnormalities, but they are seldom recognized in the neonatal period. The underlying defect in

Fanconi's anemia is an inability to repair damaged deoxyribonucleic acid (DNA). Chromosomal breakage analyses and specific molecular diagnosis have been used for prenatal diagnosis. Diamond-Blackfan and Fanconi's anemias have been successfully treated with bone marrow transplantation.

Infants with genetic hemoglobin mutations of alpha or gamma chains that result in production of hemoglobins with decreased oxygen affinity will have lower hemoglobins without signs of tissue hypoxia.

B19 parvovirus exerts an inhibitory effect on bone marrow production of red cells.[47] Infection with B19 parvovirus during pregnancy can cause hydrops fetalis, the clinical syndrome caused by severe intrauterine anemia of any cause and consisting of congestive heart failure, massive skin edema, and intrauterine demise, especially during the first two trimesters. Early detection of parvovirus infection in pregnant women and serial examinations with ultrasonography are important to diagnose and monitor the condition. Affected fetuses have been supported successfully with intrauterine transfusions of red blood cells. Postnatal infection with parvovirus does not cause anemia in most infants unless they have preexisting shortened red cell survival. Infants with congenital or acquired immunodeficiency may become anemic because of an inability to clear parvovirus.

SHORTENED RED CELL SURVIVAL

Senescent red cells are removed from the circulation by the reticuloendothelial system. Bilirubin is produced by degradation of the heme moiety of hemoglobin, and red cell iron is recycled. Many conditions accelerate removal of red cells from the circulation. ***Hemolysis*** is a term for red cell destruction that is premature in terms of expected life span of the red cells relative to post-conceptual age. Hyperbilirubinemia is evident in most cases of hemolysis. Reticulocytosis is usually found. However, in the presence of chronic illness, nutritional deficiency, or congenital infection, the reticulocyte count may be lower than expected for the degree of anemia. In the most severe cases of intrauterine hemolysis, the outcome is hydrops fetalis (Box 20-2).

BOX 20-2 CAUSES OF SHORTENED RED CELL SURVIVAL IN THE NEONATE

1. Isoimmune-mediated hemolysis
   a. Rh incompatibility
   b. ABO incompatibility
   c. Minor blood cell antigen incompatibility
2. Infection
   a. Bacterial sepsis
   b. *Campylobacter jejuni*
   c. *Clostridium welchii*
   d. Rubella
   e. Cytomegalovirus
   f. Epstein-Barr virus
   g. Disseminated herpes
   h. Malaria
   i. Toxoplasmosis
   j. Syphilis
3. Microangiopathic and macroangiopathic
   a. Cavernous hemangioma (Kasabach-Merritt)
   b. Renal vein thrombosis
   c. Disseminated intravascular coagulation
   d. Severe coarctation of the aorta
   e. Renal artery stenosis
4. Vitamin E deficiency
5. Congenital red cell membrane disorders
   a. Hereditary spherocytosis
   b. Hereditary elliptocytosis
      Hereditary poikilocytosis
      Hereditary pyropoikilocytosis
      Hereditary stomatocytosis
   c. Infantile pyknocytosis
6. Congenital red cell enzyme disorders
   a. Glucose-6-phosphate-dehydrogenase deficiency
   b. Pyruvate kinase deficiency
7. Congenital hemoglobinopathies
   a. Alpha and gamma chain defects including thalassemias; structural abnormalities; unstable hemoglobin
8. Metabolic disorders
   a. Galactosemia
   b. Organic aciduria; orotic aciduria
   c. Prolonged or recurrent acidosis
9. Liver disease

Isoimmune hemolytic anemia occurs when fetal cells, bearing antigens of paternal origin that the mother does not possess, enter the maternal circulation and stimulate production of IgG antibodies. The IgG antibodies are transferred across the placenta, coat fetal red cells, and mediate their removal from the circulation through the reticuloendothelial system.

The major fetal red cell antigens responsible for isoimmune hemolytic anemia include the Rh (also called *D*) antigen in an Rh-negative mother and the blood group A and blood group B antigens in a group O mother. Kell, Duffy, and Kidd antigens can also cause isoimmune hemolytic anemia. Sources of maternal sensitization to fetal red cell antigens include chorionic villus sampling, amniocentesis, abortion, rupture of an ectopic pregnancy, maternal blood transfusion, and fetomaternal transfusion. Anti-Rh antibodies derived from plasma of previously sensitized donors are given to Rh-negative mothers at 28 weeks' gestation, at delivery, and at the time of any of the previously mentioned events. These antibodies coat any fetal red cells present in the maternal circulation and prevent them from initiating the maternal immune response. Thus they provide a form of passive immunization. With widespread use of Rh immunoglobulin (Ig) in Rh-negative mothers, the rate of anti-Rh Ig formation dropped from 17% to 9%-13%.[3,46] The rate of Rh hemolytic disease in the United States is 1 case per 1000 live births.[9] The persistence of Rh isoimmunization may be attributed to failures in administering Rh Ig to all women at risk and incorrect dosing. Women who receive no prenatal care and women who develop silent antenatal sensitization compose two populations that are difficult to reach with prevention strategies.

ABO hemolytic anemia is more common than Rh hemolytic disease but less severe. Unlike Rh disease, hemolysis secondary to ABO incompatibility can occur during the first pregnancy because A and B antigens are ubiquitous in foods and bacteria, causing sensitization. Most isoimmune hemolytic diseases that are not related to ABO or Rh incompatibility are caused by sensitization to minor blood group antigens Kell, Duffy, Lewis, Kidd, M, or S. Mothers should be screened at 34 weeks for antibodies to these minor blood group antigens.

Congenital bacterial and viral infections may cause hemolytic anemia and bone marrow suppression with reticulocytopenia. Microspherocytes may be very prominent.

Microangiopathies and macroangiopathies are characterized by red cell fragmentation, shortened red cell survival, and thrombocytopenia. Coagulation proteins are also consumed in cavernous hemangiomas and disseminated intravascular coagulation (DIC).

Vitamin E is a fat-soluble vitamin that functions as an antioxidant. Deficiency of vitamin E manifests with hemolytic anemia, reticulocytosis, thrombocytosis, and edema of the lower extremities.[40] Diets high in polyunsaturated fatty acids and iron increase requirements for vitamin E. With current supplementation of infant formulas and parenteral nutrition with vitamin E, prevention of vitamin E deficiency using a water-soluble form of tocopherol is not currently necessary.

Shortened red cell survival secondary to an intrinsic red cell defect is a rare but important cause of shortened red cell survival in the neonate. Because even normal neonates have shortened red cell survival and hyperbilirubinemia, the presentation of these syndromes in the neonate often is more severe than in older affected family members. Affected infants usually present with anemia and hyperbilirubinemia. Splenomegaly develops later in infancy or early childhood. A preliminary diagnosis of constitutional red cell defect is made by family history and careful inspection of the peripheral smear. Abnormalities of red cell shape, including spherocytes, elliptocytes, pyknocytes, "bite cells," target cells, and other bizarre morphologic structures, are often characteristic of the specific red cell defect.

Constitutional defects in red cell membranes cause lifelong hemolytic anemia. ***Hereditary spherocytosis*** is the most common red cell membrane defect and usually is inherited as an autosomal dominant trait. Pyropoikilocytosis, an infantile form of the mild membrane defect ***hereditary elliptocytosis,*** is characterized by striking red cell pyknocytes and fragments on peripheral smear with evidence of mild hemolysis. Typical elliptocytes may not become apparent until a few months of life.

Glucose-6-phosphate dehydrogenase (G6PD) is the first rate-limiting enzyme in the pentose phosphate pathway of red cell energy metabolism. This enzyme is important in the production of nicotinamide adenine dinucleotide phosphate (NADPH), which maintains cellular systems in a reduced state. **G6PD deficiency is the most common inherited disorder of red blood cells** and is transmitted as an X-linked recessive trait. There are many isoforms of

BOX 20-3 SOME AGENTS REPORTED TO PRODUCE HEMOLYSIS IN PATIENTS WITH G6PD DEFICIENCY

Drugs and Chemicals Clearly Shown to Cause Clinically Significant Hemolytic Anemia in G6PD Deficiency

Acetanilid
Methylene blue
Nalidixic acid (NegGram)
Naphthalene
Niridazole (Ambilhar)
Phenylhydrazine
Primaquine
Pamaquine
Pentaquine
Sulfanilamide
Sulfacetamide
Sulfapyridine
Sulfamethoxazole (Gantanol)
Thiazolsulfone
Toluidine blue
Trinitrotoluene

Drugs Probably Safe in Normal Therapeutic Doses for G6PD-Deficient Individuals (Without Nonspherocytic Hemolytic Anemia)

Acetaminophen (Paracetamol, Tylenol, Tralgon, Hydroxyacetanillid)
Acetophenetidine (Phenacetin)
Acetylsalicylic acid (aspirin)
Aminopyrine (Pyramidon, Amidopyrine)
Antazoline (Antistine)
Antipyrine
Ascorbic acid (Vitamin C)
Benzhexol (Artane)
Chloramphenicol
Chlorguanidine (Proguanil, Paludrine)
Chloroquine
Colchicine
Diphenhydramine (Benadryl)
L-Dopa
Menadione sodium bisulfite (Hykinone)
Menaphthone
p-Aminobenzoic acid
Phenylbutazone
Phenytoin
Probenecid (Benemid)
Procaine amide hydrochloride (Pronestyl)
Pyrimethamine (Daraprim)
Quinidine
Quinine
Streptomycin
Sulfacytine
Sulfadiazine
Sulfaguanidine
Sulfamerazine
Sulfamethoxypyridazine (Kynex)
Sulfisoxazole (Gantrisin)
Trimethoprim
Tripelennamine (Pyribenzamine)
Vitamin K

From Beutler E: *Hemolytic anemia in disorders of red cell metabolism,* New York, 1978, Plenum.
G6PD, Glucose-6-phosphate dehydrogenase.

abnormal G6PD enzymes. The Mediterranean type produces severe hemolysis, whereas the form found in blacks usually is mild. Infants are asymptomatic until challenged with oxidant stresses from infections or drugs. Agents associated with hemolysis in G6PD-deficient infants are shown in Box 20-3.

Hemoglobinopathies are inherited disorders resulting from gene mutations that affect the quantity or quality of hemoglobin chains. The clinical expression of a hemoglobinopathy depends on the affected globin chain, the developmental stage of globin synthesis, and the amount and function of alternate hemoglobins. Hemoglobinopathies presenting at birth affect either the alpha or gamma chain of hemoglobin.[21] Hemoglobin beta chains are not produced until 3 months of postnatal age; therefore defects of beta chains, such as sickle cell anemia and beta thalassemia, do not present in the nursery. The ***thalassemias*** are disorders manifested by absence or decrease of specific globin proteins. Because four genes control alpha globin synthesis, clinical presentations may range from asymptomatic (one alpha hemoglobin gene deletion) to abnormalities incompatible with life (absence of production from all four alpha hemoglobin genes). Most infants with moderate to severe anemia related to alpha thalassemia have a three-gene deletion. Alpha globin is an essential component of both hemoglobin F and hemoglobin A. In alpha thalassemia, compensatory hemoglobins include hemoglobin Barts in the neonatal period, which is composed of four gamma chains, and later, hemoglobin H, which is composed of four beta chains.[44] In Western societies, the incidence of new births with severe thalassemia syndromes has declined dramatically because of the widespread use of molecular diagnostic techniques by couples at risk.

Methemoglobin contains an oxidized form of heme iron, Fe^{3+}, which renders it incapable of reversible binding to oxygen. Constitutional methemoglobinemia presenting in the neonatal period is caused either by deficiency of the red cell enzyme ***methemoglobin reductase*** or by an M hemoglobinopathy of the gamma chain of hemoglobin. Infants

Critical Findings

SIGNS AND SYMPTOMS OF ANEMIA IN THE NEONATE

1. Acute anemia (with hemorrhage, anemia may not be present initially; hemodilution develops over 3 to 4 hours)
   a. Hypovolemia, hypotension
   b. Hypoxemia, tachypnea
   c. Tachycardia
2. Chronic anemia (may be well compensated)
   a. Pallor, metabolic acidosis, poor growth
   b. High-output congestive heart failure
   c. Persistent or increased oxygen requirement
   d. Iron deficiency with hypochromia, microcytosis

with either of these disorders present with cyanosis of the skin and mucous membranes but are otherwise usually asymptomatic. **Acquired methemoglobinemia can be life threatening because of severe hypoxemia.** Normal newborn infants are susceptible to acquired methemoglobinemia from oxidative stresses because neonatal red blood cells contain lower levels of the enzyme ***NADH-methemoglobin reductase.***

Data Collection

HISTORY

Information obtained should include maternal history of illness and dietary intake during pregnancy, delivery type, hemorrhage, transfusion or iron therapy, and any abnormal occurrences during birth. A careful family history includes specific questioning about anemia, iron or transfusion therapy, pallor, jaundice, splenomegaly, splenectomy, gallstones, cholecystectomy, or congenital malformations in the parents, grandparents, siblings, aunts, uncles, and cousins of the infant.

SIGNS AND SYMPTOMS

In performing a physical examination of a newborn with anemia, attention should be paid to the infant's cardiovascular function, general vigor, and signs of pallor, jaundice, skin lesions, hepatosplenomegaly, lymphadenopathy, and congenital malformations (see the Critical Findings box above).

LABORATORY DATA

The diagnosis of anemia is based on the hemoglobin and hematocrit compared with normal values established for post-conceptual and postnatal age. The peripheral blood smear should be carefully examined in all cases of abnormal hemoglobin and hematocrit, and the red cell indices should be evaluated. The characterization of anemia depends on additional laboratory testing (Table 20-3). A clinical decision tree in the evaluation of anemia is shown in Figure 20-1.

Treatment

If acute blood loss is suspected and the infant is pale and limp at birth, blood pressure should be obtained and monitored, perfusion assessed, intravenous (IV) fluids started at 20 mL/kg, and oxygen administered. A catheter should be inserted into the umbilical artery to measure blood gases. Blood should be obtained for complete blood count (CBC), reticulocyte count, Coombs' test, blood type, fractionated bilirubin, and serum screen for blood group antibodies. Because infants younger than 4 months rarely produce antibodies against blood group antigens, maternal serum can be used in the antibody screen.

Once the infant's condition stabilizes, a decision can be made about transfusion based on clinical status. **If the infant is anemic with signs of hypoxemia or has underlying pulmonary or cardiac disease, transfusion of 10 mL/kg of red blood cells over 2 to 3 hours may be given to increase oxygen-carrying capacity.** Normally, larger quantities of blood should not be given in one transfusion. Most blood banks in institutions with neonatal intensive care units have protocols for neonatal blood transfusion and will give leukodepleted, either type-specific or O-negative, un-crossmatched red cells if the antibody screen is negative. **Blood used for transfusion should be less than 7 days old and negative or reduced for cytomegalovirus (CMV).** Irradiation of red blood cells and other blood cell products to prevent graft-versus-host disease is recommended for intrauterine transfusions or neonatal exchange transfusion and for infants with congenital or acquired immunodeficiency. For infants with continuing hemorrhage requiring massive transfusion exceeding one blood volume, transfusions of fresh frozen plasma (FFP) are necessary to

TABLE 20-3 CHARACTERIZATION OF ANEMIA

CHARACTERIZATION	TEST
Blood loss	Kleihauer-Betke on maternal sample Apt test on gastric blood from infant as indicated
Bone marrow production	Reticulocyte count Platelet and white blood cell count Erythropoietin level T_3, T_4, TSH Bone marrow aspirate and biopsy Fetal hemoglobin iAg, MCV
Iron deficiency	Ferritin, iron, and iron-binding capacity
Antibody mediated	Maternal and infant blood type Direct and indirect Coombs' test
Hemolysis	Bilirubin Coagulation tests (if sepsis or liver disease is suspected) Osmotic fragility, specific determinations of red cell membrane proteins, enzymes, hemoglobin, and as indicated
Infection	Culture and serologies as appropriate
Microangiopathy, macroangiopathy	DIC screen
Vitamin E deficiency	Vitamin E level
Metabolic disorder	pH, lactate, pyruvate Galactosemia screen

DIC, Disseminated intravascular coagulation; *iAg*, i antigen; *MCV*, mean corpuscular volume; *TSH*, thyroid-stimulating hormone.

replace clotting factors and prevent the consumptive coagulopathy that results from massive transfusion of stored blood. Platelet transfusions also may be needed.

An order from a physician or nurse practitioner is necessary for any blood transfusion. Parental consent should be obtained by the physician before transfusion. In the neonatal intensive care nursery, a policy of **"double checking" blood is essential to ensure that the proper blood is being administered to the infant. Blood should be warmed and administered through a blood filter of 40 mcm or finer. Fresh blood can be administered through a 25-gauge needle without significant hemolysis.**

Directed donor programs are used in hospitals for nonemergent blood transfusions, especially in small preterm infants. In most cases, biologic parents are able to serve as directed donors for their neonates. Preparation of directed donations is more costly than standard blood units and does require the same time for testing. At this time, no scientific data suggest directed donor programs increase blood safety. Some immunologic incompatibilities may exist between maternal and paternal donors; therefore the following guidelines should be considered for parental donors[13]:

- Mothers should not provide blood components containing plasma. If maternal red cells are transfused, they should be washed.
- Fathers are not recommended as blood cell (red, white, or platelet) donors for their newborns unless maternal serum is shown to lack cytotoxic antibodies.
- All parental blood components should be irradiated before transfusion to the infant.

Equipment necessary for blood transfusion includes a filter, extension tubing, and a pump. Except in extreme emergencies, blood should be administered through a peripheral catheter rather than through an umbilical artery catheter (UAC).

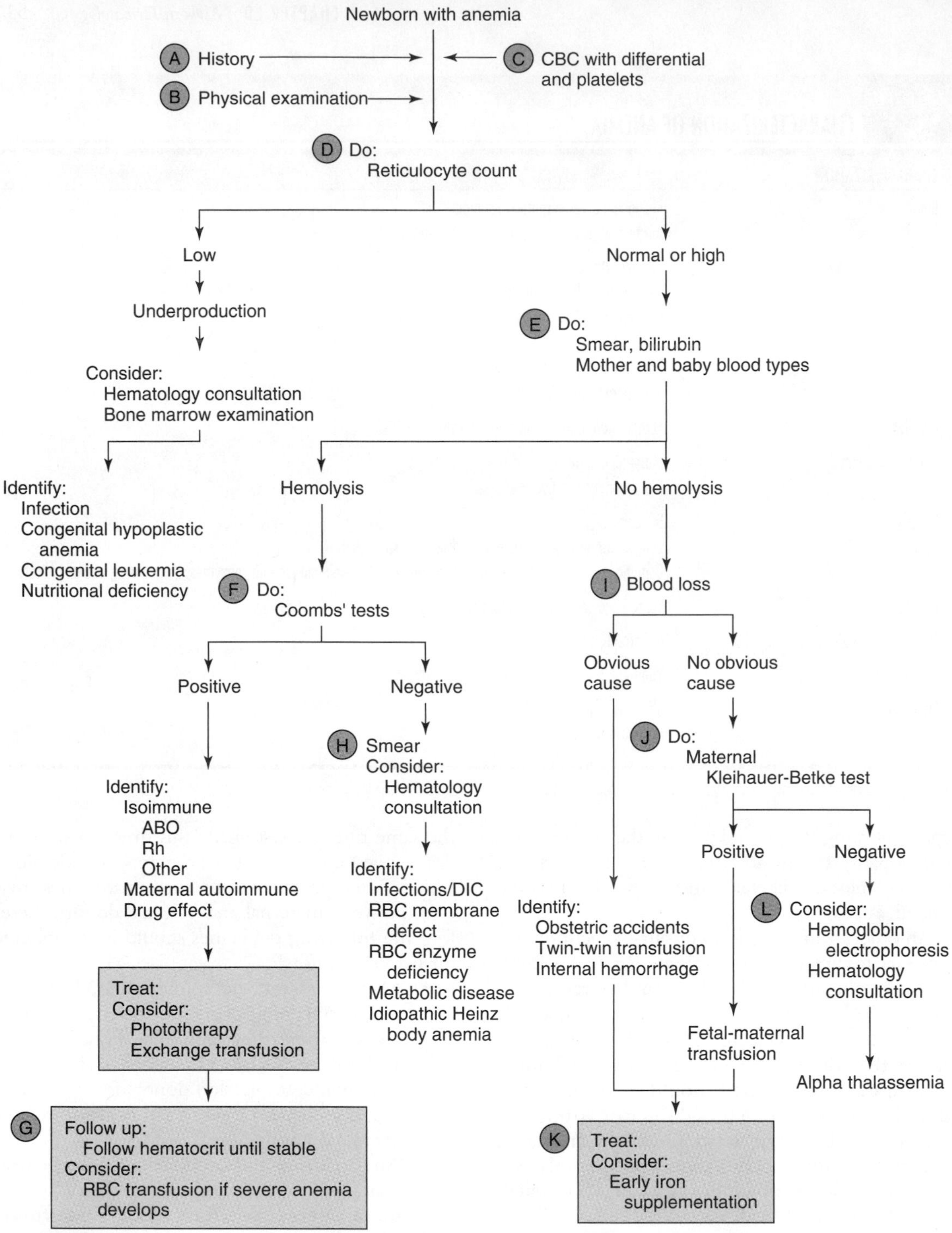

FIGURE 20-1 Clinical decision tree in evaluation of anemia. *CBC*, Complete blood count; *DIC*, disseminated intravascular coagulation; *RBC*, red blood cell. (From Lane PA, Nuss R: Anemia in the newborn. In Berman S, editor: *Pediatric decision making*, ed 3, St Louis, 1996, Mosby.)

A. In the history, document any prenatal infections or drug use. Also note any history of maternal vaginal bleeding, placenta previa, abruptio placentae, or umbilical cord rupture, constriction or velamentous insertion, as well as cesarean, breech, or traumatic delivery. Obtain a family history of neonatal jaundice, anemia, splenomegaly, and unexplained gallstones.

B. In the physical examination, note tachypnea, tachycardia, peripheral vasoconstriction (acute blood loss), and hepatosplenomegaly (chronic anemia, intrauterine infection, congenital malignancy). Jaundice appearing before 24 hours of age suggests significant hemolysis.

C. A hematocrit less than 45% during the first 3 days of life is abnormal and requires explanation. The mean corpuscular volume (MCV) at birth is normally above 95. An MCV below 95 suggests alpha thalassemia or chronic intrauterine blood loss (as with fetal maternal transfusion). Rarely, a low MCV may be seen with hemolytic disease caused by hereditary elliptocytosis or pyropoikilocytosis. The presence of neutropenia or thrombocytopenia suggests the possibility of infection. Except in an emergency, no anemic newborn should receive a blood transfusion before adequate diagnostic studies.

D. Normal reticulocyte values are 3% to 7% during the first day of life and 1% to 3% during the second and third days. A low reticulocyte count in the presence of significant anemia suggests bone marrow failure.

E. An indirect hyperbilirubinemia, abnormal peripheral blood smear, or ABO or Rh incompatibility between the mother and infant suggests hemolysis.

F. Perform direct and indirect Coombs' tests. ABO isoimmunization is usually associated with a negative direct and a positive indirect Coombs' test.

G. Infants with immune hemolysis have varying degrees of hemolysis, which may continue for 3 months. Severe, life-threatening anemia may develop in infants with Rh sensitization; such infants require close follow-up with serial hematocrit measurements until the hemolysis resolves.

H. Examine the peripheral blood smear. Spherocytes suggest ABO isoimmunization, hereditary spherocytosis, or infection (e.g., cytomegalovirus). Red cell fragmentation suggests intravascular hemolysis (infection, disseminated intravascular coagulation [DIC]). Consider infection or DIC in any ill newborn with hemolysis, particularly if thrombocytopenia is also present.

I. Review the obstetric history and examine the placenta for clues to the cause of fetal blood loss.

J. Perform a Kleihauer-Betke test to detect fetal red cells in the maternal circulation. False-negatives occur when an ABO incompatibility results in the rapid clearance of the infant's red cells from the maternal circulation.

K. Newborns with significant prenatal or perinatal blood loss are at risk for iron deficiency during the first 6 months of life.

L. Anemic infants without evidence of hemolysis or blood loss whose mothers have a negative Kleihauer-Betke test may have alpha thalassemia, especially if the MCV is below 95. Ethnic groups affected most often include South and Southeast Asians, Mediterraneans, and Africans. The diagnosis of alpha thalassemia may be confirmed with a hemoglobin electrophoresis that shows hemoglobin Barts.

REFERENCES

Ballin A, Brown EJ, Zipursky A: Idiopathic Heinz body hemolytic anemia in newborn infants, *Am J Pediatr Hematol Oncol* 11:3, 1989.

Blanchettte VS, Zipursky A: Assessment of anemia in newborn infants, *Clin Perinatol* 11:489, 1984.

Oski FA: Anemia in the neonatal period. In Oski FA, Naiman JL, editors: *Hematologic problems in the newborn*, ed 3, Philadelphia, 1982, Saunders.

Oski FA: The erythrocyte and its disorders. In Nathan DG, Oski FA, editors: *Hematology of infancy and childhood*, ed 4, Philadelphia, 1993, Saunders.

FIGURE 20-1 cont'd For legend, see opposite page.

It is essential to confirm that the unit of blood infused matches the typed blood bank form and assigned number, patient name, and patient hospital number. The expiration date and time must be respected. IV tubing used for blood transfusion should be flushed with 0.45% normal saline solution before it is used for infusing blood products.

Blood bags should not be used for longer than 4 to 6 hours after opening. Vital signs should be obtained and recorded every 15 minutes during blood transfusion. Careful observations should be made for reactions including increased temperature, diaphoresis, irregular respiration, bradycardia, restlessness, and pallor. Transfusions should be stopped promptly if any of these signs are present. All materials used for blood transfusion should be disposed of properly.

Infants who are anemic because of chronic blood loss or acute blood loss who do not require transfusion therapy should be **treated with iron replacement 6 mg/kg/day until the blood count is normal and for 2 additional months to replace stores.**

Infants who are born with isoimmune hemolytic anemia are often treated with exchange transfusion. In this procedure, catheters placed in central and peripheral veins are used to remove the infant's blood in small aliquots and replace it with packed red cells usually reconstituted with FFP. General guidelines for aliquot volumes are as follows:

- 3 kg (infant's weight): 20 mL per aliquot
- 2 kg (infant's weight): 15 mL per aliquot
- 1 kg (infant's weight): 5 mL per aliquot

Infants who are treated for isoimmune hemolytic anemia with intrauterine transfusions may be born with normal or near-normal hematocrit and bilirubin levels. Exchange transfusion is often used early after delivery to remove antibody and decrease postnatal hemolysis. Hyperbilirubinemia can be managed using phototherapy (see Chapter 21).

Prevention

Many forms of neonatal anemia are preventable. Improved fetal monitoring and obstetric care may prevent anemia caused by blood loss during delivery.

Administering Rh Ig to Rh-negative mothers within 72 hours of delivery of an Rh-positive infant prevents most cases of hydrops fetalis in subsequent pregnancies. For previously sensitized Rh-negative mothers carrying Rh-positive fetuses, amniocentesis performed between 20 and 22 weeks' gestation may allow for intrauterine transfusion of Rh-negative red blood cells and possible early delivery of a nonhydropic infant. For severe thalassemia syndromes and sickle cell anemia, prenatal diagnosis is possible. Intrauterine transfusions are also appropriate for infants with alpha-thalassemia major.

Hemolysis may be prevented in infants with significant G6PD deficiency by avoiding administration of drugs known to present an oxidative stress to the red cells.

Low-birth-weight premature infants are at high risk for late-onset anemia because of low endogenous production of erythropoietin, which is exacerbated by phlebotomy losses for laboratory surveillance. Inadequate nutrition and other factors also may play a significant role. **Recombinant human erythropoietin (r-HuEPO) has been successfully used to decrease the severity of anemia and lessen the use of blood transfusion in small premature infants.** Long-term risks are unknown but appear to be minimal. Benefits of therapy other than decreased exposure to blood transfusion are also unknown. Potential improvements in organ maturation or infant growth because of higher sustained levels of hemoglobin and improved neural development are speculative at present. The cost of a 6-week course of therapy with r-HuEPO is comparable in most institutions with that of conventional therapies with blood replacement.

Treatment with erythropoietin (EPO) should be considered in all infants of birth weight 800 to 1300 g. Infants with a birth weight of less than 800 g may receive so many transfusions early in their hospital course that treating with r-HuEPO may confer no substantial additional benefit. Infants with a birth weight of more than 1300 g rarely require blood transfusion.

Treatment with r-HuEPO can begin when infants are stable and can tolerate iron supplementation, usually when tolerating approximately 60% of caloric requirements by enteral feedings. **The recommended dose is 200 to 250 units/kg r-HuEPO given IV or subcutaneously (sub-Q), three times weekly.** The reticulocyte count should be monitored to document an adequate response. **Oral iron supplementation should be initiated at the time of therapy, beginning with 2 mg/kg/day of elemental iron and increasing to 6 mg/kg/day as tolerated.** A baseline hematocrit measurement and reticulocyte count should be obtained and followed weekly. Dosing should be adjusted to maintain a reticulocyte count above 6%. **Supplemental vitamin E, 15 to 25 international units/day, and folic acid, 100 mcg/kg/day, may be given at the start of therapy.** Treatment is continued for 6 weeks or until 36 weeks' post-conceptual age. Once treatment is discontinued, hematocrit levels should be monitored every other week until stable.[30,31]

The ***treatment of methemoglobinemia*** is methylene blue, 1 to 2 mg/kg given IV over 5 to 10 minutes, or orally; this therapy is ineffective in infants with deficient NADPH or G6PD, as well as M-hemoglobinopathies. Treatment of methemoglobinemia in G6PD-deficient infants consists of ascorbic acid, 200 to 500 mg/kg/day.[20,37]

POLYCYTHEMIA AND HYPERVISCOSITY

Physiology

Neonatal polycythemia is most commonly defined by a venous hematocrit greater than 65%.[17] Viscosity is related to but not identical to hematocrit. The viscosity of blood increases logarithmically in relation to the hematocrit.[26] Although viscosity may be measured directly, hematocrit is often used as an indicator of viscosity. Blood sampling at 12 hours postnatal age seems ideal to determine hematocrit and viscosity for diagnosis of polycythemic hyperviscosity.[45] **Capillary hematocrit can be used as a screening test, but a venous sample should be analyzed to confirm an abnormally high capillary hematocrit.**[24]

Pathophysiology

Hyperviscosity is a syndrome of circulatory impairment resulting from increased resistance to blood flow. Complications of polycythemia and hyperviscosity include respiratory distress, congestive heart failure, hypoglycemia, hyperbilirubinemia, neurologic signs, and sequelae such as significant motor and mental retardation and cerebral palsy. Thromboemboli, arterial ischemic stroke, necrotizing enterocolitis (NEC), and acute tubular necrosis are additional complications. Polycythemia can result from a large number of perinatal complications, as shown in Box 20-4.

In up to one third of monochorionic twins there is a significant transfusion of blood from one twin into the other defined as a discrepancy in the infants' blood counts of greater than 5 g/dL of hemoglobin. Usually, the recipient twin is larger and prone to cardiorespiratory symptoms, hyperviscosity, and hyperbilirubinemia, whereas the donor twin is smaller and at risk for congestive heart failure.[49] Blood viscosity correlates better with symptoms than does hematocrit.[35] In addition, clinical signs and symptoms may be related to an underlying condition instead of polycythemia per se.

BOX 20-4 CAUSES OF NEONATAL POLYCYTHEMIA

1. Placental transfusion
   a. Delayed cord clamping (may increase the blood volume and red cell mass of the infant by as much as 55%)
   b. Twin-to-twin transfusion
2. Intrauterine hypoxia/placental vascular insufficiency
   a. Intrauterine growth restriction syndrome
   b. Maternal diabetes
   c. Maternal smoking
   d. Maternal hypertension syndromes
   e. Maternal cyanotic heart disease
3. Fetal factors
   a. Trisomy 13, 18, 21
   b. Hyperthyroidism
   c. Neonatal thyrotoxicosis
   d. Congenital adrenal hyperplasia
   e. Beckwith-Wiedemann syndrome
4. High altitude
5. Idiopathic

Data Collection

HISTORY

In addition to a complete history of the pregnancy and delivery, questions should be directed to pertinent maternal medical conditions, including insulin-dependent diabetes mellitus, hypertension, and heart disease. Additional maternal risk factors include cigarette smoking and living at high altitude. Fetal risk factors include documented intrauterine growth restriction and delayed cord clamping.

SIGNS AND SYMPTOMS

Newborn infants with hematocrit values of greater than 65% to 70% may manifest symptoms because of increased viscosity.[45] Physical examination may be normal except for plethora and, occasionally, cyanosis. Neurologic findings may include lethargy, irritability, hypotonia, tremor, and poor suck. Tachypnea, tachycardia, and respiratory distress may be present. Poor GI function is common with abdominal distention, decreased bowel sounds, and poor feeding.

LABORATORY DATA

The diagnosis of polycythemia is based on hemoglobin and hematocrit in comparison with normal values for post-conceptual and postnatal age. The diagnosis of hyperviscosity may be based on direct viscosity measurement but usually is assigned based on polycythemia in the presence of consistent clinical signs and symptoms. Affected infants often have thrombocytopenia, hyperbilirubinemia, and hypoglycemia. Tests of thyroid and adrenal function to rule out hyperthyroidism and adrenal hyperplasia should be performed with appropriate clinical indication. Chromosome analysis should be considered for babies with dysmorphic features.

Treatment

Therapy of polycythemia is generally based on the presence of consistent signs and symptoms. Therapy, when indicated, is aimed at decreasing the hematocrit and includes removal of red cells by simple phlebotomy, as well as partial exchange transfusion with replacement of removed red cell volume with volume expanders. FFP has not shown greater efficacy than saline in initial correction in hematocrit or viscosity or in improvement in outcome. In a randomized controlled trial,

Roithmaier et al[36] showed that partial exchange transfusion using crystalloid solution (Ringer's solution) was as effective as partial exchange transfusion using a colloid (plasma) in decreasing the hematocrit of polycythemic neonates. Crystalloid solutions are preferable to colloids because they are less expensive and are infection free. Exchange transfusion often requires placement of an umbilical venous catheter (UVC). Risks of umbilical catheterization in polycythemic infants include portal vein thrombosis, phlebitis of the portal vein, and decreased plasma volume (if phlebotomy is used alone). In addition, infants with polycythemia and hyperviscosity are at increased risk for spontaneous large vessel thrombosis, especially renal vein thrombosis, and stroke.

There is evidence that treating all infants with polycythemia may not improve outcome. In a study by Bada et al,[4] symptomatic infants received partial plasma exchange transfusion, which reduced blood viscosity, improved cerebral blood flow, and ameliorated symptoms. Infants who were asymptomatic before therapy showed little or no improvement in cerebral blood flow with partial exchange transfusion. Neurologic sequelae in babies with hyperviscosity appear to be related to prenatal risk factors for fetal asphyxia as much as or more than hematocrit per se.[38]

COAGULATION

Physiology

When a blood vessel is torn, blood clots at the site of vessel injury through a series of carefully controlled enzymatic reactions. First, platelets, which are small, platelike blood cells without nuclei, adhere to the damaged endothelium both directly and by linkage through the von Willebrand protein (von Willebrand factor [vWF]) to collagen, which is exposed beneath the blood vessel lining. The platelets release adenosine diphosphate (ADP), which, in addition to collagen, recruits more platelets to the activation process. Activated platelets express a receptor for the blood protein fibrinogen, glycoprotein IIb/IIIa (GPIIb/IIIa), which binds to adjoining platelets and links them. Fibrinogen is a contractile protein that pulls platelets together, forming a tightly woven net over the vessel tear. vWF, fibronectin, and thrombospondin similarly link activated platelets through the GPIIb/IIIa receptor. This is known as a ***platelet plug*** and is responsible for the initial cessation of bleeding, especially in mucous membranes of the nose, mouth, throat, and GI and genitourinary tracts. At the same time, thromboxanes produced by the platelet prostaglandin pathway stimulate platelet aggregation, vasoconstriction, and decreased local blood flow.

Figure 20-2 shows the sequential reactions in activation of coagulation known as the "clotting cascade."[28] The coagulation proteins in blood are inert proenzymes called ***zymogens*** until they are activated. The primary activation process involves exposure of a potent membrane glycoprotein receptor for clotting activation called ***tissue factor,*** for which the tissue factor pathway of coagulation activation is named. Tissue factor is normally hidden in the subendothelium and becomes exposed by vascular injury or is presented on the intact surface of monocytes and endothelial cells through the inflammatory process. Small amounts of circulating activated factor VII (FVIIa) in the plasma bind to exposed tissue factor and form a complex that results in the sequential activation first of factor X and then of factor II (also called ***prothrombin***). These biochemical reactions are similar in that they take place preferentially on procoagulant phospholipid surfaces of endothelial cells and platelets at the site of injury, involve calcium-dependent binding to the surface, and can be accelerated by cofactors (activated factors VIII [FVIIIa] and V [FVa]).

The contact activation pathway is an alternative route to factor X activation. In this pathway, factor XII is activated by contact with negatively charged subendothelial collagen or by acidosis, cold, or heat injury. Activated factor XII subsequently activates factors XI and IX. Prekallikrein and high-molecular-weight kininogen serve as cofactors for activation. Contact activation initiates clot lysis and also many inflammatory pathways, including the complement system, which is important for host defense. There is cross-activation between the tissue factor and contact pathways, and thus each generally is not functioning completely independently.

Procoagulant factors II, VII, IX, and X and regulatory proteins, protein C and protein S, are biochemically related. They are all produced in the liver and require vitamin K to become functional. Vitamin K catalyzes the transfer of carboxyl groups to certain glutamic acid residues of vitamin K–dependent proteins; only after carboxylation can these unique proteins then bind to surfaces via calcium.

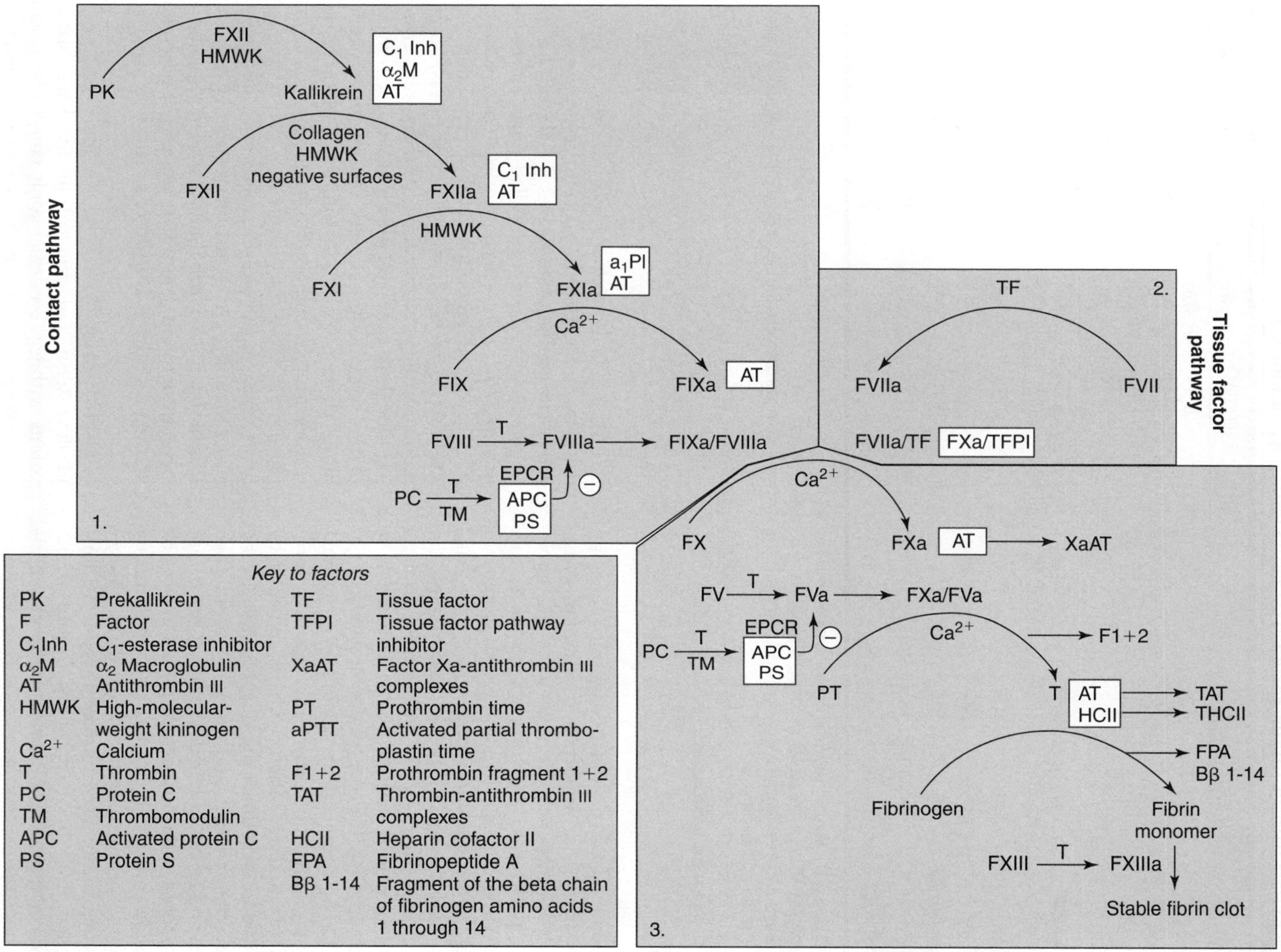

FIGURE 20-2 The clotting cascade. The aPTT screening test and coagulation tests factors are included in panels *1* and *3*. The PT test factors are shown in panels *2* and *3*. Proteins encased in boxes inhibit the procoagulant reactions. *EPCR,* Endothelial protein C receptor.

TABLE 20-4 COAGULATION FACTOR VALUES* FOR FETUS AND NEWBORN INFANT

AGE-GROUP	I (mg/dL)	II	V	VII	VIII:C	vWF:Ag	IX	X	XI
Fetus (≈20 wk)	96 (40)	0.16 (0.10)	0.70 (0.40)	0.21 (0.12)	0.50 (0.23)	0.65 (0.40)	0.10 (0.05)	0.19 (0.15)	— —
Preterm newborn (25-32 wk)	250 (100)	0.32 (0.18)	0.80 (0.43)	0.37 (0.24)	0.75 (0.40)	1.50 (0.90)	0.22 (0.17)	0.38 (0.20)	0.20 (0.12)
Preterm newborn (33-36 wk)	300 (120)	0.45 (0.26)	0.82 (0.48)	0.59 (0.34)	0.93 (0.54)	1.66 (1.35)	0.41 (0.20)	0.44 (0.21)	— —
Term newborn (37-41 wk)	240 (150)	0.52 (0.25)	1 (0.54)	0.57 (0.35)	1.50 (0.55)	1.60 (0.84)	0.35 (0.15)	0.45 (0.30)	0.42 (0.20)
Older infant (age and level when adult value is approximated)	340 (21 days)	0.97 (45-60 days)	1 (1 day)	0.90 (21 days)	0.93 (1-2 days)	1.13 (1 wk)	0.7 (6 mo)	0.55 (6 wk)	0.52 (6 wk)

From Hathaway WE, Bonnar J: *Hemostatic disorders of the pregnant woman and newborn infant,* New York, 1987, Elsevier Science.

AT-III, Antithrombin III; *HMWK,* high-molecular-weight kininogen; *PK,* prekallikrein; *vWF,* von Willebrand factor.

Values (data taken from references discussed in text) are expressed in units per milliliter as compared with normal adult subject reference plasma (100% = 1 unit/mL); the mean and lower limit of range (or −2 SD) are shown.

*Clotting activity or chromogenic substrate methods (except protein C:Ag, protein S:Ag) in subjects in the first 24 hours of life.

†Cord blood. All other values are venous. All subjects received vitamin K at birth.

Thrombin is the terminal coagulation enzyme and functions as an important regulator of coagulation. It is a potent platelet activator. Thrombin provides positive feedback activation of factors VIII and V. Thrombin when complexed to the cell receptor ***thrombomodulin*** changes from a procoagulant to an anticoagulant protein and initiates the inactivation of factors VIIIa and Va through activation of protein C (APC). The endothelial protein C receptor (EPCR) enhances the activation of protein C and complements the important protein C system.[12] Thrombin cleaves fibrinogen to form a sticky fibrin strand. Factor XIII is activated by thrombin and cross-links the fibrin strand, greatly increasing its strength and stability. Fibrin then contracts and forms a tight, dense clot. A fibrin clot holds opposed surfaces together for about a week as thrombin and other growth factors stimulate fibroblasts to grow. Ultimately, scar tissue bridges the original injury. When a blood clot is no longer needed, it is dissolved by an enzyme system called ***fibrinolysis.*** The blood zymogen plasminogen is activated by tissue plasminogen activator (TPA) or urokinase-type plasminogen activator (UPA), which is released from vascular endothelial cells or renal epithelial cells, respectively. The active enzyme plasmin cleaves the fibrin clot into fragments of various sizes, called ***fibrin split products (FSPs).*** Split products that contain factor XIII–mediated cross-linked fibrin are called the ***D-dimer fragments***. Several proteins are responsible for regulating the coagulation process and ensuring that these powerful enzymes are not activated in the systemic circulation, causing uncontrolled blood clotting. The most important of these regulatory proteins are antithrombin, protein C, and the protein C cofactor protein S. Heparin cofactor II, alpha$_2$-macroglobulin, and alpha$_1$-antitrypsin also function as coagulation regulatory proteins. Plasminogen activator inhibitor (PAI), histamine-rich glycoprotein, and fibrin binding of plasminogen regulate the activation of fibrinolysis.

NORMAL VALUES

Healthy term and preterm infants have platelet counts within the normal adult range. The coagulation system of the newborn infant is unique in that blood clotting proteins mature at different rates

XII	PK	HMWK	XIII	PLASMINOGEN	ALPHA2-ANTIPLASMIN	AT-III	PROTEIN C:Ag	PROTEIN S:Ag
—	—	—	≈0.30	—	—	0.23	0.10	—
—	—	—	—	—	—	(0.12)	(0.06)	—
0.22	0.26	0.28	0.11-0.40	0.35	74	0.35	0.29	—
(0.09)	(0.14)	(0.20)	—	(0.20)	(≈50)	(0.20)	(0.21)	—
0.25	0.33	—	—	0.38	73	0.40	0.38	—
(0.09)	(0.23)	—	—	(0.26)	(≈50)	(0.25)	(0.23)	—
0.44	0.35	0.64	0.61	0.49	83	0.56	0.50†	0.24†
(0.16)	(0.16)	(0.50)	(0.36)	(0.25)	(≈65)	(0.32)	(0.30)	(0.10)
1	0.86	0.82	1	1	1	0.82	0.82	—
(14 days)	(6 mo)	(6 mo)	(1 mo)	(6 mo)	(1wk)	(3-6 mo)	(24 mo)	—

(Table 20-4).[19] Mean levels of factors V and VIII and fibrinogen are within the normal adult range by 20 weeks of fetal development. Very low levels of these clotting proteins are never normal. The level of the vWF is elevated above adult normal values at birth, and the neonatal vWF protein subunits, called ***multimers,*** include ultra-large forms, which makes the protein more adherent to platelets and vessel walls. Fetal fibrinogen differs from the adult molecule in its increased content of sialic acid. This prolongs the thrombin time (TT) of the neonate. Vitamin K–dependent factors II, VII, IX, and X and protein C and protein S develop very slowly. Factor IX does not reach its full adult potential until 9 months of age; protein C may not reach adult levels until puberty. It is very difficult to determine if these proteins are genetically deficient during the neonatal period.

The clotting system is evaluated using a hemostasis screen, which includes testing for the activated partial thromboplastin time (aPTT), prothrombin time (PT), TT, fibrinogen concentration, platelet count, and a test of platelet function, such as the platelet function analyzer (PFA-100). The aPTT may be within the adult range at term birth or may be slightly prolonged and achieve the adult range by 2 months. The aPTT of a stable preterm infant with a birth weight of less than 1000 g is often extremely prolonged, without signs of excessive bleeding. The PT is usually near normal at birth, may prolong slightly by day 3, and reaches adult normal values by day 5. The TT is slightly prolonged because of fetal fibrinogen until 3 weeks of age. The fibrinogen and platelet concentration are within the normal adult range at birth in stable term and preterm infants. The PFA-100 is a whole blood test that estimates platelet function. Certain tests of specific platelet activities including aggregation give somewhat decreased values at birth and for the first 3 weeks of age. However, platelet adhesion to collagen, mediated via the vWF, is increased at birth compared with well adults, and the PFA-100, which measures global platelet function, demonstrates shorter closure time in a term neonate than in an adult. Global coagulation assays demonstrate that neonatal plasma generates less thrombin than adult plasma, but thrombin activity is generated after a shorter lag time than that determined in adult plasma.

Pathophysiology

THROMBOCYTOPENIA

***Thrombocytopenia* is a general term that denotes a decreased number of platelets in the blood.** Thrombocytopenia is the most common coagulation disorder in the neonate. Determine whether the infant appears well or ill. The causes of thrombocytopenia in an otherwise well infant differ from those in an acutely ill neonate (Box 20-5).

BOX 20-5 CAUSES OF THROMBOCYTOPENIA IN THE NEWBORN INFANT

1. Well infant
   a. Immune
      Alloimmune thrombocytopenia (NAIT)
      Maternal idiopathic thrombocytopenia purpura
   b. Constitutional
      Thrombocytopenia—absent radius
      Amegakaryocytic thrombocytopenia
      Wiskott-Aldrich syndrome
      Fanconi's anemia
      Bernard-Soulier syndrome
      Autosomal dominant thrombocytopenia
2. Sick infant
   a. Respiratory distress syndrome
   b. Bacterial sepsis
   c. Viral infection
   d. Necrotizing enterocolitis
   e. Hyperviscosity
   f. Disseminated intravascular coagulation
3. Infant appearing either well or sick
   a. Kasabach-Merritt (giant hemangioma) syndrome
   b. Trisomy 21, 18, 13
   c. Leukemia
   d. Thrombosis

NAIT, Neonatal alloimmune thrombocytopenia.

A well-appearing infant is likely to suffer from neonatal alloimmune thrombocytopenia (NAIT), in which the platelets are coated by circulating antibody and rapidly cleared from the circulation by the spleen and liver. Alloimmune thrombocytopenia develops when the mother is negative for a platelet antigen, usually PLA-1, for which the father is positive. Fifty percent of recognized cases of alloimmune thrombocytopenia occur in a mother's first infant. Subsequent infants can be more severely involved. Presentations of alloimmune thrombocytopenia range from asymptomatic infants in whom a low platelet count is detected coincidentally on a blood count to fatal cases of intracranial hemorrhage with onset in utero. Infants of mothers with ***idiopathic thrombocytopenic purpura (ITP)*** may have a low platelet count because the maternal antibody crosses the placenta to the infant but usually do not develop life-threatening hemorrhage.

Constitutional thrombocytopenia is rare. Affected infants often manifest congenital skeletal malformations of the hands and arms. ***Thrombocytopenia–absent radius (TAR)*** is a rare but well-characterized syndrome. A bone marrow examination is important to evaluate the megakaryocyte pool, which produces platelets. In Bernard-Soulier syndrome, the platelet number is moderately decreased and giant platelets are seen on the peripheral smear. Infants with trisomy 21 (Down syndrome), 18, or 13 can manifest abnormal platelet counts without apparent illness. The bone marrow of infants with Down syndrome is highly reactive. Other features of trisomy 21 should be present.

Giant, cavernous hemangiomas often trap platelets in a syndrome known as ***Kasabach-Merritt,*** resulting in accelerated destruction. Clues to this syndrome include skin hemangiomas; bruits over the liver, spleen, or brain; and high-output congestive heart failure with a structurally normal heart.

Thrombocytopenia develops in most infants with respiratory distress severe enough to require mechanical ventilation. The lowest platelet counts are usually found about day 3 of life, and normal counts recover by day 10 if the infant's course is not complicated by infection or thrombosis. Infants of less than 32 weeks' gestation with respiratory distress syndrome (RDS) and severe thrombocytopenia are at increased risk for intracranial hemorrhage.

Bacterial and viral infections must be excluded in any thrombocytopenic neonate. The infant of a mother with chorioamnionitis often demonstrates thrombocytopenia in the cord blood.

Thrombosis in a neonate often presents with an idiopathic falling platelet count. Thromboses are most commonly found at the tips of umbilical artery and venous catheters and can be diagnosed with ultrasound. An infected clot should be suspected in an infant with diagnosed catheter-related thrombosis and alterations in temperature, respiratory stability, or cardiovascular stability.

Heparin-induced thrombocytopenia (HIT) has been described in neonates, especially babies with significant heparin exposure associated with cardiac surgery, cardiopulmonary bypass, or extracorporeal membrane oxygenation (ECMO). HIT is caused by antibodies that develop against a complex of heparin with platelet factor 4 on the platelet surface. When HIT is suspected, all heparin must be promptly removed, including solutions used to flush catheters.

DISSEMINATED INTRAVASCULAR COAGULATION

Thrombocytopenia in an ill infant is often part of the larger syndrome of disseminated intravascular coagulation (DIC).[29] In DIC, activation of blood-clotting proteins is initiated by tissue factor from bacterial products (endotoxin) or inflammation or through the contact system. The activation of clotting proteins leads to a hypercoagulable state, and thromboses form, especially in the small vessels of the liver, spleen, brain, lungs, kidneys, and adrenal glands. The bone marrow and liver partially compensate by releasing platelets and clotting factors into the circulation. However, the regulatory system of coagulation is immature in term and preterm neonates. The capacity to neutralize activated clotting proteins is quickly exhausted, and the resulting deficiencies of platelets and clotting factors are called ***consumptive coagulopathy.*** Depletion of procoagulant proteins leads to bleeding, and paradoxic bleeding and thrombosis can occur simultaneously. DIC predisposes a preterm infant to intracranial hemorrhage. Venous thrombosis of the germinal matrix occurs as the initial lesion, followed by postthrombotic hemorrhage. Bleeding is also seen in the skin, around indwelling catheters and endotracheal and chest tubes, into the lungs and other parenchyma, and in the urine and stool.

LIVER FAILURE

The coagulopathy of liver failure is complex and includes thrombocytopenia, platelet dysfunction, decrease in synthesis of coagulation proteins in the liver, and enhanced fibrinolysis. Severe liver disease is characterized by a markedly abnormal PT, in excess of aPTT prolongation. Liver failure in the neonatal period can result from viral hepatitis or rare metabolic disorders such as infantile hemochromatosis. Other signs of liver dysfunction, such as hepatomegaly, jaundice, and elevated liver enzymes, are present. Infants with liver dysfunction manifest bleeding into the skin, GI tract, retroperitoneum, and cranium. Invasive procedures, such as liver biopsy, can provoke severe bleeding.

CONGENITAL PLATELET DYSFUNCTION

Genetic platelet function defects causing severe bleeding in the neonatal period are rare. Glanzmann's thrombasthenia is an autosomal recessive disorder resulting from a severe deficiency or dysfunction in the platelet fibrinogen receptor, GPIIb/IIIa. Severe neonatal bleeding, including intracranial hemorrhage, can occur. Platelet number is normal in this syndrome. Absent receptors can be determined by flow cytometry, and genetic mutations have been determined, but all cases can be diagnosed by severe abnormalities on platelet aggregation studies or PFA-100. Platelet storage pool disorders can be suspected from abnormal granule staining on the peripheral smear. Hermansky-Pudlak syndrome is a recessively inherited syndrome characterized by absence of platelet-dense granules and oculocutaneous albinism. Chédiak-Higashi disease is characterized by large, dysfunctional platelet granules. In gray platelet syndrome, the alpha granules are absent and the platelets have a pale appearance on the peripheral smear. Acquired platelet dysfunction can cause bleeding in the first several days of life in an infant after maternal use of aspirin or other drugs affecting platelet function shortly before delivery.

VITAMIN K DEFICIENCY

The most important bleeding syndrome in the otherwise stable neonate is hemorrhagic disease of the newborn, caused by vitamin K deficiency.[23] There is a tenfold gradient in vitamin K concentration between the maternal and fetal plasma. Marginal fetal vitamin K levels are further compromised by maternal use of anticonvulsants or warfarin. Approximately 3% of cord blood samples from normal term pregnancies show biochemical evidence of noncarboxylated clotting proteins related to vitamin K deficiency.[41] ***Early hemorrhagic disease of the newborn*** presents within the first 24 hours of life with skin bruising, massive cephalhematoma, GI tract bleeding, or intracranial hemorrhage. ***Classic hemorrhagic disease of the newborn*** presents between 1 and 7 days of life; late vitamin K deficiency occurs between 1 week and 2 months of life. **The recommendation of the American Academy of Pediatrics is to give every neonate 1 mg of vitamin K by intramuscular injection[5]; this is adequate to prevent bleeding in most infants** (see Chapter 5).Vitamin K prophylaxis can be achieved with use of an oral vitamin K preparation. However, because oral therapy requires multiple doses over the first 6 weeks of life, it is difficult to ensure compliance and protect all infants using this formulation. Vitamin K concentrations are physiologically very low in human breast milk; cow's milk contains 10 times the amount of vitamin K (1.5 and 15 mg/L, respectively). Infants fed breast milk are at increased risk for vitamin K deficiency. In addition, infants with fat malabsorption caused by cystic fibrosis, alpha$_1$-antitrypsin deficiency, or biliary atresia and infants treated with prolonged courses of antibiotics are at increased risk for vitamin K deficiency.

HEMOPHILIA AND OTHER CONGENITAL BLEEDING DISORDERS

The hemophilias are a group of lifelong bleeding disorders caused by genetic deficiencies of one or more coagulation proteins. Factor VIII deficiency causes 80% of the hemophilias, and factor IX deficiency causes most of the remainder. Both factors VIII and IX are encoded on the X chromosome; thus deficiency states are manifested in carrier mothers and affected sons. Deficiencies of other coagulation factors are inherited as autosomal traits with severe bleeding manifested with homozygous deficiency. Most infants with hemophilia appear to tolerate labor and a routine vaginal delivery with no undue problems. However, intracranial hemorrhage has been documented in approximately 1% to 4% of infants with hemophilia as a result of birth trauma.[8] Current recommendations call for vaginal delivery in the absence of complications; however, cesarean section should be elected if needed to avoid prolonged or difficult labor. Use of vacuum extraction or forceps to assist delivery should be avoided. **Approximately 50% of male infants with severe hemophilia will hemorrhage from a circumcision.** The absence of procedure-related bleeding in the neonatal period does not exclude hemophilia, because hemostasis can be supported by physiologically increased platelet function around birth. Prolonged bleeding from the umbilical cord stump is suggestive of factor XIII deficiency. Spontaneous intracranial hemorrhage also occurs in infants with homozygous deficiency of factors V, VII, X, or XIII or fibrinogen.

Data Collection

HISTORY

A history of maternal bleeding, medical and obstetric diagnoses, and medications should be elicited for every infant at birth. A careful family history for bleeding disorders in the parents, grandparents, siblings, aunts, uncles, and cousins should be taken as part of every admission evaluation. Specific questions must be asked about excessive bleeding with surgeries, menses, childbirth, and traumas and about spontaneous bleeding events. Efforts should be made to obtain confirmatory medical records for any positive response. **Procedures, including circumcision, should not be performed until the possibility of a bleeding disorder in the infant is excluded.** The administration of vitamin K to the infant should be confirmed by review of the nursing notes.

SIGNS AND SYMPTOMS

Thrombocytopenia usually manifests with small, flat hemorrhages into the skin called ***petechiae*** that do not blanch with pressure. Petechiae may be concentrated in skin creases of the neck and axillae and around the site of a tourniquet or may be scattered over the entire body. More severe thrombocytopenia results in large ecchymoses, which are flat bruises. Infants with severe thrombocytopenia may hemorrhage into the central nervous system or GI tract.

Bleeding with coagulation disorders causes palpable ***hematomas*** of the skin and scalp. Intracranial, retroperitoneal, intraperitoneal, GI, and genitourinary bleeding may occur. Bleeding with surgeries or procedures may be immediate or delayed.

LABORATORY DATA

Any infant with bleeding signs should be evaluated with a hemostasis screen and a platelet count. The results of the hemostasis screen in the healthy infant and during many states of illness are shown in Table 20-5. The possibility of hemophilia should be excluded by specific factor assays. In addition, factors XIII, alpha$_2$-antiplasmin, and PAI-1 should be assayed in a term infant with unexplained significant hemorrhage, such as intracranial hemorrhage. Platelet function should be assessed with a screening test, such as the PFA-100, bleeding time, or aggregation studies, if Glanzmann's or a similar congenital platelet dysfunction is suspected. Tests should be sent for HIT for infants who develop thrombocytopenia or a decrease in platelet count by 50% on heparin therapy in the absence of other obvious cause.

Treatment

THROMBOCYTOPENIA

Therapy for thrombocytopenia depends on the overall health and stability of the neonate, as well

TABLE 20-5 COAGULATION RESULTS IN NORMAL NEONATES AND NEONATES WITH BLEEDING SYNDROMES

DESCRIPTION	PTT	PT	TT	FIB	D-DIMER	Plt Ct
Healthy term	N-↑	N-↑	↑	NL	Neg	NL
Healthy preterm	↑↑	N-↑	↑	NL	Neg	NL
Vitamin K deficiency	↑↑	↑↑↑	↑	NL	Neg	NL
Liver disease	↑↑	↑↑↑	↑↑-↑↑↑	↓	Pos	↓
Hemophilia	↑↑↑	N-↑	↑	NL	Neg	NL
DIC	↑↑↑	↑↑	↑↑	↓	Pos	↓↓

Fib, Fibrogen; *N*, normal; *Plt Ct*, platelet count; *PT*, prothrombin time; *PTT*, partial thromboplastin time; *TT*, thrombin time; ↑, mildly prolonged; ↑↑, moderately prolonged; ↑↑↑, severely prolonged; ↓, decreased.

as the cause of the thrombocytopenia. In immune thrombocytopenia, antibodies that are affecting neonatal platelets also may cause rapid destruction of transfused platelets. Platelet antibodies in infants with NAIT do not react against maternal platelets, and washed maternal platelets are an effective therapy for affected infants with severe bleeding. Thrombocytopenia in this disorder, as well as maternal autoimmune thrombocytopenia, responds well to intravenous immunoglobulin (IVIG). Infants with alloimmune thrombocytopenia are likely to receive incompatible platelets from a random donor, and platelet transfusions, when needed, must be from a donor who shares maternal antigen profile. If HIT is suspected, heparin should be stopped promptly, a blood sample should be sent for HIT testing, and alternative anticoagulation (e.g., with argatroban or bivalirudin) should be substituted until test results are obtained. Infants with Kasabach-Merritt syndrome may respond to steroid therapy, antifibrinolytic agents, or interferon.

The primary support of most other thrombocytopenic infants is replacement transfusions of platelets, which are derived from CMV-reduced donor units. A stable, otherwise healthy infant can tolerate a platelet count as low as 20,000/mcL without undue risk for serious bleeding. However, an infant who is less than 30 weeks' gestation, mechanically ventilated, on ECMO therapy, with indwelling UACs or UVCs and chest tubes, septic, or otherwise unstable will require a platelet count of 50,000/mcL to prevent or treat bleeding.

BOX 20-6 THERAPY OF DISSEMINATED INTRAVASCULAR COAGULATION

1. Reverse the trigger: Treat the underlying disorder.
2. In bleeding infants, maintain hemostatic levels of fibrinogen (>100 mg/dL) and platelets (>50,000/mcL) using cryoprecipitate, FFP, and platelet concentrates (10 mL/kg). FFP is also indicated to treat bleeding infants with PT >3 seconds above the upper limit of normal.
3. If necessary, replace regulatory proteins; antithrombin or protein C concentrate (50 to 150 units/kg).
4. Consider low-dose heparin therapy 10 units/kg/hr if survival of infused fibrinogen and platelets is <12 hours.

FFP, Fresh frozen plasma.

DISSEMINATED INTRAVASCULAR COAGULATION

Transfusion of platelets into infants with thrombosis or DIC may aggravate the platelet consumption unless specific therapy of the underlying condition also is administered. **The primary treatment of DIC is reversal of the trigger (Box 20-6).** Adequate ventilation, support of circulation and perfusion, treatment of sepsis, and general supportive care usually interrupt the DIC process within 48 hours. Routine infusion of FFP into infants with DIC does not improve infant outcomes, although infants with active bleeding require replacement of coagulation proteins and platelets to maintain minimal hemostatic levels.[16] Replacement of coagulation regulatory proteins in FFP or antithrombin (AT) concentrate or inhibition of coagulation activation with low-dose heparin is helpful in some cases.

BLEEDING DISORDERS

Infants with vitamin K deficiency are treated with vitamin K, 1 mg by slow IV push or subcutaneous injection. FFP, 10 to 15 mL/kg, may be given to control active bleeding.

Neonates with severe liver disease can be treated for active bleeding or prepared for liver biopsy using transfusions of FFP and platelet concentrates. **Parenteral administration of vitamin K should be confirmed;** ongoing replacement may be necessary if there is fat malabsorption. There is no benefit to treating babies with liver disease and abnormal clotting tests but no clinical bleeding signs. A recombinant preparation of activated factor VII (rFVIIa, NovoSeven, Novo Nordisk [Copenhagen, Denmark]) has been used to control bleeding in the neonate with encouraging results. Concentrates of vitamin K–dependent clotting factors purified from human plasma and subjected to viral inactivation techniques are also available. **Consultation with a regional hemophilia treatment center about use and availability of these specialized products is strongly recommended.**

Treatment of congenital coagulation factor deficiencies is based on the deficient factor. The most specific and viral-safe product available should be used. Factor VIII or IX should be replaced in a bleeding neonate (or for surgery) using recombinant proteins. Viral-inactivated, human plasma–derived concentrates are available for vWF; similar concentrates are pending Food and Drug Administration (FDA) approval for fibrinogen and FXIII. Factor XIII and fibrinogen may be replaced in cryoprecipitate. Replacement of other clotting proteins usually requires FFP. DDAVP, a synthetic vasopressin that stimulates release of endothelial stores of factor VIII and the von Willebrand protein, is generally not used in the neonate because of the possibility of seizures related to hyponatremia in this age-group. The hemophilia center should be involved in the diagnosis and management of all infants with congenital bleeding disorders.

Prevention and Parent Teaching

Mothers should be instructed during pregnancy that vitamin K deficiency is routinely prevented with an intramuscular (IM) injection of vitamin K to the neonate. Primary care providers should be careful to document administration of vitamin K, especially for infants born at home.

Bleeding in an infant with a bleeding disorder can be minimized by preventing undue trauma. IM injections and other invasive procedures should be avoided if possible, although vitamin K may be safely administered to infants with severe hemophilia if a small-bore needle is used and it is not Z-tracked under the skin. The infant should be handled as gently as possible. Pressure for holding and placement of a tourniquet should be minimized. Extreme care should be taken with arterial puncture.

Replacement platelet or clotting factor infusions should be considered before any necessary invasive procedure. Parents should be educated about the nature of the bleeding disorder and its cause in their infant. They should know whether this is a time-limited complication of the neonatal course or a long-term concern. Infants with constitutional thrombocytopenia or coagulopathy are at lifelong risk for bleeding. The risk for platelet sensitization and the consequent aim to minimize platelet exposure must be conveyed to the parents. Any other family member at risk for having a genetic thrombocytopenia or bleeding disorder should be identified, screened, and counseled.

Education of families about hemophilia or constitutional thrombocytopenia begins as soon as the diagnosis is established. Nurses, in coordination with the hemophilia nurse coordinator, should instruct parents about routine infant care and recognition of possible bleeding events.

THROMBOSIS

Pathophysiology

Thrombosis is an uncommon problem in pediatric patients, with increased incidence noted both in the neonatal period and after puberty. Physiologic correlates of the neonate's increased predisposition to thrombosis are shown in Boxes 20-7 and 20-8.

BOX 20-7 PROTHROMBOTIC CHARACTERISTICS OF NEONATAL BLOOD

- Increased hematocrit values
- Increased concentration and size of von Willebrand factor multimers
- Increased concentration of circulating tissue factor in preterm infants
- Low concentrations of physiologic anticoagulants, antithrombin, protein C, protein S, and tissue factor pathway inhibitor
- Low concentration of the fibrinolytic protein plasminogen
- Small-caliber, reactive blood vessels

BOX 20-8 PATHOLOGIC CONDITIONS PREDISPOSING TO THROMBOSIS IN THE NEONATE

- Hypotension
- Hyperviscosity
- Severe genetic and acquired deficiencies of antithrombin, protein C, protein S, and plasminogen
- Genetic mutations in factor V and prothrombin; elevations in homocysteine and lipoprotein(a)
- Mechanical obstruction by catheters
- Maternal diabetes mellitus

The most common sites of spontaneous thrombosis in the neonate are the renal veins, the central nervous system (CNS), the superior vena cava and inferior vena cava, and the aorta. **Catheters placed for critical care support are associated with an increased risk for thrombosis.**

PURPURA FULMINANS

Purpura fulminans is a syndrome of skin necrosis from venous thrombosis caused by severe deficiencies of protein C or protein S.[18,27] Most cases are caused by homozygous or compound heterozygous genetic defects. Rarely, acquired deficiencies from maternal lupus anticoagulants can mimic the genetic syndromes. Consumption of protein C and protein S during bacterial sepsis usually manifests at a later age and is less fulminant than the genetic syndromes.

THROMBOCYTOSIS

Thrombocytosis occurs with iron-deficiency anemia. An iron-deficient neonate may have suffered from chronic blood loss in utero, either by hemorrhage into the placenta, blood loss to a twin, or with GI bleeding. Neuroblastoma, a malignancy of neural crest cells, and Down syndrome may also be associated with thrombocytosis.

Data Collection

HISTORY

A history of thrombosis, including deep vein thrombosis, pulmonary embolism, heart attack, or stroke in persons younger than 50 years in the parents, grandparents, siblings, aunts, uncles, and cousins of the infant, raises suspicion of genetic thrombophilia. Many family members affected with heterozygous deficiencies of protein C or S are asymptomatic. A history of fetal or neonatal death with thrombosis is helpful. Maternal obstetric complications have been linked to thrombophilia. A maternal history of severe or recurrent preeclampsia, severe intrauterine growth restriction, three first-trimester losses, or any fetal death beyond 10 weeks' gestation indicates potential genetic thrombophilia. Maternal diabetes mellitus is a cause of acquired neonatal thrombophilia.

SIGNS AND SYMPTOMS

Thrombosis. **Signs of decreased organ perfusion and subsequent dysfunction indicate the possibility of a thrombosis.** The classic presentation of renal vein thrombosis includes hematuria, thrombocytopenia, and hypertension. Palpably enlarged kidneys may be noted on physical examination. The presence of unilateral or bilateral flank masses on the initial physical assessment indicates prenatal occurrence of renal vein thrombosis. Stroke usually presents with seizures during the first 24 hours of life. Aortic thromboses present with cool, pale extremities, decreased pulses and capillary refill, and upper extremity hypertension. Confirmation of thrombosis is made with ultrasound examination of the renal veins and other abdominal vasculature, inferior vena cava, and aorta; renal scan; and computed tomography (CT) or magnetic resonance imaging (MRI) of the brain. Classic signs of arterial emboli include purple toes or fingers.

Purpura Fulminans. Purpura fulminans is a dramatic syndrome that usually manifests within hours of birth. Infants develop patchy areas of skin thromboses over the trunk and buttocks, usually in dependent areas. The lesions are palpable and initially dark red and quickly become dusky purple and then black; an eschar forms. The lesions are exquisitely painful. Most infants with severe protein C deficiency manifest a white light reflex of the eyes from in utero thrombosis of the primary vitreal veins with subsequent retinal detachment, hemorrhage, and blindness. Imaging studies of the brain show evidence of CNS infarction in many infants. Renal vein thrombosis is not uncommon.

Thrombocytosis. Infants rarely manifest signs of thrombocytosis. Occasionally, platelet counts of greater than 2,000,000/mcL are associated with cerebral ischemia.

TREATMENT

Thrombosis. The optimal therapy for neonatal thrombosis has not been determined. Two approaches include anticoagulation with unfractionated or low-molecular-weight heparin to prevent propagation of the clot or fibrinolytic therapy to dissolve the clot, as shown in Box 20-9. **Anticoagulation remains the standard of care for most neonatal thromboses.** Fibrinolytic therapy may restore blood flow more rapidly. However, **the risk for hemorrhage is greater with fibrinolytic therapy, especially in preterm infants.** Oozing around catheters is the most common bleeding complication of thrombolytic therapy, but the most important complication is CNS bleeding, which occurs most often in infants with brain ischemia from a previous episode of asphyxia or hypotension. Fibrinolytic therapy, if deemed acceptably safe, may be indicated for renal vein thrombosis, especially bilateral renal vein thrombosis with functional renal insufficiency, and for life-threatening or limb-threatening aortic thrombosis. Long-term anticoagulation with warfarin or low-molecular-weight heparin is necessary only in the small proportion of infants who have an ongoing trigger for thrombosis.

Purpura Fulminans. The treatment of neonatal purpura fulminans resulting from genetic thrombophilia is replacement of deficient regulatory proteins. Viral inactivated, human plasma–derived concentrates of protein C and antithrombin are FDA-approved for severe deficiencies. Protein S for replacement is available only in FFP. The hemophilia center staff members are the best resources for information on the availability and safety of existing replacement proteins. **FFP may be administered while confirmatory laboratory assays are being performed, using 10 mL/kg every 8 to 12 hours.** Prophylactic replacement with protein C concentrate is currently available for infants with severe genetic protein C

BOX 20-9 ANTITHROMBOTIC THERAPY IN THE NEONATE

Anticoagulant Therapy

Unfractionated Heparin

Term infants: 100 units/kg bolus
25 to 50 units/kg/hr maintenance; adjusted to maintain anti-Xa activity level of 0.3 to 0.7 unit/mL

Preterm infants: 50 units/kg bolus
15 to 35 units/kg/hr maintenance; adjusted to maintain anti-Xa activity level of 0.3 to 0.7 unit/mL

Low-Molecular-Weight Heparin (Enoxaparin)

1.7 mg/kg Sub-Q every 12 hour; adjusted to maintain anti-Xa activity level of 0.5 to 1 unit/mL 4 hour after injection

Consider FFP 10 mL/kg or AT concentrate 50 to 150 units/kg q 24 to 48 hr to enhance heparin effect, if heparin resistant.

Fibrinolytic Therapy

Tissue Plasminogen Activator (TPA)

0.1 to 0.5 mg/kg/hr for 4 to 12 hr (bleeding risk is greater at the higher doses) or 0.06 to 0.12 mg/kg/hr for 12 to 48 hr

Fibrinolytic therapy has been given to neonates both as higher-dose, shorter-term infusions and lower-dose, longer-term infusions. The higher-dose infusions may be more effective in thromboses that are acute, arterial, and smaller in volume (e.g., aortic or cardiac). Lower, longer infusions may be more efficacious in larger, older, or venous thromboses (e.g., subclavian or extensive vena cava).

Contraindications to TPA: Intracranial hemorrhage, surgery, or ischemia (poor Apgar scores) in previous 10 days; surgery within 7 days; invasive procedures within 72 hours; seizures within 48 hours; active bleeding.

Concomitant with TPA, may give heparin 10 units/kg/hr (no bolus) or enoxaparin 0.5 mg/kg q 12 hr Sub-Q.

Consider FFP 10 mL/kg q 24 hr to replace plasminogen.

Term infants show the highest dose requirements for unfractionated and low-molecular-weight heparin with increased volume of distribution and more rapid plasma elimination. Extremely preterm infants show the lowest dose requirements.

AT, Antithrombin; *FFP,* fresh frozen plasma; *Sub-Q,* subcutaneous; *TPA,* tissue plasminogen activator.

deficiency, although some infants may be medically managed with anticoagulation after the neonatal period.

Infants with acquired deficiencies of protein C or S caused by autoantibodies may respond to IVIG or steroids in addition to plasma replacement. **Infants with sepsis require FFP or protein concentrate until antibiotics have successfully controlled their infection.**

Prevention and Parent Teaching

Parents of infants with severe genetic deficiencies of protein C or S require intensive teaching about administration and monitoring of anticoagulation therapy, observation for early lesions of purpura fulminans, as well as care and rehabilitation of early lesions, which may lead to blindness, skin necrosis, and other lesions.

WHITE BLOOD CELLS

Physiology

White cell production in the fetus begins relatively late in human gestation (14 to 16 weeks) and appears to be limited to the bone marrow, in contrast to erythropoiesis, which is found earlier in liver, spleen, and lymph nodes. Neutrophil reserve pool size is extremely small during the second trimester and increases slowly during gestation. At 18 to 20 weeks, the fetal total white count is approximately 4000 with 5% neutrophils.[28] This increases to 8.5%, or 350 absolute neutrophil count, by 26 to 30 weeks. **Developmental levels of total granulocytes and neutrophils are shown in Figure 20-3.** Thus the baby born at extreme prematurity has severely limited neutrophil capacity and is at increased risk for overwhelming bacterial infection.

White cell counts rise after normal delivery with a peak at 12 hours and a gradual decline over the subsequent 48 hours, as shown in Figure 20-4. Neutrophil counts must be evaluated with respect to post-conceptual and postnatal age.

Pathophysiology of Neutropenia

As with anemia, etiology of neutropenia in the neonate can be divided into decreased production and shortened survival. Decreased production of neutrophils can result from maternal hypertension. Constitutional disorders causing neutropenia are rare, but all result in a predisposition to infections. Reticular dysgenesis is a severe defect leading to absent production of all myeloid cells, including neutrophils, monocytes, macrophages, and lymphocytes. Kostmann's syndrome is an autosomal recessive disorder resulting in severe neutropenia with monocytosis and eosinophilia. Shwachman-Diamond is another autosomal recessive syndrome of neutropenia associated with short stature, metaphyseal dysostoses, and

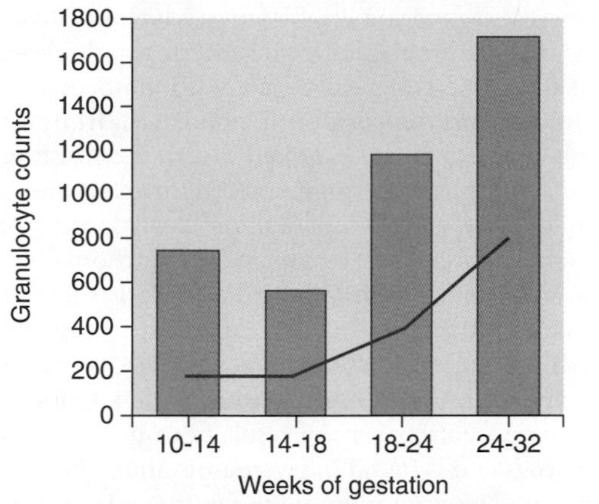

FIGURE 20-3 Mean and range of neutrophil counts at 10 to 14, 14 to 18, 18 to 24, and 24 to 32 weeks gestational age. (From Thomas DB, Yoffey JM: The cellular composition of foetal blood, *Br J Haematol* 8:290, 1962.)

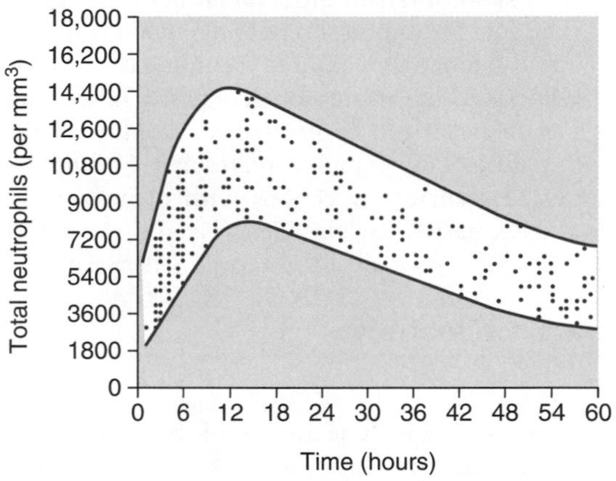

FIGURE 20-4 The total neutrophil count reference range in the first 60 hours of life. (From Manroe BL, Weinberg AG, Rosenfeld CR, et al: The neonatal blood count in health and disease. I. Reference values for neutrophilic cells, *J Pediatr* 95:89, 1979.)

pancreatic exocrine insufficiency. Myelokathexis is a disorder of intramedullary destruction and release of small numbers of neutrophils with abnormal morphology into the peripheral circulation. In dyskeratosis congenital, an X-linked disorder consisting of nail dystrophy, hyperpigmented dystrophic skin, and leukoplakia, one third of children develop neutropenia. In cartilage-hair hypoplasia, an autosomal recessive syndrome of short-limbed dysostosis, one fourth of children develop neutropenia or lymphopenia.

Increased destruction of neutrophils is mediated by antibodies, infection, or inflammation. Congenital acquired neutropenia can result from maternal lupus or drugs and is found in severe isoimmune hemolytic anemia. Neonatal isoimmune neutropenia, similar to NAIT, occurs in about 1 in 1000 live births and often is an incidental finding on the CBC. **Most neutropenia developing in the neonatal nursery results from infection or other stresses, including respiratory distress syndrome and intracranial hemorrhage.**

The most common severe congenital disorder of neutrophil function is chronic granulomatous disease (CGD). CGD has an autosomal recessive inheritance and is characterized by normal neutrophil number but a failure of the granulocytic respiratory burst and results in recurrent infections with organisms that produce catalase, such as *Staphylococcus, Escherichia coli, Candida, Serratia marcescens*, and *Salmonella*.

Data Collection

HISTORY

History should include questioning about maternal gestational complications, hypertension, collagen vascular disorders, and medications. Family history of previously affected infants and information about predisposition to or death during childhood from infections are important.

SIGNS AND SYMPTOMS

Signs and symptoms of neutropenia follow, primarily from related secondary infections. Although older infants may manifest fevers and aphthous ulcers with neutropenia, these are rarely apparent in newborn infants.

LABORATORY DATA

The CBC should be obtained with attention to all cell lines. The peripheral smear should be carefully inspected for evidence of abnormal neutrophil morphology.

TREATMENT

Infants with neutropenia must be evaluated for sepsis and other infections and treated with appropriate antimicrobial agents while cultures are pending. Immune neutropenia responds to IVIG and steroids. CGD can be treated with granulocyte colony-stimulating factor (G-CSF) and γ-interferon. Replacement IVIG has a role in defects that also affect lymphocyte production of antibodies. The role of transfused granulocytes is controversial, and its use is most indicated for overwhelming infections with gram-negative organisms in severely neutropenic babies.

Prevention and Parent Teaching

The sequelae of some severe genetic neutropenias can be prevented with bone marrow transplantation. Important adjuvant approaches for all neutropenic babies include careful attention to hygiene when touching babies, infant skin care to prevent infections, and recognition of early signs. Most acquired neutropenias in neonates are of short duration. Parents of babies with congenital neutropenia must be instructed about the diagnosis, underlying defect, available treatments, and long-term prognosis.

REFERENCES

1. Alter BP: Fanconi's anemia: current concepts, *Am J Pediatr Hematol Oncol* 14:170, 1992.
2. Apt L, Downey WS: "Melena" neonatorum: the swallowed blood syndrome—a simple test for the differentiation of adult and fetal hemoglobin in bloody stools, *J Pediatr* 47:6, 1955.
3. Ascari WQ, Levine P, Pollack W: Incidence of maternal Rh immunization by ABO compatible and incompatible pregnancies, *BMJ* 1:399, 1969.
4. Bada HS, Korones SB, Pourcyrous M, et al: Asymptomatic syndrome of polycythemic hyperviscosity: effect of partial plasma exchange transfusion, *J Pediatr* 120:579, 1992.
5. Barness LA: *Vitamins in pediatric nutrition handbook,* Evanston, Ill, 1979, American Academy of Pediatrics.
6. Boria I, Quarello P, Avondo F, et al: A new database for ribosomal protein genes which are mutated in Diamond-Blackfan anemia, *Huma Mutat* e263:29, 2008.
7. Boussios T, Bertles JF, Goldwasser E: Erythropoietin: receptor characteristics during the ontogeny of hamster yolk sac erythroid cells, *J Biol Chem* 148:443, 1989.

8. Bray GL, Luban NLC: Hemophilia presenting with intracranial hemorrhage, *Am J Dis Child* 141:1215, 1987.
9. Chavez GF, Mulinare J, Edmonds LD: Epidemiology of Rh hemolytic disease of the newborn in the United States, *JAMA* 265:3270, 1991.
10. Clapp DW, Shannon KM: Embryonic and fetal erythropoiesis. In Feig SA, Freedman MH, editors: *Clinical disorders and experimental models of erythropoietin failure,* Boca Raton, Fla, 1993, CRC Press.
11. Cohen A, Manno C: Anemia, intensive care of the fetus and neonate. In Spitzer AR, editor: *Intensive care of the fetus and neonate,* St Louis, 1996, Mosby.
12. Dahlbäck B, Villoutreix BO: Regulation of blood coagulation by the protein C anticoagulant pathway, *Arterioscler Thromb Vasc Biol* 25:1, 2005.
13. Dallman PR: Anemia of prematurity, *Annu Rev Med* 32:143, 1981.
14. Finne PH, Halvorsen S: Regulation of erythropoiesis in the fetus and newborn, *Arch Dis Child* 47:683, 1972.
15. Gilmore JR: Normal hematopoiesis in intra-uterine and neonatal life, *J Pathol Bacteriol* 52:25, 1941.
16. Goldenberg NA, Manco-Johnson MJ: Pediatric hemostasis and use of plasma components, *Best Prac Res Clin Haematol* 19(1):143, 2006.
17. Gross GP, Hathaway WE, McGaughey HR: Hyperviscosity in the neonate, *J Pediatr* 82:1004, 1973.
18. Hartman KP, Manco-Johnson M, Rawlings J, et al: Homozygous protein C deficiency: early treatment with warfarin, *Am J Pediatr Hematol Oncol* 11:395, 1989.
19. Hathaway WE, Bonnar J: *Hemostatic disorders of the pregnant woman and newborn infant,* New York, 1987, Elsevier Science.
20. Jaffe ER: The reduction of methemoglobin in erythrocytes of a patient with congenital methemoglobinemia, subjects with glucose-6-phosphate dehydrogenase deficiency, and normal individuals, *Blood* 21:561, 1963.
21. Kan YW, Forget BG, Nathan DG: Gamma-beta thalassemia: a cause of hemolytic disease of the newborn, *N Engl J Med* 286:129, 1972.
22. King PJ: Iron supplementation in prematurity: how much is too much?, *J Pediatr* 151:3, 2007.
23. Lane PA, Hathaway WE: Vitamin K deficiency, *J Pediatr* 106:351, 1985.
24. Linderkamp O, Versmold HT, Strohhacker I, et al: Capillary-venous hematocrit differences in newborn infants, *Eur J Pediatr* 127:9, 1977.
25. Lipton JM, Alter BP: Blackfan-Diamond anemia. In Feig SA, Freedman MH, editors: *Clinical disorders and experimental models of erythropoietic failure,* Boca Raton, Fla, 1993, CRC Press.
26. MackIntosh TF, Walker CHM: Blood viscosity in the newborn, *Arch Dis Child* 48:547, 1973.
27. Mahasandana C, Suvatte V, Chuansumrit A, et al: Homozygous protein S deficiency in an infant with purpura fulminans, *J Pediatr* 117:750, 1990.
28. Maheshwari A, Christensen RD: *Fetal and neonatal physiology,* ed 2, Philadelphia, 2004, Saunders.
29. Manco-Johnson MJ: Disseminated intravascular coagulation and other hypercoagulable syndromes, *Int J Pediatr Hematol Oncol* 1:1, 1994.
30. Mentzer WC Jr, Shannon KM, Phibbs RH: Recombinant human erythropoietin (epoetin alpha) in patients with the anemia of prematurity. In Erslev AJ, editor: *Erythropoietin, molecular cellular, and clinical biology*, Baltimore, 1991, Johns Hopkins University Press.
31. Meyer MP, Meyer JH, Commerford A, et al: Recombinant human erythropoietin in the treatment of the anemia of prematurity: results on a double-blind, placebo controlled study, *Pediatrics* 93:918, 1994.
32. Oh W, Lind J: Venous and capillary hematocrit in newborn infants and placental transfusion, *Acta Paediatr* 55:38, 1966.
33. Oski FA: Iron deficiency anemia in infancy and childhood, *N Engl J Med* 329:190, 1993.
34. Paludetto R: Neonatal complications specific to twin (multiple) births (twin transfusion syndrome, intrauterine death of cotwins), *J Perinatal Med* 19:246, 1964.
35. Ramamurthy RD, Brans YW: Neonatal polycythemia. I. Criteria for diagnosis and treatment, *Pediatrics* 68:168, 1981.
36. Roithmaier A, Arlettaz R, Bauer K, et al: Randomized controlled trial of Ringer solution versus serum for partial exchange transfusion in neonatal polycythemia, *Eur J Pediatr* 154:53, 1995.
37. Rosen PJ, Johnson C, McGehee WG, et al: Failure of methylene blue treatment in toxic methemoglobinemia associated with glucose-6-phosphate dehydrogenase deficiency, *Ann Intern Med* 75:83, 1971.
38. Rothenberg T: Partial plasma exchange transfusion in polycythemic neonates, *Arch Dis Child* 86:60, 2002.
39. Shannon KM: Anemia of prematurity: progress and prospects, *Am J Pediatr Hematol Oncol* 12:14, 1990.
40. Shannon KM, Naylor GS, Torkildson JC, et al: Circulating erythroid progenitors in the anemia of prematurity, *N Engl J Med* 317:728, 1987.
41. Shapiro AD, Jacobson LJ, Armon ME, et al: Vitamin K deficiency in the newborn infant: prevalence and perinatal risk factors, *J Pediatr* 109:675, 1986.
42. Shohat M, Reisner SH: Neonatal polycythemia. I. Early diagnosis and incidence relating to time of sampling, *Pediatrics* 73:7, 1984.
43. Tan KL, Tan R, Tan SH, et al: The twin transfusion syndrome: clinical observation of 35 affected pairs, *Clin Pediatr* 18:111, 1979.

44. Todd D, Lai MC, Beaven GH, et al: The abnormal haemoglobins in homozygous alpha-thalassemia, *Br J Haematol* 20:9, 1970.
45. Villalta IA, Pramanik AK, Diaz-Blanco J, et al: Diagnostic errors in neonatal polycythemia based on method of hematocrit determination, *J Pediatr* 115:460, 1989.
46. Woodrow JC, Donohue WTA: Rh-immunization by pregnancy: results of a survey and their relevance to prophylactic therapy, *BMJ* 4:139, 1968.
47. Yaegashi N, Shiraishi H, Takeshita T, et al: Propagation of human parvovirus B19 in primary culture of erythroid lineage cells derived from fetal liver, *J Virol* 63:2422, 1989.
48. Zipursky A, Hull A, White FD, et al: Foetal erythrocytes in the maternal circulation, *Lancet* 1:451, 1959.
49. Zivny J, Kobilkova J, Neuwirt J, et al: Regulation of erythropoiesis in fetus and mother during normal pregnancy, *Obstet Gynecol* 60:77, 1982.

SUGGESTED READINGS

Bizzarro MJ, Colson E, Ehrenkranz RA: Differential diagnosis and management of anemia in the newborn, *Pediatr Clin North Am* 51:1087, 2004.

Bussel JB: Fetal and neonatal cytopenias: what have we learned?, *Am J Perinatol* 20:425, 2003.

Chalmers EA: Neonatal coagulation problems, *Arch Dis Child Fetal Neonatal Ed* 89:F475, 2004.

Christensen RD, Calhoun DA: Congenital neutropenia, *Clin Perinatol* 31:29, 2004.

Golomb MR: The contribution of prothrombotic disorders to peri- and neonatal ischemic stroke, *Semin Thromb Hemost* 29:415, 2003.

Harkness UF, Spinnato JA: Prevention and management of RhD isoimmunization, *Clin Perinatol* 31:721, 2004.

Heller C, Nowak-Göttl U: Maternal thrombophilia and neonatal thrombosis, *Best Pract Res Clin Haematol* 16:333, 2003.

Isarangkura P, Mahasandana C, Chuansumrit A, et al: Acquired bleeding disorders: the impact of health problems in the developing world, *Haemophilia* 10(Suppl 4):188, 2004.

Kulkarni R: Bleeding in the newborn, *Pediatr Ann* 30:548, 2001.

Kulkarni R, Lusher J: Perinatal management of newborns with haemophilia, *Br J Haematol* 112:264, 2001.

Lee LA: Neonatal lupus: clinical features and management, *Paediatr Drugs* 6:71, 2004.

Monagle P, Chan A, Massicotte P, et al: Antithrombotic therapy in children: the seventh ACCP conference on antithrombotic and thrombolytic therapy, *Chest* 645S:126, 2004.

Nowak-Göttl U, Kosch A, Schlegel N: Neonatal thromboembolism, *Semin Thromb, Hemost* 29:227, 2003.

Petaja J, Manco-Johnson MJ: Protein C pathway in infants and children, *Semin Thromb, Hemost* 29:349, 2003.

Rabe H, Reynolds G, Diaz-Rosello J: Early versus delayed umbilical cord clamping in preterm infants, *Cochrane Database Syst Rev* 4:CD003248, 2004.

21

JAUNDICE

BEENA D. KAMATH, ELIZABETH H. THILO, AND JACINTO A. HERNANDEZ

Jaundice, or hyperbilirubinemia, is an almost universal occurrence in neonates. All infants have a rise in their bilirubin levels after birth because of excessive bilirubin formation and an immature liver that cannot clear the bilirubin from the blood. Sixty percent of normal newborns become noticeably jaundiced sometime during the first week of life.[19]

Severe hyperbilirubinemia, defined as total serum bilirubin above the 95th percentile for age in hours, occurs in 8% to 9% of infants during the first week of life.[5] Experiences have shown the dangers of excessive levels of unconjugated bilirubin, such as the development of bilirubin encephalopathy and the devastating and irreversible effects of kernicterus. Although the severe sequelae remain rare, a resurgence of kernicterus was seen in the 1990s.[8,14] The increasing incidence of kernicterus was attributed to several causes: the advent of early postnatal discharge before establishment of effective breast feeding, a lack of recognition for the signs of bilirubin encephalopathy, a lack of appropriate follow-up for discharged infants, and a delay in the measurement of bilirubin levels. Therefore an understanding of the pathophysiology and clinical significance of hyperbilirubinemia is critical in the care of newborn infants.

This chapter provides the reader with a basic overview of the multiple causes and contributing factors in the development of hyperbilirubinemia; describes the diagnosis, clinical significance, and complications of hyperbilirubinemia; and discusses current treatment modalities and their complications.

PHYSIOLOGY

To understand the pathophysiology and clinical significance of hyperbilirubinemia, normal bilirubin metabolism in the newborn must be reviewed (Figure 21-1). A newborn has a rate of bilirubin production of 8 to 10 mg/kg/24 hr, which is 2 to 2½ times the production rate in adults. Red blood cells in newborns have a shortened life span of 70 to 90 days, compared with 120 days in adults. As the catabolism of **1 g of hemoglobin yields 35 mg of bilirubin,** this accelerated red blood cell breakdown produces most of the bilirubin (75% to 85%) in newborns. The remaining 15% to 25% of bilirubin is derived from non-erythroid heme proteins found principally in the liver and heme precursors in the marrow and extramedullary hematopoietic areas that do not go on to form red blood cells (early peak or shunt bilirubin).

Bilirubin metabolism is initiated in the reticuloendothelial system, principally in the liver and spleen, as old or abnormal red blood cells are removed from the circulation. The enzyme ***microsomal heme oxygenase*** will act on heme to produce biliverdin, and ***biliverdin reductase*** will convert this biliverdin into bilirubin. This bilirubin, in its unconjugated or indirect-reacting form, is released into the plasma. Exhaled carbon monoxide is an end product of these pathways.

At a normal plasma pH, bilirubin is very poorly soluble and binds tightly to circulating albumin, which serves as a carrier protein. Albumin contains one high-affinity site for bilirubin and one or more sites of lower affinity. **Bilirubin binds to albumin in a molar ratio of between 0.5 and 1 mole of bilirubin per mole of albumin. A bilirubin/albumin molar ratio of 1 corresponds to approximately 8.5 mg bilirubin/g of albumin. This ratio may be somewhat lower in a sick very-low-birth-weight (VLBW) infant.**[7]

Bilirubin bound to albumin is carried to the liver and transported into the hepatocyte by carrier-mediated diffusion. Intracellularly, bilirubin is bound to ligandin (Y protein) and, to a lesser extent, the Z protein. Conjugation occurs within the smooth

Please note that the PURPLE type in each chapter is intended to make it easier to identify clinically applicable material.

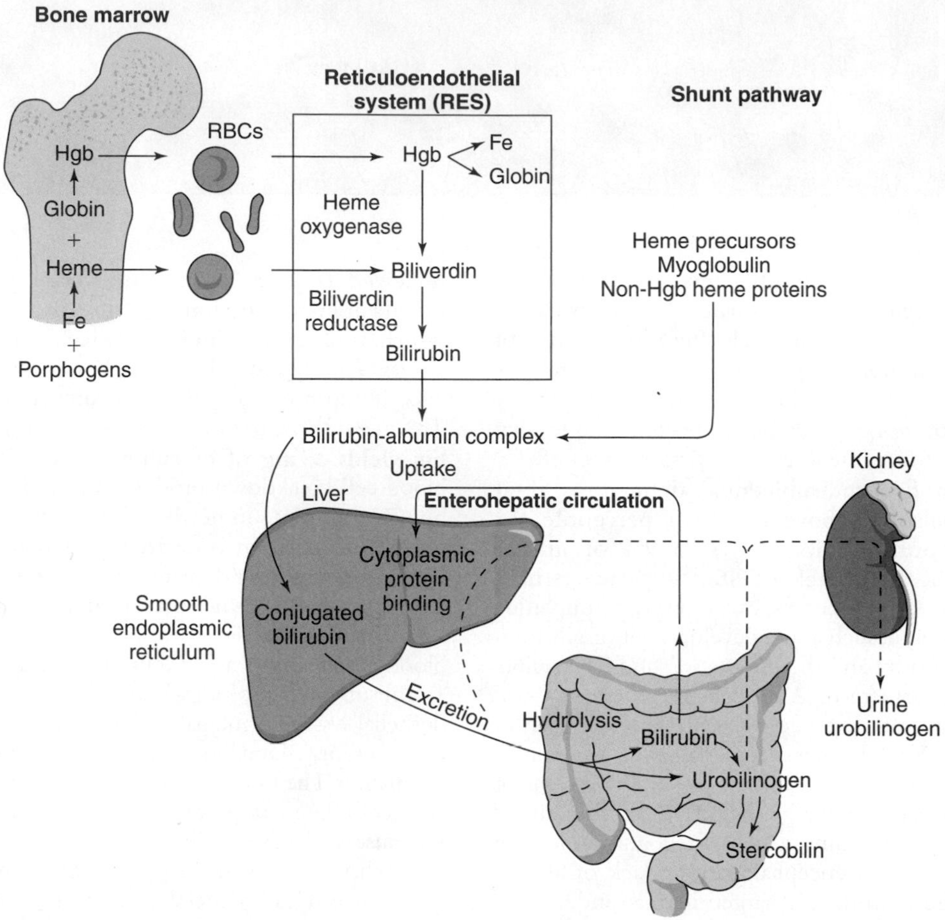

FIGURE 21-1 Pathways of bilirubin synthesis, transport, and metabolism. *Fe,* Iron; *Hgb,* hemoglobin; *RBC,* red blood cells. (From Gartner LM, Hollander M: Disorders of bilirubin metabolism. In Assali NS, editor: *Pathophysiology of gestation,* vol 3, New York, 1972, Academic Press.)

endoplasmic reticulum of the cell. This reaction, catalyzed by the enzyme bilirubin ***uridine diphosphate glucuronosyl transferase (UDPGT),*** leads to the formation of water-soluble compounds called ***bilirubin glucuronides.*** In addition to UDPGT, conjugation requires glucuronic acid synthesized from glucose. Conjugated bilirubin is then actively secreted into bile and passes into the small intestine.

Conjugated bilirubin is not reabsorbed from the intestine, but the bowel lumen of the newborn contains the enzyme ***beta-glucuronidase,*** which can convert conjugated bilirubin back into glucuronic acid and unconjugated bilirubin, which may be absorbed. **This pathway constitutes the enterohepatic circulation of bilirubin and contributes significantly to an infant's bilirubin load.**[22]

Factors That Affect Bilirubin Levels

The ability of albumin to bind bilirubin is affected by a number of different factors, including plasma pH, free fatty acid levels, and certain drugs (Table 21-1). Albumin binding of unconjugated bilirubin may be important in the prevention of toxicity (bilirubin encephalopathy or kernicterus). Once the high-affinity site is saturated, there is a rapid increase in potentially toxic free (nonbound) unconjugated bilirubin. Kernicterus has been clinically associated with administration of sulfisoxazole to newborns as a result of displacement of bilirubin from the primary binding site on albumin. Other drugs, such as ceftriaxone, also appear to displace bilirubin from this binding site. The effect on bilirubin-albumin binding

TABLE 21-1 FACTORS AFFECTING BILIRUBIN-ALBUMIN BINDING

FACTOR	MECHANISM
pH (acidosis)	Decreases binding by decreasing affinity at the binding site and increasing tissue affinity
Hematin	Competitively inhibits binding at primary site
Free fatty acid (intralipid)*	Competitively inhibits binding at primary site
Infection	Mechanism not established
Drugs such as sulfa compounds, sodium salicylate, phenylbutazone, and ceftriaxone	Primarily competitive binding; principally at secondary site; and best established for sulfisoxazole
Stabilizers for albumin preparations	Competitively inhibit binding at primary site
X-ray contrast media for cholangiography	Competitively inhibit binding at primary site

*From Hargreaves T: Effects of fatty acids on bilirubin conjugation, *Arch Dis Child* 48:446, 1973.

of some but not all drugs used in newborn medicine has been studied in vitro.[23]

Newborn monkeys have been shown to be deficient in the intracellular Y and Z proteins for the first few days of life, and this also may occur in the human newborn. The hormonal (estrogen) environment of the infant may inhibit liver function and bilirubin secretion. A rise in bilirubin levels shortly after birth is also partially attributable to a relative deficiency of UDPGT activity (0.1% of adult levels at 30 weeks' gestation). Enzyme activity increases rapidly after birth independent of the infant's gestational age.

Certain ethnic groups, including Eskimo, Asian, and Native American, have an increased incidence and severity of hyperbilirubinemia for reasons that are not clearly understood. In a hypoglycemic infant, glucuronide production may be limited and thus conjugation is impaired. The presence of beta-glucuronidase in the bowel lumen during fetal life enables bilirubin to be reabsorbed and transported across the placenta for excretion by the maternal liver.

BOX 21-1 CAUSES OF HYPERBILIRUBINEMIA

Overproduction

- Hemolytic disease of the newborn
- Hereditary hemolytic anemias
    - Membrane defects
    - Hemoglobinopathies
    - Enzyme defects
- Polycythemia
- Extravascular blood
    - Swallowed
    - Bruising or enclosed hemorrhage (e.g., cephalohematoma)
- Increased enterohepatic circulation

Slow Excretion

- Decreased hepatic uptake
    - Decreased sinusoidal perfusion
    - Ligandin deficiency
- Decreased conjugation
    - Enzyme deficiency
    - Enzyme inhibition, such as the Lucey-Driscoll syndrome
- Inadequate transport out of hepatocyte
- Biliary obstruction

Combined (Overproduction and Slow Excretion)

- Bacterial infection
- Congenital intrauterine infection

Breast Feeding

- Breast feeding jaundice
- Breast milk jaundice

Physiologic

Miscellaneous

- Hypothyroidism
- Galactosemia
- Infant of diabetic mother

ETIOLOGY

Bilirubin levels rise in newborn infants by three main mechanisms: increased production (accelerated red blood cell breakdown), decreased removal (transient liver enzyme insufficiency), and increased reabsorption (enterohepatic circulation) (Box 21-1). The normal pathways of bilirubin metabolism described earlier account for much of the increase in bilirubin levels in newborn infants; however, the following circumstances deserve special attention for infants who have prolonged or marked increases in bilirubin levels than would otherwise be expected.

From a management perspective, it is helpful to describe severe hyperbilirubinemia according to its time of onset, early or late, to determine its specific etiology. In general, early-onset severe hyperbilirubinemia is associated with increased bilirubin production, whereas late-onset hyperbilirubinemia is often associated with delayed bilirubin elimination with or without increased bilirubin production (Figure 21-2).[25]

Overproduction of Bilirubin

HEMOLYTIC DISEASE OF THE NEWBORN

Hemolytic disease of the newborn may occur when blood group incompatibilities such as Rh, ABO, or minor blood groups exist between a mother and her fetus. The classic example of hemolytic disease of the newborn has been erythroblastosis fetalis occurring as a result of Rh incompatibility. Fifteen percent of the white population is Rh negative. When an Rh-negative mother is sensitized to the Rh antigen by an improperly matched blood transfusion or the occurrence of fetal-maternal blood transfusion during pregnancy, delivery, abortion, or amniocentesis, the presence of the Rh antigen induces maternal antibody production. Because prior sensitization with the Rh antigen is necessary for antibody production, the first Rh-positive infant usually is not affected. **Once a mother is sensitized, maternal immunoglobulin G (IgG) crosses the placenta into the fetal circulation where it reacts with the Rh antigen on fetal erythrocytes. These antibody-coated cells are recognized as abnormal and destroyed by the spleen.** This results in increased amounts of

<table>
<tr><th colspan="2">Early-onset hyperbilirubinemia
(age < 72 hours)</th><th colspan="2">Late-onset hyperbilirubinemia
(age >72 hours and <2 weeks)</th></tr>
<tr><th>First 24 hours of life</th><th colspan="2">First week of life</th><th>>1 week of life</th></tr>
<tr><td rowspan="3">Direct Coombs' positive:
• Isoimmune erythroblastosis fetalis
• Rhesus disease
• Minor blood group incompatibilities
• ABO (often the direct Coombs' is negative)</td><td colspan="2">Benign idiopathic jaundice (physiologic; <40th percentile)</td><td>Prolonged idiopathic jaundice (breast milk jaundice; TSB <13 mg/dL)</td></tr>
<tr><td colspan="2">Sepsis (viral or bacterial)</td><td>Sepsis (viral or bacterial)</td></tr>
<tr><td colspan="2">Increased enterohepatic circulation</td><td>Functional gastrointestinal tract abnormality</td></tr>
<tr><td rowspan="2">Direct Coombs' negative:
• G6PD deficiency
• Intrinsic red blood cell defect
• Spherocytosis
• Elliptocytosis
• Hemoglobinopathies</td><td colspan="3">Disorders of bilirubin metabolism:
• UGT1A1 gene polymorphisms (delayed conjugation)
• Co-inheritance of UGT1A1 polymorphism with G6PD deficiency, ABO incompatibility, spherocytosis
• Crigler-Najjar syndrome: I and II
• Gilbert syndrome
• Others
Metabolic disorders:
• Galactosemia
• Alpha$_1$-antitrypsin deficiency
• Storage diseases
• Others</td></tr>
<tr><td colspan="2">Enclosed hemorrhages:
• Cephalhematoma
• Subaponeurotic hemorrhage
• Bruising</td><td>Cystic fibrosis
Hypothyroidism</td></tr>
</table>

FIGURE 21-2 Differential diagnosis of severe neonatal hyperbilirubinemia based on pathophysiology and timing at presentation. *G6PD,* Glucose-6-phosphate dehydrogenase; *TSB,* total serum bilirubin. (Modified from Smitherman H, Stark AR, Bhutani VK: Early recognition of neonatal hyperbilirubinemia and its emergent management, *Semin Fetal Neonatal Med* 11:214, 2006.)

hemoglobin, requiring metabolic degradation. As the destruction of erythrocytes and production of bilirubin progress, the ability of the fetus to compensate may be surpassed. **Fortunately, the use of anti-D gamma globulin (RhoGAM), particularly antenatal administration at 26 to 28 weeks' gestation to non-sensitized pregnant women, has markedly decreased the incidence of Rh isoimmunization and the resulting hyperbilirubinemia in newborn infants.**

With the widespread use of RhoGAM, **the most frequent cause of hemolytic disease of the newborn is now ABO blood group incompatibility.** ABO incompatibility is limited to mothers of blood group O and affects infants of blood group A or B. All group O individuals have naturally occurring anti-A and anti-B (IgG) antibodies, so specific sensitization is not necessary. The resulting hyperbilirubinemia in the newborn is very variable and generally milder than that seen with Rh incompatibility.

HEREDITARY HEMOLYTIC ANEMIAS

Erythrocytes with abnormal membranes or containing abnormal hemoglobin variants have increased rates of red blood cell destruction. Individuals with enzyme defects, such as spherocytosis and elliptocytosis, cannot maintain the integrity of red blood cells because of abnormal osmotic fragility (generally increased) and an increased rate of splenic destruction. Glucose-6-phosphate dehydrogenase (G6PD) deficiency is the most common enzyme defect and is more commonly found in certain racial and ethnic groups, including Chinese, Greeks, and blacks. Pyruvate kinase deficiency is less common.

Individuals with hemoglobinopathies, which can be diagnosed by hemoglobin electrophoresis, also have increased splenic destruction. Often, the precipitating factor for the hemolysis cannot be found in infants. A family history is important, however, since it may be positive in as many as 80% of cases.

POLYCYTHEMIA

Polycythemia (with a central venous hematocrit value >65) is the condition in which an increased red blood cell mass, coupled with the shortened life span of these cells found in all newborns, results in an increased bilirubin load. Polycythemia may be idiopathic or may occur as a result of a maternal-fetal transfusion, twin-to-twin transfusion, chronic in utero hypoxia, or delayed clamping of the umbilical cord at the time of delivery.

EXTRAVASCULAR BLOOD

Enclosed hemorrhage includes cephalohematoma, subgaleal hemorrhage, cerebral hemorrhage, intra-abdominal bleeding, and any occult internal bleeding, as well as extensive bruising. As these enclosed hemorrhages resolve, red blood cells trapped within are broken down and add to bilirubin production. Swallowed maternal blood is another possible source of increased bilirubin load.

INCREASED ENTEROHEPATIC CIRCULATION

As mentioned, the intestinal brush border contains the enzyme ***beta-glucuronidase,*** which can convert conjugated bilirubin back into its unconjugated (absorbable) form and glucuronic acid. **Meconium contains a substantial amount of bilirubin, estimated at 1 mg of bilirubin per 1 g of meconium, or a total load of 100 to 200 mg. Any delay in the passage of meconium, as can occur with prematurity or bowel obstruction, increases the bilirubin load that must be metabolized.** Hyperbilirubinemia requiring treatment due to these causes is rarely evident in the first 24 to 48 hours of life.

Slow Excretion of Bilirubin

Infants with normal bilirubin production rates may be unable to remove this load for a variety of reasons, as described in the following conditions.

DECREASED HEPATIC UPTAKE OF BILIRUBIN

Diminished hepatic uptake of bilirubin may be a result of inadequate perfusion of hepatic sinusoids or deficient carrier proteins (Y and Z). Certain drugs and compounds (e.g., steroid hormones, free fatty acids, chloramphenicol) may competitively bind to these proteins, creating a functional deficiency.

Inadequate perfusion of hepatic sinusoids occurs when there is a shunt through a persistent ductus venosus or extrahepatic portal vein thrombosis or with hyperviscosity and hypovolemia, as seen in infants with severe congestive heart failure. Although Y and Z proteins are decreased in some newborn primates, no actual deficiency has yet been demonstrated in the human newborn.

DECREASED BILIRUBIN CONJUGATION

Decreased bilirubin conjugation may be a result of UDPGT deficiency, as in the Crigler-Najjar syndromes or Gilbert syndrome. These disorders are caused by defects in the *UDPGT1* gene complex recently identified on chromosome 2. ***Crigler-Najjar syndrome*** is rare and exists in two forms with either complete (type I) or partial (type II) absence of enzymatic activity. Type I is an autosomal recessive disorder. Phototherapy becomes ineffective in preventing excessive bilirubin levels, and liver transplantation is the only possible cure. Type II is inherited as an autosomal dominant disorder and responds to enzyme induction with phenobarbital. ***Gilbert syndrome*** is a milder and very common autosomal dominant disorder with partial enzyme activity generally becoming apparent beyond the newborn period with mild bilirubin elevation during times of stress or intercurrent illness. It may well be an important contributing factor, however, in cases of late-onset severe hyperbilirubinemia.

INADEQUATE TRANSPORT OUT OF THE HEPATOCYTE

Dubin-Johnson and ***Rotor syndromes*** are genetically inherited conditions (autosomal recessive and dominant, respectively) in which individuals can conjugate bilirubin normally but cannot excrete it, resulting in direct (conjugated) hyperbilirubinemia. These conditions, in addition to causing generalized hepatocellular damage, require specialized evaluation, including liver biopsy.

BILIARY OBSTRUCTION

Biliary obstruction often is seen as a diagnostic dilemma requiring differentiation between generalized hepatocellular damage and mechanical obstruction.

A variety of disorders can cause hepatocellular damage, including infections such as hepatitis and metabolic disorders such as galactosemia. In the neonatal intensive care unit (NICU), the most common cause of hepatocellular damage is the use of parenteral nutrition. The mechanism is not well established, but the damage takes at least 2 weeks to develop and is especially prominent in VLBW infants. Biliary atresia or, much less frequently, a choledochal cyst can cause mechanical obstruction to bile flow, resulting in a conjugated hyperbilirubinemia with light-colored stools.

Combined Overproduction and Slow Excretion

INFECTIONS

Bacterial infections (sepsis neonatorum, especially necrotizing enterocolitis [NEC] caused by toxin-producing organisms such as certain strains of *Escherichia coli [E. coli]*) or intrauterine viral infections can result in increased bilirubin production and decreased hepatic clearance.

Intrauterine infections, including syphilis, toxoplasmosis, rubella, cytomegalovirus, herpes simplex, Coxsackie B virus, and hepatitis virus, cause clinical jaundice with evidence for hepatocellular damage. Infants with these infections often have additional clinical stigmata of their infection such as thrombocytopenia and rash.

INFANT OF A DIABETIC MOTHER

The cause of hyperbilirubinemia in an infant of a diabetic mother (IDM) appears to be multifactorial. In addition to prematurity and a tendency to feed poorly, an IDM may have an increased bilirubin load as a result of an expanded red blood cell mass. Erythrocyte membrane composition may be altered, and macrosomic infants often are bruised during labor and delivery.

Jaundice Associated with Breast Feeding

Ideally, a trained observer should evaluate all breast-fed infants within 48 to 72 hours of discharge in either a home or office setting.[6] Early discharge of breast-fed infants with inadequate follow-up may result in excessive levels of bilirubin and the possibility of kernicterus. Thus promotion and support of successful breast feeding constitutes a key element of the American Academy of Pediatrics (AAP) clinical practice guideline on the management of hyperbilirubinemia.[1]

BREAST-FEEDING JAUNDICE

In general, breast-fed infants have higher bilirubin levels than bottle-fed infants, especially in the first days of life. It has been postulated that this early jaundice is related to decreased caloric and fluid intake from colostrum and increased enterohepatic circulation resulting from low stool output and breast milk beta-glucuronidase.[1] Many studies show a relationship between the degree of hyperbilirubinemia and the amount of weight lost by the infant after birth.

Because of concern for breast-fed infants being underfed, it once was common practice in some institutions to supplement with glucose water or electrolyte solutions after nursing. Such supplementation should be avoided because it reduces breast-feeding frequency and maternal milk production, without improving the infant's intestinal motility, leading to higher peak bilirubin levels. **Optimal management of a breast-feeding mother and infant includes early and frequent nursing: 8 to 12 times each day.** If the infant is unable to feed this frequently, the mother should be instructed in the use of a mechanical breast pump, and the infant supplemented with expressed breast milk or formula to improve both the milk supply and the infant's nutritional status and intestinal motility.

BREAST MILK JAUNDICE

A small percentage (1% to 2%) of breast-fed infants exhibit prolonged and exaggerated jaundice possibly related to an inhibitor or inhibitory substance found in their mother's breast milk that prolongs and increases enterohepatic circulation. The rate of recurrence in families approaches 70%.

Such infants have an unconjugated hyperbilirubinemia (>12 mg/dL) that becomes exaggerated and persistent toward the end of the first week of life.[10] Other causes of excessive hyperbilirubinemia should be ruled out. Elevated bilirubin levels may persist for 4 to 14 days, followed by a very gradual decline. For the vast majority of infants, it is not necessary to interrupt breast feeding, even if the bilirubin increases to a level that may require phototherapy.

Miscellaneous Causes

The following causes of hyperbilirubinemia are uncommon but important to consider in infants who have no other clear etiology to explain their elevated bilirubin levels. These conditions include hypothyroidism and galactosemia. States now require routine screening for these conditions, since early detection allows intervention before permanent adverse neurologic outcomes. Hyperbilirubinemia, unconjugated or mixed, may be the initial sign of these conditions.

HYPOTHYROIDISM

A prolonged period of unconjugated hyperbilirubinemia can be seen in infants with hypothyroidism. The mechanism of hyperbilirubinemia in hypothyroidism is not well understood, but in some animal studies, thyroxine was needed for the hepatic clearance of bilirubin.

GALACTOSEMIA

Galactosemia is an autosomal recessive disorder characterized by increased jaundice in infants fed breast milk or lactose-containing formulas. The mechanism of hyperbilirubinemia in galactosemia may be related to a lack of substrate for glucuronidation and the accumulation of abnormal hepatotoxic by-products. The presence of non–glucose-reducing substances in the urine suggests galactosemia.

INTERPRETATION OF HIGH BILIRUBIN LEVELS

Identification of those infants at risk for hyperbilirubinemia enables clinicians to provide timely treatment to prevent neuronal injury. The AAP has described risk factors for hyperbilirubinemia, which can be seen in Box 21-2.

The most important determinants of brain injury caused by hyperbilirubinemia are the concentrations of unconjugated bilirubin and free bilirubin, the concentration of serum albumin and its ability to bind unconjugated bilirubin, the concentration of hydrogen ion (pH), and neuronal susceptibility.[24] The blood-brain barrier allows free bilirubin to pass; however, the blood-brain interface, consisting of capillary endothelium and astrocytic foot processes, and the choroid plexus have specific transporters that can pump free bilirubin out of the central nervous system, thereby protecting the brain from exposure to high bilirubin. Timing of exposure to excess bilirubin during neurodevelopment is important in determining the pattern of the neurologic damage; for example, because auditory pathways mature earlier than motor pathways, patterns of damage in premature infants may differ from those in mature infants.[24] Unconjugated bilirubin is fat soluble and can cross cell membranes; however, because most unconjugated bilirubin is bound to albumin, toxicity is avoided.[25] Therefore development of toxicity may also depend on albumin-bilirubin binding. Factors that interfere with albumin-bilirubin binding appear to predispose to the development of kernicterus (see Table 21-1). Once toxicity has occurred, it appears to be irreversible.

BOX 21-2 RISK FACTORS FOR HYPERBILIRUBINEMIA IN NEWBORNS

Major Risk Factors

- Pre-discharge TSB or TcB level in the high-risk zone
- Jaundice observed in the first 24 hours of life
- Blood group incompatibility with positive direct antiglobulin test, other known hemolytic disease (e.g., G6PD deficiency), elevated ETcoc
- Gestational age 35 to 36 weeks
- Previous sibling received phototherapy
- Cephalohematoma or significant bruising
- Exclusive breast feeding, especially if nursing is not going well and weight loss is excessive
- East Asian race*

Minor Risk Factors

- Pre-discharge TSB or TcB level in the high intermediate-risk zone
- Gestational age 37 to 38 weeks
- Jaundice observed before discharge
- Previous sibling with jaundice
- Macrosomic infant of a diabetic mother
- Maternal age ≥25 years
- Male gender

Decreased Risk (these factors are associated with decreased risk for significant jaundice, listed in order of decreasing importance)

- TSB or TcB level in the low-risk zone
- Gestational age ≥41 weeks
- Exclusive bottle feeding
- Black race*
- Discharge from the hospital after 72 hours

From American Academy of Pediatrics, Subcommittee on Hyperbilirubinemia: Clinical Practice Guideline: Management of hyperbilirubinemia in the newborn infant 35 or more weeks of gestation, *Pediatrics* 114:297, 2004.

ETcoc, End-tidal carbon monoxide corrected; *G6PD,* glucose-6-phosphate dehydrogenase; *TcB,* transcutaneous bilirubin; *TSB,* Total serum bilirubin.

*Race as defined by mother's description.

Although elevated levels of bilirubin occur in virtually all newborns, precise identification of what constitutes a "safe" level for an individual newborn, especially if sick or premature, remains elusive and is the subject of much ongoing investigation. A "pathologic" level for one infant may be a "physiologic" level for another infant; therefore it has been suggested that these terms be done away with altogether.

All bilirubin levels should be interpreted according to the infant's age in hours. The AAP recommends a nomogram that designates risk for newborn infants at 35 weeks or greater, according to bilirubin level obtained at varying postnatal ages in hours. **The nomogram (Figure 21-3), based on earlier work by Bhutani et al, designates whether an infant is at high, intermediate, or low risk for requiring further intervention for hyperbilirubinemia.**[1,5] This hour-specific bilirubin nomogram has been shown to be more accurate than a clinical risk factor scoring system for assessing risk for significant hyperbilirubinemia,[16] although the addition of gestational age to the risk assessment strategy can increase accuracy further.[17]

PREVENTION

Early Feeding

The physiologic mechanism is not entirely known but may be caused by a decrease in intestinal transit time and decreased enterohepatic circulation. When

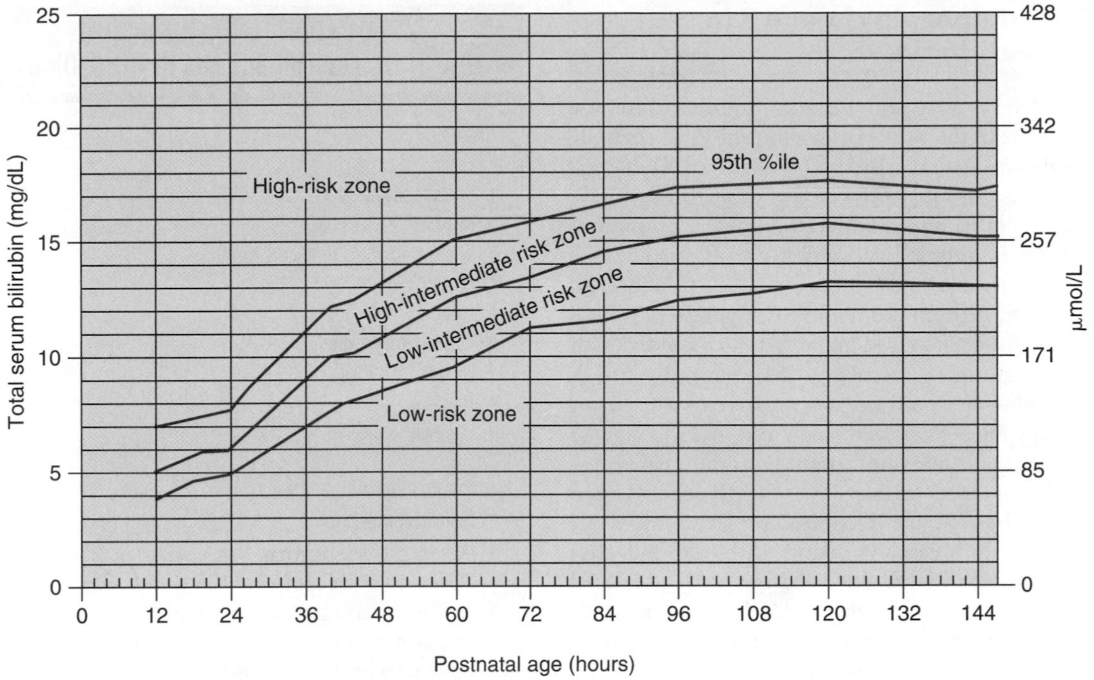

FIGURE 21-3 Nomogram for designation of risk in 2840 well newborns at 36 or more weeks gestational age with birth weight of 2000 g or more or 35 or more weeks gestational age with birth weight of 2500 g or more based on the hour-specific serum bilirubin levels. The serum bilirubin level was obtained before discharge, and the zone in which the value fell predicted the likelihood of a subsequent bilirubin level exceeding the 95th percentile (high-risk zone). (From Bhutani VK, Johnson L, Sivieri EM: Predictive ability of a predischarge hour-specific serum bilirubin for subsequent significant hyperbilirubinemia in healthy term and near-term newborns, *Pediatrics* 103:6, 1999.)

compared with infants not fed during the first 24 to 48 hours of life, infants fed earlier have lower peak bilirubin levels.

RhoGAM

Widespread use of RhoGAM has proven effective in preventing the sensitization of Rh-negative mothers after delivery or abortion of Rh-positive infants. RhoGAM, or anti-D gamma globulin, provides passive protection by preventing maternal production of anti-Rh antibodies that might affect subsequent Rh-positive pregnancies, causing destruction of fetal red blood cells.

Failures may occur if the amount of RhoGAM administered is insufficient compared with the load of fetal red blood cells received or if a significant fetal-maternal hemorrhage occurred before prophylaxis. Routine management of the Rh-negative mother now includes the administration of antenatal RhoGAM in the second trimester (26 to 28 weeks), at the time of amniocentesis, and after delivery.

Phenobarbital

Phenobarbital acts as an inducer of microsomal enzymes, increasing the levels of UDPGT. It also has a direct effect to stimulate bile secretion in infants with nonobstructive cholestasis and increases the concentration of ligandin. When used in conjunction with phototherapy, however, phenobarbital does not increase the rate of decline in bilirubin levels. Phenobarbital is effective when given to the mother before delivery. In infants with significant hemolytic disease of the newborn, it appears to slow the rate of rise of bilirubin and decrease the incidence of exchange transfusion. It is indicated in infants with Crigler-Najjar syndrome type II. Its use is not indicated on a routine prophylactic basis, because such use would overtreat many infants and other effects may be detrimental.

Tin Protoporphyrin and Tin Mesoporphyrin

Clinical trials have shown that administration of a single dose of tin protoporphyrin (SnPP) or tin mesoporphyrin (SnMP) to infants with ABO hemolytic disease or G6PD deficiency at birth effectively decreases bilirubin production. These compounds are potent competitive inhibitors of the enzyme ***heme oxygenase.***[15] Heme is excreted directly into bile when bilirubin production is suppressed. Infants receiving a single dose of SnMP (6 mcmol/kg of body weight intramuscularly [IM]) have lower peak serum bilirubin levels and a decreased need for phototherapy. Side effects have been minimal and include a transient erythema in those infants requiring phototherapy after receiving SnMP. SnMP also has been shown to be effective in controlling severe hyperbilirubinemia in breast-fed infants with high bilirubin levels between 48 and 96 hours of age.[20] Additional studies to determine what role these compounds will have in the management and prevention of neonatal jaundice are ongoing.

DATA COLLECTION

The history, physical examination, and laboratory data play an important role in the evaluation of the infant with hyperbilirubinemia (Box 21-3).

History

The evaluation of a jaundiced infant begins with a complete family, perinatal, and neonatal history. The family history should include the occurrence of disorders associated with hyperbilirubinemia in other family members, particularly siblings. The perinatal and obstetric history may provide clues or enable the clinician to anticipate possible hyperbilirubinemia. For example, hydrops fetalis is associated with Rh isoimmunization but is rarely seen with ABO incompatibility. The infant's course during labor, delivery, and thereafter may be important. Items of interest include possible infection during the pregnancy, the use of oxytocin induction for delivery, or the occurrence of an asphyxial episode during labor or delivery. A history of medications used and the infant's feeding and stooling patterns should also be obtained. **The time of onset or detection of jaundice may be important, because jaundice in the first 24 hours of life always must be considered abnormal.**

BOX 21-3 EVALUATION OF UNCONJUGATED HYPERBILIRUBINEMIA IN THE NEONATE

History
- Family
- Perinatal and obstetric
- Neonatal

Physical Examination
- Pallor
- Hepatosplenomegaly
- Enclosed hemorrhage
- Petechiae
- Congenital anomalies

Laboratory Data

All Jaundiced Infants
- Maternal and infant blood type
- Coombs' test on cord blood
- Total/direct bilirubin (serial measurements)
- Complete blood count, including hematocrit, reticulocyte and platelet counts, white blood cell differential, and peripheral smear for red blood cell morphology
- Urinalysis, test for reducing substances

Selected Cases
- Protein, total/albumin

Sepsis Evaluation
- IgM
- Urine cytology for cytomegalovirus
- Viral cultures

New Techniques
- Transcutaneous bilirubinometry
- Bilirubin-binding tests

Signs and Symptoms and Clinical Approach

A wide spectrum of signs and symptoms may occur in a jaundiced infant, often depending on the cause of the jaundice. **Jaundice in a newborn**

usually can be detected visually at a level of 6 to 7 mg/dL. Visible icterus appears first on the head and face and progresses in a cephalocaudal manner. The skin of the extremities, particularly the palmar and plantar surfaces, are the last skin surfaces to be affected. However, multiple studies show **the inaccuracy of visual estimation of jaundice, even by experienced health care workers; thus all newborns should be assessed for hyperbilirubinemia with a serum or transcutaneous measurement if concern exists. Any measurement of bilirubin needs to be interpreted based on the infant's age in hours at the time of measurement (see Figure 21-3), which allows classification into high-risk, high intermediate-risk, low intermediate-risk, and low-risk zones.** In addition, premature infants have a slightly later peak and are at risk for adverse neurologic outcomes at lower levels of bilirubin than older infants.

An infant with hemolytic disease of the newborn may show signs of jaundice and pallor in association with severe anemia and hydrops fetalis or may appear entirely normal at birth. ***Hepatosplenomegaly*** resulting from congestion and extramedullary hemopoiesis may be present. **Infants affected by hemolytic disease of the newborn may also have pancreatic islet cell hyperplasia and are at increased risk for hypoglycemia.** Careful physical examination may reveal the presence of a cephalohematoma or other lesion resulting from enclosed hemorrhage. The occurrence of petechiae or purpura raises the possibility of intrauterine infection or sepsis. Congenital anomalies or syndromic appearance should be noted, because an increased incidence of jaundice is noted in trisomic syndromes. Jaundice and umbilical hernia are also associated with congenital hypothyroidism.

SIGNS OF BILIRUBIN TOXICITY

Hyperbilirubinemia is of clinical concern because of the potential for brain injury. The spectrum of bilirubin-induced neurologic dysfunction (BIND) ranges from acute bilirubin encephalopathy to the devastating and irreversible syndrome of kernicterus.[8,10,17] Acute bilirubin encephalopathy (ABE) describes the effects of hyperbilirubinemia seen during the hyperbilirubinemia and immediately thereafter. Clinical signs of ABE include lethargy, poor feeding, poor tone, a poor Moro reflex with incomplete flexion of the extremities, and a high-pitched cry. Opisthotonos posturing and retrocollis also may occur in the later stages.[24] As the symptoms of acute bilirubin encephalopathy worsen, the infant progresses to apnea, seizures, coma, and death.

Kernicterus, or chronic bilirubin encephalopathy, is an irreversible and devastating brain injury evidenced pathologically by yellowish staining in the deep nuclei of the central nervous system (CNS), particularly in the basal ganglia, cerebellum, and hippocampus. As opposed to other forms of perinatal brain injury, in the instance of kernicterus, a clear correlation exists between etiology, pathogenesis, and symptomatology.[24] Based on multiple studies, kernicterus has a mortality of 10% and at least 70% long-term morbidity.[11] Its clinical signs include extrapyramidal movement disorder, including dystonia and choreoathetoid movements (rapid, highly complex, involuntary, spasmodic movements); gaze abnormalities (especially affecting upward gaze); auditory disturbances (deafness); dysplasia of the enamel of deciduous teeth; and mild cognitive defects. The neuromotor abnormalities may be subtle, with the auditory abnormalities most apparent because the auditory pathways are the neural system most sensitive to bilirubin injury.[24]

In later life, severely affected survivors with kernicterus may exhibit choreoathetosis, spastic cerebral palsy, mental retardation, sensory and perceptual deafness, and visual-motor incoordination. It is not likely that significant mental retardation alone, without the other features, is caused by bilirubin encephalopathy.

Whether more subtle long-term sequelae may occur in less severely affected infants and may not be apparent during the newborn period remains very controversial. There is speculation that some learning disabilities may be related to hyperbilirubinemia even at what had been previously considered "safe" levels. **High bilirubin levels have been consistently associated with hearing impairment and abnormal brainstem auditory evoked potentials.**[11] Regarding other neurodevelopmental outcomes, extensive review of the literature dealing with full-term infants without hemolytic disease has found inconsistent evidence of adverse effects of bilirubin on intelligence quotient and neurologic examination; however, many of these studies have yielded mixed results and had limitations.[11,21] A recent study compared 140 term infants without kernicterus who had total serum bilirubin levels of at least 25 mg/dL with randomly selected controls. The study found no difference in adverse neurodevelopmental outcomes in infants born at or near term when the infants with hyperbilirubinemia were treated aggressively with phototherapy or exchange transfusion.[21]

Infants with hemolytic disease and premature (especially VLBW) infants should receive phototherapy and exchange transfusion at lower bilirubin levels. Unfortunately, the "critical level" at which bilirubin toxicity occurs in either preterm or term infants has not been established.

Laboratory Data

A serum bilirubin level is the most reliable method upon which to make clinical decisions. Transcutaneous bilimeters have been used in newborn nurseries to screen for hyperbilirubinemia and work by emitting a beam of light onto the skin and measuring the light reflected, which is not absorbed by bilirubin in the skin. **Transcutaneous bilimeters have been shown to be valid[3]; however, new studies are showing that bilimeter levels may significantly underestimate the severity of hyperbilirubinemia.** Because of the uncertain accuracy of the transcutaneous bilirubin measurement, **it is not recommended to consider this device reliable at levels greater than 14 mg/dL.[18]**

Because the breakdown of bilirubin is the only chemical reaction in the body that results in formation of carbon monoxide (CO), this marker has been used to measure bilirubin production.[9] Measurement of end-tidal CO corrected for inhaled CO (ETcoc) can identify infants with unusually high rates of bilirubin production and is the only clinical test providing direct measurement of the rate of heme catabolism and bilirubin production. It is not yet clear what role measurement of ETcoc will play in clinical management. The device is not commercially available in the United States.

In addition to a bilirubin level, mother's and infant's blood types and Rh status, as well as Coombs' testing (antibody testing), both direct and indirect, are needed to evaluate for hemolytic disease. The direct Coombs' test on cord blood is positive because of the presence of IgG on the surface of the infant's red blood cells, whereas an indirect Coombs' test is positive with the presence of IgG in the infant's serum. An indirect positive only is generally less severe than a direct positive antibody screen.

In addition to measurements of hematocrit and reticulocytes, the peripheral blood smear should be carefully examined, seeking evidence of hemolysis (increased numbers of nucleated red blood cells or the presence of fragmented cells, poikilocytosis, and anisocytosis). Microspherocytosis is characteristic of ABO incompatibility and at times may be confused with hereditary spherocytosis. A knowledge of mother's and baby's blood types and the clinical course help differentiate the two.

Obtaining fractionated (total/direct) bilirubin levels and serial levels helps establish causes and enables the clinician to follow the rate of bilirubin rise, although the total bilirubin should be used for making clinical treatment decisions. Serum albumin levels should be determined and the bilirubin:albumin (B:A) ratio considered as an additional factor in deciding when to start phototherapy or perform an exchange transfusion. Clinical laboratory measurement of unbound ("free") bilirubin is not available but may be a useful test in the future.

Evaluation for other potential causes of hyperbilirubinemia is essential when the etiology is not immediately clear. An elevated direct fraction of bilirubin, abnormal white blood cell count, left shifted differential, or thrombocytopenia may suggest infection. Urinalysis, including evaluation for reducing substances, may be helpful. Infants suspected of having congenital infection should have additional tests, including immunoglobulin M (IgM) levels. Blood, cerebrospinal fluid, and/or exudate from skin vesicles should be sent for viral cultures, and urine may be tested for cytomegalovirus (CMV). Newborns should be screened for hypothyroidism and galactosemia.

Minimum laboratory evaluation of the jaundiced newborn should include the mother's and infant's blood types, Rh status, and Coombs' test (direct and indirect) on cord blood. A complete blood count (CBC) to include reticulocyte and platelet counts, white blood cell count and differential, peripheral smear for red blood cell morphology, and hematocrit should be performed. Infants suspected of having bacterial sepsis should receive antibiotic treatment and a complete sepsis evaluation, including cultures of blood, urine, and cerebrospinal fluid. Bilirubin levels (total and direct) should be measured serially and interpreted based on the infant's age in hours at the time of measurement (see Figure 21-3). Serum albumin levels may be helpful at higher bilirubin levels.

In addition to jaundice and anemia in the first few days of life, infants with hemolytic disease are at risk for late anemia after discharge from the nursery, potentially driving the infant's physiologic nadir of red blood cell count even lower than usual, requiring treatment with erythropoietin or transfusion. These infants require close follow-up for anemia from their primary care provider.

TREATMENT

Treatment is aimed at lowering the concentration of circulating bilirubin or keeping it from increasing, thereby preventing the complications of acute bilirubin encephalopathy and the irreversible damage of kernicterus. Phototherapy, in particular, and exchange transfusions, now less so, are widely used in the treatment of hyperbilirubinemia; however, decisions to use these therapies are complicated by an incomplete understanding of bilirubin toxicity, especially as applied to an individual infant (Table 21-2). The AAP Subcommittee on Hyperbilirubinemia published clinical management guidelines that lend direction regarding the use of these therapies, and the recommendations are outlined in the algorithm detailed in Figure 21-4 and in Figure 21-5 (phototherapy) and Figure 21-6 (exchange transfusion).

Phototherapy

Phototherapy is the most commonly used treatment for hyperbilirubinemia. With the widespread use of phototherapy, the need for exchange transfusion in infants with non-hemolytic hyperbilirubinemia is almost obsolete. Hospital-based studies in the United States have shown that 5 to 40 infants per 1000 term and late preterm infants receive phototherapy before discharge from the nursery and an equal number are readmitted for phototherapy after discharge.[19] The decision to initiate phototherapy must be individualized for each newborn and should be based on the recent AAP guidelines (see discussion in legend for Figure 21-5).

With effective phototherapy, the infant's bilirubin level should drop at a rate of 0.5 to 1 mg percent per hour, and by 30% to 40% after 24 hours of treatment, when applied at several days of age. The rate of decline of bilirubin in the first days (early hyperbilirubinemia, likely the result of increased bilirubin production) will not be as brisk, but the rate of rise will be significantly slowed. Bilirubin best absorbs light in the blue-green spectrum, particularly in the blue region of the spectrum near 460 nm[19]; the spectrum of light at 425 to 475 nm is therefore most effective. Phototherapy uses this light energy to change the shape and structure of bilirubin, converting it to molecules that can be excreted, even when normal conjugation is deficient.[19] The most important of these molecules is lumirubin, a stable structural photoisomer. Lumirubin does not require conjugation and is rapidly excreted in both bile and urine. The production of lumirubin is an irreversible reaction that appears to be dose-related.

The efficacy of phototherapy depends on the energy output (irradiance) of the light source (measured with a radiometer in units of watts per square centimeter or microwatts per square centimeter per nanometer over a given wavelength band), the distance of the light source from the infant, and the surface area of the infant exposed to the light. Intensive phototherapy consists of 30 $\mu W/cm^2/nm$ or more.[1] Fiberoptic blankets delivering phototherapy from a high-intensity light source are available for use by themselves or in conjunction with other sources of phototherapy but are unlikely to expose an adequate surface area on a term infant to provide intensive phototherapy.[19]

TABLE 21-2 PHOTOTHERAPY AND EXCHANGE TRANSFUSION CRITERIA FOR VERY-LOW AND EXTREMELY-LOW-BIRTH-WEIGHT INFANTS

WEIGHT (g)	INITIATE PHOTOTHERAPY (mg/dL)	CONSIDER EXCHANGE TRANSFUSION (mg/dL)
500-750	5-8	12-15
751-1000	6-10	>15
1001-1250	8-10	15-18
1251-1500	10-12	17-20

Modified from Cashore WJ: Bilirubin and jaundice in the micropremie, *Clin Perinatol* 27:178, 2000.

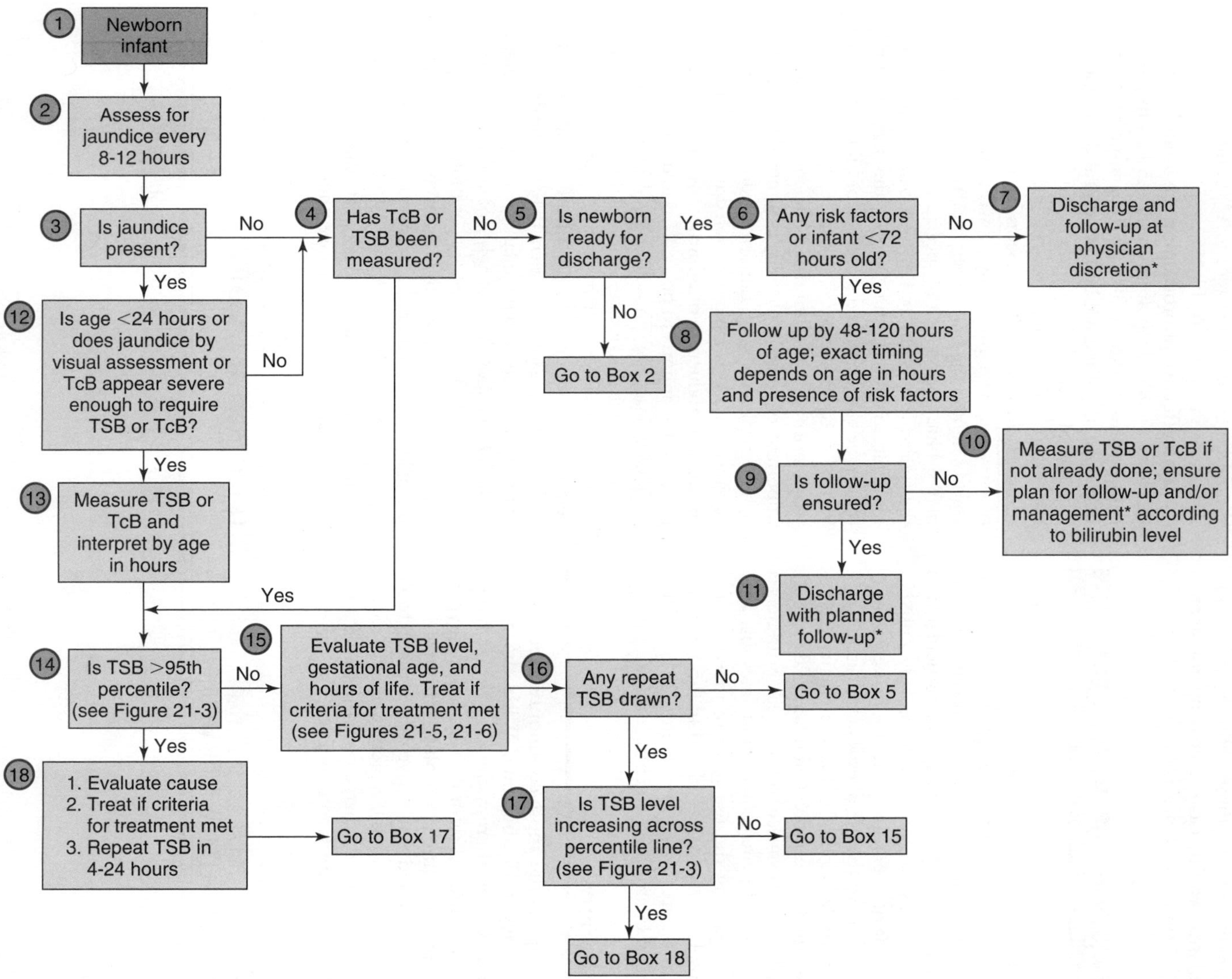

*Provide information and written guidelines about jaundice to parents of all newborns at discharge.

FIGURE 21-4 Algorithm for the management of jaundice in the newborn nursery. *TcB,* Transcutaneous bilirubin; *TSB,* total serum bilirubin. (Modified from American Academy of Pediatrics, Subcommittee on Hyperbilirubinemia: Clinical Practice Guideline: Management of hyperbilirubinemia in the newborn infant 35 or more weeks of gestation, *Pediatrics* 114:297, 2004.)

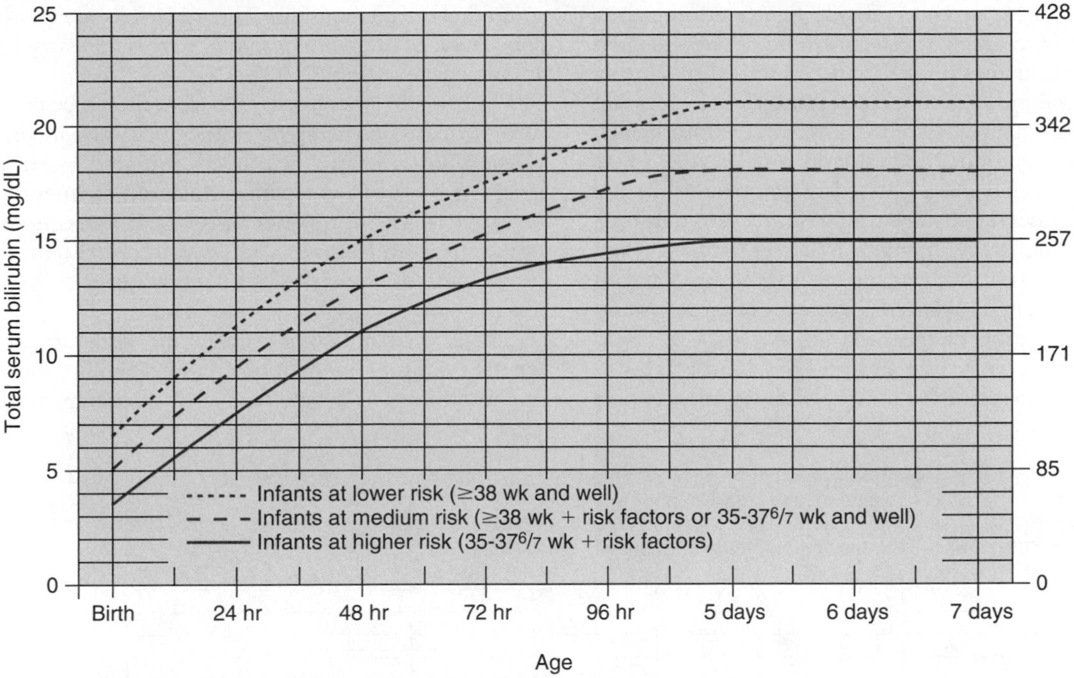

- Use total bilirubin. Do not subtract direct-reacting or conjugated bilirubin.
- Risk factors = isoimmune hemolytic disease, G6PD deficiency, asphyxia, significant lethargy, temperature instability, sepsis, acidosis, or albumin <3.0 g/dL (if measured).
- For well infants 35-37 6/7 weeks, can adjust TSB levels for intervention around the medium risk line. It is an option to intervene at lower TSB levels for infants closer to 35 weeks and at higher TSB levels for those closer to 37 6/7 weeks.
- It is an option to provide conventional phototherapy in the hospital or at home at TSB levels 2-3 mg/dL (35-50 mmol/L) below those shown, but home phototherapy should not be used in any infant with risk factors.

FIGURE 21-5 American Academy of Pediatrics (AAP) guidelines for phototherapy in hospitalized infant of 35 or more weeks' gestation. (NOTE: These guidelines are based on limited evidence, and the levels shown are approximations. The guidelines refer to the use of intensive phototherapy that should be used when the total serum bilirubin [TSB] exceeds the line indicated for each category. Infants are designated as "higher risk" because of the potential negative effects of the conditions listed on albumin binding of bilirubin, the blood-brain barrier, and the susceptibility of the brain cells to damage by bilirubin.) *G6PD*, Glucose-6-phosphate dehydrogenase. (From American Academy of Pediatrics, Subcommittee on Hyperbilirubinemia: Clinical Practice Guideline: Management of hyperbilirubinemia in the newborn infant 35 or more weeks of gestation, *Pediatrics* 114:297, 2004.)

The AAP discusses in their 2004 guidelines the most commonly used phototherapy units. These include daylight, cool white, blue, or "special blue" fluorescent tubes or tungsten-halogen lamps in different configurations, either free-standing or as part of a radiant warming device. A system using high-intensity gallium nitride light-emitting diodes has been introduced; in this model, six fiberoptic systems deliver light from a high-intensity lamp to a fiberoptic blanket. Most of these devices deliver enough output in the blue-green region of the visible spectrum to be effective for standard phototherapy use. **The most effective light sources commercially available for phototherapy are those that use special blue fluorescent tubes or a specially designed light-emitting diode light** (Natus Inc, San Carlos, Calif.). The special blue fluorescent tubes are labeled *F20T12/BB* (General Electric, Westinghouse, Sylvania) or *TL52/20W* (Phillips, Eindhoven, The Netherlands). It is important to note that special blue tubes provide much greater irradiance than regular blue tubes (labeled *F20T12/B*). Special blue tubes are most effective because they provide light predominantly in the blue-green spectrum. At these wavelengths, light penetrates skin well and is absorbed maximally by bilirubin.[1] Fiberoptic phototherapy blankets are available. These systems (Wallaby Phototherapy System, Fiberoptic Medical Products, Inc., Allentown, Pa.; and Biliblanket, Ohmeda, Columbia, Md.) use a high-intensity halogen light source for transmission of light by fiberoptic bundles. Irradiance and efficacy appear comparable with those for standard phototherapy. Purported advantages of these systems are elimination of the need for eye patches, exposure of greater surface area, and provision of phototherapy outside of the nursery with less interference in mother-infant bonding. These blankets are more convenient to use when phototherapy is necessary in an outpatient setting.

Physical and laboratory evaluation should be performed before initiating phototherapy in any infant. **Once phototherapy has been initiated, serum levels of bilirubin must be monitored frequently (every 4 to 12 hours) because visual assessment of icterus is no longer valid.** Hematocrit also must be monitored, especially in infants with hemolytic disease.

There are conflicting data in the literature on whether continuous or intermittent administration of phototherapy is most effective. Phototherapy may

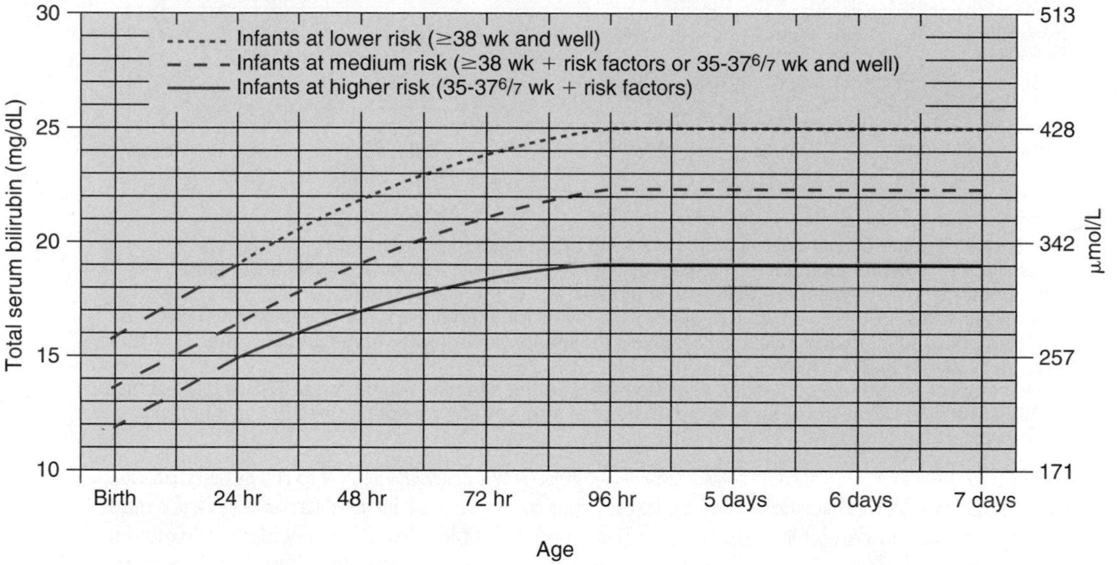

- The dashed lines for the first 24 hours indicate uncertainty due to a wide range of clinical circumstances and a range of responses to phototherapy.
- Immediate exchange transfusion is recommended if infant shows signs of acute bilirubin encephalopathy (hypertonia, arching, retrocollis, opisthotonos, fever, high-pitched cry) or if TSB is ≥5 mg/dL (85 μmol/L) above these lines.
- Risk factors: isoimmune hemolytic disease, G6PD deficiency, asphyxia, significant lethargy, temperature instability, sepsis, acidosis.
- Use total bilirubin. Do not subtract direct-reacting or conjugated bilirubin.
- If infant is well and 35-37 6/7 weeks (median risk), can individualize TSB levels for exchange based on actual gestational age.

FIGURE 21-6 American Academy of Pediatrics (AAP) guidelines for exchange transfusion in infants of 35 or more weeks' gestation. (NOTE: These suggested guidelines represent a consensus of most of the American Academy of Pediatrics Subcommittee on Hyperbilirubinemia but are based on limited evidence, and the levels shown are approximations. During birth hospitalization, exchange transfusion is recommended if the total serum bilirubin [TSB] rises to these levels despite intensive phototherapy. For readmitted infants, if the TSB level is above the exchange level, repeat TSB measurement every 2 to 3 hours and consider exchange if the TSB remains above the levels indicated after intensive phototherapy for 6 hours.) *G6PD,* Glucose-6-phosphate dehydrogenase; *TSB,* total serum bilirubin. (From American Academy of Pediatrics, Subcommittee on Hyperbilirubinemia: Clinical Practice Guideline: Management of hyperbilirubinemia in the newborn infant 35 or more weeks of gestation, *Pediatrics* 114:297, 2004.)

be interrupted during brief periods for feeding and parental contact. Table 21-3 outlines some of the nursing assessments and management to be performed in infants undergoing phototherapy.

After phototherapy ceases, bilirubin levels should be followed for at least 24 hours to rule out the occurrence of significant rebound. A rebound in the total serum bilirubin level of 1 to

TABLE 21-3 NURSING MANAGEMENT OF INFANTS UNDERGOING PHOTOTHERAPY

NURSING ASSESSMENT	
AREA	**PARAMETER**
Physical status	Intake and output Color Location of jaundice Skin integrity Stools (character, consistency) Vital signs Infant/environmental temperature Hydration status Signs of phototherapy side effects Eye discharge and tearing Position Activity
Neurobehavioral status	Sleep-wake states Sensory threshold Behavioral responsiveness Feeding behaviors Consoling abilities Stress responses Interactive capabilities
NURSING MANAGEMENT	
NURSING DIAGNOSIS	**INTERVENTION**
Deficient Fluid Volume (actual or potential)	Monitor intake and output. Monitor hydration status (weight, specific gravity, urine output). Monitor stooling pattern, character. Maintain adequate fluid intake (oral or parenteral).
Imbalanced Nutrition: Less Than Body Requirements	Assess feeding behavior and activity. Monitor fluid and caloric intake, weight, abdominal girth. Remove eye shields during feeding. Hold during oral feedings as health and thermal status permit. Bring to alert state before feeding. Feed on demand if possible.
Impaired Skin Integrity	Observe color, rashes, excoriation. Clean skin with warm water. Clean perineal area after stooling. Turn frequently (also increases skin exposure to phototherapy). Ensure Plexiglas shield is in place between light source and infant to reduce exposure to UV light.

From Blackburn S: Hyperbilirubinemia and neonatal jaundice, *Neonatal Netw* 14:15, 1995.

Continued

TABLE 21-3 NURSING MANAGEMENT OF INFANTS UNDERGOING PHOTOTHERAPY—cont'd

	NURSING MANAGEMENT
NURSING DIAGNOSIS	INTERVENTION
Risk for Injury	Observe for side effects associated with phototherapy. Observe for signs of sepsis. Provide care to minimize side effects of phototherapy. Shield eyes from lights with opaque patches. Ensure eyelids are closed when shield is applied to prevent corneal injury. Remove eye shield and observe eyes regularly. Monitor position of eye shield to prevent occlusion of nose. Avoid tight head band on eye shield to reduce risk of increased intracranial pressure especially in preterm infants. Observe for eye discharge, tearing. Shield testes and possibly ovaries (data unclear about need to do this) with diaper.
Ineffective Thermoregulation	Place in warm, thermoneutral environment. Monitor environmental and infant temperature. Observe for hypothermia and hyperthermia. Reduce heat losses from environmental sources. Use servocontrol for infants in incubator or under radiant warmer. Shield servocontrol thermistor from direct exposure to phototherapy lights.

From Blackburn S: Hyperbilirubinemia and neonatal jaundice, *Neonatal Netw* 14:15, 1995.

2 mg/dL, and occasionally more, can occur after phototherapy is discontinued. Infants at increased risk for rebound are those less than 37 weeks' gestation, those with hemolytic disease, and those treated with phototherapy during the birth hospitalization, since the bilirubin is still expected to rise at the time phototherapy is discontinued.[19]

Despite its widespread use since 1958, questions about the safety and side effects of phototherapy remain. However, reports of clinically significant toxicity are rare.[19] Animal studies have demonstrated a potential retinal toxicity of light. Although it is not established that this occurs in the human newborn, the possibility remains a concern and the infant's eyes should be covered while phototherapy is in use. Patches should completely cover the eyes without placing excessive pressure on the eyes and should be carefully positioned to avoid occluding the nares. **Eye patches should be removed every 4 hours to permit evaluation of the infant's eyes. The patches should be left off during feedings and parental visits.**

Infants exposed to phototherapy, particularly low-birth-weight infants and infants under a radiant warmer, have significant increases in their insensible water losses (IWLs). Infants in incubators or servo-controlled care centers may become overheated. The servocontrol probe should be shielded by an opaque covering. Infants treated in open cribs may become cold stressed. Fluid balance must be monitored carefully in an infant receiving phototherapy. Infants under phototherapy also have increased stool water losses and may develop temporary lactose intolerance. The infant's temperature, weight, and intake and output should be monitored frequently. The presence of reducing substances in the stool can be treated with a non–lactose-containing formula.

Infants who have an associated cholestatic jaundice and are exposed to phototherapy may develop the bronze baby syndrome, presumably caused by retention of a bilirubin breakdown product produced by phototherapy, although the mechanism is unclear. An infant with bronze baby syndrome develops a dark gray-brown discoloration of the skin, urine, and serum. There are generally no clinical symptoms with this syndrome, but at least one death has been reported. After phototherapy ceases, the bronzing gradually resolves.

Transient skin rashes and tanning resulting from increased melanin production have been reported, as have bullous skin eruptions in infants treated with tin mesoporphyrin who are subsequently exposed to sunlight or daylight fluorescent bulbs.[19] A recent study has suggested that intensive phototherapy might increase the number of melanocytic nevi identified at school age.[19] Other potential problems include interference with biologic (circadian) rhythms and maternal-infant bonding. Although there may be some transient, short-term growth effects, long-term growth effects and development appear unaffected by phototherapy.

Intravenous Immunoglobulin

When Coombs'-positive hemolysis is present and the total serum bilirubin is rising despite intensive phototherapy or is approaching the exchange level, **intravenous immunoglobulin (IVIG) should be administered to the infant to decrease the severity of hemolysis. The dose is 500 mg/kg to 1 g/kg IV over 2 to 4 hours and may be repeated one time after 12 hours.** This intervention has been shown in multiple trials to decrease the need for exchange transfusion by approximately 70% and is recommended for either Rh or ABO isoimmunization.[1,2]

Exchange Transfusion

An exchange transfusion is indicated for correction of severe anemia and removal of antibody-coated red blood cells in hemolytic disease or removal of excessive unconjugated bilirubin regardless of its cause. Phototherapy cannot be used in place of an exchange transfusion in those infants with severe hemolytic disease. A packed red blood cell exchange transfusion using type O Rh-negative blood will correct anemia and hypoxemia, as well as remove sensitized cells and bilirubin, leading to a more complete therapy for the problem.

It must be stressed that the decision to perform an exchange transfusion must be individualized for each patient. Particularly in VLBW infants, the indications to perform an exchange transfusion vary from nursery to nursery. The recent AAP guidelines for performing exchange transfusion in infants of 35 or more weeks of gestation are shown in Figure 21-6 (see discussion in legend).

Usually a double-volume exchange transfusion is performed using 160 mL/kg of appropriate whole blood product. ABO type-specific Rh-negative blood should be used in cases with Rh incompatibility. Type O Rh-specific cells are indicated when ABO incompatibility exists.

The blood bank can prepare this blood for the infant with a predetermined hematocrit, usually 50% to 55%. **An exchange transfusion will reduce bilirubin levels by approximately 45% to 85%, according to various sources.** Administration of 1 g/kg of 25% albumin 1 hour before the exchange transfusion has been shown in some studies to increase the efficiency of exchange by about 40%. **As plasma and tissue levels equilibrate post-transfusion, the bilirubin rises to about 60% of the pre-exchange level.**

Exchange transfusion trays are commercially available and include a four-way stopcock, necessary tubing and syringes, 10% calcium gluconate, and a plastic bag for discarded blood.

The infant should be in a NICU for close observation during and immediately after the procedure. The procedure is performed by removing small aliquots of the infant's blood and replacing similar small aliquots of transfused blood product while blood pressure, heart rate, and general condition are monitored. Generally, 5-mL to 20-mL aliquots of blood are used, depending on the size and condition of the infant. The initial aliquot should be withdrawn and sent to the laboratory for bilirubin, hematocrit, calcium, and cultures. The rate of exchange is usually 5 to 8 mL/min. Blood used in the exchange should be warmed and mixed in the bag after every 50 to 100 mL.

The final aliquot from an exchange should be sent for complete blood count (CBC), fractionated bilirubin, calcium ion, electrolytes, culture, and repeat type and crossmatch studies for potential additional exchange transfusion. In addition to the individuals performing the exchange, one person must keep an accurate record of time, volumes withdrawn and infused, vital signs, and medications administered.

Exchange transfusion is a procedure with many potential complications and carries a mortality risk of about 0.5%. For this reason and because so few exchange transfusions are performed today, this procedure should be done only by personnel familiar with it and its complications, preferably in a tertiary care unit. Vascular complications are related to the use of umbilical catheters (discussed in Chapter 7). Necrotizing enterocolitis has been reported as a post-exchange complication, probably as a result of bowel ischemia during the procedure.

Electrolyte and glucose disturbances are related to the blood preparation used for the exchange. Citrate used as part of the anticoagulant solution binds divalent ions such as calcium and magnesium; thus laboratory evaluation of calcium and magnesium during the procedure is essential. **The infant should be evaluated for hypocalcemia after each 100 mL of the exchange has been completed.** Clinical signs and symptoms of hypocalcemia include irritability, tachycardia, or prolongation of the Q-oTc interval. If hypocalcemia is detected, 1 mL of a 10% calcium gluconate solution is infused slowly.

Acid-citrate-dextrose and citrate-phosphate-dextrose blood have high levels of sodium and glucose and sometimes potassium. Initial hyperglycemia may be followed by reactive hypoglycemia as a result of an insulin response. Although acidic at the time of infusion, a post-exchange alkalosis may occur as citrate is metabolized to bicarbonate in the liver.

Many of the electrolyte and acid-base disturbances may be avoided by the use of fresh, heparinized blood. Bleeding may occur in an overheparinized infant but is reversible with protamine sulfate. Thrombocytopenia may occur, especially in the infant needing repeated exchange transfusions. Bacterial infection is rare, and routine antibiotic prophylaxis is not indicated. Most complications are avoidable if careful attention to technique is observed.

PARENT TEACHING

Providing parents with written information about jaundice and its therapy may be a beneficial adjunct to verbal explanations and is a key element of recent AAP guidelines on management of hyperbilirubinemia (Box 21-4). Because early discharge policies (<48 hours) have increased the need for outpatient evaluation or management of neonatal hyperbilirubinemia, it is important that parents feel empowered to ask questions about hyperbilirubinemia and its symptoms so that they can bring any concerns to the attention of health care providers. Indeed, early discharge of infants has now led to hyperbilirubinemia being the most common cause for hospital readmission in term infants.

Hyperbilirubinemia and its treatment can be disturbing to parents. Parents often feel guilty that something they did or failed to do may have resulted in their infant's jaundice. Providing parents and families with consistent information, reassurance, and support is essential. This is especially true for the nursing mother, who may be questioning her ability to provide adequate nourishment for her infant.

The use of phototherapy can be distressing for parents and should be explained to them before they see the infant under phototherapy lights for the first time. Parents often worry that the bright lights will cause permanent damage to their infant's eyes despite reassurances to the contrary.

In addition, incubators, bili-masks, and phototherapy lights can all contribute to a sense of separation between parents and their infant by creating a physical and emotional barrier. Parents may avoid coming to the nursery to be with their infant. If they do come to their infant's bedside, they may be reluctant to touch or participate in care for fear of interfering with phototherapy and potentially hindering their infant's progress. Phototherapy lights should be

BOX 21-4 KEY ELEMENTS OF AAP CLINICAL PRACTICE GUIDELINE (2004): MANAGEMENT OF HYPERBILIRUBINEMIA IN THE NEWBORN INFANT 35 OR MORE WEEKS OF GESTATION

Important Points for the Management of Jaundice

- Promote and support successful breastfeeding.
- Establish nursery protocols for the identification and evaluation of hyperbilirubinemia.
- Measure the total serum bilirubin (TSB) or transcutaneous bilirubin (TcB) level on infants jaundiced in the first 24 hours.
- Recognize that visual estimation of the degree of jaundice can lead to errors, particularly in darkly pigmented infants.
- Interpret all bilirubin levels according to the infant's age in hours.
- Recognize that infants at less than 38 weeks' gestation, particularly those who are breastfed, are at higher risk of developing hyperbilirubinemia.
- Perform a systematic assessment on all infants before discharge for the risk of severe hyperbilirubinemia.
- Provide parents with written and verbal information about newborn jaundice.
- Provide appropriate follow-up based on the time of discharge and risk assessment.
- Treat newborns, when indicated, with phototherapy or exchange transfusion.

From American Academy of Pediatrics, Subcommittee on Hyperbilirubinemia: Clinical Practice Guideline: Management of hyperbilirubinemia in the newborn infant 35 or more weeks of gestation, *Pediatrics* 114:297, 2004.

turned off and eye patches removed for brief periods during feedings and social times to facilitate face-to-face interaction with parents.

As with many disorders in newborn infants, time and energy spent providing parents with information and support can alleviate much fear, guilt, and anger. It also can help facilitate the development of a healthy family relationship in a time of crisis. Signs and symptoms of jaundice should be explained in a manner that is understandable and meaningful for parents, emphasizing that neonatal hyperbilirubinemia is usually a transient condition and one to which all infants must adapt after birth.

HEALTH SYSTEMS APPROACH TO BILIRUBIN

In the 1970s and 1980s, few health care providers had the opportunity to see a patient with kernicterus.[24] In recent times, however, rates of kernicterus have been rising and is seen as a systems failure in neonatal services.[4] For that reason, the Joint Commission on Accreditation of Healthcare Organizations issued Sentinel Event Alerts on kernicterus in 2001 and again in 2004.[12,13] However, neither hyperbilirubinemia nor kernicterus has been a reportable disease, and no reliable information source exists to produce national annual estimates.[11]

The root cause analysis for the reappearance of kernicterus revealed several factors. First, health services are provided by multiple providers at multiple sites, many of whom do not have a sufficient understanding of bilirubin and its potential for toxicity. Early discharge of newborn infants younger than 72 hours has the consequence that infants will be discharged before the natural peak of bilirubin rise in term infants and before the establishment of adequate breast feeding. A lack of knowledge by parents regarding hyperbilirubinemia and its symptoms and limitations within health care systems to provide appropriate pre-discharge screening of at-risk infants only serves to complicate issues.[4]

The AAP published guidelines on the management of hyperbilirubinemia in infants 35 weeks or more in 2004.[1] The overall aim was to promote an approach that would (1) reduce the frequency of severe hyperbilirubinemia and bilirubin encephalopathy, (2) minimize the risk for unintended harm (e.g., increased anxiety, decreased breast feeding, unnecessary treatment for the general population), and (3) avoid excessive cost and waste. These guidelines emphasize the importance of universal systematic assessment for the risk for severe hyperbilirubinemia, close follow-up, and prompt intervention when indicated. The ten key elements of the AAP practice guidelines are listed in Box 21-4. Bhutani and Johnson went further to recommend a five-step nationwide strategy to prevent severe neonatal hyperbilirubinemia as follows[4]:

- An institutional curriculum for the systems approach, including universal prenatal, pre-discharge, and post-discharge risk assessment of severe neonatal hyperbilirubinemia
- Advocacy for on-site services that promote breast feeding in the context of supervised and seamless health care delivery during the first month of life
- Effective parent-provider partnerships for safer management of neonatal jaundice
- Statewide (or regional) reporting of birthing institution outcome assessment for severe neonatal hyperbilirubinemia along with outcomes for neonatal screening for other inherited disorders
- Nationwide surveillance in which all severe cases of severe neonatal hyperbilirubinemia are reported

REFERENCES

1. American Academy of Pediatrics: Subcommittee on Hyperbilirubinemia: Clinical Practice Guideline: Management of hyperbilirubinemia in the newborn infant 35 or more weeks of gestation, *Pediatrics* 114:297, 2004.
2. Anderson D, Ali K, Blanchette V, et al: Guidelines on the use of intravenous immunoglobulin for hematologic conditions, *Transfus Med Rev* 21(2 Suppl 1):S9, 2007.
3. Bhutani VK, Gourley GM, Adler S, et al: Noninvasive measurement of total serum bilirubin in a multiracial predischarge newborn population to assess the risk of severe hyperbilirubinemia, *Pediatrics* 106:e17, 2000.
4. Bhutani VK, Johnson L: Prevention of severe neonatal hyperbilirubinemia in healthy infants of 35 or more weeks gestation: implementation of a systems based approach, *J Pediatr (Rio J)* 83:289, 2007.
5. Bhutani VK, Johnson L, Sivieri EM: Predictive ability of a predischarge hour-specific serum bilirubin for subsequent significant hyperbilirubinemia in healthy term and near-term newborns, *Pediatrics* 103:6, 1999.
6. Blackburn S: Hyperbilirubinemia and neonatal jaundice, *Neonatal Netw* 14:15, 1995.

7. Cashore WJ: Bilirubin and jaundice in the micropremie, *Clin Perinatol* 27:178, 2000.
8. Centers for Disease Control and Prevention: Kernicterus in full term infants: United States, 1994–1998, *MMWR Morb Mortal Wkly Rep* 50:494, 2001.
9. Dennery PA, Seidman DS, Stevenson DK: Neonatal hyperbilirubinemia, *N Engl J Med* 344:581, 2001.
10. Gartner LM: Jaundice and breastfeeding, *Pediatr Clin North Am* 48:389, 2001.
11. Ip S, Chung M, Kulig J, et al: An evidence-based review of important issues concerning neonatal hyperbilirubinemia, *Pediatrics* e130:114, 2004.
12. Joint Commission on Accreditation of Healthcare Organizations (JCAHO): Kernicterus threatens healthy newborns, *Sentinel Event Alert* Issue 18: April 1, 2001.
13. Joint Commission on Accreditation of Healthcare Organizations (JCAHO): Revised guidelines to help prevent kernicterus, *Sentinel Event Alert* Issue 31: August 31, 2004.
14. Juretschke LJ: Kernicterus: still a concern, *Neonatal Netw* 24:7, 2005.
15. Kappas A, Drummond GS, Henschke C, et al: Direct comparison of Sn-mesoporphyrin, an inhibitor of bilirubin production, and phototherapy in controlling hyperbilirubinemia in term and near-term newborns, *Pediatrics* 95:468, 1995.
16. Keren R, Bhutani VK, Luan X, et al: Identifying newborns at risk of significant hyperbilirubinemia: a comparison of two recommended approaches, *Arch Dis Child* 90:415, 2005.
17. Keren R, Luan X, Friedman S, et al: A comparison of alternative risk-assessment strategies for predicting significant neonatal hyperbilirubinemia in term and near-term infants, *Pediatrics* 121:e170, 2008.
18. Leite MJ, Granato V de A, Facchini FP, et al: Comparison of transcutaneous and plasma bilirubin measurement, *J Pediatr (Rio J)* 83:283, 2007.
19. Maisels MJ, McDonagh AF: Phototherapy for neonatal jaundice, *N Engl J Med* 358:920, 2008.
20. Martinez JC, Garcia HO, Otheguy LE, et al: Control of severe hyperbilirubinemia in full-term newborns with the inhibitor of bilirubin production Sn-mesoporphyrin, *Pediatrics* 103:1, 1999.
21. Newman TB: Outcomes among newborns with total serum bilirubin levels of 25 mg per deciliter or more, *N Engl J Med* 354:1889, 2006.
22. Poland RL, Odell GB: Physiologic jaundice: the enterohepatic circulation of bilirubin, *N, Engl J Med* 284:1, 1971.
23. Robertson A, Karp W, Brodersen R: Bilirubin displacing effect of drugs used in neonatology, *Acta Paediatr Scand* 80:1119, 1991.
24. Shapiro SM, Bhutani VK, Johnston L: Hyperbilirubinemia and kernicterus, *Clin Perinatol* 33:387, 2006.
25. Smitherman H, Stark AR, Bhutani VK: Early recognition of neonatal hyperbilirubinemia and its emergent management, *Semin Fetal Neonatal Med* 11:214, 2006.

SELECTED READINGS

Auerbach K, Gartner L: Breastfeeding and human milk: their association with jaundice in the neonate, *Clin Perinatol* 14:89, 1987.

Catz C, Hanson JW, Simpson L, et al: Summary of workshop: early discharge and neonatal hyperbilirubinemia, *Pediatrics* 96:743, 1995.

Kopelman AE, Brown RS, Odell GB: The "bronze" baby syndrome: a complication of phototherapy, *J Pediatr* 8:466, 1972.

Maisels MJ: Phototherapy: 25 years later. In Fanaroff AA, Klaus MH, editors: *The yearbook of neonatal and perinatal medicine*, St Louis, 1996, Mosby.

Maisels MJ: Neonatal jaundice. In Avery GB, editor: *Neonatology: pathophysiology and management of the newborn*, ed 5, Philadelphia, 1999, Lippincott.

Martin GI: Proceedings from the International Congress on Neonatal Jaundice March 16-18, 2001, *J Perinatol* 21(Suppl 1):S1-S27, 2001.

Scheidt PC, Bryla DA, Nelson KB, et al: Phototherapy for neonatal hyperbilirubinemia: six-year follow-up of the National Institute of Child Health and Human Development Clinical Trial, *Pediatrics* 85:455, 1990.

Stevenson DK, Vreman HJ: Carbon monoxide and bilirubin production in neonates, *Pediatrics* 100:252, 1997.

Volpe J: Bilirubin and brain injury. In Volpe J, editor: *Neurology of the newborn*, ed 5, Philadelphia, 2008, Saunders.

Yao TC, Stevenson DK: Advances in the diagnosis and treatment of neonatal hyperbilirubinemia, *Clin Perinatol* 22:741, 1995.

22 INFECTION IN THE NEONATE

MOHAN P. VENKATESH, KAREN M. ADAMS, AND LEONARD E. WEISMAN

A newborn infant is uniquely susceptible to infectious diseases. This chapter presents causes of infectious diseases with particular emphasis on prevention, history, presenting signs and symptoms, laboratory data, treatment, and parent teaching methods of prevention applicable to the care of the neonate. Abbreviations for this chapter are listed in Box 22-1.

PATHOPHYSIOLOGY AND PATHOGENESIS

An infection occurs when a susceptible host comes in contact with a potentially pathogenic organism. When the encountered organism proliferates and overcomes the host defenses, infection results. Sources of infection in a newborn can be divided into three categories: (1) transplacental acquisition (intrauterine infection), (2) perinatal acquisition during labor and delivery (intrapartum infection), and (3) hospital acquisition in the neonatal period (postnatal infection) from the mother, hospital environment, or hospital personnel.

In general, most infecting organisms can, under the proper circumstances, cross the placenta or ascend from the birth canal and invade the at-risk neonate. These infections may result in abortion, stillbirth, and disease present at birth or in the neonatal period.

The main goal is to prevent infections in the fetus and newborn. Unfortunately, few proven measures exist for the prevention of transplacentally or perinatally acquired infections. These measures are important, because most nonbacterial infections (except syphilis and possibly toxoplasmosis, cytomegalovirus [CMV] infection, and herpes simplex) do not respond to current therapy.

ETIOLOGY

Thorough data collection for diagnosis of infectious diseases includes a review of the perinatal history, signs and symptoms, and laboratory data. Intrauterine, intrapartum, or neonatal disease may be caused by a wide variety of organisms, many of which are discussed in this chapter.

SPECIFIC INFECTIOUS DISEASES

The following specific infectious diseases are grouped according to their source of infection.

Transplacental (Intrauterine) Acquisition

HUMAN IMMUNODEFICIENCY VIRUS INFECTION AND ACQUIRED IMMUNODEFICIENCY DISORDER

Prevention. The primary risk to infants for infection with human immunodeficiency virus (HIV), the causative agent of acquired immunodeficiency syndrome (AIDS), is intrauterine, intrapartum, and postpartum exposure to a mother with HIV infection. HIV has been isolated from blood and many body fluids. Epidemiologic evidence has implicated only blood, semen, vaginal secretions, and breast milk in transmission. In countries such as the United States, where safe alternatives exist, mothers with HIV infection should be discouraged from breast feeding.[93] HIV testing should be recommended and encouraged to all pregnant women.[5,6,114]

Acknowledgment: This is the first edition in which Gerry Merenstein has not contributed to this chapter. We miss him and dedicate this chapter to him for all his work on this chapter in the first six editions of this book.

Please note that the **PURPLE** type in each chapter is intended to make it easier to identify clinically applicable material.

BOX 22-1 ABBREVIATIONS

AIDS	Acquired immunodeficiency syndrome
CF	Complement fixation (test)
CIE	Counterimmunoelectrophoresis
CRP	C-reactive protein
CRS	Congenital rubella syndrome
CSF	Cerebrospinal fluid
DFA	Direct fluorescent antibody
DNA	Deoxyribonucleic acid
ELISA	Enzyme-linked immunosorbent assay
FA	Fluorescent antibody (test)
FAMA	Fluorescent antibody to membrane antigen
FTA-ABS	Fluorescent treponemal antibody absorption (test)
GBS	Group B *Streptococcus*
HbsAg	Hepatitis B surface antigen
HIV	Human immunodeficiency virus
IAHA	Immune adherence hemagglutination
IFA	Indirect fluorescent antibody (test)
IHA	Indirect hemagglutination inhibition (test)
IPV	Inactivated poliovirus vaccine
IUGR	Intrauterine growth restriction
LA	Latex agglutination (test)
MHA-TP	Microhemagglutination test for *Treponema pallidum* infection
NAAT	Nucleic acid amplification test
OPV	Oral poliovirus vaccine
PCP	*Pneumocystis jiroveci* pneumonia*
PCR	Polymerase chain reaction
RNA	Ribonucleic acid
RPR	Rapid plasma reagin (test)
RT-PCR	Reverse transcriptase PCR
VDRL	Venereal Disease Research Laboratory (test)

*Formerly *Pneumocystis carinii.*

Because the medical history and examination cannot reliably identify all patients infected with HIV (or other bloodborne pathogens) and because during delivery and initial care of the infant, perinatal care providers are exposed to large amounts of maternal blood, Standard Precautions (e.g., gloves) should be consistently used for all patients when handling the placenta or infant until all maternal blood has been washed away.[5,50]

Data Collection

History. HIV infection in the mother is acquired primarily sexually or by intravenous (IV) drug abuse. Infection may be asymptomatic. Transmission from an untreated infected mother to the fetus or infant occurs in 13% to 39% of births. Approximately 40% of transmissions are before birth and the rest around the time of delivery. Two thirds of infections occurring before delivery are caused by transmission within the 14 days before delivery.[5] A high maternal plasma viral load, high cervico-vaginal viral load, low $CD4^+$ lymphocyte count, advanced maternal illness, an increase in exposure of the fetus to maternal blood, premature delivery, prolonged labor, longer duration of rupture of membranes before delivery, and mode of delivery all increase perinatal transmission of HIV infection.[4,6,113]

Signs and Symptoms. Infants with perinatally acquired HIV infection uncommonly have symptoms in the neonatal period, but the majority of these infants present with clinical illness by 24 months of life (median age at onset of symptoms is 11 to 12 months). One fifth of infants infected with HIV perinatally develop serious disease or die in the first year of life.[114] Symptoms include failure to thrive, developmental disabilities, neurologic dysfunction, hepatosplenomegaly, generalized lymphadenopathy, parotitis, persistent oral candidiasis (thrush), and chronic or recurrent diarrhea. Lymphoid interstitial pneumonia is frequently seen in these infants. HIV-infected infants commonly have osteomyelitis, septic joints, pneumonia, sepsis, meningitis, and otitis media with common organisms (e.g., *Streptococcus pneumoniae, Haemophilus influenzae* type b), and these infections may be recurrent.[4,114]

Laboratory Data. HIV nucleic acid detection by polymerase chain reaction (PCR) of DNA extracted from peripheral blood mononuclear cells is the gold standard for early diagnosis of infected infants, and results are available within 24 hours.[114] About 30% of HIV-infected infants have a positive DNA PCR assay from samples obtained within 48 hours of age; 93% have detectable HIV DNA by 2 weeks; and almost all by 1 month of age. The primary serologic laboratory test for HIV antibody is the enzyme-linked immunosorbent assay (ELISA). The Western blot test is used for confirmation of positive ELISA results. Differentiation of the child with passively acquired antibody from the infant with active infection is critical but difficult. Acquired antibody is undetectable in 75% of infants by 12 months of age and in most infants by 15 to 18 months of age. Infants have also been described with negative serology but active infection.[79] Virus isolation by culture is difficult and expensive, and p24 antigen detection is less sensitive.[4,72] The plasma HIV RNA PCR assay is currently used for quantifying the viral load but not routinely used for diagnosis. Although hypogammaglobulinemia has been reported (<10% of patients), hypergammaglobulinemia usually is present.

Treatment. Antiretroviral therapy with zidovudine (ZDV) alone or in combination with other antiretroviral agents reduces HIV transmission from infected mothers to their newborns.[69,78,79] **ZDV should be given to infants of infected women beginning at 8 to 12 hours of life and should be continued for 6 weeks.**[6,69] ZDV is administered orally at 2 mg/kg body weight/dose every 6 hours.[6] If the infant is confirmed to be HIV positive, ZDV is changed to a multidrug antiretroviral regimen. Infants who are perinatally infected with HIV are at high risk for developing *Pneumocystis jiroveci* pneumonia (PCP, formerly known as *Pneumocystis carinii* pneumonia) early in the first year of life. Guidelines recommend initiating prophylaxis for the prevention of PCP for all HIV-exposed infants at 4 to 6 weeks of age, regardless of their $CD4^+$ cell count. For infants receiving ZDV, PCP prophylaxis should begin after completion of the 6-week course of ZDV. The recommended PCP prophylaxis may be provided by 150 mg/m^2/day (5 mg/kg/day) of trimethoprim (TMP) and 750 mg/m^2/day (25 mg/kg/day) of sulfamethoxazole (SMX) administered in two divided doses for three consecutive days in a week.[4,6,69] TMP/SMX prophylaxis should be continued through the first year of life or until HIV infection is reasonably excluded.[6,69]

Parent Teaching. Care of an infant at risk for HIV requires close and long-term follow-up. Involvement of the parents is essential to this process. Education of the parents will maximize the success of such a care plan, and utilization of all available community resources should provide additional support. In addition to the rationale for and importance of the medical management just outlined, the parents should be counseled concerning the need for the following:

- Immunizations following the American Academy of Pediatrics schedule
- Rapid consultation with the infant's physician if he or she is exposed to varicella (may need treatment with varicella-zoster immune globulin [VZIG] within 96 hours of exposure) or measles (needs immune globulin intramuscularly regardless of immunization status)
- Rapid consultation with the physician for tetanus-prone wounds (requires tetanus immune globulin irrespective of immunization status)
- Rapid consultation with the physician for thrush, a diaper rash, or any other signs or symptoms of illness

Prevention of infections is important, and this requires good handwashing, regular bathing, appropriate food preparation skills (wash bottles, nipples, and pacifiers), and good skin care (changing diapers and moisturizing skin in other areas to prevent drying and cracking).[4]

CYTOMEGALOVIRUS INFECTION

Prevention. There are no practical methods for preventing CMV infection. Avoiding exposure is virtually impossible because of the ubiquitous and asymptomatic nature of the infections. Avoiding unnecessary blood transfusions or using CMV-seronegative blood donors, white blood cell–depleted blood products, or frozen deglycerolized blood cells has proved to be important in minimizing the occurrence of postnatally acquired CMV, particularly in premature infants.[4,5]

The question frequently arises about assignment of staff to infants with a possible diagnosis of CMV infection. Staff members who may be pregnant have heightened concern about this issue. Staff members should be aware that many infants with CMV infection are often asymptomatic and therefore not identified while in the hospital. **To avoid any problems,**

staff members should employ good handwashing technique with all infants. Wearing gloves when handling urine and other secretions is a strategy that can also be employed by staff members who are working in the neonatal intensive care unit (NICU) and are pregnant or of childbearing age. The actual risk for an infected infant's transmitting disease to a susceptible health care worker is unknown but probably small.[4]

Data Collection

History. Congenital infections are represented by a wide spectrum of disease from asymptomatic disease to profoundly symptomatic disease. CMV infection in the mother is usually asymptomatic.[44,116]

Signs and Symptoms. **An infant with CMV infection is usually asymptomatic.** Congenital manifestations include intrauterine growth restriction (IUGR), neonatal jaundice (increased direct fraction), purpura, hepatosplenomegaly, microcephaly, seizures, intracerebral calcification, chorioretinitis, and progressive sensorineural hearing loss.[12]

Laboratory Data. CMV may be cultured from urine, pharyngeal secretions, and peripheral leukocytes. Isolation of the virus within 3 weeks of birth indicates transplacental acquisition. A paired sera demonstration of a fourfold titer rise or histopathology demonstration of characteristic nuclear inclusions in certain tissues can confirm infection. Examining the urine for intranuclear inclusions is not helpful. PCR detection of viral DNA in tissues and cerebrospinal fluid is also available.[4]

Treatment. Ganciclovir, foscarnet, valganciclovir, and cidofovir are the only licensed antiviral agents effective against CMV. These drugs are approved only for treatment of life- and sight-saving disease. In a randomized controlled trial that evaluated 42 neonates with congenital CMV infection involving the central nervous system (CNS), 6 weeks of IV ganciclovir therapy prevented hearing deterioration at 6 months. However, two thirds of neonates treated with ganciclovir had significant neutropenia.[67] More studies are necessary before ganciclovir can be routinely recommended in congenital CMV infection involving the CNS.[4,33]

Parent Teaching. The need for good handwashing technique by parents and caregivers of infants with suspected CMV should be included in discharge instructions.

RUBELLA

Prevention. Medical personnel should ensure that all mothers have a protective hemagglutination titer before conception. If the woman is susceptible, vaccinate her with rubella vaccine before conception and advise her that she should avoid conception for 28 days after receiving the vaccine.[4,74] If a woman is found to lack immunity to rubella during pregnancy, she should receive rubella immunization in the postpartum period even if she is breast feeding.[43,74]

All perinatal health care workers should have rubella titers drawn to identify immunity status, and they should be reimmunized if this is not adequate. Women of childbearing age who do not have immune titers should be encouraged to have rubella immunization.[4,5]

Data Collection

History. Rubella in the first 4 to 5 months of pregnancy is associated with a high incidence of sequelae in the infant.[5] A mother with rubella may be relatively asymptomatic or mildly ill with respiratory symptoms with or without a rash.[4]

Signs and Symptoms. Congenital manifestations of rubella include IUGR, sensorineural deafness, cataracts, neonatal jaundice (increased direct fraction), purpura, hepatosplenomegaly, microcephaly, chronic encephalitis, chorioretinitis, and cardiac defects (especially patent ductus arteriosus and peripheral pulmonic stenosis). Less frequent manifestations include bone lesions and pneumonitis.[4]

Laboratory Data. The virus may be isolated from the throat, blood, urine, and cerebrospinal fluid (CSF). A paired sera demonstration of a fourfold titer rise, such as an indirect hemagglutination (IHA) inhibition test or an indirect fluorescent antibody (IFA) test, is diagnostic. The IHA test generally has been replaced by one of several more sensitive methods including enzyme linked immunoassay, or latex agglutination, and reverse transcriptase polymerase chain reaction (RT-PCR) assays.[4,18]

Parent Teaching. **Infants with congenital rubella syndrome (CRS) may secrete the virus for many years. This requires that discharge instructions include preventive strategies that should be employed to decrease the chance of contact of susceptible pregnant women with the infant. Parents should be informed of their responsibility to ensure that potentially seronegative**

women of childbearing age avoid direct contact with the infant.[4] The challenge arises to impress this on the family and at the same time avoid ostracizing the infant or negatively affecting the parent-infant attachment process. In discharge planning with these families, a collaborative approach should be employed, using community health, medical, nursing, and social work input and support. Another challenge is to impress on parents that an infant exposed to rubella during pregnancy may appear normal at birth, but the first appearance of some CNS symptoms may extend into childhood. Thus families and clinicians should keep a watchful eye on these children during the early childhood years.[74]

SYPHILIS

Prevention. Pregnant women should avoid exposure to syphilis. Monitor the serum early and late in pregnancy, and treat the mother for the appropriate stage of disease. Erythromycin, previously used in penicillin-sensitive women, is not considered adequate treatment during gestation because of 30% treatment failure rates in adults and failure to establish a cure in newborns as a result of poor transplacental passage of erythromycin. Infants born to women treated with erythromycin should be considered high risk for infection and appropriately evaluated and treated. If penicillin allergy is confirmed in the pregnant woman, acute desensitization is necessary. Desensitization can be accomplished using increasing doses of oral penicillin over 4 to 6 hours.[106]

Data Collection

History. A congenital infection may be manifested by a multisystem disease. A primary syphilitic chancre on the cervix or rectal mucosa in a mother may be unnoticed.[106]

Signs and Symptoms. An infant exposed to syphilis may be asymptomatic at birth, or virtually all organ systems may be involved. Clinical findings may include hepatitis, pneumonitis, bone marrow failure, myocarditis, meningitis, nephrotic syndrome, rhinitis (snuffles), a rash involving the palms and soles, and pseudoparalysis of an extremity.[4,26,106]

Laboratory Data. The microscopic darkfield examination identifies spirochetes from nonoral lesions. Nonspecific, nontreponemal reaginic tests, such as Venereal Disease Research Laboratory (VDRL) tests and rapid plasma reagin (RPR) tests, followed serially with a rise or absence of fall after birth, are useful for screening.[26,106] Specific treponemal antibody serologic tests, such as a fluorescent treponemal antibody absorption (FTA-ABS) test or a microhemagglutination test for *Treponema pallidum* (MHA-TP), provide diagnostic confirmation of a reactive nontreponemal test, but an FTA-ABS IgM test is unreliable.[26,106] False-positive results may occur with nontreponemal tests secondary to other medical conditions or other spirochetal diseases. Therefore confirmation of diagnosis is necessary.[4] A long-bone x-ray examination showing metaphysitis or periostitis may help in diagnosing syphilis. VDRL tests on CSF are mandatory in all infants suspected of having congenital syphilis. When the diagnosis of active congenital syphilis is equivocal, often it is best to treat and ascertain the diagnosis by serial serologic determinations.[4,26,106]

Treatment. Table 22-1 outlines the treatment for syphilis.[4]

Parent Teaching. Adequate follow-up of both symptomatic and asymptomatic neonates is very important. A physical evaluation should be conducted at 1, 2, 3, 6, and 12 months. Serologic testing should be performed at 3, 6, and 12 months after completion of therapy regimen, or until titer decreases fourfold. Noninfected or adequately treated infants' titers should be decreased by 3 months and nonreactive by 6 months. If titers fail to decline or if they increase or are still present after 6 to 12 months of age, the infant should be reevaluated and retreated. Infants with neurosyphilis should have a repeat CSF examination every 6 months until it is normal and VDRL nonreactive. If CSF VDRL is still reactive at 6 months or CSF white cell count is not decreasing at each reexamination or is abnormal at 24 months, retreatment is indicated.[4]

TOXOPLASMOSIS

Prevention. Women should avoid unnecessary exposure to raw meat, cat feces, and eating fruits or vegetables not peeled or washed thoroughly. Using a pair of gloves when emptying the litter box may provide protection if the pregnant woman (or a woman attempting to become pregnant) must empty the litter box.[4] A pregnant woman (or woman attempting to become pregnant) should use hot soapy water to wash her hands immediately after exposure to any infectious source, even after wearing gloves.[17]

TABLE 22-1 **RECOMMENDED THERAPY FOR INDICATED CONDITIONS**

CONDITION	TREATMENT
SEPSIS AND/OR MENINGITIS	
Initial Therapy	
Early onset	Intravenous (IV) ampicillin and gentamicin or IV amikacin (if gentamicin-resistant organisms are present in nursery, ampicillin plus cefotaxime is a suitable alternative, particularly if meningitis is present).
Late onset	IV vancomycin plus cefotaxime or IV aminoglycoside (see "Early onset").
ONCE SPECIFIC ORGANISMS ARE IDENTIFIED	
Group B *Streptococcus*	IV ampicillin and gentamicin for 10 to 14 days (gentamicin may be discontinued if strain is not tolerant).
Coliform species	IV ampicillin and gentamicin for 10 to 14 days (cefotaxime may replace gentamicin).
Listeria monocytogenes	IV ampicillin and IV gentamicin for 14 to 21 days.
Enterococci	Same as for *Listeria monocytogenes.* For ampicillin resistance, use vancomycin.
Group A *Streptococcus*	IV penicillin G for 10 to 14 days.
Group D *Streptococcus* (non-enterococcus)	Same as for Group A *Streptococci.*
Staphylococcus aureus	IV nafcillin for 10 to 14 days; IV vancomycin for methicillin-resistant strains.
Staphylococcus epidermidis	IV vancomycin for 10 to 14 days.
Pseudomonas aeruginosa	IV ceftazidime and aminoglycoside for 10 to 14 days.
Anaerobes	IV metronidazole, clindamycin, or meropenem.
PNEUMONIA	
Group B *Streptococcus*	Same as for sepsis (respiratory distress syndrome may mimic pneumonitis and vice versa).
Staphylococcus aureus	Same as for sepsis.
Chlamydia trachomatis	Oral (PO) erythromycin for 14 days.
Pneumocystis jiroveci	PO or IV trimethoprim and sulfamethoxazole, or IV pentamidine isethionate.
Pertussis	PO or IV azithromycin for 5 days (clinical course is unchanged, but shedding of organism is diminished significantly).
Other organisms	Same as for sepsis.
SKIN AND SOFT TISSUE INFECTIONS	
Impetigo	IV or intramuscular (IM) nafcillin; PO cephalexin for 7 days (depending on clinical severity). For methicillin-resistance, use vancomycin. Also consider topical mupirocin.
Group A *Streptococcus* infections	IV penicillin G for 7 days.
Breast abscess	IV nafcillin and gentamicin for 7 days pending identification of etiologic agent (change to IV penicillin if *Streptococcus* is etiologic agent; IV ampicillin or gentamicin should be used for coliform species pending sensitivities); value of surgical drainage is individualized; vancomycin for methicillin-resistant strains.
Omphalitis and/or funisitis	IV nafcillin for 7 days (penicillin may be used if infection is caused by group A or B streptococci); if gram-negative rods, consider gentamicin or cefotaxime also.

Data from Bradley JS, Nelson JD: *Nelson's pocket book of pediatric antimicrobial therapy:2006-2007*, ed 16, Philadelphia, 2006, Alliance for World Wide Editing.

TABLE 22-1 RECOMMENDED THERAPY FOR INDICATED CONDITIONS—cont'd

CONDITION	TREATMENT
GASTROINTESTINAL INFECTIONS	
Salmonella species	IV ampicillin for 7 to 10 days; or IV cefotaxime or ceftriaxone for 7 to 10 days depending on sensitivities (focal complications of meningitis and arthritis should be monitored closely).
Shigella species	PO trimethoprim/sulfamethoxazole or PO or IV ampicillin, depending on sensitivities.
Necrotizing enterocolitis	IV ampicillin and IV gentamicin for 2 to 3 weeks (if *Pseudomonas* is isolated, IV ceftazidime or piperacillin/tazobactam combination may be substituted for ampicillin); supportive measures (gastrointestinal suction) are appropriate.
OSTEOMYELITIS OR SEPTIC ARTHRITIS	
Group B *Streptococcus*	IV penicillin G for 21 days minimum.
Staphylococcus aureus	IV oxacillin for 21 days minimum.
Coliform species	IV gentamicin for 21 days (IV ampicillin for 21 days minimum if organism is sensitive).
Gonococcus species	IV penicillin G for 10 days.
Unknown	IV oxacillin and gentamicin for 21 days minimum.
URINARY TRACT INFECTIONS	Suspect predisposing anatomic defect if urinary tract infection; individualize workup and follow-up.
Coliform species	Gentamicin, 3 mg/kg/day divided q 8 hr for 10 days.
Enterococcus species	Ampicillin, 30 mg/kg/day divided q 8 hr for 10 days.
MISCELLANEOUS CONDITIONS	
Congenital syphilis	If more than 1 day of treatment is missed in either of the following regimens, the entire course should be restarted.
Without central nervous system (CNS) involvement	IM procaine penicillin G (50,000 units/kg) daily for 10 to 14 days (follow-up Venereal Disease Research Laboratory [VDRL] test results should revert to negative if treatment is adequate by 1 year).
With CNS involvement	IV aqueous crystalline penicillin G 100,000-150,000 units/kg/day, administered as 50,000 for a total units/kg/dose q 12 hr for the first 7 days of life and q 8 hr thereafter for 10 days. Repeat lumbar puncture about every 6 months until results are normal.
Toxoplasmosis	PO sulfadiazine, 100-120 mg/kg/day divided q 12 hr and PO pyrimethamine, 1 mg/kg/day divided q 12 hr (duration of treatment is debatable but should be long [i.e., months]; supplemental folic acid, 1 mg/day, should be added). Ocular, CNS, or human immunodeficiency virus (HIV) involvement may require additional therapy.
Herpes simplex infections	IV acyclovir, 20 mg/kg/dose q 8 hr, for 14 days if skin or mucous membrane involvement; 21 days if CNS involvement.
Conjunctivitis	
Chlamydia species	PO erythromycin for 10 days (topical may be ineffective).
Gonococcus species	IV penicillin G for 10 days; cefoxitin for penicillin-resistant strains.
Otitis media	
In otherwise normal neonate	PO amoxicillin/clavulanic acid (Augmentin), 40 mg/kg.
In neonate with nosocomial infection	PO or IV ampicillin and IV gentamicin (if there is no response to treatment, consider diagnostic tympanocentesis; *Staphylococcus aureus* and coliform species may be present).

Data Collection

History. Congenital infections are represented by a wide range of disease, from asymptomatic disease to profound symptomatic disease, and all require treatment.[4,111] Mothers may have noted an influenza-like illness, posterior cervical adenitis, or chorioretinitis but usually lack accompanying signs or symptoms. A history of exposure to cat feces or ingestion of raw meat occasionally may be obtained.[5,60,111]

Signs and Symptoms. Manifestations in a newborn may be prematurity, IUGR, hydrocephalus, chorioretinitis, seizures, cerebral calcifications, hepatosplenomegaly, thrombocytopenia, jaundice, generalized lymphadenopathy, and a rash.[4,111]

Laboratory Data. Isolating *Toxoplasma gondii* from blood or body fluids is difficult and tedious. Cysts may be found in the placenta or tissues of a fetus or newborn.[81] Most congenitally infected infants have a Sabin-Feldman dye test titer greater than 1:1000 at birth.

Treatment. Table 22-1 outlines the treatment of toxoplasmosis.[4]

Perinatal Acquisition During Labor and Delivery

CHLAMYDIA TRACHMOMATIS INFECTION

Prevention. Eye prophylaxis with erythromycin (preferred) or tetracycline ophthalmic ointment minimizes the development of conjunctivitis but has no effect on the subsequent development of pneumonitis.[4,118]

Data Collection

History. A mother with a *Chlamydia trachomatis* infection is usually asymptomatic during her pregnancy.[5,118]

Signs and Symptoms. Conjunctivitis may be manifested as congestion and edema of the conjunctiva, with minimal discharge developing 1 to 2 weeks after birth and lasting several weeks with recurrences, particularly after topical therapy. Infants with pneumonitis usually do not have a fever but have a prolonged staccato cough, tachypnea, mild hypoxemia, and eosinophilia. Otitis media and bronchiolitis also may occur.[4,118]

Laboratory Data. Definitive diagnosis is made by isolating the organism in tissue culture and by nucleic acid amplification tests (NAATs) (e.g., PCR). Demonstrating chlamydial antigen in clinical specimens by the direct fluorescent antibody method or enzyme immunoassay is very reliable. To enhance the likelihood of obtaining an adequate sample, scrape the lower conjunctiva (for conjunctivitis) or obtain deep tracheal secretions or a nasopharyngeal aspirate (for pneumonia). NAATs are not recommended for nasopharyngeal aspirates. Scraping conjunctival epithelial cells and demonstrating characteristic intracytoplasmic inclusion bodies by a Giemsa stain is diagnostic. Although serologic tests for conjunctivitis are unreliable, a significant titer rise in IgM specific antibody may be reliable in cases of pneumonia. Eosinophilia (>300 eosinophils/mm^3) may suggest Chlamydial pneumonia.[4,118]

ENTEROVIRUS (COXSACKIEVIRUS A, COXSACKIEVIRUS B, ECHOVIRUS, AND POLIOMYELITIS) INFECTIONS

Enterovirus infections are the most commonly diagnosed viral infections in the neonatal intensive care unit, and coxsackievirus B1 was the most common in 2007 by the National Enterovirus Surveillance System.[23,65,119]

Prevention. To prevent poliomyelitis, it is essential to maintain poliomyelitis immunity with active immunization before conception. Passive protection with pooled human serum globulin may help in selected exposures (0.2 mL/kg body weight, given intramuscularly). **Routine nursery infection control procedures must be observed. It is recommended that only inactivated poliovirus vaccine (IPV) be used in the nursery.** The IPV is administered intramuscularly and contains no live virus, whereas oral poliovirus vaccine (OPV) (OPV is no longer available in the United States) is administered orally and contains live but attenuated virus, which has been reported to cause infection in immunocompromised patients.[4]

Data Collection

History. Infection may occur year-round but is more prevalent from June to December in temperate climates. Most enterovirus infections are asymptomatic. Poliomyelitis is rare because of a high level of vaccine-induced immunity in most of the world.[4]

Signs and Symptoms. Mothers with enteroviral infections are usually mildly ill, with fever or diarrhea. Infants may be asymptomatic or have fever or diarrhea. Infants who acquire the infection without maternal antibody have severe disease and high mortality. Fever, irritability, lethargy, and rash are common. Severe disease with sepsis, meningoencephalitis, myocarditis, pneumonia, hepatitis, or coagulopathy may occur.[1] Prematurity, early onset of illness (<7 days), maternal history of illness, high white blood cell count ($\geq$15,000/mm^3), and low hemoglobin (<10.7 g/dL) have been shown to be risk factors of severe infection.[73]

Laboratory Data. The virus may be isolated from the throat, rectum, or CSF. Isolating coxsackievirus A may require suckling mouse inoculation. Serologic screening is impractical because of the large number of serotypes. PCR assay for enterovirus RNA in CSF and other specimens is available and is more sensitive than viral isolation.[4]

Treatment. **The antiviral agent *pleconaril* is undergoing clinical evaluation in neonates to treat enteroviral infections.**[98] Pleconaril has a novel mechanism of action by preventing the viral attachment and entry into the host cells and seems to be well tolerated in neonates.[2,99] Hand hygiene is paramount to control spread of enteroviral infections.[4]

GROUP B *STREPTOCOCCUS* INFECTION

Prevention. **Intrapartum (during labor) treatment of the mother with penicillin significantly decreases disease caused by group B *Streptococcus* (GBS) in the neonate and maternal postpartum endometritis.**[4,15,76,83] Neonatal sepsis has been reported with less than 4 hours of maternal antibiotics at term and with up to 48 hours in preterm infants.[121] Five to fifteen percent of clinical GBS isolates are resistant to clindamycin and 16% to 22% to erythromycin, and antibiotic prophylaxis with clindamycin in penicillin-allergic women may not prevent neonatal GBS disease.[32,34,58,77]

Data Collection. See the section on bacterial infections and bacterial sepsis on pp. 565, 568-569, 571-572, and 574-575.

Treatment. Table 22-1 outlines the treatment of group B *Streptococcus* infection.

Parent Teaching. See the section on bacterial infections and bacterial sepsis on pp. 571-572 and 575.

HEPATITIS B

Prevention. Prenatal screening of women for hepatitis B surface antigen (HBsAg) is indicated and is cost effective. **Use of active and passive immunization in infants born to HBsAg-positive mothers is indicated (Tables 22-2 and 22-3).**[4] **Use of active immunization for infants born to HBsAg-negative women is recommended at birth** by the Advisory Committee on Immunization Practices. However, the Centers for Disease Control and Prevention (CDC) analyzed data from the 2006 National Immunization Survey (for the years 2003 to 2005) showed only 50.1% of newborns had hepatitis B vaccine by day 3 of life with a considerable geographical variation.[24]

TABLE 22-2 ACCEPTABLE METHODS OF PASSIVE IMMUNIZATION IN NEWBORNS

DISEASE	INDICATIONS	WHEN TO USE	PRODUCT	DOSE
Hepatitis A	Active infection in mother or close family contacts	As soon as possible	HSIG	0.02-0.04 mL/kg body weight, give intramuscularly (IM)
Hepatitis B	Mothers with acute type B infection or who are antigen (+)	As soon as possible (within 12 hr)	HBIG*	0.5 mL/kg body weight IM
Tetanus	Inadequately immunized mothers with contaminated infant (e.g., dirty cord)	As soon as possible	TIG	250 units given IM (optimal dose not established)
Varicella	Infant born to a mother who develops lesions <5 days before delivery or within 2 days after delivery	Within 72 hours of birth	ZIG	2 mL given IM

Modified from Remington JS, Klein JO, editors: *Infectious diseases of the fetus and newborn infant,* ed 5, Philadelphia, 2001, Saunders.
*Should be used in conjunction with active immunization with hepatitis B virus (HBV) vaccine (see Table 22-3).
HBIG, Hepatitis B immune globulin; *HSIG,* human serum immune globulin; *TIG,* tetanus immune globulin (human); *ZIG,* zoster immune globulin.

TABLE 22-3 ACCEPTABLE METHODS OF ACTIVE IMMUNIZATION IN NEWBORNS

DISEASE	INDICATION	WHEN TO USE	PRODUCT	DOSE
Hepatitis B	HBsAg-positive or HBsAg-negative	3 separate doses: at birth*; at 1 month; and at 6 months	Recombivax HB® Engerix-B®	0.5 mL intramuscularly (IM) 0.5 mL IM
Pertussis	To control outbreak in nursery	As soon as possible	Pertussis vaccine	0.25-0.5 mL administered subcutaneously
Tuberculosis	Selected infants at risk for contracting tuberculosis	As soon as possible	Calmette-Guérin bacillus (CGB)	0.1 mL given intradermally and divided into 2 sites over deltoid muscle

HBsAg, Hepatitis B surface antigen.
*As soon as possible.

Data Collection

History. Mothers who are HBsAg positive because of the chronic carrier state or acute disease before delivery may pass the infection to their infants at delivery.[5] Women at high risk include those of Asian, Pacific Island, or Alaskan Eskimo descent; women born in Haiti or sub-Saharan Africa; and those with a history of liver disease, IV drug abuse, or frequent exposure to blood in a medical-dental setting.

Signs and Symptoms. A neonate with hepatitis B is usually asymptomatic. Occasionally, infected infants demonstrate elevated liver enzymes or acute fulminating hepatitis.[4] Neonatal infection with subsequent chronic carriage has been implicated in the development of primary hepatocellular carcinoma later in life.

Laboratory Data. Most infants at risk for acquiring hepatitis from their mother are HBsAg negative at birth. Many untreated infants become HBsAg positive 4 to 12 weeks after birth and become lifelong asymptomatic carriers or develop hepatitis B.[4]

HEPATITIS C

Prevention. Neonates acquire hepatitis C virus (HCV) infection mostly through vertical transmission from the mother and rarely through transfusion of hepatitis C–contaminated blood products. Vertical transmission rates from the mother to the infant vary (≈5%), and risk factors associated with increased transmission are HCV viral load, co-infection with HIV, rupture of membranes more than 6 hours, and internal fetal monitoring.[31,75,87,88] Reducing viral load by maternal antiviral therapy, especially in HIV co-infected women, and avoiding internal fetal monitoring are interventions that can reduce transmission but have not been evaluated. Breast feeding is not associated with increased rates of transmission and is not contraindicated.[4] Screening of blood products for HCV is mandatory for prevention of transfusion-related HCV infection.

Data Collection

History. One to two percent of pregnant women in the United States are seropositive for HCV, but vertical transmission occurs only if the mother is HCV RNA positive at the time of delivery.[4] HCV RNA titers rise many weeks after birth in infants, indicating a perinatal acquisition rather than an intrauterine transmission.[31]

Signs and Symptoms. Neonates with perinatal acquisition of HCV infection are usually asymptomatic without jaundice and with normal or only mildly elevated liver transaminase levels.[88,95,115] Progression to chronic hepatitis is common and occurs in approximately 80% of infected infants. Liver biopsies in infants with perinatally acquired HCV during follow-up show evidence of chronic inflammation. A small percentage (20%) of infants may spontaneously resolve their infection.[40]

Laboratory Data. The essential diagnostic feature is HCV RNA positivity on at least two occasions by PCR. Sensitivity of the PCR is 22% in infants younger than 1 month and 97% after 1 month of age.[37] Maternal antibodies may persist in the infant for 13 to 18 months and are not useful for diagnosis. Following liver transaminase levels may help monitor the course of hepatic inflammation.

Treatment. Ribavirin and interferon alfa are used in the treatment of adults. Small studies in children indicate efficacy of ribavirin with interferon alfa or pegylated interferon alfa combinations producing approximately 45% viral clearance rates.[53,125,126]

HERPES SIMPLEX (TYPES 1 AND 2) INFECTION

Prevention. The key to preventing herpes simplex is avoiding exposure. Mothers with active lesions or prodrome should have a cesarean section preferably within 4 to 6 hours of membrane rupture. **Treatment with acyclovir should begin at the first sign of neonatal disease or when infants have been exposed to an active lesion.**[4,5]

Communication is necessary between obstetric and neonatal staff to determine the status of a family with a history of herpes. Unnecessary restrictions should not be placed on postpartum mothers who are not actively infected.[5] Health professionals should employ all family-centered strategies used in their institutions with families unless such strategies are precluded by the need for the infant's treatment.

Data Collection

History. Disease caused by type 1 herpes simplex usually is spread by the oral route, whereas disease caused by type 2 herpes simplex is usually spread by the genital route.[4] **Many mothers who transmit herpes simplex to their newborn infants are asymptomatic.**[68] The risk to the infant from recurrent lesions is minimal.[4,46]

Signs and Symptoms. Infants with herpes simplex have a spectrum of illnesses ranging from localized skin lesions to generalized infections involving the liver, lungs, and CNS. This disseminated disease has high morbidity and mortality rates.[66,68,82]

Laboratory Data. A cytologic examination of the base of skin vesicles with a Giemsa stain (Tzanck test) may reveal characteristic but nonspecific giant cells and eosinophilic intranuclear inclusions. The virus may be readily identified on a tissue culture within 48 hours from the respiratory and genital tracts, blood, urine, and CSF.[82] Rapid viral diagnosis by direct fluorescent antibody tests is widely available.[4] Detection of virus in CSF by PCR assay is preferred, if available.[19] Although tests of paired serology such as complement fixation (CF) test, ELISA, and neutralization are available, they are of little value in an acute clinical situation.[4] Elevated liver transaminases and thrombocytopenia may indicate herpes infection.[16]

Treatment. Table 22-1 outlines the treatment of herpes simplex infection.

Parent Teaching. Families with herpes simplex require consistent and detailed teaching about prevention of transmission of herpes to the infant. **Breast-feeding mothers can be reassured that they may continue to breast feed as long as no lesions are on their breasts. Emphasis should be placed on the need for breast-feeding mothers to check their breasts for lesions.**[5]

Parents with active herpes simplex should employ good handwashing technique while caring for their infants. Parents with oral herpes should avoid kissing their infants while lesions are open and draining.[4]

LISTERIA MONOCYTOGENES INFECTION

Prevention. Pregnant women should avoid drinking unpasteurized milk to prevent *Listeria monocytogenes* infection.[39,91]

Data Collection. See the section on bacterial infections and bacterial sepsis on pp. 565, 568-569, 571-572, and 574-575.

Treatment. Table 22-1 outlines the treatment of *Listeria monocytogenes* infection.

Parent Teaching. See the section on bacterial infections and bacterial sepsis on pp. 571-572 and 575.

MYCOBACTERIUM TUBERCULOSIS INFECTION

Prevention. Mothers at risk for *Mycobacterium tuberculosis* infection may be identified with a tuberculin test during pregnancy. If the mother is a tuberculin converter (has had a positive skin test result within the past 2 years), a radiographic examination of the chest and lungs should be performed. If the mother has active tuberculosis, she should be treated with isoniazid plus rifampin and ethambutol for at least 9 months. Safety of pyrazinamide in pregnancy is not well established, and this drug is not used routinely in pregnant women. Pyridoxine (vitamin B_6) always should be given with isoniazid during pregnancy and breast feeding because of the increased requirements for this vitamin. If the mother does not have active tuberculosis, household contacts should be screened. If the disease is identified in the mother or household contacts, the infant is at high risk for developing tuberculosis.[4]

Separate infants of mothers with active disease from the mother until the mother is not contagious (usually negative sputum). Treat high-risk infants with isoniazid (10 mg/kg/day) or a tuberculosis vaccine (Calmette-Guérin bacillus) (see Table 22-3).[4,5]

Data Collection

History. A strong history of maternal contact with tuberculosis favors the diagnosis. This is especially true in high-risk populations (Southeast Asians, American Indians, and families with a known cavitary disease). Mothers with HIV infection are at an increased risk for developing active tuberculosis.[4,112]

Signs and Symptoms. Mothers may be relatively asymptomatic or have signs and symptoms that are generalized (fever and weight loss) or localized to the respiratory tract.[4] A congenital infection is extremely rare.[5] **Nonspecific signs and symptoms such as failure to thrive and unexplained hypothermia or hyperthermia are the most common manifestations in the neonatal period.**

Laboratory Data. Acid-fast organisms found on smears of gastric aspirates, sputum, CSF, or infected tissues strongly suggest tuberculosis in the neonate. Isolating *Mycobacterium tuberculosis* by culture is diagnostic and should be sought aggressively. The tuberculin test result usually is positive (>10-mm induration) in active tuberculosis. However, a positive skin test result requires 3 to 12 weeks after infection to manifest itself, and the test result usually is negative in a neonate. A chest radiograph examination also usually yields a negative result in a neonate.[4]

Treatment. Because congenital tuberculosis is such a rare condition, optimal therapy has not been established. However, most recommendations suggest four-drug therapy (isoniazid, rifampin, pyrazinamide, and streptomycin or kanamycin).[4]

Parent Teaching. Infants who are treated with isoniazid or breast-fed infants whose mothers are treated with isoniazid should receive pyridoxine supplementation.[4]

NEISSERIA GONORRHOEAE INFECTION

Prevention. Screening high-risk mothers before delivery may identify asymptomatic gonorrhea. Treating positive mothers before delivery or exposed infants at delivery is necessary.[4]

Administering silver nitrate, erythromycin, or tetracycline in the eyes is mandatory in all vaginal deliveries.[4]

Data Collection

History. Mothers with previous venereal disease are a high-risk group, because 80% of the infected women may be asymptomatic.

Signs and Symptoms. The predominant manifestation of gonorrhea is ophthalmia neonatorum, although a systemic bloodborne infection may rarely occur involving the joints, lungs, endocardium, and CNS. Conjunctivitis usually begins 2 to 5 days after birth. Eye prophylaxis minimizes but does not guarantee freedom from infection. Scalp abscess resulting from fetal monitoring has been reported.[4]

Laboratory Data. A Gram stain of purulent eye discharge revealing gram-negative intracellular diplococci is diagnostic. Culture confirmation using fermentation or fluorescence establishes the diagnosis of gonorrhea. The organism is labile, so specimens for culture should be taken to the laboratory and plated immediately. When gonorrhea is diagnosed, other sexually transmitted diseases may be present concomitantly (especially chlamydial infection).[4]

Treatment. Table 22-1 outlines the treatment of *Neisseria gonorrhoeae* infection.

VARICELLA

Prevention. Table 22-2 outlines prevention of infection.[4]

Data Collection

History. A history of varicella in the mother before conception virtually excludes the diagnosis. Varicella manifests in the mother with a fever, respiratory symptoms, and characteristic vesicular rash primarily on the trunk. If this occurs within 5 days of delivery, the newborn is at risk for infection.[4] Preventive measures should be instituted as soon as possible.[5] Acute perinatal varicella is frequently a devastating systemic disease. Nosocomially acquired transmission of varicella is a potentially significant problem for high-risk infants: premature infants born to susceptible mothers; infants who are severely premature regardless of maternal status; and immunocompromised patients of all ages (Table 22-4).

Signs and Symptoms. Congenital varicella is rare but has followed maternal varicella in the first trimester of pregnancy. Congenital manifestations include limb atrophy, skin scars, and CNS and eye abnormalities.[4]

Laboratory Data. The demonstration of multinucleated giant cells containing intranuclear inclusions in skin scrapings on Giemsa stain is nonspecific but helpful.

Virus can be isolated from scrapings of vesicle base during the first 3 to 4 days of the eruption by direct fluorescent antibody (DFA) test, or isolation of virus in tissue culture.[22,25] Isolating the virus from the respiratory tract is difficult. A number of serologic tests such as the fluorescent antibody to membrane antigen (FAMA) test, immune adherence hemagglutination (IAHA) test, ELISA, and neutralization test are available but are not helpful in the acute clinical situation. CF serologic tests are relatively insensitive.[4]

Critical Findings

ORGANISMS CAUSING EARLY-ONSET BACTERIAL SEPSIS

Common Organisms

Group B *Streptococcus*
Escherichia coli
Coagulase-negative *Staphylococcus*

Unusual Organisms

Staphylococcus aureus
Neisseria meningitidis
Streptococcus pneumoniae
Haemophilus influenzae (type B and nontypable)

Rare Organisms

Klebsiella pneumoniae
Pseudomonas aeruginosa
Enterobacter species
Serratia marcescens
Group A *Streptococcus*
Anaerobic species

EARLY-ONSET BACTERIAL DISEASE

Prevention. For GBS only, see p. 561.

Data Collection

History. Early-onset disease is almost always acquired perinatally and is discussed here. Late-onset disease is discussed in the "Postnatal Acquisition Late-Onset Bacterial Disease" section. **Early-onset disease presents as a fulminant multisystem illness during the first days of life (<72 hours of age).** Significant risk factors for early-onset disease include prematurity, low birth weight, premature onset of labor, rupture of membranes more than 18 hours, maternal intrapartum temperature higher than 37.5° C, and chorioamnionitis.[90] Bacteria responsible for early-onset disease are acquired from the birth canal before or during delivery and are listed in the Critical Findings box above. Although the advent of intrapartum antibiotic prophylaxis for GBS infections has generally reduced early-onset disease of this pathogen, it has not been universally experienced and black preterm infants remain at considerably greater risk than do white preterm infants and both black and white term infants.[21]

Also, since the practice of intrapartum prophylaxis began, a predominance of gram-negative organisms has been noted in infants weighing less than 1500 grams at birth, and concern for this continued trend remains.[9,107] **Gram-negative infections now account for more than half of the instances of early-onset sepsis.**[108,110] Data from the National Institute of Child Health and Human Development (NICHD) Neonatal Research Network, which comprises 16 major neonatal units, showed an increase in *Escherichia coli (E. coli)* infections in very-low-birth-weight (VLBW) infants during the period 1998 to 2000 compared with 1991 to 1993 that persisted during the 2002-2003 period.[110] Data from the Norwegian National Cohort demonstrated that in infants born at less than 28 weeks gestational age and with birth weight less than 1000 g, *E. coli* was the most common organism isolated on the first day of life.[97] Early-onset bacterial disease is associated with a high mortality and significant morbidity.[102,107,108]

Signs and Symptoms. Neonatal bacterial sepsis is characterized by systemic signs of infection associated with bacteremia. Meningitis in a neonate can be a sequela of bacteremia. In addition, bloodborne bacteria may localize in other tissues, causing focal disease. Both patterns of bacterial disease, early onset and late onset, have been associated with systemic infections during the neonatal period.[4,94]

In general, signs, particularly in early-onset disease, are nonspecific and nonlocalizing. Signs and symptoms may include temperature instability (hypothermia or hyperthermia), respiratory distress (apnea, cyanosis, and tachypnea), lethargy, feeding abnormalities (vomiting, increased residuals, and abdominal distention), jaundice (particularly increased direct fraction), seizures, or purpura (Figure 22-1).[94]

Newborn Scale of Sepsis (SOS) is an objective, reliable, and validated scoring tool for the assessment of neonatal infection. By using both clinical indicators (e.g., color, perfusion, muscle tone, response to pain, respiratory distress and rate, temperature, and

TABLE 22-4 INFECTION CONTROL MEASURES AND ISOLATION TECHNIQUES FOR SPECIFIC DISEASES

	RECOMMENDED PRECAUTIONS				
DISEASE/ORGANISMS	WASH HANDS	PRIVATE ROOM OR COHORT	MASK	GOWN	GLOVE
AIDS/HIV	X	D	No	(X)	(X)
Adenovirus	X	X	No	(X)	(X)
Conjunctivitis					
Gonococcal (ophthalmia neonatorum)	X	X	No	No	(X)
Chlamydia	X	No	No	No	(X)
Coxsackievirus	X	D	No	(X)	(X)
Cytomegalovirus	X	No	No	No	(X)
Diarrhea	X	D	No	(X)	(X)
Echovirus	X	D	No	(X)	(X)
Gastroenteritis	X	X	No	(X)	(X)
Hepatitis—type A	X	D	No	(X)	(X)
Hepatitis—type B	X	No	No	(X)	(X)
Herpes simplex	X	X	No	(X)	(X)
Influenza A or B	X	X	No	(X)	(X)
Meningitis					
Aseptic	X	D	No	(X)	(X)
Bacterial	X	No	No	No	No
Necrotizing enterocolitis	X	No	No	(X)	(X)
Respiratory syncytial virus	X	X	X	(X)	(X)
Rubella	X	X	X	No	No
Staphylococcal disease *(Staphylococcus aureus)*	X	D	No	(X)	(X)
Streptococcal disease					
Group A	X	D	No	(X)	(X)
Group B	X	D	No	(X)	(X)
Syphilis	X	No	No	No	(X)
Toxoplasmosis	X	No	No	No	No
Varicella	X	X	X	X	X
Vancomycin-resistant organisms	X	X	No	X	X

AIDS, Acquired immunodeficiency syndrome; D, desirable but optional; *HIV, human immunodeficiency virus; X,* recommended at all times; *(X),* recommended if soiling is likely or if touching infective materials.

INFECTIVE MATERIAL	DURATION OF ISOLATION/PRECAUTION	COMMENTS
Blood and body fluids	Duration of illness	Utmost care needed to avoid needle sticks
Respiratory secretions and feces	Duration of hospitalization	During outbreaks, cohort patients suspected of having adenovirus infection
Purulent exudates	Until 24 hr after initiation of effective therapy	
Purulent exudates	Duration of illness	
Feces and respiratory secretions	For 7 days after onset of illness	
Urine and respiratory secretions		Counsel pregnant personnel
Feces	Duration of illness	Identify colonized or infected infants by culture; institute cohorting
Feces and respiratory secretions	For 7 days after onset of illness	
Feces	Duration of illness	
Feces	For 7 days after onset of illness	Most contagious before symptoms
Blood and body fluids	Duration of positivity	Avoid needle sticks
Lesions, secretions, urine, and stool	Duration of illness	
Respiratory secretions	Duration of illness	Cohort patients suspected of having influenza during outbreak; staff should receive yearly influenza vaccine
Feces	Duration of illness	Cohort colonized or infected infants during a nursery outbreak
(?) Feces	Duration of illness	Cohort ill infants
Respiratory secretions	Duration of illness	Cohort suspected infants, especially premature infants, during outbreaks
Respiratory secretions	Duration of hospitalization	Infants may shed virus for as long as 2 years; seronegative women should avoid contact
Purulent exudate	Duration of illness	
Respiratory secretions	24 hr after initiation of effective therapy	
Respiratory and genital secretions		Cohort ill and colonized infants during a nursery outbreak
Lesion secretion and blood	24 hr after initiation of effective therapy	
	None	
Respiratory and lesion secretions	Until lesions are crusted	Neonates born to mothers with active chickenpox should be placed in isolation precautions at birth; persons who are not susceptible do not need to mask
Secretions	Duration of illness	

apnea) and laboratory findings (e.g., white blood cell count [WBC], ratio of immature to total neutrophils [I:T ratio], platelet count, pH, and absolute neutrophil count), the health care provider assigns a score for each parameter. A score less than 10 indicates that the newborn does not have sepsis—a negative predictive value of 97%. The SOS (see Resource Materials for Professionals and Parents on p. 580) awaits testing in a large cohort of neonates.

Laboratory Data. **Isolating bacteria from a nonpermissive site (blood, CSF, urine, closed body space) is the most valid method of establishing the diagnosis of bacterial sepsis.**[127] Surface cultures (including ear and gastric aspirates) do not establish the presence of active systemic infection but merely indicate colonization. Bacterial antigens or endotoxins may be demonstrated in sera, CSF, urine, or body fluids by a variety of methods (counterimmunoelectrophoresis [CIE], latex agglutination [LA], and limulus lysate test). Such a demonstration is not totally definitive, nor does it allow the determination of the antibiotic sensitivity of the offending organism.[94] False-positive reactions may be caused by skin surface contamination or gastrointestinal absorption of antigen.[8] **The CSF is examined in most infants suspected of sepsis, because meningitis is a frequent manifestation of sepsis in neonates, especially in symptomatic infants and infants with GBS sepsis and with late-onset disease (Table 22-5).** It has been suggested that, because of the low yield and potential adverse effects from lumbar puncture, examination of CSF be deferred in asymptomatic infants being evaluated for maternal risk factors or respiratory distress.[43,59,94,103,123] **The CSF is examined in most infants suspected of sepsis, because meningitis is difficult to exclude without a lumbar puncture and its diagnosis affects therapy and follow-up in a neonate.**[94,107]

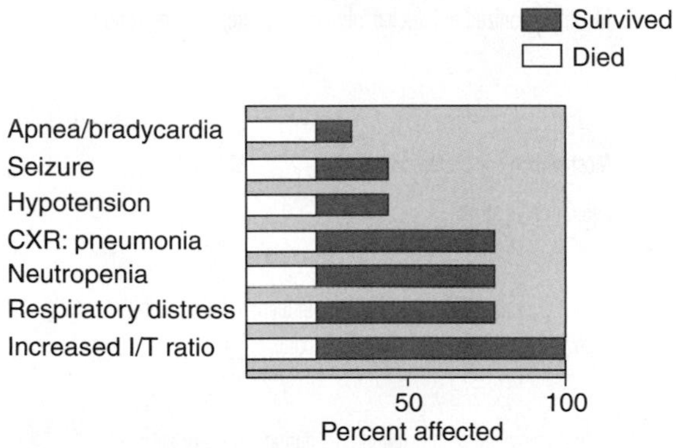

FIGURE 22-1 Clinical and laboratory findings in nine infants with signs and symptoms of early-onset group B streptococcal disease. *CXR*, Chest x-ray; *I/T*, ratio of immature to total neutrophils. (From Nelson SN, Merenstein GB, Pierce JR: Early onset group B streptococcal disease, *J Perinatol* 6:234, 1986.)

Several laboratory aids are used in assessing neonatal sepsis, but it must be realized that these tests are not sensitive or specific enough to influence clinical decisions on their own.[4,28,38] ***Leukocyte indices*** predict sepsis with sensitivities ranging from 17% to 90% and specificities from 31% to 100%.[28] ***C-reactive protein (CRP)*** is an acute-phase reactant synthesized in the liver in the first 6 to 8 hours of the infective process with a low sensitivity (60%) early in sepsis. However, serial CRP measurements at 24 and 48 hours improve sensitivity to 82% and 84% and

TABLE 22-5 NORMAL CEREBROSPINAL FLUID VALUES IN NEONATES*

	WHITE BLOOD CELLS	POLYMORPHONUCLEAR NEUTROPHILS	PROTEIN (mg/dL)	GLUCOSE (mg/dL)
PREMATURE INFANTS				
Reported means	2-27		75-150	79-83
Reported ranges	0-112		31-292	64-106
TERM INFANTS				
Reported means	3-5	2-3	47-67	51-55
Reported ranges	0-90	0-70	17-240	32-78

*Modified from Remington JS, Klein JO, editors: *Infectious diseases of the fetus and newborn infant,* ed 5, Philadelphia, 2001, Saunders. See also Mhanna MJ, Alessah H, Gori A, et al: Cerebrospinal fluid values in very low birth weight infants with suspected sepsis at different ages, *Pediatr Crit Care Med* 9:294, 2008.

specificity and positive predictive value range from 83% to 100%.[84] Negative predictive values for CRP are extremely high. Serial CRP patterns have been found to be useful to follow resolution of infection and guide antibiotic therapy.[35,45,64,120,124] CRP levels do not seem to be affected by gestational age and have better sensitivity and negative predictive values when compared with leukocyte indices.[30,124] CRP response has been found to be better in gram-negative infections when compared with infections with coagulase-negative *Staphylococcus* (CoNS).[92,96] ***Procalcitonin,*** another acute-phase reactant, which rises within 4 hours of exposure to bacterial endotoxin, has a sensitivity and specificity ranging from 83% to 100%. The serum profile of procalcitonin has been claimed to be superior to that of CRP in the diagnosis of sepsis, after resolution of infection, and may differentiate between sepsis and other inflammatory processes (e.g., trauma).[7,70,117]

Evaluation of a composite set of markers (e.g., CRP and interleukin-6 [IL-6][86]; CRP and leukocyte indices[51]) involving acute phase reactants, leukocytes, and cytokines/chemokines may increase sensitivity and specificity in the diagnosis of sepsis. Serial measurements may be more useful, as is a combination of tests.[84] Radiographic examination of the chest and other specific areas indicated by clinical concerns may also be helpful.[94]

Several other nonspecific laboratory abnormalities may accompany neonatal sepsis, including hyperglycemia, hypoglycemia, and unexplained metabolic acidosis. Molecular techniques for diagnosis of infection are fast and reliable and may be very useful, especially in infants whose mothers have received intrapartum antibiotics. In a study of 548 paired neonatal blood samples that compared the utility of PCR for the bacterial *16S rRNA* gene with that of microbial culture by BACTEC 9240 instrument, sensitivity, specificity, positive predictive values, and negative predictive values were 96.0%, 99.4%, 88.9%, and 99.8%, respectively. This required a 9-hour turnaround time with blood volumes as little as 200 mcL.[61] Real-time PCR assay targeting the highly conserved 380 bases of *16S rDNA* requires less than 4 hours with excellent agreement with blood culture results.[62] PCR with microarray hybridization not only detects bacteremia but also can identify the infecting organism rapidly and reliably.[104] It may be that using PCR assays with microarray hybridization will become the future for diagnosing bacteremia in an accurate and rapid way.

Treatment. Antibiotics are the cornerstone of the treatment for presumed or confirmed infections in neonates. The indiscriminate or inappropriate use of systemic antibiotics may cause undesirable side effects, favor the emergence of resistant strains of bacteria, and alter the normal flora of the newborn.[20] Adequate and appropriate specimens for culture should be obtained before antibiotic therapy is initiated. Emergence of antibiotic resistance in gram-negative organisms is a major clinical concern.[10] In the data from the NICHD Neonatal Research Network, 85% and 75% of early-onset *E. coli* infections were ampicillin resistant in the 1998-2000 and the 2002-2003 cohorts, respectively.[108,110] Plasmid-mediated extended-spectrum beta-lactamases (ESBLs) (produced by *Klebsiella* spp., *E. coli,* and *Serratia*) that confer resistance to a variety of β-lactam agents (penicillins and cephalosporins) and chromosomally mediated AmP-C–type β-lactamase (*Enterobacter* and *Citrobacter* spp.)–producing gram-negative organisms have been isolated from the NICU.[54,55,89] Exposure to third-generation cephalosporins (e.g., cefotaxime) and being a VLBW infant are noted risk factors for the acquisition of resistant organisms.

Broad-spectrum antibiotic coverage, usually with ampicillin and an aminoglycoside for early-onset sepsis, is commonly initiated pending culture and sensitivity results. Once causative organisms are identified and antibiotic sensitivities established, the most appropriate and least toxic antibiotic or antibiotic combination should be continued for an appropriate period by a suitable route. If adequate cultures are negative after a reasonable period (24 to 48 hours), antibiotic therapy may be discontinued in most situations.

Antibiotics are not the entire solution to treating the infected newborn.[42,47] Meticulous attention to the treatment of associated conditions, such as shock, hypoxemia, thermal abnormalities, electrolyte or acid-base imbalance, inadequate nutrition, anemia, or presence of pus or foreign bodies, may be as important as choosing the proper antibiotic. Further investigation is necessary before newer adjunctive therapies such as IV immunoglobulin and non-antibiotic therapies or preventive regimens can be recommended.[56,80,86,122] Table 22-1 provides guidelines for choosing the proper antibiotic for indicated conditions; Table 22-6 gives the proper dose, route, and frequency of administration of commonly used antibiotics in the newborn nursery. Table 22-7 describes the passage of antibiotics across the placenta, and Table 22-8 describes their passage into breast milk.

TABLE 22-6

ANTIBIOTIC, ANTIVIRAL, AND ANTIFUNGAL AGENTS: DOSAGES FOR NEONATES

ANTIBIOTIC, ANTIVIRAL, OR ANTIFUNGAL	ROUTE	DAILY DOSAGES AND INTERVALS: 0 TO 7 DAYS OF AGE	DAILY DOSAGES AND INTERVALS: MORE THAN 7 DAYS OF AGE
Acyclovir†	IV	20 mg/kg/dose q 8-12 hr depending on gestation and age	Same
Amikacin sulfate	IV, IM	7.5-10 mg/kg/dose q 12 hr depending on gestation and age	Same
Amoxicillin	PO	50 mg/kg/day divided q 12 hr	50 mg/kg/day divided q 8 hr
Amoxicillin/Clavulanic acid	PO	Not recommended	30 mg/kg/day divided q 12 hr
Ampicillin			
Meningitis	IV	100 mg/kg/day divided q 12 hr	150-200 mg/kg/day divided q 6-8 hr
Other indications	IV, IM, PO	50 mg/kg/day divided q 12 hr	75 mg/kg/day divided q 8 hr
Azithromycin	IV, PO	5 mg/kg/day q 24 hr	10 mg/kg/day q 24 hr
Cefazolin*	IV, IM	50 mg/kg/day divided q 12 hr	50-75 mg/kg/day divided q 8-12 hr
Cefotaxime	IV, IM	100 mg/kg/day divided q 12 hr	150 mg/kg/day divided q 8 hr
Ceftazidime*	IV	100 mg/kg/day divided q 12 hr	150 mg/kg/day divided q 8 hr
Clindamycin	IV, PO	10-15 mg/kg/day divided q 8-12 hr	15-20 mg/kg/day divided q 6-8 hr
Erythromycin ethyl succinate (EES)	PO	20 mg/kg/day divided q 12 hr	30-40 mg/kg/day divided q 8 hr
Ganciclovir†	IV	6 mg/kg/dose q 12-24 hr depending on gestation and age	
Gentamicin	IV, IM	2.5 mg/kg/dose q 8-24 hr depending on gestation and age	Same
Meropenem*	IV	40 mg/kg/day divided q 12 hr	60 mg/kg/day divided q 8 hr (higher doses may be needed in meningitis)
Metronidazole	IV, PO	7.5-15 mg/kg/day divided q 12-24 hr	15-30 mg/kg/day divided q 12 hr
Nafcillin	IV	50-75 mg/kg/day divided q 8-12 hr	75-150 mg/kg/day divided q 6-8 hr
Nystatin‡	PO	400,000 units/day divided q 6 hr	Same
Penicillin G			
Meningitis	IV	100,000-150,000 units/kg/day divided q 8-12 hr	200,000-225,000 units/kg/day divided q 6-8 hr
Other indications	IV	50,000 units/kg/day divided q 12 hr	75,000 units/kg/day divided q 6-8 hr
Penicillin G, benzathine	IM	50,000 units/kg (1 dose only)	Same
Penicillin G, procaine	IM	50,000 units/kg/day once daily	Same
Pentamidine isethionate*	IV	4 mg/kg/day for 14 days (available from CDC, Atlanta, Georgia)	Same
Piperacillin/Tazobactam	IV	100-200 mg/kg/day divided q 12 hr	300 mg/kg/day divided q 8 hr
Rifampin	IV, PO	10 mg/kg/day q 24 hr	Same
Ticarcillin	IV, IM	150-225 mg/kg/day divided q 8-12 hr	225-300 mg/kg/day divided q 6-8 hr
Tobramycin	IV, IM	2.5 mg/kg/dose q 12-24 hr depending on gestation and age	2.5 mg/kg/dose q 8-18 hr
Trimethoprim/sulfamethoxazole (TMP/SMX)	IV, PO	10-20 mg/kg/day TMP and 50-100 mg/kg/day SMX	Same

CDC, Centers for Disease Control and Prevention; *IM,* intramuscularly; *IV,* intravenously; *PO,* orally.

*Pharmacokinetics in newborns not well characterized. These drugs should be used with extra caution in neonates (pediatric infectious disease consultation recommended).

†Antiviral agent.

‡Antifungal agent.

TABLE 22-6 ANTIBIOTIC, ANTIVIRAL, AND ANTIFUNGAL AGENTS: DOSAGES FOR NEONATES—cont'd

ANTIBIOTIC, ANTIVIRAL, OR ANTIFUNGAL	ROUTE	DAILY DOSAGES AND INTERVALS: 0 TO 7 DAYS OF AGE	DAILY DOSAGES AND INTERVALS: MORE THAN 7 DAYS OF AGE
Vancomycin	IV	15 mg/kg/dose q 12-24 hr depending on gestation and age	15 mg/kg/dose q 8-18 hr depending on gestation and age
Zidovudine†	IV	1.5 mg/kg/dose q 6-12 hr depending on gestation and age	Same
	PO	2 mg/kg/dose q 6-12 hr depending on gestation and age	Same

TABLE 22-7 PASSAGE OF ANTIBIOTICS ACROSS THE PLACENTA*

PERCENTAGE OF ANTIBIOTIC IN INDICATED CATEGORY	ANTIBIOTIC
Equal to serum concentration	Amoxicillin Ampicillin Carbenicillin Chloramphenicol Methicillin Nitrofurantoin Penicillin G Sulfonamides
50% of serum concentration	Aminoglycosides
10%-15% of serum concentration	Amikacin Cephalosporins Clindamycin Nafcillin Tobramycin
Negligible (<10% of serum concentration)	Dicloxacillin Erythromycin

*Several factors determine the degree of transfer of antibiotics across the placenta, including lipid solubility, degree of ionization, molecular weight, protein binding, placental maturation, and placental and fetal blood flow.

TABLE 22-8 PASSAGE OF ANTIBIOTICS INTO BREAST MILK*

PERCENTAGE OF ANTIBIOTIC IN INDICATED CATEGORY	ANTIBIOTIC
Equal to serum concentration	Isoniazid Metronidazole Sulfonamides Trimethoprim
50% of serum concentration	Chloramphenicol Erythromycin Tetracyclines
<25% of serum concentration	Cefazolin Kanamycin Nitrofurantoin Oxacillin Penicillin G Penicillin V

*Data on concentrations of antibiotics in human breast milk are sparse. Because most antibiotics are present in breast milk in microgram amounts, they are normally not ingested by the infant in therapeutic amounts.

Parent Teaching. Transplacental infection often results in fetal abnormality or death. Newborns who survive may have long-term sequelae such as developmental, neurologic, motor, sensory, growth, and physical abnormalities.

Before antibiotic use, the mortality from bacterial sepsis was 95% to 100%, but antibiotics and supportive care have reduced the mortality rate to less than 50%, but survival is highly variable and depends on the organism and underlying or associated conditions. Debilitated infants (preterm and sick neonates) are at greater risk and have a higher incidence of morbidity and mortality than term healthy neonates. **The most common complications of bacterial sepsis are**

meningitis and septic shock. The outcome is influenced by early recognition and vigorous treatment with appropriate antibiotics and supportive care.

POSTNATAL ACQUISITION LATE-ONSET BACTERIAL DISEASE

Prevention. The CDC defines ***nosocomial*** as all neonatal infections acquired in the intrapartum period or during hospitalization. Infants requiring the specialized care of NICUs are highly susceptible to infections. Prematurity, stress, immature immune systems, and complicated medical and surgical problems contribute to their increased susceptibility. In addition, most infants in the NICU require a variety of invasive diagnostic, therapeutic, and monitoring procedures; many of these procedures bypass natural physical barriers, which may allow colonization to occur and a nosocomial (late-onset) infection to develop.[48]

Infection control principles and practices for the prevention of these nosocomial infections are outlined in Table 22-9. Table 22-4 outlines infection control measures and isolation techniques for specific diseases.[4,13,49,105]

TABLE 22-9 INFECTION CONTROL PRINCIPLES AND PRACTICES TO PREVENT NOSOCOMIAL INFECTION

PRINCIPLE	PRACTICE
HANDWASHING	
Handwashing is the most important procedure for controlling infection in the NICU.	1. Before each shift, wash hands, wrists, forearms, and elbows with antiseptic. Scrub hands with a brush or pad for 2-3 min and rinse thoroughly. Chlorhexidine, hexachlorophene, and iodophors are the preferred products. 2. Wash hands for 10-15 sec between infant contacts. Soap and water are adequate unless the infant is infected or contaminated objects have been handled. 3. Use an antiseptic for handwashing before surgical or similar invasive procedures. 4. Alcohol-based disinfectants are increasingly employed and are effective when used before and after patient contact.
PATIENT PLACEMENT	
Overcrowding in the NICU increases risk for cross-contamination.	1. Provide 4- to 6-ft intervals between infants.
SKIN AND CORD CARE	
The skin, its secretions, and its normal flora are natural defense mechanisms that protect against invading pathogens (see Chapter 19)	1. The American Academy of Pediatrics suggests using a dry technique: a. Delay initial cleansing until temperature is stable. Manipulating an infant's skin must be minimized. b. Use sterile cotton sponges and sterile water or mild soap to remove blood from face and perineal area. c. Do *not* touch other areas unless they are grossly soiled.
No single method of cord care has been identified to prevent colonization or limit disease.	2. Local application of alcohol, triple dye, and various antimicrobial is currently used.
MEDICAL DEVICES	
Medical devices facilitate infections by the following: 1. Bypassing normal defense mechanisms, providing direct access to blood and deep tissues 2. Supporting growth of microorganisms and becoming reservoirs from which bacteria can be transmitted with the device to another patient	1. Intravenous (IV) infusion devices predispose infants to phlebitis and bacteremia. Preventive measures include preparing the site with tincture of iodine (2% iodine in 70% alcohol), an iodophor, or 70% alcohol; anchoring the IV securely; performing site assessment and care every 24 hr (routine site care is not necessary with polyurethane dressing); rotating the IV site every 48-72 hr; changing the IV tubing every 24-48 hr on regular IVs; and discontinuing the IV at the first sign of complication.

NICU, Neonatal intensive care unit.

TABLE 22-9 INFECTION CONTROL PRINCIPLES AND PRACTICES TO PREVENT NOSOCOMIAL INFECTION—cont'd

PRINCIPLE	PRACTICE
MEDICAL DEVICES—cont'd	
3. Providing a "protected site" when placed in deeper tissue, so phagocytosis or defense mechanisms cannot eradicate the organisms 4. Using sterile medical devices that are occasionally contaminated from the manufacturer or central supply	2. Arterial lines predispose infants to bacteremia. Preventive measures include aseptically inserting the catheter using gloves, inspecting the site and performing site care every 24 hr, treating the catheter and stopcocks as sterile fields, and minimizing manipulation by drawing all blood specimens at the same time. 3. Intravascular pressure–monitoring systems predispose infants to septicemia. Preventive measures include replacing the flush solution every 24 hr, replacing the chamber dome, and replacing the tubing and continuous flow device (if used) at 48-hr intervals and between each patient. 4. Respiratory therapy devices increase the risk for contamination. Preventive measures include using aseptic technique during suctioning; dating opened solution for irrigation, humidification, and nebulization, and discarding after 24 hr; ensuring routine replacement and cleaning of all respiratory equipment, including Ambu bags, cascade nebulizers, endotracheal tube adaptors, and tubing; and checking sputum cultures and Gram stains every several days to assess the degree of colonization or infection in the intubated patient.
SPECIMEN COLLECTION	
Improperly collected specimens cause infection at the site of collection or erroneous diagnosis, leading to the administration of the wrong antibiotic or delayed administration of the appropriate antibiotic.	1. Wash hands before collecting specimen. 2. Observe aseptic technique to reduce risk for infection and to avoid contamination of specimen. 3. Deliver specimens to the laboratory immediately. 4. Do not use femoral sticks.
NURSERY ATTIRE	
Personal clothing and unscrubbed skin areas of personnel should not touch infants.	1. Short-sleeved scrub gowns accommodate washing elbows. 2. Long-sleeved gowns should be worn and changed between handling of infected or potentially infected infants. 3. Sterile gowns are necessary for sterile procedures.
EMPLOYEE HEALTH	
Transmission of disease among patients and employees can occur bidirectionally. Each NICU must establish reasonable guidelines for restriction of assignments based on the employee's potential to transmit disease and the potential risk for acquiring disease.	1. Conditions that commonly restrict personnel from patient care in the NICU are skin lesions and draining wounds, acute respiratory infections, fever, gastroenteritis, active herpes simplex (oral, genital, or paronychial), and herpes zoster. 2. Conditions that are transmitted from infants to personnel are the following: a. Rubella: Obtain rubella titers from women of childbearing age; if a protective level is not present, they should be vaccinated. b. Cytomegalovirus is a potential threat to pregnant women. Adherence to good infection control practices may reduce this threat. c. Hepatitis B is usually not a major problem in the NICU, because host vaccine is available and may be considered for high-risk individuals (see Tables 22-2 and 22-3). d. Use of gloves with body fluid contact will decrease the risk for transmission of hepatitis B virus and human immunodeficiency virus.
COHORTING	
Cohorting is an important infection control measure used primarily during outbreaks or epidemics in the NICU. The object of cohorting is to limit the number of contacts of one infant with other infants and personnel.	1. Group together infants born within the same time frame (usually 24-48 hr) or who are colonized or infected with the same pathogen. These infants should remain together until discharged. 2. Provide nursing care by personnel who do not care for other infants. 3. After all infants in cohort are discharged, clean the room before admittance of a new group of infants.

Critical Findings

ORGANISMS CAUSING LATE-ONSET BACTERIAL SEPSIS

- Coagulase-negative *Staphylococcus*
- *Escherichia coli*
- *Klebsiella* species
- *Enterobacter* species
- *Candida* species
- *Malassezia furfur*
- Other enteric organisms
- Group B *Streptococcus*
- Methicillin-resistant *Staphylococcus aureus*

Data Collection

History. **Late-onset disease may occur as early as 3 days of age but is more common after the first week of life.** Affected infants may have a history of obstetric complications, but they are less common than obstetric complications in early-onset disease. Bacteria responsible for late-onset sepsis and meningitis include those acquired from the maternal genital tract and organisms acquired after birth from human contact or from contaminated equipment or material (see the Critical Findings box above).[5] Gram-positive organisms predominate in late-onset sepsis, and gram-negative organisms account for about one third of late-onset cases of sepsis in VLBW infants.[109] Although prematurity remains the most significant factor, invasive procedures performed on a neonate, such as intubation, catheterization, and surgery, also increase the risk for bacterial infection.[47,71,109]

Signs and Symptoms. Similar to those of early-onset sepsis, they are nonspecific.

Laboratory Data. A complete set of culture specimens should be obtained, but limitations are similar to those in early-onset infection.[43,103]

Treatment. **Broad-spectrum antibiotic coverage, usually vancomycin and an aminoglycoside or a third-generation cephalosporin, is commonly initiated pending culture and sensitivity results.** However, vancomycin resistance remains a potential problem in the care of sick neonates.[20,52,100] To minimize the development of these resistant organisms, the CDC has recommended prudent vancomycin use, education of medical personnel about the problem of vancomycin resistance, early detection and prompt reporting of organisms, and immediate implementation of appropriate infection control measures (see Table 22-4).

FUNGAL INFECTION

Fungal infections have been a significant cause of neonatal morbidity and mortality. They are the second most common infection after 72 hours of life in infants weighing less than 1500 g.[109] *Candida* species are the most common. In addition, they are usually seen in infants with congenital anomalies requiring surgery or infants who require multiple or prolonged vascular catheterization.

Prevention. Because these infants are often colonized at birth, strict adherence to aseptic technique when dealing with central catheters is essential. Antibiotic use should be minimized and limited to treatment of specific illnesses.

Data Collection

History. Prematurity (<32 weeks' gestation), Apgar score less than 5 at 5 minutes, shock, antibiotic therapy, parenteral nutrition for longer than 5 days, use of lipids for longer than 7 days, presence of a central catheter, length of stay in hospital longer than 7 days, use of histamine-2 (H_2) blockers, and intubation are risk factors for fungal infections.[101]

Signs and Symptoms. **Signs and symptoms may be nonspecific, nonlocalizing, and difficult to differentiate from those of bacterial sepsis.** Skin infections in high-risk infants, especially in VLBW infants, can become invasive and should be treated.[27]

Laboratory Data. Routine laboratory data, as may be collected based on clinical signs and symptoms, are rarely helpful in differentiating fungal from bacterial infection. A positive culture result from urine, blood, or a skin biopsy indicates systemic infection. Urine for analysis and culture, ophthalmologic examination, echocardiogram for endocarditis, and renal ultrasound for fungal mycetomas are mandatory in disseminated fungal infections.[85]

Treatment. The treatment of fungal infection varies from infant to infant. Very few infants will respond to simple interventions such as stopping broad-spectrum antibiotics, stopping lipid infusions, or removing central catheters. **Almost all require treatment with antifungal agents such as amphotericin B or 5-fluorocytosine (5-FC) for synergistic effect or for CSF penetration (Table 22-10).**[41] Lipid formulations of amphotericin are available that are

TABLE 22-10 ANTIFUNGAL THERAPY

DRUG	DOSAGE	COMMENTS
Amphotericin B	0.1-1 mg/kg/day IV; begin at 0.1 mg/kg and increase daily as tolerated	Nephrotoxic
Amphotericin B lipid complex	1-5 mg/kg/dose IV over 2 hr; begin at 1 mg/kg and increase daily as tolerated	Thrombocytopenia Anemia Hypokalemia
5-Fluorocytosine (5-FC)	50-100 mg/kg/day PO q 6 hr	Hepatotoxic Bone marrow suppression
Fluconazole	12 mg/kg IV loading dose; then 6 mg/kg per dose over 30 min every 24 to 72 hr depending on postnatal and gestational age	Liver toxicity

IV, Intravenously; *PO,* orally.

less toxic and may be the choice in infants who cannot tolerate standard amphotericin.[3] Fluconazole therapy may have efficacy similar to amphotericin but without the toxicity.[11,36] **Intravenous fluconazole prophylaxis may help prevent invasive fungal infection in neonates and reduce mortality during hospital stay in neonates whose birth weight is less than 1500 g.[29,63] However, resistance to fluconazole remains a potentially serious concern.[11]** In a meta-analysis of four trials of 536 VLBW infants that compared prophylactic fluconazole with placebo, fluconazole prophylaxis compared with placebo reduced invasive fungal infection (relative risk [RR] 0.23, 95% confidence interval [CI] 0.11 to 0.46) but without statistically significant difference in mortality before hospital discharge (RR 0.61, 95% CI 0.37 to 1.03).[29] There appeared to be no increased risk for the emergence of resistant *Candida* species with prophylactic fluconazole; however, the follow-up periods were probably not sufficient to detect changes in the resistance pattern. Retrospective studies have reported conflicting results regarding the emergence of fluconazole-resistant *Candida* species. Recent evidence from the United States and Italy suggests that with commonly used fluconazole prophylaxis regimens in the NICU, emergence of resistance is an unlikely event but still warrants tracking.[14,57] In summary, **fluconazole prophylaxis may be effective in reducing invasive fungal infections and mortality in high-risk patients** (e.g., extremely-low-birth-weight [ELBW] infants, neonates on multiple antibiotics, and those in neonatal units in which the baseline rate of systemic fungal infections is high).

PARENT TEACHING

Parents who have infants with viral or bacterial infection require support and information about their infant's condition. Questions arise about treatment and prognosis, as well as possible long-range effects of the infection. Parents experience significant guilt feelings based on misperceptions about what role they had in causing the infection. Health care professionals should remain sensitive to the crisis that parents are experiencing and address the issues of etiology, as well as treatment and prognosis. Valid and factual data, as well as information about complications and long-term effects, should be shared with parents in a timely manner.

Controlling infection in the nursery is of prime importance but does not include excluding the parents from caring for their sick infant. Everyone must adhere to proper handwashing, gowning, and isolation techniques.[105] Educating the parents and siblings about the importance of these procedures, along with appropriate reminders, ensures cooperation. With proper precautions, there is no evidence of increased incidence of infection with parent and sibling visits.

All those entering the nursery must be screened for the presence of illness. Anyone (including staff) with a fever, respiratory symptoms (cough, runny nose, sore throat), gastrointestinal symptoms (nausea, vomiting, diarrhea), or skin lesions should not come in contact with the infant. People with communicable disease (e.g., varicella) or recent exposure to a communicable disease also should not come in contact with the sick neonate.[13,105] Daily cord care should be demonstrated, and a demonstration by the parents should be observed before discharging the infant. ***Every* parent should be taught the signs and symptoms of neonatal illness, because early recognition of signs and symptoms expedites prompt treatment (see Resource Materials for Professionals and Parents on p. 580).** Parents must be taught to take axillary temperatures and to read a thermometer. They should be aware that both hypothermia and hyperthermia may be signs of neonatal illness.[13,105]

REFERENCES

1. Abzug MJ: Presentation, diagnosis, and management of enterovirus infections in neonates, *Paediatr Drugs* 6:1, 2004.
2. Abzug MJ, Cloud G, Bradley J, et al: Double blind placebo-controlled trial of pleconaril in infants with enterovirus meningitis, *Pediatr Infect Dis J* 22:335, 2003.
3. Adler-Shohet F, Waskin H, Lieberman JM: Amphotericin B lipid complex for neonatal invasive candidiasis, *Arch Dis Child Fetal Neonatal Ed* 84:F131, 2001.
4. American Academy of Pediatrics: *Red Book: Report of the Committee on Infectious Disease,* ed 27, Elk Grove Village, Ill, 2006, The Academy.
5. American Academy of Pediatrics and American College of Obstetricians and Gynecologists: *Guidelines for perinatal care,* ed 6, Elk Grove Village, Ill, 2007, The Academy/The College.
6. American Academy of Pediatrics: Committee on Pediatric AIDS: HIV testing and prophylaxis to prevent mother-to-child transmission in the United States, *Pediatrics* 122:1127, 2008.
7. Arkader RE, Troster J, Lopes MR, et al: Procalcitonin does discriminate between sepsis and systemic inflammatory response syndrome, *Arch Dis Child* 91:117, 2006.
8. Ascher DP, Wilson S, Mendiola J, et al: Group B streptococcal latex agglutination testing in the neonate, *J Pediatr* 119:458, 1991.
9. Baltimore RS: Consequences of prophylaxis for Group B streptococcal infections of the neonate, *Semin Perinatol* 31:33, 2007.
10. Bizzarro MJ, Gallagher PG: Antibiotic-resistant organisms in the neonatal intensive care unit, *Semin Perinatol* 31:26, 2007.
11. Bliss JM, Wellington M, Gigliotti F: Antifungal pharmacotherapy for neonatal candidiasis, *Semin Perinatol* 27:365, 2003.
12. Boppana SB, Fowler KB, Britt WJ, et al: Symptomatic congenital cytomegalovirus infection in infants born to mothers with preexisting immunity to cytomegalovirus, *Pediatrics* 104(1 Pt 1):55, 1999.
13. Borghesi A, Stronati M: Strategies for the prevention of hospital-acquired infections in the neonatal intensive care unit, *J Hosp Infect* 68:e293, 2008.
14. Borg-von Zepelin M, Kunz L, Rüchel R, et al: Epidemiology and antifungal susceptibilities of *Candida* spp. to six antifungal agents: results from a surveillance study on fungaemia in Germany from July 2004 to August 2005, *J Antimicrob Chemother* 60:424, 2007.
15. Boyer SM, Gotoff SP: Prevention of early onset group B streptococcal disease with selected intrapartum chemoprophylaxis, *N Engl J Med* 31:1655, 1986.
16. Caviness AC, Demmler GJ, Selwyn BJ: Clinical and laboratory features of neonatal herpes simplex virus infection: a case-control study, *Pediatr Infect Dis J* 27:425, 2008.
17. Centers for Disease Control and Prevention: Preventing congenital toxoplasmosis, *MMWR Morb Mortal Wkly Rep* 49(RR2):57, 2000.
18. Centers for Disease Control and Prevention: Control and prevention of rubella: evaluation and management of suspected outbreaks, rubella in pregnant women, and surveillance for congenital rubella syndrome, *MMWR Morb Mortal Wkly Rep* 50(Suppl):12, 2001.
19. Centers for Disease Control and Prevention: Sexually transmitted diseases: treatment guidelines, 2006, *MMWR Morb Mortal Wkly Rep* 55(RR11):6, 2006.
20. Centers for Disease Control and Prevention: In Siegel JD, Rhinehart E, Jackson M, et al: *for the Healthcare Infection Control Advisory Committee: Guideline: Management of multidrug resistant organisms in healthcare settings,* (pp. 1-74), 2006. Atlanta, 2009, The Centers. Accessed June 3, from www.cdc.gov/ncidod/dhqp/pdf/ar/mdroGuideline2006.pdf.
21. Centers for Disease Control and Prevention: Perinatal group B streptococcal disease after universal screening recommendations—United States, 2003-2005, *MMWR Morb Mortal Wkly Rep* 56(28):701, 2007.
22. Centers for Disease Control and Prevention: Prevention of varicella: recommendations of the Advisory Committee on Immunization Practices (ACIP), *MMWR Morb Mortal Wkly Rep* 56(RR4):1, 2007.
23. Centers for Disease Control and Prevention: Increased detections and severe neonatal disease associated with coxsackievirus B1 infection—United States, 2007, *MMWR Morb Mortal Wkly Rep* 57:553, 2008.
24. Centers for Disease Control and Prevention: Newborn hepatitis B vaccination coverage among children born January 2003–June 2005—United States, *MMWR Morb Mortal Wkly Rep* 57:825, 2008.
25. Centers for Disease Control and Prevention: National Immunization Program: Epidemiology and prevention of vaccine-preventable diseases: Varicella. In *The Pink Book*, ed 10 Bethesda, Md, 2008, U.S. Department of Health and Human Services, pp 283-304. Accessed September 20, 2009, from www.cdc.gov/vaccines/pubs/pinkbook/downloads/varicella.pdf.
26. Chakraborty R, Luck S: Syphilis is on the increase: the implications for child health, *Arch Dis Child* 93:105, 2008.
27. Chapman RL, Faix RG: Invasive neonatal candidiasis: an overview, *Semin Perinatol* 27:352, 2003.
28. Christensen RD, Rothstein G, Hill HR, et al: Fatal early onset group B streptococcal sepsis with normal leukocyte counts, *Pediatr Infect Dis J* 4:242, 1985.

29. Clerihew L, Austin N, McGuire W: Prophylactic systemic antifungal agents to prevent mortality and morbidity in very low birth weight infants, *Cochrane Database Syst Rev* 4:CD003850, 2007
30. Da Silva O, Ohlsson A, Kenyon C: Accuracy of leukocyte indices and C-reactive protein for diagnosis of neonatal sepsis: a critical review, *Pediatr Infect Dis J* 14:362, 1995.
31. Davison SM, Mieli-Vergani G, Sira J, et al: Perinatal hepatitis C virus infection: diagnosis and management, *Arch Dis Child* 91:781, 2006.
32. de Azavedo JC, McGavin M, Duncan C, et al: Prevalence and mechanisms of macrolide resistance in invasive and noninvasive group B *Streptococcus* isolates from Ontario, Canada, *Antimicrob Agents Chemother* 45:3504, 2001.
33. Demmler GJ: Congenital cytomegalovirus infection treatment, *Pediatr Infect Dis J* 22:1005, 2003.
34. DiPersio LP, DiPersio JR: High rates of erythromycin and clindamycin resistance among OBGYN isolates of group B *Streptococcus*, *Diagn Microbiol Infect Dis* 54:79, 2006.
35. Dollner H, Vatten L, Austgulen R: Early diagnostic markers for neonatal sepsis: comparing C-reactive protein, interleukin-6, soluble tumour necrosis factor receptors and soluble adhesion molecules, *J Clin Epidemiol* 54:1251, 2001.
36. Driessen M, Ellis B, Cooper PA, et al: Fluconazole vs. amphotericin B for the treatment of neonatal fungal septicemia: a prospective randomized trial, *Pediatr Infect Dis J* 15:1107, 1996.
37. Dunn DT, Gibb DM, Healy M, et al: Timing and interpretation of tests for diagnosing perinatally acquired hepatitis C virus infection, *Pediatr Infect Dis J* 20:715–716, 2001.
38. Engle WD, Rosenfeld CR: Neutropenia in high risk neonates, *J Pediatr* 105:982, 1984.
39. Enocksson E, Wretlind B, Sterner G, et al: Listeriosis during pregnancy and in neonates, *Scand J Infect Dis* 71(Suppl):89, 1990.
40. European Paediatric Hepatitis C Virus Network: Three broad modalities in the natural history of vertically acquired hepatitis C virus infection, *Clin Infect Dis* 41:45, 2005.
41. Faix RG, Chapman RL: Central nervous system candidiasis in the high-risk neonate, *Semin Perinatol* 27:384, 2003.
42. Fakler CR, Weisman LE: Currently available nonantibiotic approaches to the prevention or adjunct therapy of neonatal bacterial infections, *Semin Pediatr Infect Dis* 10:97, 1999.
43. Fielkow S, Reuter S, Gotoff SP: Cerebrospinal fluid examination in symptom free infants with risk factors for infection, *J Pediatr* 119:971, 1991.
44. Fowler KB, Stagno S, Pass RF: Maternal immunity and prevention of congenital cytomegalovirus infection, *JAMA* 289:1008, 2003.
45. Franz AR, Steinbach G, Kron M, et al: Reduction of unnecessary antibiotic therapy in newborn infants using interleukin-8 and C-reactive protein as markers of bacterial infections, *Pediatrics* 104:447, 1999.
46. Freedman E, Mindel A: Epidemiological, clinical and laboratory aids for the diagnosis of neonatal herpes: an Australian perspective, *Herpes* 11:2, 2004.
47. Freeman J, Platt R, Epstein MF, et al: Birth weight and length of stay as determinants of nosocomial coagulase negative staphylococcal bacteremia in neonatal intensive care unit populations: potential for confounding, *Am J Epidemiol* 132:1130, 1991.
48. Fryklund B, Tullu K, Burman LG: Epidemiology of enteric bacteria in neonatal units: influence of procedures and patient variables, *J Hosp Infect* 18:15, 1991.
49. Garner JS: The Hospital Infection Control Practices Advisory Committee: Guideline for isolation precautions in hospitals. Part I. Evolution of isolation practices, *Am J Infect Control* 24:24, 1996.
50. Garner JS: The Hospital Infection Control Practices Advisory Committee: Guideline for isolation precautions in hospitals, *Infect Control Hosp Epidemiol* 17:53, 1996.
51. Gerdes JS: Clinicopathologic approach to the diagnosis of neonatal sepsis, *Clin Perinatol* 18:361, 1991.
52. Golan Y, Doron S, Sullivan B, et al: Transmission of vancomycin-resistant enterococcus in a neonatal intensive care unit, *Pediatr Infect Dis J* 24:566, 2005.
53. Gonzalez-Peralta RP, Kelly DA, Haber B, et al: Interferon alfa-2b in combination with ribavirin for the treatment of chronic hepatitis C in children: efficacy, safety, and pharmacokinetics, *Hepatology* 42:1010, 2005.
54. Gupta A: Hospital-acquired infections in the neonatal intensive care unit—*Klebsiella* pneumonia, *Semin Perinatol* 26:340, 2002.
55. Gupta A, Ampofo K, Rubenstein D, et al: Extended spectrum beta lactamase-producing *Klebsiella pneumoniae* infections: a review of the literature, *J Perinatol* 23:439, 2003.
56. Haque K, Mohan P: Pentoxifylline for neonatal sepsis, *Cochrane Database Syst Rev* 4:2003 CD004205.
57. Healy CM, Campbell JR, Zaccaria E, et al: Fluconazole prophylaxis in extremely low birth weight neonates reduces invasive candidiasis mortality rates without emergence of fluconazole-resistant *Candida* species, *Pediatrics* 121:703, 2008.
58. Heelan JS, Hasenbein ME, McAdam AJ: Resistance of group B *Streptococcus* to selected antibiotics, including erythromycin and clindamycin, *J Clin Microbiol* 42:1263, 2004.
59. Johnson CE, Whitwell JK, Pethe K, et al: Term newborns who are at risk for sepsis: are lumbar punctures necessary? *Pediatrics* 99:e10, 1997.

60. Jones JL, Kruszon-Moran D, Wilson M: *Toxoplasma gondii* infection in the United States, 1999-2000, *Emerg Infect Dis* 9:1371, 2003. Accessed January 20, 2009, from www.cdc.gov/ncidod/EID/vol9no11/03-0098.htm.
61. Jordan JA, Durso MB: Comparison of *16S rRNA* gene PCR and BACTEC 9240 for detection of neonatal bacteremia, *J Clin Microbiol* 38:2574, 2000.
62. Jordan JA, Durso MB: Real-time polymerase chain reaction for detecting bacterial DNA directly from blood of neonates being evaluated for sepsis, *J Mol Diagn* 7:575, 2005.
63. Kaufman D, Boyle R, Hazen KC, et al: Fluconazole prophylaxis against fungal colonization and infection in preterm infants, *N Engl J Med* 345:1660, 2001.
64. Kawamura M, Nishida H: The usefulness of serial C-reactive protein measurement in managing neonatal infection, *Acta Paediatr* 84:10, 1995.
65. Khetsuriani N, Lamonte A, Oberste MS, et al: Neonatal enterovirus infections reported to the national enterovirus surveillance system in the United States, 1983-2003, *Pediatr Infect Dis J* 25:889, 2006.
66. Kimberlin DW: Neonatal herpes simplex infection, *Clin Microbiol Rev* 17:1, 2004.
67. Kimberlin DW, Lin CY, Sánchez PJ, et al: Effect of ganciclovir therapy on hearing in symptomatic congenital cytomegalovirus disease involving the central nervous system: a randomized, controlled trial, *J Pediatr* 143:16, 2003.
68. Kimberlin DW, Whitley RJ: Neonatal herpes: what have we learned, *Semin Pediatr Infect Dis* 16:7, 2005.
69. King SM: Evaluation and treatment of the human immunodeficiency virus-1-exposed infant, *Pediatrics* 114:497, 2004.
70. Koksal N, Harmanci R, Cetinkaya M, et al: Role of procalcitonin and CRP in diagnosis and follow-up of neonatal sepsis, *Turk J Pediatr* 49:21, 2007.
71. Landers S, Moise AA, Fraley JK, et al: Factors associated with umbilical catheter-related sepsis in neonates, *Am J Dis Child* 145:675, 1991.
72. Lewis DE, Adu-Oppong A, Hollinger FB, et al: Sensitivity of immune complex-dissociated p24 antigen testing for early detection of human immunodeficiency virus in infants, *Clin Diagn Lab Immunol* 2:87, 1995.
73. Lin TY, Kao HT, Hsieh SH, et al: Neonatal enterovirus infections: emphasis on risk factors of severe and fatal infections, *Pediatr Infect Dis J* 22:889, 2003.
74. March of Dimes, Professionals and Researchers, Medical References: *Quick reference and fact sheets: Rubella*, White Plains, NY, 2007, March of Dimes. Accessed September 20, 2009, from www.marchofdimes.com/professionals/14332_1225.asp.
75. Mast EE, Hwang LY, Seto DS, et al: Risk factors for perinatal transmission of hepatitis C virus (HCV) and the natural history of HCV infection acquired in infancy, *J Infect Dis* 192:1880, 2005.
76. McNanley AR, Glantz JC, Hardy DJ, et al: The effect of intrapartum penicillin on vaginal group B *Streptococcus* colony counts, *Am J Obstet Gynecol* 197:583e1, 2007.
77. Merino-Diaz L, Torres-Sanchez MJ, Aznar-Martin J: Prevalence and mechanisms of erythromycin and clindamycin resistance in clinical isolates of beta-haemolytic streptococci of Lancefield groups A, B, C and G in Seville, Spain, *Clin Microbiol Infect* 14:85, 2008.
78. Mofenson LM: Technical report: perinatal human immunodeficiency virus testing and prevention of transmission, Committee on Pediatric AIDS, *Pediatrics* e88:106, 2000.
79. Mofenson LM: U.S. Public Health Service Task Force recommendations for use of antiretroviral drugs in pregnant HIV-1-infected women for maternal health and interventions to reduce perinatal HIV-1 transmission in the United States, *MMWR Recomm Rep* 51(RR-18):1, 2002 quiz CE1.
80. Mohan P, Brocklehurst P: Granulocyte transfusions for neonates with confirmed or suspected sepsis and neutropenia, *Cochrane Database Syst Rev* 4:CD003956, 2003.
81. Montoya JG, Remington JS: Management of *Toxoplasma gondii* infection during pregnancy, *Clin Infect Dis* 47:554, 2008.
82. Nahmias AJ: Neonatal HSV infection. Part I. Continuing challenges, *Herpes* 11:2, 2004.
83. Nandyal RR: Update on group B streptococcal infections: perinatal and neonatal periods, *J Perinat Neonatal Nurs* 22(3):230, 2008.
84. Ng PC: Diagnostic markers of infection in neonates, *Arch Dis Child Fetal Neonatal Ed* 89:F229, 2004.
85. Noyola DE, Fernandez M, Moylett EH, et al: Ophthalmologic, visceral, and cardiac involvement in neonates with candidemia, *Clin Infect Dis* 32:1018, 2001.
86. Ohlsson A, Lacy JB: Intravenous immunoglobulin for suspected or subsequently proven infection in neonates, *Cochrane Database Syst Rev* 1:CD001239, 2004.
87. Ohto H, Terazawa S, Sasaki N, et al: Transmission of hepatitis C virus from mothers to infants. The Vertical Transmission of Hepatitis C Virus Collaborative Study Group, *N Engl J Med* 330:744, 1994.
88. Palomba E, Manzini P, Fiammengo P, et al: Natural history of perinatal hepatitis C virus infection, *Clin Infect Dis* 23:47, 1996.
89. Pessoa-Silva CL, Meurer-Moreira B, Camara-Almeida V, et al: Extended-spectrum beta-lactamase-producing *Klebsiella pneumoniae* in a neonatal intensive care unit: risk factors for infection and colonization, *J Hosp Infect* 53:198, 2003.

90. Pettersson K: Perinatal infection with Group B streptococci, *Semin Fetal Neonatal Med* 12:193, 2007.
91. Posfay-Barbe KM, Wald ER: Listeriosis, *Pediatr Rev* 25:151, 2004.
92. Pourcyrous M, Bada HS, Korones SB, et al: Significance of serial C-reactive protein responses in neonatal infection and other disorders, *Pediatrics* 92:431, 1993.
93. Read JS: Human milk, breastfeeding, and transmission of human immunodeficiency virus type 1 in the United States. American Academy of Pediatrics, Committee on Pediatric AIDS, *Pediatrics* 112:1196, 2003.
94. Remington JS, Klein JO, editors: *Infectious diseases of the fetus and the newborn infant,* ed 6, Philadelphia, 2006, Saunders.
95. Resti M, Jara P, Hierro L, et al: Clinical features and progression of perinatally acquired hepatitis C virus infection, *J Med Virol* 70:373, 2003.
96. Ronnestad A, Abrahamsen TG, Gaustad P, et al: C-reactive protein (CRP) response patterns in neonatal septicaemia, *APMIS* 107:593, 1999.
97. Ronnestad A, Abrahamsen TG, Medbo S, et al: Septicemia in the first week of life in a Norwegian national cohort of extremely premature infants, *Pediatrics* 115:e262, 2005.
98. Rotbart HA: Antiviral therapy for enteroviral infections, *Pediatr Infect Dis J* 18:632, 2000.
99. Rotbart HA, Webster AD: Treatment of potentially life-threatening enterovirus infections with pleconaril, *Clin Infect Dis* 32:228, 2001.
100. Rupp ME, Marion N, Fey PD, et al: Outbreak of vancomycin-resistant *Enterococcus faecium* in a neonatal intensive care unit, *Infect Control Hosp Epidemiol* 22:301, 2001.
101. Saiman L, Ludington E, Pfaller M, et al: Risk factors for candidemia in neonatal intensive care unit patients. The National Epidemiology of Mycosis Survey Study Group, *Pediatr Infect Dis J* 19:319, 2000.
102. Schrag SJ, Stoll BJ: Early-onset neonatal sepsis in the era of widespread intrapartum chemoprophylaxis, *Pediatr Infect Dis J* 25:939, 2006.
103. Schwerenski J, McIntyre L, Bauer CR: Lumbar puncture frequency and cerebrospinal fluid analysis in the neonate, *Am J Dis Child* 145:54, 1991.
104. Shang S, Chen G, Wu Y, et al: Rapid diagnosis of bacterial sepsis with PCR amplification and microarray hybridization in *16S rRNA* gene, *Pediatr Res* 58:143, 2005.
105. Siegel JD, Rhinehart E, Jackson M, et al: *and the Healthcare Infection Control Practices Advisory Committee: 2007 Guideline for isolation precautions: preventing transmission of infectious agents in healthcare settings,* June 2007. Accessed September 20, 2009, www.cdc.gov/ncidod/dhqp/gl_isolation.html.
106. Singh AE, Romanowsski B: Syphilis: review with emphasis on clinical, epidemiologic, and some biologic features, *Clin Microbiol Rev* 12:187, 1999.
107. Smith PB, Cotton CM, Garges HP, et al: A comparison of neonatal Gram-negative rod and Gram-positive cocci meningitis, *J Perinatol* 26:111, 2006.
108. Stoll BJ, Hansen N, Fanaroff AA, et al: Changes in pathogens causing early-onset sepsis in very-low-birth-weight infants, *N Engl J Med* 347:240, 2002.
109. Stoll BJ, Hansen N, Fanaroff AA, et al: Late-onset sepsis in very low birth weight neonates: the experience of the NICHD Neonatal Research Network, *Pediatrics* 110(2 Pt 1):285, 2002.
110. Stoll B, Hansen N, Higgins R, et al: Very low birth weight preterm infants with early onset neonatal sepsis, *Pediatr Infect Dis J* 24:635, 2005.
111. Tama P, Serwint JR: Toxoplasmosis, *Pediatr Rev* 28:470, 2007.
112. Thillagavathie P: Current issues in maternal and perinatal tuberculosis: impact of the HIV-1 epidemic, *Semin Neonatol* 5:189, 2000.
113. Thorne C, Newell ML: Mother-to-child transmission of HIV infection and its prevention, *Curr HIV Res* 1:447, 2003.
114. Thorne C, Newell ML: HIV, *Semin Fetal Neonatal Med* 12:174, 2007.
115. Tovo PA, Pembrey LJ, Newell ML: Persistence rate and progression of vertically acquired hepatitis C infection. European Paediatric Hepatitis C Virus Infection, *J Infect Dis* 181:419, 2000.
116. Trincado DE, Rawlinson WD: Congenital and perinatal infections with cytomegalovirus, *J Paediatr Child Health* 37:187, 2001.
117. Vazzalwar R, Pina-Rodrigues E, Puppala BL, et al: Procalcitonin as a screening test for late-onset sepsis in preterm very low birth weight infants, *J Perinatol* 25:397, 2005.
118. Venkatesh M, Hammerschlag M: *Chlamydia trachomatis* infections in the newborn. In Rose B, editor: *UpToDate*, Waltham, Mass, 2009, UptoDate, Inc. Accessed February 5, from www.utdol.com/online/content/topic.do?topicKey=neonatol/20765&selectedTitle=3~76&source=search_result.
119. Verboon-Maciolek MA, Krediet TG, Gerards LJ, et al: Clinical and epidemiologic characteristics of viral infections in a neonatal intensive care unit during a 12-year period, *Pediatr Infect Dis J* 24:901, 2005.
120. Wasunna A, Whitelaw A, Gallimore R, et al: C-reactive protein and bacterial infection in preterm infants, *Eur J Pediatr* 149:424, 1990.
121. Weisman LE, Stoll BJ, Cruess DF, et al: Early onset group B streptococcal sepsis: a current assessment, *J Pediatr* 121:428, 1992.
122. Weiss MD, Burchfield DJ: Adjunct therapies to bacterial sepsis in the neonate, *Newborn Infant Nurs Rev* 4(1):46, 2004.

123. Weiss MG, Ionides SP, Anderson CL: Meningitis in premature infants with respiratory distress: role of admission lumbar puncture, *J Pediatr* 119:973, 1991.
124. Weitkamp JH, Aschner JL: Diagnostic use of C-reactive protein (CRP) in assessment of neonatal sepsis, *NeoReviews* 6:e508, 2005.
125. Wirth S, Lang T, Gehring S, et al: Recombinant alfa-interferon plus ribavirin therapy in children and adolescents with chronic hepatitis C, *Hepatology* 36:1280, 2002.
126. Wirth S, Pieper-Boustani H, Lang T, et al: Peginterferon alfa-2b plus ribavirin treatment in children and adolescents with chronic hepatitis C, *Hepatology* 41:1013, 2005.
127. Wiswell TE, Hachey WE: Multiple site blood cultures in the evaluation for neonatal sepsis during the first week of life, *Pediatr Infect Dis J* 10:365, 1991.

RESOURCE MATERIALS FOR PROFESSIONALS AND PARENTS

Gardner SL, Brown VD: *Clinical practice tool: Newborn Scale of Sepsis (SOS),* © Rubarth, 2005 and ©NPDPA, 2009, Available at www.npdpa.com.

Gardner SL, Brown VD: *How will I know if my baby is sick?* ©NPDPA, 2008, Written discharge teaching tool for parents to recognize newborn infection. Available at www.npdpa.com.

Gardner SL, Brown VD: *Newborn Scale of Sepsis (SOS) assessment sheet,* ©NPDPA, 2008, Documentation forms for SOS scale. Available at www.npdpa.com.

23 RESPIRATORY DISEASES

SANDRA L. GARDNER, MARY ENZMAN-HINES, AND LORRAINE A. DICKEY

Despite the marked improvement over the past years in the survival of premature newborns with respiratory distress, significant mortality and high morbidity rates persist. Much of the improvement in neonatal mortality has been the result of successful treatment and management of respiratory diseases in the neonate.

This chapter presents an overview of some of the common respiratory diseases, their treatments, and outcomes. General principles and concepts related to respiratory physiology, etiologic factors, and symptomatology are presented, followed by specific disease processes and their management.

GENERAL PHYSIOLOGY

Any discussion of general respiratory physiology must include some elements of anatomy and embryology and their significance to the clinician (Table 23-1).

Surface-active compounds such as phosphatidylcholine and phosphatidylglycerol stabilize the alveoli. Surface tension forces act on air-fluid interfaces, causing a water droplet to "bead up." The surface-active compound (e.g., soap added to a water droplet) reduces the surface tension and allows the droplet to spread out in a thin film. In the lung, surface tension forces tend to cause alveoli to collapse. A compound such as surfactant reduces surface tension and allows the alveoli to remain open.

However, the situation is more complicated than just described. Laplace detailed the magnitude of the pressure *(p)* exerted at the surface of an air-liquid interface as equaling twice the surface tension *(st)* divided by the radius *(r)* of curvature of the surface ($p = 2\ st \div r$). In the absence of surfactant, an alveolus with a small radius of curvature has a greater magnitude of pressure at its surface (tending to collapse it) than does an alveolus with a larger radius of curvature. Therefore smaller alveoli tend to collapse and empty contained gas into larger alveoli.

Surfactant modifies surface tension by decreasing surface tension when the radius of curvature is small and increasing surface tension when the radius of curvature is greater. An alveolus with a larger radius of curvature has a greater-than-expected pressure (tending to reduce its volume), and an alveolus with a smaller radius of curvature has less-than-expected pressure. Therefore the alveoli are stabilized at a uniform radius of curvature (uniform volume).

Surfactant provides a number of useful properties in addition to reducing surface tension, which increases lung compliance, provides alveolar stability, and decreases opening pressure. It also enhances alveolar fluid clearance, decreases precapillary tone, and plays a protective role for the epithelial cell surface. Surfactant is constantly being formed, stored, secreted, and recycled. Conditions that interfere with surfactant metabolism include acidemia, hypoxia, shock, overinflation, underinflation, pulmonary edema, mechanical ventilation, and hypercapnia. **Surfactant production is delayed in infants of diabetic mothers (IDMs) of classes A, B, and C; infants with erythroblastosis fetalis; and infants who are the smaller of twins.** Surfactant production is accelerated in the following:

- IDMs of classes D, F, and R
- Infants of heroin-addicted mothers
- Premature rupture of membranes of greater than 48 hours' duration

Please note that the **PURPLE** type in each chapter is intended to make it easier to identify clinically applicable material.

TABLE 23-1 LUNG DEVELOPMENT

STAGE AND MAJOR EVENTS	SIGNIFICANCE
EMBRYONIC (UP TO 5 WEEKS)	
Single ventral outpocketing quickly divided into two lung buds.	Airways begin to differentiate.
Mesenchyme surrounds endodermal lung buds, which continue to divide and extend into the mesenchyme.	
Branching of the airways begins.	Branching anomalies (e.g., pulmonary agenesis and sequestered lobe) occur early in fetal life.
Pulmonary arteries invade lung tissue, following the airways, and divide as the airways divide.	
Pulmonary veins arise independently from the lung parenchyma and return to the left atrium, thus completing the pulmonary circuit.	
PSEUDOGLANDULAR (5-16 WEEKS)	
Progressive airway branching begins; bronchi and terminal bronchioles form.	All subdivisions that will form airways are complete by the sixteenth week.
Muscle fibers, elastic tissue, and early cartilage formation can be seen along the tracheobronchial tree.	
Mucous glands are found at 12 weeks and increase in number until 25-26 weeks, when cilia begin to develop.	
Diaphragm develops.	Herniation of the diaphragm occurs.
CANALICULAR (13-25 WEEKS)	
Airway changes from glandular to tubular and increases in length and diameter.	Air-conducting portion (bronchi and terminal bronchioli) continues luminal development.
20 WEEKS	
Fetal airways end in blind pouches lined with cuboid epithelium; a relatively large amount of interstitial mesenchyme is present; few pulmonary capillaries are present, and they are not closely associated with the respiratory epithelium.	
22-24 WEEKS	
Rapid proliferation of the pulmonary capillary bed, an increase of the surface area of the respiratory epithelium, and formation of alveolar ducts and sacculi occur.	Development of gas exchange portion (the respiratory bronchi and alveolar ducts) begins; pulmonary vasculature develops most rapidly.
Respiratory epithelium contains cells that become differentiated into type I and type II pneumocytes.	
Type I pneumocytes produce an extremely thin squamous epithelial layer that lines the alveoli and fuses to the underlying capillary endothelial cells.	By the late fetal period, the resulting membrane between the alveoli and capillaries allows sufficient gas exchange to support independent life.
Type II pneumocytes (cuboid cells) are the site of surfactant synthesis and storage.	At 22 weeks, surface-active phospholipids (lecithin) can first be detected.

TABLE 23-1 LUNG DEVELOPMENT—cont'd

STAGE AND MAJOR EVENTS	SIGNIFICANCE
TERMINAL (24-40 WEEKS)	
Lung differentiation: proliferation of the pulmonary vascular bed, creation of new respiratory units (alveolar ducts and alveoli), decrease in amount of mesenchyme, and fusion of the gas-exchange epithelium to the pulmonary capillary epithelium occur.	Before this time, the fetal lungs are incapable of supporting adequate gas exchange because of insufficient alveolar surface area and inadequate pulmonary vasculature.
34-36 WEEKS	
Phosphatidylglycerol appears, and a dramatic increase in the principal surfactant compound phosphatidylcholine occurs.	Adequate amounts of surface-active material protect against the development of respiratory distress syndrome.
ALVEOLAR (POSTNATAL LUNG DEVELOPMENT: LATE FETAL LIFE TO 8-10 YEARS OF AGE)	
At term, the number of airways is complete; there is sufficient respiratory surface for gaseous exchange, and the pulmonary capillary bed is sufficient to carry the gases that have been exchanged.	Although the infant is capable of sustaining respiratory effort and the lung is able to provide oxygenation and ventilation at birth, lung development is still incomplete.
Alveoli continue to increase in number, size, and shape; they enlarge and become deeper to maximize the exposed surface area for gas exchange.	Ongoing lung development implies that infants who have suffered severe lung disease at birth need not become life-long pulmonary cripples.

- Infants of mothers with hypertension
- Infants subjected to maternal infection
- Infants suffering from placental insufficiency
- Infants affected by administration of corticosteroids
- Infants affected by abruptio placentae

The fetal lung is filled with a volume of liquid (20 to 30 mL/kg) equal to the functional residual capacity. This fluid is not amniotic fluid but, rather, a liquid that has been produced in the lung and discharged through the larynx and mouth into the amniotic fluid. Lung fluid is continuously produced at a rate of approximately 2 to 4 mL/kg/hr.

Because of the movement of lung fluid and its components (notably lecithin) into amniotic fluid, the lecithin-sphingomyelin (L/S) ratio has become a notable clinical tool. Noting a sharp increase in the L/S ratio, Gluck and Kulovich[138] found they could predict which infants were at risk for respiratory distress syndrome (RDS). In general, **L/S ratios of more than 2:1 are not associated with RDS, whereas ratios of less than 2:1 are associated with it.** Phosphatidylglycerol (PG), the second most common phospholipid in surfactant, appears at about 36 weeks' gestation and increases until term. **The presence of PG is associated with a very low risk for RDS, whereas its absence is associated with the development of RDS.** Unlike the L/S ratio, PG determination is valid in the presence of blood-contaminated amniotic fluid.

During vaginal delivery, approximately one third of the lung fluid may be removed during the thoracic "squeeze" as the infant passes through the birth canal; the remainder of the fluid is removed mainly by the pulmonary lymphatics, although pulmonary capillaries may play a role. After a cesarean section, all of the lung fluid will be removed by the pulmonary lymphatic system and the capillaries.

The first breath of life, a response to tactile, thermal, chemical, and mechanical stimuli, initiates respiratory effort. The fluid-filled lungs, surface forces, and tissue-sensitive forces are obstacles to the first breath. At birth, gas is substituted for liquid to expand the alveoli. After the alveoli are "opened" during the first few breaths, a film of surface-active material stabilizes the alveoli.

The first breath of life requires an opening pressure of 60 to 80 cm of water to overcome the effects of the surface tension of the air-liquid interface, particularly the small airways and alveoli. Thus on each subsequent breath, less pressure is necessary to allow for a similar increase in air volume in the lung. The effort of breathing is lessened with subsequent breaths.

GENERAL ETIOLOGIC FACTORS

Respiratory disease may be defined as a progressive impairment of the lungs to exchange gas at the alveolar level. Although the pathologic process causing respiratory disease in the neonate may occur in any portion of the respiratory system (or in other organ systems), the final common pathway in respiratory disease is impairment of gas exchange.

Prematurity is the single most common factor in the occurrence of RDS. Its incidence is inversely proportional to gestational age and occurs most frequently in infants of less than 1200 g and 30 weeks' gestation. RDS occurs in male infants twice as frequently as in female infants (2:1). **The principal factor operating in the development of RDS in very premature infants is surfactant deficiency.**

Multiple gestations increase the risk for respiratory disease related to lung maturity in the second, third, or more siblings. The second and subsequent infants may experience perinatal asphyxia, malpresentation, or mode of delivery (e.g., cesarean section) that contributes to respiratory disease. A recent study shows a significantly increased risk for respiratory disease associated with being the second-born preterm twin, especially at 30 to 31 weeks' gestation.[152] Grand multiparity is associated with increased risk for respiratory disease, particularly when other siblings have had RDS.

Prenatal maternal complications increase the risk for respiratory disease in the infant. Maternal illnesses such as cardiorespiratory disease, hypoxia, hemorrhage, shock, hypotension, or hypertension result in decreased uterine blood flow with subsequent hypoxia or ischemia at the placental level. Severe maternal anemia causes fetal cardiac depression and respiratory depression. Maternal diabetes may result in preterm delivery because of fetal and maternal indications. There is also a greater incidence of false-positive L/S ratios in diabetic populations. There has been a propensity of IDMs to develop RDS despite documentation of L/S ratios greater than 2:1. (A combination of an L/S ratio of 2:1 or greater and the presence of PG confirms fetal lung maturity.) Abnormal placental conditions (compressed umbilical cord caused by prolapse or breech delivery, placental disease such as infarcts or syphilis, or hemorrhage as a result of placenta previa or abruptio placentae) affect oxygen transfer from mother to fetus and result in an asphyxial insult to the developing fetal lung. Premature rupture of the membranes predisposes the fetus or newborn to the development of infections such as pneumonia, sepsis, or meningitis. Premature or prolonged rupture of the membranes not associated with neonatal infection accelerates fetal lung development and thereby lessens the incidence of RDS. Maternal toxemia and maternal heroin addiction also hasten fetal lung maturation. Antenatal administration of glucocorticoids[260] results in less severe RDS and fewer doses of surfactant, fewer cases of patent ductus arteriosus (PDA) and intraventricular hemorrhage (IVH), and less mortality.[314] The benefits of antenatal steroids are dose-dependent,[314] but even an incomplete course benefits the preterm infant.[111]

Factors affecting the fetus during the birth process may lead to respiratory distress. Depression of the respiratory center can occur as a result of maternal medications that cross the placenta. An infant delivered shortly after an analgesic or anesthetic is administered to the mother may have only minimal respiratory efforts at birth. Excessive uterine activity, usually as a result of oxytocin induction or augmentation of labor, results in decreased uterine blood flow, late fetal heart deceleration, and respiratory depression in the infant at birth. Respiratory disease may be the result of direct trauma to the respiratory center or a cerebral hemorrhage in proximity to it. Fetal shock caused by difficult labor or dystocia, tight nuchal cord, cerebral hemorrhage, or hemorrhage from the fetal side of the placenta results in central nervous system (CNS) depression and hypoxia. Bleeding results in a generalized hypovolemic condition characterized by decreased oxygen-carrying capacity. Fetal or neonatal asphyxia and blood loss lead to progressive respiratory distress. Delivery by cesarean section prevents one third of the lung fluid from being expelled by the thoracic squeeze of vaginal birth. Thus after cesarean birth, all lung fluid must be absorbed through circulatory and lymphatic channels; therefore a greater incidence of transient tachypnea of the newborn may occur as the increased volume of retained fluid is absorbed.

The timing of cesarean section influences the incidence of RDS. Recent studies noting the increased risk of late preterm infants and RDS in elective cesarean sections are cited in Chapter 5.

Obstruction of the airway caused by aspiration of meconium or amniotic fluid occurs either spontaneously at birth or during resuscitative efforts. Although the lungs initially fill with air, subsequent atelectasis occurs as complete airway obstruction prevents further entrance of air. Conversely, a "ball-valve" or "air-trapping" effect may occur as air is allowed in but is unable to escape because of intermittent obstruction. The presence of amniotic debris, vernix, lanugo, and meconium in the respiratory tract increases the incidence and severity of pulmonary infection. Diaphragmatic paralysis occurs after phrenic nerve injury during birth (usually in a large-for-gestational-age [LGA] infant) and is often associated with Erb's palsy. The paradoxic movement of the paralyzed diaphragm during inspiration and expiration results in inadequate tidal volume and impaired gaseous exchange.

Existing neonatal conditions increase the risk for respiratory disease. Congenital defects that prevent transmission of the stimulus to or from the respiratory center, prevent normal respiratory effort, reduce gas-exchange surface area, or hamper the delivery of oxygen to the site of exchange will predispose the infant to respiratory embarrassment. Such defects include heart or great vessel anomalies, diaphragmatic hernia and hypoplastic lung, respiratory tract anomalies (e.g., choanal atresia or tracheoesophageal fistula), chest wall deformities, and CNS defects.

Diseases of the infant also can lead to respiratory disease. Hemolytic disease, such as ABO and Rh incompatibility, results in anemia and, if severe, in hypovolemic shock. Blood incompatibilities increase respiratory distress by decreasing the oxygen-carrying capacity of the blood. Infections stress the body's systems, increase oxygen requirements, and contribute to an impairment of surfactant production. Chronic lung disease in the form of bronchopulmonary dysplasia (BPD) occurs in 17% to 54% of very-low-birth-weight (VLBW) infants.[168] Prolonged treatment of RDS may be necessitated by the severity of the disease but may increase the risk for developing chronic lung disease.

GENERAL PREVENTION

Antepartum

Prevention of respiratory disease begins with prevention of conditions that predispose to respiratory distress. These conditions that constitute "reproductive risks" have been identified and can be categorized as psychosocial, genetic, biophysical, or economic in nature. Once an individual is identified as being in a high-risk category, comprehensive prenatal care with immediate attention given to maternal complications that arise is crucial (see Chapter 2).

Intrapartum

Fetal well-being is assessed by using electronic monitoring of uterine activity, fetal heart rate, and fetal scalp blood sampling. Electronic fetal heart rate monitoring enables instantaneous fetal heart rate tracings as opposed to the previous method of intermittent evaluation by stethoscope. Fetal heart rate monitoring allows coincident correlation between uterine contractions and fetal response. These tools enable the practitioner to evaluate how well the fetus withstands the stresses of labor and to make decisions about the laboring course.

Fetal cardiac response to stress is unlike an older child's or adult's response to hypoxia, hypercapnia, and acidosis with tachycardia from sympathetic nervous system discharge. A fetus responds to these same stresses with an initial increase in heart rate. This is quickly followed by bradycardia from parasympathetic stimulation when the hypoxia, hypercapnia, and acidosis persist (see Chapter 2).

Postpartum

After delivery, an infant should be maintained in an environment that minimizes stress and thereby minimizes oxygen requirement. All infants, but particularly at-risk infants, should be maintained within the narrow parameter of physiologic homeostasis (as outlined in Unit Two, Support of the Neonate).

GENERAL DATA COLLECTION

Because the clinical manifestations of many neonatal illnesses include respiratory symptoms (cardiac, metabolic, neurologic, and hematologic), a systematic and thorough approach to data collection is essential in evaluating an infant in respiratory distress.

History

The perinatal history (antepartum, intrapartum, and postpartum) should be reviewed for risk factors (see Chapter 2).

Signs and Symptoms

Vital signs such as temperature, pulse, respiration, and blood pressure should be evaluated. Hypothermia and hyperthermia increase oxygen requirements by altering the basal metabolic rate. Hypotension often is associated with respiratory disease.

RESPIRATORY EXAMINATION

Respiratory effort is normally irregular in rate and depth and is chiefly abdominal, rather than thoracic, with a **rate of 30 to 60 breaths/min.** Bradypnea is characterized by a rate below 30 breaths/min that is regular (as opposed to periodic or apneic) and may be caused by an insult to the respiratory center of the CNS. **Tachypnea, a rate above 60 breaths/min after the first hour of life, is the earliest sign of respiratory (and often other) diseases.** As a compensatory mechanism, tachypnea attempts to maintain alveolar ventilation and gaseous exchange. As a decompensatory mechanism, tachypnea increases oxygen demand, energy output, and the "work" of breathing.

Periodic respirations are cyclic respirations of apnea (5 to 10 seconds) and ventilation (10 to 15 seconds). The average respiratory rate is 30 to 40 breaths/min. Periodic breathing is a common occurrence in small preterm infants as a result of an immature CNS. **Apnea is a nonbreathing episode lasting longer than 20 seconds and accompanied by physiologic alterations.** The syndrome of apnea is discussed in the "Apnea" section on pp. 657-661.

Use of accessory muscles of respiration is indicative of a marked increase in the work of breathing. **Retractions reflect the inward pull of the thin chest wall on inspiration.** Retracting is best observed in relation to the sternum (substernal and suprasternal) and the intercostal, supracostal, and subcostal spaces. The increased negative intrathoracic pressure necessary to ventilate the stiff, noncompliant lung causes the chest wall to retract. This further compromises the lung's expansion. The degree of retraction is directly proportional to the severity of the disease.

Nasal flaring is a compensatory mechanism that attempts to take in more oxygen by increasing the size of the nares and thus decreasing the resistance (by as much as 40%) of the narrow airways. **Grunting is forced expiration through a partially closed glottis.** The audible grunt may be heard with or without the aid of a stethoscope. As a compensatory mechanism, grunting stabilizes the alveoli by increasing transpulmonary pressure and increases gaseous exchange by delaying expiration.[160]

Color is normally pink after the first breaths of life. **Acrocyanosis,** which is peripheral cyanosis of the hands and feet in the first 24 hours of life, is normal. **Pallor** with poor peripheral circulation may indicate systemic hypotension. **Ruddy, plethoric skin color** may indicate hyperviscosity, polycythemia, or both as the cause of respiratory symptoms. However, the lack of a deep-red coloring does not rule out polycythemia or hyperviscosity.

Cyanosis, a late and serious sign, is a blue discoloration of the skin, nail beds, and mucous membranes. Differentiation between **peripheral cyanosis** (of hands and feet) and **central cyanosis** (of mucous membranes of mouth and generalized body cyanosis) is essential. **Because a large decrease in Pa_{O_2} may be tolerated without detectable cyanosis, the lack of cyanosis does not ensure a healthy infant.** When hypoxemia reaches a level that produces frank cyanosis, the insufficiency is usually in advanced stages (see Chapter 8). Therefore cyanosis or its lack is not a reliable sign in neonates.

Symmetry of the newborn chest is characterized by a relatively round or barrel shape, because the anteroposterior diameter equals the transverse diameter. With prolonged respiratory distress, there is an increase in the anteroposterior diameter, so the neonate becomes pigeon-chested.

Auscultation of a newborn's chest includes comparing and contrasting one side with the other and noting the quality of breath sounds and the presence or absence of rales, rhonchi, or other abnormal sounds. Because of the relatively small size of the newborn's chest, it is **hyperresonant,** so breath sounds are widely transmitted. **Therefore one cannot always rely on auscultation to detect pathologic conditions (e.g., pneumothorax).** Percussion of the chest to determine the presence of air, fluid, or solids may not be useful in the neonate because of small chest size and hyperresonance. Palpation of the neonatal chest wall while the infant is crying may detect gross changes in sound transmission through the chest. Palpation of crepitus in the neck, around the clavicles, or on the chest wall suggests the complication of air leak.

NONRESPIRATORY EXAMINATION

Hypotonia is characterized by a froglike positioning and a lax, open mouth. Progressing from flexion to flaccidity indicates progression of hypoxia and exhaustion from the work of breathing. Cardiac and related findings such as a murmur, absence of pulses, bounding pulses, palmar or calf pulses, weight gain, hepatosplenomegaly, cyanosis, edema, bradycardia, or tachycardia indicate congestive heart failure or congenital heart defects. A **scaphoid abdomen** indicates a diaphragmatic hernia.

Laboratory Data

Because the clinical presentation of many respiratory and nonrespiratory diseases is the same, a **chest x-ray examination** may be the only way to differentiate cause and establish the proper diagnosis. X-ray evaluation helps eliminate congenital anomalies (e.g., diaphragmatic hernia with lung hypoplasia, masses, and obstruction) as the cause when acquired respiratory disease (e.g., RDS, transient tachypnea of the newborn, and pneumonia) is the cause of the distress. X-ray films confirm the presence of pneumothorax or other pulmonary air leaks.

Measurement of arterial blood gases is used to demonstrate alterations in oxygenation and acid-base balance and to differentiate between respiratory and metabolic components. Initial baseline values are followed by serial observations at least every 15 to 30 minutes after any change in therapy during the acute phase of illness. Pulse oximetry enables immediate evaluation of oxygenation status and is an adjunct to arterial blood gas sampling.[9] **A shunt study may differentiate between lung origin and cardiac origin of respiratory distress.** The symptoms of pulmonary disease (cyanosis and low PaO_2) are often alleviated with crying, increased FIO_2, or continuous positive airway pressure. If the same symptoms are cardiac in origin, they remain unchanged or worsen with these interventions. Administration of 100% FIO_2 for 10 minutes or longer may result in an increased PaO_2 (>100 mm Hg), whereas in cardiac disease caused by right-to-left shunting, there is no change in PaO_2 after 100% FIO_2 administration. **CAUTION:** In the presence of severe lung disease with significant right-to-left shunting, cyanosis and PaO_2 may not be changed with 100% FIO_2.

The **hematocrit value is used to rule out anemia or polycythemia** as the cause of the respiratory distress. In anemia, inadequate oxygen content promotes tissue hypoxia. In polycythemia, increased viscosity and sludging of blood flow adversely affect tissue oxygenation.

The white blood cell count, differential, and C-reactive protein (CRP) (see Chapter 22) aid in diagnosing sepsis as the cause of distress. A blood culture is an invaluable aid when infection is suspected and should be obtained before antibiotic therapy is initiated. **Blood glucose** determination to rule out hypoglycemia as a cause is particularly important in IDMs, small-for-gestational-age (SGA) infants, LGA infants, and preterm appropriate-for-gestational-age (AGA) infants. An **electrocardiogram (ECG), echocardiogram, and cardiac catheterization** are used to rule out cardiac abnormalities.

An electroencephalogram (EEG) and ultrasonographic examination of the brain help rule out CNS abnormalities. **Serum electrolytes** (calcium, sodium, and potassium) aid in eliminating metabolic aberration as the cause of the distress.

GENERAL TREATMENT STRATEGIES

Treatment of any condition should be directed at correction of its underlying cause. In meconium aspiration syndrome, the presence of meconium damages the neonatal lung. No therapeutic measure is available at present to augment the healing process. Therapy is thus directed at preventing or alleviating the consequences of neonatal lung diseases, such as hypoxemia and acidemia, allowing healing to take place and reducing the potential for iatrogenic complications.

Respiratory support is the hallmark of treatment of neonatal respiratory disease. Respiratory support involves increasing inspired oxygen tensions and providing ventilation if necessary.

Supplemental Oxygen

Oxygen is a *drug,* the most commonly used drug in neonatal care. Historically, the policy of unrestricted and unmonitored oxygen therapy was accompanied by potential harm (e.g., RDS, chronic lung disease [CLD]/BPD, retinopathy of prematurity [ROP], PDA [see "Patent Ductus Arteriosus" section], necrotizing enterocolitis [NEC] [discussed in Chapter 28], and IVH/periventricular leukomalacia, hypoxic-ischemic encephalopathy [PVL, HIE] [discussed in Chapter 26]) from oxygen free radicals without clear benefits.[15]

Free radicals are continuously produced in all cells as a by-product of cell metabolism. Free radicals have positive effects in normal physiologic processes as follows: (1) biologic defense against bacteria, viruses, and cancer cells; (2) vasodilation; (3) neurotransmission; and (4) the up-regulation of some genes.[19] However, free radicals may also have harmful effects. **Free radicals, highly reactive atomic molecules with unpaired electrons, regain their stability by quickly reacting with other molecules in proximity to obtain the molecules they need. Reaction with free radicals causes damage to these close molecules by changing their structure and function.** To maintain homeostasis, the human body either uses or counters free radical activity with endogenous and exogenous antioxidants. Neonates, especially preterms, have maturational deficiencies in endogenous antioxidant systems, nutritional issues altering exogenous dietary intake of antioxidants, and diseases/conditions requiring interventions that preclude control of free radical–generating stimuli in their environment.[19] **Therefore the neonatal period is an especially vulnerable time for free radical damage and injury.**[316] **The neonate, especially preterms and sick term infants, depend on care providers to use strategies that emphasize the prudent use of oxygen therapy (e.g., use of the minimum amount of oxygen to provide the desired therapeutic effect)**[19,145,205,341] **because the proper concentration of supplemental oxygen, especially for extremely preterm infants, remains to be established.**[171]

When the neonate cannot maintain adequate oxygenation, supplemental oxygen must be provided. Because oxygen is a drug, it must be treated as such and given only for specific indications. **Biochemical criteria (Pa_{O_2} <60 mm Hg) and clinical criteria such as respiratory distress, central cyanosis, apnea, asphyxia, hypotonia, and low oxygen saturation are indications to prescribe oxygen.** Institutional protocol for ordering, delivering, monitoring, and documenting oxygen therapy is recommended.[9]

Regardless of the mode of delivery (hood, nasal cannula or prongs, endotracheal tube, bag, or mask), safe and effective oxygen administration follows certain principles:

- **No concentration of oxygen has been proved to be "safe."** A concentration (e.g., 30%, 40%, 80%, 100%) that is therapeutic for one infant may be toxic for another. **Oxygen blenders** must be available wherever oxygen is being administered (e.g., delivery room, transition nursery, level I, II, or III nursery) so that delivery of different amounts of inspired oxygen concentration is possible.[19,145,189,293,341]
- To titrate inspired oxygen concentrations to the individual infant's need, arterial P_{O_2} should be measured and maintained in a normoxic state (Pa_{O_2} between 60 and 80 mm Hg)[9]; **both hypoxia and hyperoxia should be avoided.**[205,293] Acutely ill neonates requiring supplemental oxygen therapy also should have blood pH and Pa_{CO_2} measured.[9]
- **To titrate inspired oxygen concentration to the individual neonate's need, oxygen saturation (using continuous noninvasive pulse oximetry [PO]) should be measured and maintained in the appropriate range for birth weight, gestational/chronologic age, and disease process** wherever oxygen is being administered (e.g., delivery room, transition nursery, level I, II, or III nursery).[293,341] Oxygen targeting for the VLBW preterm is discussed in the "Retinopathy of Prematurity" section.
- Oxygen administration without some form of continuous monitoring of the infant's oxygenation (e.g., arterial blood gases, pulse oximetry) is dangerous and not recommended.[9]
- **Delivered oxygen should be humidified (30% to 40%),** because dry gases are irritating to the airways and humidity decreases insensible water losses. To prevent respiratory therapy equipment from becoming a source of infection, humidifiers and tubing should be replaced per institutional and product protocol.
- **Oxygen should be warmed (31° to 34° C [87.8° to 93.2° F])** so temperature at the delivery site is the same as the incubator temperature. **Oxygen delivered by endotracheal tube should be warmed to core temperature (i.e., 36.5° to 37° C [97.7° to 98.6° F]).**[145] This prevents cold stress and increased oxygen consumption from blowing cold air in the infant's face.[350]
- Oxygen concentration must be monitored by continuous or intermittent sampling (at least every hour) and recorded. In addition, **hourly documentation** of the following parameters should be recorded: (1) pulse oximetry (PO)

saturation values; (2) mode of oxygen delivery (e.g., hood, nasal cannula, continuous positive airway pressure [CPAP], ventilator); and (3) amount of oxygen being administered (e.g., F_{IO_2}, liter flow/min).[9]

- **Oxygen monitors and analyzers should be calibrated** according to the manufacturer's recommendations.[9]
- **A stable concentration of oxygen is necessary to maintain Pa_{O_2} within normal limits.** A sudden increase or decrease in oxygen concentration may result in a disproportionate increase or decrease in Pa_{O_2} caused by vasodilation or vasoconstriction in response to oxygen.[350] Adjust F_{IO_2} in small increments (2% to 5%) to avoid hypoxia and/or hyperoxia.[67,293] **Adjustment of supplemental oxygen (particularly lowering F_{IO_2}) must be done slowly to avoid the *flip-flop phenomenon.*** Hypoxic insult initiates pulmonary vasoconstriction, which causes hypoperfusion and increased pulmonary vascular resistance. **The infant should be weaned from supplemental oxygen cautiously.**[350] (Refer to Chapter 8) for a discussion of the "rule of seven," which states that the estimated percentage change in inspired oxygen is equal to the desired change in Pa_{O_2} divided by 7.)
- Observing color, respiratory effort, activity, and circulatory response and monitoring arterial oxygen concentration aid in determining the need for oxygen therapy and for appropriate adjustments.
- Clinical observations, F_{IO_2} concentrations, and time of adjustments must be described, documented, and reported.
- Oxygen concentration should be returned to previous levels if clinical observations of distress and inability to tolerate decreased levels of oxygen occur.

DELIVERY METHODS

For instructions on the bag-and-mask resuscitation method, see Chapter 4. **An oxygen hood is a clear plastic hood that fits over the infant's head to deliver a constant concentration of oxygen.** If the infant has sufficient ventilation to maintain a normal arterial carbon dioxide tension, oxygenation by increased inspired oxygen tensions through an oxygen hood may be the only respiratory support that is necessary. This degree of support is particularly applicable in cases of mild RDS, transient tachypnea of the newborn (TTN), meconium aspiration, or neonatal pneumonia.

A **blender system** is the most reliable way to administer a fixed oxygen concentration via a hood. An appropriate-size hood should be used. If it is too large, the infant may slip out of the hood and F_{IO_2} may be diluted by leaks; if it is too small, pressure points may develop, especially around the neck. **Another source of oxygen must be provided when the infant's head is removed from the hood because of feeding, being held, or suctioning.** This secondary source may be set up from the blender source so that the infant's Pa_{O_2} remains constant during suctioning or feedings. The infant may need increased F_{IO_2} from the secondary source, and this can be adjusted easily according to assessments made with pulse oximetry; these changes should be recorded.

For both home and hospital use, a **nasal cannula** is used to administer oxygen to the dependent infant who is developing social and motor skills:

- Choose the appropriate-size cannula for the infant—a cannula that is too large obstructs the nares, prevents air leak thus enabling an increase in CPAP, irritates the nasal mucosa, and is uncomfortable for the baby.[210]
- Position the cannula across the infant's upper lip. Secure it to the infant's face by first applying Stomahesive or Tegaderm (OpSite) directly to the infant's cheeks and taping the cannula to it to prevent skin irritation.
- Oxygen tubing should be long enough to provide opportunities for social and gross motor skill development.

CAUTION: Neonates are obligatory nasal breathers, so nasal obstruction (mucus or milk) will decrease the amount of oxygen actually received. Therefore nares should be suctioned as needed. Because the exact concentrations of oxygen delivered by cannula cannot be measured, flow rates are titrated by monitoring Pa_{O_2} or pulse oximetry readings and by evaluating the clinical course.

Without studies to establish safety and efficacy, many centers (64%)[334] have adopted heated, humidified, high-flow (>1 L/min) nasal cannula (HHHFNC) therapy as primary support for preterms with RDS, apnea of prematurity, and post-extubation respiratory care.[210] One study comparing the use of high-flow nasal cannula (e.g., up to 2.5 L/min) with nasal CPAP (NCPAP) for treatment of apnea found that the nasal cannula high-flow oxygen was as effective as NCPAP. Preterm infants with high-flow nasal cannula oxygen tolerated it well and had no drying of the nares, and no ventilation was necessary.[344] Use of nasal cannulas with oxygen rates above 0.5 L/min may result in inadvertent administration of continuous distending (positive) pressure, causing increased respiratory effort (i.e., tachypnea, retractions, thoracoabdominal asynchrony, exaggerated periodic breathing, and increased work of breathing.).[229] Use of high-flow oxygen cannulas in extremely-low-birth-weight (ELBW) infants increases (1) nasal secretions, (2) nasal erosion and bleeding, (3) nasal suctioning, (4) nasal obstruction/work of breathing, and (5) risk for staphylococcal sepsis.[209] **HHHFNC generates CPAP to the preterm airway that may be excessive** given the conditions of (1) closed mouth, (2) tightly fitting nasal cannula (NC), (3) rate of flow, and (4) infant size (<1500 g).[210] Commercial HHHFNC devices currently in use can achieve flow rates of 4 to 8 L/min.[123] Unlike CPAP devices that are equipped with a pressure gauge and a pop-off safety valve, HHHFNC devices do not have a direct measure of the pressure applied to the infant's airway or a pop-off valve to prevent the accumulation of excessive pressure; flow rates as high as 6 L/min have been used without measurement of the level of CPAP delivered.[61,123] Recently it was found that measurements of oral cavity pressures closely estimate the delivered CPAP of the HHHFNC devices.[210] These researchers found that CPAP generated with HHHFNC depends on flow rate and weight; the smallest infants with the highest flow rates and a completely closed mouth may achieve clinically significant and unpredictable levels of CPAP. Their recommendation was that HHHFNC should not be used as a replacement device for delivering CPAP.[210]

Continuous Distending Pressure

Application of a continuous distending pressure (CDP) to the lungs increases functional residual capacity and Pa_{O_2}. Oxygenation is improved by decreasing intrapulmonary shunting and by improving the match of ventilation and perfusion. The application of CDP improves compliance of the lung and lessens the work of breathing.[146] Early application of CDP in preterms with RDS reduces the subsequent use of intermittent positive pressure ventilation (IPPV) with its accompanying adverse effects.

In RDS, in which the functional residual capacity is reduced, increased respiratory oxygen tensions through an oxygen hood (oxyhood) may not be sufficient to maintain an adequate arterial oxygen tension. More invasive techniques may be necessary.

CPAP and continuous negative pressure (CNP) are two methods of delivery of CDP. If the infant cannot maintain a Pa_{O_2} of 60 mm Hg in 0.6 F_{IO_2}, a trial of CPAP through the nasal route is indicated. Initial levels of CPAP should be in the range of 4 to 5 cm of water. CPAP should be increased to 8 to 10 cm of water by 1- to 2-cm increments if necessary to raise the infant's Pa_{O_2} (as measured by arterial blood gas determinations, noninvasive monitoring, or both).

Not all CPAP application techniques are equal. Neonates receiving "bubble" CPAP experience chest wall vibrations (similar to those seen in high-frequency ventilation [HFV]) that contribute to gaseous exchange. ***Bubble CPAP*** reduces minute volume by 39% and respiratory rate by 7% when compared with CPAP provided through a ventilator.[69] In one center, use of bubble CPAP from birth in 401-g to 1000-g preterms has resulted in (1) fewer delivery room intubations, (2) fewer days on mechanical ventilation, (3) less use of postnatal steroids, (4) better weight gain, and (5) no increase in complications, including the incidence of CLD/BPD.[259] In a randomized controlled trial (RCT), larger preterms (mean gestational age [GA] 36 wks; mean birth weight [BW] 2900 g) with respiratory distress were treated with either supplemental oxygen in an oxyhood or with bubble CPAP through nasal prongs.[56] Only 23% of the larger preterms who were treated with CPAP were transported to a higher-level neonatal intensive care unit (NICU) compared with 40% of the preterms who were treated with oxygen in a hood. Also, cost savings were realized and there was no increase in oxygen use or mortality. However, there was a clinically, not statistically, significant increase in the incidence of pneumothorax in the CPAP group; the **24-hour presence of a neonatal nurse practitioner or physician to relieve air leaks is mandatory with the use of CPAP.**

Indications and complications in the use of CPAP are listed in Table 23-2. If the infant can maintain ventilation as indicated by normal arterial carbon dioxide tension, no further respiratory support may be necessary. Comparison of 9 years of records from a single tertiary center and matched Vermont Oxford Network (VON) sites found that

TABLE 23-2 CONTINUOUS POSITIVE AIRWAY PRESSURE

INDICATIONS	COMPLICATIONS
Infant who breathes spontaneously yet has mild to moderate respiratory distress syndrome	Respiratory difficulty secondary to narrowing of the nasal passage with prongs, of the trachea with the presence of an endotracheal tube
Very-low-birth-weight infant with primary or secondary apnea	Pneumothorax and other air leaks
Support during weaning from mechanical ventilation	Nasal and/or septal irritation, trauma, deformity, infection, obstruction[343,411]; gastric and abdominal distention; perforation[66]

early use of NCPAP in VLBW infants is associated with decreased rates of BPD/CLD and ROP.[202] The COIN trial[251] compared NCPAP with intubation and ventilation of 25 to 28 weeks' gestation preterms who breathed spontaneously by 5 minutes of age and had respiratory distress. Within the first 5 days of life, 46% of those randomized to NCPAP were intubated, at a median of 6.6 hours of life. Outcomes at 36 weeks were no different for either group in the combined outcome of death or oxygen dependence. A non-significant trend toward less CLD/BPD occurred in the more mature preterms, whereas there was a trend toward increased mortality in the less mature preterms randomized to NCPAP. Unlike other studies, only 77% of the infants randomized to intubation received surfactant and surfactant use was halved in the NCPAP group.[251] **Although early institution of NCPAP in the management of respiratory insufficiency may reduce the need for mechanical ventilation, combining early NCPAP with early surfactant therapy further reduces treatment failures.** (See "Surfactant Replacement Therapy" discussion in the "Respiratory Distress Syndrome" section.)

CPAP may be delivered by facemask, nasal pharyngeal tubes, nasal prongs, or endotracheal (ET) tube. Delivery of CPAP by nasal prongs is the most common method used; use of short binasal prongs is the most effective.[98,102] However, in much of the research literature, nasal prongs are compared with nasal pharyngeal tubes for administration of CPAP. Advantages to the use of nasal CPAP include the following[17,98,145,239,384]:

- Less invasive than endotracheal tube
- Decreased incidence, duration, and complications of intubation and mechanical ventilation
- Earlier extubation
- Decreased incidence and morbidity of BPD/CLD
- Improved oxygenation and decreased work of breathing
- Decreased need for surfactant and second doses of surfactant
- Reduced mortality

Disadvantages include (1) gaseous distention of the bowel[182] or gastrointestinal (GI) perforation[134] (both are rare occurrences), (2) increased rate of pneumothorax,[56,98,250] (3) difficulties keeping prongs in the nose and maintaining patency; infant agitation, and (4) alteration in appearance (dilation of the nares).[343] **CPAP is labor-intensive for the neonatal nurse. Choosing the correct size of nasal prong is important to avoid movement and erosion of nasal tissue. Box 23-1 lists important aspects of care of the neonate on NCPAP to optimize safety and efficacy.**

Criteria that indicate improvement on CPAP are listed in the Critical Findings box on p. 592. When the infant's $Pa{O_2}$ is consistently over 70 mm Hg, inspired oxygen concentration or CDP may be lowered. Oxygen concentration is usually lowered in 5% to 10% increments to a level of 40% to 60%. CDP is lowered in increments of 1 cm of water to a level of 2 cm of water before discontinuation. The infant may then be placed into an oxygen hood with the same $F{IO_2}$. Neonates should be monitored closely with pulse oximetry and arterial blood gases.

Pulmonary Hygiene

Pulmonary hygiene is normally maintained by ciliary activity, a covering of mucus, and narrowing and dilation of the bronchi with respiration and coughing. Anatomic and physiologic variations in the neonate alter these normal pulmonary mechanisms.

BOX 23-1

CARE OF INFANTS RECEIVING NCPAP TO OPTIMIZE SAFETY AND EFFICACY

Prongs

- Nasal prongs should fill the entire nares without distending or causing blanching of the nares
- Presence of a small space (at least 2 mm) between the nares and prong base
- Lateral straps are used to secure the prongs by providing gentle, equal tension
- Assess prongs and NCPAP device at least every hour to ensure proper positioning and functioning
- Remove NCPAP device q 2-4 hr to assess skin integrity (e.g., color, perfusion, pressure, excoriation) and massage nasal septum

Hat

- Use the appropriate-size hat to avoid prong movement; change hat size with neonatal head growth
- Position just above the eyebrows, with the back of the hat extending to the base of the neck, and completely covering the infant's ears
- Use ties on the hat to secure tubing, thus decreasing movement and/or upward pull of CPAP system

Nose

- Suction nares only PRN to maintain nasal patency
- Avoid deep nasal suctioning, unless absolutely necessary for individual infant
- Use a hydrocolloid dressing over the nose and philtrum to provide a barrier layer for skin protection

Mouth

- Place orogastric tube for decompression of the stomach
- Encourage closed mouth by use of pacifier and/or prone positioning

Comfort Measures

- Positioning prone, swaddled, or contained (to promote flexion) (see Chapter 13) decreases movement and pulling/dragging of the device on the nares
- Minimal handling and position change q 2-4 hr and/or with infant agitation
- Skin-to-skin care with parents (see Chapters 12 and 13)
- Pacifier, nonnutritive sucking, sucrose
- Environmental management—decrease light/noise (see Chapter 13)
- Use neonatal pain scale and administer pharmacologic sedation and/or pain relief (see Chapter 12)

Adapted from McCoskey L: Nursing care guidelines for prevention of nasal breakdown in neonates receiving nasal CPAP, *Adv Neonatal Care* 8:116, 2008; Squires AJ, Hyndman M: Prevention of nasal injuries secondary to NCPAP application in the ELBW infant, *Neonatal Netw* 28:13, 2009.

CPAP, Continuous positive airway pressure; *NCPAP,* nasal CPAP; *PRN,* as needed.

Critical Findings

CRITERIA THAT INDICATE IMPROVEMENT ON CONTINUOUS POSITIVE AIRWAY PRESSURE

Blood Gases

- Decrease or stabilization of oxygen requirement F_{IO_2} ≤0.60 with Pa_{O_2} >50 mm Hg or pulse oximetry >90%
- Maintenance of adequate ventilation
  - Pa_{CO_2} ≤50 to 60 mm Hg
  - pH 7.25-7.45

Clinical

- Decreased work of breathing—decreased respiratory rate, grunting, flaring, and retracting
- Improved lung volumes and appearance on chest x-ray films
- Improved patient comfort

The small airway of the neonate has a diameter that is four times smaller than that of the normal adult. Debris that causes only a moderate obstruction for the adult airway causes a disproportionately greater obstruction of the smaller airway of the neonate. Also, a neonate normally has an underdeveloped cough reflex. A sick neonate with insufficient respiratory effort and a weak or nonexistent cry has underventilated lungs. If a neonate who is attached to multiple life-support systems is cared for in the same position, secretions localize in the dependent pulmonary tree and predispose to hypostatic pneumonia.

Pulmonary hygiene consists of two major components: chest physiotherapy (CPT) and suctioning. The goals of pulmonary hygiene are the following:

- To maintain a patent airway by clearing secretions
- To promote optimal pulmonary oxygenation and ventilation

- To prevent pulmonary infection from accumulated secretions
- To facilitate removal of pulmonary debris by loosening and mobilizing secretions into the mainstem bronchi for suctioning

Pulmonary hygiene has been used as a treatment for intubated patients with conditions associated with atelectasis, increased secretions, and pulmonary debris (pneumonia, meconium aspiration, RDS, and BPD).

CHEST PHYSIOTHERAPY

CPT consists of positioning, percussion, and vibration. Postural changes use gravity to facilitate the movement of pulmonary debris from smaller to larger bronchi. Postural changes used with pediatric and adult respiratory patients have been used for neonatal CPT. **However, most ill neonates, especially VLBW and ELBW infants, do not tolerate multiple positioning and repositioning.** Periodic (every 2 to 4 hours with care) repositioning changes the ventilation-perfusion matching in dependent lung areas and improves oxygenation. Prone positioning improves lung mechanics and lung volumes and improves oxygenation (see Chapter 13).

Percussion of the chest wall creates a suction action that loosens secretions. Percussion should occur through gently tapping over the affected lung. **In infants with BPD, rib fractures have been documented that resulted from vigorous percussion[296] and vibrator use.[403]** Vibration of the neonate's chest may follow percussion. Even though vibration must be done on expiration to move secretions with the exhalation of air, this is very difficult to accomplish with the neonate's rapid, shallow breathing cycle.

Any manipulation of the sick neonate has the potential for decreasing oxygenation and precipitating hypoxia (see Chapter 13). During CPT, bradycardia, cyanosis, hypotonia, fighting, struggling, and alterations in oxygenation are signs of stress. There is also an increase in plasma epinephrine and norepinephrine levels with CPT and endotracheal suctioning; this stress response is decreased in sedated preterm infants.[147] CPT is no better than standard care for clearing secretions in ventilated neonates and is accompanied by hypoxia and increased oxygen requirements. Post-extubation CPT has also shown no differences in preventing atelectasis, decreasing the number of apnea/bradycardia episodes, the need for reintubation, or the duration of supplemental oxygen.[20]

The most severe complications reportedly resulting from CPT are an increased risk for IVH (see Chapter 26) and cerebral encephalopathy. An increased incidence of severe intraventricular/periventricular hemorrhage has been reported in preterm infants treated with early CPT.[305] In 1992, a previously unrecognized and distinct pattern of severe, late-onset brain injury was reported in 15 neonates (24 to 32 weeks GA; 600 to 1270 g BW). The pattern of brain injury was of extensive, dense, and cystic lesions involving the periphery of the brain bilaterally. This full-thickness cortical necrosis, called ***encephaloclastic porencephaly,*** resulted in 14 deaths and severe neurologic deficit in the only survivor.[86] This nursery changed its protocol to include holding the baby's head steady during CPT; no further cases of brain injury have occurred.[304]

Another study of 454 babies found 13 babies (24 to 27 weeks GA; 680 to 1100 g BW) with lesions similar to the encephaloclastic porencephaly just described. The lesions in these infants were described as cystic with cortical and subcortical destruction, and peripheral rather than periventricular; they occurred between 2 and 3 weeks of life. These hemorrhagic infarcts are consistent with the pathologic changes in older infants from ***shaken baby syndrome***.[206,207,313,399] The extremely immature brain of the VLBW infant may be particularly vulnerable to the shaking movements of CPT. Five of these infants died; seven of the eight surviving infants had handicaps (e.g., mild hemiplegia to severe spastic quadriplegia; cognitive delay) at 6 to 16 months of age. For longer than 3 years, no VLBW infant in this NICU has received CPT in the first month of life; no further cases of this brain injury have occurred.[77,158]

The techniques, efficacy, complications, outcomes, safety, and frequency of CPT have not been studied sufficiently.[177] Given the lack of data, the lack of clear evidence of benefit, and the concerns of safety for VLBW infants, recommendations include the following:

- Use CPT cautiously.
- Do not use CPT on VLBW infants in the first month of life.[158]
- Keep the infant's head steady during CPT.[304]
- CPT should be used only for definite indications when the infant is fit and able to tolerate the procedure.[304]
- CPT should never be done "routinely" but should be applied on an individual basis after careful and thorough assessment.[304]

- Percussion should be used only when secretions are not cleared by suction alone.[304]
- Use of CPT in the delivery room lacks evidence-based research.
- CPT should not be included in pulmonary hygiene until research clearly substantiates its benefits.[405]

SUCTIONING

Once secretions are loosened and mobilized, they must be removed through the nose, mouth, or trachea with suctioning.

Naso-oropharyngeal Suctioning. When an infant has no artificial airway, suctioning the naso-oropharynx serves two purposes: removing secretions and initiating a cough reflex that mobilizes secretions. With either a suction bulb or catheter, the infant is suctioned when secretions are produced. Providing an oxygen source during the procedure is necessary. **Because stimulation of the nares causes reflex inspiration with possible inhalation of oropharyngeal contents, first the *mouth* and then the *nose* should be suctioned.** The results should be documented.

CAUTION: Suctioning should be avoided for 30 minutes to 1 hour after feeding unless it is necessary to establish a patent airway. The catheter should be gently inserted upward and back into the nares, never forced. If the catheter is hard to pass or the nares seem blocked, this procedure should be abandoned to prevent swelling or trauma. **Frequent nasal suction creates trauma and edema. The catheter may initiate vasovagal stimulation with resultant bradycardia.**

Endotracheal Suctioning. An artificial airway prevents normal warming, humidifying, and cleansing of the air by the upper airway. The presence of the foreign body (the tube) also increases pulmonary secretions. To **maintain a patent airway, sterile endotracheal suction should be performed on an individual basis, *never* on a routine basis** (e.g., on a schedule of every 2, 3, or 4 hours). **Individual assessment criteria to establish that the infant "needs" suction are listed in the Critical Findings box above.** Knowledge of the infant's respiratory diagnosis suggests the need and the frequency of suction. The acute phase (first 72 hours) of RDS is a restrictive disease; few secretions are produced, so minimal suctioning (every 12 to 24 hours) is necessary. Studies have found no increase in occluded tubes when suction frequency was changed from every 6 to every 12 hours (during the first 72 hours of RDS)[401] and from every 4 to every 8 hours.[82] Disease processes noted for secretion production (e.g., the chronic phase of RDS, CLD/BPD, meconium aspiration syndrome, or pneumonia) may require early and frequent suctioning.

Endotracheal tube (ETT) suctioning is not an innocuous procedure. **ETT suction is associated with numerous physiologic alterations and complications (Box 23-2).** Hypoxia and changes in heart rate and blood pressure alter cerebral blood flow, increase intracranial pressure, and predispose the preterm to an increased risk for IVH (see Chapter 26). Pulse oximetry is a valuable tool in assessing oxygenation status during and after suctioning. The infant may be preoxygenated before suctioning, or if oxygen saturation falls (<90%) during suctioning, the infant may be hyperventilated. **Preoxygenation** is the increase of FIO_2 above baseline concentration before ETT suction to prevent/reduce hypoxemia. To avoid

Critical Findings

INDIVIDUAL ASSESSMENT CRITERIA FOR SUCTION

Evidence of Secretions

- Visible secretions in tube
- Audible coarse, wet, or decreased breath sounds
- Palpation of wet, coarse vibrations through chest wall

Alterations in Vital Signs

- Changes in respiratory pattern:
  - Increased work of breathing (retractions, grunting, flaring)
  - Tachypnea or apnea
- Change in cardiac pattern; tachycardia or bradycardia

Alterations in Neonatal State

- Increased agitation, irritability, restlessness
- Hypertonic or hypotonic
- Listless, lethargic

Alterations in Oxygenation and Ventilation

- Desaturations (<90%) or labile saturations on pulse oximeter
- Skin color changes—pale, dusky, cyanotic
- Changes in arterial blood gas values—increased Pco_2, decreased Pao_2, respiratory acidosis
- Increased peak inspiratory pressure on mechanical ventilation and increased high-pressure alarms
- Decreased chest wall vibration with high-frequency ventilation (HFV)

BOX 23-2 PHYSIOLOGIC ALTERATIONS AND COMPLICATIONS ASSOCIATED WITH ENDOTRACHEAL TUBE SUCTION

- Hypoxia/hypoxemia[120,295]
  - Caused by disconnection from the ventilator and oxygen, as well as presence of suction catheter and application of negative pressure, which partially occludes the airway; handling during the procedure; desaturations on the PO
- Alterations in heart rate[120,311]
  - Bradycardia, dysrhythmias, and asystole are precipitated by hypoxemia
- Alterations in blood pressure
  - Hypertension/hypotension
- Alterations in cerebral blood flow[280,311]
  - Changes in oxygenation, heart rate, and blood pressure increase cerebral blood flow, both during and after the procedure (late [6 minutes]/prolonged [25 minutes] elevations of CBF),[186] and intracranial pressure, which increase the risk for intraventricular hemorrhage
- Increase in plasma epinephrine and norepinephrine levels[147]
- Tissue damage[54,203]
  - Granuloma formation within airways; increased severity of CLD/BPD associated with colonization of lungs with gram-negative bacilli; lobar emphysema and atelectasis; bronchial stenosis
- Atelectasis
  - Marked increase in opening (inflation) pressures of the lungs; adequate lung recruitment and PEEP may prevent lung collapse and deterioration in arterial oxygenation; atelectasis
- Pneumothorax
  - From aggressively ventilating neonate above baseline pressures
- Infection[81,154]
  - Airway colonization with gram-positive cocci and gram-negative bacilli by 2 weeks of life despite the method of suction
- Unplanned extubation

CBF, Cerebral blood flow; *CLD/BPD,* chronic lung disease/bronchopulmonary dysplasia; *PEEP,* positive end-expiratory pressure; *PO,* pulse oximetry.

exposing the preterm to hyperoxic events that may predispose to ROP, the FIO_2 is increased by 10% to 20% above baseline when clinically indicated for an individual infant. For ELBW/VLBW infants, FIO_2 increases may be from 2% to 5%. Using 100% oxygen only if it is clinically indicated for the individual infant prevents hyperoxia. **Hyperventilation** (e.g., increasing respiratory rate) with a bag or the manual breaths on the ventilator after each catheter pass minimizes hypoxia and contributes to shortened time of stabilization and recovery. More research is needed on the optimal timing of increasing the FIO_2 and the amount of oxygen to use.[295]

Administration of intermittent doses of morphine during endotracheal suctioning has not been shown to reduce pain scores in ventilated preterms. In this same RCT, multisensory stimulation after suctioning also was not associated with reduced pain scores.[68] Comfort measures (e.g., nonnutritive sucking, sucrose, swaddling, facilitated tucking) have been used during suction to provide pain relief,[389] as well as to reduce bradycardia and desaturations (see Chapter 12).

Most of the physiologic alterations and complications of ETT suction are the result of decreases in positive end-expiratory pressure (PEEP), lung volume, and oxygen during disconnection of the ETT from the ventilator for use of the open suction procedure. Use of closed suction systems (e.g., an adapter to suction without disconnection from the ventilator) decreases associated hypoxemia and bradycardia by enabling oxygenation and ventilation to continue during suction.[81,404] Closed suction is associated with smaller decreases in cerebral oxygenation, smaller variations in cerebral blood volume, and related hemodynamic changes, particularly in ventilated preterms.[187,253] A recent study comparing the effects of open versus closed suction for mechanically (conventional and high frequency) ventilated ELBW preterms (n = 19) found decreases in cerebral blood flow and heart rate during suction and return to baseline after suctioning ceased; both of these changes were independent of the kind of ventilation and the type of suction used.[311]

Closed suction removes secretions as effectively as open suction with no increase in the rate of bacterial airway colonization (with catheter change every 24 hours), suction frequency, reintubation, duration of mechanical ventilation, length of hospitalization, incidence of nosocomial pneumonia or sepsis, severity of CLD/BPD, or mortality in 175 low-birth-weight (LBW) infants.[81] Enclosure of the catheter in a clear sheath decreases the possibility of cross-contamination and environmental pollution of objects and personnel with bacterial and viral pathogens. Closed suction systems are easier to use, less time consuming, better tolerated by the neonate, cost-effective, and well accepted by neonatal nurses.[81] **Closed ETT suction has been identified as "best practice" in reducing nosocomial sepsis in the NICU.**[71]

The actual procedures used in closed and open suction are often not supported by research

data. Table 23-3 outlines common suction techniques, research data, and recommendations to alter clinical practice.

Procedure for Closed Suction

Equipment To Be Prepared

- Inline suction catheter (changed daily)
- Sterile normal saline (without preservative)
- Suction canister and tubing (60 to 80 mm Hg negative pressure)

Procedure

- Unlock the inline suction catheter. Press suction control valve and check suction pressure.
- Place saline solution syringe on the proximal port of the adapter to irrigate the catheter before suction, place normal saline syringe or bullet at the distal port or adapter and squeeze saline solution into the port while applying suction.

TABLE 23-3 SUCTION PROCEDURE: RESEARCH BASIS AND RECOMMENDATIONS

COMMON TECHNIQUES	RECOMMENDATIONS	RESEARCH DATA
Instillation of 0.25-0.5 mL sterile NS before suction *Purpose:* Mobilize and thin secretions; aid in catheter passage	Mucus is not miscible with saline solution so bolus saline does not thin or liquefy secretions;[101] vaporized or nebulized NS thins secretions.[101] Bolus saline accumulates at the end of the ETT; <20% of the saline solution is retrieved with suction, and remainder is absorbed by the body.[157] Use of NS associated with increased hypoxia, deterioration of lung mechanics, and infection.[33,154] Maintenance of adequate humidification (100%) and warming oxygen to core temperature keep secretions loose and lubricate the ETT and the surrounding tissues.	*Closed suction:* Irrigate catheter before suction; place NS syringe at distal port adapter and squeeze saline solution into port while simultaneously applying suction. *Open suction:* Dip or moisten catheter tip in sterile NS or water-soluble jelly to facilitate sliding down the small-diameter ETT.
Head turned from side-to-side with suction *Purpose:* To advance catheter down contralateral bronchus	Suction causes fluctuations in cerebral blood flow, which increases ICP and the risk for intraventricular hemorrhage.[280,281] Sharply turning head to the side occludes the jugular vein and increases ICP, which is at its lowest when the head is in the midline or slightly elevated.[204]	*Turned head position:* Contraindicated because of data on increased ICP, jugular vein occlusion, and anatomic impossibility of passing catheter into bronchi using this strategy Do not turn the infant's head during suction; keep head in midline for suction.
Catheter inserted until resistance (touching the carina) is met, withdrawn slightly; then suction applied	Application of negative pressure with suction and touching the bronchial mucosa with catheter cause irritation, tissue damage, and significant oxygen desaturations.[54,145,203]	Shallow suction does not touch the carina with the catheter tip; using the ETT markings and the length of the adapter, insert the catheter no more than 1 cm beyond the total distance (e.g., if the ETT is inserted 10 cm and the length of the adapter is 1.5 cm, the suction catheter should be inserted 11.5 cm to no farther than 12.5 cm).
Catheter is inserted and removed several times	One small study (n = 16) evaluated nurses' subjective reports of amount of secretions obtained with one and two suction passes; no difference was noted.[1]	Limit number of catheter passes to the number needed to adequately remove secretions. Do not use up-and-down motion while removing the catheter, since this decreases oxygenation and promotes hypoxia and tissue damage. Only one suction attempt should be made before the neonate is again ventilated; every catheter passage is considered a suction event; occlude ETT with catheter for no longer than 5-10 sec.
No use of developmental care adjustments during the stressful procedure of suction	Body containment significantly decreases the magnitude of the preterm's response (e.g., pain, desaturations, and bradycardia) to suctioning.[120,362,389]	Use the developmental care technique of containment during suction (see Chapter 13).

ETT, Endotracheal tube; *ICP,* intracranial pressure; *NS,* normal saline.

- Slide the catheter through the plastic cover down the endotracheal tube to the predetermined distance.
- Apply suction while withdrawing the catheter tip to the catheter window (the plastic cover will inflate from ventilation if the catheter is pulled back too far; the catheter will completely or partially occlude the ventilatory circuit if not pulled back far enough). Only one suction attempt should be made before the infant is again ventilated. Assess tolerance of the procedure by observing pulse oximeter and infant's color, heart rate, tone, and activity. Hyperventilate the lungs with appropriate FIO_2 for 6 to 8 breaths or until adequate oxygenation has been established.
- To irrigate the catheter after suction, place a normal saline syringe at the distal port adapter and squeeze saline solution into the port while simultaneously applying suction. Remove the saline solution and close the port when the catheter has been thoroughly rinsed.
- Rotate and lock the suction control cap to discontinue suction.
- Suction the nasopharynx and oropharynx as needed with a suction bulb or separate suction catheter and tubing. *Do not* disconnect the closed suction catheter from its suction line—this contaminates the setup for ETT suction.
- Check respirator settings, including alarm system in "on" position. Check tube position to be sure the tracheal tube is not strained or bent.
- Note amount and type of secretions obtained.

Procedure for Open Suction

Equipment To Be Prepared

- Sterile suction catheter of appropriate size (discard after each suctioning)
- Sterile gloves
- Sterile normal saline solution (without preservative)
- Stethoscope
- Suction machine and tubing (60 to 80 mm Hg negative pressure)

Procedure

- The sterile catheter and glove package are opened. Sterile normal saline solution (0.25 to 0.5 mL) is drawn up in a 1-mL syringe. The resuscitation bag is connected to oxygen, and the patency is checked so that, if the neonate becomes apneic or bradycardic during the procedure, resuscitation equipment is immediately available. If the infant is on a ventilator equipped with a bag, this may be used for resuscitation if necessary.
- Disconnect and dip the suction catheter in/or wet the tip of the suction catheter with the sterile normal saline.
- Put gloves on and attach sterile catheter to suction tubing. With nondominant hand, disconnect ETT from ventilator.
- Gently pass catheter down endotracheal tube to premeasured length.
- Occlude suction hole in catheter and withdraw. Use continuous suction so that secretions are not "released" with intermittent suction. Only one suction attempt should be made before the infant is again ventilated. Assess tolerance of procedure by observing pulse oximeter and infant's color, heart rate, tone, and activity.
- Reconnect ETT to ventilator and hyperventilate with appropriate FIO_2 for 6 to 8 breaths or until adequate oxygenation has been established. Check ventilator settings including alarm system in "on" position. Check tube position to ensure that the tube is not bent or strained. Note amount and type of secretions obtained.

NOTE: When two persons are available for suction, one remains "sterile" and does the suctioning while the other detaches the ETT from the ventilator and hyperventilates the infant between suctionings.

Because ETT suctioning compromises the neonate's physiologic homeostasis, adequate recovery time is necessary after the procedure.[120] For ETT suction, an average of 4.4 minutes of recovery time is necessary (6 of 25 infants in one study never returned to baseline during the observation). Use of containment, such as facilitated tucking, has been shown to decrease pain response and improve oxygenation after suctioning.[389] **These infants may need a significant rest period after suctioning before other aspects of care such as feeding are attempted.**

Endotracheal Intubation

Endotracheal intubation may be accomplished by the orotracheal route or the nasotracheal route. An endotracheal tube diameter that approximates the diameter of the infant's fifth digit generally fits snugly into the trachea. To measure for an endotracheal tube, the distance from the oral orifice to midway between the glottis and carina may be calculated by multiplying the crown-heel length by 0.2. In an emergency, the distance from the lips to midway between the glottis and carina may be approximated by the *7-8-9-10 rule*. The distance is 7 cm in a 1-kg infant, 8 cm in a 2-kg infant, 9 cm in a 3-kg infant, and 10 cm in a 4-kg infant.

Premedication for intubation should be strongly considered for any non-emergent intubation. Intubation has been identified as a painful procedure associated with unfavorable physiologic side effects such as bradycardia, desaturation, increased blood pressure, and increased intracranial pressure. Increases in intracranial pressure in the ELBW infant are of particular concern because this population already is predisposed to IVH. The neonate should be pretreated for pain with an opiate such as morphine or fentanyl. Midazolam may be used for additional sedation or to potentiate the effect of the opiate so smaller doses of each medication can be administered. In addition, it has been suggested that atropine may be useful as a pre-intubation medication.[99] Atropine increases the heart rate, blocks the vagal response to placement of the laryngoscope blade and ETT, and minimizes oral secretions, allowing for easier visualization of the glottis and making securing of the ETT easier.[99] The suggested dose of atropine for this use is 0.01 to 0.03 mg/kg/dose IV over 1 minute with onset of action expected in 2 minutes.[99]

INTUBATION PROCEDURE

ETT placement must be immediately verified by auscultation and confirmed by a chest x-ray examination; ultrasound imaging may also be used for secondary confirmation. **Findings on auscultation and what they suggest are listed in the Critical Findings box above. End-tidal carbon dioxide ($ETco_2$) detectors are available to immediately verify tube placement** and have been tested in the delivery room and NICU.[18] In the presence of exhaled CO_2 (after six breaths), the $ETco_2$ detector changes color from purple to yellow. The time necessary to detect proper ETT placement with these detectors is 4 to 12 seconds versus 0 to 90 seconds by clinical evaluation. This significantly faster time enables quicker extubation and reintubation if the ETT is in the esophagus.[18] **Use of $ETco_2$ detection devices to confirm proper ETT placement is suggested by the American Academy of Pediatrics (AAP) in the Neonatal Resuscitation Program (NRP) Guidelines.**[190] This device also is useful for ongoing assessment of ETT placement.[100] Other available devices are capnometry, with a numeric display, and capnography, with both a numeric and waveform display (see Chapter 7).[100]

Critical Findings

CHEST AUSCULTATION FOR ENDOTRACHEAL TUBE PLACEMENT

FINDING	CAUSE
No air entry bilaterally	Esophagus intubated; air leak
Air entry over left upper abdominal quadrant	Esophagus intubated; air entry heard over stomach
Diminished air entry	Endotracheal tube too high; air leak
Air entry unequal; right chest better aerated than left chest	Endotracheal tube too low; down right mainstem bronchus

For long-term stability, commercially available ETT anchors prevent accidental extubation. Some nurseries still prefer fixing tubes with tape or sutures.

EXTUBATION PROCEDURE

Assess the infant's condition by observing the heart rate, color, and respiratory rate and effort and by auscultating the chest. If the infant's condition is stable, proceed with extubation. Extubate before feeding or empty the stomach to prevent vomiting. Because neonates are obligatory nasal breathers, the nasopharynx also must be suctioned and patent for extubation.

Hyperinflate with deep breaths with the infant's head in the midline and remove the tube (1) on inflation (to provide adequate lung expansion and prevent atelectasis), (2) on expiration[146] (so that secretions that have accumulated around the tracheal tube are "blown away" on exhalation and tube removal), or (3) while suctioning (to remove secretions that have accumulated around the tube). Place the neonate in a warm, humidified oxygen hood at FIO_2 to keep pulse oximeter at 92% to 94%.

Reassess the infant's condition, especially for signs of increased work of breathing and distress. Document tube removal and the infant's tolerance. Check arterial blood gases 15 to 20 minutes after extubation to assess oxygenation and ventilation status. Perform a chest x-ray examination to document atelectasis or fully expanded lungs. Observe for complications of intubation (Table 23-4).

MECHANICAL VENTILATION

Mechanical ventilation is used in neonates to correct abnormalities in oxygenation ($\downarrow Pao_2$), alveolar ventilation ($\uparrow Paco_2$), or respiratory effort (apnea,

TABLE 23-4 COMPLICATIONS OF ENDOTRACHEAL INTUBATION

COMPLICATIONS	COMMENTS
IMMEDIATE	
Malposition	
Too low	Usually in right mainstem bronchus; no or diminished breath sounds in left chest or upper right lobe; asymmetric chest movement; atelectasis (withdraw tube until breath sounds are heard bilaterally and equally).
Too high	Inadequate ventilation bilaterally; especially at lung bases.
Esophageal	Air movement auscultated in stomach with no or inadequate breath sounds.
Obstruction	
Plug	Partial—no change or diminished breath sounds audible. Complete—distant or no breath sounds audible.
Kinking of the tube	
Head position	Flexion or extension of the head results in diminished or blocked airflow.
Perforation	
Vocal cords	
Trachea	
Pharynx	
Esophagus/gastric	
Pulmonary hemorrhage	
Infection	Colonization in the neonatal airway increases with the duration of intubation; presence of ETT longer than 72 hours is associated with colonization; this biofilm may contribute to the chondritis that precedes subglottic stenosis; MRSA tracheal infection causes subglottic stenosis.[406] Late-onset sepsis is more common in VLBW infants with prolonged ventilation[353]; mechanical ventilation is a risk factor for nosocomial infection.[192]
Air leak	ETT displacement (e.g., into the right mainstem bronchus or to the level of the carina) is a major factor in the development of air leaks.[267]
Increased intracranial pressure	Suctioning increases mean BP, which increases cerebral blood flow velocity and intracranial pressure, which increases the risk for IVH/PVL (see Box 23-2).
Post-extubation	
Migratory lobar collapse	Prevent and treat with pulmonary hygiene.
Diffuse microatelectasis	In VLBW infants may be associated with apnea; treatable by pulmonary hygiene or nasal CPAP, or both.
LONG-TERM	
General	Vocal cord inflammation, stenosis, and eventual dysfunction; tracheobronchial fistula; subglottic stenosis; tracheal inflammation and stenosis; necrotizing tracheobronchitis; contributes to CLD/BPD.
Specific to the type of tube	
Orotracheal	Abnormal dentition; gingival and palatal erosion; palatal grooves.
Nasotracheal	Otitis media; erosion of alae nasi and nasal septum; nasal stenosis.

BP, Blood pressure; *CLD/BPD,* chronic lung disease/bronchopulmonary dysplasia; *CPAP,* continuous positive airway pressure; *ETT,* endotracheal tube; *IVH,* intraventricular hemorrhage; *MRSA,* methicillin-resistant *Staphylococcus aureus; PVL,* periventricular leukomalacia; *VLBW,* very-low-birth-weight.

Critical Findings

CRITERIA THAT QUALIFY NEWBORNS FOR ASSISTED VENTILATION

Blood Gases

- Severe hypoxemia (Pao_2 <50-60 mm Hg with Fio_2 ≥0.60 or Pao_2 <60 mm Hg with Fio_2 >0.40 in infant weighing <1250 g)
- Severe hypercapnia ($Paco_2$ >55-65 mm Hg with pH <7.20-7.25)

Clinical

- Apnea and bradycardia requiring resuscitation in infants with lung disease or unresponsive to CPAP or requiring theophylline therapy in preterm infants with normal lungs
- Inefficient respiratory effort, such as gasping respirations from asphyxia, narcosis, or primary cardiopulmonary disease
- Shock and asphyxia with hypoperfusion and hypotension
- RDS in infants weighing <1000 g, frequently making them incapable of maintaining ventilation

CPAP, Continuous positive airway pressure; *RDS,* respiratory distress syndrome.

ineffectual respirations, or increased work of breathing). It may not be used to treat the primary disease but frequently is used to support the infant until the disease is treated or resolved (see the Critical Findings box above.

Ventilator Settings. To individualize assisted ventilation, knowledge of the ventilator capabilities is essential.

Intermittent Mandatory Ventilation. Most mechanical ventilators in common use today allow for intermittent mandatory ventilation (IMV). **IMV provides a continuous flow of gas that is available to the infant during spontaneous respirations. Periodic occlusion of the system diverts gas under pressure to the infant.** Because IMV provides for spontaneous and mechanical ventilation, only the amount of ventilatory assistance that is needed by the individual infant is provided.

Continuous Distending Pressure. CDP is expressed in centimeters of water. CDP may be given without IMV (CPAP) or with it (PEEP). The effects of CDP include increased alveolar stability, increased functional residual capacity, decreased risk for atelectasis, increased intrathoracic pressure, and impeded passage of fluid from lung capillaries to alveolar spaces, aiding in the prevention or treatment of pulmonary edema. Effects of changes in PEEP depend on severity of lung disease and degree of lung inflation. High PEEP in the presence of relatively compliant lungs will cause overdistention, worsen Pao_2, and increase pulmonary vascular resistance. In addition, overdistention may increase the risk for barotrauma. However, the use of levels of PEEP that are too low contributes to hypoxia and pulmonary hypertension because of low lung volumes. Acute lung injury is actually worsened by the failure to recruit adequate lung volume by using insufficient PEEP.

Peak Inspiratory Pressure. Peak inspiratory pressure (PIP) is the maximum pressure measured during the delivery of gas (inspiration) during conventional mechanical ventilation. PIP reflects the effects of the amount of gas delivered to the lungs in a given breath (tidal volume: 4-6 mL/kg in preterms; 8-10 mL/kg in term infants) and the underlying mechanical properties of the lungs. For example, if the same PIP is used in neonates with severe RDS (with stiff, noncompliant lungs) as in neonates ventilated for apnea with minimal lung disease, the tidal volume will be much greater in the latter group. Recent studies suggest that **overdistention of the lungs caused by excessive tidal volumes, and not pressure itself, worsens acute lung injury (so-called *volutrauma*).** Thus adverse effects of high PIP depend on the degree of lung disease.

When questioning whether PIP or PEEP is more likely to cause air leaks, the answer is PIP. Both PIP and PEEP cause air leak if they are excessive and is influenced by the lung compliance of the infant. Evidence strongly suggests that lung injury results from excessive tidal volume (excessive PIP).[252] It would be difficult to overexpand the lungs with PEEP to the point of air leak. Too little PEEP is far more often the cause of air leak.[193]

Rate. The rate reflects how often a volume of gas in the system is delivered to the infant. It is expressed as breaths per minute. Too rapid a rate, especially with a poorly inflated lung, can cause lung injury caused by gas trapping ("inadvertent PEEP").

Inspiratory/Expiratory Ratio. The inspiration/expiration ratio (I/E ratio) reflects the relationship between time spent in inspiration and time spent in expiration. When the rate is 60 breaths/min and the total respiratory cycle is 1 second, an I/E ratio of

1:1 means 0.5 second is inspiration and 0.5 second is expiration. If the I/E ratio is 1:2 with a rate of 60 and the total respiratory cycle is 1 second, inspiration is 0.33 second and expiration is 0.66 second.

Prolonged inspiration may be associated with more efficient ventilation, optimal arterial oxygenation, a higher risk for air leak, and impeding venous return. Prolonged expiration also improves oxygenation, especially in air-trapping conditions (e.g., rapid-rate ventilation or airway disease).[47]

Mean Airway Pressure. **Mean airway pressure (MAP) is the amount of pressure transmitted to the airway throughout an entire respiratory cycle.**[47] Any change in ventilator settings affects the MAP. MAP is most affected by changes in PEEP, inspiratory time, or I/E ratio.[47] MAP is associated with optimal oxygenation (↑$Pa{O_2}$) and ventilation (↓$Pa{CO_2}$) when pressures range between 6 and 14 cm of water.[47] When MAP exceeds 14 cm of water, there is a progressive deterioration of the blood gases (↓$Pa{O_2}$, ↑$Pa{CO_2}$).[47] The effects of any given level of MAP depend on the changes in mechanical properties of the lung caused by the primary disease. For example, high MAP may be needed to improve oxygenation in severe RDS or meconium aspiration syndrome, especially in term neonates. Low MAP in this setting causes sustained hypoxemia and atelectasis. In contrast, use of high MAP in neonates in the presence of minimal lung disease causes overdistention and deterioration of arterial blood gas tensions. In general, the goal of increasing MAP is to improve $Pa{O_2}$ and usually is achieved by small increases in PEEP or prolongation of inspiratory time. Repeat chest x-ray examination and continuous monitoring of blood pressure and oxygenation (by pulse oximeter) help determine the optimal level of MAP.

Usual starting pressures for beginning ventilatory support are listed in Table 23-5. The inspired oxygen tension is adjusted to provide an adequate arterial oxygen tension. If the infant still has difficulty maintaining an adequate carbon dioxide tension, a faster rate or greater inspiratory pressure would be indicated. **Table 23-6 lists the usual effects to be expected from changing specific ventilator settings.**

To evaluate the efficacy of mechanical ventilation and any adjustments made with the system, continuous monitoring with pulse oximeters (see Chapter 8) must be maintained or blood gases obtained. During the acute phase of illness, blood gases should be obtained 15 to 30 minutes after beginning ventilatory support or after any change in settings, every 4 to 6 hours if no change is made in ventilator settings, and as needed based on the clinical condition of the infant.

TABLE 23-5 STARTING PRESSURES FOR BEGINNING VENTILATORY SUPPORT

PARAMETER	RANGE
$F{IO_2}$	At previous level or 10% higher than previously required concentration
PEEP	4-6 cm water
PIP	16-20 cm water
Rate	40-60
I/E ratio	1:1-1:2

I/E, Inspiration to expiration; *PEEP,* Positive end-expiratory pressure; *PIP,* peak inspiratory pressure.

Arterial blood gases should be maintained in the following range (see Chapter 8):

$Pa{O_2}$	**60 to 80 mm Hg**
$Pa{CO_2}$	**35 to 45 mm Hg**
pH	**7.35 to 7.45**

Optimal arterial blood gas tensions are somewhat controversial. To decrease the risk for acute lung injury by minimizing lung overdistention and barotrauma, some investigators advocate strategies that **target lower $Pa{O_2}$ and higher $Pa{CO_2}$ ("permissive hypercapnia").**[234,364] The risks and benefits of such strategies depend on the specific clinical setting. If excessive ventilator settings are necessary to lower $Pa{CO_2}$, allowing $Pa{CO_2}$ to rise (to 50 to 60 mm Hg) (as long as the pH is greater than 7.25) often is accepted in an attempt to avoid lung injury. In addition, because the goal of respiratory care is to optimize oxygen delivery to tissues, the effect of a given $Pa{O_2}$ depends partly on cardiac function (see Chapter 24) and hemoglobin level (see Chapter 20). Accepting lower $Pa{O_2}$ and O_2 saturation may lead to worse outcomes in the setting of systemic hypotension and poor cardiac function (e.g., sepsis).

Recognizing that aggressive ventilator management (e.g., intubation, high PIP, high MAP) is associated with increased lung injury and CLD/BPD,

TABLE 23-6 USUAL EFFECTS OF CHANGING CONVENTIONAL MECHANICAL VENTILATOR SETTINGS

	CAUSES			
INCREASING	PaO_2	$PaCO_2$	pH	COMPLICATIONS
FIO_2	↑	0	0	Oxygen toxicity (CLD/BPD, ROP); absorption atelectasis; FIO_2 may have no effect on oxygenation in the presence of severe R→L (right to left) shunt (PPHN), congenital heart disease, or marked intrapulmonary shunting as a result of severe parenchymal lung disease
CPAP/PEEP	↑	0/↑	0/↓	Hypoventilation with respiratory acidosis; decreased cardiac output with metabolic acidosis; air leaks
PIP	↑	↓	↑	Barotrauma with air leaks and CLD/BPD; respiratory alkalosis
Rate	↓	↓	↑	Respiratory alkalosis
I/E ratio (1:1-1:2)	↑	0	0	Increased intrapleural pressure; decreased venous return

CLD/BPD, Chronic lung disease/bronchopulmonary dysplasia; *CPAP,* continuous positive airway pressure; *I/E ratio,* Inspiration to expiration ratio; *PEEP,* positive end-expiratory pressure; *PIP,* peak inspiratory pressure; *PPHN,* persistent pulmonary hypertension of the newborn; *ROP,* retinopathy of prematurity.

gentler ventilator techniques and management have been developed and are being used.[229,252] Many gentler strategies incorporate relinquishment of traditional ventilator controls (from the health care provider) to patient control of ventilator parameters. Facilitated by computer-assisted technology, newer types of ventilators are being used. Volume-targeted versus pressure-limited ventilation results in significant reductions in duration of ventilation, rates of pneumothorax, and rates of severe IVH (grades 3 and 4) but no significant difference in the rates of CLD/BPD or death.[238]

Patient-Triggered Ventilation. Asynchrony between the infant's respiratory efforts and the ventilator is uncomfortable for the neonate and causes increased barotrauma, which contributes to lung injury (e.g., CLD/BPD).[252] Altered cerebral blood flow may contribute to IVH. **Patient-ventilator synchrony occurs when patient-triggered ventilation (PTV) responds to the neonate's signal representing spontaneous respiratory effort and delivers a mechanical breath, timed to the onset of inspiration.** PTV has been demonstrated to do the following[105,339]:

- Decrease asynchrony
- Improve gaseous exchange (e.g., oxygenation and carbon dioxide elimination)
- Create respiratory support that is more synergistic with the neonate's respiratory efforts
- Increase comfort for the infant, thus reducing the need for use of sedatives, narcotics, and paralyzing medications
- Decrease the need for ventilatory support

Studies comparing PTV with conventional mechanical ventilation (CMV) have found no proven decrease in the following[31,38]:

- Incidence and severity of CLD/BPD
- Mortality
- Head ultrasound abnormalities

These studies did show an increased rate of pneumothorax, worsening arterial blood gas values, more frequent desaturations, and increased need for increased ventilatory support.[31,38]

Modes of PTV include the following:

- Synchronized intermittent mandatory ventilation (SIMV)
- Assist-control ventilation (ACV)—oxygenation, volume guarantee ventilation (VGV), and minute ventilation (V_{min})
- Pressure-support ventilation (PSV)
- Pressure-regulated volume control (PRVC)
- Proportional assist ventilation (PAV)

Synchronized Intermittent Mandatory Ventilation. SIMV, a commonly used form of PTV, delivers mechanical breaths at a fixed rate.[308] SIMV enables

synchronization of ventilation breaths by sensing (through an airway or diaphragmatic sensor) the neonate's initiation of respiration and then triggering a mechanical breath. Synchronized ventilation prevents the generation of excessive pressure within the respiratory tract when infant exhalation coincides with mechanical ventilation. Use of SIMV is associated with a decrease in (1) oxygen need, (2) duration of ventilator therapy, (3) incidence of BPD, and (4) severity of IVH and is more comfortable for the infant.[39,143,308,339] Use of SIMV is also associated with fewer episodes of hypoxia and better oxygenation as a result improved ventilation-perfusion and increased resting lung volume (functional residual capacity [FRC]) when compared with IMV ventilation of VLBW infants.[126]

Assist-Control Ventilation. Newer neonatal ventilators are equipped with computer technology with rapid digital feedback circuits. Computer-assisted control enables adjustments of FIO_2, PIP to control tidal volume, and ventilatory rate to control minute ventilation. ACV is used in preterms with RDS, infants with a strong respiratory drive, and infants who are not heavily sedated. ACV is also more comfortable for the infant but may result in difficulty weaning from the ventilator because of diaphragmatic muscle atrophy.[339] Small studies have reported that computer-assisted maintenance of target oxygen saturation is as effective as manual FIO_2 adjustments. Larger RCTs on safety and efficacy are warranted.

In volume-guarantee ventilation, a preset target tidal volume is maintained by the ventilator because the pressure limit varies inversely with lung compliance and the neonate's respiratory effort. In preliminary studies, VLBW infants had lower MAP on volume-guarantee when compared with VLBW infants treated with SIMV.[62,168] Less ventilator support for the VLBW infant was necessary, because volume-guarantee enables an increase in the infant's respiratory effort while guaranteeing a physiologic tidal volume (about 4 to 5 mL/kg) in contrast to SIMV, which delivers a constant PIP regardless of tidal volume delivered.[168] Use of SIMV with volume-guarantee results in automatic weaning from mechanical support, enhances spontaneous respiratory effort, and maintains gaseous exchange similar to conventional SIMV.[168] Other small studies of volume-guarantee show (1) minimal changes in cardiovascular and lung function, cerebral hemodynamics, and oxygenation, (2) shortened duration and severity of hypoxemic episodes,[292] and (3) accelerated recovery from forced exhalation episodes.[194] Larger RCTs are necessary.[168]

Minute ventilation (i.e., the volume of gas moving in and out of the lungs over time, expressed in milliliters per kilogram per minute) is a successful predictor of readiness to wean, extubate, and establish optimal pulmonary mechanics.[137] Mandatory minute ventilation (MMV), a new ventilator mode in the NICU, provides mechanically generated breaths only if the neonate's spontaneous breathing does not meet a minimum level of minute ventilation (chosen by the health care provider). If the infant's spontaneous pressure-supported breaths exceed the minimum minute ventilation, no additional breaths are delivered by the ventilator. If the infant fails to meet the specified minute ventilation, intermittent mandatory breaths are delivered at the preset tidal volume. MMV enables the infant to control the rate, flow, and inspiratory time of the ventilator, which enhances synchrony and ensures a "backup" system to assume the work of breathing if the infant cannot maintain adequate minute ventilation.[151]

Pressure-Support Ventilation. **PSV complements the infant's respiratory effort by triggering a mechanical breath, preset to a specific pressure.** PSV decreases the work of breathing created by airway resistance (e.g., narrowed diameter of neonatal ETT) and ventilator circuit resistance. PSV also decreases work of breathing by assisting the activity of the infant's respiratory muscles. PSV is used alone (if the infant has effective respiratory drive) or in conjunction with SIMV. PSV is useful in chronic and acute situations, as well as weaning chronically ventilator-dependent infants. When PSV was compared with SIMV, preterms exhibited better respiratory function (e.g., lower respiratory rates and less work of breathing), so PSV is effective for fatigued or weaning infants.[246] Another study comparing two levels of PSV with SIMV found that PSV increased total minute ventilation, stabilized breathing for preterms less than 32 weeks' gestation, and may be a useful strategy to wean preterms from mechanical ventilation.[149]

Pressure-Regulated Volume Control. PRVC delivers four breaths and modifies the ventilator's pressure to attain the prescribed tidal volume; breaths are both volume and pressure regulated.[339] Studies show conflicting results: (1) safe and a lower incidence of air leaks and IVH[289] and (2) no benefit when compared with SIMV in the treatment of RDS in preterm infants.[90]

Proportional-Assist Ventilation. **In PAV, ventilator pressure increases in proportion to inspiratory volume (e.g., inspiratory flow varies to match the neonate's respiratory effort).** Both volume and flow proportional assist relieve the neonate of both elastic (e.g., respiratory muscles) and resistive work of breathing. During PAV, the infant's breathing completely controls all variables of the ventilator breathing pattern through exceptionally fast computer-controlled feedback circuitry. In the initial trial using PAV in infants, lower MAP and transpulmonary pressure were used to effectively oxygenate and ventilate infants with mild to moderate respiratory insufficiency.[321] Respiratory rates were 50 to 80/min with a fast and shallow pattern and tidal volumes less than 5 mL/kg. A more recent RCT comparing PAV and PTV in ELBW preterms found that PAV safely maintained gaseous exchange at lower MAP when compared with PTV. Although there were no adverse effects, the researchers concluded that backup conventional ventilation breaths must be provided during PAV to prevent apnea-related oxygen desaturations.[322]

High-Frequency Ventilation. Barotrauma/volutrauma is a major contributing factor to the development of chronic lung disease or death from progressive lung injury in newborns treated with conventional mechanical ventilation. **The goal of HFV is to reduce barotrauma by the application of HFV early in the course of RDS or to reduce the progression of injury in infants who already have pulmonary interstitial emphysema, recurrent pneumothorax, or bronchopleural fistula.** In addition to minimizing lung injury, the goal of HFV is to effectively enhance oxygenation over conventional ventilation.

HFV differs from conventional modes of ventilator support, using smaller tidal volumes (less than anatomic dead space) at supraphysiologic frequencies and allowing for generation of lower intrathoracic pressure. At high frequencies, the calculated tidal volume is less than dead space. Thus the physics of gas flow and exchange are different from the traditional teaching of lung mechanics and are related to augmented diffusion. Reduction in barotrauma occurs by allowing for ventilation with very small pressure amplitude around the mean airway pressure in the distal airway. Therefore at high frequencies (commonly 10 to 15 Hz), the peak inspiratory and expiratory pressures approach MAP (i.e., lower downstream pressures). Because of this effect, higher MAP can be used to improve oxygenation without worsening lung injury.

HFV can be achieved by jet ventilators, oscillators, or high-frequency flow interrupters. The only U.S. Food and Drug Administration–approved device for jet ventilations is the Bunnell Life Pulse High Frequency Jet Ventilator (HFJV). Jet ventilators and HFV deliver short bursts of high-flow gases directly into the proximal airway via a small cannula and have a passive exhalation cycle. This ventilatory mode usually is augmented with a back-up rate by a conventional ventilator that gives sigh breaths. The frequency range of the HFJV is 240 to 660 breaths/min (4 to 11 Hz).[105] Early use of HFJV results in (1) decreased incidence of CLD/BPD and neurologic injury,[195] (2) reduction of pulmonary interstitial emphysema without producing a higher incidence of CLD,[105] (3) no significant difference in overall mortality, and (4) no significant increase in adverse effects (e.g., IVH, air leaks, necrotizing tracheobronchitis).[185]

Oscillators vibrate columns of air and have active exhalation cycles. The usual frequency is 600 to 900 breaths/min (10 to 15 Hz). Oscillators (high-frequency oscillatory ventilation [HFOV]) are used both as a rescue therapy when CMV is unsuccessful and electively as a primary mode of ventilation. The HFOV ventilator most commonly used is the SensorMedics 3100A, which uses a piston with a diaphragm to actively move gas into and out of the lung. Early elective use of HFOV (compared with CMV) results in the following:

- Decrease in mortality[161]
- Decrease in surfactant replacement requirements[250]
- Decrease in days on oxygen and ventilation[84]
- Significant decrease in the risk for severe air leak
- Decrease in the incidence of CLD/BPD[84,195]
- No increase in the risk for periventricular leukomalacia (PVL),[84,195] NEC, ROP, hearing loss, or sepsis[84]
- No association with an increase in IVH rate in preterm infants[84]

Studies have also shown HFOV to (1) fail to decrease the incidence of CLD/BPD, (2) have a similar incidence of air leak,[84] (3) be associated with an increased incidence of severe (grade III or higher) IVH,[170,250] and (4) result in better neuromotor outcomes.[374] When HFOV was compared with PSV plus volume guarantee (VG), early use of HFOV treatment was associated with a reduction in lung inflammation in preterms less than 30 weeks' gestation[92]; another study found VG to result in lower inflammation markers than HFOV.[227] Discordance in study findings may be attributed to (1) maturity/immaturity of preterm infants, (2) time to initiation of HFOV, (3) use of antenatal steroids, (4) use of surfactant replacement, (5) differences in techniques used (e.g., presence or absence of lung volume recruitment strategy), (6) level of MAP, (7) duration of use, and (8) variations in cerebral blood flow (CBF) secondary to changes in Pco_2.[250] Some researchers recommend that CMV be the first choice in treatment of preterm infants with RDS and HFOV be reserved for rescue therapy if CMV is unsuccessful.[250] Further research is needed to clarify which ventilator should be used initially.

Remember that the rate of carbon dioxide removal is determined by minute ventilation. **Minute ventilation is the product of tidal volume and respiratory rate** (TV × RR). In CMV, the tidal volume and rate can both be adjusted by increasing or decreasing the breaths per minute (rate) and by increasing or decreasing the PIP or PEEP for tidal volume (TV = PIP − PEEP). In HFV, the same minute ventilation equation holds true but the rate is set by breaths/min (hertz) and the tidal volume is determined by the amplitude (Box 23-3).

In HFOV, tidal volume is adjusted primarily by changing the amplitude setting. Amplitude is the amount of pressure oscillation that occurs around the MAP. **Increasing the amplitude will increase the tidal volume and therefore decrease Pco_2.** Conversely, decreasing the amplitude will decrease the tidal volume and therefore increase the Pco_2. Amplitude is initially set when chest rise is adequate and then slowly adjusted up or down in increments of one or two.

The respiratory rate in HFV is determined by the hertz setting. One hertz equals 60 breaths per minute. Therefore 10 Hertz equals 600 breaths/min. The rate is initially set between 10 and 15 Hz. There is a paradoxic effect of high-frequency breaths in the bronchi of the lungs so that when the hertz setting is increased, the Pco_2 increases. The opposite is also true. Whereas HFOV has an active expiration phase, HFJV has a passive expiration phase and therefore uses a low CMV back-up rate to deliver intermittent sigh breaths to prevent air trapping and augment Pco_2 removal.

Oxygenation in CMV and HFV is determined by the Fio_2 and the MAP. With use of HFOV in the rescue mode, the MAP is initially set 1 to 2 cm H_2O above the previous CMV setting. Chest x-ray studies are helpful in determining optimal lung volume. **As lung compliance improves, and it can improve quite rapidly after surfactant administration, there is a risk for overinflating the lungs with too much MAP.** This increase in MAP leads to an increase in intrathoracic pressure that may result in air leaks or IVH or may impede venous return, which can in turn lead to hypotension. MAP is generally slowly increased or decreased in increments of one or two. Chest x-ray studies, blood gases, and blood pressure should be monitored closely during HFV.

Adjustments for oxygenation (MAP, Fio_2) and ventilation (Amplitude, Hz) can be made independently and therefore can be done simultaneously. (See the Critical Findings box on p. 606.) A Cochrane Review in 2007 demonstrated that HFOV had no significant effect on death in the studies that were reviewed and was associated with only a small reduction in chronic lung disease.[161]

Synchronized mechanical ventilation, delivered as high frequency positive pressure ventilation (HFPPV), is another mode of oxygenation and ventilation in which positive airway pressure and spontaneous inspiration occur simultaneously. Adequate gas exchange should be achievable at lower peak airway pressures. HFPPV results in a reduction of air leaks and ventilator duration.[143]

BOX 23-3 MINUTE VENTILATION (V_{min})

CV: $V_{min} = TV \times RR$

HFOV*: $V_{min} = fx\ (\text{Amplitude, } Hz^{-1})$

Data from Donn SM, Sinha S: Invasive and noninvasive neonatal mechanical ventilation. *Respir Care* 48(4):426, 2003; Tarczy-Hornoch P, Mayock DE, Jones D, et al: Mechanical ventilators. Revised July 2008. Accessed October 3, 2009, from http://neonatal.peds.washington.edu/NICU-WEB/vents.

CV, Conventional ventilation; *HFOV,* high-frequency oscillating ventilation; *Hz,* hertz; *RR,* respiratory rate; *TV,* tidal volume (PIP-PEEP).

*There is a paradoxic effect with HFOV in which an increase in the frequency (Hz) actually decreases ventilation and therefore increases Pco_2. Conversely, decreasing Hz increases ventilation and decreases Pco_2.

Critical Findings

COMPARISON OF VENTILATOR OPTIONS

	LOW O_2	HIGH O_2	LOW CO_2	HIGH CO_2
CMV/SIMV	Increase PEEP Increase PIP Increase FIO_2	Wean PIP Wean PEEP Wean FIO_2	Decrease rate Decrease TV	Increase rate Increase TV
HFOV	Increase MAP Increase FIO_2	Decrease MAP Decrease FIO_2	Decrease Amp Increase Hz	Increase Amp Decrease Hz
HFJV	Increase MAP Increase FIO_2 Adjust CMV back-up IMV breaths →	Decrease MAP Decrease FIO_2	Decrease Amp Increase Hz	Increase Amp Decrease Hz

Data from Donn SM, Sinha S: Invasive and noninvasive neonatal mechanical ventilation. Respir Care 48(4):426, 2003; Tarczy-Hornoch P, Mayock DE, Jones D, et al: Mechanical ventilators. Revised July 2008. Accessed October 3, 2009, from *http://neonatal.peds.washington.edu/NICU-WEB/vents.*

Amp, Amplitude; *CMV,* conventional mechanical ventilation; *Hz,* hertz; *HFJV,* high-frequency jet ventilation; *HFOV,* high-frequency oscillatory ventilation; *IMV,* intermittent mandatory ventilation; *MAP,* mean airway pressure; *PEEP,* positive end expiratory pressure; *PIP,* peak inspiratory pressure; *SIMV,* synchronized intermittent mandatory ventilation; *TV,* tidal volume.

Inhaled Nitric Oxide. Vascular endothelial cells endogenously produce a potent vasodilator substance ("endothelium-derived relaxing factor"), later identified as nitric oxide. **Nitric oxide (NO), delivered as a gas, causes potent, selective, and sustained pulmonary vasodilation in the perinatal pulmonary circulation.**[200] The vasodilator response occurs as a result of inhaled nitric oxide (iNO) stimulation of soluble guanylate cyclase activity, increasing cyclic guanosine monophosphate (cGMP) in vascular smooth muscle and causing vasorelaxation. Selectivity of iNO for the pulmonary circulation is based on direct delivery of NO into the lung; because NO is avidly bound by hemoglobin in red blood cells and inactivated after metabolism to nitrite and nitrate, there are no direct effects on systemic arterial pressure.[200] Potential toxicities include decreased platelet aggregation, hemorrhage, and methemoglobinemia.

Inhaled NO has been approved by the FDA for treatment for late preterm (>34 weeks GA) and term neonates with persistent pulmonary hypertension of the newborn (PPHN).[200] **(See "Persistent Pulmonary Hypertension of the Newborn" section.) Use of iNO in preterm infants (<34 weeks GA) remains investigational.**[200] **(See "Respiratory Distress Syndrome" section.)**

Extracorporeal Membrane Oxygenation/Extracorporeal Life Support. Extracorporeal membrane oxygenation/extracorporeal life support (ECMO/ECLS) is a modification of cardiopulmonary bypass that allows more prolonged therapy that is traditionally performed in the operating room for cardiac surgery.[376] **ECMO/ECLS establishes a pulmonary bypass circuit, allowing gas exchange to occur outside of the lung by perfusion of blood through a membrane oxygenator.** Blood is drawn from a catheter in the right internal jugular vein or right atrium, oxygenated as it crosses the membrane, and then returned to the patient via the right common carotid artery (venoarterial ECMO/ECLS) or the femoral vein (venovenous ECMO/ECLS). The pump produces a continuous, nonpulsatile flow through the membrane oxygenator as the patient is kept heparinized and continues to be ventilated at low pressures, rates, and oxygen tensions. **The goal of this therapy is to "buy time" for the severely injured lung to heal while attenuating ongoing lung injury by decreasing exposure to hyperoxia and barotrauma.** Therapy can be continued for several days, until lung recovery appears sufficient to maintain adequate gas tension without ECMO/ECLS.

ECMO/ ECLS therapy improves survival in term neonates with severe hypoxemic respiratory failure and PPHN. **ECMO/ECLS is used as a treatment of last option when neonates are unresponsive to maximum conventional support.**[300] ECMO/ ECLS criteria include the following[121,300]:

- Gestational age 34 weeks or older, weight 2000 g or more
- No more than 7 to 10 days of assisted ventilation
- Reversible lung disease
- No CNS or multisystem disease, no lethal congenital anomalies
- No intracranial hemorrhage above grade I or uncorrectable coagulopathy
- No cardiac disease (unless ECMO/ECLS is to be used for the preoperative/postoperative period for cardiac surgery)
- No severe asphyxia
- Failure of maximal medical management
- A ventilatory index (MAP × Rate) of 1500 or above or an oxygenation index (MAP × FIO_2 × 100/PaO_2) of 40 or more

Use of ECMO/ECLS for severe respiratory failure is beneficial in improving survival rates, especially in congenital diaphragmatic hernia, without increasing the risk for severe disability.[258] **Conditions treated with ECMO/ECLS and their survival rates are listed in Table 23-7.**

In the past decade, the number of neonates being treated with ECMO/ECLS has declined by 50%.[276,300] Because ECMO/ECLS is invasive, labor intensive, and costly and involves risks associated with systemic anticoagulation (e.g., intracranial hemorrhage), alternative therapies (e.g., surfactant replacement, iNO, and HFV) are used initially and have reduced the need for ECMO.[300] These therapies have changed the population being treated with ECMO/ECLS, shortened length of stay, reduced costs, and raised concerns in delay of use of ECMO/ECLS.[300] A recent study from the United Kingdom showed poor respiratory outcomes for infants older than 2 weeks when ECMO/ECLS was started and for infants needing ECMO/ECLS for respiratory distress syndrome.[32] Considerable variability exists between centers, however, suggesting that the use of these techniques depends partly on the clinical strategy and other issues in patient management.

Complications of ECMO/ECLS depend on initial disease process, pre–ECMO/ECLS factors (e.g., asphyxia, coagulopathy, hypoventilation, hyperventilation), and type of ECMO/ECLS used (e.g., venoarterial vs. venovenous).[300] The most common complications are hemorrhagic (e.g., intracranial [incidence 4.6%; survival 50%]) and non-hemorrhagic (e.g., infarctions [incidence 10.7%; survival 50%]) CNS insults. Neonates who develop intracranial hemorrhage are at highest risk for mortality and poor neurodevelopmental outcomes. Recent follow-up studies showed abnormalities in (baseline and after exercise) pulmonary function representing lung injury lasting into childhood that was correlated with the duration of oxygen use after ECMO decannulation[48] and prolonged use of supplemental oxygen and duration of tube feedings.[128]

TABLE 23-7 CONDITIONS TREATED WITH EXTRACORPOREAL MEMBRANE OXYGENATION/EXTRACORPOREAL LIFE SUPPORT

TYPE/CONDITION	PERCENTAGE SURVIVAL
Meconium aspiration syndrome	94
Congenital diaphragmatic hernia	51
Respiratory distress syndrome	84
Sepsis/pneumonia	73
Persistent pulmonary hypertension of the newborn	78
Air leak syndromes	74
Others	64

Data from Extra Corporeal Life Support Organization registry reports at http://neonatal.peds.washington.edu/NICU-WEB/ecmo2.stm and http://www.med.umich.edu/ecmo/referrals.htm.

Partial Liquid Ventilation. Although prenatal administration of steroidal agents, use of surfactant, and HFOV therapies have improved the clinical course of sick preterm newborns with respiratory failure, the morbidity of severe RDS persists. Based on 40 years of experimental (animal) studies, perfluorocarbon (PFC) liquids have been found to improve gaseous exchange, lung mechanics, and cardiopulmonary stability in various respiratory diseases.[85,145] PFC liquids are suitable for liquid ventilation because of their high solubility of respiratory gases, easy elimination by evaporation from the lungs, and lack of metabolism by the body.[144] Instillation of an FRC of PFC liquid into the lungs during gaseous ventilation constitutes partial liquid ventilation (PLV). The best ventilator management during PLV has not been determined and may differ with underlying lung pathology.[144]

PLV is applicable to the surfactant and structurally deficient preterm lung because it reduces or eliminates surface tension forces, optimizes lung recruitment, and reexpands atelectatic lung. In a term infant, PLV is applicable to structural lung disease (e.g., diaphragmatic hernia) or lung disease associated with airway debris (e.g., aspiration syndromes or pneumonia). A nonrandomized, nonblinded clinical study of 13 preterm infants with severe RDS who failed to improve with CMV showed improved oxygenation within 1 hour of initiation of PLV.[218] A recent case report of partial liquid ventilation accompanying HFV showed improved gas exchange with a decrease in oxygenation index.[245] In infants with respiratory failure, a combination of PLV, iNO, and surfactant may produce optimal response. Currently the safety and efficacy of PLV are undergoing phase III trials in adults in the United States; trials are contemplated in infants and children in Europe.

WEANING FROM THE VENTILATOR

When the infant's condition improves, ventilatory support is slowly removed. **Evidence of improvement includes biochemical, clinical, and pulmonary function parameters as follows:**

- Arterial blood gases are stable and physiologic.
- Spontaneous respiratory efforts occur in addition to ventilator-generated respirations and if the infant is disconnected from the ventilator for suctioning.
- There is increased activity and muscle tone and progressively decreasing FIO_2 requirement.
- Pulmonary function studies (in LBW preterms with RDS) include (1) tidal volume values >6 mL/kg, (2) minute ventilation >309 mL/kg/min, (3) work of breathing <0.172 J/L, (4) dynamic compliance ≥1 mL/cm H_2O/kg, and (5) airway resistance ≤176 cm H_2O/L/sec.[358]

Weaning an infant as soon as possible from intubation and the ventilator is associated with a decrease in the complications of intubation (see Table 23-4) and the incidence of CLD/BPD resulting from barotrauma, volutrauma, and oxygen toxicity.[17] With IMV, there is a gradual decrease in mechanical ventilation with a corresponding increase in spontaneous respiration. **One ventilator setting at a time is changed, and arterial blood gases and pulse oximetry values are evaluated to determine the infant's response before another adjustment is made.** Because each ventilator parameter has risks and benefits, each parameter must be evaluated before the decision is made as to which one will be lowered. **Because high concentrations of oxygen are toxic to lungs and hyperoxia damages eyes, oxygen is usually lowered first to a level below 80% in 5% to 10% increments. PIP is lowered in 1- to 2-cm increments to a level of 16 to 18 cm of water, and respiratory rate is lowered in increments of 1 to 5 breaths/min until the infant has a rate of 15 to 20 breaths/min.**

Failure of extubation results in a reintubation rate of 25% to 40% in ELBW/VLBW infants.[349] **Nasal CPAP is effective in preventing extubation failure and decreasing CLD/BPD by preventing atelectasis, improving oxygenation, decreasing apnea/bradycardia, and improving thoracoabdominal motion synchrony, which indicates improved breathing strategy.**[196] Weaning an intubated neonate to ventilator CPAP increases the work of breathing associated with endotracheal tube resistance and dead space (e.g., breathing through a straw). A meta-analysis of three RCTs comparing use of ventilator CPAP with extubation to nasal CPAP showed a significant advantage (e.g., decreased the risk for reintubation and ventilation) for extubation to nasal CPAP, especially using nasal prongs.[96]

Extubation directly to nasal CPAP has also been shown to be more effective than extubation directly to supplemental oxygen in a hood. A meta-analysis of six RCTs comparing nasal CPAP (by any method) with use of an oxyhood after extubation found that nasal CPAP (1) decreases adverse clinical events (e.g., apnea, bradycardia, respiratory acidosis, hypoxia), (2) decreases the incidence of CLD/BPD, and (3) decreases the incidence of reintubation.[97] These positive effects increase when nasal prong CPAP is used, compared with nasopharyngeal CPAP, and the benefits are consistent across ranges of weight and gestational age.[97]

For weaning preterm infants from mechanical ventilation, prophylactic use of nasal CPAP (with nasal prongs) has been defined as the standard of care. However, variations in therapeutic methods and devices are associated with variations in outcomes. Although RCTs demonstrate a clear advantage of nasal prongs over nasopharyngeal administration, differences in design of nasal prongs may alter effectiveness. Use of binasal prongs is more effective than a single nasal prong in weaning ELBW infants from the ventilator.[102]

Various clinical strategies for initiation, management, and weaning of nasal CPAP are used. Use of nasal CPAP with the Aladdin/Infant Flow System (i.e., residual gas pressure is provided by the constant flow of gas) decreases the work of breathing by a more stable volume recruitment in the lungs and has been shown to facilitate extubation in VLBW infants compared with nasal pharyngeal CPAP.[83] Other studies show equal efficacy (e.g., no differences in apnea, bradycardia, or desaturation) when nasal prong CPAP is compared with nasal synchronized IMV[103] or nasal CPAP on a ventilator compared with the Infant Flow System.[349] A recent RCT comparison of bubble CPAP versus Infant Flow Driver CPAP for post-extubation support found that use of bubble CPAP reduced the mean duration of CPAP use by 50% and in preterms ventilated for 14 days or less, there was a higher rate of successful extubation.[150]

If nasal CPAP fails, the nasal route may also be used to administer mechanical ventilation, which augments the effectiveness of NCPAP, reduces the inspiratory work of breathing, improves rates of successful extubation, and is even being used as the initial method of respiratory support.[98] In two studies, both preterm infants (34 weeks GA) and VLBW preterm infants extubated to synchronized nasal intermittent positive-pressure ventilation (SNIPPV) had a significantly higher success rate at 72 hours after extubation when compared with an NCPAP group.[27,196] The first study of SNIPPV as the primary method of respiratory support compared the outcomes of 600- to 1250-gram preterms who were randomized to CMV or SNIPPV after their initial dose of surfactant.[41] Only 20% of the preterms receiving SNIPPV versus 52% receiving CMV had the primary outcome of BPD/CLD/death with no difference in the groups on mental/psychomotor indices.[41]

Once adequate oxygenation and ventilation on CPAP alone have been maintained, the infant may be placed in an oxygen hood. **Oxygen should be adjusted with the use of pulse oximetry.**

During the recovery phase of RDS (approximately 72 hours), changes in lung compliance occur rapidly. Hyperoxia, air leaks, increased intracranial pressure, and decreased cardiac output easily occur if high pressures and high oxygen concentrations are not decreased as rapidly as the lung is recovering.

Infants who are difficult or impossible to wean from the ventilator may have CLD/BPD, PDA, or CNS damage that affects the respiratory control center.

GENERAL COMPLICATIONS

Acute Complications

Acute and chronic complications are the result of the disease process, treatment, or both. Beginning with the least invasive therapy and progressing to more complicated ones only as needed accomplishes two goals: it individualizes therapy, and it minimizes the risk for complications. Continuous monitoring of the individual infant's progress is vital to decrease complications from the disease and from the interventions used to support the infant or treat the primary condition. **Complications of respiratory diseases are listed in Box 23-4.**

Sudden deterioration of the infant's condition is an emergency, and the cause must be found and corrected as soon as possible to minimize further damage. **Causes of sudden deterioration are listed in Box 23-5.**

RESPIRATORY

Management of an infant who has suddenly deteriorated begins with a visual inspection. The oxygen

BOX 23-4 COMPLICATIONS OF RESPIRATORY DISEASE

1. Acute
   a. Sudden deterioration of condition
   b. Air leaks
   c. Central nervous system
      Hypoxic-ischemic injury
      Increased intracranial pressure
      Hemorrhage
   d. Cardiac
      Patent ductus arteriosus
      Decreased cardiac output
   e. Infection
   f. Bleeding diathesis
   g. Tube
   h. Pulmonary hemorrhage
2. Chronic
   a. Oxygen toxicity and barotraumas (CLD/BPD)
   b. Hyperoxia (retinopathy of prematurity)
   c. Hypoxia
   d. Tube

CLD/BPD, Chronic lung disease/bronchopulmonary dysplasia.

BOX 23-5 CAUSES OF SUDDEN DETERIORATION

1. Tube
   a. Accidental extubation
   b. Accidental disconnection
   c. Plug
2. Machine malfunction
   a. Ventilator or continuous positive airway pressure device
   b. Oxygen blender
   c. Tubing and connections
3. Alarm system "off"
4. Severe hypoxia
5. Metabolic factors
6. Air leak
7. Intraventricular hemorrhage

TABLE 23-8 CHEST AUSCULTATION ABNORMALITIES AND UNDERLYING CAUSES

FINDING	POSSIBLE CAUSE
No air entry bilaterally	Air leak Plugged endotracheal tube
Diminished air entry	Air leak Endotracheal tube too high
Air entry over stomach	Unplanned extubation
Air entry unequal	Air leak Endotracheal tube too low
Cardiac point of maximum intensity shifted	Air leak with tension

hood, CPAP, or ventilator must be properly connected and free of water. If all connections are intact, the infant must be disconnected from assisted ventilation and connected to a resuscitation bag (which is connected to an oxygen source and kept at the bedside). Manual ventilation matching pressure, rates, and F_{IO_2} to ventilator settings must be maintained. **If the infant improves with these interventions, mechanical failure of the ventilator should be suspected.** Assistance should be summoned to find the mechanical problem or replace the system. The infant's respiratory effort must be manually assisted until the problem is solved.

If the infant does not improve with manual ventilation, there is probably a problem with the tube. The infant's condition can be assessed by auscultating the chest for quality of breath sounds. Findings and what they suggest are listed in Table 23-8.

The ETT should be suctioned quickly. If there is no improvement in clinical condition or air entry, the tube should be replaced while supporting the infant with bag-and-mask ventilation. **If the tube is too low, it can be repositioned by pulling it back 0.5 to 1 cm. If air entry and clinical condition improve with auscultation, the tube must be secured in the new position and a chest x-ray examination done to confirm tube placement. If assessment of the chest leads to suspicion of accidental extubation, the tube must be removed, ventilation with bag and mask administered, and reintubation performed.** If the infant does not improve with manual ventilation and the tube is in place, an air leak or IVH could be the cause.

Monitors and ventilators are equipped with alarm systems to warn care providers of sudden changes in the infant's condition or supportive systems. **It is imperative that all alarm systems be maintained in the "on" position.** Turning the alarms "off" during care for such procedures as suctioning and weighing creates the risk for forgetting to turn them on again. In a busy NICU, the compromised infant may not be visually noticed until the hypoxia is so severe that resuscitation is more difficult or impossible. Monitor parameters (both high and low alarm settings) must be individualized for each infant and recorded (see Chapter 7).

A sick neonate may experience a severe hypoxic insult when oxygen is too rapidly altered during caregiving procedures. **Feeding, weighing, or turning without an alternative oxygen source may cause a sudden decrease in Pa_{O_2}, pulmonary vasoconstriction, hypoperfusion, and an iatrogenic worsening of the condition.** Prolonged ETT suctioning (15 to 20 seconds) causes hypoxia and atelectasis. Care must be organized to conserve energy, minimize hypoxic insults, and maintain the infant in physiologic homeostasis. **Alternative oxygen sources must be provided when the usual method of oxygen delivery is disrupted for giving care.** Small alterations in F_{IO_2} prevent rapid increases or decreases in oxygen tension.

METABOLIC FACTORS

Hypoglycemia must never be overlooked as the cause of sudden collapse. Undetected infiltration or disconnection of intravenous fluids may cause a precipitous drop in blood glucose, with respiratory irregularity, apnea, or seizures. Quickly checking the blood glucose with a glucometer is always warranted. If low blood glucose is not the cause of the sudden deterioration, it may be a complication of the asphyxial episode. After the infant is stabilized, screening for hypoglycemia and providing adequate fluids and glucose are appropriate (see Chapter 15).

Hypothermia and overwhelming sepsis with their associated metabolic derangements may be the cause of sudden deterioration. Muted response to cold stress is a consequence of asphyxial insult, and cold stress must be avoided after the acute episode. A high level of suspicion for infection should accompany sudden deterioration (see Chapters 6 and 22).

AIR LEAKS

Physiology. When air dissects from an alveolus, it follows the tracheobronchial tree and may accumulate in the mediastinum (pneumomediastinum), in the pleural space (pneumothorax), in the space surrounding the heart (pneumopericardium), in the peritoneal cavity (pneumoperitoneum), or subcutaneously (subcutaneous emphysema). **Air leaks are complications of respiratory diseases and treatment strategies.** When air continues to accumulate, pressure builds in the pleural space, compresses the lung, and pushes the mediastinum toward the unaffected side; a tension pneumothorax results.

The free air released from ruptured alveoli may lead to pulmonary interstitial emphysema (PIE) (Figure 23-1). This free air intravasates into interstitial tissue and can compromise pulmonary vascular circulation and ventilation. Localized pulmonary interstitial emphysema sometimes resolves spontaneously. Frequently it can continue for weeks or even months. Use of HFV has improved the outcome of these infants.

Etiology. Infants at increased risk for the development of air leaks fall into three specific categories: healthy term neonates, neonates with pulmonary diseases, and neonates receiving positive-pressure support (CPAP and IMV).

Healthy term neonates generate pressures of 40 to 80 cm of water for their first breath of life.

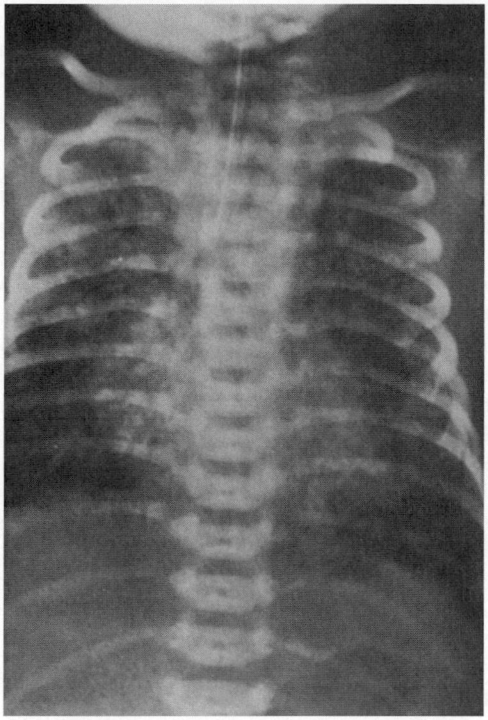

FIGURE 23-1 Pulmonary interstitial emphysema.

Therefore a spontaneous air leak is more common in the neonatal period (2% to 10%) than at any other time of life.

Pulmonary diseases such as RDS result in stiff, noncompliant lungs requiring higher pressures for alveolar ventilation. Aspiration syndromes cause a ball-valve obstruction of debris with distal air trapping (meconium, milk, amniotic fluid, blood, and mucus). Hypoplastic lungs create a risk for air leaks because lung growth and development are abnormal and the lungs are stiff and noncompliant (diaphragmatic hernia and oligohydramnios syndrome). In either congenital lobar emphysema or PIE, alveolar rupture is associated with positive-pressure ventilation.

Positive-pressure ventilation, especially with excessive pressure, results in overdistention with alveolar rupture and air dissection. Air leaks occur in 16% to 36% of infants who are ventilated by CPAP or IMV or are resuscitated with a bag and mask or with an endotracheal tube and bag. ETT displacement is a major factor in the development of air leaks (see Table 23-4). Administration of surfactant lowers the levels of ventilatory support necessary to adequately ventilate the preterm infant's lungs and results in a reduced incidence of pneumothorax.

Prevention. Using the least amount of positive pressure to obtain physiologic results decreases the chances of air leaks. The incidence of pneumothorax is reduced in surfactant-treated prematures and with the use of HFV. Scrupulously clearing the airway before resuscitation and using pressure gauges on resuscitation equipment may prevent aspiration and the possibility of inadvertently using pressure that is too high. Vigilance in positioning, securing, and maintaining ETT position may significantly reduce the incidence of air leaks.[267] Because air leaks alter systemic hemodynamics, they are associated with the development of IVH (see Chapter 26). Rapid recognition of at-risk infants, recognition of clinical manifestations and diagnosis, and rapid emergency treatment improve survival and decrease the long-term sequelae of hypoxia and ischemia.

Data Collection

History. Pneumothorax or other air leaks should be suspected when any one of the following infants takes a sudden turn for the worse:

- A preterm infant with RDS either with or without positive-pressure support
- A term or postterm infant with meconium-stained amniotic fluid
- An infant with a chest x-ray showing interstitial or lobar emphysema
- An infant requiring resuscitation at birth
- An infant receiving CPAP or positive-pressure ventilation

Signs and Symptoms. Asymptomatic air leaks occur in term neonates; these frequently require no treatment and resolve spontaneously in 24 to 48 hours. Gradual onset of symptoms is characterized by increasing difficulty in ventilation, oxygenation, and perfusion. Early clinical manifestations may include restlessness and irritability, lethargy, tachypnea, and use of accessory muscles including grunting, flaring, and retractions. These subtle clinical changes may be unnoticed until the infant progresses to a sudden, profound collapse.

Sudden and severe deterioration in clinical course is characterized by the following:

- Profound generalized cyanosis
- Bradycardia
- Decrease in the height of the QRS complex on the monitor
- Air hunger including gasping and anxious facies
- Diminished or shifted breath sounds
- Chest asymmetry
- Diminished, shifted, or muffled cardiac sounds and point of maximal intensity (PMI)
- Severe hypotension and poor peripheral perfusion
- Easily palpable liver and spleen
- Subcutaneous emphysema
- Cardiorespiratory arrest

Laboratory Data. Arterial blood gas determinations reveal increasing hypoxemia (↓Pa_{O_2}), increasing hypercapnia (↑Pa_{CO_2}), and a persistent metabolic acidosis with gradual onset of symptoms. Transillumination of the chest with a fiberoptic probe may reveal hyperlucency of the affected side when compared with the other side. **A chest x-ray examination is the definitive diagnostic technique in air leaks.** Because clinical manifestations of many other diseases may be similar to air leaks, the only way to be sure of the diagnosis is to perform a chest x-ray examination. Anteroposterior and lateral films must be obtained. Occasionally a decubitus lateral x-ray film may be of value. X-ray findings in pneumothorax, the most common air leak, include the following:

- Increased lucency, overall increase in size, and flattened diaphragm on the affected side
- Widened intercostal spaces
- Decreased or absent pulmonary vascular markings
- Sharp contrast of the cardiac border and diaphragm (sharp edge sign)

Tension pneumothorax results in mediastinal shifts with decreased volume, increased opacity of opposite lung, and deviation of heart and trachea to the other side.

Treatment. An air leak is a surgical emergency of the chest. Tension within the chest cavity compromises lung excursion and cardiac output; without prompt treatment, the infant will not survive. Trained care providers must be available immediately to provide emergency management in any institution that provides positive-pressure ventilatory support.

Evacuation of trapped air to decrease tension and allow proper organ function is the goal of treatment. Pneumomediastinum rarely needs to be treated, but pneumopericardium often results in cardiac tamponade and requires needle aspiration or tube drainage. Pneumoperitoneum must be differentiated from a perforated viscus.

A suggested conservative treatment is endotracheal intubation of the unaffected lung. The tube is advanced 1 to 2 cm beyond the carina to occlude the involved lung. This procedure is difficult to perform if the left lung is involved. If the pulmonary interstitial emphysema is localized to one lung or lobe of the lung, differential ventilation or surgical removal of the lobe may be curative. **Pneumothorax may be treated with needle aspiration of air. Tube thoracotomy with suction drainage is frequently necessary.**

Use of fibrin glue to treat persistent pneumothorax has been reported, with resolution within 24 hours of treatment.[315] Complications included (1) bradycardia requiring manual ventilation, (2) significant hypercalcemia, (3) diaphragmatic paralysis, (4) contralateral pneumothorax, and (5) localized tissue necrosis.

Immediate Supportive Care. **The head of the bed is elevated 30 to 40 degrees.** This decreases the work of breathing by using gravity to localize the air in the upper chest and to push the abdominal organs downward away from the diaphragm.

Oxygen at 100% concentration is administered. The two goals for using 100% oxygen for immediate care are to improve oxygenation in a severely compromised infant and to increase by as much as sixfold the rate of absorption of the trapped air by means of a nitrogen washout technique.

CAUTION: Prolonged administration of 100% oxygen to treat an air leak in term infants has been used. Because of new understanding about the effects of oxidative stress from use of 100% oxygen, prolonged use for "nitrogen washout" should be used with caution (see "Supplemental Oxygen" section). Exclusive use of 100% oxygen to treat trapped air is contraindicated in preterm infants because of the risk for developing retinopathy of prematurity and the length of time necessary to obtain complete resolution.

A severely compromised infant requires immediate emergency procedures. A diagnostic and therapeutic thoracentesis may be necessary in life-threatening situations in which there is not time to wait for x-ray examination.

Needle Aspiration. A scalp vein needle (23- to 25-gauge) or an Angiocath (24-gauge), a three-way stopcock, and a 10- to 20-mL syringe may be used for needle aspiration. The equipment is connected (syringe-stopcock-needle/Angiocath), the chest is aseptically prepared, and the needle is inserted into the third intercostal space in the anterior axillary line. A slight pop may be felt when the pleura is entered. Air is withdrawn into the syringe and evacuated into the room by turning the stopcock. This procedure is repeated until no more air can be aspirated or a chest tube can be placed.

Chest Tube. Chest tube thoracotomy is the definitive treatment for pneumothorax. The insertion of a chest tube is an invasive procedure that requires strict surgical technique, with each operator wearing a gown, gloves, mask, and cap. The infant should be appropriately positioned, restrained, provided with a sucrose pacifier, and monitored before the chest is prepared for asepsis. Ideally, the anterior chest wall should be prepared with a scrub solution for a minimum of 3 minutes. If a special tray is not available, a minor suture tray will usually contain the necessary instruments. Necessary equipment is as follows:

- Chest tube (8- to 12-Fr Argyle)
- Iodine or povidone-iodine (Betadine) scrub solution
- Gloves, gown, mask, hat
- Sterile drapes
- Syringes
- Sterile sponges (gauze)
- Medicine cups
- Lidocaine 1% without epinephrine
- Scalpel blades (No. 11 or 15)
- Hemostat (mosquito and Kelly clamps)
- Scissors
- Needle holder
- Sterile suture
- Sterile connectors (straight)
- Tubing
- Infant disposable underwater seal drainage system (two- or three-bottle or Pleur-evac system)
- Wall suction
- Sterile saline solution
- Tape, Tegaderm, or OpSite
- Chest tube clamp for emergency disconnection

The insertion site depends on the clinician's preference. In the lateral approach, the site is the fourth to sixth intercostal space on or lateral to the anterior axillary line. In the superior approach, the site is the second or third intercostal space on or just lateral to the midclavicular line (Figure 23-2). A case report of breast deformity, psychological distress, and

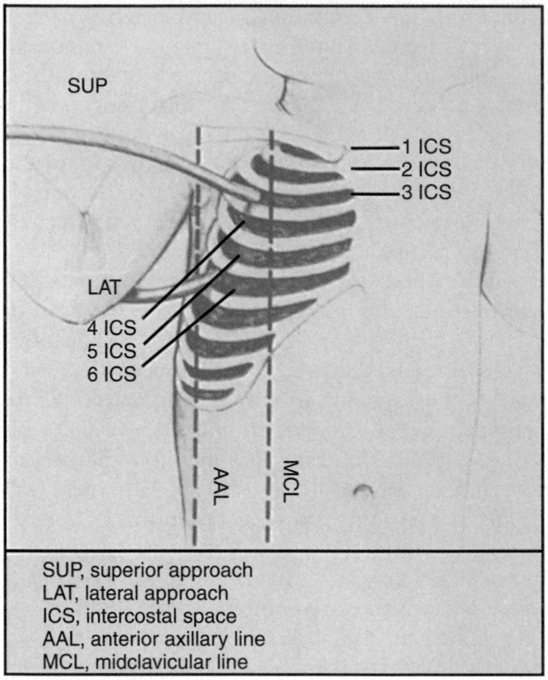

FIGURE 23-2 Chest tube insertion site. (From Oellrich RG: Pneumothorax: chest tubes and the neonate, *MCN Am J Matern Child Nurs* 10:31, 1985.)

need for corrective surgery (in adolescent preterm girls) as a result of chest tube insertion for multiple pneumothoraces recommends a preventive strategy of using the anterior axillary line, maintaining a distance of 4 to 5 cm inferior to the nipple, and inserting the tube through the fifth or sixth intercostal space.[299]

After infiltration of the area with 1% lidocaine for pain control, a small incision is made. A pursestring suture should be placed around the incision with ends left loose. A curved hemostat is inserted into the incision and opened. The catheter is advanced through the interspace and into the pleural space. The most frequent error by an inexperienced operator is applying too little force to enter the pleural cavity. The pursestring is tightened and tied and then tied to the chest tube. The tube is connected to the underwater drainage system, which may then be connected to a continuous suction device (10 to 20 cm of water is most commonly recommended). The tube should be secured with tape. An x-ray examination is used to confirm placement of the tube and evaluate the effectiveness of the therapy. **After the procedure, attention to pain control with opioids and/or nonnarcotic analgesics is necessary** (see Chapter 12).

Complications. In some instances, complications have arisen from the placement of chest tubes in neonates. These include hemorrhage, lung perforation, infarction, and phrenic nerve injury with eventration of the diaphragm. Clinical signs of eventration (elevation of the diaphragm into the thoracic cavity) include a shift of the umbilicus upward and toward the affected side.[235]

Care of Chest Tube and Drainage System. The chest tube drainage system removes air and fluid material from the pleural space to restore negative pressure and expand the lung. Care providers must be familiar with the operation of the drainage system used in the nursery. The single-bottle water seal system drains air and fluid by gravity and blocks atmospheric air from being drawn into the pleural space. In addition to the water seal, the multiple-bottle systems allow suction to be applied to facilitate drainage and expansion. The Pleur-evac system is a single plastic unit divided into three chambers: the collection, water seal, and suction chambers.

Oscillation of fluid in the tube demonstrates effective communication between the pleural space and drainage bottle. In the small, sick infant, intrapleural pressure may cause only fluctuation in the tube at the chest wall. Fluctuation in either the tube or bottle should be observed. Fluctuation may cease as a result of fibrin or blood clots obstructing the tube, kinked or compressed tubing, or the suction apparatus not working properly. Milking and stripping the chest tube generally are unnecessary if only air is being removed. Presence of clots or debris may require gentle kneading of the tube. Milking and stripping generate tremendously high pressures that may entrap and damage the lung in the chest tube eyelets.

Bubbling in the drainage bottle indicates that air is being removed from the pleural space. Continuous bubbling may indicate an air leak in the system. To locate the source of the leak, the tube is momentarily clamped (beginning close to the chest and working toward the bottle) with a rubber-tipped hemostat. When the clamp is placed between the air leak and the water seal, the bubbling will stop. Patency of the tube, fluctuation, and bubbling should be observed and charted hourly.

Excessive or insufficient fluid in the drainage bottles may interfere with proper function of the drainage system. The bottle may have to be changed, or sterile saline may have to be added.

Frequent turning is important for maximum drainage and lung expansion. Proper stabilizing and positioning of the chest tube is necessary for function, comfort, and prevention of accidental removal. The tubing may be secured by encircling it with an adhesive tab, placing a safety pin through the tape (not the tube), and securing it to the bed. **If the tube becomes dislodged, the opening should be covered with sterile gauze and pressure applied until the tube can be replaced.**

When the infant is moved for such procedures as x-ray examination and weighing, the tube must be stabilized by holding it close to the chest. **If the closed system is disturbed (e.g., because of a broken bottle), the tube should be clamped with a rubber-tipped hemostat that always should be kept at the bedside.** The chest tube should be clamped for as short a time as possible. **After necessary clamping, vital signs and clinical conditions should be closely monitored.**

Bottles should be stabilized by being taped to an incubator or warmer so that they are not accidentally broken or picked up. **The bottles must always be below the level of the infant's chest to prevent water from being pulled into the pleural space.**

Removal of Chest Tubes. When bubbling has ceased for at least 24 hours and the chest x-ray films show no free air for 12 to 24 hours, the chest tube may be removed. **Attention to pain relief during the removal process includes a sucrose pacifier and pharmacologic pain relief (see Chapter 12).** Rapid, sterile removal of the tube is followed by application of a petrolatum gauze pressure dressing.

CENTRAL NERVOUS SYSTEM INSULT

Acute insult to the CNS may result in increased intracranial pressure, hemorrhage, or hypoxic ischemic brain injury (see Chapter 26).

CARDIAC COMPLICATIONS

CDP or IMV may exert sufficient pressure on the pulmonary capillary bed to raise pulmonary artery pressure and interfere with cardiac output. The effect of CDP or IMV on the pulmonary vascular bed and cardiac output may be alleviated by lowering the PIP or PEEP, or both. At times, a fluid infusion to increase the intravascular volume may overcome the resistance to the pulmonary blood flow. The effect of MAP on cardiac output is difficult to monitor in most NICUs, because pulmonary artery or pulmonary wedge pressures are not routinely obtained. Until such time as these measurements are routinely obtained, the best CPAP is determined only on clinical grounds.

PDA is the most common cardiac complication in neonates with respiratory disease. Most often it is manifested by an increasing oxygen requirement or increased dependency on ventilatory support (see Chapter 24).

INFECTION AND BLEEDING

Procedures such as intubation expose the neonate to the risk for acquired (nosocomial) infection. Scrupulous attention to technique when caring for respiratory equipment and performing procedures such as sterile suctioning of the endotracheal tube minimizes the risks for infection. **Handwashing before and after every contact with the neonate is the best method of preventing hospital-acquired infection in an already compromised, sick neonate.** Neonates who are severely ill with respiratory disease may exhibit bleeding diathesis at birth or during the acute phase of their disease. Early recognition and treatment are important (see Chapter 20).

Chronic Complications

CHRONIC LUNG DISEASE/ BRONCHOPULMONARY DYSPLASIA

Despite improvements in neonatal respiratory care, the incidence of CLD/BPD continues to be high and is the direct result of the survival of extremely premature infants.[368] The survival of these extremely premature infants may be contributing to the static incidence of CLD/BPD reported by investigators. Several authors have reported an atypical type of CLD/BPD occurring in infants less than 1000 g at birth with mild or absent initial respiratory distress. A recent retrospective study of preterms with atypical CLD/BPD found that they were (1) born in hospital, (2) received natural surfactant therapy, (3) had fewer days of mechanical ventilation, and (4) were larger, more mature preterms.[277] The primary pathology of CLD is related to lung injury, it is in fact a multisystem disease, and most of the treatment is supportive.

CLD/BPD was first described by Northway and Rosan[271] as serial roentgenographic changes occurring in the lungs of premature infants who survived hyaline membrane disease (HMD). CLD/BPD also occurs in a variety of conditions, including esophageal atresia, aspiration pneumonia, congenital heart disease, PDA, and MAS. The clinical course of CLD/BPD is one of increasing respiratory distress and often is described as the chronic phase of RDS.

Recent changes in neonatal care have modified the classic stages of BPD as first described by Northway and Rosan.[69,271] In comparison with the infants in earlier studies, today neonates with CLD are far more premature, have lower birth weights, and generally lack many of the radiographic changes of cystic lung disease. The "new BPD" is characterized by arrested lung development resulting from interference with alveolarization and vascularization.[69] VLBW neonates who require supplemental oxygen at 28 to 30 days of life or at 36 weeks post-menstrual age (PMA) have CLD.[387] Despite these changes, the incidence of chronic lung disease in infants after NICU care remains a significant clinical problem, with an incidence of 23% to 85% in VLBW infants. Although atypical CLD/BPD is common in preterms less than 1250 g, a recent retrospective study found that the majority of preterms with CLD/BPD still have classic CLD/BPD.[277]

The incidence of CLD/BPD varies among NICUs because of variations in respiratory management associated with oxygen toxicity and barotrauma and volutrauma.[310] Although use of nasal CPAP is associated with lower CLD/BPD rates,[17,384] increased use of intubation, mechanical ventilation, and high pressures (PIP and MAP) is associated with increased CLD/BPD rates. When mechanical ventilation is used, the shorter the duration, the less often CLD/BPD occurs.[57]

Pathophysiology. CLD/BPD is a disorder of premature infants that is characterized by respiratory distress and impaired gas exchange. **The pathogenesis of CLD/BPD is one of chronic and constant and recurring lung injury, with ongoing repair and healing of the injury.** Chronic injury and repair may in itself prolong the need for the very factors that contribute to the development of BPD: oxygen therapy and mechanical ventilation. In RDS, there is injury to the alveolar mucosa, airway mucosa, serum exudation membranes, and fibrin coagulation-forming hyaline membranes. If sufficient hypoxia occurs with resultant damage, the alveolar and airway epithelium and its basement membrane will hemorrhage and round cell infiltration will begin. Cellular and noncellular debris fill the alveoli and small airways. The obstruction causes microatelectasis, and unobstructed airways become hyperexpanded and emphysematous.

In the healing and repair process, type II alveolar cells or their precursors multiply and differentiate into type I pneumocytes, which provide alveolar epithelium. Cells of the basal layer of the pseudostratified, ciliated, columnar epithelium lining the airways multiply and migrate to cover the injured airway and rejuvenate the epithelium. During this healing phase, the rapidly multiplying and differentiating transitional cells are squamous or cuboidal and therefore appear "metaplastic." Epithelial metaplasia is one of the characteristics of BPD.

As healing occurs, increased inspired oxygen tensions, barotrauma, and infection continue to injure the cells that are taking part in the healing process.

Etiology. CLD/BPD is an iatrogenic disease caused by oxygen toxicity and barotrauma resulting from pressure ventilation. Even preterm infants with mild respiratory distress in the first week of life may develop CLD/BPD.[368] CLD/BPD is multifactorial, and prenatal predictors include prematurity (e.g., early gestational age and low birth weight) and male gender.[163] A recent study showed that an elevated placenta growth factor (P1GF) level in cord blood at birth was correlated with an increased risk for premature infants to develop CLD/BPD.[375] This may be a biologic marker for predicting CLD/BPD. In addition, another study revealed that levels of trypsinogen-2 are higher during the postnatal days of infants who develop CLD/BPD.[59] Plasma concentration of soluble L-selectin (sL-selectin), soluble E-selectin (sE-selectin) and soluble intercellular adhesion molecule-1 may also be indicators for treatment with dexamethasone. The arterial plasma level of sL-selectin in infants who had RDS and did not develop CLD/BPD was significantly decreased when they were treated with dexamethasone.[21]

Oxygen Toxicity. CLD/BPD has been documented in both long-term and short-term exposure to oxygen at both low and high levels (>60% to 80%), as well as in infants treated with mechanical ventilation without supplemental oxygen. As a result of these findings, many units have instituted guidelines for oxygen use and monitoring of levels with pulse oximetry. **Avoidance of excessive oxygen exposure and careful attention to oxygen saturations and arterial Pao_2 may help reduce lung injury resulting from oxygen exposure.**[145,365,367]

Barotrauma/Volutrauma. Development of CLD/BPD is a result of barotrauma and volutrauma. CLD/BPD has been described in infants who have received high peak inspiratory pressures (PIPs) and high PEEP[145] and neonates with pneumothorax and PIE. A decrease in the incidence of CLD/BPD has been noted when lower PIPs are used.[145] Although PIPs should be limited whenever possible, some infants with very noncompliant lungs require the use of high pressure for survival. Volutrauma (e.g., increased lung volume [stretch]) results in regional overdistention of lung units or airways, which may promote lung injury more than pressure itself. **Using the smallest possible tidal volumes to inflate the lung avoids the overdistention and volutrauma that causes CLD/BPD.**[145]

Use of surfactant therapy and newer ventilatory techniques[234,247,310,364] has decreased the pressures necessary to adequately oxygenate and ventilate the neonate's lungs, as well as resultant air leaks. A ventilator strategy of low tidal volume and adequate PEEP minimizes lung injury.[364] **A gentler ventilator strategy has been used to decrease exposure of preterm lungs to barotrauma/volutrauma necessary to maintain Pco_2 in the normal range.** A strategy of **"permissive hypercapnia"** (e.g., accepting a $Paco_2$ of 45 to 58 mm Hg) using lower PIP, MAP, and ventilator rate reduces the duration of assisted ventilation and of supplemental oxygen (at 28 days of life and total days) and rate of reintubation.[234,247,364]

Although alterations in $Paco_2$ are associated with fluctuations in cerebral blood flow, in one study there was no difference in IVH and PVL, mortality, air leaks, ROP, or PDA compared with the control group.[234] Permissive hypercapnia may protect against cerebral hypoperfusion and subsequent PVL associated with hypocapnia; extreme hypercapnia, however, is associated with an increased risk for intracranial hemorrhage.[364] Therefore large fluctuations of $Paco_2$ values should be avoided and further studies of the relationship between hypocarbia/hypercarbia and brain injury are needed. **Even though mild permissive hypercapnia is safe and has modest benefit, the optimal $Paco_2$ level has not been determined, so current evidence does not support a general recommendation for its use in preterm infants.**[364]

Use of HFV, HFV with surfactant replacement, and HFV with "high volume" technique are all associated with a decreased incidence of CLD/BPD (see "High-Frequency Ventilation" section).

Patent Ductus Arteriosus. There is a high incidence of BPD among infants with PDA and congestive heart failure. The amount of oxygen and peak inspiratory pressure necessary to support a neonate through the pulmonary complications of PDA may result in damage from oxygen toxicity and barotrauma. The increased pulmonary blood flow that occurs may also contribute to pulmonary damage. Very preterm infants (<29 weeks' gestation) with a PDA have a higher mortality rate compared with preterms with a closed ductus (70.7% vs. 11.2%).[270] Because of these findings, medical closure of the ductus with indomethacin or ibuprofen or surgical ligation is advocated (see Chapter 24) but has not affected the incidence of BPD.

Nutrition. SGA infants who were undernourished in utero have been shown to have an increased risk for CLD/BPD.[215] Inadequate nutrition caused by poor intake or increased nutritional requirements resulting in catabolism may potentiate the effects of oxygen and barotrauma on the neonatal lung. A recent retrospective review of the nutritional status of 30 preterms with BPD/CLD found that they received significantly less protein and calories (e.g., by 28 days of life, 98.63 kcal/kg/day instead of the recommended 120 kcal/kg/day for growth), resulting in a significant energy and protein deficit.[188] **This undernutrition may be contributing to the development of BPD/CLD by altering the growth of immature lungs.** Inadequate intake of antioxidants, trace elements, vitamins, and polyunsaturated fatty acids also may predispose the lung to injury.

Fluids. CLD/BPD is common in preterms who have developed symptoms of fluid overload within the first few days of life. Fluid balance in a VLBW infant is complicated by huge insensible water loss and often intolerance for enteral feedings. Intake, output, and changes in weight must be closely monitored to calculate the fluid needs. Furthermore, clinical research indicates that careful restriction of water intake so that physiologic needs are met without allowing for significant dehydration is indicated. This practice also decreases the risk for PDA and NEC and might decrease the overall risk for death without significantly increasing the risk for adverse consequences.[36]

Family History of Asthma. Infants who develop BPD may have relatives with asthma who require periodic hospitalization. The lungs of these infants may be less tolerant of the insults of pulmonary disease, oxygen, pressure, and fluids.

Prematurity. **Developmental immaturity is of principal importance in the etiologic picture of CLD/BPD.** Premature births alone may have a significant effect on pulmonary development, because prematurity results in differences in the development of small airways. As a result, premature infants are more susceptible to additional damage to the small airways from oxygen, ventilator pressure, fluids, and circulatory overload. As the survival rate of VLBW infants born at less than 28 weeks' gestation increases, the occurrence of CLD/BPD is increasing (e.g., the lower the gestational age, the higher the risk).[163] However, the current form of CLD/BPD is less severe, with fewer infants requiring tracheostomies and long-term ventilation therapy (6 months or more).[69]

Oxygen and Antioxidants. Oxygen accepts free electrons generated by oxidative metabolism within the cell and produces free radicals, molecules that are toxic to living cells or tissues.[365] Normally, antioxidants protect cells against free radicals, but this balance may be upset by increased free radical production or decreased antioxidant defense. **A preterm neonate is deficient in antioxidants and thus more susceptible to lung damage from free radicals and oxidative stress.**[23,69]

Inflammation. Oxygen radicals, barotrauma, infection, and other factors initiate the inflammatory process,[69] resulting in the infiltration of leukocytes, with release of other inflammatory mediators, resulting in pulmonary damage (e.g., decrease in capillary endothelial integrity, albumin leakage in the alveoli resulting in pulmonary edema). Neonates whose lungs are mechanically ventilated have increased pulmonary cytokine and phagocyte levels within 1 to 3 hours after the onset of mechanical ventilation.[69,377] Activated neutrophils release enzymes that directly destroy the elastin and collagen of the lung. **Lung inflammation and injury predispose the lung to increased susceptibility to volutrauma and oxidant-induced lung injury.**[69] This inflammatory cycle produces significant pulmonary injury during a critical period of rapid lung growth and development (24 to 40 weeks) (see Table 23-1). Increasingly, studies show that preterm infants exposed to antenatal inflammation and infection (e.g., chorioamnionitis) are at increased risk for developing CLD/BPD.[64,306] Postnatal nosocomial infection is associated with an increased risk for CLD/BPD.[107,353] Variation in nosocomial infection rates may be a factor in the variation in inter-NICU CLD/BPD rates.

Preterm infants with increased lung inflammation who subsequently develop CLD/BPD have been shown to have early adrenal insufficiency.[392,394] Even very early preterm infants (24 to 25 weeks) have been shown to have an increase in cortisol levels after birth, reaching maximum levels at 24 hours, with a gradual decrease in 14 to 28 days.[392] Low cortisol levels may be associated with an increased risk for developing CLD/BPD.[394] A multicenter, randomized trial to test early low-dose hydrocortisone therapy was halted because of an increase in spontaneous GI perforations in the treated preterms, especially those also receiving indomethacin.[393] Prophylaxis of early adrenal insufficiency decreased mortality and improved survival without CLD/BPD only in the chorioamnionitis-exposed preterms.[393] The 18- to 22-month follow-up of these infants showed no difference in growth, no increase in cerebral palsy, and indicators of improved neurodevelopmental outcome in those treated with early, low-dose hydrocortisone.[395] Another RCT of early administration (within the first 36 hours of life) of hydrocortisone to prevent CLD/BPD was terminated early because of the increased incidence of GI perforations and found lower rates of CLD/BPD.[283] Current evidence does not show a clear advantage of hydrocortisone versus dexamethasone use for CLD/BPD on long-term neurodevelopmental outcomes.[298]

Prevention. **Potentially better practices to reduce the CLD/BPD in VLBW infants are listed in Box 23-6.** Widespread use of antenatal steroids and surfactant administration have not reduced the rate of CLD/BPD or the NICU disparities in CLD/BPD rates. Use of surfactant does reduce the severity of CLD/BPD,[69] and use of a new synthetic surfactant recently has been shown to reduce the incidence of CLD/BPD.[255] A single course of antenatal steroid therapy decreases the incidence and severity of CLD/BPD.[260] Widespread use of both antenatal and postnatal steroid therapy has not improved the outcome in ELBW infants. Premature and full-term infants (with pneumonia or MAS) treated with surfactant replacement have a lower incidence of CLD/BPD because of (1) better ventilation and pressure distribution in the alveoli, (2) stabilization

BOX 23-6

POTENTIALLY BETTER PRACTICES TO REDUCE THE INCIDENCE OF CLD/BPD IN THE VERY-LOW-BIRTH-WEIGHT PRETERM INFANT

- Improved use of surfactant in the delivery room
- Use of the antioxidant *vitamin A*
- Increased use of permissive hypercapnia
- Use lower target oxygen saturation levels (PO) than traditionally used adult saturation norms
- Decrease the incidence of sentinel events such as air leaks and unplanned extubations
- Minimize exposure in the delivery room to supplemental oxygen by titrating F_{IO_2} and monitoring oxygen saturations with PO
- Early closure of PDA, either medically or surgically
- Monitor and minimize tidal volumes on mechanically ventilated preterms
- Extubate from assisted ventilation as soon as possible
- Improve team work in the delivery room
- Use Neopuff™, instead of hand ventilation, to minimize overinflation of the preterm lung
- Provide consistent respiratory management and consistent ventilator weaning
- Provide blended F_{IO_2} in the delivery room and during transport to the NICU to minimize exposure to unnecessary levels of supplemental oxygen

Adapted from Geary C, Caskey M, Fonseca R, et al: Decreased incidence of bronchopulmonary dysplasia after early management changes, including surfactant and nasal continuous positive airway pressure treatment at delivery, lowered oxygen saturation goals, and early amino acid administration: a historical cohort study, *Pediatrics* 121:89, 2008; Payne NR, LaCorte M, Sun S, et al and the Breathsavers Group: Evaluation and development of potentially better practices to reduce bronchopulmonary dysplasia in very low birth weight infants, *Pediatrics* 118: S65, 2006.

NICU, Neonatal intensive care unit; *PDA,* patent ductus arteriosus; *PO,* pulse oximeter.

of the alveoli, (3) prevention of overdistention, and (4) decreased cytokines and inflammatory response.

A recent review of 10 years of neonatal ventilation of VLBW preterms showed that noninvasive ventilatory support now accounts for greater than 50% of ventilation hours.[310] This increased use of noninvasive strategies has not been associated with an increase in respiratory morbidities.[310] Use of nasal CPAP may reduce or eliminate the need for intubation and mechanical ventilation, as well as assist in successful extubation.[17,96,97] In an attempt to prevent re-injury and allow healing, **inspired oxygen tensions should be kept as low as is reasonable to provide adequate arterial oxygen tension. Pressures on the ventilator should be reduced when possible to prevent barotrauma.** Although the collaborative HFV trial did not demonstrate a difference in the incidence of BPD between HFV and conventional ventilation,[170] early use of HFV or use of HFV with surfactant may decrease lung damage and resultant CLD/BPD.[195]

Use of inhaled nitric oxide in care of preterms with RDS results in a reduction in the incidence of CLD/BPD (see the "Treatment" discussion in the "Respiratory Distress Syndrome" section). iNO therapy in the preterm infant at risk for CLD/BPD does not alter plasma biomarkers of oxidative stress, which supports the safety of iNO as well as indicating that the benefits of iNO on pulmonary outcomes does not involve reduced levels of oxidative stress.[23] At 1-year follow-up, preterms randomized to iNO therapy used fewer bronchodilators, inhaled/systemic steroids, diuretics, and supplemental oxygen.[169]

In a multicenter trial, administration of vitamin A (e.g., 5000 international units intramuscularly [IM] three times a week for 4 weeks) to VLBW infants reduced the risk for CLD/BPD.[378] Monitoring of serum levels (the desired range of plasma vitamin A concentrations is 30 to 60 mcg/dL; the desired plasma retinol-binding protein [RBP] concentration is >25 mg/dL)[330] and assessment for manifestations of toxicity (e.g., lesions on skin/mucous membranes, bone and joint abnormalities, jaundice, hepatomegaly, and increased intracranial pressure) should accompany vitamin A administration.[330] Concurrent dexamethasone therapy increases serum blood levels of fat-soluble vitamins (e.g., A and E) independent of intake.[11,331] In a more recent study, oral supplementation of vitamin A (e.g., 5000 international units/day for 28 days) in ELBW infants did not significantly alter the incidence of CLD/BPD.[390] Supplementing VLBW infants with vitamin A is associated with a reduction in death, oxygen requirement at 1 month of age, and oxygen requirement at 36 weeks PMA in preterms less than 1000 g BW.[93] Furthermore, vitamin A supplementation to ELBW neonates resulted in a similar if not modestly improved neurodevelopmental outcome when followed up at 18 to 22 months of age.[7]

Prevention of oxygen free radical injury to the pulmonary tree and CNS (e.g., CLD/BPD and IVH/PVL)[316] occurs with intratracheal injection of recombinant human CuZn superoxide dismutase (rhSOD). A significant decrease in markers of pulmonary inflammation occurred in rhSOD-treated preterm infants without short-term or long-term abnormalities.[94] A systematic review of clinical trials revealed that evidence is still insufficient to draw conclusions about the efficacy of superoxide dismutase in preventing CLD.[356]

Data Collection

History. A history of prematurity, moderate to severe RDS, intubation with oxygen and positive-pressure ventilation in the first week of life, inability to be weaned from the ventilator, and increasing oxygen requirement at the end of the first week of life are associated with CLD/BPD. Long-term features include tachypnea, rales, retractions, abnormal chest x-ray examination results, and the need for supplemental oxygen for more than 28 to 30 days of life or at 36 weeks PMA.

Signs and Symptoms. Tachypnea, exercise intolerance (feeding and handling), oxygen dependence, and respiratory distress (retractions, nasal flaring, fine rales at the bases or throughout the lung fields) are associated with CLD/BPD.

Laboratory Data. X-ray findings (Figure 23-3) correlate with the stage of disease; however, the pathologic changes are often more severe than the chest x-ray findings indicate[271]:

- Stage I: Reticulogranular pattern and air bronchogram or RDS (first 3 days of life)
- Stage II: Coarse granular infiltrates that are dense enough to obscure the cardiac markings (first 3 to 10 days of life)
- Stage III: Multiple small cyst formation within the opaque lungs and visible cardiac borders (first 10 to 20 days of life)
- Stage IV: Irregular larger cyst formation that alternates with areas of increased density (after 28 days of life)

Mild hyperinflation as demonstrated on a chest x-ray film is a common finding in VLBW infants with CLD/BPD.

Cardiovascular changes include (1) right ventricular hypertrophy on ECG, (2) elevated right ventricular systolic time intervals or left ventricular and septal wall thickening on echocardiogram, or (3) elevated pulmonary vascular pressures and resistance at cardiac catheterization.

Treatment. The therapeutic goal is to reduce those factors that produce re-injury and to allow the lung to heal so that normal function can resume. This process may take weeks, months, or even years in severe lung injuries or in small infants under 1000 g.

Concurrent supportive therapies include (1) maintenance of adequate oxygenation and ventilation, (2) adequate nutrition and fluid restriction, (3) early PDA closure, and (4) pharmacologic management. Sufficient PIP should be used to prevent atelectasis while maintaining the lowest F_{IO_2} (if possible, 0.5 or lower) to maintain adequate

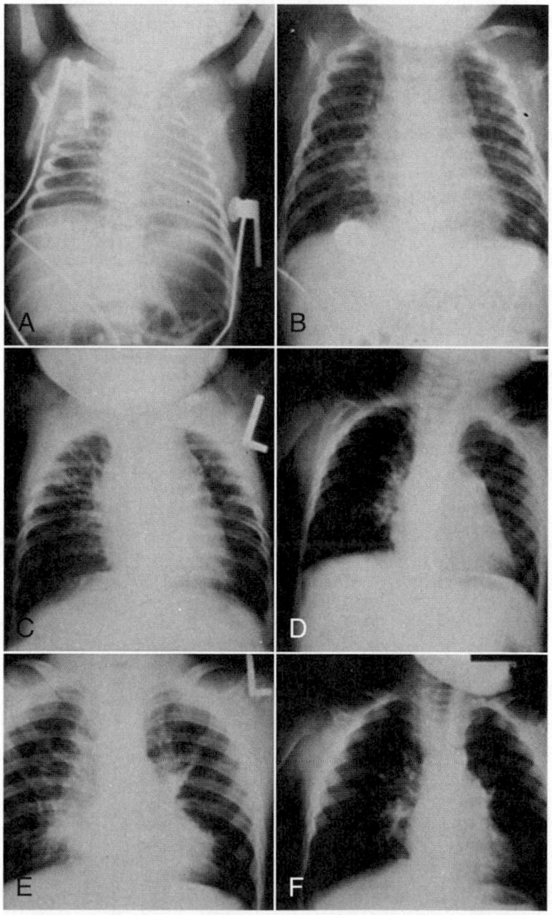

FIGURE 23-3 Serial chest x-ray films of premature infant with bronchopulmonary dysplasia over 2-year period. **A,** Newborn. **B,** 2 months. **C,** 3 months. **D,** 1 year. **E,** 2 years. Infant's disease process was characterized by multiple hospitalizations for reactive airway disease and pulmonary hypertension. Note progressive lung disease characterized by hyperinflation and eventual clearing of infiltrate by 2 years of age **(F)**.

oxygenation (i.e., PaO_2 60 to 80 mm Hg; O_2 saturation 90% to 95%). Weaning from mechanical ventilation is done slowly and may be facilitated by (1) use of SIMV that reduces the work of breathing, (2) use of methylxanthines before extubation, and (3) use of nasal CPAP after extubation.[17,96,97] **Usually in CLD/BPD, the infant's ability to maintain ventilation develops before the ability to maintain adequate oxygenation.** Often infants are discharged from the NICU on home oxygen therapy. **Infants with CLD/BPD who require oxygen at a rate of 20 mL/kg/min or less and those who can maintain oxygen saturations of 92% or above after 40 minutes of breathing room air are ready to begin successful weaning from supplemental oxygen.**[336]

Neonates with CLD/BPD have an increased resting metabolic expenditure as the major reason for growth failure, especially in the smallest, sickest infants.[212] These infants may require 150 to 200 kcal/kg/day to support adequate growth (i.e., 10 to 30 g/day weight gain). Without adequate protein or caloric intake, damaged pulmonary tissue cannot heal, and provision of appropriate nutrition to the neonate with BPD is essential (see Chapters 14 through 18).

Pharmacologic management of CLD/BPD includes the use of bronchodilators, steroids, and diuretics (Table 23-9). Inhaled and systemic bronchodilators improve lung mechanics and gaseous exchange by relaxation of bronchial smooth muscle.[95]

TABLE 23-9 PHARMACOLOGIC AGENTS USED IN TREATMENT OF CHRONIC LUNG DISEASE/BRONCHOPULMONARY DYSPLASIA

DRUG	DOSAGE	COMMENTS
I. Bronchodilators		Further clinical trials are needed to assess the role of bronchodilators and diuretics in the treatment and prevention of CLD/BPD.[265]
A. Inhaled		
1. $Beta_2$-agonists		
a. Albuterol (Proventil; Ventolin)	0.1 mg/kg up to 5 mg in 2 mL of NS solution q 4-6 hr Max dose: 0.5 mL or 2.5 mg/treatment; up to six treatments/24 hr Onset: 5-15 min Peak action: 30 min to 2 hr Duration: 3-4 hr	Drug of choice for bronchospasm—improves pulmonary resistance and lung compliance by bronchial smooth muscle relaxation; tachycardia, tremors, nausea and vomiting; can cause paradoxical bronchoconstriction, irritability. MDI dosage improves lung function as well as nebulization, is faster and more cost effective.
b. Terbutaline (Brethine)	0.03-0.3 mg/kg/day Onset: 5-30 min Duration: 3-4 hr	Same as for albuterol.
2. Histamine inhibitor (Cromolyn: 20 mg/2 mL solution for nebulizer)	10-20 mg TID	Prevents release of inflammatory mediators and reduces airway hypersensitivity; urticaria, rash, and throat irritation; dosage may need adjusting in patients with hepatic or renal dysfunction. A systematic review showed no significant evidence that cromolyn has a role in the treatment or prevention of CLD/BPD.[266]
B. Systemic		
1. Methylxanthines		
a. Caffeine citrate	Loading: 20 mg/kg Maintenance: 5 mg/kg/day IV or PO Half-life: as long as 100 hr	Promotes weaning from low rates of ventilatory support by reduction of pulmonary resistance, improved lung compliance, and improved skeletal muscle and diaphragmatic contractility, has diuretic effect; excreted unchanged in urine; safer drug with fewer side effects than theophylline. Side effects rare but include tachycardia, diuresis, dysrhythmias, glucosuria, seizures, ketonuria, vomiting, hyperglycemia, jitteriness, hemorrhagic gastritis.

BID, Two times/day; *BUN*, blood urea nitrogen; *CLD/BPD*, chronic lung disease/bronchopulmonary dysplasia; *CNS*, central nervous system; *GFR*, glomerular filtration rate; *GI*, gastrointestinal; *IV*, intravenously; *KCl*, potassium chloride; *LOS*, length of stay; *MDI*, metered dose inhaler; *NS*, normal saline; *PO*, per os, orally; *PVR*, pulmonary vascular resistance; *TID*, three times/day.

Continued

TABLE 23-9 PHARMACOLOGIC AGENTS USED IN TREATMENT OF CHRONIC LUNG DISEASE/ BRONCHOPULMONARY DYSPLASIA—cont'd

DRUG	DOSAGE	COMMENTS
b. Theophylline (PO)	4-6 mg of active theophylline, which should produce a serum level of 10-20 mcg/mL Maintenance: calculated by rate of plasma clearance, usually 3-7 mg/kg/day q 12 hr Half-life: 30-40 hr	Metabolized to caffeine in the liver and excreted in urine; multisystem effect; CNS stimulant; increases respiratory rate, inspiratory drive, and surfactant production; increases GFR; increases heart rate, contractility, and output; decreases GI motility and increases GI secretions; increases glucose levels, ketonuria, and glycosuria; increases muscle contractility; increases catecholamine and insulin levels. Side effects: same as for caffeine citrate.
2. Beta$_2$-agonists		
a. Terbutaline	5 mcg/kg Sub-Q q 4-6 hr	Improves pulmonary mechanics; side effects same as for albuterol on p. 621; adjunct to methylxanthines.
b. Albuterol	0.15 mg/kg/dose PO q 8 hr	Reduces pulmonary resistance; adjunct to methylxanthines; side effects same as albuterol on p. 621.
II. Steroids		
A. Inhaled		
1. Corticosteroids (dexamethasone [Decadron])	100 mcg/inhalation from MDI	30%-60% systemic bioavailability versus 53%-78% from oral intake; majority removed from lung within 20 min after administration; anatomic, physiologic, and pathophysiologic variations in the neonate, coupled with the aerosol delivery system and its use, influence the amount of drug actually administered and the aerosol's efficacy. Side effects: oral candidiasis, bronchospasm, and pituitary-adrenal suppression, tongue hypertrophy. No evidence that early (<2 weeks of age) administration to ventilated preterms is effective in reducing CLD/BPD.[327] No evidence of a difference in side effects or effectiveness in inhaled vs. systemic steroids.[326]
2. Glucocorticoids		
a. Flunisolide (Nasalide)	250 mcg/inhalation	Unknown stability—do not mix with other drugs; bronchospasm may result from buffers and/or preservatives. Side effects: same as for dexamethasone.
b. Beclomethasone (Beconase; Vancenase)	42 mcg/inhalation	
B. Systemic (corticosteroids—dexamethasone [Decadron])	0.5 mg/kg/day IV or PO q 12 hr for 3 days; decrease to 0.3 mg/kg/day for 3 days Taper 10%-20% q 3 days	Hyperglycemia; hypothalamic-pituitary-adrenal axis suppression; renal calcification; protein depletion and/or tissue catabolism (increase BUN; failure to gain weight); gastric irritation, perforation, bleeding; restlessness and/or irritability; myocardial hypertrophy; hypertension; increased risk for infection (see Box 23-7).
	Initial dose: 0.1 to 0.2 mg/kg/day for 3 days[184] If extubated, taper dose over 3-6 days (total treatment 6-9 days) If unable to extubate after initial 3 days of therapy, discontinue therapy[184]	Use for ventilator-dependent infant at 14-28 days of age who is developing CLD/BPD to accomplish extubation. Lower dose for shorter treatment period. Avoids hyperglycemia and hypertension seen in the higher doses of longer duration.[184]

BID, Two times/day; *BUN,* blood urea nitrogen; *CLD/BPD,* chronic lung disease/bronchopulmonary dysplasia; *CNS,* central nervous system; *GFR,* glomerular filtration rate; *GI,* gastrointestinal; *IV,* intravenously; *KCl,* potassium chloride; *LOS,* length of stay; *MDI,* metered dose inhaler; *NS,* normal saline; *PO,* per os, orally; *PVR,* pulmonary vascular resistance; *TID,* three times/day.

TABLE 23-9 PHARMACOLOGIC AGENTS USED IN TREATMENT OF CHRONIC LUNG DISEASE/BRONCHOPULMONARY DYSPLASIA—cont'd

DRUG	DOSAGE	COMMENTS
III. Diuretics		
A. Furosemide (Lasix)	1-2 mg/kg/dose IV BID or 2-4 mg/kg/dose PO BID Onset: 5 min IV; 1 hr PO Duration: 2-4 hr	Acute and chronic administration of furosemide in preterm infants >3 weeks of age with CLD/BPD improves lung compliance. Chronic administration of IV or PO furosemide also improves oxygenation. Routine or sustained use of systemic loop diuretics in infants with or developing CLD/BPD cannot be recommended based on current evidence.[51] Treatment of choice for fluid overload in CLD/BPD—decrease interstitial edema and PVR; daily or alternate-day administration improves pulmonary mechanics and facilitates weaning from ventilator. Side effects: metabolic acidosis, hypokalemia, hypocalcemia, hypochloremia, hyponatremia, renal calcifications, gallstones, ototoxicity, requires KCl supplementation. For preterms >3 weeks of age with CLD/BPD, administration of distal diuretics improves pulmonary mechanics.[51] Further study is needed to assess whether thiazide administration reduces mortality, decreases duration of oxygen and ventilator dependency, shortens LOS, and improves long-term outcomes of infants with CLD/BPD.[52]
B. Thiazide		
1. Chlorothiazide (Diuril)	5-20 mg/kg/dose IV or PO BID	Less potent than furosemide; promotes potassium and bicarbonate excretion with sodium and chloride; spares calcium given with spironolactone. Combination of thiazide and spironolactone results in improved lung mechanics and increased urine output. Side effects: electrolyte imbalance, hypercalcemia, hyperglycemia, decreased magnesium level, hypersensitivity, GI upset, glycosuria.
2. Hydrochlorothiazide (HydroDIURIL)	1-2 mg/kg/dose PO BID Onset: 1-2 hr Duration: 6-12 hr	Side effects: electrolyte imbalance, hypercalcemia, hyperglycemia, metabolic alkalosis, increased urinary losses of sodium, potassium, magnesium, chloride, phosphorus, and bicarbonate; spares calcium.
3. Spironolactone (Aldactone)	1.5 mg/kg/dose PO BID Onset: 2-3 days	Weak diuretic; causes increased sodium chloride and water loss; spares potassium. Side effects: irritability, lethargy, vomiting, diarrhea, rash.
4. Bumetanide (Bumex)	0.015 mg/kg/day up to 0.1 mg/kg/day PO	40 times the potency of furosemide; used in neonates and infants with CLD/BPD refractory to furosemide therapy. Side effects: same as for furosemide plus hypophosphatemia.

However, bronchodilators may fail to relieve airway obstruction because of relatively poor development of bronchial smooth muscle in preterm infants.

Methylxanthine therapy promotes weaning of infants with RDS from low rates of ventilatory support.[162] A meta-analysis of six trials evaluating the prophylactic use of methylxanthine treatment for successful intubation observed a 27% absolute reduction in the incidence of failed extubation. This benefit was observed in infants less than 1000 g and those younger than 1 week. The advantages were lost if the infants were less than 1000 g and older than 1 week or 1000 to 1250 g who had failed extubation once.[162]

Diuretics alone and diuretics combined with methylxanthines improve lung mechanics, clinical respiratory status, and ability to wean from mechanical ventilation (see Table 23-9). Aerosolized diuretics (e.g., a single dose of furosemide at 1 mg/kg) transiently improve lung mechanics in preterms older than 3 weeks with CLD/BPD. RCTs are needed to evaluate the effects of aerosolized diuretics on oxygen dependence, mortality, duration of ventilator use, length of stay, and long-term outcomes.[53]

Use of antenatal steroid therapy is associated with improved survival, more rapid ventilator weaning because of decreased severity of RDS, and decreased need for supplemental oxygen (e.g., CLD/BPD) in at-risk neonates and lowers the incidence of IVH and PDA.[260,314] **Steroids reduce lung inflammation and improve pulmonary function in severe RDS.**[240] Even the choice of which glucocorticoid to use antenatally may be significant. Betamethasone, rather than dexamethasone, is associated with reduced risk for neonatal death and trends toward risk reduction for other adverse neonatal outcomes (e.g., IVH, severe IVH, and ROP).[220] A National Institutes of Health consensus statement[260] discourages multiple courses of antenatal steroids because of (1) impaired head/fetal growth, (2) impaired brain development and behavior and psychomotor development,[118] (3) increased incidence of IVH, (4) increased sepsis, mortality, and lung disease,[283,385] (5) associated gastroesophageal reflux,[63] and (6) an increased severity of ROP. Two recent studies of 2-year-olds and 2- to 3-year-olds exposed to multiple courses of antenatal steroids found no significant differences in somatic growth or neurocognitive measures.[87,388] However, in the U.S. study, there was a non–statistically significant difference in the incidence of cerebral palsy (e.g., 2.9% in the repeated-doses group vs. 0.5% in the placebo group) that is concerning and requires further study.[388]

Postnatal steroid use became widespread in the 1990s without properly conducted RCTs for safety and efficacy,[125] despite warnings from researchers in the 1970s about serious potential dangers. Steroid use has been enthusiastically accepted because of the dramatic, short-term improvements in respiratory status (e.g., facilitates extubation, more rapid ventilator weaning, reduces the risk for CLD/BPD and PDA).[40,106,155,156] Two large RCTs of postnatal steroid use were halted because of serious short-term complications—intestinal perforation, growth retardation, PVL, hyperglycemia, hypertension, and infection.[141,347] **Adverse long-term outcomes are listed in Box 23-7. Adverse developmental outcomes are the result of the effects of steroids on the developing nervous system.**[26,30,261,407] Two meta-analyses caution that the short-term benefits of early (<7 days) and late (>7 days) **postnatal steroids may not outweigh the actual or potential adverse effects.**[232,234] In a recent report, decreased use of postnatal steroids (23.5% to 11%) resulted in an increase in CLD/BPD (12.9% to 18.7%).[333] A more recent retrospective analysis of decreasing postnatal steroid use in extremely preterm infants found no increase in CLD/BPD or home oxygen use and a (nonsignificant) reduction in the incidence of CP with a decrease in dexamethasone use.[325]

The efficacy of inhaled steroids in decreasing pulmonary inflammation and CLD/BPD while decreasing the incidence and severity of complications of systemic steroid usage is being studied. Using surfactant as a vehicle for administration, early intratracheal instillation of corticosteroid has been shown in a pilot study to significantly improve the outcomes of death and chronic lung disease in small preterms without short-term adverse effects.[408] In a

BOX 23-7 LONG-TERM ADVERSE EFFECTS OF STEROID USE

Slower Growth[30,347]

- Somatic and head growth
- Arrested lung development caused by interference in pulmonary alveolarization and vascularization

"Neurotoxic" Substances[26,30,261,386]

- Further reduces size/cerebral tissue/gray matter volume of premature brain[278]
- Increased rate of cerebral palsy (CP)[107,407]
- Increased risk for CP significantly related to the total cumulative doses of dexamethasone[294]
- Increased cognitive deficits[352,386,407]: at school age, children had lower scores on verbal or written language skills, math, perceptual organization, freedom from distractibility, and processing speed[407]
- Increased severity of retinopathy of prematurity[386]

Contributes to Long-Term

- Cardiovascular disease[274]
- Immune system disorders/autoimmune diseases
- Renal calcifications
- Neurologic and behavioral deficits[261,386]

small (n = 10) study, inhaled corticosteroid therapy was associated with a reduction in cytokine levels (≥2 weeks after therapy) in the sputum of very preterm infants with CLD/BPD; cytokines were significantly lower in the HFV versus CMV group.[174] Meta-analysis of the early administration (in first 2 weeks of life) of inhaled steroids to ventilated preterms does not decrease the incidence of CLD/BPD.[327] Meta-analysis of inhaled versus systemic steroid use found no difference in the incidence of CLD/BPD and the duration of intubation or oxygen dependence and no follow-up data regarding neurodevelopmental outcomes from inhaled steroid use.[326] Delivery of therapeutic levels of drug to the lungs is problematic and may account for the lack of efficacy of inhaled steroids.[184] **Based on available evidence, the use of inhaled steroids for preterm infants cannot be recommended.**[326,327]

Historically, steroids have been "routinely" used with widely varying practices about type of medication (e.g., natural hormone [hydrocortisone] or synthetic hormones [dexamethasone; betamethasone]), dosage (e.g., standard or low dose), timing (e.g., early or late), and duration (e.g., weaning after 7 to 10 days or 42-day treatment).[125,184] Considered "routine practice," parents were rarely asked to give informed consent. Parents (in addition to health care providers)[26,347] must be honestly informed about the experimental nature of steroid use and its short-term and long-term complications, so that they are able to participate in giving or withholding their fully informed consent.[25,159] A recent RCT (DART Study)[106] of low-dose steroid use was halted because infants could not be recruited; fully informed parents concerned about risks to their infant refused permission to be part of the study.

After reviewing the short-term and long-term effects of systemic and inhaled corticosteroid use for the prevention and treatment of CLD/BPD in the VLBW infant, the AAP and Canadian Pediatric Society have published joint recommendations[10]:

- Routine use of systemic dexamethasone to prevent or treat CLD/BPD in VLBW infants is not recommended.
- Postnatal use of systemic dexamethasone should be limited to carefully designed RCTs.
- Long-term neurodevelopmental assessment is strongly encouraged.
- The use of alternative anti-inflammatory corticosteroids, both systemic and inhaled, awaits RCTs before additional recommendations.
- Outside of RCTs, use of corticosteroids should be limited to exceptional clinical circumstances and written informed parental consent.

Use of postnatal steroids has declined from its peak in 1997 (28% use in Vermont Oxford Network [VON]; 23% use in Neonatal Research Network) to a rate in 2006 of 8% of VLBW infants in VON, and 23% of these infants were at highest risk for CLD/BPD (e.g., 501 to 750 g).[184] Recent research shows benefits (e.g., better lung function at school age; improved neurodevelopmental outcome)[148,268] and no adverse effects (e.g., no difference in neurodevelopmental impairment, growth, fat mass, blood pressure, incidence of cerebral palsy [CP], or death when compared with controls at school age)[275,391,402] of postnatal steroid use when compared with older research.[184] Other recent research still shows adverse effects of postnatal steroids: (1) reduced cerebral tissue/gray matter volume, (2) increased incidence of CP, (3) increased risk for CP that is significantly related to the total cumulative dose of dexamethasone, and (4) poorer neurodevelopmental outcomes.[107,261,278,294] Doyle et al used a meta-regression analysis and found that postnatal corticosteroids actually decreased the risk for CP and death when used in the population of infants having a more than 50% risk for developing CLD/BPD.[107] "Routine use" (e.g., treating every preterm, including those with a low risk for CLD/BPD) may increase the risk for adverse outcomes.[107,184] Postnatal steroids continue to be administered to the smallest, sickest (ELBW/VLBW) ventilated preterms who are developing CLD/BPD.[184] **The dose and duration of use of late postnatal corticosteroids should be minimized and reserved for preterms who cannot wean from the ventilator.**[155,184,261] Table 23-9 gives a proposed (expert opinion rather than evidence-based) dosing regimen for low-dose, short-duration treatment with dexamethasone.[184]

Complications. Complications of CLD/BPD are **most common in the smallest, sickest infants (Box 23-8).**

RESPIRATORY SYNCYTIAL VIRUS INFECTION

More than 50% of infants with CLD/BPD are rehospitalized within the first 2 years of life, usually with viral respiratory infections. Respiratory syncytial virus (RSV) is the major cause of pneumonia, bronchiolitis, and otitis media in young

BOX 23-8

COMPLICATIONS OF CHRONIC LUNG DISEASE/BRONCHOPULMONARY DYSPLASIA[70,386]

Increased Mortality

Increased Morbidity

Pulmonary

- *Acute:* pulmonary interstitial emphysema, air leaks, pulmonary hypertension, cyst formation
- *Chronic:* altered pulmonary function, respiratory infections, rehospitalizations, home oxygen

Cardiac

- Cor pulmonale and right-sided heart failure

Growth Restriction

- Somatic growth (weight)
- Head growth

Orthopedic

- Fractures, rickets

Neurodevelopmental Delay

- Cognitive impairment/impaired intelligence/increased need for special education services
- Cerebral palsy/delays in gross motor skills
- Behavior/attention/school problems
- Cerebral ventriculomegaly

Sensory Deficits

- Sensorineural hearing loss
- Increased severity (stage 3) retinopathy of prematurity

Long-Term Effects of Steroid Use

- See Box 23-7

children.[291] There is increased morbidity and mortality in preterm infants younger than 6 months and in young children (2 years of age or younger) with CLD/BPD or congenital heart disease.[291] **RSV risk factors are found in Box 23-9.** RSV is a seasonal infection that occurs from winter (October to December) to early spring (March to May).

RSV infection may be prevented by educating parents and by pharmacologic prophylaxis. Parents should be taught the following principles of infection control:

- Practice good hand hygiene (washing; use of hand rubs).
- Clean infant bedding, toys, play area frequently; do not allow the infant's personal items (e.g., cups, bottles, pacifiers) to be shared.
- Restrict contacts with the infant (no one with a cold).
- Avoid crowds (e.g., day care, shopping areas, church nurseries, children's parties).
- Reduce or eliminate day care, or use day care with only one or two children.
- Eliminate exposure to secondhand tobacco smoke.
- Vaccinate all high-risk infants for influenza beginning at 6 months of age, as well as all of their contacts.
- Vaccinate monthly for RSV according to the recommendations in Box 23-9.

Palivizumab (Synagis), a humanized monoclonal antibody, results in a hospitalization rate for RSV infection of 1.3% and an even lower rate with home-care prophylaxis with palivizumab.[133] Higher rates of hospitalization are associated with gender, gestational age less than 32 weeks, chronic lung disease, congenital heart disease, congenital airway abnormality, severe neuromuscular disease, Medicaid, and more than two other children in the household.[133] **RSV prophylaxis (Table 23-10) should be initiated at the beginning and terminated at the end of RSV season, taking into account regional differences.** Palivizumab is costly and studies report conflicting cost-effectiveness of treatment.[110,396] However, cost-effectiveness research does not often study the impact of RSV infection and hospitalization on the family. A recent study showed that significant stress (e.g., health and functional status of the child; more caregiver stress, poorer health, anxiety, and poorer family functioning) occurred at hospitalization and for as long as 60 days after discharge.[222]

RETINOPATHY OF PREMATURITY

Since the 1950s, researchers have recognized the association among oxygen administration, prematurity, and subsequent retinal changes often resulting in blindness.[335] Severe restriction in the use of oxygen with premature infants resulted in less ROP but also in increased morbidity and mortality rates. ROP develops in 84% of preterm survivors of less than 28 weeks GA.[363] Incidence rates and severity of ROP vary among NICUs. In 80% of cases, ROP spontaneously regresses without visual loss.[88,363] Some centers report unchanged or decreased incidence and severity of ROP despite increasing survival of

BOX 23-9 RISK FACTORS FOR RESPIRATORY SYNCYTIAL VIRUS INFECTION AND RECOMMENDATIONS FOR PROPHYLAXIS

Eligible for a Maximum of 5 Doses of Palivizumab Prophylaxis

- Infants with major risk factors: gestational age and post-conceptual age
  - Preterm infants less than 32 weeks GA ($31\frac{6}{7}$ weeks)
    - Preterm infants less than 28 weeks GA: Give prophylaxis during RSV season (whenever it occurs in the first 12 months of life)
    - Preterm infants 29-32 weeks GA ($31\frac{6}{7}$ weeks): Benefit most if less than 6 months of age at the start of RSV season
- Infants with chronic lung disease of prematurity (CLD)
  - Preterm infants less than 24 months of age who receive medical therapy for their CLD within 6 months of the start of RSV season (for severe CLD, preterms may also benefit from prophylaxis in their second RSV season)
- Infants less than or equal to 24 months of age with hemodynamically significant cyanotic or acyanotic CHD
  - Most likely to benefit are infants with CHF (if medications are required), moderate to severe pulmonary hypertension, or cyanotic CHD
  - These infants are not at increased risk for RSV and should not be given prophylaxis:
    - Infants with hemodynamically insignificant CHD (such as ASD, VSD, PDA, uncomplicated AS, PS, and mild coarctation of the aorta)
    - Infants with surgically corrected CHD (unless CHF medications are needed)
    - Infants with mild cardiomyopathy
- Infants with immunodeficiency disease (either acquired or congenital) or treatment causing immunosuppression at any age
- Infants with congenital abnormalities of the airway or neuromuscular disease
  - Infants born less than 35 weeks GA
  - Infants with conditions that compromise their handling of respiratory secretions (e.g., CP, Down syndrome[46])

Eligible for Maximum of 3 Doses of Palivizumab Prophylaxis

Risk Factors

- Infants with major risk factors: gestational age and post-conceptual age
  - Eligibility for prophylaxis is defined as $32\frac{0}{7}$ weeks to $34\frac{6}{7}$ weeks GA
- Infants must have one of two risk factors:
  - Attendance at child care
  - Siblings less than 5 years of age

Age Cut-Off

- Eligibility criteria of less than 3 months of age at the start of RSV season or born during RSV season

Dosing

- A maximum of 3 doses is to be given
- Stop dosing once the infant is 3 months (90 days) of age (whenever that occurs in RSV season)

Modified from American Academy of Pediatrics: Red Book: Report of the Committee on Infectious Diseases, ed 29, Elk Grove Village, Illinois, 2009.

AS, Aortic stenosis; *ASD,* atrial septal defect; *CP,* cerebral palsy; *CHD,* congenital heart disease; *CHF,* congestive heart failure; *CLD,* chronic lung disease; *GA,* gestational age; *PDA,* patent ductus arteriosus; *PS,* pulmonary stenosis; *VSD,* ventricular septal defect.

TABLE 23-10 PHARMACOLOGIC PROPHYLAXIS FOR RESPIRATORY SYNCYTIAL VIRUS INFECTION

DRUG	DOSE	COMMENTS
Palivizumab (Synagis)	15 mg/kg IM once a month during RSV season First dose administered before onset of RSV season Use open vial within 6 hours	Does not interfere with MMR/varicella vaccines. *Adverse effects:* mild/transient erythema at the injection site; pain, induration, and swelling; bruising; fever; rash; URTI; otitis media, rhinitis; hernia; increased SGOT. Monitor vital signs, blood pressures, and oxygen saturation before and after administration.

IM, intramuscular; *MMR,* measles, mumps, rubella; *RSV,* respiratory syncytial virus; *SGOT,* serum glutamate oxaloacetate transaminase; *URTI,* upper respiratory tract infection.

ELBW infants, whereas others report an increased incidence in severity of ROP with decreased gestational age, decreased birth weight, and decreased number of days fed breast milk.[108]

Pathophysiology. The pathophysiologic process in the development of ROP is not completely understood. **Many factors, not just oxygen, are involved in the pathogenesis of ROP (Box 23-10).** Abnormal growth and development of retinal vessels that results in ROP depends on the immaturity of retinal vasculature and exposure of these immature retinal vessels to injury or an abnormal environment. **The degree of retinal vascularization at birth determines the individual's susceptibility to the insults listed in Box 23-10.** The majority of retinal vascularization is complete by 32 weeks' gestation. However, even at 40 weeks, the temporal periphery of the retina may still not be completely vascularized.

In response to hyperoxia, the retinal vessels constrict. They may permanently constrict and become necrotic (vaso-obliteration). The resultant hypoxia of the inner retina stimulates the vessels (by vascular endothelial growth factor [VEGF]) that have not been obliterated to proliferate in an attempt to reestablish retinal circulation. Proliferating vessels may extend into the vitreous, causing fluid leakage or hemorrhage, with retinal scar formation, traction on the retina, detachment, and blindness.

BOX 23-10 FACTORS ASSOCIATED WITH RETINOPATHY OF PREMATURITY

Pregnancy Complications

- Primary hypertension
- Pregnancy-induced hypertension
- Diabetes
- Bleeding
- Smoking

Prematurity—Low Birth Weight and Low Gestational Age

- Babies with the lowest birth weights (<1000 g) and lowest gestational ages (<29 weeks) have the highest risk for the development of ROP and blindness.[108]
- Multiple gestation

Supplemental Oxygen

- Vascular endothelial growth factor (VEGF), necessary for normal angiogenesis, is stimulated by hypoxia and decreases in the presence of hyperoxia. Both single episodes and repeated cycles of hypoxia/hyperoxia stimulate VEGF expression.[332]
- Hypoxia causes increase of VEGF factor and protein in the retina within 30 minutes to 2 hours after hypoxic insult. When retinal cells are exposed to normoxic environment, there is a gradual decrease in vascular endothelial growth factor but not in protein levels. Desaturations of oxygen (decreased pulse oximeter readings) are associated with increased severity of ROP.
- Hyperoxia causes oxidant stress-induced vaso-obliteration of ROP. Risk for ROP from increased oxygen saturations (e.g., 96% to 99%) is a concern in preterms in the earlier postnatal period (before 34 weeks postmenstrual age). This earlier postnatal use of high oxygen saturations (hyperoxia) may worsen ROP.[363]
- Oxygen radicals are a major causative factor in oxygen-induced retinopathy.[316]

Growth Hormone Deficiency

- Vascular low serum concentrations of insulin-like growth factor I (IGF-1) after preterm birth is associated with the development of ROP by preventing the normal survival of vascular endothelial cells.[328]
- IGF-1 deficit results in a parallel growth deficit in the head circumference of preterms with ROP.[230]

Ventilator Support

- Increased risk for ROP with more complex medical problems, prolonged oxygen requirements, lower overall arterial oxygen levels, and more episodes of fluctuating blood levels. Prolonged ventilatory support with episodes of hypoxia, hyperoxia, hypocapnia/hypercapnia.

Surfactant Therapy

- Administration of surfactant may be associated with hypoxemia as a result of obstruction of the ETT.[262]
- Significant improvements in supplemental oxygen needs and ventilator requirements occur within 10 to 15 minutes because of a change in lung compliance that may result in hypocarbia and/or hyperoxia.

Apnea/Bradycardia

- Causes repeated cycles of hypoxia/hyperoxia and hypocapnia/hypercapnia with stimulation to breathe and increasing oxygen concentrations and need for cardiopulmonary resuscitation, exposing retinal vessels to alternating ischemia and hyperoxic toxicity.[198]

BOX 23-10 FACTORS ASSOCIATED WITH RETINOPATHY OF PREMATURITY—cont'd

Hypercapnia/Hypocapnia

- Prolonged exposure to carbon dioxide impairs developmental retinal neovascularization through increasing endothelial nitric oxide synthesis and inducing nitrative stress.[219]

Asphyxia/Acidosis/Shock

Blood Transfusion/Anemia

- Anemia, a decrease in oxygen-carrying capacity, results in increased FiO_2 to maintain adequate oxygenation, thus exposing the lung/retina to more oxygen/oxygen toxicity.[37]
- Blood transfusions and the use of recombinant human erythropoietin (rhEPO) in preterms of lower gestational age are associated with increased risk for ROP.[55,355]

Sepsis

- Fungal sepsis significantly and independently associated with ROP in ELBW and only with threshold ROP.[233]
- Cytokines that are released during sepsis may be involved in neovascularization of the retina.

Steroids

Antenatal

Conflicting study results:

  - Significant increased risk for ROP
  - No effect of antenatal steroids on increased risk for ROP

Postnatal

Conflicting study results:

  - Increased risk for stage 3 ROP with decreasing gestational age and increased number of courses of steroids
  - Increased risk for ROP because of increased vascular tortuosity; steroids have an angiogenic effect on retinal vascular development
  - Increased risk for ROP: 15% without versus 48% with postnatal steroid use; 8% without and 32% with steroid use[303]
  - Use of postnatal steroids associated with increased risk for severe ROP requiring cryotherapy
  - Late postnatal systemic steroid use more common in the ROP group[338]
  - No significant association with severe ROP[10]

Intraventricular Hemorrhage/Seizures

- Infants with severe IVH and PVL are at increased risk for development of ROP and prethreshold disease.
- Preterm infants with ROP requiring laser surgery are at significantly increased risk for nonvision neurodevelopmental impairments.

Hyperglycemia

- Hyperglycemia in the first month of life in VLBW infants is associated with the development of ROP.[116]

Nutritional Deficiency (e.g., Antioxidants)

- Preterms have low antioxidant (vitamin E) reserves and are vulnerable to tissue damage as a result of necessary supplemental oxygen. Plasma vitamin E levels are positively correlated with vitamin E intakes; early nutrient intervention may decrease susceptibility to tissue damage from oxygen exposure.
- Low plasma vitamin A concentrations.[232]
- Poor postnatal weight gain; poor enteral intake of antioxidants.[19,316]

Ethnicity/Genetics

- White infants develop severe ROP and require laser therapy more often than black infants,[359] whose fundal pigmentation may modify the risk for ROP.
- Black infants are less likely to develop ROP and have a significant protective effect in slowing the progression to threshold ROP.[359,363]
- Strong genetic predisposition to the development of ROP.[45]

Exposure to Bright Light

- May contribute to free radical–induced oxidative retinal vascular damage and ROP.
- Multicenter study of light reduction not associated with decrease in ROP or morbidity for VLBW infants[309]; ocular protection did not reduce the incidence of ROP.[49]

Photopic Adaptation

- Exposure of the eye to room light decreases oxygen consumption of the retina, thus decreasing retinal ischemia; retinal oxygen consumption increases in the dark, rather than in light exposure.

Bilirubin/Phototherapy

- Retrospective study of 128 infants (≤800 g; ≤27 weeks' gestational age)—severe visual loss as a result of ROP significantly associated with low peak serum bilirubin concentrations (<9.4 mg/dL), low gestational age, and longer duration of phototherapy.[409]
- Elevated peak serum bilirubin levels may be a risk factor in VLBW infants.[249]

ELBW, Extremely low birth weight; *ETT,* Endotracheal tube; *IVH,* intraventricular hemorrhage; *PVL,* periventricular leukomalacia; *RCTs,* randomized controlled trials; *ROP,* retinopathy of prematurity; *VLBW,* very low birth weight.

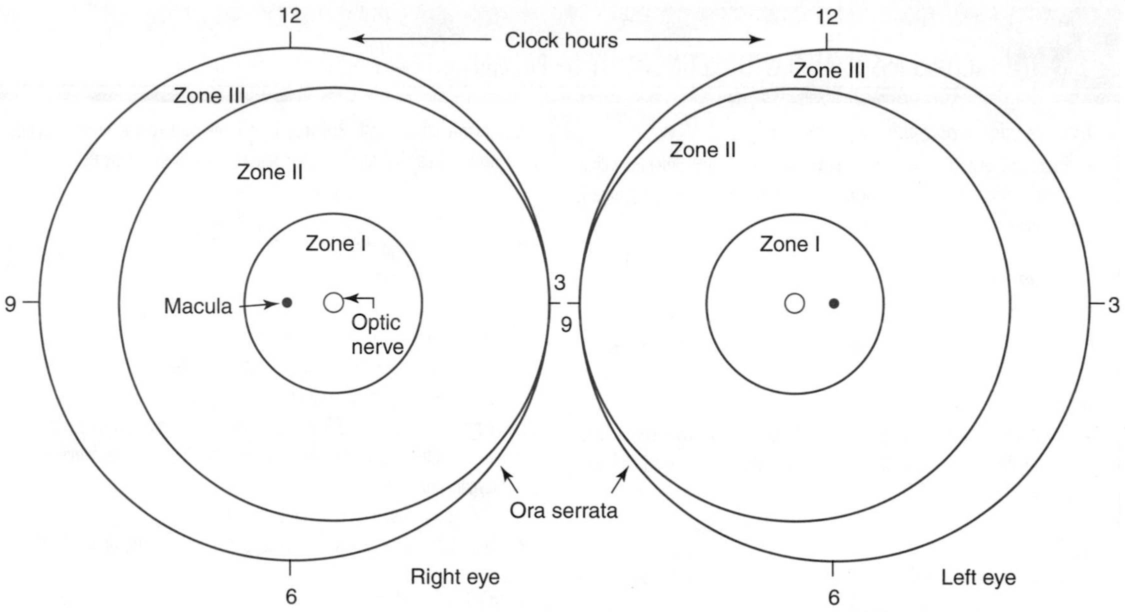

FIGURE 23-4 International classification of retinopathy of prematurity. (Courtesy Ross Laboratories, Columbus, Ohio.)

Early changes may first be evident at the temporal periphery, because this area is the last to be completely vascularized. Proliferation of new vessels may remain localized and spontaneously resolve or may progress to cause total retinal detachment.

ROP is classified by location of disease in the retina (zone), by degree (stage) of vascular abnormality, and by extent of developing vasculature (clock hour) (Figure 23-4 and Table 23-11).[181] When excessive vessels are reabsorbed and normal vascularization is reestablished, the central retinal regression of ROP occurs.

Etiology. **ROP is considered primarily a disease of prematurity,** because once vascularization is complete, the retinal vessels are no longer susceptible to injury. **The incidence is inversely proportional to birth weight and gestational age.** Damage may occur in any preterm infant and has its highest incidence in infants younger than 28 weeks' gestation. Infants weighing less than 1500 g (appropriate weight for gestational age) have the highest incidence of disease and the highest incidence of blindness.[108]

Prevention. Preventing prematurity is the best way to prevent ROP. Because multiple gestation is associated with babies of low birth weight and shorter gestation, higher order multiples should be avoided.

Decreasing light levels and the vulnerable preterm infant's exposure to bright light has not been shown to decrease the incidence of ROP.[287,309] However, in one study, the eye protection (goggles) was placed within the first 24 hours of life, after the infant had already been exposed to the bright lights at birth, during NICU admission, and during the ophthalmoscopic examination.

Intravenous D-penicillamine, used to treat hyperbilirubinemia in Europe, has been shown to significantly lower the incidence of acute ROP; these findings justify further studies on a broader population with careful attention to possible side effects.[286]

A Cochrane review of 26 RCTs of supplementation with vitamin E to prevent morbidity and mortality in preterm infants states that the evidence does not support the routine use of IV vitamin E at high doses or attempting to achieve serum tocopherol levels greater than 3.5 mg/dL.[50] **The current recommendation is a routine intake of 2 mL/kg/day of MVI Pediatric in VLBW infants (maximum of 5 mL/day or 7 international units/day).**[50]

Oxygen Targeting for the VLBW Preterm. Because an infant who is hyperoxic (Pao_2 >80 mm Hg)[9] clinically looks no

TABLE 23-11 STAGES OF RETINOPATHY OF PREMATURITY (ROP)

STAGES	DESCRIPTION
Stage 1: Demarcation line	A thin white line separates the avascular retina anteriorly from the vascularized retina posteriorly. Abnormal branching vessels lead to the demarcation line, which is flat and lies in the plane of the retina.
Stage 2: Ridge	The ridge has a definite height and width, occupies a volume, and extends up out of the plane of the retina. Its color may change from white to pink. Small, isolated tufts of new vessels may appear posterior to the structure.
Stage 3: Extraretinal fibrovascular proliferations	To the ridge of stage 2 is added the presence of extraretinal fibrovascular proliferative tissue. Characteristic locations: 1. Continuous with the posterior aspect of the ridge (ragged ridge) 2. Immediately posterior to the ridge but not always appearing to be connected to it 3. Into the vitreous perpendicular to the retinal plane
Stage 4: Partial retinal detachment	To stage 3 is added unequivocal detachment of the retina caused by exudative effusion of fluid, traction, or both.
Stage 4A: Extrafoveal	Detachment of the retina does not include the macula; vision may be good.
Stage 4B: Foveal	Macula is detached: visual potential markedly reduced.
Prethreshold disease[181]	Zone I, any ROP less than threshold. Zone II: • Stage 2 ROP with "plus" disease • Any amount of stage 3 ROP without "plus" disease • Stage 3 with "plus" disease
Threshold disease	Occurs with stage 3 ROP and the presence of "plus" disease.
Aggressive posterior ROP (AP-ROP) (Rush disease)	A rapid progression (in days rather than weeks) to severe ROP (without the usual progression through stages 1-3) and retinal detachment. ROP in zone I with "plus" disease: poorer prognosis for sight; usually occurs in the smallest, sickest preterms.
Stage 5: Total detachment	Complete retinal detachment: the retina is pulled into a funnel-shaped configuration by the fibrovascular scar tissue. Complete blindness in affected eye.

different from an infant whose Pao_2 is normal, **monitoring of oxygen saturations and partial pressure of oxygen with arterial blood gases is mandatory whenever oxygen is administered.** Because pulse oximetry (PO) gives immediate and continuous data, fewer Pao_2 values are obtained, so interpretation of PO readings and their relationship to Pao_2 values is critical. Because PO saturations higher than 92% can often be associated with hyperoxia (e.g., Pao_2 >80 mm Hg),[366] NICUs that accept higher PO saturations and targets have a higher incidence of ROP. Some NICUs use "higher" oxygen saturations (>90%), whereas others use "lower" saturations (<90%) both in acute and chronic phases of respiratory disease.[14]

Several observational studies have shown a decrease in the incidence of ROP (and less CLD/BPD) in the VLBW infant when oxygen saturation targets and oxygen saturation alarms are decreased in this vulnerable population at increased risk for the results of oxidative stress. **A national survey of NICUs documented a wide range of oxygen saturation guidelines.** Eighty-seven percent of the responding NICUs had guidelines requiring oxygen saturation ranges for preterms weighing 1500 g or less; 58% of the NICUs maintained oxygen saturation guidelines for preterms in the first 2 weeks of life that were different from the oxygen saturation guidelines for preterms older than 2 weeks.

The range of oxygen saturations was 82% to 100% with an average minimum saturation of 89% and an average maximum of 95% in the first 2 weeks of life.[12] When the maximum acceptable oxygen saturation was less than 89% in the first 2 weeks of life, there was less retinal ablation surgery in infants weighing 1500 g or less; conversely, when the maximum saturation was at least 98% in the first 2 weeks of life, there was a higher rate of retinal surgery. When the maximum acceptable oxygen saturation was less than 92% after the first 2 weeks of life, there was a significantly lower rate of stage 3 or higher ROP and retinal ablation surgery; conversely, when the maximum saturation was greater than 92% after 2 weeks of age, there was a high rate of stage 3 or higher ROP.[12]

A retrospective review of **NICUs with policies that maintained oxygen saturations (Spo_2) from 88% to 98% in preterms during their first 8 weeks of life found a fourfold increase in the rate of threshold ROP when compared with oxygen saturations from 70% to 90%.**[367] This study also showed no increase in CP rates between the two groups; there was an increase in adverse pulmonary sequelae (e.g., CLD/BPD; prolonged assisted ventilation) in the higher oxygen saturation group. Collated data from the Vermont Oxford Network on 1544 ELBW preterms (with oxygen saturations ≤95% and >95%) found a significantly lower incidence of stages 3 and 4 ROP (10% vs. 29%) and CLD/BPD (27% vs. 53%) among those preterms cared for with the lower targeted oxygen saturation. Another study showed a decline in severe ROP from 12.5% to 2.5% over a 5-year period after education and contracting with the staff, strict management of oxygen delivery, and monitoring to maintain strict oxygen saturation guidelines (e.g., 85% to 95% for infants >32 weeks; 85% to 93% for preterms born at 32 week or less) while on supplemental oxygen.[67] This decline in ROP may the result of lower oxygen saturations or tighter oxygen control in titrating/weaning oxygen (e.g., fewer fluctuations of oxygen saturations when oxygen was increased/decreased by only 2% to 5%) in VLBW infants (e.g., 500 to 1500 g). The ongoing evaluation of development in this cohort of infants shows that the rate of CP has not significantly changed.

Another NICU decreased PO saturations (85% to 93%) for infants 1250 grams or less or 28 weeks or less GA until these preterms had reached 32 weeks PMA or they were breathing room air. Their study compared the rate of prethreshold ROP for the 3 preceding years with the rate during the study year and found a significant decrease of 17.5% to 5.6%.[380] A nonrandomized retrospective study of all infants in one level III NICU from 2005 to 2007 evaluated the effects of strictly monitored oxygen supplementation (e.g., <34 weeks corrected GA: oxygen limits 80% to 95% and oxygen saturation targets 85% to 92%; >34 weeks corrected GA: oxygen limits 85% to 100% and oxygen saturation targets 92% to 97%).[323] The study found that use of lower oxygen targets at early gestational age and higher oxygen targets at older gestational age reduced the incidence and severity of ROP (13% [stage 3 ROP 2%] in the restricted oxygen vs. 35% [stage 3 ROP 11%] in the standard oxygen supplementation group).[323]

Even though observational studies show an association between lower target oxygen saturations and improved outcomes, they do not show a causal relationship, which must be established in RCTs such as the STOP-ROP and BOOST trials. The STOP-ROP trial was a randomized, multicenter controlled study to test the safety and efficacy of administering supplemental oxygen (to keep pulse oximetry saturations at 96% to 99%) to infants with prethreshold ROP to decrease progression to ROP. The study reported that ROP progression rates were decreased with supplemental oxygen (48.5% to 40.9% [not statistically significant]).[363] In a subset analysis in infants without "plus" disease, the progression to threshold ROP was 32% in the supplemented group versus 46% in the conventional use group (saturations 89% to 94%). The progression to ROP took longer in the supplemental group (2.5 weeks) than in the conventional group (2.4 weeks). Diagnosis of threshold ROP was at 37.3 weeks PMA in the supplemented group and 36.8 weeks PMA in the conventional group. Administering oxygen to keep saturations at 96% to 99% does not increase the severity of ROP in infants with prethreshold ROP.[363] Infants in the higher saturation, oxygen-supplemented group did not gain weight faster, and those infants with the worst lung disease had more pulmonary complications than infants on conventional oxygen supplementation.[363] The data of the STOP-ROP trial apply to infants well beyond the initial weeks after birth and do *not* show the safety of supplemental oxygen levels (saturations 96% to 99%) at younger ages.[363]

The BOOST Trial[16] randomized ELBW infants to standard (e.g., 91% to 94%) or higher (e.g., 95%

to 98%) oxygen saturations and found a reduction in the need for retinal ablative surgery in infants from higher saturation levels after 32 weeks PMA. There were no differences in the BOOST Trial in short-term or long-term growth or major developmental abnormality rates between the higher versus lower oxygen saturation ranges. However, there was an increase in infants requiring home oxygen for CLD/BPD in the higher saturation group.

Determination of appropriate oxygen saturations (Spo_2) for preterms is a balance between the risk:benefit ratio of hypoxia versus hyperoxia. Hyperoxia is associated with retinal damage and lung developmental arrest or remodeling. Hypoxia is associated with increased mortality, permanent damage to brain structures necessary for neurologic, motor, and cognitive development, damage to organ systems (e.g., heart, kidney, intestine), poor weight gain, and pulmonary hypertension. **Fluctuations of Pao_2 (e.g., hypoxemia and hyperoxemia episodes) in the VLBW preterm may be a more significant risk factor than hyperoxia for the development of threshold ROP.**[412] These episodes of hyperoxia and/or hypoxia may result from the underlying respiratory pathology or the result of care providers' interventions (e.g., positioning; suction; "chasing desaturations by increasing Fio_2"; surfactant administration). A recent systematic review[15] shows a **highly significant reduction in the incidence and severity of ROP and no differences in mortality in infants randomized to restricted rather than liberal oxygen exposure.** The reviewers concluded that unrestricted and unmonitored oxygen therapy has potential harms without clear benefits and that the reviewed data did not answer the question "What is the optimal target range for maintenance of blood oxygen levels in preterm and LBW infants?"[15]

Controversy, uncertainty, and a lack of consensus exist about the appropriate or optimal oxygen saturation for the most vulnerable preterms (e.g., <28 weeks' gestation).[12,14,365-367] Currently, multicenter, international, masked RCTs of (n = 5000) preterms (e.g., <28 weeks' gestation) who will be randomized (from birth) to clinically acceptable oxygen saturation ranges (e.g., 85% to 89% vs. 91% to 95%) are being conducted.[366]

Use of lower oxygen saturation levels may be a strategy to prevent rather than treat ROP. Changing the NICU culture to accept and comply with lower saturation levels for preterms in the first few weeks of life has been proven to be a challenge with various measures of success in keeping babies in the recommended ranges (e.g., 22%[74]; 35%[130]; 16% to 64%[153]; 57% to 59%[216]). Establishing new oxygen targeting for preterms requires knowledge about oxygen and oxygen toxicity, multidisciplinary "buy in," parental involvement, wider saturation targets, leadership, and process-improvement principles.[130,140,293] To illustrate that higher PO saturations are not better, a recent study evaluated 976 matched PO saturation levels and Pao_2 values from seven NICUs (at sea level) to evaluate whether PO values of 85% to 93% were associated with Pao_2 levels of less than 40 mm Hg.[58] When supplemental oxygen is used and the PO saturation range is maintained between 85% and 93%, high Pao_2 values very rarely occur and low Pao_2 values are infrequent. PO saturation values above 93% were frequently associated with Pao_2 values above 80 mm Hg so that **accepting an oxygen saturation greater than 93% exposes vulnerable preterm infants to the risk for hyperoxemia and subsequent oxygen toxicity to their eyes (ROP) and lungs (CLD/BPD).**[58]

Data Collection. **Because treatment with laser/cryotherapy is associated with a 50% decrease in retinal detachment, screening examinations of preterm infants for ROP are essential.** Evidence-based screening criteria have been developed based on the natural history of ROP as determined from analysis of the data of the CRYO-ROP study[128] and the LIGHT-ROP study (Box 23-11).[8]

Eye examinations are stressful and painful for the preterm infant.[34] Swaddling or nesting and providing an external heat source to prevent cold stress are useful. The infant should be positioned supine and swaddled with the head immobilized. The infant may exhibit crying or struggling, hypertonia or hypotonia, apnea, tachycardia or bradycardia, oxygen desaturation, increased blood pressure, transient paralytic ileus, feeding intolerance, necrotizing enterocolitis, and bronchospasm as a result of the use of mydriatic (Cyclomydril) eye drops and ocular stimulation during the examination. Provide monitoring with pulse oximetry and cardiorespiratory monitoring, an oxygen source, cardiopulmonary resuscitation (CPR) equipment, and rest periods as needed. Topical anesthesia, use of nonnutritive sucking, and sucrose are all strategies of pain relief for ROP examinations (see Chapter 12). Provision of eye examinations with RetCam imaging instead of indirect ophthalmoscopy is being studied.

BOX 23-11 SCREENING EXAMINATION OF PREMATURE INFANTS FOR RETINOPATHY OF PREMATURITY[8]

Target Population

- Infants with birth weight <1500 g or gestational age ≤30 weeks
- Selected infants with birth weight 1500 to 2000 g and >30 weeks gestational age with unstable clinical course who are thought to be at increased risk by their pediatricians/neonatologists
- Initial examination: at 4 to 6 weeks chronologic age OR 31 to 33 weeks PMA

Initial Eye Examination Based on Gestational Age at Birth*:

Gestational Age at Birth (week)	Age of Initial Examination (weeks)	
	Postmenstrual	Chronologic
22†	31	9
23†	31	8
24	31	7
25	31	6
26	31	5
27	31	4
28	32	4
29	33	4
30	34	4
31‡	35	4
32‡	36	4

*Schedule shown is for detecting prethreshold ROP with 99% confidence, usually long before any required treatment.
†This is a tentative, rather than evidence-based, guideline for 22 to 23 weeks gestational age–newborns because of the small numbers of survivors at these gestational-age categories.
‡If necessary.

- Follow-up examinations: Determined by findings on first examination
- Retinal findings that require strong consideration of ablative therapy within 72 hours of diagnosis:
  - Zone I ROP: any stage with plus disease
  - Zone I ROP: stage 3, no plus disease
  - Zone II ROP: stage 2 or 3 with plus disease
- Transfer to another facility and/or discharge to home within the period of susceptibility for development or progression of ROP, requires monitoring examinations by experienced ophthalmologist to continue.
- Because treatment is time-sensitive, a systematic program of scheduling and tracking ophthalmology examinations of premature infants at risk for ROP is strongly recommended.

PMA, Post-menstrual age (gestational age plus chronologic age); *ROP,* retinopathy of prematurity.

Treatment. The best treatment is prevention. NOTE: Even strict adherence to all principles of good care may still not prevent ROP in VLBW infants.

Early treatment of prethreshold ROP with peripheral retinal ablation (with laser or cryotherapy) has been shown to significantly improve anatomic structure and visual outcomes.[108] As in the earlier CRYO-ROP study, the ETROP study[108] showed more benefit for retinal reattachment than for visual acuity. **Revised indications for treatment of ROP are listed in Table 23-12.** The importance of these revised indications is demonstrated in a retrospective chart review of outcomes before and after use of the new treatment guidelines. With the adoption of the revised indications for treatment (see Table 23-12), one study found a decrease from 10.3% to 1.9% of eyes developing stage 5 retinal detachment, even though the group of study preterms had a lower average birth weight and gestational age.[4]

Use of laser therapy is the standard treatment for ROP. The laser is directed through the infant's pupil so that the light photocoagulates retinal tissue, stops abnormal vessel growth, and halts the progression of ROP. Laser surgery is less invasive, requires no anesthesia, enables deeper tissue penetration and more predictable tissue interaction, and results in less

TABLE 23-12 REVISED INDICATIONS FOR THE TREATMENT OF RETINOPATHY OF PREMATURITY (ROP)

TYPE 1 ROP* (NEW THRESHOLD)	TYPE 2 ROP†
ADMINISTER PERIPHERAL ABLATION THERAPY	***WAIT AND WATCH FOR PROGRESSION***
Zone II	Zone II
"Plus" disease with stage 2 or 3	Stage 3 without "plus" disease
Zone I	Zone I
"Plus" disease with stage 1, 2, or 3 Stage 3 with or without "plus" disease	Stage 1 or 2 without "plus" disease

Data from Early Treatment for ROP Cooperative Group: Revised indications for the treatment of ROP, *Arch Ophthalmol* 121:684, 2003; Phelps D: The Early Treatment for ROP study: better outcomes, changing strategy, *Pediatrics* 114:490, 2004.
*Type 1 ROP = eyes with a 15% or greater risk for progression to an unfavorable outcome without treatment.
†Type 2 ROP = eyes with less than a 15% risk for progression to an unfavorable outcome without treatment.

inflammation and pain postoperatively than with cryosurgery.[3]

When retinal detachment has occurred, surgical procedures known as *scleral buckling* and *vitrectomy* may be performed; even if anatomic results (e.g., retinal reattachment) after these surgeries are good, visual results (e.g., light perception, ambulatory vision) are poor.[117] Recently, a retrospective chart review was conducted to evaluate the outcomes of intravitreal injection of bevacizumab, an anti-angiogenic, as an initial treatment for severe ROP at risk for progression to retinal detachment despite laser therapy. Intravitreal injection of bevacizumab reduced neovascular activity in 14 of 15 eyes with ROP, resulted in tractional retinal detachment in 3 of the treated eyes, and had no other ocular or systemic adverse effects. In this pilot study, intravitreal injection of bevacizumab reduced retinal neovascularization and was beneficial for treating severe ROP refractory to laser therapy.[213] Another case series reported neovascular regression in 17 of 18 treated eyes, 1 spontaneous retinal detachment after injection, and no serious ocular or systemic adverse effects.[297] RCTs of this therapy to determine safety and long-term efficacy are needed.

Complications. Long-term visual consequences of laser surgery for ROP include decreased peripheral vision and myopia, which is less severe in laser therapy. Complications of laser surgery include choroidal hemorrhage; scarring; increased risk for cataracts; burns of the cornea, iris, or lens; and (rarely) pain. In several follow-up studies of preterm infants, 5% to 43% of the survivors had some ocular disorder, indicating a significant relationship between ocular disorders and ROP, and there was also an increased incidence of ocular disorders in preterm infants without ROP.[88,381] Disorders include decreased visual acuity, myopia, hypermyopia, astigmatism, refractive errors, and strabismus.[79,183] Severe myopia may develop as early as 6 months of age; myopia occurs in 80% of infants with ROP.[183] Early detection and correction with lenses is essential to save the child's remaining sight. The presence of threshold ROP is associated with higher incidence of motor, developmental, cognitive, educational, and social sequelae in childhood; preservation of more favorable visual status results in more children performing at grade level.[79,257] Glaucoma, strabismus, amblyopia, and late retinal detachment (in teens or early twenties) may develop.[183]

Parent Teaching. At discharge, parents must be educated about the importance of timely follow-up visits for the management of ROP (see the Parent Teaching box below).

Blindness is defined by many in our society as one of the worst handicaps. Parents experience grief over this devastating loss and need help to cope before they can bond to their blind child. Parents must be taught to care for their blind or visually impaired child. Blind infants cannot communicate with care providers through the signs and signals of facial expressions.[131] Because of the absence of eye language, no cues to infant needs and no feedback of preference, recognition, and delight can be given. Absence of a smile from the blind infant connotes a negative response to the care provider. When care providers understand these behavioral differences, they can assist parents to understand the lack of facial expression. Instead of facial expression, parents are taught to read the special hand language of their infants as an expression of emotions, intentions, preference, and recognition.[131] Appropriate referrals to occupational therapy, physical therapy, and community agencies that are resources for the blind and their families may help avoid developmental delays from insufficient or inappropriate stimulation.

Acute Respiratory Diseases

RESPIRATORY DISTRESS SYNDROME

Pathophysiology. RDS is a disease of immature lung anatomy and physiology. Anatomically, the preterm lung cannot support oxygenation and ventilation, because alveolar saccules are insufficiently

Parent Teaching

RETINOPATHY OF PREMATURITY

- Receive information, both verbally and in writing, about retinopathy of prematurity (ROP).
- Understand the time-sensitive nature of ROP and the need for timely follow-up visits after discharge so that prethreshold ROP is identified and treated early.
- Understand the importance to the child's development of wearing corrective lens.
- Schedule the ophthalmology appointment for follow-up before discharge, and review with the parents.

developed, causing a deficient surface area for gas exchange. Also, the pulmonary capillary bed is deficient and the interstitial mesenchyme is present to a greater extent, increasing the distance between the alveolar and the endothelial cell membranes.

Physiologically, the volume of surfactant is insufficient to prevent collapse of unstable alveoli. Because the alveoli collapse with each breath, normal functional residual capacity (FRC) is not established. Because of alveolar collapse, oxygenation and ventilation are insufficient and each breath requires increased energy output.

Compliance is related to the volume achieved during a given application of pressure. Compliance of the lung is equal to the ratio of the change in volume to the change in pressure. The lung in RDS has low compliance (i.e., little change in volume is achieved with a relatively great application of pressure), thereby contributing to increased work of breathing. However, the chest wall of the neonate unfortunately is very compliant; a slight application of pressure results in a large change in volume. The infant may not be able to create enough inspiratory pressure to open the alveoli as the chest wall retracts and collapses about the relatively stiff lung. Thus in RDS, the diaphragm contracts, creating an inspiratory pressure that moves less volume into the lung than expected and simultaneously causes large sternal and intercostal retractions of the chest wall.

The increased effort of these opposing forces usually results in hypoxemia and acidemia, which cause constriction of the pulmonary vascular (arterial) musculature, severely limiting pulmonary capillary blood flow. The integrity of pulmonary capillary blood flow is critical for the integrity of the alveolar epithelial membrane and the production of surfactant. Without adequate pulmonary capillary blood flow, the type II pneumocytes become deficient in the precursor material necessary for production of surfactant. Lack of surfactant production compounds the deficiency and leads to low compliance. **These physiologic factors (surfactant deficiency and decreased lung compliance) promote increased work of breathing, fatigue, atelectasis, reduced FRC, and ventilation-perfusion ($\dot{V}/\dot{Q}$) mismatch.**

In the fetus, pulmonary vascular resistance is high and pulmonary artery blood pressure is greater than systemic blood pressure, causing blood flow from the main pulmonary artery to travel through the open ductus arteriosus to the descending aorta. A second right-to-left shunt occurs across the foramen ovale in the fetus. The high pulmonary vascular resistance is "reactive" to the normal fetal "hypoxemia," because the pulmonary vascular resistance and the pulmonary artery blood pressure decrease as the $Pa{O_2}$ of the neonate increases. At birth, the ductus arteriosus actively constricts in response to the increase in $Pa{O_2}$ ($Pa{O_2}$ >50 mm Hg), eliminating blood flow across the ductus and completing the transition to neonatal circulation.

The fetal circulatory pattern may persist from birth or be initiated by a transient hypoxemic episode. **In the instance of neonatal hypoxemia, the pulmonary vasculature "reacts" by vasoconstriction, raising pulmonary vascular resistance, and the ductus arteriosus "reacts" by relaxing, once again allowing blood flow from the pulmonary artery to the descending aorta, as normally occurs in the fetus.** Pulmonary vascular resistance is increased with shunting through the ductus arteriosus. Fetal circulatory patterns are perpetuated by hypoxemia and acidemia and produce systemic hypoxemia that aggravates and perpetuates the condition.

Endothelial damage and alveolar necrosis aggravate the already existing surfactant deficiency. A cyclic deterioration is established, and hypoxia and acidosis persist unless treatment is initiated.

Microscopically, the events that occur in the lung include injury to and death of the alveolar epithelial cells and airway epithelial cells. This injury and death are followed by sloughing of the cells from the respiratory basement membrane, leaving the basement membrane denuded, followed by exudation of serum. Fibrin in the serum clots, and hyaline membranes are formed, covering the denuded basement membranes in the airways and alveolar spaces. If there is sufficient hypoxic damage to the cells and basement membranes, frank hemorrhage may fill the alveolar spaces. These factors decrease the total surface area of the gas exchange membrane. The end result is hypoxemia, acidemia, and increasing respiratory distress.

The entire sequence of events in RDS is related to the inability to maintain lung expansion and alveolar stability as a result of surfactant deficiency. **RDS evolves from two interrelated problems: atelectasis and persistence of pulmonary hypertension (Figures 23-5 and 23-6).**

Etiology. **RDS occurs in infants born prematurely and is a consequence of immature lung anatomy and physiology.** In premature or stressed

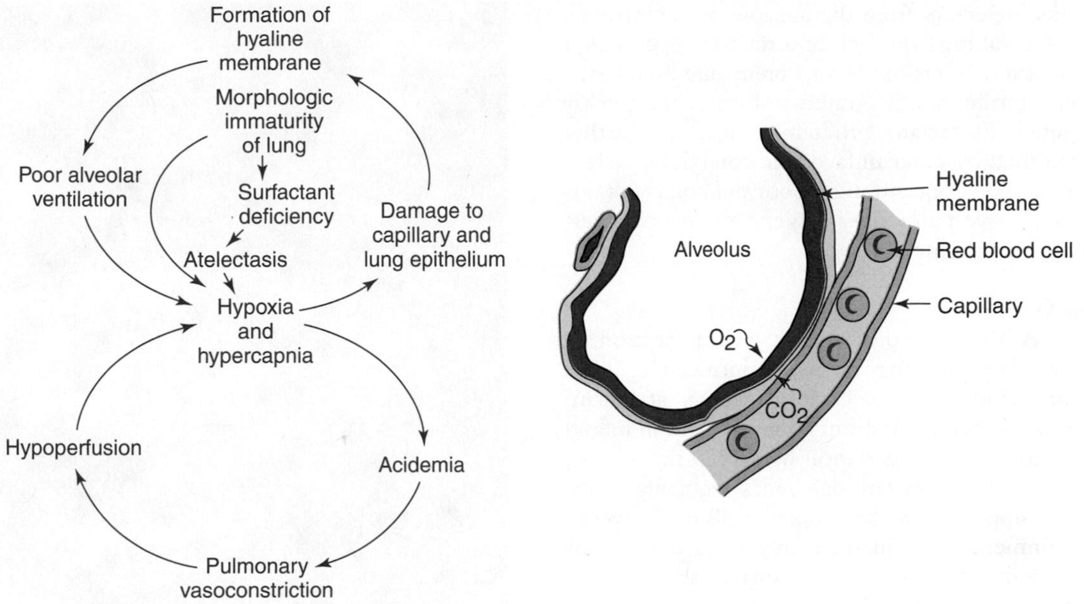

FIGURE 23-5 Interdependent relationship of factors involved in pathology of respiratory distress syndrome. (From Pierog SH, Ferrara A: *Medical care of the sick newborn,* ed 2, St Louis, 1976, Mosby.)

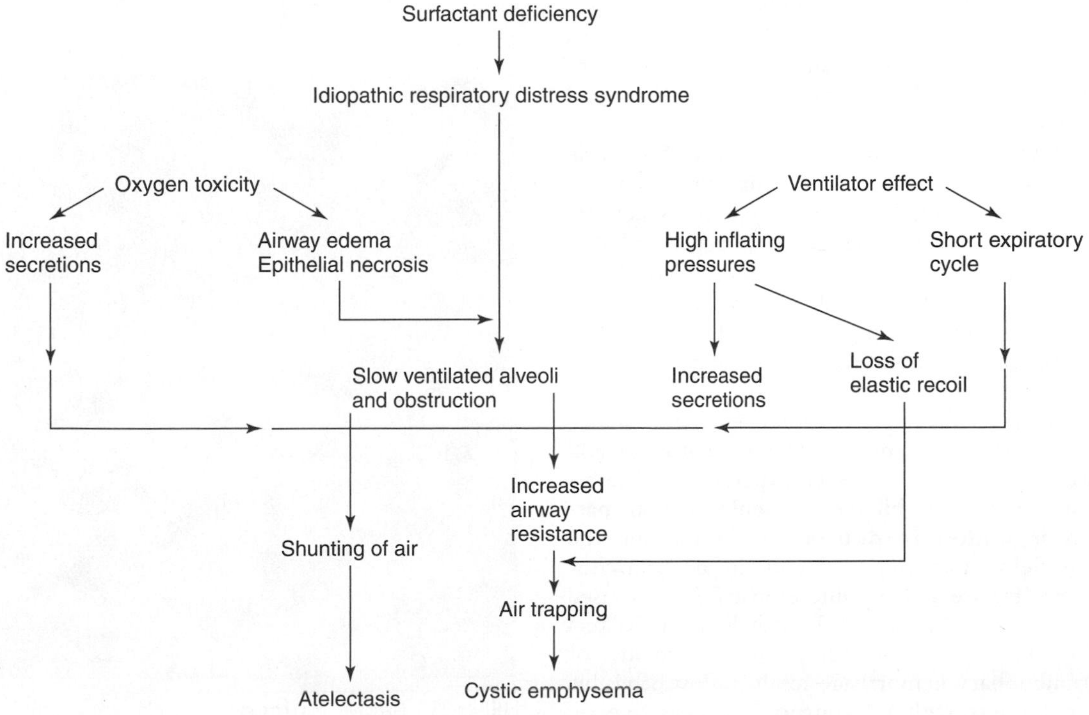

FIGURE 23-6 Schematic representation of pathogenesis of respiratory distress syndrome.

infants, atelectasis from the collapse of the terminal alveoli resulting from lack of surfactant appears after the first few hours of life. In a premature infant, surfactant production is limited and stores are quickly depleted. Surfactant production may be further diminished by other unfavorable conditions such as high oxygen concentration, poor pulmonary drainage, excessive pulmonary hygiene, or effects of respirator management.

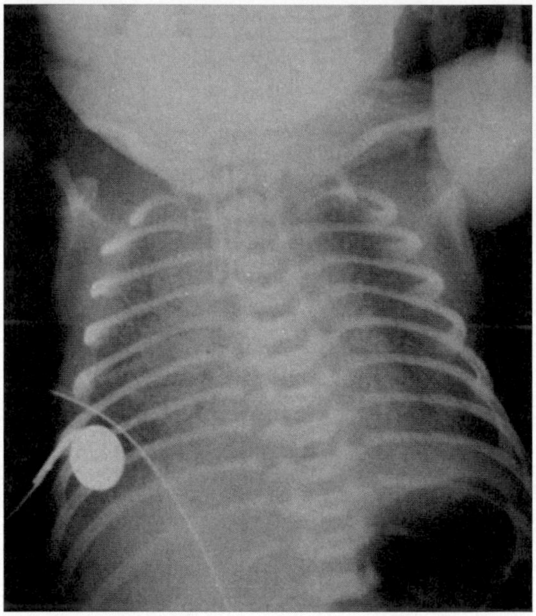

FIGURE 23-7 Chest x-ray film of a preterm infant (27 weeks' gestation) with respiratory distress syndrome. Note characteristic infiltrate pattern with air bronchograms.

Data Collection

History. A history of prematurity, cesarean section, or asphyxial episodes may be seen in infants with RDS. In one study, elective cesarean section at "term" (e.g., 34 weeks' gestation or older) resulted in infants of 37 to 38 weeks' gestation being 120 times more likely to have surfactant deficiency requiring ventilatory support than those born at 39 to 41 weeks. Recommendations include only using delivery by elective induction or elective cesarean section at 39 weeks' gestation (see Chapter 5).

Physical Examination. **Infants with RDS are often tachypneic and demonstrate grunting, nasal flaring, and chest retractions within the first few minutes to hours of life. Pallor or cyanosis also may be present.** The trachea is midline, and the apical pulse is normal. **Auscultation of the chest reveals decreased breath sounds and often rales. Many of these infants may be hypotensive with prolonged capillary refill.**

Laboratory Data. **Chest x-ray findings in RDS include (1) reduced lung volume, (2) air bronchograms, (3) reticulogranularity, and (4) lung opacification.** Surfactant deficiency results in diffuse atelectasis, a reduction in lung volume, and decreased lung expansion as demonstrated on x-ray examination. Atelectasis increases lung density and results in visible outlines of air-filled bronchi (e.g., air bronchograms) against opaque lung tissue. Chest x-ray examination also reveals a ground-glass appearance that represents areas of atelectatic respiratory alveoli adjacent to expanded or even hyperexpanded respiratory units. **This bilateral reticulogranular pattern is uniformly distributed throughout the lung fields and may also contain air bronchograms (Figure 23-7).** Diffuse opacification caused by (1) nonexpanded alveoli with little or no terminal airway aeration, (2) pulmonary edema, or (3) pulmonary hemorrhage results in loss of visible heart borders, with a **"white out" appearance on chest x-ray films (Figure 23-8).**

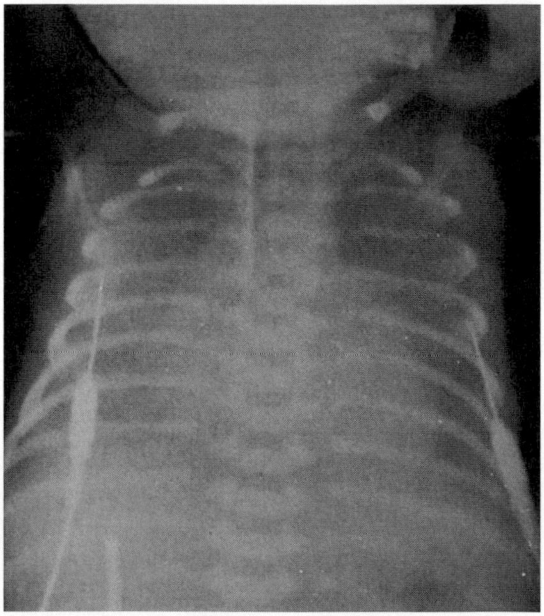

FIGURE 23-8 Chest x-ray film of a preterm infant (28 weeks' gestation) with severe respiratory distress syndrome. Note "white out" appearance.

Arterial blood gases reveal hypoxemia and often acidemia that may be metabolic, respiratory, or a combination of both (see Chapter 8).

Prevention. A single course of antenatal steroids has decreased the incidence and severity of RDS, comorbid conditions (e.g., NEC, intracranial hemorrhage, CLD), and mortality in infants of less than 32 weeks' gestation. Even a partial course appears to be beneficial.[260]

A meta-analysis of prophylactic use of NCPAP (regardless of respiratory status) after the birth of VLBW preterms found an increased use of IPPV and incidence of CLD/BPD, death, and IVH.[354]

Prophylactic use of surfactant in animal studies is associated with more uniform and homogenous distribution when administered to a fluid-filled lung.[324] **Delayed surfactant administration (even by 15 minutes after the onset of assisted ventilation) may offset the benefits of surfactant.**[324] Studies comparing timing of administration found increased survival, decreased mortality, less pneumothorax and PIE (especially in infants <26 weeks' gestation), and less CLD/BPD associated with prophylactic versus rescue usage.[351] Because 30% to 40% of preterm infants of less than 30 weeks GA will not have RDS, prophylactic use is associated with overtreatment[351] so it is reserved for the smallest, most immature infants at increased risk for RDS (e.g., ≤29 weeks' gestation).

Treatment

Surfactant Replacement Therapy. Because surfactant deficiency is the primary abnormality of RDS, the development of an effective clinical strategy for administering exogenous surface-active material to premature infants has been the focus of research efforts for many years. Administration of surfactant leads to the following[342,351]:

- Reduction in surface tension
- Dramatic and rapid improvement in gas exchange
- Decreased need for high levels of supplemental oxygen and ventilatory support
- Less barotrauma
- Improved chest x-ray findings because of improved lung compliance and lung volume

The use of lower levels of ventilatory support decreases the mortality rate and the incidence of pneumothorax. However, surfactant administration does not fully correct lung abnormalities of the VLBW infant with RDS.[191] Comorbid conditions (e.g., NEC, nosocomial infections, PDA, IVH, and CLD/BPD) in the VLBW infants have not been affected by surfactant therapy.[113]

Optimal clinical strategies—the type of surfactant to use, the timing and method of administration, and the number of doses—affect surfactant safety and efficacy.[342,351] Several studies have documented the **safety and efficacy of INSURE (i.e., INtubation, early SURfactant therapy, followed by Extubation to nasal CPAP)** in preterms of varying gestational ages (25 to 35 weeks); birth weights (1250 to 2500 g); degrees (mild to severe) of RDS; and timing after birth. Benefits from this approach include (1) decreased need for intubation and mechanical ventilation (10% to 40%), (2) delayed onset of mechanical ventilation, (3) decreased incidence (2% vs. 9%)[312] of air leaks (pneumothorax), (4) fewer rescue surfactant doses (12% vs. 26%),[312] (5) decreased CLD/BPD (49% vs. 59%)[312] (6) decreased length of oxygen therapy, (7) shortened length of stay, and (8) more cost-effective.* The most recent of these studies randomized 27 to 31$^{6}/_{7}$ weeks' gestation preterms to intubation, very early (within 15 to 60 minutes of age) treatment with surfactant, and extubation to NCPAP (n = 141) versus use of NCPAP alone (n = 138). In addition to the outcomes just mentioned, this study also found a significant decrease in need for mechanical ventilation and incidence of CLD/BPD in the more mature (30 to 31$^{6}/_{7}$ weeks) but not in the younger (27 to 29 weeks) gestation group.[312] It is important to note that this study also demonstrated a lower rate of treatment failure in the control group (39%) when compared with treatment failures in two other studies: 68%[384] and 70%.[307]

The Avoid Mechanical Ventilation (AMV) trial is a multicenter study of surfactant therapy without intubation. Through a thin catheter passed into the trachea of spontaneously breathing preterms (26 to 28$^{6}/_{7}$ weeks' gestation; <1500 g BW), the surfactant dose (100 mg/kg) is administered on the first day of life. If repeated doses of surfactant are needed, they will also be administered without intubation until the third day of life. The primary study hypothesis is that giving surfactant without intubation will reduce the frequency of mechanical ventilation. This trial will be complete at the end of 2010.

*References 91,135,307,312,351,384.

Numerous studies comparing surfactants have documented more rapid improvement in respiratory status, decreased incidence of pneumothorax, lower mortality rates, improved survival, and less ROP and CLD/BPD with natural than with synthetic surfactant.[112] Use of animal-derived surfactants entail the risks of infection, immunogenicity, proinflammatory mediators, and variability of concentration of active ingredients in different aliquots. A next-generation synthetic surfactant, lucinactant, has been developed and is as safe and effective as the natural surfactants without the potential risks (Table 23-13). This synthetic surfactant contains a peptide, sinapultide, that mimics surfactant protein B (SP-B) and its effects on lung tissue. Multicenter RCTs of lucinactant administered within 30 minutes of birth to ELBW/VLBW preterms born at 32 weeks' gestation or less found (1) a significantly lower incidence of RDS at 24 hours of age, (2) significantly reduced RDS-related mortality at 14 and 28 days, and (3) significantly lower incidence of CLD/BPD and all-cause mortality through 36 weeks' PMA when compared with the use of natural surfactants.[255,256] A meta-analysis of two RCTs using protein-containing synthetic surfactant compared with natural surfactant found no statistically significant difference in CLD/BPD and death.[285]

Various methods of surfactant administration have been studied, **with bolus injection improving the homogenous distribution of surfactant in lungs when compared with slow injection or ultrasonic nebulization.** Aerosolized surfactant therapy may prevent the need for intubation and needs to be studied in RCTs to establish safety and efficacy.[237] There is a potential for the new synthetic surfactant (i.e., lucinactant) to be available in a formulation for nasal or nasopharyngeal aerosolization or nebulization, thus avoiding intubation and mechanical ventilation. **Rapid bolus injection has been associated with alteration in CBF (which may increase the risk for IVH).**[317] A study of bolus administration showed no alteration in CBF (with careful attention to FIO_2 and pressures); however, alterations in CBF were related to changes in mean systolic blood pressure.[272] Studies of the number of doses document (1) decreased severity of RDS but no improvement of survival with a single dose and (2) increased survival, decreased mortality, and decreased incidence of pneumothorax with multiple doses.[416]

The incidence of BPD/CLD is lower in surfactant treated preterms 30 weeks' or more gestation; the incidence for preterms less than 30 weeks' gestation is unchanged.[113] Even early use of surfactant, extubation, and early use of NCPAP results in a significant decrease in the incidence of CLD/BPD in the more mature (30 to 31⁶⁄₇ weeks) but not in the younger (27 to 29 weeks) gestation group.[312] **The incidence of CLD/BPD is lower in the prophylactic use of surfactant (decreases the incidence and severity of RDS) when compared with a rescue strategy—treating preterms after they develop RDS.** Prophylactic use is also associated with fewer complications of RDS: (1) pneumothorax and pulmonary interstitial emphysema; (2) death; and (3) the combined outcomes of BPD/CLD and death.[113] Methods of resuscitation, types of ventilators (nasal CPAP vs. CMV vs. HFOV),[351] and ventilation style[351] (e.g., as few as six large tidal volume breaths in a surfactant-deficient lung causes lung injury)[180] also contribute to lung injury resulting in CLD/BPD.

Other outcomes of surfactant use include PDA, pulmonary hemorrhage, and long-term outcomes. Studies have documented an increased incidence of significant PDA after birth among surfactant-treated preterm infants.[351] Another study found a 50% increase in pulmonary hemorrhage after surfactant treatment especially in LBW preterm infants and when synthetic surfactant had been administered.[301] Long-term outcome studies of preterm infants who have received surfactant therapy show no significant effects on the rates of neurologic, developmental, behavioral, medical, or educational outcomes.[113]

Recommendations for surfactant replacement therapy for RDS are outlined in Box 23-12. Surfactant preparations are commercially available as (1) organic solvent extract of minced bovine lung, (2) artificial or synthetic surfactant, (3) modified porcine-derived minced lung extract, and (4) natural surfactant extracted from calf lung by lavage. **Table 23-13 summarizes the commercially available products for surfactant replacement. Other treatment is directed toward the indications in Box 23-13.**

Inositol Therapy. Inositol, an essential nutrient, promotes maturation of several components of surfactant. A systematic review of inositol supplementation for RDS found significant reductions in (1) CLD/BPD, (2) mortality, (3) ROP, and (4) grade III to grade IV IVH with no increase in sepsis or NEC.[178] A multicenter RCT to confirm these findings is recommended.[178]

Inhaled Nitric Oxide Therapy. Inhaled nitric oxide (iNO) therapy not only is a selective pulmonary vasodilator but also improves oxygenation by redirecting blood from poorly aerated (atelectatic) and diseased lung (with RDS) regions to better aerated distal air spaces.[200] Low-dose iNO (<20 ppm) optimizes ventilation-perfusion matching (thus treating ventilation-perfusion mismatch) by preferentially vasodilating lung units that are well ventilated.[200] Other therapeutic effects of iNO include the following[200,236,242]:

- Reduction of lung inflammation and edema
- Antioxidant effect on lung injury
- Protective effects on surfactant function
- Potential beneficial effects on pulmonary vascular and alveolar development
- Neuroprotection (e.g., decreased incidence of brain injury and improved long-term neurodevelopmental outcomes for preterm infants with moderately severe RDS)

Early RCTs of iNO in preterm infants found improved oxygenation, decreased need for mechanical ventilation, improved survival without increase in IVH, and a trend toward a decrease in CLD/BPD.[263] Two newer studies of preterms with moderate RDS demonstrated that iNO reduced the combined endpoint of death and CLD.[201,320] These studies also noted a significant reduction in severe (grade III/IV) IVH, PVL, and ventriculomegaly in treated preterms when compared with those not receiving iNO.[201,320] Prospective follow-up of 82% of preterms from the earlier study found an improvement in neurodevelopmental outcomes (24% disability and delay vs. 46% in placebo group) at 2 years of age.[243]

BOX 23-12 RECOMMENDATIONS FOR SURFACTANT REPLACEMENT THERAPY[113]

- Target population: High-risk, LBW infants with multisystem disorders.
- Directed by physicians qualified and trained in use and administration, including management of mechanical ventilation of LBW infants.
- Nursing and respiratory therapy personnel experienced in management of LBW infants, including mechanical ventilation available at the bedside during administration.
- Equipment available to manage and monitor LBW infants being mechanically ventilated; support services (e.g., radiology, laboratory) available.
- Used only in institutions with facilities and personnel experienced in and available for the management of multisystem disorders of LBW infants.
- Existence of an institutionally approved surfactant therapy protocol.
- In situations in which timely transfer cannot be achieved, surfactant may be administered by a physician skilled in endotracheal intubation, after consultation with tertiary center and transfer to tertiary center arranged as soon as possible.

LBW, Low-birth-weight.

TABLE 23-13 SURFACTANT REPLACEMENT THERAPY

DRUG/SOURCE	INDICATIONS	ADMINISTRATION AND DOSAGE	ADVERSE EVENTS
Beractant* (Survanta) Exogenous surfactant from bovine lung extract	Prophylaxis and treatment ("rescue") of RDS in preterm infants; significantly reduces the incidence of RDS, mortality, and air leak complications Prophylaxis: In preterm infants <1250 g BW or with evidence of surfactant deficiency, give as soon as possible, preferably within 15 min of birth Rescue: To treat infants with RDS confirmed by x-ray examination and requiring mechanical ventilation, give as soon as possible, preferably by 8 hr of age	Administration: For *intratracheal* administration only; instillation through a 5-Fr end-hole catheter inserted into the infant's ETT and above the infant's carina; each dose is 100 mg of phospholipids/kg BW (4 mL/kg; 100 mg/kg); four doses can be administered in the first 48 hr of life; give doses no more frequently than every 6 hr; repeat doses are based on the infant's BW	The most commonly reported adverse experiences are associated with the dosage procedure: transient bradycardia, oxygen desaturation, alterations in BP, drug reflux

*Use of bovine and porcine products may be objectionable to persons of Jewish, Islamic, and/or Hindu beliefs; informed consent from parents is essential.

Continued

TABLE 23-13 SURFACTANT REPLACEMENT THERAPY—cont'd

DRUG/SOURCE	INDICATIONS	ADMINISTRATION AND DOSAGE	ADVERSE EVENTS
Poractant alpha* (Curosurf) Modified porcine-derived minced lung extract	Prophylaxis and treatment ("rescue") of RDS in preterm infants	For *intratracheal* administration, see procedure on p. 641 Dosage: *Initial dose:* 2.5 mL/kg divided into aliquots *Subsequent dose:* Up to two doses of 1.25 mL/kg/dose given 12 hr apart, if needed	As for beractant
Calfactant* (Infasurf) Natural surfactant extracted from calf lung lavage	Prophylaxis and treatment ("rescue") of RDS in preterm infants	Administration: For *intratracheal* administration, see p. 641 Dosage: *Initial dose:* 3 mL/kg (105 mg/kg) divided into two aliquots *Subsequent dose:* Up to three doses of 3 mL/kg/dose given 12 hr apart, if needed	As for beractant
Lucinactant (Surfaxin)† Synthetic surfactant containing a peptide, sinapultide, that mimics surfactant protein B (SP-B)[255,256]	Prophylaxis and treatment ("rescue") of RDS in preterm infants	For *intratracheal* administration, see procedure for beractant Dosage: *Initial dose:* 5.8 mL/kg (175 mg/kg) dosing q 6 hr based on clinical response. Gels when stored at 4° C; requires up to 15 min of warming at 44° C in a heating block to liquefy; rapidly cools to body temperature when removed from heating block	As for beractant

*Use of bovine and porcine products may be objectionable to persons of Jewish, Islamic, and/or Hindu beliefs; informed consent from parents is essential.
†FDA issued Approvable Letter on Feb. 14, 2005. (www.discoverylabs.com)
BP, Blood pressure; *BW,* birth weight; *C,* centigrade; *ETT,* endotracheal tube; *RDS,* respiratory distress syndrome.

Another RCT that started iNO later (at 7 to 21 days of life) and treated longer (24 days) using gradually decreasing doses (after starting at 20 ppm) found significantly better survival without CLD in preterms (<1250 g) treated with iNO.[22] Two other multicenter trials of iNO have been completed: in the United Kingdom, the INNOVA trial[122]; in the United States, the NICHD trial.[382] The multicenter non-blinded and nonrandomized INNOVA trial enrolled preterms (n = 108) with a mean gestational age of 27 weeks with severe respiratory disease to iNO beginning at 5 ppm and in a step-wise method doubling the dose to a maximum of 40 ppm. Outcomes in the INNOVA trial included (1) improved oxygenation, (2) no effect on death or neurologic disability at 1 year corrected age (CA) and at 4 to 5 years of age, and (3) significantly increased cost with iNO use.[122,179]

The multicenter NICHD study, a double-blind RCT, of iNO (5 to 10 ppm) in preterms (n = 420) with severe respiratory failure was terminated early because of increased rates of severe IVH in treated infants.[382] A secondary analysis of the data showed that only treated preterms less than 1000 g had the increase in IVH and mortality; preterms more than 1000 g had a significant decrease in combined outcomes of death and CLD. Follow-up of these preterms

BOX 23-13 TREATMENT FOR RESPIRATORY DISTRESS SYNDROME

1. Reducing hypoxemia (see "General Treatment Strategies" section in this chapter and in Chapter 8)
   a. Maintain in thermoneutral environment (see Chapter 6)
   b. Maintain blood pressure and hematocrit (see Chapters 5 and 20)
   c. Decrease stimuli from the neonatal intensive care environment (see Chapter 13)
   d. Recognize and relieve pain or agitation (see Chapter 12)
2. Correcting acidemia (see Chapter 8)
3. Increase the functional residual capacity (see "General Treatment Strategies" section)
   a. Maintain appropriate temperature (see Chapter 6)
   b. Monitor vital signs and arterial blood gases (see Chapters 7 and 8)
   c. Provide appropriate fluid, electrolytes, glucose, and calories (see Unit Three)
   d. Observe for complications of disease and treatments (see "General Complications" section)
4. Monitoring for complications (see "General Complications"—sections on "Acute Complications" and "Chronic Complications")

(both <1000 g and >1000 g) at 18 to 22 months CA found no significant increase in neurodevelopmental impairment in either group.[172] A small (n = 61) 3-year follow-up study of preterms (mean BW: 820 g; mean GA: 25.5 weeks) with PPHN who were treated with iNO found a significantly lower incidence of cerebral palsy (12.5%) when compared with pre-iNO period (46.7%).[361] Use of iNO reduces the incidence of CLD, IVH/PVL in preterm infants, thus contributing to better neurodevelopmental outcomes[243]; iNO may also have an independent neuroprotective effect on the developing brain.[236,242]

Variations in use of iNO include (1) administration, (2) duration, (3) early versus later use, (4) best candidates, and (5) outcomes.[248,264,340] Systematic reviews of iNO use in preterms have found the following[28,29]:

- Early rescue (0 to 3 days) of preterms based on oxygenation index demonstrated no significant effect of iNO on mortality or BPD.
- Studies of routine use of iNO in intubated/ventilated preterms showed a barely significant reduction in the combined outcomes of death and BPD.
- Later use of iNO (after 3 days) based on an increased risk of BPD showed no significant benefit for BPD.

BOX 23-14 RECOMMENDATIONS: BEST PRACTICE GUIDELINES FOR INHALED NITRIC OXIDE IN THE TREATMENT OF PRETERM INFANTS

- Clinical trials have not yet consistently shown reproducible improvements in long-term outcomes (CLD/BPD, mortality, neurodevelopment).
- Possible benefits in selected preterms (BW >1000 g; GA >29 weeks) who have a better response to iNO. To reduce CLD/BPD, routine prolonged use of iNO may be more beneficial than rescue use (e.g., when severe respiratory failure has already occurred).
- Preterms with pulmonary hypoplasia secondary to oligohydramnios and PPROM may benefit.
- More research is necessary to determine which preterms will respond to iNO and which will benefit.
- Uncertainties about the dose, timing, duration, initiation criteria, and long-term outcomes exist and must be studied before iNO is used routinely with preterm infants.

Data from Miller S, Rhine W: Best Practice Guideline: Inhaled nitric oxide in the treatment of preterm infants, *Early Hum Dev* 84:703, 2008.

BW, Birth weight; *CLD/BPD,* chronic lung disease/bronchopulmonary dysplasia; *GA,* gestational age; *iNO,* inhaled nitric oxide; *PPROM,* prolonged preterm rupture of membranes.

Use of iNO in preterm infants remains experimental. Preterms with pulmonary hypertension are better responders to iNO if they are more than 1000 g BW and more than 29 weeks GA.[211] **Recommendations from best practice guidelines are contained in Box 23-14.**

TRANSIENT TACHYPNEA OF THE NEWBORN (RESPIRATORY DISTRESS SYNDROME TYPE 2)

Pathophysiology. TTN is the result of delayed reabsorption of normal lung fluid, and thus an alternative name is *wet lung syndrome,* or *RDS type 2.* Lung fluid accumulates in the peribronchiolar lymphatics and the bronchovascular spaces. **Thus TTN is an "obstructive" lung disease, whereas RDS is a "restrictive" lung disease.** Abnormalities in lung function of neonates with TTN include high total ventilation, high breathing frequency, low tidal volume, high dead space, prolonged nitrogen clearance, and low dynamic compliance. Reabsorption of lung fluid occurs by the following: (1) lung liquid production slows; (2) pulmonary epithelium changes from chloride-secreting to sodium-absorbing barrier; (3) air intake at birth shifts fluid from alveoli to interstitium and perivascular spaces; and (4) a higher protein content and osmotic pressure of blood/lymph facilitates flow of lung fluid.

Etiology. **TTN generally occurs in term or late preterm infants with a history of cesarean section** (especially elective section in the late preterm infant—see Chapter 5), low Apgar scores, pulmonary artery hypertension, poor left ventricular function, and precipitous delivery.[360] In these situations, there is a lack of the gradual compression of the chest that eliminates some fluid during a normal vaginal delivery. Accumulation of interstitial fluid interferes with the forces that hold the bronchioli open, causing collapse and air trapping.

Data Collection

History. Term or late preterm male infants with a history of cesarean section, precipitous delivery, prenatal exposure to methamphetamine, or other abnormalities of labor and transition are predisposed to TTN. Onset is usually 2 to 6 hours after birth.

Physical Examination. Evidence for respiratory distress, including tachypnea, mild retractions, grunting, and flaring, may be seen. Cyanosis in room air also may be present.

Laboratory Data. Mild hypoxemia (requiring <40% oxygen) and mild acidemia are usually present. A significant degree of hypoxemia or acidemia tends to constrict the pulmonary vasculature and aggravate the problem. Chest x-ray examination reveals hyperexpansion with streaky infiltrates radiating from the hilum. These infiltrates are thought to represent interstitial fluid along the bronchovascular spaces. Air trapping causes the appearance of mild to moderate hyperaeration or inflation on the chest x-ray film. Visible fluid in the pulmonary fissures and cardiomegaly also may be seen on chest x-ray film. Use of lung sonography in infants with TTN shows a difference in echogenicity between the upper and lower lung fields—specifically the presence of comet-tail artifacts ("double lung point") in the inferior lung fields.[80]

Treatment. In general, **support of the neonate with TTN requires only provision of sufficient supplemental oxygen to maintain an arterial oxygen tension of more than 70 to 80 mm Hg and maintenance of usual supportive neonatal care.** Although diuretic agents have been advocated, usually little more than general support is necessary while the normal absorption of lung fluid through the lymphatics takes place. As the lung fluid clears, both the x-ray abnormalities and clinical presentation resolve within 72 hours.

Complications. TTN is independently and significantly associated with the development of childhood wheezing and asthma, especially in male infants.[44,224]

MECONIUM ASPIRATION SYNDROME

Pathophysiology. Before meconium aspiration can occur, meconium must find its way into the amniotic fluid. A hypoxic event before birth stimulates intestinal peristalsis and relaxation of the anal sphincter. Colonic peristalsis ensues, resulting in the expelling of meconium into the amniotic fluid and, in severe cases, gasping in utero that leads to meconium aspiration. Respirations after birth draw meconium first into major airways and subsequently into the smaller airways, causing obstruction, atelectasis, air trapping, and pneumothorax. Meconium can also cause chemical pneumonitis and inactivation of surfactant, further impairing gas exchange and potentiating barotrauma. This condition occurs more often in term or postterm infants when a hypoxic episode is experienced in utero.[383] These movements open the glottis so that meconium flows into the oropharynx and on into the lung. Thus the pathophysiology of lung disease in meconium aspiration syndrome (MAS) is related to the mechanisms causing fetal stress, as well as the direct adverse effects of meconium in the lung. MAS is a common reason for lung disease in neonates. Meconium staining of amniotic fluid occurs in 10% of deliveries at term.

Etiology. Meconium aspiration produces disease by several mechanisms: (1) meconium physically obstructs the glottis, trachea, or any number of smaller airways, resulting in atelectasis, air trapping, alveolar collapse, and ventilation-perfusion mismatching; (2) it promotes an inflammatory response known as *chemical pneumonitis;* (3) it inhibits surfactant function; and (4) it increases pulmonary vascular resistance, caused by asphyxial episodes, resulting in increased right-to-left shunting and the development of PPHN (Figure 23-9).[136] **Of the 8% to 19% of infants born through meconium-stained amniotic fluid, 2% to 33% develop MAS.**[136]

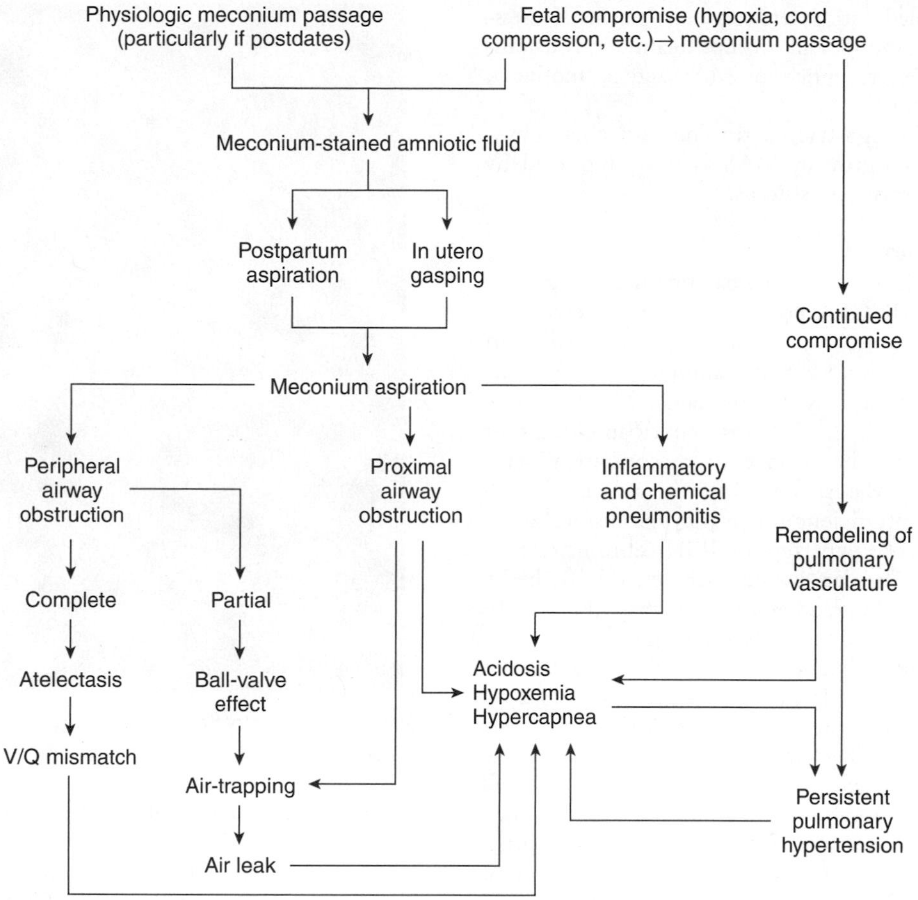

FIGURE 23-9 Pathophysiology of meconium passage and the meconium aspiration syndrome. $\dot{V}/\dot{Q}$, Ventilation-perfusion. (From Wiswell T, Bent R: Meconium staining and the meconium aspiration syndrome: unresolved issues, *Pediatr Clin North Am* 40[5]:957, 1993.)

Prevention. Before an infant is born, meconium aspiration may be prevented by early recognition of the compromised fetus, appropriate intervention, and prevention of cesarean delivery (which is associated with the development of MAS).[244,329,410] Amnioinfusion to dilute meconium in amniotic fluid has recently been studied in a multicenter RCT of 1998 pregnant women in labor at 36 or more weeks' gestation who had thick meconium-stained amniotic fluid. **Amnioinfusion did not reduce the risk for moderate to severe MAS or perinatal death** (4.5% vs. 3.5% control group) and is not recommended to prevent MAS.[132]

A large multicenter (i.e., 12-hospital) RCT of intrapartum oropharyngeal or nasopharyngeal suctioning for term infants born through meconium-stained amniotic fluid showed **no significant difference in the incidence of MAS (e.g., 4% for both the suction and the no-suction group),** the need for mechanical ventilation, mortality, or the duration of oxygen use, days of ventilation, and length of stay.[379] The study conclusion, that routine suctioning does not prevent MAS, has resulted in revision of present recommendations for care of these infants (see Chapter 4). **Routine tracheal suction is recommended *only* for depressed infants (e.g., non-vigorous infants with depressed tone and respirations and/or heart rate <100 beats/min) and those with respiratory symptoms.**[383] An interdisciplinary health care team for "rapid response" prepared and credentialed (e.g., NRP) for management of the neonate born through meconium-stained amniotic fluid, coupled with interdisciplinary postnatal assessment, observation, and prompt treatment, is recommended for prevention of MAS and its morbidity and mortality.[43]

Use of orogastric suctioning and chest physiotherapy to prevent MAS is not supported by evidence from any studies.

Data Collection

History. A history of asphyxia, intrauterine growth restriction (IUGR), postterm delivery, meconium-stained amniotic fluid, non-reassuring fetal heart tracing, low Apgar (<5 at 5 minutes), and African-American race may be present.[197,346] There is a positive association between chorioamnionitis or infection and the passage of meconium at term gestation.[372] Maternal risk factors associated with placental insufficiency (e.g., hypertension, pregnancy-induced hypertension [PIH], chronic respiratory/cardiovascular disease, diabetes, IUGR, heavy cigarette smoking, and postterm) may also lead to fetal asphyxia and meconium passage.[397]

Physical Examination. Tachypnea, rales, and cyanosis are seen in mild cases. In moderately severe cases, grunting, retractions, and nasal flaring also may be seen. In severe cases, the infant is asphyxiated and severely depressed at birth. There is profound cyanosis and pallor, irregular gasping respirations, and an increased anteroposterior diameter of the chest (a barrel chest) as a result of gas trapping and alveolar overdistention.

Laboratory Data. The chest x-ray examination shows marked air trapping, hyperexpansion, and hyperinflation. There are bilateral, diffuse, coarse, patchy infiltrates (Figure 23-10). Complete occlusion by debris results in atelectatic areas. Air leaks are frequently seen. Pleural effusion may occur as a result of the inflammatory process in the lung. Cardiomegaly may be present; this results from intrauterine asphyxia or cardiac hypoxia.

Severe hypoxemia and hypercapnia as a result of ventilation-perfusion mismatching and right-to-left shunting caused by pulmonary hypertension are present. Severe acidosis usually is combined respiratory and metabolic acidosis. Infants with MAS have elevated serum cytokines and chemokines.[273]

Treatment. Because the major problem in meconium aspiration is hypoxemia, treatment should be directed at improving oxygenation. Mildly affected infants will frequently require only warmed, humidified oxygen by hood. Increasing severity of meconium aspiration will require increased levels of intervention. About 30% to 50% of infants with MAS require CPAP or mechanical ventilation.[139] **Some infants respond to CPAP (4 to 6 cm of water), but others require full ventilator support. Because these infants are usually term or postterm, they resist assisted ventilation and may require paralyzation (Table 23-14), sedation, and/or analgesia (see Chapter 12) to ventilate and oxygenate the lungs adequately.** With paralysis, these infants may require rapid rates, high peak inspiratory pressure, and PEEP for adequate oxygenation and ventilation. Even though the majority of MAS infants are able to be treated with CPAP and CMV, use of other treatment modalities (e.g., HFV, iNO, ECMO/ECLS) may become necessary with accompanying PPHN and severe respiratory failure.[139]

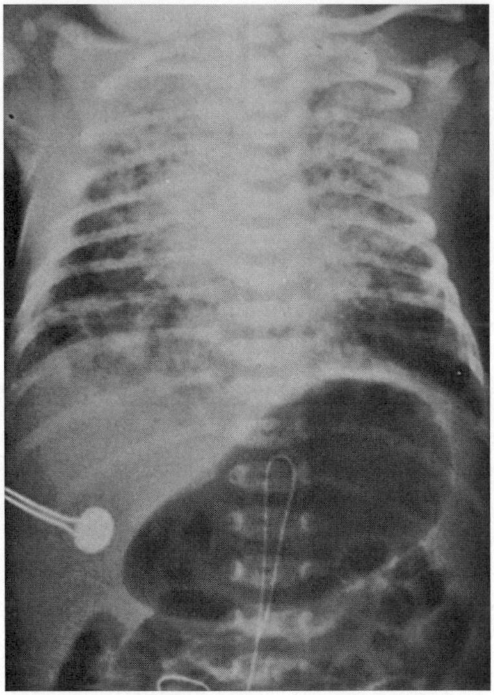

FIGURE 23-10 Chest x-ray film of infant with meconium aspiration. Note diffuse infiltrates.

Because meconium inhibits surfactant function in a dose-dependent manner, studies of **surfactant replacement to infants with MAS suggest improvement in some neonates with severe respiratory failure and MAS.**[199] Improved oxygenation/ventilation, decreased severity of respiratory compromise, no

TABLE 23-14 DRUGS FOR PARALYZATION

DRUG	DOSAGE	COMMENTS
Pancuronium (Pavulon)	0.1 mg/kg IV push (0.04-0.15 mg/kg) q 1-2 hr based on duration of paralysis Onset: 1-2 min	*Indications:* Paralysis for mechanical ventilation to improve oxygenation/ventilation; reduce barotrauma and alteration in cerebral blood flow Although paralyzed, neonate still feels pain—analgesia necessary for painful procedures and to accompany paralysis (see Chapter 12) *Adverse effects:* corneal drying (lubricate eyes); tachycardia; increased salivation; blood pressure changes (hypotension and hypertension) *Reversed by:* Neostigmine: 0.04-0.08 mg/kg IV Atropine: 0.02 mg/kg
Vecuronium	0.1 mg/kg IV push (0.03-0.15 mg/kg) q 1-2 hr based on duration of paralysis Onset: 1-2 min	*Indications:* same as above *Adverse effects:* corneal drying (lubricate eyes); decreases in heart rate and blood pressure when used with narcotics; special sensitivity in preterms (that diminishes with age); duration of effect prolonged in preterms *Reversed by:* same as above

increase in air leaks, and less use of ECMO have been observed in some studies.[112] Variable study results of surfactant use in MAS may result from timing, type, amount, and method of surfactant administration.

Surfactant lavage has been shown to improve oxygenation/ventilation and pulmonary function measurements (e.g., increased lung compliance and decrease in airway resistance) and has shown trends for earlier weaning from assisted ventilation and need for less oxygen in several small studies.[199,357] Complications of lung lavage include severe hypoxemia and systemic hypotension.[199] Surfactant lavage versus routine management of infants with moderate to severe MAS is being studied; **surfactant lavage remains an experimental therapy.**

Mucosal irritation and increased mucosal secretion hamper respiratory and mucociliary clearance efforts. Frequent pulmonary hygiene (every 2 to 3 hours) may help alleviate this problem.

As with any sick infant, close attention must be given to physiologic support and homeostasis. (See "General Treatment Strategies" section; see also Chapters 6, 7, and 8 and Unit Three.)

Complications. Use of new treatments has decreased the mortality rate to less than 5%.[383] Persistent pulmonary hypertension frequently complicates MAS, potentiates the difficulties in oxygenation, and contributes to a large portion of the mortality associated with MAS.[136,199] Air leaks are complications of both the disease (ball-valve obstruction causing air trapping) and the treatment. Infants with MAS are at increased risk for adverse neurologic outcomes (e.g., CP and global delays)[35] and long-term pulmonary problems (e.g., increased airway reactivity, abnormal pulmonary function).[414]

NEONATAL PNEUMONIA

Neonatal pneumonia occurs perinatally or postnatally in about 1% of term neonates and 10% of preterm neonates and may be as high as 28% for ventilated ELBW infants in the NICU.[13] **Neonates requiring prolonged hospitalization in the NICU are at risk for developing pneumonia from nosocomially acquired organisms.** The organisms most often causing neonatal pneumonia are mainly group B streptococci and gram-negative organisms (e.g., *Escherichia coli, Klebsiella, Pseudomonas,* and *Serratia marcescens*) but also include *Staphylococcus aureus, Staphylococcus epidermidis, Streptococcus pneumoniae,* and *Candida.* Less commonly acquired viral infections include herpes, cytomegalovirus, varicella-zoster, and syphilis. Community-acquired viral infections also occur in the NICU setting and include respiratory syncytial virus, enterovirus, adenovirus, and parainfluenza virus infections (Table 23-15).

TABLE 23-15 ETIOLOGIC FACTORS AND CHEST X-RAY FINDINGS IN NEONATAL PNEUMONIA

CAUSATIVE AGENT	CHEST X-RAY FINDINGS
BACTERIAL	
Group B beta-hemolytic streptococci (GBS)	Diffuse reticulogranular pattern, opacity ("white out"), patchy infiltrates, and pleural effusion
Streptococcus pneumoniae	Patchy infiltrates (lobar), pleural effusion
Staphylococcus aureus	Diffuse infiltrates; pneumatocele
Methicillin-resistant *Staphylococcus aureus* (MRSA)	Diffuse infiltrates; abscess formation
Staphylococcus epidermidis	Hazy lung fields; infiltrates
Listeria monocytogenes	Bilateral patchy infiltrates
Escherichia coli	Lobular consolidation; pneumatocele
Klebsiella	Bilateral consolidation; lung abscess, pneumatocele
Pseudomonas and *Serratia*	Parenchymal consolidation (patchy or basilar); pneumatocele
Haemophilus influenzae	Nonspecific; x-ray findings similar to those of GBS (above) or respiratory distress syndrome
VIRAL	
Herpes virus	Perihilar infiltrates; streaky, lobar consolidation; pleural effusion (late onset)
Cytomegalovirus	Nonspecific, perihilar streaking; hazy lung fields; infiltrates; opacification
Rubella virus	Interstitial infiltrates; hazy lung fields
Respiratory syncytial virus	Hyperexpansion; patchy consolidation
Adenovirus, enterovirus	Hyperexpansion; patchy consolidation
FUNGAL	
Candida albicans	Diffuse granularity; coarse infiltrates; opacification
MYCOPLASMA	
Ureaplasma urealyticum	Fine reticular pattern progressing to opacification and consolidation
Mycoplasma hominis	Diffuse reticular pattern, opacity, and pleural effusion
OTHER	
Treponema pallidum (syphilis)	Diffuse opacification; consolidation
Chlamydia trachomatis	Hyperinflation; streaky infiltrates
Pneumocystis jiroveci (formerly *carinii*)	Diffuse haziness; granularity; opacity

Modified from Carey B, Trotter C: Neonatal pneumonia, *Neonatal Netw* 19:46, 2000.

Pathophysiology. In bacterial pneumonia, alveoli are often more edematous and inflamed than in viral infections. Protein-rich fluid may partially or completely fill the alveoli. This is often followed by an influx of polymorphonuclear leukocytes and RBCs. Macrophages enter the alveoli and remove intraalveolar debris, restoring normal lung functioning.[69] *S. aureus* and *Klebsiella* organisms often cause severe damage to alveoli and often destroy lung tissue by causing necrosis of the septum between the alveoli. In some cases, abscesses form.

Viruses and *Mycoplasma* organisms also may be acquired transplacentally, during the delivery, or postnatally. Viral and mycoplasmal pneumonias commonly involve the bronchi and peribronchial interstitium more often than the alveoli. Viral and mycoplasmal organisms cause loss of epithelial ciliary appendages and sloughing into the airways. This results in stasis of mucus and secretions and bronchial obstruction with atelectasis. A secondary inflammatory response is characterized by mononuclear infiltration into the submucosa and perivascular areas causing narrowing of the airway lumen. Another response to this inflammatory process is smooth muscle constriction, which leads to increased airway obstruction and bronchospasm. In severe cases of viral and mycoplasmal infection, the inflammatory process involves the alveoli.

Fungal infections, the most common being *Candida* infection, may be acquired in utero, during the birth process, or in the postnatal period. Congenitally acquired pneumonia can be diffuse resulting from the inflammatory process at birth. *Candida* often invades the pharynx and larynx and may produce a thick layer of hyphae that lines the upper and lower respiratory tract. Ulceration of the pharynx, larynx, and the lower respiratory tract can occur.

Etiology. Predisposing factors that lead to the development of neonatal infections and pneumonia include, in part, the immaturity of the immune system, colonization of the mother's genital and vaginal tracts with pathogens, amnionitis, prolonged rupture of membranes, prematurity requiring intubation and assisted ventilation, and nosocomial infections acquired in the NICU. Bacterial pneumonia can be secondary to the spread of pathogens from the mother to the baby in utero. Pneumonia acquired in utero often leads to stillbirth and premature delivery.

Neonates who require NICU care are at particularly high risk for colonization of their upper respiratory tract with pathogenic organisms and the passage of pathogens from caregivers or contaminated equipment.[13] Risk factors that are independently predictive of ventilator-associated pneumonia (VAP) in the NICU include reintubation, duration (prolonged) of mechanical ventilation, use of opiates, and endotracheal suctioning.[345,413]

Primary ciliary dyskinesia, an autosomal recessively inherited condition, should be suspected in any infant with unexplained respiratory distress or recurrent pneumonias/atelectasis, especially if situs inversus is present (e.g., Kartagener syndrome).[176]

Prevention. Prevention begins with identifying mothers at risk for infection (e.g., group B *Streptococcus* [GBS], herpes, chlamydial infection, syphilis, gonorrhea); early management of infections with antibiotic therapy; meticulous equipment disinfection and handwashing practices by health care providers in the NICU; and restricting the entry of *anyone* with respiratory infections into the NICU (see Chapter 22). A recent RCT of 60 intubated infants (half in supine position and the other half in side-lying) investigated whether positioning would decrease VAP. Despite no significant difference in the number of positive tracheal cultures after 2 days, **after 5 days, cultures were positive in 87% of the supine versus 30% of the side-lying group.**[6] There is no evidence to support interventions used in adults (e.g., head-of-bed [HOB] elevation and oral care) as preventive of VAP in neonates.

Data Collection

History. The clinical presentation of neonatal pneumonia varies, depending on the infecting organism and the incidence of acquisition. Acute respiratory distress is frequently seen in intrauterine and intrapartally acquired secondary infections. Neonates with pneumonia often have a history of low Apgar scores, temperature instability, and poor tone and activity. **The clinical signs and symptoms of pneumonia are similar to those of respiratory distress, TTN/retained lung fluid, or sepsis.** Late-acquired pneumonia may have a gradual or abrupt onset, depending on the organism. Infants with chlamydial pneumonia frequently present with a characteristic staccato cough.

Physical Examination. The infant with pneumonia often presents with respiratory distress (e.g., tachypnea, low pulse oximetry readings, respiratory deterioration, apnea, temperature instability). **The signs and symptoms of pneumonia often are nonspecific and difficult to differentiate from other neonatal respiratory problems** without the aid of chest x-ray evaluation.

Laboratory Data. The appearance of pneumonia varies depending on the duration of infection, cause of the pneumonia, and presence of respiratory disease (e.g., RDS, BPD). **Serial x-ray films are more valuable than one isolated x-ray examination** in making the diagnosis and following the course of the disease. Infiltration patterns on chest x-ray films include lobar consolidation; patchy alveolar infiltrates; hilar and peribronchial infiltrates; reticulogranular, nodular, or miliary infiltrates; and hazy or opaque lungs (see Table 23-15).

Tracheal aspiration and blood culture also are useful tools in identifying the organisms of pneumonia. A **workup for sepsis** is often part of the diagnostic evaluation for these neonates (see Chapter 22).

Treatment. **Treatment of neonatal pneumonia includes supportive care** (e.g., thermoregulation, nutrition, oxygenation, ventilation if necessary, and parenteral support). If the **causative agent is bacterial, antibiotic therapy must be instituted after a**

sepsis workup; if viral, an antiviral agent is considered; if fungal, an antifungal agent is used (see Chapter 22). Neonatal pneumonia may be accompanied by surfactant inactivation, and **surfactant rescue therapy has resulted in improved oxygenation** and decreased need for ECLS/ECMO.[113]

Complications. The mortality rate for perinatally acquired pneumonia is variable but has been estimated at 20%, with a higher mortality rate, 50%, for postnatally acquired pneumonia. In a recent review of perinatally acquired neonatal infections, the overall mortality rate for pneumonia was 10%.[173] The decline in mortality is the result of perinatal antibiotic use. VAP in the NICU results in longer length of stay, higher cost, and higher mortality.[13,345,413]

PERSISTENT PULMONARY HYPERTENSION OF THE NEWBORN

PPHN manifests as severe pulmonary hypertension with pulmonary artery pressure elevation to levels equal to systemic pressure or higher and large right-to-left shunts through the foramen ovale and the ductus arteriosus. PPHN manifests early in life: 77% of cases are diagnosed in the first 24 hours of life, 93% in the first 48 hours, and 97% by 72 hours of age. The incidence of PPHN is 1 in 1000 live births.[276]

Pathophysiology. Once the placental blood source is severed, adequate oxygenation of the newborn depends on inflation of the lungs, closure of the fetal shunts, a decrease in pulmonary vascular resistance, and an increase in pulmonary blood flow (an eightfold to tenfold increase at the first breath). Normally, pulmonary vascular resistance decreases with the first breath of life. When it remains high, successful transition from fetal to neonatal circulation is impaired. In an infant manifesting PPHN, high pulmonary vascular resistance and pulmonary hypertension impede pulmonary blood flow. **Factors that increase and decrease pulmonary vascular resistance are listed in Table 23-16.**

Increased PVR leads to hypoxemia, acidemia, hypercarbia, and eventually lactic acidosis. The pulmonary arterioles respond to this process with further constriction, promoting an additional decrease in blood flow; thus a cyclic pattern is established. Pulmonary vascular resistance also maintains higher right-sided pressures in the heart that equal or exceed systemic pressures, resulting in right-to-left shunting, which is characteristic of PPHN. PPHN also produces direct and indirect effects on myocardial function. A combination of pressure alterations, hypoxia, and acidemia leads to a cyclic pattern of decreased cardiac output, decreased pulmonary blood flow, and further vasoconstriction (Figure 23-11).

TABLE 23-16 FACTORS THAT ALTER PULMONARY VASCULAR RESISTANCE (PVR)

LOWERS PVR	INCREASES PVR
Endogenous mediators and mechanisms:	Endogenous mediators and mechanisms:
Oxygen	Hypoxia
Nitric oxide	Acidosis
PGI_2, PGE_2, PGD_2	Endothelin-1
Adenosine, ATP, magnesium	Leukotrienes
Bradykinin	Thromboxanes
Atrial natriuretic factor	Platelet-activating factor
Alkalosis	Ca^{2+} channel activation
K+ channel activation	Alpha-adrenergic stimulation
Histamine	$PGF_{2\alpha}$
Vagal nerve stimulation	
Acetylcholine	
Beta-adrenergic stimulation	
Mechanical factors:	Mechanical factors:
Lung infection	Overinflation or underinflation
Vascular cell structural changes	Excessive muscularization, vascular remodeling
Interstitial fluid and pressure changes	Altered mechanical properties of smooth muscle
Shear stress	Pulmonary hypoplasia
	Alveolar capillary dysplasia
	Pulmonary thromboemboli
	Main pulmonary artery distention
	Ventricular dysfunction, venous hypertension

From Kinsella J, Abman S: Recent developments in the pathophysiology and treatment of PPHN, *J Pediatr* 126:855, 1995.

ATP, Adenosine triphosphate; *$PGF_{2\alpha}$,* prostaglandin $F_{2\alpha}$; *PGI_2, PGE_2, PGD_2,* prostaglandins I_2, E_2, and D_2; *PVR,* pulmonary vascular resistance.

Etiology. Pulmonary vascular resistance (PVR) remains high after birth because of underdevelopment, maldevelopment, or maladaptation of pulmonary vasculature (see the Critical Findings box below). In utero, development of increased vascular smooth muscle or perinatal factors that cause or

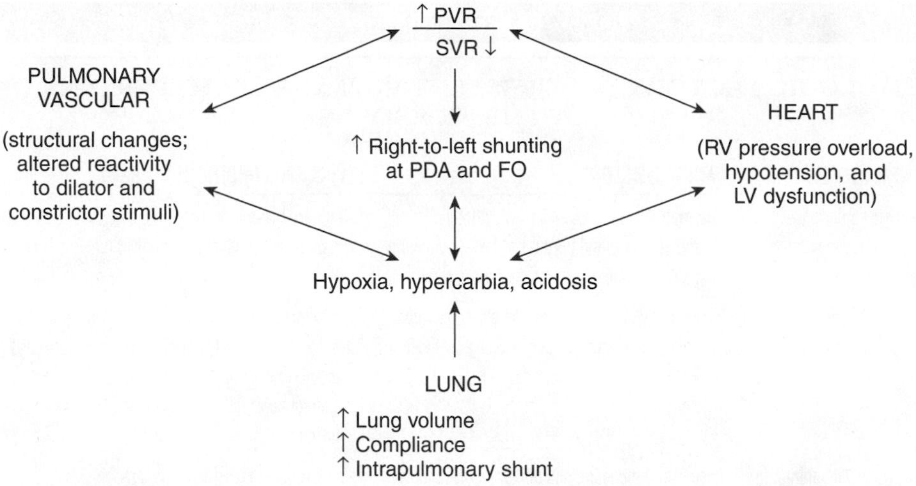

FIGURE 23-11 Cardiopulmonary interactions in persistent pulmonary hypertension of the newborn. *FO,* Foramen ovale; *LV,* left ventricle; *PDA,* patent ductus arteriosus; *PVR,* pulmonary vascular resistance; *RV,* right ventricle; *SVR,* systemic vascular resistance. (From Kinsella J, Abman S: Recent developments in the pathophysiology and treatment of PPHN, *J Pediatr* 126:855, 1995.)

contribute to vasospasm are thought to be prime mechanisms of PPHN. Independent predictors of pulmonary hypertension in the preterm infant include (1) low Apgar scores, (2) preterm premature rupture of membranes (PPROM), (3) oligohydramnios, (4) pulmonary hypoplasia, and (5) sepsis.[211]

An uncommon autosomal recessive lung disorder in term infants called *surfactant protein B (SP-B) deficiency* causes progressive, fatal hypoxemic respiratory failure.[398]

Prevention. Prevention of PPHN includes minimizing intrauterine and perinatal risk factors when possible, maintaining postnatal physiologic homeostasis, and detecting and correcting any underlying abnormality.

Data Collection

History. In addition to the risk factors listed in the Critical Findings box on p. 651 and above, **maternal tobacco use, maternal obesity, premature rupture of membranes, maternal lack of private or use of public insurance, cesarean delivery, late preterm or postterm birth, LGA infant, race (black, Asian), maternal diabetes, and maternal asthma are associated with an increased risk for PPHN.**[167]

There are two major considerations in the history of these infants: (1) the recognition of major disease processes or syndromes that are highly associated with pulmonary hypertension and (2) the timing of the onset of cyanosis and the deterioration of the infant.

Physical Examination. The initial clinical presentation is usually a late preterm (34 weeks or greater GA), term, or postterm infant with worsening cyanosis within the first 24 hours of life. Tachypnea is a common finding and, when accompanied by retractions, is indicative of decreased pulmonary compliance. Cyanosis may be either intense at birth or progressively worsen in association with increased right-to-left shunting.

Despite increasing F_{IO_2}, the infant continues to have low Pa_{O_2} (hypoxemia) as a result of right-to-left shunting. Milder cases of PPHN feature minimal tachypnea and cyanosis, frequently associated with stress from crying or feeding. Severe cases are characterized by marked cyanosis, tachypnea, low systemic blood pressure, and decreased peripheral perfusion.

Increased pulmonary artery pressure results in the following signs:

- Pulmonic systolic ejection clicks
- A second heart sound that is single, loud, or narrowly split with a loud pulmonary component
- A prominent right ventricular impulse that is visible or palpable at the lower left sternal border
- A soft systolic murmur in the pulmonary area

Laboratory Data. The laboratory evaluation of an infant with suspected PPHN should include a **complete blood count (CBC) with differential, platelet count, chest x-ray examination, and serum glu-**

Critical Findings

ETIOLOGIC FACTORS IN PERSISTENT PULMONARY HYPERTENSION OF THE NEWBORN

DEVELOPMENTAL PROCESS	PATHOPHYSIOLOGY	ASSOCIATED CONDITIONS
Underdevelopment, a decreased number of pulmonary vessels	Interruption in lung development, resulting in shunting of blood because of fewer pulmonary vessels and less area for gaseous exchange	Pulmonary hypoplasia (e.g., diaphragmatic hernia, premature rupture of membranes, oligohydramnios, Potter syndrome)
Maldevelopment, abnormally developed pulmonary vessels	Hypertrophy of musculature and extension into nonmuscularized arteries resulting in smaller lumen size, which increases PVR	Intrauterine asphyxia/hypoxia,[214] MAS, and maternal smoking Intrauterine fetal ductus arteriosus closure increases pulmonary blood flow Congenital heart defects that result in abnormal pulmonary vessel formation
Maladaptation (from intrauterine to extrauterine life) as a result of transient or persistent vasoconstriction	Results in remodeling and abnormal muscularization of small pulmonary arteries Results in pulmonary vasospasm and vascular remodeling	Hypoxia/acidosis/asphyxia Asphyxia may result in persistent vasospasm Pulmonary parenchymal disease
	Pulmonary vasospasm and decreased cardiac output resulting from release of endotoxins and reaction to systemic inflammatory response	Bacterial sepsis Prenatal pulmonary hypertension (e.g., fetal systemic hypertension or premature closure of the ductus arteriosus) associated with maternal ingestion of NSAIDs (e.g., ibuprofen, naproxen, indomethacin), salicylates, phenytoin, lithium, prostaglandin inhibitors, or selective serotonin reuptake inhibitors[2,60,127,214,279]
	Prevents normal circulatory transition at delivery	Delayed or ineffective resuscitation, narcosis, other central nervous system depression, hypothermia, hypotension
	Potentiation of vasoconstriction	Hypothermia, hypoglycemia, hypocalcemia, acidosis, hypoxia, myocardial dysfunction, and ischemia
	Functional obstruction of pulmonary vascular bed	Polycythemia, hyperviscosity

Data from VanMarter L: Persistent pulmonary hypertension of the newborn. In Cloherty J, Stark A, editors: *Manual of neonatal care,* ed 4, Philadelphia, 1998, Lippincott-Raven; Weardon M, Hansen T: Persistent pulmonary hypertension of the newborn. In Hansen T, Cooper T, Weisman L, editors: *Contemporary diagnosis and management of neonatal respiratory diseases,* ed 2, Newton, Pa, 1998, Handbook of Health Care.
MAS, Meconium aspiration syndrome; *NSAIDs,* nonsteroidal anti-inflammatory drugs; *PVR,* pulmonary vascular resistance.

cose, calcium, electrolytes, and arterial blood gas determinations. The CBC is used to detect anemia, which could contribute to systemic hypertension; detect polycythemia, which could lead to increased pulmonary vascular resistance; and detect an infectious process such as group B streptococcal sepsis or pneumonia.

Arterial blood gases demonstrate acidosis, hypoxia, and increased $Paco_2$. If blood gas specimens are obtained simultaneously in the right radial artery (preductal) and the descending aorta (postductal), the right-to-left shunt can be documented (preductal Pao_2 greater than postductal). Simultaneous preductal and postductal pulse oximetry or transcutaneous oxygen measurements may also be useful in the diagnosis. Other diagnostic tests are outlined in Table 23-17.

The most common chest x-ray findings associated with PPHN include the following:
- Prominent main pulmonary artery segment
- Mild to moderate cardiomegaly
- Variable pulmonary vasculature (increased, decreased, or normal)
- Signs of left ventricular dysfunction that include pulmonary venous congestion and cardiomegaly

The ECG is usually normal but may demonstrate right ventricular hypertrophy, evidence of pulmonary hypertension, and signs of myocardial

TABLE 23-17 DIAGNOSTIC TESTS FOR PERSISTENT PULMONARY HYPERTENSION OF THE NEWBORN (PPHN)

TEST	USE
Hyperoxia test	If Po_2 does not increase in 100% oxygen, a right-to-left shunt is demonstrated (may be secondary to either PPHN or congenital heart defect)
Comparison of preductal and postductal arterial Pao_2	Demonstrates ductal shunting; if negative, it does not rule out PPHN; most infants with congenital heart disease have no ductal shunting
Contrast echocardiography "bubble echo"	Demonstrates foramen ovale shunting but should be present in most cases of PPHN
Hyperoxia-hyperventilation	Most definite test; if Po_2 <50 mm Hg prehyperventilation and rises above 100 mm Hg is almost always PPHN

From Duara S, Gewitz MH, Fox WW: Use of mechanical ventilation for clinical management of persistent pulmonary hypertension of the newborn, *Clin Perinatol* 11:641, 1984.
PPHN, Persistent pulmonary hypertension of the newborn.

ischemia. Echocardiography is essential in (1) evaluating cardiac structures, (2) ruling out cyanotic cardiac lesions, (3) diagnosing the right-to-left shunting at the foramen ovale and/or ductus arteriosus, (4) estimating pulmonary artery pressure, (5) determining therapy, and (6) evaluating response to therapy.[200]

Treatment. Historically, treatment of PPHN included hyperventilation, IV infusions (e.g., systemic vasodilators, sedatives, narcotics, paralysis, alkali, and inotropes), surfactant administration, high-frequency ventilation, and ultimately ECMO/ECLS as a last resort. These treatments were widely used without RCTs to test safety and efficacy, and none of these treatments improved survival in infants with PPHN.

Treatment of PPHN focuses on preventing or intervening in the development of the cyclic pattern illustrated in Figure 23-11. Goals of current therapy include (1) treating associated pathology (e.g., antibiotics for sepsis/pneumonia; partial exchange transfusion for polycythemia/hyperviscosity; volume expanders),[276] (2) providing adequate oxygenation, (3) reducing PVR by pulmonary vasodilation that improves pulmonary blood flow, (4) increasing and maintaining systemic vascular resistance (SVR) (e.g., systemic blood pressure), and (5) preventing right-to-left shunting by decreasing PVR and increasing SVR. Pulmonary blood flow should increase if PVR is decreased or if SVR is increased.

Adequate Oxygenation. **Maintaining adequate oxygenation is a prime goal of care of infants with PPHN; alterations in "routine" care and handling are essential.** Because handling a sick newborn for any reason causes a fall in Pao_2, the benefits of handling for routine care such as changing linens, weighing, suctioning, and taking vital signs must be balanced against the risk for iatrogenic hypoxia. **Pao_2 variations in the newborn are as follows[89,119]:**

At rest	±15 mm Hg variation
While crying	↓Pao_2 by as much as 50 mm Hg
With routine care	↓Pao_2 by as much as 30 mm Hg

Maintaining organized, coordinated care and minimizing disturbances are therefore very important. Keeping the infant calm is important because severe hypoxia accompanies crying. Using pacifiers and decreasing noxious stimuli (e.g., invasive procedures) keep struggling and crying to a minimum. **Continuously monitoring vital signs, blood pressure, and pulse oximetry decreases the need for physical manipulation and disturbance. These large, vigorous infants require sedation and analgesia** (see Chapter 12) or paralysis (see Table 23-14) to promote effective oxygenation and ventilation and decrease air leaks.

Ventilation Therapy. **Conventional mechanical ventilation uses hyperventilation to produce hypocarbia (↓$Paco_2$) and respiratory alkalosis.** Both metabolic and respiratory alkalosis have a direct vasodilator effect on pulmonary vasculature that decreases PVR and improves oxygenation. **The neonate's lungs should be ventilated with whatever combination of rate, pressure, and oxygen is needed to lower $Paco_2$ and raise pH.** Hyperventilation has not improved the clinical outcomes of PPHN, has been associated with adverse neurologic sequelae (e.g., CP and cystic PVL), and exposes the lung to barotrauma/volutrauma, CLD/BPD, and air leaks.[276]

HFV, both oscillator and jet, is used to treat PPHN. Use of HFOV optimizes lung inflation and oxygenation, improves ventilation, and achieves respiratory alkalosis. HFOV is an effective rescue treatment for some neonates meeting ECMO/ECLS criteria who were unresponsive to CMV.[72] A discussion of the combination of HFOV and inhaled nitric oxide follows. In the only prospective RCT comparing HFJV with CMV, HFJV acutely improved oxygenation and ventilation without a significant increase in mortality and morbidity.[114] Because of the small samples, a multicenter RCT is needed.[114]

Inhaled Nitric Oxide. Endogenous NO production dilates the fetal pulmonary vascular bed and is essential in decreasing PVR after birth.[76] **Because endogenous production of NO in the pulmonary vasculature of neonates with PPHN is reduced, treatment with iNO is beneficial because iNO is a selective pulmonary vasodilator (e.g., decreases pulmonary hypertension and increases oxygenation without reducing systemic blood pressure).**[200] Early clinical studies of iNO demonstrated brief exposure actually improved oxygenation and lowered pulmonary artery pressure. RCTs from multicenters have confirmed that prolonged iNO treatment for PPHN (1) results in sustained improvement of oxygenation,[124,263] (2) decreases the need for ECMO/ECLS treatment,[92,263] and (3) is an adjunct to CMV[263] and that combined therapy (e.g., iNO, HFOV) is more effective than either therapy alone. The Neonatal Inhaled Nitric Oxide Study Group (NINOSG)[263] found that iNO had no effect on mortality, length of stay, number of days of ventilatory support, incidence of air leak, CLD/BPD, IVH/PVL, seizures, and pulmonary and GI hemorrhages. The effectiveness of iNO depends on (1) the initial degree of pulmonary vasoconstriction and hypoxemia, (2) the severity of parenchymal lung disease, and (3) the recruitment of adequate lung volume/inflation that decreases intrapulmonary shunting and improves iNO delivery to the pulmonary system.[200] In the ECMO/ECLS population, iNO use has increased from 0% to 24%.

Inhaled NO is an effective treatment for PPHN but "should be considered a part of the overall clinical strategy that cautiously manages parenchymal lung disease, cardiac performance, and systemic hemodynamics."[200] **Inhaled NO has been approved by the U.S. Food and Drug Administration for treatment of near-term (>34 weeks GA) and term neonates with PPHN. Recommendations for use of iNO are listed in Table 23-18.** Use of iNO in moderate PPHN improves oxygenation, decreases the amount of ventilation needed, and prevents progression to severe PPHN. A recent retrospective study comparing the use of HFOV and HFJV with iNO found similar short-term effects of decreasing the need for ECMO, improving oxygenation and ventilation of infants with PPHN regardless of which type of ventilator was used.[75]

Use of HFOV and iNO to treat PPHN has decreased the number of neonates meeting ECMO/ECLS criteria who subsequently require ECMO/ECLS treatment, has shortened length of hospital stay, and has decreased costs. Survival is increased and short-term morbidity is decreased in neonates 34 weeks GA or older with PPHN who are treated with ECMO/ECLS versus conventional therapies.

Pharmacologic Therapy. Surfactant replacement therapy is used when significant parenchymal lung disease (e.g., MAS) is the cause of PPHN. Secondary surfactant deficiency also may exist in PPHN. Surfactant replacement in the early phase of PPHN significantly decreases the need for ECMO/ECLS in term newborns without increasing the risk for complications.[113]

Use of inotropic support (e.g., vasopressors) (Table 23-19) increases SVR, which decreases right-to-left shunting through the foramen ovale and ductus arteriosus. Cardiac output, cardiac contractility, and systemic blood pressure are all increased. Recently, a small study of newborns (n = 18) treated with iNO for PPHN (but with symptoms of circulatory failure [despite adequate fluids]) showed that IV norepinephrine improved lung function by decreasing the ratio between pulmonary and systemic artery pressures and improving cardiac performance.[371]

Systemic vasodilators (e.g., tolazoline, sodium nitroprusside, prostaglandin E_1) have been used to decrease PVR. These medications have resulted in variable and unpredictable results and are associated with systemic hypotension, the need for volume expansion and fluid resuscitation, and an inability to achieve and maintain pulmonary vasodilation. When vasodilators are infused in dosages sufficient to decrease pulmonary hypertension, there is increased venous admixture as a result of right-to-left shunting of venous blood and pulmonary ventilation-perfusion mismatch. **Because of these adverse effects, use of systemic vasodilators is no longer recommended.**

Use of phosphodiesterase inhibitors (e.g., milrinone, sildenafil) has been reported in several case series, retrospective data analysis, and one small

TABLE 23-18 RECOMMENDATIONS FOR USE OF INHALED NITRIC OXIDE (iNO)

RECOMMENDATION	RESEARCH BASIS
GESTATIONAL AGE	
≥34 weeks' gestation	Clinical trials[73,263] and FDA approval support use of iNO in late preterm/term newborns.[200]
POSTNATAL AGE	
Within the first week of life; postnatal age alone should not define the duration of therapy when prolonged therapy could be beneficial	Clinical trials support iNO use within the first week of life; may also be used as adjunct therapy after ECMO/ECLS treatment.
SEVERITY OF ILLNESS	
Oxygenation index (OI) = (MAP × F_{IO_2} × 100 ÷ Pa_{O_2}) >25 with echocardiographic evidence of extrapulmonary right-to-left shunting	Mean OI in multicenter trials was 40; earlier use of iNO at lower OI has not resulted in reduction of mortality or ECMO/ECLS use.
DOSE	
Initial: 20 ppm in term newborns with PPHN	Increasing dose to 40-80 ppm does not improve response to 20 ppm.
Brief exposure to 40-80 ppm is safe	Initial treatment with low dose (1-2 ppm) does not compromise responses to higher doses (10-20 ppm); a majority of low doses require dose increases.
Sustained treatment with 80 ppm increases the risk for methemoglobinemia	The lowest effective starting dose has not been determined.
DURATION	
Typically <5 days	Longer usage may be necessary in pulmonary hypoplasia. For therapy >5 days, other causes of pulmonary hypertension should be investigated.
WEANING AND DISCONTINUATION	
Differing approaches toward weaning have been studied with few differences in outcomes until iNO is discontinued:	Withdrawal of iNO can be associated with life-threatening elevations in PVR, profound oxygen desaturation, and systemic hypotension because of decreased cardiac output.
After 4 hours at 20 ppm, iNO reduced to 6 ppm without change in oxygenation;	Dose-response relationship between iNO given and a drop in Pa_{O_2}. A decrease in iNO to 1 ppm before discontinuation minimizes decrease in Pa_{O_2}, and compensatory changes in F_{IO_2} and ventilator parameters are unnecessary.
iNO decreased by 20% increments in stepwise fashion to dose of 1 ppm before discontinuation	
VENTILATOR MANAGEMENT	
High-frequency oscillatory ventilation (HFOV)	Inadequate lung inflation results in less response to iNO therapy.
With significant parenchymal lung disease	Combination of HFOV and iNO results in best improvement in oxygenation because of improved lung inflation during HFOV that augments response to iNO by reducing intrapulmonary shunting and improving iNO delivery to pulmonary circulation.
Without significant parenchymal lung disease	Combination of HFOV and iNO and iNO alone are more effective than HFOV alone.
CONGENITAL DIAPHRAGMATIC HERNIA	
Routine use in CDH not recommended	CDH infants are poor responders to iNO. Limited to CDH infants with supra-systemic PVR (after establishing optimal lung inflation and echocardiography determination of adequate LV function).
Late pulmonary hypertension in CDH infants	Late pulmonary hypertension is clinically evident when PVR becomes supra-systemic with right-to-left venoarterial admixture across the FO and/or ductus arteriosus measured on echocardiography.

Modified from Kinsella, JP: Inhaled nitric oxide in the term neonate, *Early Hum Dev* 84:709, 2008.

CDH, Congenital diaphragmatic hernia; *CLD/BPD,* chronic lung disease/bronchopulmonary dysplasia; *ECMO/ECLS,* extracorporeal membrane oxygenation/extracorporeal life support; *FDA,* Food and Drug Administration; *FO,* foramen ovale; *IVH,* intraventricular hemorrhage; *LV,* left ventricular; *PPHN,* persistent pulmonary hypertension of the newborn; *PVR,* pulmonary vascular resistance.

Continued

TABLE 23-18 RECOMMENDATIONS FOR USE OF INHALED NITRIC OXIDE (iNO)—cont'd

RECOMMENDATION	RESEARCH BASIS
USE IN ECMO/ECLS CENTERS	
Use to stabilize before cannulation for ECMO	Lower mortality for iNO-treated group than for infants not treated with iNO.[129]
Use of iNO has not adversely affected outcome by delaying ECMO	iNO treatment associated with improved short-term pulmonary outcomes,[73] and decreased ECMO use is not associated with increased late-term morbidity.[70,264]
USE IN NON–ECMO/ECLS CENTERS AND TRANSPORT WITH iNO	
If progressive deterioration in oxygenation occurs in centers without ECMO/ECLS, transport to ECMO/ECLS center without interruption of iNO therapy must be accomplished[231]	Withdrawal of iNO to transport to an ECMO/ECLS center may result in acute and life-threatening deterioration.

Data from Kinsella, JP: Inhaled nitric oxide in the term neonate, *Early Hum Dev* 84:709, 2008.

CDH, Congenital diaphragmatic hernia; *CLD/BPD,* chronic lung disease/bronchopulmonary dysplasia; *ECMO/ECLS,* extracorporeal membrane oxygenation/extracorporeal life support; *FDA,* Food and Drug Administration; *FO,* foramen ovale; *IVH,* intraventricular hemorrhage; *LV,* left ventricular; *PPHN,* persistent pulmonary hypertension of the newborn; *PVR,* pulmonary vascular resistance.

TABLE 23-19 VASOPRESSOR RESPONSE IN THE NEONATE

DRUG DOSE	DISADVANTAGE
DOPAMINE	
<4 mcg/kg/min: renal vasodilation, mesenteric and cerebral vasodilation (effects unknown) plus increase in cardiac output	May decrease systemic arterial pressure
5-20 mcg/kg/min: increase in cardiac output depending on myocardial norepinephrine	Loss of renal and mesenteric perfusion
>20 mcg/kg/min: systemic arterial pressure increases more than pulmonary artery pressure	Cardiac output may decrease Myocardial oxygen consumption increases Marked increase in left ventricular afterload Dysrhythmias noted
DOBUTAMINE	
10 mcg/kg/min: increases cardiac contractility directly; cardiac output increases depending on myocardial catecholamine stores	No selective renal or mesenteric vasodilation Tends to increase skeletal blood flow at the expense of viscera Increase in pulmonary artery pressure
ISOPROTERENOL	
0.05-1 mcg/kg/min: lowers pulmonary vascular resistance in pulmonary hypotensive and vascular disease in child and adult; lowers hypoxemia-induced pulmonary vascular resistance in animal models	Dysrhythmias No specific vasodilation effects
NITROPRUSSIDE	
0.4-5 mcg/kg/min: cardiac output increases because of decreased left ventricular afterload; systemic vascular resistance (indicated by blood pressure) decreases because of decreased left ventricular afterload	Systemic vascular resistance remains constant if CO_2 increases

Modified from Drummond W: The use of cardiotonic therapy in the management of infants with PPHN, *Clin Perinatol* 11:715, 1984.

RCT.[241,254,269,373] Use of sildenafil has the following effects[24,254,269,373]:

- It is as effective as iNO in improving pulmonary vasodilation.
- It has been helpful in weaning from iNO.
- It does/does not decrease systemic blood pressure.
- It improves cardiac output.
- It is more effective when used together with iNO than either used separately.
- Chronic use is safe, effective, and well tolerated.

Intravenous (IV) milrinone improves oxygenation without compromising systemic blood pressure.[241] One case report of severe ROP in a preterm treated with sildenafil for pulmonary hypertension has been reported.[361] RCTs are needed to establish the safety, efficacy, side effects, and outcomes of sildenafil and milrinone use in PPHN; until then, use is experimental.[24,241,269,373]

Complications. Follow-up at 18 to 24 months of age of the neonates in the NINOSG trial found no increase in neurodevelopmental or behavioral abnormality; the children in the control group experienced a higher incidence of seizures after discharge than did the iNO treated group.[264] Two other studies also showed no increase in adverse neurodevelopmental or pulmonary outcomes as a result of treatment with iNO and avoidance of ECMO treatment.[70,226] A recent follow-up study of term newborns (at 1 year postnatal age) treated with iNO for PPHN found a lower incidence of respiratory morbidity (26%) when compared with the respiratory morbidity after ECMO treatment (37%) or CMV (56%).[175]

A recent follow-up study of 85 children (at 5 to 11 years of age) who had been treated for PPHN compared with a matched reference group found (1) sensorineural hearing loss (11%), (2) increase in chronic health problems (42% vs. 17%), (3) use of bronchodilators (21% vs. 8%), and (4) increased use of remedial education (19% vs. 5%).[115] Survivors of PPHN may have significant pulmonary and neurodevelopmental impairment whether treated with conventional methods or with ECMO/ECLS and should have long-term follow-up.

APNEA

Pathophysiology. The two major control mechanisms that regulate pulmonary ventilation are the neural and chemical systems. The cerebral cortex and brainstem are the governing agents for the neural control system, which regulates respiratory rate and rhythm. The peripheral components of this system are found in the upper airway and lung. The chemical control center is found in the medulla and is sensitive to changes in $Paco_2$. The peripheral portion of the chemical system lies in the carotid and aortic vessels and is sensitive to changes in $Paco_2$. Alveolar ventilation is controlled by the chemical system, and this system is the principal defense against hypoxia. Neonates have a unique response to hypoxemia and carbon dioxide retention. Unlike adults, who have sustained increase in ventilation, infants have a brief period of increased ventilation followed by respiratory depression.

Carbon dioxide responsiveness is less developed in the preterm infant, which may be the result of decreased sensitivity in the chemical center or mechanical factors that prevent an increase in ventilation. Apnea of prematurity or primary apnea is not associated with other specific disease entities. **The younger the gestational age, the greater is the incidence of apnea, so at least 85% of preterms less than 34 weeks' gestation have apnea of prematurity.**[319] Apnea and bradycardia episodes usually begin within the first week after birth and spontaneously resolve at 36 weeks PMA.[288] In infants born at 27 weeks' gestation or earlier, 58% to 60% have persistent apnea at 36 weeks' postconceptual age (PCA).[109] Apnea may be associated with hypoxemia, neuronal immaturity, sleep, catecholamine deficiency, and respiratory muscle fatigue.

Etiology. Causes of apnea in the premature are characterized as *central apnea* (absence of breathing effort), *obstructive apnea* (breathing efforts occur but the airway is blocked), or, most commonly, *mixed apnea* (an initial central apnea followed by obstruction of the airway).[277] Various conditions may cause apnea in the premature infant by producing hypoxia and/or altering the sensitivity of peripheral or central chemoreceptors (Table 23-20). Neuronal immaturity is a plausible cause for apnea because respiratory efforts are more unstable at younger gestational ages. The decreased response appears to be the result of a general lack of dendritic formation and limited synaptic connections, thereby decreasing the excitatory drive. Another hypothesis is that apneic episodes are manifestations of synaptic

TABLE 23-20 CAUSES OF APNEA IN THE PREMATURE INFANT

CAUSE	SPECIFICS
Infection	Pneumonia, sepsis, meningitis
Respiratory distress	Immaturity of respiratory development, RDS, airway obstruction, CPAP application, post-extubation, congenital anomalies of the upper airways
Cardiovascular disorders	Patent ductus arteriosus, congestive heart failure
Gastrointestinal disorders	Vomiting, necrotizing enterocolitis, deglutition syncope
Central nervous system disorders	Depressant drugs, intraventricular hemorrhage, seizure, elevated bilirubin levels, bilirubin encephalopathy/kernicterus, infection, tumors/ischemia
Metabolic disorders	Hypoglycemia, hypocalcemia, hyponatremia/hypernatremia
Environmental	Rapid increase of environmental temperature, hypothermia, vigorous suctioning, feeding, stooling, stretching/movement; fatigue/stress, prenatal exposure to maternal cigarette smoking, position, sleep state (e.g., active vs. quiet) First immunization (DTP/IPV/Hib): increase in apnea, bradycardia, and desaturations within 72 hours of immunizations[221]
Hematopoietic	Polycythemia, anemia

DTP, Diphtheria-tetanus-pertussis; *CPAP,* continuous positive airway pressure; *Hib, Haemophilus influenzae* type B; *IPV,* inactivated polio virus; *RDS,* respiratory distress syndrome.

disorders that occur without a motor component. Such phenomena have been confirmed on EEG. Infants depend on alternating excitation and inhibition to establish rhythmic breathing; therefore imbalances (e.g., hypoxia, hypoglycemia, hypocalcemia) may cause respiratory arrest.

Apnea is more frequent during sleep and especially during rapid eye movement (REM) or active sleep in both term and preterm infants.[370] Apnea associated with sleep becomes more significant in that premature infants, particularly those of less than 32 weeks' gestation, spend 80% of their time asleep. Equally significant is the time spent in REM sleep, the predominant sleep state of premature infants. Apnea is uncommon in non-REM sleep, but periodic breathing may be observed. The effects of REM sleep are inhibition of spinal motor neurons, increase in brain activity causing increasing eye movements and muscular twitching, and changes in brain temperature and cerebral blood flow and CNS arousal, shown by EEG changes.

A premature infant has a more compliant chest cage and less compliant lungs, resulting in greater respiratory workload. Respiratory muscle fatigue occurs easily in the absence of fatigue-resistant fibers.

Secondary apnea may be associated with a particular disease entity or in response to special procedures. Many disorders leading to secondary apnea may exert their influence through hypoxemia and subsequent respiratory center depression.

The majority of cases of secondary apnea arise from four conditions. In RDS, apnea is related to the degree of parenchymal disease and may result from muscle fatigue. With CNS hemorrhage and seizures, apnea arises from asphyxia with subsequent hypoxemia and respiratory center depression or actual brain injury. Apnea is related to central depression in sepsis. In addition, carbon dioxide retention and hypoxemia associated with the left-to-right shunting of a PDA may cause apnea.

Iatrogenic causes of apnea include increased environmental temperature, sudden increases in environmental temperature, vagal response to suctioning of the nasopharynx or to a gavage tube, vomiting, and obstruction of the airway. Reflex apnea occurs when foreign material (milk or secretions) is present in the oropharynx. This laryngeal chemoreflex is protective in that it prevents inhalation of the substance into the airway and has been documented in preterm and hospitalized infants. Obstruction may occur from improper neck positioning or aspiration.

Cerebral blood flow (CBF) velocity decreases with apnea and bradycardia[282] and is directly correlated with the severity of bradycardia,[302] and an increase in CBF may occur on recovery.[228] Decreased oxygen saturation also correlates with the duration of apnea, regardless of type. Obstructive apnea is associated with significantly greater maximum fall in cerebral blood volume than central or mixed apneic episodes. Because alteration of CBF may cause or exacerbate IVH, obstruction of upper airways with resultant apneic episodes should be prevented.

Prevention. All infants assessed as being at high risk for apneic spells should be carefully monitored for at least 10 to 12 days. Impedance apnea monitors do not distinguish normal respiratory efforts from gasping movements associated with obstruction. Both heart and respiratory rates should be monitored. Alarm systems should be used at all times. A qualified observer is essential.

Apneic episodes are frequently associated with alterations in heart rate and oxygen saturation—the degree of these changes is related to the duration of apnea. Apnea generally precedes a drop in heart rate and oxygen desaturation. Changes in oxygen saturation are distinct from heart rate changes, so the desaturation cannot be predicted from changes in heart rate patterns. Because episodes of apnea and bradycardia are associated with a decrease in CBF and because oxygen desaturation (as little as 5% to 10%) is associated with alteration of cerebral circulation,[228] **oxygen saturation monitoring should accompany cardiorespiratory monitoring** (both in-hospital and home monitoring).

Pulse oximetry monitors may detect hypoxemic conditions that may lead to apneic spells. In a premature infant younger than 32 weeks' gestation, this type of apnea is common. Care should be organized to decrease stressful, hypoxic episodes.

Apneic episodes may be prevented or decreased by several means. **Reducing environmental stress by providing adequate rest** has resulted in a faster rate of decline in apneic episodes.[369] **Gentle tactile stimulation** alone has been shown to be effective in decreasing and preventing apneic spells in most premature infants. Noxious stimuli such as shaking or banging on the incubator should be avoided. If tactile stimulus is ineffective and **temporary bag-and-mask ventilation is necessary,** attention should be paid to preventing undue pressure on the lower chin and neck so that the airway remains open. Bagging that is too vigorous also may stimulate pulmonary stretch receptors and induce apnea; therefore it should be avoided. **Waterbed flotation** may decrease the frequency of apnea but generally does not completely eliminate it. Recent systematic reviews have concluded that (1) prophylactic use of kinesthetic stimulation (e.g., waterbed, oscillating mattress) to reduce apnea or bradycardia cannot be recommended,[164] (2) prophylactic use of methylxanthine for prevention of apnea is not supported by data,[165] and (3) prophylactic use of methylxanthines increases the chances of successful extubation of preterm infants within 1 week.[162] **Apneic episodes are decreased when twins are co-bedded,** because of either a change in sleep patterns (e.g., more frequent arousal by the co-bedded twin) or a more regular breathing pattern, reflecting a positive physiologic response to skin-to-skin contact between the twins (see Chapter 13).

Because increased environmental temperature and sudden changes in temperature have resulted in apneic episodes, prevention includes maintaining the environmental temperature at the lower end of the normal spectrum, particularly if an apneic episode already has occurred. Incubator temperature may require a 0.5° to 1.0° C (1° to 2° F) decrease to counter the problem. The frequency of apnea during active sleep is influenced by temperature: more apnea occurs in a warmer environment, whereas apnea is less frequent in cooler conditions.[370] Phototherapy may provide sufficient radiant energy to increase an infant's temperature and contribute to the incidence of apnea. **Care should be taken to avoid sudden changes in temperature.** An infant should not be placed on a cold scale; he or she should be placed in a prewarmed incubator or bed. Oxygen should be warmed and humidified before administration.

Careful attention must be paid to prevent airway obstruction. Small neck rolls under the neck and shoulders have been used to decrease neck flexion and prevent airway obstruction when in the supine position. A recent study comparing supine with prone positioning of preterm infants (n = 21) found no clinically significant increase in acid gastroesophageal reflux (GER) or obstructive apnea episodes associated with GER in asymptomatic convalescent preterms.[42] Close monitoring should be done during procedures such as lumbar puncture in which accidental airway obstruction may occur.

Data Collection. Evaluation of apnea should include studies to rule out treatable causes.

History. Evaluation of the prenatal and birth history may give a clue to the causes and also provide a basis for further study.

Physical Examination. A thorough physical and neurologic examination rules out grossly apparent abnormalities. **Observation and documentation of apneic and bradycardic episodes and any relationship to precipitating factors help differentiate primary from secondary apnea.**

Laboratory Data. A CBC and CRP assay assess for infection and anemia as causes of apnea. Measurements of serum glucose, calcium, phosphate, magnesium, sodium, potassium, and chloride levels assess metabolic causes. Arterial blood gas measurements assess hypoxemia and metabolic and respiratory contributions to apnea. Blood, urine, and cerebral spinal fluid (CSF) cultures rule out sepsis as the cause of apnea. The CSF culture usually is performed only when other signs and symptoms of infection are present. Chest x-ray examinations assess cardiac and respiratory causes. The examinations may also rule out aspiration of gastric contents caused by vomiting or gastroesophageal reflux. Ultrasonographic examination of the head and an EEG may be used to rule out IVH or other neurologic causes of apnea.

Treatment. **Treatment of secondary apnea is aimed at the diagnosis and management of the specific causes. In the treatment of primary apnea (apnea of prematurity), initial efforts should begin with the least invasive intervention possible. Gentle tactile stimulation** is frequently successful, especially with early recognition and intervention. When infants do not immediately respond to external stimuli, bag-and-mask ventilation must be initiated. Generally, an FiO_2 approximating that used before the spell but not exceeding a 10% increase will alleviate hypoxemia and avoid marked elevations in the arterial PaO_2. The use of pulse oximetry monitoring allows closer evaluation of PaO_2 fluctuation and helps prevent complications of oxygen toxicity. Elevation in ambient oxygen concentrations, although decreasing the frequency of apnea, causes prolongation of apnea spells.

Apnea responds to low-pressure (3 to 5 cm of water) nasal CPAP. Mechanical ventilation may be necessary if the infant fails to respond to lesser measures and continues to have repeated and prolonged apneic episodes. It also may be necessary in extremely immature, unstable, or debilitated infants. **Mechanical ventilation for apnea may be administered with nasal prongs or nasotracheal tube to avoid intubation.** Synchronized nasal intermittent positive-pressure ventilation (SNIPPV) is useful in augmenting the beneficial effects of nasal CPAP in preterms with frequent or severe apnea.[223]

Methylxanthines (e.g., caffeine, theophylline, aminophylline) are used to treat apnea of prematurity (Table 23-21). They are used only in primary apnea (i.e., when pathologic causes have been eliminated). Methylxanthines are potent cardiac, respiratory, and CNS stimulants and smooth muscle relaxers. Their effect on decreasing the frequency of

TABLE 23-21 METHYLXANTHINES USED TO TREAT APNEA OF PREMATURITY

DRUG	DOSAGE	THERAPEUTIC LEVELS	SIDE EFFECTS
Caffeine citrate	Route: PO Loading: 20-40 mg/kg Maintenance: 5-8 mg/kg/day administered 24 hr after the loading dose Route: IV Dose: Cafcit 20 mg/mL Administer IV over 15-30 min to avoid cardiac dysrhythmias	Afterload: 8-14 mcg/mL Maintenance: 5-25 mcg/mL Toxic: >40-50 mcg/mL	Administer orally with feedings: administer in morning so infant's sleep pattern is less disrupted than pm administration Tachycardia (withhold dose if >180/min), dysrhythmias, diuresis, glucosuria, ketonuria, hyperglycemia, jitteriness, seizures, vomiting, hemorrhagic gastritis, NEC
Theophylline	Route: PO Loading: 4-6 mg/kg Maintenance: 1.5 mg/kg q 8 hr to 3 mg/kg q 12 hr IV: Aminophylline 4-6 mg/kg over 30 min	5-15 mcg/mL, although levels of 3-4 mcg/mL have been shown to be effective in decreasing apnea	See above. IV theophylline delays gastric emptying in VLBW infants[142] Aminophylline is effective in preventing apnea that is associated with prostaglandin E1 (PGE1) injection in infants with ductal-dependent lesions[225]

Data from Young T, Magnum B: *Neofax* 2008, Raleigh, NC, 2008, Acorn Publishing.
IV, Intravenous; *NEC*, necrotizing enterocolitis; *PO*, per os, by mouth; *VLBW*, very low birth weight.

apnea is related to central stimulation[180] rather than to changes in pulmonary function. Caffeine citrate is considered the drug of choice because (1) administration is once a day, (2) there is an earlier onset of action, (3) it has a wide therapeutic range, requiring fewer serum blood level evaluations, and (4) there are fewer side effects than with theophylline.[166,348] Although methylxanthines reduce the frequency of apnea and are associated with a decrease in the use of mechanical ventilation, there is no evidence that they decrease hypoxemia.[165,166,348] A large (n = 2006 preterms with BW of 500 to 1250 g) multisite, international RCT of caffeine use for apnea of prematurity found that caffeine (1) reduced the incidence of CLD/BPD (36% in the treated group vs. 47% in the placebo group), (2) reduced the use of positive airway pressure by 1 week, and (3) temporarily (in the first 2 weeks of the study) reduced weight gain.[318]

Theophylline has been shown to significantly decrease CBF velocity. A recent RCT comparing theophylline with inhalation of (0.8%) CO_2 to treat apnea of prematurity found equal efficacy in decreasing the number and duration of apneic episodes, with fewer side effects, and no alteration of CBF with the inhalation therapy.[5]

Although gastroesophageal reflux is frequent in preterm infants because of lower esophageal sphincter relaxation, recent studies do not find an association between pre-discharge apnea and reflux.[42,104,208,284,290] Reflux events are unrelated to apneic events; apneic events are not a frequent marker of reflux, and when there is a temporal association, there is no effect on apnea duration, desaturation, or bradycardia.[104] A recent study measured cardiorespiratory and GER event rates during prefeeding and post-feeding intervals and found that the frequency, height, and pH of GER are significantly altered by feedings in preterms but that apnea, bradycardia, and desaturations were not more prevalent after feeding.[337]

Medications to improve gastric emptying (e.g., metoclopramide) have been used to treat reflux and decrease apnea secondary to reflux, although a relationship between gastric emptying and reflux in preterm infants has not been supported by research.[208,284,290] Antireflux medications have not been found to decrease the incidence of apnea and bradycardia in preterms, so their efficacy requires testing. Because a large proportion of preterm infants have abnormally high degrees of esophageal acid, administration of acid-reducing agents (e.g., ranitidine, omeprazole) may be beneficial, and these have fewer side effects and drug interactions.

Complications. Side effects of xanthines include gastric irritation, hyperactivity (restlessness, irritability, wakefulness), myocardial stimulation (tachycardia, hypotension), and increased urinary output.

The prognosis for apnea arising from an underlying cause depends on the outcome of the disease process itself. The prognosis for apnea is generally good in infants who are otherwise well and healthy and for whom the apnea is not prolonged. Delayed resolution of apnea (>36 weeks PMA) and increased frequency and duration of episodes are associated with an increased risk for neurodevelopmental disturbance at 13 months CA.[288] Long-term follow-up of the preterms in the randomized multicenter trial of caffeine use for apnea of prematurity study found improved rates of survival without neurodevelopmental disability at 18 to 21 months of age among the caffeine-treated group.[319] Prompt recognition and intervention decrease the possibility of severe complications from hypoxia.

PARENT TEACHING

Parental attachment to an infant with respiratory disease is especially difficult. It is made more difficult if the infant is also premature. Normal interaction is curtailed by the infant's condition and appearance, the environment, and the parent's reaction to these factors. An infant who is in an oxygen hood or receiving ventilation therapy to the lungs may give inadequate cues to arouse parental attachment and instead may arouse feelings of grief and loss (see Unit Six).

The goal of discharge planning is the best possible outcome with the least family disruption. Evaluation of parental readiness to care for their infant is essential to effective teaching and learning (see the Parent Teaching box on p. 662). **Physical surroundings and preparations for the infant are assessed when possible by a home visit. Parental concerns at bringing home an infant with special care needs must be assessed and discussed.** The parents learn to be comfortable in handling and caring for their infant gradually throughout hospitalization. A specially designated or decorated room is used for family visiting and caregiving. Before discharge, the mother and/or father spends the night caring for the infant. Positive reinforcement and praise from the professional staff should be freely given to parents who attend classes and successfully master the tasks of caregiving for their infant.

Special equipment such as oxygen tanks, nasal cannulas, a ventilator, and suction equipment for home use must be acquired before discharge. Sources, mode of delivery, and use of equipment must all be taught to parents before discharge. Pulmonary hygiene for infants with prolonged difficulty in handling secretions also must be taught. Written protocols and instructions should be provided to parents whenever possible. **Parents must be informed of dosage, route of administration, side effects, and planned duration of use of all medications.**

Because fluid and nutritional status is so important to any infant with a chronic condition, nutritional information for parents is necessary. Infants with tachypnea (CLD/BPD) often have difficulty with coordinating suck and swallow. Often smaller, more frequent feedings are necessary with use of supplemental oxygen. Alternative feeding methods such as gavage or gastrostomy feeding may be necessary to safely provide enough calories with a minimum of work.

Parent Teaching

IMPORTANT ASPECTS FOR PARENTS OF INFANTS WITH RESPIRATORY DISEASE

- Individualize parent teaching and evaluate parental readiness to care for an infant with ongoing respiratory care needs (e.g., home oxygen, tracheostomy, or ventilator care).
- Involve and teach parents care of their infant throughout hospitalization.
- Provide parents with written instructions for home care (e.g., tracheostomy care; suction; gastrostomy tube [g-tube] care).
- Provide parents with written instructions about all medications (dose, route of administration, side effects).
- Teach parents how to feed their infant, and encourage frequent feeding opportunities; teach parents how to feed with alternative feeding methods such as gastrostomy tube.
- Teach parents and other care providers how to perform cardiopulmonary resuscitation.
- Instruct parents in use of apnea monitors and other equipment for home use.
- Instruct parents to notify emergency personnel about their infant; posting emergency phone numbers.
- Instruct parents about the importance of follow-up care.

Apnea is especially distressing to parents because of their fears of recurrence once the infant goes home. If apnea is related to an underlying disease, treatment of the cause should result in resolution of the apneic episodes. Parents can be assured reliably that recurrence is unlikely unless the disease recurs. With apnea of prematurity, assurance can be offered that infants do grow into a regular ventilatory pattern as their respiratory center matures and that all means to protect the infant will be used until that time. Also, the parents can be assured that the infant will not go home until he or she is ready and the parents are adequately prepared to handle situations that may arise.

Before an infant needing a home monitoring system is discharged from the hospital, the parents must be given adequate support and instruction. Classes on the use of the apnea monitors must include demonstration of the equipment and return demonstrations. Minor equipment checks and repairs should be mastered before discharge.

Support by the primary care providers after discharge is essential. Parents must have telephone numbers of the medical facility and personnel they can call 24 hours a day in case of problems or equipment failure.

Anticipatory support includes discussion of potential stress factors related to having an infant on a monitor and oxygen at home: sibling rivalries, marital stresses, scheduling problems, potential problems with babysitters, and the parents' own fears of the situation.[415] An apnea monitor in the home may provoke anxiety despite discussion and instruction. **When infants are discharged with apnea monitors, there is a marked increase in maternal fatigue 1 month after discharge** when compared with a similar group discharged without monitors.[400] Increased fatigue interferes with activities of daily living and ability to parent and increases caregiver stress.[400] Interventions to alleviate fatigue after discharge may include spousal support, household help, child care for siblings, and opportunities for increasing sleep.

The parents of every infant who has apneic episodes or serious respiratory disease must be taught CPR. This set of skills is learned over the course of time by reading written materials and seeing and returning the demonstration. Learning CPR cannot be done on the day of discharge but, rather, must be a staged process of individual and class instruction. Supplying instructional pamphlets written just for parents aids in initial learning and provides a quick reference. If other family members or babysitters will provide child care during work or evening hours, they too must be able to resuscitate the infant.

Other emergency actions for which parents must be prepared include clearing the infant's airway, calling for help (having emergency phone numbers easily accessible), planning for an alternative communication source (e.g., neighbor's phone), and notifying the community rescue squad of the infant's presence in the home.

Parents must be taught how to recognize signs of illness or significant deterioration in the condition of their infant. In addition to information about special care needs, parents need information about normal newborn care. Developing realistic expectations and positive parenting skills is as important to these parents as to all new parents.

For the parents of an infant with special respiratory problems, the importance of continuous follow-up care must be emphasized. Follow-up visits should coincide with developmental stages, the natural course of the disease, and expected complications of the disease.

The parents whose child has special respiratory needs must learn a myriad of involved technical information. The primary care provider (frequently the primary nurse) is responsible for organizing, teaching, coordinating, and documenting the information. This nurse is also responsible for ensuring that the parents have not only been taught but in fact understand these concepts.

REFERENCES

1. Abrams C, Johnson B: Endotracheal tube suctioning of the neonate: an informal procedural study, *Neonatal Netw* 3:18, 1984.
2. Alano M, Ngougmna E, Ostrea E, et al: Analysis of non-steroidal anti-inflammatory drugs in meconium and its relation to PPHN, *Pediatrics* 107:519, 2001.
3. Allegaert K, Van de Velde M, Debeer A, et al: Cryotherapy versus laser photocoagulation for threshold retinopathy of prematurity: impact on early postoperative clinical recovery, *Bull Soc Belge Ophthalmol* 300:7, 2006.
4. Alme AM, Mulhern ML, Hejkal TW, et al: Outcome of retinopathy of prematurity patients following adoption of revised indications for treatment, *BMC Ophthalmol* 8:23, 2008.
5. Al-Saif S, Alvaro R, Manfreda J, et al: A randomized controlled trial of theophylline versus CO_2 inhalation for treating apnea of prematurity, *J Pediatrics* 153:513, 2008.
6. Aly H, Badawy M, El-Kholy A, et al: Randomized, controlled trial on tracheal colonization of ventilated infants: can gravity prevent ventilator-associated pneumonia? *Pediatrics* 122:770, 2008.
7. Ambalavana N, Tyson J, Kennedy N, et al: Vitamin A supplementation for extremely low birth weight infants: outcomes at 18-22 months, *Pediatrics* 115:e249:2005.
8. American Academy of Pediatrics; Section on Ophthalmology; American Academy of Ophthalmology; American Association for Pediatric Ophthalmology and Strabismus: Screening examination of premature infants for retinopathy of prematurity, *Pediatrics* 117:572, 2006.
9. American Academy of Pediatrics and American College of Obstetricians and Gynecologists: *Guidelines for perinatal care*, ed 6, Evanston, Ill, 2007, American Academy of Pediatrics.
10. American Academy of Pediatrics and Canadian Pediatric Society: Postnatal corticosteroids to treat or prevent chronic lung disease in preterm infants, *Pediatrics* 117:1846, 2006.
11. Amin S, Laroia N, Sinkin R, et al: Effect of dexamethasone therapy on serum vitamin E concentrations in premature infants with BPD, *J Perinatol* 23:552, 2003.
12. Anderson C, Benitz W, Madan A: Retinopathy of prematurity and pulse oximetry: a national survey of recent practices, *J Perinatol* 24:164, 2004.
13. Apisarnthanarak A, Holzmann-Pazgal G, Hamvas A, et al: Ventilator-associated pneumonia in extremely preterm neonates in a neonatal intensive care unit: characteristics, risk factors, and outcomes, *Pediatrics* 112:1283, 2003.
14. Askie L: Appropriate levels of oxygen saturation for preterm infants, *Acta Paediatr Suppl* 444:26, 2004.
15. Askie L, Henderson-Smart D: Restricted versus liberal oxygen exposure for preventing morbidity and mortality in preterm or LBW infants, *Cochrane Database Syst Rev* 1: CD001077, 2009.
16. Askie L, Henderson-Smart D, Irwing L, et al: Oxygen-saturation targets and outcomes in extremely preterm infants, *N Engl J Med* 349:959, 2003.
17. Avery ME, Tooley WH, Keller JB, et al: Is chronic lung disease in low birth weight infants preventable? A survey of eight centers, *Pediatrics* 79:26, 1987.
18. Aziz H, Martin J, Moore J: The pediatric disposable end-tidal carbon dioxide detector role in endotracheal intubation in newborns, *J Perinatol* 19:110, 1999.

19. Baba L, McGrath J: Oxygen free radicals: effects in the newborn period, *Adv Neonatal Care* 8:256, 2008.
20. Bagley CE, Gray PH, Tudehope DI, et al: Routine postextubation chest physiotherapy: a randomized controlled trial, *J Paediatr Child Health* 41:592, 2005.
21. Ballabh P, Kumari J, Krauss A, et al: Soluble E-selectin, soluble L-selectin and soluble ICAM-1 in bronchopulmonary dysplasia, and changes with dexamethasone, *Pediatrics* 111:461, 2003.
22. Ballard R, Truog W, Cnaan A, et al: Inhaled nitric oxide in preterm infants undergoing mechanical ventilation, *N Engl J Med* 355:343, 2006.
23. Ballard P, Truog W, Merrill J, et al: Plasma biomarkers of oxidative stress: relationship to lung disease and inhaled nitric oxide therapy in premature infants, *Pediatrics* 121:555, 2008.
24. Baquero H, Soliz A, Neira F, et al: Oral sildenafil in infants with persistent pulmonary hypertension of the newborn: a pilot randomized blinded study, *Pediatrics* 117:1077, 2006.
25. Barrington K: Hazards of systemic steroids for ventilator-dependent preterm infants: what would the parents want? *J Can Med Assoc* 165:33, 2001.
26. Barrington K: The adverse neuro-developmental effects of postnatal steroids in the preterm infant: a systematic review of RCTs, *BMC Pediatr* 1:1, 2001.
27. Barrington K, Bull D, Finer N: Randomized trial of nasal synchronized intermittent mandatory ventilation compared with continuous positive airway pressure after extubation of very low birth weight infants, *Pediatrics* 107:638, 2001.
28. Barrington K, Finer N: Inhaled nitric oxide for respiratory failure in preterm infants, *Cochrane Database Syst Rev* 3: CD000509, 2007.
29. Barrington K, Finer N: Inhaled nitric oxide for preterm infants: a systematic review, *Pediatrics* 120:1088, 2007.
30. Baud O: Postnatal steroid treatment and brain development, *Arch Dis Child Fetal Neonatal Ed* 89:F96, 2004.
31. Baumer J: International randomized controlled trial of patient triggered ventilation in neonatal respiratory distress syndrome, *Arch Dis Child Fetal Neonatal Ed* 82:F5, 2000.
32. Beardsmore CS, Westaway J, Killer H, et al: How does the changing profile of infants who are referred for extracorporeal membrane oxygenation affect their overall respiratory outcome? *Pediatrics* 120:e762, 2007.
33. Beeram M, Dhanireddy R: Effects of saline instillation during tracheal suction on lung mechanics in newborn infants, *J Perinatol* 7:120, 1992.
34. Belda S, Pallas C, Dela Cruz J, et al: Screening for ROP: is it painful? *Biol Neonate* 86:195, 2004.
35. Beligere N, Roa R: Neurodevelopmental outcome of infants with meconium aspiration syndrome: report of a study and literature review, *J Perinatol* 28(Suppl 3):S93, 2008.
36. Bell E, Acarregui M: Restricted versus liberal water intake for preventing morbidity and mortality in preterm infants, *Cochrane Database Syst Rev* 1: CD000503, 2008.
37. Bell FE, Strauss RG, Widness JA, et al: Randomized trial of liberal versus restrictive guidelines for red blood cell transfusion in preterm infants, *Pediatrics* 115:1685, 2005.
38. Beresford MW, Shaw NJ, Manning D: Randomised controlled trial of patient triggered and conventional fast rate ventilation in neonatal respiratory distress syndrome, *Arch Dis Child Fetal Neonatal Ed* 82:F14, 2000.
39. Bernstein G, Mannino F, Heldt G, et al: Randomized multicenter trial comparing synchronized and conventional intermittent mandatory ventilation (SIMV vs. IMV) in neonates, *J Pediatr* 128:4, 1996.
40. Bhandari A, Schramm CM, Kimble C, et al: Effect of a short course of prednisolone in infants with oxygen-dependent bronchopulmonary dysplasia, *Pediatrics* 121:e344, 2008.
41. Bhandari V, Gavino RG, Nedrelow JH, et al: A randomized controlled trial of synchronized nasal intermittent positive pressure ventilation in respiratory distress syndrome, *J Perinatol* 27:697, 2007.
42. Bhat RY, Rafferty GF, Hannam S, et al: Acid gastroesophageal reflux in convalescent preterm infants: effects of posture and relationship to apnea, *Pediatric Res* 62:620, 2007.
43. Bhutani VK: Developing a systems approach to prevent meconium aspiration syndrome: lessons learned from multinational studies, *J Perinatol* 28:S30, 2008.
44. Birnkrant DJ, Picone C, Markowitz W, et al: Association of transient tachypnea of the newborn and childhood asthma, *Pediatr Pulmonol* 41:978, 2006.
45. Bizzarro MJ, Hussain N, Jonsson B, et al: Genetic susceptibility to retinopathy of prematurity, *Pediatrics* 118:1858, 2006.
46. Bloemers BL, van Furth AM, Weijerman ME, et al: Down syndrome: a novel risk factor for respiratory syncytial virus bronchiolitis—a prospective birth-cohort study, *Pediatrics* e1076:120, 2007.
47. Boros SJ, Matalon SV, Ewald R, et al: The effect of independent variations in inspiratory-expiratory ratio and end expiratory pressure during mechanical ventilation in hyaline membrane disease: the significance of mean airway pressure, *J Pediatr* 91:114, 1977.
48. Boykin A, Quivers E, Waganhoffer K, et al: Cardiopulmonary outcome of neonatal extracorporeal membrane oxygenation at ages 10-15 years, *Crit Care Med* 31:2380, 2003.

49. Braz RR, Noreira ME, de Carvalho M, et al: Effect of light reduction on the incidence of retinopathy of prematurity, *Arch Dis Child Fetal Neonatal Ed* 91:F443, 2006.
50. Brion L, Bell E, Raghuveer T: Vitamin E supplementation for prevention of morbidity and mortality in preterm infants, *Cochrane Database Syst Rev* 4: CD003665, 2003.
51. Brion L, Primhak R: Intravenous or enteral loop diuretics for preterm infants with (or developing) chronic lung disease, *Cochrane Database Syst Rev* 1: CD001453, 2002.
52. Brion L, Primhak R, Ambrosio-Perez I: Diuretics acting on the distal renal tubule for preterm infants with (or developing) chronic lung disease, *Cochrane Database Syst Rev* 1:CD001817, 2002.
53. Brion L, Primhak R, Yong W: Aerosolised diuretics for preterm infants with (or developing) chronic lung disease, *Cochrane Database Syst Rev* 3:CD001694 2006.
54. Brodsky L, Reidy M, Stanievich J: The effects of suctioning techniques on the distal tracheal mucosa in intubated low birth weight infants, *Int J Pediatr Otorhinolaryngol* 14:1, 1987.
55. Brown MS, Baron AE, France EK, et al: Association between higher cumulative doses of recombinant erythropoietin and risk for retinopathy of prematurity, *JAAPOS* 10:143, 2006.
56. Buckmaster AG, Arnolda G, Wright IM, et al: Continuous positive airway pressure therapy for infants with respiratory distress in non-tertiary care centers: a randomized, controlled trial, *Pediatrics* 120:509, 2007.
57. Carlo WA, Stark A, Wright L, et al: Minimal ventilation to prevent BPD in extremely-low-birth-weight infants, *J Pediatr* 141:370, 2002.
58. Castillo A, Sola A, Baquero H, et al: Pulse oxygen saturation levels and arterial oxygen tension values in newborns receiving oxygen therapy in the neonatal intensive care unit: is 85% to 93% an acceptable range? *Pediatrics* 121:882, 2008.
59. Cederqvist K, Haglund C, Heikkila P, et al: Pulmonary trypsin-2 in the development of bronchopulmonary dysplasia in preterm infants, *Pediatric* 112:570, 2003.
60. Chambers CD, Hernandez-Diaz S, Van Marter LJ, et al: Selective serotonin reuptake inhibitors and persistent pulmonary hypertension of the newborn, *New Engl J Med* 354:579, 2006.
61. Chang GY, Cox CC, Shaffer TH: Nasal cannula, CPAP and vapotherm: effect of flow on temperature, humidity, pressure and resistance, *Pediatr Acad Soc* 57:1231, 2005.
62. Cheema I, Ahluwalia J: Feasibility of tidal volume-guided ventilation in newborn infants: a randomized, crossover trial using the volume guarantee modality, *Pediatrics* 107:1323, 2001.
63. Chin S, Brodsky N, Bhandari V: Antenatal steroid use is associated with increased gastroesophageal reflux in neonates, *Am J Perinatol* 20:205, 2003.
64. Choi CW, Kim BI, Koh YY, et al: Clinical characteristics of chronic lung disease without preceding respiratory distress syndrome in preterm infants, *Pediatr Int* 47:72, 2005.
65. Reference deleted in proofs
66. Chouteau W, Green D: Neonatal gastric perforation, *J Perinatol* 23:345, 2003.
67. Chow L, Wright K, Sola A: and the CSMC Oxygen Administration Study Group: Can changes in clinical practice decrease the incidence of severe ROP in VLBW infants? *Pediatrics* 111:339, 2003.
68. Cignacco E, Humers JP, van Lingen RN, et al: Pain relief in ventilated preterms during endotracheal suctioning: a randomized controlled trial, *Swiss Med Weekly* 138:635, 2008.
69. Clark R, Gerstmann D, Jobe A, et al: Lung injury in neonates: causes, strategies for prevention, and long-term consequences, *J Pediatr* 139:478, 2001.
70. Clark R, Huckaby J, Kueser T, et al: Low-dose nitric oxide therapy for PPHN: 1-year follow-up, *J Perinatol* 23:300, 2003.
71. Clark R, Powers R, White R, et al: Prevention and treatment of nosocomial sepsis in the NICU, *J Perinatol* 24:446, 2004.
72. Clark R, Yoder B, Sell M: Prospective, randomized comparison of high-frequency oscillation and conventional ventilation in candidates for extracorporeal membrane oxygenation, *J Pediatr* 124:447, 1994.
73. Clark RH, Kueser TJ, Walker MW, et al: Low-dose nitric oxide therapy for persistent pulmonary hypertension of the newborn, *N Engl J Med* 342:469, 2000.
74. Clucas L, Doyle LW, Dawson J, et al: Compliance with alarm limits for pulse oximetry in very preterm infants, *Pediatrics* 119:1056, 2007.
75. Coates EW, Klinepeter ME, O'Shea TM: Neonatal pulmonary hypertension treated with inhaled nitric oxide and high-frequency ventilation, *J Perinatol* 28:675, 2008.
76. Colnaghi M, Condo V, Pugni L, et al: Endogenous nitric oxide production in the airways of preterm and term infants, *Biol Neonate* 83:113, 2003.
77. Coney S: Physiotherapy technique banned in Auckland, *Lancet* 345:510, 1995.
78. Reference deleted in proofs
79. Cooke R, Foulder-Hughes L, Newsham D, et al: Ophthalmic impairment at 7 years of age in children born very preterm, *Arch Dis Child Fetal Neonatal Ed* 89:F249, 2004.
80. Copetti R, Cattarossi L: The 'double lung point': an ultrasound sign diagnostic of transient tachypnea of the newborn, *Neonatology* 91:203, 2007.

81. Cordero L, Sananes M, Ayers L: Comparison of a closed (Trach Care MAC) with an open endotracheal suction system in small premature infants, *J Perinatol* 3:151, 2000.
82. Cordero L, Sananes M, Ayers L: A comparison of two airway suctioning frequencies in mechanically ventilated, very-low-birthweight infants, *Respir Care* 46:783, 2001.
83. Courtney S, Aghai Z, Saslow J, et al: Changes in lung volume and work of breathing: a comparison of variable-flow nasal continuous positive airway pressure devices in low birth weight infants, *Pediatr Pulmonol* 36:248, 2003.
84. Courtney S, Durand D, Asselin J, et al: High-frequency oscillatory ventilation versus conventional mechanical ventilation for very-low birthweight infant, *N Engl J Med* 347:643, 2002.
85. Cox C, Wolfson M, Shafer T: Liquid ventilation: a comprehensive overview, *Neonatal Netw* 15:31, 1996.
86. Cross JH, Harrison CJ, Preston PR, et al: Postnatal encephaloclastic porencephaly: a new lesion? *Arch Dis Child* 67:307, 1992.
87. Crowther CA, Doyle LW, Haslam RR, et al: and the ACTORDS Study Group: Outcomes at 2 years of age after repeat doses of antenatal corticosteroids, *New Engl J Med* 357:1179, 2007.
88. CRYO-ROP Cooperative Group: Multicenter trial of cryotherapy for ROP: natural history ROP—ocular outcome at 5½ years in premature infants with birth weights less than 1251 g, *Arch Ophthalmol* 120:595, 2002.
89. Dangeman BC, et al: The variability of Pa_{O_2} in newborn infants in response to routine care, *Pediatr Res* 10:149, 1976.
90. D'Angio CT, Chess PR, Kovacs SJ, et al: Pressure-regulated volume control ventilation vs. synchronized intermittent mandatory ventilation for very-low-birth weight infants, *Arch Ped Adolesc Med* 159:868, 2005.
91. Dani C, Bertini G, Pezzati M, et al: Early extubation and nasal continuous positive airway pressure after surfactant treatment for RDS among preterm infants <30 weeks' gestation, *Pediatrics* 113:e560, 2004.
92. Dani C, Bertini G, Pezzati M, et al: Effects of pressure support ventilation plus volume guarantee vs. high-frequency oscillatory ventilation on lung inflammation in preterm infants, *Pediatr Pulmonol* 41:242, 2006.
93. Darlow B, Graham P: Vitamin A supplementation to prevent mortality and short- and long-term morbidity in very low birthweight infants, *Cochrane Database Syst Rev* 4:2007, CD000501.
94. Davis J, Parad R, Michele T, et al: Pulmonary outcome at 1 year corrected age in premature infants treated at birth with recombinant human CuZn Superoxide Dismutase, *Pediatrics* 111:469, 2003.
95. Davis JM, Bhutani VK, Stefano JL, et al: Changes in pulmonary mechanics following caffeine administration in infants with bronchopulmonary dysplasia, *Pediatr Pulmonol* 6:49, 1989.
96. Davis P, Henderson-Smart D: Extubation from low-rate intermittent positive airways pressure vs. extubation after a trial of endotracheal CPAP in intubated preterm infants, *Cochrane Database Syst Rev* 4: CD001078, 2001.
97. Davis P, Henderson-Smart D: Nasal continuous positive airways pressure immediately after extubation for preventing morbidity in preterm infants, *Cochrane Database Syst Rev* 2:CD000143, 2003.
98. Davis PG, Morley CJ, Owen LS: Non-invasive respiratory support of preterm neonates with respiratory distress: continuous positive airway pressure and nasal intermittent positive pressure ventilation, *Semin Fetal Neonatal Med* 14:14, 2009.
99. DeBoer S, Peterson L: Sedation for nonemergent neonatal intubation, *Neonatal Netw* 20:19, 2001.
100. DeBoer S, Seaver M: End tidal CO_2 verification of endotracheal tube placement in neonates, *Neonatal Netw* 23:29, 2004.
101. Demers R, Saklad M: Minimizing the harmful effects of mechanical aspiration, *Heart Lung* 2:542, 1973.
102. DePaoli A, Davis P, Faber B, et al: Devices and pressure sources for administration of nasal continuous positive airway pressure (NCPAP) in preterm neonates, *Cochrane Database Syst Rev* 4:CD002977, 2008.
103. DePaoli A, Davis P, Lemyre B: Nasal continuous positive airway pressure vs. nasal intermittent positive pressure ventilation for preterm neonates: a systematic review and meta-analysis, *Acta Paediatr* 92:70, 2003.
104. DiFiore J, Arko M, Whitehouse M, et al: Apnea is not prolonged by acid gastroesophageal reflux (GER) in preterm infants, *Pediatrics* 116:1059, 2005.
105. Donn S, Sinha S: Invasive and noninvasive neonatal mechanical ventilation, *Respir Care* 48:426, 2003.
106. Doyle LW, Davis PG, Morley CJ, et al: Low-dose dexamethasone facilitates extubation among chronically ventilator-dependent infants: a multicenter, international, randomized, controlled trial, *Pediatrics* 117:75, 2006.
107. Doyle LW, Halliday HL, Ehrenkranz RA, et al: Impact of postnatal systemic corticosteroids on mortality and cerebral palsy in preterm infants: effect modification by risk for chronic lung disease, *Pediatrics* 115:655, 2005.
108. Early Treatment for ROP (ETROP) Cooperative Group: Revised indications for the treatment of ROP: results of the Early Treatment for ROP randomized trial, *Arch Ophthalmol* 121:1684, 2003.

109. Eichenwald E, Abimbola A, Stark A: Apnea frequently persists beyond term gestation in infants delivered at 24-28 weeks, *Pediatrics* 100:354, 1997.
110. Elhassan NO, Sorbero ME, Hall CB, et al: Cost-effectiveness analysis of palivizumab in premature infants without chronic lung disease, *Arch Pediatr Adolesc Med* 160:1070, 2006.
111. Elimian A, Figueroa R, Spitzer A, et al: Antenatal corticosteroids: are incomplete courses beneficial? *Obstet Gynecol* 102:352, 2003.
112. El Shahed AI, Dargaville P, Ohlsson A, et al: Surfactant for meconium aspiration syndrome in full term/near term infants, *Cochrane Database Syst Rev* 3:CD002054, 2007.
113. Engle W: and the Committee on Fetus and Newborn: Surfactant-replacement therapy for respiratory distress in the preterm and term neonate, *Pediatrics* 121:419, 2008.
114. Engle W, Yoder M, Andreali S, et al: Controlled prospective randomized comparison of HFJV and conventional ventilation in neonates with respiratory failure and PPHN, *J Perinatol* 17:3, 1997.
115. Eriksen V, Nielsen LH, Klokker M, et al: Follow-up of 5- to 11-year-old children treated for persistent pulmonary hypertension of the newborn, *Acta Paediatr* 98:304, 2009.
116. Erti T, Gyarmati J, Gaal V, et al: Relationship between hyperglycemia and retinopathy of prematurity in very low birth weight infants, *Biol Neonate* 89:56, 2006.
117. Ertzbischoff L: A systematic review of anatomical and visual function outcomes in preterm infants after scleral buckle and vitrectomy for retinal detachment, *Adv Neonatal Care* 4:10, 2004.
118. Esplin M, Fausett M, Smith S, et al: Multiple courses of antenatal steroids are associated with delay in long-term psychomotor development in children with birth weight 1,500 grams, *Am J Obstet Gynecol* 182:S24, 2000.
119. Evans J: Incidence of hypoxia associated with caregiving in premature infants, *Neonatal Netw* 10:17, 1991.
120. Evans J: Reducing the hypoxemia, bradycardia and apnea associated with suctioning in low birthweight infants, *J Perinatol* 7:137, 1992.
121. Extracorporeal Life Support Organization: *Neonatal ECMO Registry*, Ann Arbor, Mich, 2004, The Organization.
122. Field D, Elbourne D, Truesdale A, et al: Neonatal ventilation with inhaled nitric oxide versus ventilatory support without inhaled nitric oxide for preterm infants with severe respiratory failure: The INNOVA multicenter randomised controlled trial (ISRCTN17821339), *Pediatrics* 115:926, 2005.
123. Finer N: Nasal cannula use in the preterm infant: oxygen or pressure? *Pediatrics* 116:1216, 2005.
124. Finer N, Barrington K: Nitric oxide for respiratory failure in infants born at or near term, *Cochrane Database Syst Rev* 4:CD000399, 2006.
125. Finer N, Craft A, Vaucher Y, et al: Postnatal steroids: short-term gain, long term pain?, *J Pediatr* 137:9, 2000.
126. Firme S, McEvoy C, Alconcel C, et al: Episodes of hypoxemia during synchronized intermittent mandatory ventilation in ventilator-dependent very low birth weight infants, *Pediatr Pulmonol* 40:9, 2005.
127. Fittenberg J: Persistent pulmonary hypertension after lithium intoxication in the newborn, *Eur J Pediatr* 138:321, 1982.
128. Flamant C, Lorino E, Nolent P, et al: Newborn infants supported by extracorporeal membrane oxygenation: survival and clinical outcome, *Arch Pediatr* 14:354, 2007.
129. Fliman PJ, deReigner RA, Kinsella JP, et al: Neonatal extracorporeal life support: impact of new therapies on survival, *J Pediatr* 148:595, 2006.
130. Ford SP, Leick-Rude MK, Meinert KA, et al: Overcoming barriers to oxygen saturation targeting, *Pediatrics* 118:S117, 2006.
131. Fraiberg S: Blind infants and their mothers: an examination of the sign system. In Lewis M, Rosenblum L, editors: The effect of the infant on its caregiver, New York, 1974, John Wiley & Sons.
132. Fraser W, Hotmeyr J, Lede R, et al: Amnioinfusion for the prevention of the meconium aspiration syndrome, *N Engl J Med* 353:946, 2005.
133. Frogel M, Newton C, Cohen A, et al: Prevention of hospitalization due to respiratory syncytial virus: results from the Palivizumab Outcomes Registry, *J Perinatol* 28:511, 2008.
134. Garland J, Nelson D, Rice T, et al: Increased risk of gastrointestinal perforations in neonates mechanically ventilated with either face mask or nasal prongs, *Pediatrics* 76:406, 1985.
135. Geary C, Caskey M, Fonseca R, et al: Decreased incidence of bronchopulmonary dysplasia after early management changes, including surfactant and nasal continuous positive airway pressure treatment at delivery, lowered oxygen saturation goals, and early amino acid administration: a historical cohort study, *Pediatrics* 121:89, 2008.
136. Gelfand S, Fanaroff J, Walsh M: Controversies in the treatment of meconium aspiration syndrome, *Clin Perinatol* 31:445, 2004.
137. Gillespie LM, White SD, Sinha SK, et al: Usefulness of the minute ventilation test in predicting successful extubation in newborn infants: a randomized controlled trial, *J Perinatol* 23:205, 2003.
138. Gluck L, Kulovich M: Fetal lung development, *Pediatr Clin North Am* 20:367, 1973.
139. Goldsmith J: Continuous positive airway pressure and conventional mechanical ventilation in

the treatment of meconium aspiration syndrome, *J Perinatol* 28(Suppl 3):S49, 2008.
140. Goldsmith J, Greenspan JS: Neonatal intensive care unit oxygen management: a team effort, *Pediatrics* 119:1195, 2007.
141. Gordon P, Rutledge J, Sawin R, et al: Early postnatal dexamethasone increases the risk of focal small bowel perforation in extremely low birth weight infants, *J Perinatol* 19:573, 1999.
142. Gounaris A, Kokori P, Varchalama L, et al: Theophylline and gastric emptying in VLBW neonates: a randomized controlled trial, *Arch Dis Child Fetal Neonatal Ed* 89:F297, 2004.
143. Greenough A, Dimitriou G, Prendergast M, et al: Synchronized mechanical ventilation for respiratory support in newborn infants, *Cochrane Database Syst Rev* 1:CD000456, 2008.
144. Greenspan J, Wolfson M, Shaffer T: Liquid ventilation, *Semin Perinatol* 24:396, 2000.
145. Greenspan JS, Shaffer TH: Ventilator-induced airway injury: a critical consideration during mechanical ventilation of the infant, *Neonatal Netw* 25:159, 2006.
146. Gregory G: Respiratory care of newborn infants, *Pediatr Clin North Am* 19:311, 1972.
147. Greisen G, Frederiksen P, Hertel J, et al: Catecholamine response to chest physiotherapy and endotracheal suctioning in preterm infants, *Acta Paediatr Scand* 74:525, 1985.
148. Gross SJ, Anbar RD, Mettleman BB: Follow-up at 15 years of preterm infants from a controlled trial of moderately early dexamethasone for the prevention of chronic lung disease, *Pediatrics* 115:681, 2005.
149. Gupta S, Sinha SK, Donn SM: The effect of two levels of pressure support ventilation on tidal volume delivery and minute ventilation, *Arch Dis Child Fetal Neonatal Ed* 94:F80, 2009.
150. Gupta S, Sinha SK, Tin W, et al: A randomized controlled trial of post-extubation bubble continuous positive airway pressure versus Infant Flow Driver continuous positive airway pressure in preterm infants with respiratory distress syndrome, *J Pediatr* 154:645, 2009.
151. Guthrie SO, Lynn C, Lafleur BJ, et al: A crossover analysis of mandatory minute ventilation compared to synchronized intermittent mandatory ventilation in neonates, *J Perinatol* 25:643, 2005.
152. Hacking D, Watkins A, Fraser S, et al: Respiratory distress syndrome and birth order in premature twins, *Arch Dis Child Fetal Neonatal Ed* 84:F117, 2001.
153. Hagadorn JI, Furey AM, Nghiem TH, et al: Achieved versus intended pulse oximeter saturation in infants born less than 28 weeks' gestation: the AVIOx study, *Pediatrics* 118:1574, 2006.
154. Hagler D, Travner G: ET saline and suction catheters: sources of lower airway contamination, *Am J Crit Care* 3:444, 1994.
155. Halliday H, Ehrenkranz R, Doyle L: Late (>7 days) postnatal corticosteroids for chronic lung disease in preterm infants, *Cochrane Database Syst Rev* 1:CD001145, 2009.
156. Halliday H, Ekrenkranz R, Doyle L: Early (<8 days) postnatal corticosteroids for preventing chronic lung disease in preterm infants, *Cochrane Database Syst Rev* 1:CD001146, 2009.
157. Hanley M, Rudd T, Butler J: What happens to intratracheal saline instillations? *Am, J Resp Dis* 117(Suppl):S124, 1978.
158. Harding JE, Miles FK, Becroft DM, et al: Chest physiotherapy may be associated with brain damage in extremely premature infants, *J Pediatr* 132:440, 1998.
159. Harrison H: Preemies on steroids: a new iatrogenic disaster? *Birth* 28:57, 2001.
160. Harrison VC, Heese H, Klein M: The significance of grunting in hyaline membrane disease, *Pediatrics* 41:549, 1968.
161. Henderson-Smart D, Cools F, Bhuta T, et al: Elective high frequency oscillatory ventilation versus conventional ventilation for acute pulmonary dysfunction in preterm infants, *Cochrane Database Syst Rev* 3:CD000104, 2007.
162. Henderson-Smart D, Davis P: Prophylactic methylxanthines for extubation in preterm infants, *Cochrane Database Syst Rev* 1:CD000139, 2003.
163. Henderson-Smart DJ, Hutchinson JL, Donoghue DA, et al: Prenatal predictors of chronic lung disease in very preterm infants, *Arch Dis Child Fetal Neonatal Ed* 91:F40, 2006.
164. Henderson-Smart D, Osborn D: Kinesthetic stimulation for preventing apnea in preterm infants, *Cochrane Database Syst Rev* 2:CD000373, 2002.
165. Henderson-Smart D, Steer P: Prophylactic methylxanthine for prevention of apnea in preterm infants, *Cochrane Database Syst Rev* 2:CD000432, 2000.
166. Henderson-Smart D, Steer P: Methylxanthine treatment for apnea in preterm infants, *Cochrane Database Syst Rev* 3:CD000140, 2001.
167. Hernandez-Diaz S, Van Marter LJ, Werler MM, et al: Risk factors for persistent pulmonary hypertension of the newborn, *Pediatrics* 120:e272, 2007.
168. Herrera C, Gerhardt T, Claure N, et al: Effects of volume-guaranteed synchronized intermittent mandatory ventilation in preterm infants recovering from respiratory failure, *Pediatrics* 110:529, 2002.
169. Hibbs AM, Walsh MC, Martin RJ, et al: One-year respiratory outcomes of preterm infants enrolled in the Nitric Oxide (to prevent) Chronic Lung Disease trial, *J Peds* 153:525, 2008.
170. HiFi Study Group: High-frequency oscillatory ventilation compared with conventional mechanical ventilation in the treatment of respiratory failure in preterm infants, *N Engl J Med* 320:88, 1989.

171. Higgins RD, Bancalari E, Willinger M, et al: Executive summary of the workshop on oxygen in neonatal therapies: controversies and opportunities for research, *Pediatrics* 119:790, 2007.
172. Hintz S, Van Meurs K, Perritt R, et al: Neurodevelopmental outcomes of premature infants with severe respiratory failure enrolled in a randomized controlled trial of inhaled nitric oxide, *J Pediatr* 151:16, 2007.
173. Hoffman J, Mason E, Schutze G, et al: *Streptococcus pneumoniae* infections in the neonate, *Pediatrics* 112:1095, 2003.
174. Honda R, Ichiyama T, Sunagawa S, et al: Inhaled corticosteroid therapy reduces cytokine levels in sputum from very preterm infants with chronic lung disease, *Acta Paediatr* 98:118, 2009.
175. Hoskote A, Castle R, Hoo A, et al: Airway function in infants treated with inhaled nitric oxide for persistent pulmonary hypertension, *Pediatr Pulmonol* 43:224, 2008.
176. Hossain T, Kappelman M, Perez-Atayde A, et al: Primary ciliary dyskinesia as a cause of neonatal respiratory distress: implications for the neonatologist, *J Perinatol* 23:684, 2003.
177. Hough JL, Flenady V, Johnson L, et al: Chest physiotherapy for reducing respiratory morbidity in infants requiring ventilatory support, *Cochrane Database Syst Rev* 3:CD006445, 2008.
178. Howlett A, Ohlsson A: Inositol for respiratory distress syndrome in preterm infants, *Cochrane Database Syst Rev* 4:CD000366, 2003.
179. Huddy CL, Bennett CC, Hardy P, et al: The INNOVA multicentre randomised controlled trial: neonatal ventilation with inhaled nitric oxide versus ventilatory support without nitric oxide for severe respiratory failure in preterm infants—follow up at 4-5 years, *Arch Dis Child Fetal Neonatal Ed* 93:F430, 2008.
180. Ingimarsson J, Bjorklund L, Curstedt T, et al: Incomplete protection by prophylactic surfactant against the added effects of large lung inflations at birth in immature lambs, *Intensive Care Med* 30:1446, 2004.
181. International Committee for the Classification of Retinopathy of Prematurity: The international classification of retinopathy of prematurity, *Arch Ophthalmol* 123:991, 2005.
182. Jaille J, Levin T, Wung J, et al: Benign gaseous distension of the bowel in premature infants treated with NCPAP, *Am J Rheumatol* 158:125, 1992.
183. Jandeck C, Kellner U, Foerster M: Late retinal detachment in patients born prematurely: outcome of primary pars plana vitrectomy, *Arch Ophthalmol* 122:61, 2004.
184. Jobe AH: Postnatal corticosteroids for bronchopulmonary dysplasia, *Clin Perinatol* 36:177, 2009.
185. Joshi VH, Bhuta T: Rescue high frequency jet ventilation versus conventional ventilation for severe pulmonary dysfunction in preterm infants, *Cochrane Database Syst Rev* 1:CD000437, 2006.
186. Kaiser J, Gauss C, Williams D: Tracheal suctioning is associated with prolonged disturbances of cerebral hemodynamics in very low birth weight infants, *J Perinatol* 28:34, 2008.
187. Kalyn A, Blatz S, Feuerstake S, et al: Closed suctioning of intubated neonates maintains better physiologic stability: a randomized controlled trial, *J Perinatol* 23:218, 2003.
188. Karn CM, Steward DK: Nutrition and weight gain before the diagnosis of bronchopulmonary dysplasia, *Newborn Infant Nurs Rev* 5:149, 2005.
189. Kattwinkel J, editor: *Textbook of neonatal resuscitation,* ed 5, Elk Grove Village, Ill, 2006, American Academy of Pediatrics and American Heart Association.
190. Kattwinkel J, editor: Endotracheal intubation. In Kattwinkel J, *Neonatal resuscitation provider textbook,* ed 5, Elk Grove, Ill, 2006, American Academy of Pediatrics and American Heart Association.
191. Kavvadia V, Greenough A, Itakura Y, et al: Neonatal lung function in very immature infants with and without RDS, *J Perinat Med* 27:382, 1999.
192. Kawagoe J, Segre C, Pereira C, et al: Risk factors for nosocomial infections in critically ill newborns: a 5 year prospective cohort study, *Am J Infect Control* 29:109, 2001.
193. Keszler M: Strategy matters, *Am J Perinatol* 24:147, 2007.
194. Keszler M, Abubakar K: Volume guarantee accelerates recovery from forced exhalation episodes, *Pediatr Res* 55:545A, 2004.
195. Keszler M, Modanlou HD, Brudno DS, et al: Multicenter controlled clinical trial of high-frequency jet ventilation in preterm infants with uncomplicated respiratory distress syndrome, *Pediatrics* 100:593, 1997.
196. Khalof N, Brodsky N, Hurley J, et al: A prospective randomized, controlled trial comparing synchronized nasal intermittent positive pressure ventilation vs. nasal continuous positive airway pressure as modes of extubation, *Pediatrics* 108:13, 2001.
197. Khazardoost S, Hantoushzadeh S, Khooshideh M, et al: Risk factors for meconium aspiration in meconium stained amniotic fluid, *J Obstet Gynecol* 27:577, 2007.
198. Kim T, Sohn J, Pi S, et al: Postnatal risk factors of retinopathy of prematurity, *Ped Perinatal Epidemiol* 18:130, 2004.
199. Kinsella J: Meconium aspiration syndrome: is surfactant lavage the answer? *Am J Respir Crit Care Med* 168:113, 2003.
200. Kinsella J: Inhaled nitric oxide in the term newborn, *Early Human Dev* 84:709, 2008.

201. Kinsella J, Cutter G, Walsh W, et al: Early inhaled nitric oxide therapy in premature newborns with respiratory failure, *N Engl J Med* 355:354, 2006.
202. Kirchner L, Weninger M, Unterasinger L, et al: Is the use of early nasal CPAP associated with lower rates of chronic lung disease and retinopathy of prematurity? Nine years of experience with the Vermont Oxford Neonatal Network, *J Perinatal Med* 33:60, 2005.
203. Kleiber C, Krutzfield N, Rose EF: Acute histologic changes in the tracheobronchial tree associated with different suction catheter insertion techniques, *Heart Lung* 17:10, 1988.
204. Kling P: Nursing intervention to decrease the risk of periventricular-intraventricular hemorrhage, *J Obstet Gynecol Neonatal Nurs* 18(6):457, 1989.
205. Klinger G, Beyene J, Shah P, et al: Do hyperoxaemia and hypocapnia add to the risk of brain injury after intrapartum asphyxia? *Arch Dis Child Fetal Neonatal, Ed* 90:F49, 2005.
206. Knight D: Neonatal shaken baby syndrome: lessons to be learned, *Arch Dis Child Fetal Neonatal Ed* 87:F161, 2002.
207. Knight D, Bevan C, Harding J, et al: Chest physiotherapy and porencephalic lesions in very preterm infants, *J Paediatr Child Health* 37:554, 2001.
208. Kohelet D, Boaz M, Serour F, et al: Esophageal pH study and symptomatology of gastroesophageal reflux in newborn infants, *Am J Perinatol* 21:85, 2004.
209. Kopelman A, Holbert D: Use of oxygen cannulas in ELBW infants is associated with mucosal trauma and bleeding, and possibly with coagulase-negative Staphylococcal sepsis, *J Perinatol* 23:94, 2003.
210. Kubicka ZJ, Limauro J, Darnall RA: Heated, humidified, high-flow nasal cannula therapy: yet another way to deliver continuous positive airway pressure?, *Pediatrics* 121:82, 2008.
211. Kumar VH, Hutchison AA, Lakshminrusimha S, et al: Characteristics of pulmonary hypertension in preterm neonates, *J Perinatol* 27:214, 2007.
212. Kurzner SI, Garg M, Bautista DB, et al: Growth failure in infants with bronchopulmonary dysplasia: nutrition and elevated resting metabolic expenditure, *Pediatrics* 81:379, 1988.
213. Kusaka S, Shima C, Wada K, et al: Efficacy of intravitreal injection of bevacizumab for severe retinopathy of prematurity: a pilot study, *Br J Ophthalmol* 92:1450, 2008.
214. Lakshminrusimha S, Steinhorn R: Pulmonary vascular biology during neonatal transition, *Clin Perinatol* 26:601, 1999.
215. Lal M, Manktelow B, Draper E, et al: Chronic lung disease of prematurity and intrauterine growth retardation: a population based study, *Pediatrics* 111:483, 2003.
216. Laptook AR, Salhab W, Allen J, et al: Pulse oximetry in very low birth weight infants: can oxygen saturation be maintained in the desired range? *J Perinatol* 26:337, 2006.
217. Larsson E, Martin L, Holmstrom G: Peripheral and central visual fields in 11-year-old children who were born prematurely and at term, *J Pediatr Ophthalmol Strabismus* 41:39, 2004.
218. Leach CL, Greenspan JS, Rubenstein SD, et al: Partial liquid ventilation with perflubron in premature infants with severe respiratory distress syndrome, *N Engl J Med* 335:761, 1996.
219. Leduc M, Kermorvant-Duchemin E, Checchin D, et al: Hypercapnia- and trans-arachidonic acid-induced retinal microvascular degeneration: implications in the genesis of retinopathy of prematurity, *Semin Perinatol* 30:129, 2006.
220. Lee BH, Stoll BJ, McDonald SA, et al: Adverse neonatal outcomes associated with antenatal dexamethasone versus antenatal betamethasone, *Pediatrics* 117:1503, 2006.
221. Lee J, Robinson JL, Spady DW: Frequency of apnea, bradycardia, and desaturations following first diphtheria-tetanus-pertussis-inactivated polio-*Haemophilus influenzae* type B immunizations in hospitalized preterm infants, *BMC Pediatr* 6:20, 2006.
222. Leidy NK, Margolis MK, Marcin JP, et al: The impact of severe respiratory syncytial virus on the child, caregiver, and family during hospitalization and recovery, *Pediatrics* 115:1536, 2005.
223. Lemyre B, Davis P, DePaoli A: Nasal intermittent positive pressure ventilation (NIPPV) vs. nasal continuous positive airway pressure (NCPAP) for apnea of prematurity, *Cochrane Database Syst Rev* 1:CD002272, 2002.
224. Liem JJ, Huq SI, Ekuma O, et al: Transient tachypnea of the newborn may be an early clinical manifestation of wheezing symptoms, *J Pediatr* 151:29, 2007.
225. Lim D, Kulik T, Kim D, et al: Aminophylline for the prevention of apnea during prostaglandin E_1 infusion, *Pediatrics* e27:112, 2003.
226. Lipkin P, Davidson D, Spivak L, et al: Neurodevelopmental and medical outcomes of PPHN in term newborns treated with nitric oxide, *J Pediatr* 140:306, 2002.
227. Lista G, Castoldi F, Bianchi S, et al: Volume guarantee versus high-frequency ventilation: lung inflammation in preterm infants, *Arch Dis Child Fetal Neonatal Ed* 93:F252, 2008.
228. Livera L, Spencer S, Thorniley M, et al: Effects of hypoxaemia and bradycardia on neonatal cerebral haemodynamics, *Arch Dis Child* 66:376, 1991.
229. Locke R, Wolfson M, Shaffer T, et al: Inadvertent administration of positive end-distending pressure during nasal cannula flow, *Pediatrics* 91:135, 1993.
230. Lofqvist C, Engstrom E, Sigurdsson J, et al: Postnatal head growth deficit among premature infants parallels

retinopathy of prematurity and insulin-like growth factor-1 deficit, *Pediatrics* 117:1930, 2006.
231. Lutman D, Petros A: Inhaled nitric oxide in neonatal and paediatric transport, *Early Hum Dev* 84:725, 2008.
232. Mactier H, Weaver LT: Vitamin A and preterms infants: what we know, what we don't know and what we need to know, *Arch Dis Child Fetal Neonatal Ed* 90:F102, 2005.
233. Manzoni P, Maestri A, Leonessa M, et al: Fungal and bacterial sepsis and threshold ROP in preterm very low birth weight neonates, *J Perinatol* 26:23, 2006.
234. Mariani G, Cifuentes J, Carlo W: Randomized trial of permissive hypercapnia in preterm infants, *Pediatrics* 104:1082, 1999.
235. Marinelli P, Ortiz A, Alden E: Acquired eventration of the diaphragm: a complication of chest tube placement in neonatal pneumothorax, *Pediatrics* 67:552, 1981.
236. Marks JD, Schreiber MD: Inhaled nitric oxide and neuroprotection in preterm infants, *Clin Perinatol* 35:793, 2008.
237. Mazela J, Merritt TA, Finer NN: Aerosolized surfactants, *Curr Opin Pediatrics* 19:155, 2007.
238. McCallion N, Davis PG, Morley CJ: Volume-targeted versus pressure-limited ventilation in the neonate, *Cochrane Database Syst Rev* 3:2005 CD003666.
239. McCoskey L: Nursing care guidelines for prevention of nasal breakdown in neonates receiving nasal CPAP, *Adv Neonatal Care* 8:116, 2008.
240. McEvoy C, Bowling S, Williamson K, et al: Randomized, double-blinded trial of low-dose dexamethasone. II. Functional residual capacity and pulmonary outcome in VLBW infants at risk for BPD, *Pediatr Pulmonol* 38:55, 2004.
241. McNamara PJ, Laique F, Muang-In S, et al: Milrinone improves oxygenation in neonates with severe persistent pulmonary hypertension of the newborn, *J Crit Care* 21:217, 2006.
242. Mercier JC, Olivier P, Loron G, et al: Inhaled nitric oxide to prevent bronchopulmonary dysplasia in preterm neonates, *Sem Fetal Neonatal Med* 14:28, 2009.
243. Mestan K, Marks J, Hecox K, et al: Neurodevelopmental outcomes of premature infants treated with inhaled nitric oxide, *N Engl J Med* 353:82, 2005.
244. Meydanli M, Dilbaz B, Caliskan E, et al: Risk factors for meconium aspiration syndrome in infants born through thick meconium, *Int J Gynecol Obstet* 72:9, 2001.
245. Migliori C, Bottino R, Angeli A, et al: High-frequency partial liquid ventilation in two infants, *J Perinatol* 24:118, 2004.
246. Migliori C, Cavazza A, Motta M, et al: Effect of respiratory function of pressure support ventilation versus synchronized intermittent mandatory ventilation in preterm infants, *Pediatr Pulmonol* 35:364, 2003.
247. Miller JD, Carlo WA: Safety and effectiveness of permissive hypercapnia in the preterm infant, *Curr Opin Pediatr* 19:142, 2007.
248. Miller S, Rhine W: Inhaled nitric oxide in the treatment of preterm infants, *Early Human Dev* 84:703, 2008.
249. Milner J, Aly H, Ward L, et al: Does elevated peak bilirubin protect from ROP in VLBW infants? *J Perinatol* 23:208, 2003.
250. Moriette G, Paris-Llado J, Walti H, et al: Prospective randomized multicenter comparison of high-frequency oscillatory ventilation and conventional ventilation in preterm infants of less than 30 weeks with RDS, *Pediatrics* 107:363, 2001.
251. Morley CJ, Davis PG, Doyle LW, et al: Nasal CPAP or intubation at birth for very preterm infants, *New Engl J Med* 358:700, 2008.
252. Morris CJ, Choong K: Ventilatory management of extremely low birth weight infants, *McGill J Med* 9:95, 2006.
253. Mosca F, Colnaghi M, Lattanzio M, et al: Closed versus open endotracheal suctioning in preterm infants: effects on cerebral oxygenation and blood volume, *Biol Neonate* 72:9, 1997.
254. Mourani PM, Sontag MK, Ivy DD, et al: Effects of long-term sildenafil treatment for pulmonary hypertension in infants with chronic lung disease, *J Pediatr,* Epub ahead of print: *Oct* 23, 2008.
255. Moya F, Gadzinowski J, Bancalari E, et al: A multicenter, randomized, masked, comparison trial of lucinactant, colfosceril palmitate, and beractant for the prevention of respiratory distress syndrome among very preterm infants, *Pediatrics* 115:1018, 2005.
256. Moya F, Sinha S, Gadzinowski J, et al: One-year follow-up of very preterm infants who received lucinactant for prevention of respiratory distress syndrome: results from 2 multicenter randomized, controlled trials, *Pediatrics* 119:e1361, 2007.
257. Msall M, Phelps D, Hardy R, et al: Educational and social competencies at 8 years in children with threshold ROP in the CRYO-ROP multicenter study, *Pediatrics* 113:790, 2004.
258. Mugford M, Elbourne D, Field D: Extracorporeal membrane oxygenation for severe respiratory failure in newborn infants, *Cochrane Database Syst Rev* 3:CD001340, 2008.
259. Narandran V, Donovan E, Hoath S, et al: Early bubble CPAP and outcomes in ELBW preterm infants, *J Perinatol* 23:195, 2003.
260. National Institutes of Health: Antenatal corticosteroids revisited: repeat courses, *NIH Consens Statement* 2000(17):1, 2000.
261. Needelman H, Evans M, Roberts H, et al: Effects of postnatal dexamethasone exposure on the developmental outcome of premature infants, *J Child Neurol* 23:421, 2008.

262. Nelson M, Nicks JJ, Becker MA, et al: Comparison of two methods of surfactant administration and the effect on dosing-associated hypoxemia, *J Perinatol* 17:450, 1997.
263. Neonatal Inhaled Nitric Oxide Study Group: Inhaled nitric oxide in full-term and nearly full-term infants with hypoxic respiratory failure, *N Engl J Med* 336:597, 1997.
264. Neonatal Inhaled Nitric Oxide Study Group: Inhaled nitric oxide in term and near-term infants: neurodevelopmental follow-up of the Neonatal Inhaled Nitric Oxide Study Group (NINOS), *J Pediatr* 136:611, 2000.
265. Ng G, Da Silva O, Ohlsson A: Bronchodilators for the prevention and treatment of chronic lung disease in preterm infants, *Cochrane Database Syst Rev* 3: CD003214, 2001.
266. Ng G, Ohlsson A: Cromolyn sodium for the prevention of chronic lung disease in preterm infants, *Cochrane Database Syst Rev* 2: CD003059, 2001.
267. Niwas R, Nadroo AM, Sutija V, et al: Malposition of endotracheal tube: association with pneumothorax in ventilated neonates, *Arch Dis Child Fetal Neonatal Ed* 92:F233, 2007.
268. Nixon PA, Washburn LK, Schechter MS, et al: Follow-up study of a randomized controlled trial of postnatal dexamethasone therapy in very low birth weight infants: effects on pulmonary outcomes at age 8 to 11 years, *J Pediatr* 150:345, 2007.
269. Noori S, Friedlich P, Wong P, et al: Cardiovascular effects of sildenafil in neonates and infants with congenital diaphragmatic hernia and pulmonary hypertension, *Neonatology* 91:92, 2007.
270. Noori S, McCoy M, Friedlich P, et al: Failure of ductus arteriosus closure is associated with increased mortality in preterm infants, *Pediatrics* 123:e138, 2009.
271. Northway W, Rosan R: Radiographic features of pulmonary oxygen toxicity in the newborn: bronchopulmonary dysplasia, *Radiology* 91:49, 1968.
272. Nuntnarumit P, Bada H, Yang W, et al: Cerebral blood flow velocity changes after bovine natural surfactant instillation, *J Perinatol* 4:240, 2000.
273. Okasaki K, Kondo M, Kato M, et al: Serum cytokine and chemokine profiles in neonates with meconium aspiration syndrome, *Pediatrics* 121:e748, 2008.
274. Ortiz L, Quan A, Weinberg A, et al: Prenatal dexamethasone programs: hypertension and renal injury in the rat, *Hypertension* 41:328, 2003.
275. O'Shea T, Washburn LK, Nixon PA, et al: Follow-up of a randomized, placebo-controlled trial of dexamethasone to decrease the duration of ventilator dependency in very low birth weight infants: neurodevelopmental outcomes at 4 to 11 years of age, *Pediatrics* 120:594, 2007.
276. Ostrea EM, Villanueva-Uy ET, Natarajan G, et al: Persistent pulmonary hypertension of the newborn, *Pediatr Drugs* 8:179, 2006.
277. Panickar J, Scholefield H, Kumar Y, et al: Atypical chronic lung disease in preterm infants, *J Perinat Med* 32:162, 2004.
278. Parikh N, Lasky RE, Kennedy KA, et al: Postnatal dexamethasone therapy and cerebral tissue volumes in extremely low birth weight infants, *Pediatrics* 119:265, 2007.
279. Perkin R, Levin D, Clark R: Serum salicylate levels and right to left ductus shunts in newborn infants with persistent pulmonary hypertension of the newborn, *J Pediatr* 96:721, 1980.
280. Perlman J, Goodman S, Kreusser K, et al: Reduction in intraventricular hemorrhage by elimination of fluctuating cerebral blood flow velocity in preterm infants with respiratory distress syndrome, *N Engl J Med* 312:1353, 1985.
281. Pearlman J, Volpe J: Suctioning in the preterm infant: effects on cerebral blood flow velocity, intracranial pressure and arterial blood pressure, *Pediatrics* 72:329, 1983.
282. Pearlman J, Volpe J: Episodes of apnea and bradycardia in the preterm newborn: impact on cerebral circulation, *Pediatrics* 76:33, 1985.
283. Peltoniemi OA, Lano A, Puosi R, et al: Trial of early neonatal hydrocortisone: two-year follow-up, *Neonatology* 95:240, 2007.
284. Peter C, Sporodowski N, Bohnhorst B, et al: Gastroesophageal reflux and apnea of prematurity: no temporal relationship, *Pediatrics* 109:8, 2002.
285. Pfister RH, Soll RF, Wiswell T: Protein containing surfactant versus animal derived surfactant extract for the prevention and treatment of respiratory distress syndrome, *Cochrane Database Syst Rev* 4:CD006069, 2007.
286. Phelps D, Lakatos L, Watts J: D-Penicillamine for preventing ROP in preterm infants, *Cochrane Database Syst Rev* 1: CD001073, 2001.
287. Phelps D, Watts J: Early light reduction for preventing ROP in VLBW infants, *Cochrane Database Syst Rev* 1:CD000122, 2001.
288. Pillekamp F, Hermann C, Keller T, et al: Factors influencing apnea and bradycardia of prematurity: implications for neurodevelopmental delay, *Neonatology* 91:155, 2007.
289. Piotrowski A, Sobala W, Kawczynski P: Patient-initiated, pressure-regulated, volume-controlled ventilation compared with intermittent mandatory ventilation in neonates: a prospective, randomized study, *Intensive Care Med* 23:975, 1997.
290. Poets C: Gastroesophageal reflux: a critical review of its role in preterm infants, *Pediatrics* 113:128, 2004.
291. Polak M: Respiratory syncytial virus (RSV): overview, treatment and prevention strategies, *Newborn Infant Nurs Rev* 4:15, 2004.

292. Polimeni V, Claure N, D'Ugard C, et al: Effects of volume-targeted synchronized intermittent mandatory ventilation on spontaneous episodes of hypoxemia in preterm infants, *Biol Neonate* 89:50, 2006.
293. Pollan C: Retinopathy of prematurity: an eye toward better outcomes, *Neonatal Netw* 28:93, 2009.
294. Powell K, Kerkering KW, Barker G, et al: Dexamethasone dosing, mechanical ventilation and the risk of cerebral palsy, *J Matern Fetal Neonatal Med* 19:43, 2006.
295. Pritchard M, Flenady V, Woodgate P: Systematic review of the role of preoxygenation for tracheal suctioning in ventilated newborn infants, *J Paediatr Child Health* 39:163, 2003.
296. Purohit D, Caldwell C, Levkoff A: Multiple fractures due to physiotherapy in a neonate with hyaline membrane disease, *Am J Dis Child* 129:1103, 1975.
297. Quiroz-Mercado H, Martinez-Castellanos MA, Hernandez-Rojas ML, et al: Antiangiogenic therapy with intravitreal bevacizumab for retinopathy of prematurity, *Retina* 28(Suppl 3):S19, 2008.
298. Rademaker KJ, deVries LS, Uiterwaal CS, et al: Postnatal hydrocortisone treatment for chronic lung disease in the preterm newborn and long-term neurodevelopmental follow-up, *Arch Dis Child Fetal Neonatal Ed* 93:F58, 2008.
299. Rainer C, Gardetto A, Fruhwirth M, et al: Breast deformity in adolescence as a result of pneumothorax drainage during neonatal intensive care, *Pediatrics* 111:80, 2003.
300. Rais-Bahrami K, Short B: The current status of neonatal ECMO, *Semin Perinatol* 24:406, 2000.
301. Raju T, Langenberg P: Pulmonary hemorrhage and exogenous surfactant therapy: a meta analysis, *J Pediatr* 123:603, 1993.
302. Ramaekers V, Casaer P, Daniels H: Cerebral hyperperfusion following episodes of bradycardia in the preterm infant, *Early Hum Dev* 34:199, 1993.
303. Ramanathan R, Siassi B, deLemos RA: Severe retinopathy of prematurity in extremely low birth weight infants with short-term dexamethasone therapy, *J Perinatol* 15:178, 1995.
304. Ramsay S: The Birmingham experience, *Lancet* 345:510, 1995.
305. Raval D, Yeh T, Mora A, et al: Chest physiotherapy in preterm infants with RDS in the first 24 hours of life, *J Perinatol* 7:301, 1987.
306. Redline R, Wilson-Costello D, Hack M: Placental and other perinatal risk factors for chronic lung disease in very low birthweight infants, *Pediatr Res* 52:713, 2002.
307. Reininger A, Khalak R, Kendig JW, et al: Surfactant administration by transient intubation in infants 29 to 35 weeks' gestation with respiratory distress syndrome decreases the likelihood of later mechanical ventilation: a randomized controlled trial, *J Perinatol* 25:703, 2005.
308. Reyes ZC, Claure N, Tauscher MK, et al: Randomized, controlled trial comparing synchronized intermittent mandatory ventilation and synchronized intermittent mandatory ventilation plus pressure support in preterm infants, *Pediatrics* 118:1409, 2006.
309. Reynolds J, Hardy R, Kennedy K, et al: Lack of efficacy of light reduction in preventing retinopathy of prematurity, *N Engl J Med* 338:1572, 1998.
310. Rich W, Finer N, Vaucher Y: Ten year trends of neonatal ventilation of very low birth weight infants, *J Perinatol* 23:660, 2003.
311. Rieger H, Kuhle S, Ipsiroglu OS, et al: Effects of open vs. closed system endotracheal suctioning on cerebral blood flow velocities in mechanically ventilated extremely low birth weight infants, *J Perinatol Med* 33:435, 2005.
312. Rojas MA, Lozano JM, Rojas MX, et al: Very early surfactant without mandatory ventilation in premature infants treated with early continuous positive airway pressure: a randomized, controlled trial, *Pediatrics* 123:137, 2009.
313. Rushton D: Neonatal shaken baby syndrome: historical inexactitudes, *Arch Dis Child Fetal Neonatal Ed* 87:F161, 2003.
314. Salhab W, Hynan L, Perlman J: Partial or complete antenatal steroids treatment and neonatal outcome in ELBW infants ≤1000 g: is there a dose-dependent effect? *J Perinatol* 23:668, 2003.
315. Sarkar S, Hussain N, Herson V: Fibrin glue for persistent pneumothorax in neonates, *J Perinatol* 23:82, 2003.
316. Saugstad O: Oxygen radical disease in neonatology, *Biol Neonate* 88:228, 2005.
317. Schipper J, Mohammad G, van Straaten H, et al: The impact of surfactant replacement therapy on cerebral and systemic circulation and lung function, *Eur J Pediatr* 156:224, 1997.
318. Schmidt B, Roberts RS, Davis P, et al: for the Caffeine for Apnea of Prematurity Trial Group: Caffeine therapy for apnea of prematurity, *New Engl J Med* 354:2112, 2006.
319. Schmidt B, Roberts RS, Davis P, et al: Long-term effects of caffeine therapy for apnea of prematurity, *New Engl J Med* 357:1893, 2007.
320. Schreiber M, Gin-Mestan K, Narks J, et al: Inhaled NO in premature infants with RDS, *N Engl J Med* 349:2099, 2003.
321. Schulze A, Gerhardt T, Musante G, et al: Proportional assist ventilation in low birth weight infants with acute respiratory disease: a comparison to assist/control and conventional mechanical ventilation, *J Pediatr* 135:339, 1999.
322. Schulze A, Rieger-Fackeldey E, Gerhardt T, et al: Randomized crossover comparison of proportional assist ventilation and patient-triggered ventilation in extremely low birth weight infants with evolving chronic lung disease, *Neonatology* 92:1, 2007.

323. Sears JE, Pietz J, Sonnie C, et al: A change in oxygen supplementation can decrease the incidence of retinopathy of prematurity, *Ophthalmol* 116:513, 2009.
324. Seidner SR, Ikegami M, Yamada T, et al: Decreased surfactant dose-response after delayed administration to preterm rabbits, *Am J Respir Crit Care Med* 152:113, 1995.
325. Seth R, Gray PH, Tudehope DI: Decreased use of postnatal corticosteroids in extremely preterm infants without increasing chronic lung disease, *Neonatology* 95:172, 2009.
326. Shah S, Ohlsson A, Halliday H, et al: Inhaled versus systemic corticosteroids for the treatment of chronic lung disease in ventilated very low birth weight preterm infants, *Cochrane Database Syst Rev* 4: CD002057, 2007.
327. Shah V, Ohlsson A, Halliday H, et al: Early administration of inhaled corticosteroids for preventing chronic lung disease in ventilated very low birth weight preterm neonates, *Cochrane Database Syst Rev* 4:CD001969, 2007.
328. Shaw L, Grant M: Insulin-like growth factor-I and insulin-like growth factor binding proteins: their possible roles in both maintaining normal retinal vascular function and in promoting retinal pathology, *Rev Endocr Metab Disord* 5:199, 2004.
329. Sheiner E, Hadar A, Shoham-Vardi I, et al: The effect of meconium on perinatal outcome: a prospective analysis, *J Matern Fetal Neonatal Med* 11:54, 2002.
330. Shenai J: Vitamin A supplementation in VLBW neonates: rationale and evidence, *Pediatrics* 104:1369, 1999.
331. Shenai J, Mellen B, Chytil F: Vitamin A status and postnatal dexamethasone treatment in BPD, *Pediatrics* 106:547, 2000.
332. Shih S, Ju M, Lin N, et al: Selective stimulation of VEGFR-1 prevents oxygen-induced retinal vascular degeneration in ROP, *J Clin Invest* 112:50, 2003.
333. Shinwell ES, Lerner-Geva L, Lusky A, et al: Less postnatal steroids, more bronchopulmonary dysplasia: a population-based study of very low birthweight infants, *Arch Dis Child Fetal Neonatal Ed* 92:F30, 2007.
334. Shoemaker MT, Pierce MR, Yoder BA, et al: High flow nasal cannula versus nasal CPAP for neonatal respiratory disease: a retrospective study, *J Perinatol* 27:85, 2007.
335. Silverman W: A cautionary tale about supplemental oxygen: the albatross of neonatal medicine, *Pediatrics* 113:1, 2004.
336. Simoes E, Rosenberg A, King S, et al: Room air challenge: prediction for successful weaning of oxygen-dependent infants, *J Perinatol* 17:125, 1997.
337. Slocum C, Arko M, DiFiore J, et al: Apnea, bradycardia and desaturation in preterm infants before and after feeding, *J Perinatol* 29:209, 2009.
338. Smolkin T, Steinberg M, Sujov P, et al: Late postnatal systemic steroids predispose to retinopathy of prematurity in very-low-birth-weight infants: a comparative study, *Acta Paediatr* 97:322, 2008.
339. Snow TM, Brandon DH: A nurse's guide to common mechanical ventilation techniques and modes used in infants, *Adv Neonatal Care* 7:8, 2007.
340. Sokol G, Ehrenkranz R: Inhaled nitric oxide therapy in neonatal hypoxic respiratory failure: insights beyond primary outcomes, *Semin Perinatol* 27:311, 2003.
341. Sola A: Oxygen for the preterm newborn: one infant at a time, *Pediatrics* 121:1257, 2008.
342. Soll R: Multiple versus single doses of exogenous surfactant extract for the prevention or treatment of neonatal respiratory distress syndrome, *Cochrane Database Syst Rev* 1:CD000141, 2009.
343. Squires AJ, Hyndman M: Prevention of nasal injuries secondary to NCPAP application in the ELBW infant, *Neonatal Netw* 28:13, 2009.
344. Sreenan C, Lemke R, Hudson-Mason A, et al: High-flow nasal cannulae in the management of apnea of prematurity: a comparison with conventional nasal continuous positive airway pressure, *Pediatrics* 107:1081, 2001.
345. Srinivasan R, Asselin J, Gildengorin G, et al: A prospective study of ventilator-associated pneumonia in children, *Pediatrics* 123:1108, 2009.
346. Sriram S, Wall S, Khoshnood B, et al: Racial disparity in meconium-stained amniotic fluid and meconium aspiration syndrome in the United States, 1989-2000, *Obstet Gynecol* 102:1262, 2003.
347. Stark AR, Carlo WA, Tyson JE, et al: Adverse effects of early dexamethasone treatment in extremely-low-birth-weight infants, *N Engl J Med* 344:95, 2001.
348. Steer P, Henderson-Smart D: Caffeine versus theophylline for apnea in preterm infants, *Cochrane Database Syst Rev* 2:CD000273, 2000.
349. Stefanescu B, Murphy W, Hansell B, et al: A randomized, controlled trial comparing two different continuous positive airway pressure systems for the successful extubation of ELBW infants, *Pediatrics* 112:1031, 2003.
350. Stern L: Therapy of the respiratory distress syndrome, *Pediatr Clin North Am* 19:221, 1972.
351. Stevens T, Blennow M, Soll R: Early surfactant administration with brief ventilation vs selective surfactant and continued mechanical ventilation for preterm infants with or at risk for respiratory distress syndrome, *Cochrane Database Syst Rev* 4:CD003063, 2007.
352. Stoelhorst G, Rijken M, Martens S, et al: Developmental outcome at 18 and 24 months of age in very preterm children: a cohort study from 1996 to 1997, *Early Human Dev* 72:83, 2003.

353. Stoll B, Hansen N, Fanaroff A, et al: Late-onset sepsis in VLBW neonates: the experience of the NICHD Neonatal Research Network, *Pediatrics* 110:285, 2002.
354. Subramanian P, Henderson-Smart D, Davis P: Prophylactic nasal continuous positive airways pressure for preventing morbidity and mortality in very preterm infants, *Cochrane Database Syst Rev* 3:CD001243, 2005.
355. Suk KK, Dunbar JA, Liu A, et al: Human recombinant erythropoietin and the incidence of retinopathy of prematurity: a multiple regression model, *JAAPOS* 12:233, 2008.
356. Suresh G, Davis J, Soll R: Superoxide dismutase for preventing chronic lung disease in mechanically ventilated preterm infants, *Cochrane Database Syst Rev* 1:CD001968, 2001.
357. Szymankiewicz M, Gadzinowski J, Kowalska K: Pulmonary function after surfactant lavage followed by surfactant administration in infants with severe meconium aspiration syndrome, *J Matern Fetal Neonatal Med* 16:125, 2004.
358. Szymankiewicz M, Vidyasagar D, Gadzinowski J: Predictors of successful extubation or preterm low-birth-weight infants with respiratory distress syndrome, *Pediatr Critical Care Med* 6:44, 2005.
359. Tadesse M, Dhanireddy R, Mittal M, et al: Race, *Candida* sepsis, and ROP, *Biol Neonate* 81:86, 2002.
360. Takaya A, Igarashi M, Nakajima M, et al: Risk factors for transient tachypnea of the newborn in infants delivered vaginally at 37 weeks or later, *J Nippon Med Sch* 75:269, 2008.
361. Tanaka Y, Hayashi T, Kitajima H, et al: Inhaled nitric oxide therapy decreases the risk of cerebral palsy in preterm infants with persistent pulmonary hypertension of the newborn, *Pediatrics* 119:1159, 2007.
362. Taquino L, Blackburn S: The effects of containment during suction and heelstick on physiological and behavioral responses of preterm infants, *Neonatal Netw* 13:55, 1994.
363. The STOP-ROP Multicenter Study Group: Supplemental therapeutic oxygen for prethreshold retinopathy of prematurity (STOP-ROP), a randomized controlled trial I: primary outcomes, *Pediatrics* 105:295, 2000.
364. Thome UH, Ambalavanan N: Permissive hypercapnia to decrease lung injury in ventilated preterm neonates, *Semin Fetal Neonatal Med* 14:21, 2009.
365. Tin W: Oxygen therapy: 50 years of uncertainty, *Pediatrics* 110:615, 2002.
366. Tin W, Gupta S: Optimum oxygen therapy in preterm babies, *Arch Dis Child Fetal Neonatal Ed* 92:F143, 2005.
367. Tin W, Milligan W, Pennefather P, et al: Pulse oximetry, severe retinopathy, and outcome at one year in babies of less than 28 weeks' gestation, *Arch Dis Child Fetal Neonatal Ed* 84:F106, 2001.
368. Tin W, Wiswell T: Adjunctive therapies in chronic lung disease: examining the evidence, *Semin Fetal Neonatal Med* 13:44, 2008.
369. Torres C, Holditch-Davis D, O'Hale A, et al: Effect of standard rest periods on apnea and weight gain in preterm infants, *Neonatal Netw* 16:35, 1997.
370. Tourneux P, Cardot V, Museaux N, et al: Influence of thermal drive on central sleep apnea in the preterm neonate, *Sleep* 31:549, 2008.
371. Tourneux P, Rakza T, Bouissou A, et al: Pulmonary circulatory effects of norepinephrine in newborn infants with persistent pulmonary hypertension, *J Pediatr* 153:345, 2008.
372. Tran S, Caughey A, Musci T: Meconium-stained amniotic fluid is associated with puerperal infections, *Am J Obstet Gynecol* 189:746, 2003.
373. Travadi J, Patole S: Phosphodiesterase inhibitors for PPHN: a review, *Pediatr Pulmonol* 36:529, 2003.
374. Truffert P, Paris-Llado J, Escande B, et al: Neuromotor outcome at 2 years of very preterm infants who were treated with high-frequency oscillatory ventilation or conventional ventilation for neonatal respiratory distress syndrome, *Pediatrics* 119:e860, 2007.
375. Tsao P, Wei S, Su Y, et al: Placenta growth factor elevation in the cord blood of premature neonates predicts poor pulmonary outcome, *Pediatrics* 113:1348, 2004.
376. Tulenko D: An update on ECMO, *Neonatal Netw* 23:11, 2004.
377. Turunen R, Nupponen I, Siitonen S, et al: Onset of mechanical ventilation is associated with rapid activation of circulating phagocytes in preterm infants, *Pediatrics* 117:448, 2006.
378. Tyson JE, Wright LL, Oh W, et al: Vitamin A supplementation for extremely-low-birth-weight infants, *N Engl J Med* 340:1962, 1999.
379. Vain N, Szyld E, Prudent L, et al: Oropharyngeal and nasopharyngeal suctioning of meconium-stained neonates before delivery of their shoulders: multicenter, randomized controlled trial, *Lancet* 364:597, 2004.
380. Vanderveen DK, Mansfield TA, Eichenwald EC: Lower oxygen saturation alarm limits decrease the severity of retinopathy of prematurity, *JAAPOS* 10:445, 2006.
381. Vanhaesebrouck P, Allegaert K, Bottu J, et al: The EPIBEL study: outcomes to discharge from hospital for extremely preterm infants in Belgium, *Pediatrics* 114:663, 2004.
382. Van Meurs K, Wright L, Ehrenkranz R, et al: Inhaled nitric oxide for premature infants with severe respiratory failure, *N Engl J Med* 353:13, 2005.

383. Velaphi S, Vidayasagar D: Intrapartum and postdelivery management of infants born to mothers with meconium-stained amniotic fluid: evidence-based recommendations, *Clin Perinatol* 33:29, 2006.
384. Verder H, Albertsen P, Ebbesen F, et al: Nasal continuous positive airway pressure and early surfactant therapy for respiratory distress syndrome in newborns of less than 30 weeks' gestation, *Pediatrics* 103:e241, 1999.
385. Vermillion S, Soper D, Newman R: Neonatal sepsis and death after multiple doses of antenatal betamethasone, *Am J Obstet Gynecol* 182:S24, 2000.
386. Vohr BR, Wright LL, Dusick AM, et al: Neurodevelopmental and functional outcomes of extremely low birth weight infants in the National Institute of Child Health and Human Development Neonatal Research Network, 1993-1994, *Pediatrics* 105:1216, 2000.
387. Walsh M, Yao Q, Gettner P, et al: Impact of a physiologic definition on bronchopulmonary dysplasia rates, *Pediatrics* 114:1305, 2004.
388. Wapner RJ, Sorokin Y, Mele L, et al: for the National Institutes of Child Health and Human Development Maternal-Fetal Medicine Units Network: Long-term outcomes after repeat doses of antenatal corticosteroids, *New Engl J Med* 357:1190, 2007.
389. Ward-Larson C, Horn R, Gosnell F: The efficacy of facilitated tucking for relieving procedural pain of endotracheal suctioning in very low birthweight infants, *MCN Am J Matern Child Nurs* 29:151, 2004.
390. Wardle S, Hughes A, Chen S, et al: Randomized controlled trial of oral vitamin A supplementation in preterm infants to prevent chronic lung disease, *Arch Dis Child Fetal Neonatal Ed* 84:F9, 2001.
391. Washburn LK, Nixon PA, O'Shea TM: Follow-up of a randomized, placebo-controlled trial of postnatal betamethasone: blood pressure and anthropometric measurements at school age, *Pediatrics* 118:1592, 2006.
392. Watterberg K: Adrenocortical function and dysfunction in the fetus and newborn, *Semin Neonatol* 9:13, 2004.
393. Watterberg K, Gerdes J, Cole C, et al: Prophylaxis of early adrenal insufficiency to prevent BPD: a multicenter trial, *Pediatrics* 114:1649, 2004.
394. Watterberg KL, Scott SM, Backstrom C, et al: Links between early adrenal function and respiratory outcome in preterm infants: airway inflammation and patent ductus arteriosus, *Pediatrics* 105:320, 2000.
395. Watterberg KL, Shaffer ML, Mishefske MJ, et al: Growth and neurodevelopmental outcomes after early low-dose hydrocortisone treatment in extremely low birth weight infants, *Pediatrics* 120:40, 2007.
396. Wegner S, Vann J, Liu G, et al: Direct cost analyses of palivizumab treatment in a cohort of at-risk children: evidence from the North Carolina Medicaid Program, *Pediatrics* 114:1612, 2004.
397. Wiedemann JR, Saugstad AM, Barnes-Powell L, et al: Meconium aspiration syndrome, *Neonatal Netw* 27:81, 2008.
398. Wilder M: Surfactant protein B deficiency in infants with respiratory failure, *J Perinat Neonatal Nurs* 18:61, 2004.
399. Williams A, Sunderland R: Neonatal shaken baby syndrome: an aetiological view from Down Under, *Arch Dis Child Fetal Neonatal Ed* 86:F29, 2002.
400. Williams PD, Press A, Williams AR, et al: Fatigue in mothers of infants discharged to the home on apnea monitors, *Appl Nurs Res* 12:69, 1999.
401. Wilson G, Hughes G, Rennie J, et al: Evaluation of two endotracheal suction regimes in babies ventilated for respiratory distress syndrome, *Early Hum Dev* 25:87, 1991.
402. Wilson TT, Waters L, Patterson CC, et al: Neurodevelopmental and respiratory follow-up results at 7 years for children from the United Kingdom and Ireland enrolled in a randomized trial of early and late postnatal corticosteroid treatment systemic and inhaled (the Open Study of Early Corticosteroid Treatment), *Pediatrics* 117:2196, 2006.
403. Wood B: Infant ribs: generalized periosteal reaction resulting from vibrator chest physiotherapy, *Radiology* 162:811, 1987.
404. Woodgate P, Flenady V: Tracheal suctioning without disconnection in intubated ventilated neonates, *Cochrane Database Syst Rev* 2: CD003065, 2001.
405. Wrightson D: Suctioning smarter: answers to eight common questions about endotracheal suctioning in neonates, *Neonatal Netw* 18:51, 1999.
406. Yamada Y, Sugai M, Woo M, et al: Acquired subglottic stenosis caused by methicillin resistant *Staphylococcus aureus* that produce epidermal cell differentiation inhibitor, *Arch Dis Child Fetal Neonatal Ed* 84:F38, 2001.
407. Yeh T, Lin Y, Lin H, et al: Outcomes at school age after postnatal dexamethasone therapy for lung disease of prematurity, *N Engl J Med* 350:1304, 2004.
408. Yeh TF, Lin HC, Chang CH, et al: Early intratracheal instillation of budesonide using surfactant as a vehicle to prevent chronic lung disease in preterm infants: a pilot study, *Pediatrics* 121:e1310, 2008.
409. Yeo KL, Perlman M, Hao Y, et al: Outcomes of extremely preterm infants related to their peak serum bilirubin concentrations and exposure to phototherapy, *Pediatrics* 102:1426, 1998.
410. Yoder B, Kirsch E, Barth W, et al: Changing obstetric practices associated with decreasing incidence of meconium aspiration syndrome, *Obstet Gynecol* 99:731, 2002.
411. Yong SC, Chen SJ, Boo NY: Incidence of nasal trauma associated with nasal prong versus nasal mask during continuous positive airway pressure treatment in very low birthweight infants: a randomized control study, *Arch Dis Child Fetal Neonatal Ed* 90:F480, 2005.

412. York J, Landers S, Kirby R, et al: Arterial oxygen fluctuation and ROP in VLBW infants, *J Perinatol* 24:82, 2004.
413. Yuan TM, Chen LH, Yu HM: Risk factors and outcomes for ventilator-associated pneumonia in neonatal intensive care unit patients, *J Perinatol Med* 35:334, 2007.
414. Yuksel B, Greenough A, Gamsu H: Neonatal MAS and respiratory morbidity during infancy, *Pediatr Pulmonol* 16:358, 1993.
415. Zanardo V, Freato F: Home oxygen therapy in infants with bronchopulmonary dysplasia: assessment of parental anxiety, *Early Hum Dev* 65:39, 2001.
416. Zola ME, Gunkel JH, Chan RK, et al: Comparison of three dosing procedures for administration of bovine surfactant to neonates with respiratory distress syndrome, *J Pediatr* 122:453, 1993.

RESOURCE MATERIALS FOR PROFESSIONALS AND PARENTS

Bonner KM, Mainous RO: The nursing care of the infant receiving bubble CPAP therapy, *Adv Neonatal Care* 8:78, 2008.

Bracht M, Heffer M, O'Brien K: Preventing respiratory syncytial virus (RSV) infection, *Adv Neonatal Care* 5:50, 2005.

de Klerk A: Humidified high-flow nasal cannula, *Adv Neonatal Care* 8:98, 2008.

Fiske E: Effective strategies to prepare infants and families for home tracheostomy care, *Adv Neonatal Care* 4:42, 2004.

Fiske E: Tracheostomy home care guide, *Adv Neonatal Care* 4:54, 2004.

Gracey K, Talbot D, Lankford R, et al: The changing face of BPD: Part I, *Adv Neonatal Care* 2:327, 2002.

Gracey K, Talbot D, Lankford R, et al: What is bronchopulmonary dysplasia?, *Adv Neonatal Care* 2:339, 2002.

Gracey K, Talbot D, Lankford R, et al: The changing face of BPD. II. Discharging an infant home on oxygen, *Adv Neonatal Care* 3:88, 2003.

Gracey K, Talbot D, Lankford R, et al: Nasal cannula home oxygen, *Adv Neonatal Care* 3:99, 2003.

Stokowski LA: A primer on apnea of prematurity, *Adv Neonatal Care* 5:155, 2005.

Stokowski LA: Family Teaching Toolbox: A parents' guide to understanding apnea, *Adv Neonatal Care* 5:175, 2005.

24 CARDIOVASCULAR DISEASES AND SURGICAL INTERVENTIONS

PATRICIA M. KENNEY, DEANDRA HOOVER, LUTHER C. WILLIAMS, AND VICTOR ISKERSKY

Congenital heart disease (CHD) is the most common life-threatening birth defect encountered in the neonatal intensive care unit (NICU). Although the incidence of these conditions has remained constant at approximately 1% of all infants born in the United States, the methods of diagnosis and treatment have undergone tremendous change over the past several decades.[37] It is the responsibility of the practitioner to recognize the presence of CHD and to provide an accurate diagnose and treatment. This chapter reviews the physiology of neonatal circulation, the pathophysiology of congenital heart disease, and the most current evidence-based treatments.

CONGENITAL HEART DISEASE: OVERVIEW

History

In 1892, Dr. William Osler wrote that congenital heart disease was of "limited clinical interest as in a large proportion of cases the anomaly is not compatible with life, and in others, nothing can be done to remedy the defect or even relieve the symptoms."[8] Osler encouraged Dr. Maude Abbott in her CHD finding, and she, along with Dr. Helen Taussig and Dr. Alfred Blalock, suggested surgery to help these "blue babies."[35] This opened up the field of surgical treatment of cyanotic malformations of the heart. In 1938, Dr. Robert Gross was the first to successfully ligate a patent ductus arteriosus (PDA) in a 7-year-old girl at Boston's Children's Hospital. The first successful United States heart transplant was done at Stanford University by Dr. Norman Shumway in 1968.[7] What remarkable progress has been made in the area of congenital heart disease. This is the direct result of advances in pediatric and fetal cardiology, cardiac surgery, neonatology, and neonatal intensive care nursing.

Incidence and Survival

Each year, approximately 40,000 babies, or just under 1% of all babies born in the United States, are diagnosed with congenital heart disease.[3] Highly sensitive echocardiography has led to the detection of more trivial forms of congenital heart disease such as tiny ventricular septal defects. This inclusion has led to the higher incidence figures in recent years. The incidence of moderate to severe structural congenital heart defects (in liveborn infants) is 6 to 8 per 1000 live births.[8] Of these infants, approximately 3 per 1000 live births will have CHD that results in death or requires cardiac surgery during the first year of life.[25] Advances in diagnostic imaging, cardiac surgery, and neonatal intensive care have led to significant decreases in mortality rates. The death rate from all congenital heart defects declined nearly 32% between 1994 and 2004.[37]

Embryology

The heart is one of the earliest differentiating and functioning organs. In human embryos, the heart begins to

ACKNOWLEDGMENT: We would like to dedicate this chapter to the memory of Dr. Leslie Shelton for his contribution and dedication to pediatric cardiology.

Please note that the PURPLE type in each chapter is intended to make it easier to identify clinically applicable material.

beat at about 22 to 23 days of life. Blood begins flowing through the heart in the fourth week of life. The heart develops from the cardiogenic mesoderm that originally lies above the cranial end of the neural tube. The heart forms initially as a simple paired tube inside the pericardial cavity. When the embryonic disk folds, the heart is carried into the correct anatomic position in the chest cavity. A key aspect of heart development is the septation of the heart into separate chambers. This complex process converts this simple tube into a four-chambered heart. Cardiogenesis is such as intricate, complex process that it is of little wonder that congenital heart defects occur.

Physiology

The physiologic changes that occur during the transition from intrauterine to extrauterine life have been well documented. To develop a clear understanding of the various congenital heart defects, knowledge of the basic principles of fetal circulation must be established.

FETAL CIRCULATION

Fetal circulation is intended to use the placenta for gas exchange, whereas postnatal circulation uses the lungs for gas exchange (Figure 24-1). Highly oxygenated blood from the mother enters the fetal circulation

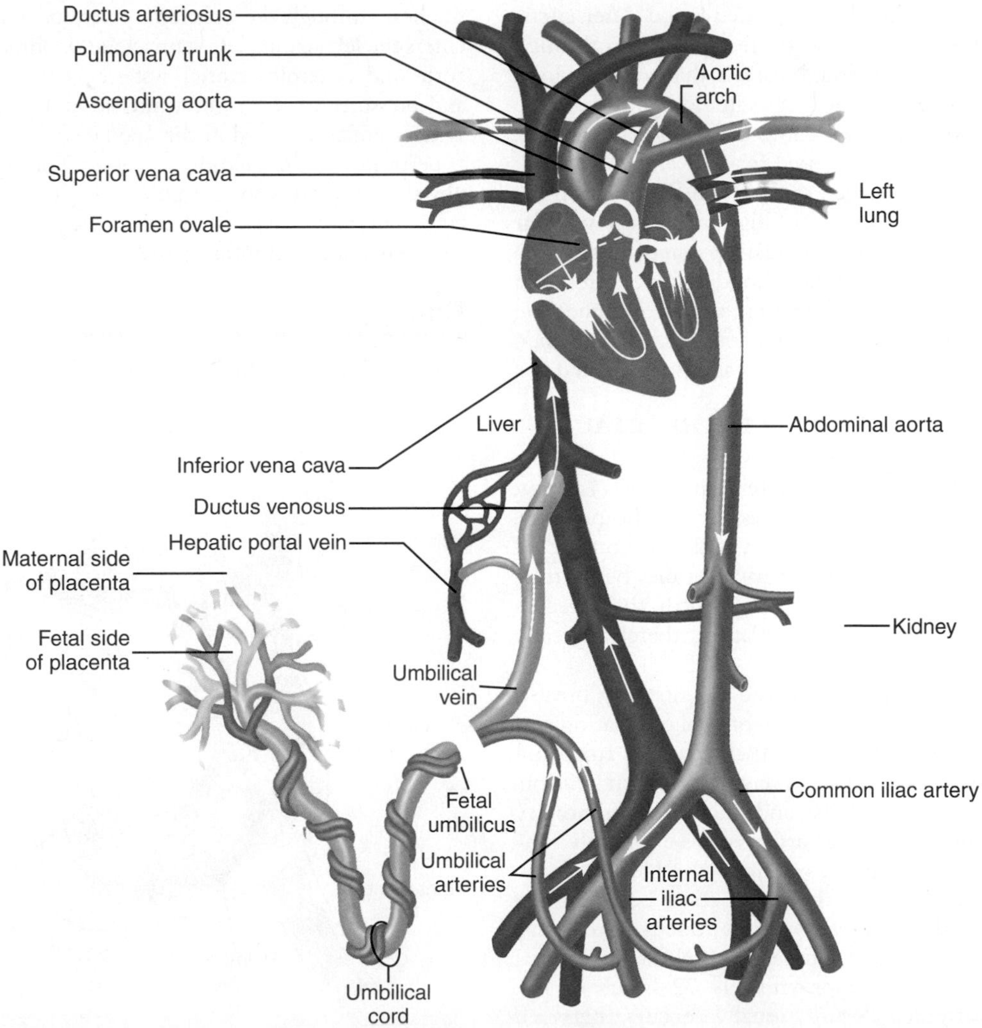

FIGURE 24-1 Fetal circulation. *LA,* Left atrium; *LV,* left ventricle; *RA,* right atrium; *RV,* right ventricle. (Modified from Patton KT, Thibodeau GA: *Anatomy and physiology,* ed 7, St Louis, 2010, Mosby.)

through the vein in the umbilical cord. This blood enters the inferior vena cava via the ductus venosus. Nearly one half of the umbilical venous blood goes through the liver and reaches the inferior vena cava via the hepatic veins. Inside the fetal heart, blood enters the right atrium, the chamber on the upper right side of the heart. Most of the blood flows to the left side through the foramen ovale, a special fetal opening between the left and right atria. Blood then passes into the left ventricle and then to the aorta, the large artery coming from the heart. From the aorta, blood is sent to the head and upper extremities. Therefore the brain (via the brachiocephalic vessels) and the heart (via the coronary arteries) are perfused with relatively highly oxygenated blood. After circulation, the blood returns to the right atrium through the superior vena cava. Nearly a third of the blood entering the right atrium stays in the right side of the heart, eventually flowing into the pulmonary artery.

Fetal lungs are not used for breathing. The work of exchanging oxygen and carbon dioxide is done by the placenta. Because of high pulmonary vascular resistance (PVR), fetal circulation shunts most of the blood away from the lungs. Blood is shunted from the pulmonary artery to the aorta through a connecting blood vessel called the *ductus arteriosus.*[29] Blood then enters the placental circulation and is resaturated.

CHANGES THAT OCCUR IN THE FETAL CIRCULATION WITH BIRTH

In utero, systemic vascular resistance (SVR) is low, primarily because of low resistance in the placenta. Conversely, the PVR is high, with the constricted and hypertrophied pulmonary arterioles being relatively resistant to blood flow. At birth, the placenta is removed from the circulation, thereby greatly increasing the SVR.

Both the labor process and the first few breaths of life begin the termination of fetal circulation and the transition to newborn circulation. Initiation of respirations produces increased oxygen tension, which decreases PVR and increases pulmonary blood flow. The ductus arteriosus is extremely sensitive to the oxygen content of the blood. As the neonatal Pa_{O_2} rises, the connection between the aorta and the pulmonary artery (ductus arteriosus) is no longer needed and begins to close. Functional closure occurs at approximately 72 hours of life, and anatomic closure usually occurs between 1 and 2 weeks after birth. The circulation in the lungs then increases, and more blood flows into the left atrium of the heart. This increased pressure in the left atrium causes the foramen ovale to close. Anatomic closure of the foramen ovale can take several months. Finally, with the clamping of the umbilical cord, umbilical venous flow ceases and the ductus venosus begins to close, with anatomic closure taking approximately 1 to 2 weeks.[29]

Once these changes occur, the newborn's circulation resembles that of an adult (Figure 24-2). Desaturated blood returns to the heart by the inferior and superior venae cavae and enters the right atrium, right ventricle, pulmonary artery, and pulmonary circulation in which oxygen and carbon dioxide are exchanged. The saturated blood then returns to the heart through the pulmonary venous system and enters the left atrium, left ventricle, and ultimately the aorta and systemic arterial system. However, PVR and pressures in the right ventricle and pulmonary system remain elevated in the neonate because of the hypertrophy of the pulmonary vessels. This hypertrophy slowly resolves so that pulmonary vascular resistance and right heart pressures decrease to lower levels between 1 and 2 months of age.

Etiology

The development of the cardiovascular system represents a complicated interaction between form and

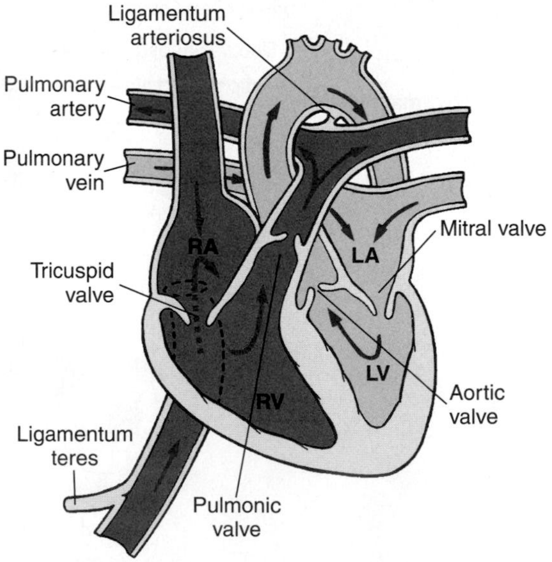

FIGURE 24-2 Postnatal circulation. (Modified from Hockenberry MJ, Wilson D: *Wong's essentials of pediatric nursing,* ed 8, St Louis, 2009, Mosby.)

function. In most cases, the cause(s) of abnormal cardiac development is unknown. Traditionally, the **etiology of congenital heart defects has been viewed as multifactorial, involving a complex interaction between genetic and environmental factors.** Studies are being done on maternal zinc deficiency and its association with an increased risk for fetal heart malformations. These studies postulate that the mechanism of action is the suppression of HNK-1 expression.[19] Table 24-1 lists the most common environmental risk factors and their associated cardiac malformations. Box 24-1 lists less common risk factors associated with CHD. Certain chronic illnesses in the mother contribute to the risk for CHD. For example, women with diabetes are at increased risk for having an infant with a heart defect. However, this risk can be greatly reduced by strict control of maternal blood sugar levels. More recent studies have found that the single greatest risk factor for congenital heart defects is genetic. Table 24-2 shows chromosomal syndromes and their associated congenital heart defects.

Since the 1990s, much progress has been made in understanding the genetics of heart disease. Studies in recent years have brought an explosion of information on the identification of potential candidate genes regulating heart development.[5] An example is the relationship between *TBX-1* and cardiovascular defects seen in DiGeorge syndrome.[16] Mutations in *NOTCH-1* have been found to cause aortic valve disease.[37] Although research defining the signaling cascades that lead to specific forms of congenital heart defects still needs to be done,[27] some information is well established (e.g., 50% of congenital heart defects involve a ventricular septal defect (VSD) alone or in combination with other abnormalities). Studies also demonstrate that **preterm infants are two and a half times more likely to have cardiovascular (CV) malformations.**[32] Table 24-3 shows the most common congenital heart defects and their time of presentation.

TABLE 24-1 MOST COMMON ENVIRONMENTAL TRIGGERS AND SPECIFIC DEFECTS ASSOCIATED WITH EACH

POTENTIAL TERATOGEN	FREQUENCY OF CARDIOVASCULAR DISEASE (%)	MOST COMMON MALFORMATIONS
DRUGS		
Alcohol	25-30	Ventricular septal defect, patent ductus arteriosus, atrial septal defect
Amphetamines	5-10	Ventricular septal defect, patent ductus arteriosus, atrial septal defect, transposition of the great vessels
Anticonvulsants	2-3	Pulmonary stenosis, aortic stenosis, coarctation of aorta, patent ductus arteriosus
Trimethadione	15-30	Transposition of great arteries, tetralogy of Fallot, hypoplastic left heart syndrome
Lithium	10	Ebstein's anomaly, tricuspid atresia, atrial septal defect
Sex hormones	2-4	Ventricular septal defect, transposition of great arteries, tetralogy of Fallot
INFECTIONS		
Rubella	35	Peripheral pulmonary artery stenosis, ventricular septal defect, patent ductus arteriosus, atrial septal defect
MATERNAL CONDITIONS		
Diabetes	3-5	Transposition of great arteries, ventricular septal defect, coarctation of aorta
	30-50	Cardiomegaly, myopathy
Lupus erythematosus	?	Heart block

TABLE 24-2 CHROMOSOMAL ABERRATIONS EVIDENT IN NEONATAL PERIOD THAT ARE ASSOCIATED WITH CONGENITAL HEART DISEASE

POPULATION	INCIDENCE OF CONGENITAL HEART DISEASE (%)	MOST COMMON LESIONS		
		1	2	3
Trisomy 21 syndrome	50	Ventricular septal defect, endocardial cushion defect	Atrial septal defect	Patent ductus arteriosus
Trisomy 18 syndrome	99+	Ventricular septal defect	Patent ductus arteriosus	Pulmonary stenosis
Trisomy 13 syndrome	90	Ventricular septal defect	Patent ductus arteriosus	Dextrocardia
Turner syndrome	35	Coarctation of the aorta	Aortic stenosis	Atrial septal defect
DiGeorge syndrome 22q deletion syndrome	50	Truncus arteriosus	Tetralogy of Fallot	Interrupted aortic arch

BOX 24-1 LESS COMMON RISK FACTORS ASSOCIATED WITH CONGENITAL HEART DEFECTS

Exposure to Environmental Agents During Work and/or Hobby

- Paternal exposure to cold temperature
- Maternal exposure to various solvents, hair dyes, auto body repair work

Drug Exposure

- Diazepam, phenothiazines
- Corticosteroids
- Gastrointestinal drugs
- Paternal exposure to cocaine

Maternal Reproductive History

- Genetic risk factor (family history of congenital heart disease), more than three prior pregnancies and an increased number of miscarriages
- Without genetic risk but with premature births and previous induced abortion

Syndromic Association

- 27.7% of all cases had chromosomal anomalies, heritable syndromes, or an additional major organ system defect (see Table 24-2)

PRENATAL DIAGNOSIS

Because of the widespread use of antenatal ultrasound, it is increasingly common for the fetus to be diagnosed with congenital heart disease. Fetal echocardiography has proven to be a valid, reliable, and accurate tool in the prenatal diagnosis of CHD.[9] The recommended timing of a fetal echocardiogram is between 18 to 20 weeks' gestation, although reasonable images can be obtained as early as 16 weeks. Physical examination alone picks up 30% of cases of CHD.[20] Pulse oximetry is not an accurate screening tool for CHD because of its relatively high false-positive rate, especially when used shortly after birth when the Spo_2 in neonates is low.[20] Recent studies are investigating serum high-sensitivity C-reactive protein (hs-CRP) and brain natriuretic protein (BNP) levels as markers of CHD. Thus far, hs-CRP and BNP levels are useful only as indicators of hypoxia.[33]

Pregnant women are encouraged to undergo fetal echocardiography if (1) genetic evaluation determines that the fetus has a chromosomal or genetic syndrome associated with CHD, (2) the mother or a previous child has CHD, or (3) there is a family history of CHD. Box 24-2 lists CHDs that are diagnosed and CHDs that may be missed on fetal echocardiogram. Magnetic resonance angiography is also an important diagnostic tool, especially for lesions that may be missed by fetal echocardiography. Detailed postnatal examinations are critical in determining the full extent of cardiac malformation.

Data Collection

HISTORY

A family history of congenital heart disease is significant, since a sibling with CHD increases the

TABLE 24-3 **DIAGNOSIS OF HEART DISEASE IN INFANTS AT SELECTED AGES***

0-6 DAYS	(%)	7-13 DAYS	(%)	13-20 DAYS	(%)
Transposition of great arteries	(17)	Coarctation of the aorta	(19)	Ventricular septal defect	(20)
Hypoplastic left ventricle	(12)	Ventricular septal defect	(15)	Transposition of great arteries	(17)
Lung disease	(10)	Hypoplastic left ventricle	(11)	Coarctation of the aorta	(16)
Tetralogy of Fallot	(9)	Transposition of great arteries	(9)	Tetralogy of Fallot	(8)
Coarctation of the aorta	(7)	Tetralogy of Fallot	(6)	Endocardial cushion defect	(6)
Ventricular septal defect	(7)	Heterotaxia	(4)	Heterotaxia	(6)
Pulmonary atresia (with intact ventricular septum)	(7)	Truncus arteriosus	(4)	Patent ductus arteriosus	(4)
		Single ventricle	(4)	Total anomalous pulmonary venous return	(3)
Heterotaxia	(6)				
Other	(25)	Other	(28)	Other	(20)
Total 896	(100)	Total 210	(100)	Total 116	(100)

From Flyer DC et al: Report of the New England Regional Infant Cardiac Program, *Pediatrics* 65:377, 1980.

*These numbers are intended as a rough guideline because there is considerable overlap. Infants with congenital heart disease are often active initially and appear well for several hours or days after birth. In contrast, infants with respiratory distress often have characteristic symptoms within the first several hours after birth.

BOX 24-2 **FETAL ECHOCARDIOGRAPHY AND CARDIAC LESIONS**[18]

Accurately Diagnosed

- Hypoplastic left heart syndrome
- Tricuspid atresia
- Pulmonary atresia
- Truncus arteriosus
- Tetralogy of Fallot
- Atriovenous septal defects
- Large ventricular septal defect (VSD)
- Transposition of the great arteries

May Be Missed

- Coarctation of the aorta
- Small VSD/atrial septal defect (ASD)
- Total anomalous pulmonary venous return (TAPVR)
- Mild aortic or pulmonary stenosis

recurrence risk threefold. Viral exposure during pregnancy (rubella, Coxsackie B, and enteroviruses) and maternal ingestion of alcohol or drugs should be evaluated. Pregnancy, labor, and delivery complications should be carefully examined as risk factors that could affect the cardiovascular system. For example, intrauterine hypoxia and perinatal hypoxia are risk factors for the development of myocardial dysfunction, as well as persistent pulmonary hypertension of the newborn (PPHN). The timing of the onset of symptoms may indicate the type of anomaly (see Table 24-3).

CLINICAL PRESENTATION OF INFANTS WITH SEVERE CARDIAC DISEASE

In many neonates, congenital heart disease is not suspected until after birth when the newborn presents with one or more signs or symptoms (see the Critical Findings box on p. 684).[36] Timing of presentation of signs or symptoms depends on severity of the defect, in utero effects of the defect, and alterations in cardiovascular physiology during transitional circulation (i.e., closure of the ductus arteriosus and the fall in PVR). Despite the presence of many heterogeneous forms of heart disease, a surprisingly limited number of signs and symptoms present in the neonate.

Murmurs. Heart murmurs are a common finding in neonates. Estimates of prevalence of heart murmurs

Critical Findings

SEVERE CARDIAC DISEASE

- Cyanosis
- Respiratory distress
- Congestive heart failure
- Diminished cardiac output
- Abnormal cardiac rhythm
- Cardiac murmurs

in neonates range from 1% to 70% depending on the study.[8] Although cardiac murmurs in the neonatal period do not necessarily indicate heart disease, they must be carefully evaluated. The absence of a murmur does not exclude severe life-threatening cardiac anomalies. Pathologic murmurs tend to appear at characteristic ages (e.g., murmurs associated with semilunar valve stenosis and atrioventricular valve insufficiency tend to be noted very shortly after birth). In contrast, murmurs caused by left-to-right shunt lesions (PDA, VSD) may not be heard until the second to fourth week of life. Therefore the age of the neonate when the murmur is first noted and the character of the murmur give important clues about the nature of the cardiac defect.

Cyanosis. Cyanosis (a bluish discoloration of the skin, nail beds, and mucous membranes) is one of the most common presenting signs of congenital heart disease in the neonate. Depending on the underlying skin complexion, clinically apparent cyanosis is usually not visible until there is more than 3 gm/dL of desaturated hemoglobin in the arterial system.[20] Cyanosis depends on both the severity of hypoxemia (which determines the percent of oxygen saturation) and the hemoglobin concentration. True central cyanosis should be differentiated from acrocyanosis, blueness of the hands and feet only, which is a normal finding in the neonate.

Cyanosis in the newborn must be differentiated between cardiac and respiratory causes. Pulmonary disorders cause cyanosis in the neonate because of intrapulmonary right-to-left shunting. Varying degrees of hypoxemia manifest as cyanosis and can be to the result of primary lung disease (see Chapter 23) and central nervous system abnormalities. Clinical cyanosis can occur without hypoxemia in a neonate with methemoglobinemia and polycythemia.

Respiratory Distress. Most infants with cyanosis from CHD do not have respiratory distress (e.g., tachypnea, intercostal retractions, grunting, nasal flaring, dyspnea, rales, cyanosis). Often the degree of cyanosis is not proportional to the degree of respiratory distress evaluated from the physical and chest x-ray examinations. If cyanosis is present and is caused by a fixed right-to-left shunt (cardiac lesion), increasing inspired oxygen will have little effect on the arterial blood gases. However, if the cyanosis is caused by a diffusion defect in the lungs (pulmonary disorder), the degree of cyanosis often decreases with increasing inspired oxygen.

The hyperoxia test is beneficial in differentiating respiratory disease from cyanotic heart disease. This single test is perhaps the most sensitive and specific tool in the initial evaluation of the neonate with suspected congenital heart disease and is used to investigate the possibility of a fixed (intracardiac) right-to-left shunt. The hyperoxia test is performed by obtaining arterial blood gas measurements (preferably from the right radial artery) when the infant is in room air and then after the infant has been in 100% oxygen for 5 to 10 minutes. If the Pao_2 is greater than 150 mm Hg, the presence of a right-to-left shunt and cyanotic congenital heart disease as the cause of cyanosis is unlikely. Pulse oximetry cannot be used for documentation.

Congestive Heart Failure. Congestive heart failure (CHF) occurs when the heart cannot meet the metabolic demands of the tissues. Signs and symptoms of congestive heart failure reflect decreased cardiac output and decreased tissue perfusion. In the early stages, the neonate may be tachypneic and tachycardic with an increased respiratory effort, rales, hepatomegaly, and delayed capillary refill. Edema caused by CHF is rarely seen in neonates. Diaphoresis, feeding difficulties, and growth failure later become apparent. Finally, congestive heart failure may present acutely with cardiorespiratory collapse, particularly with obstructive defects. Birth asphyxia and anemia must also be considered as causes of congestive heart failure in neonates.

The common symptoms associated with congestive heart failure (see the Critical Findings box on p. 685) can be understood using the physiologic principles previously outlined.

Critical Findings

CONGESTIVE HEART FAILURE

- Tachycardia
- Cardiac enlargement
- Tachypnea
- Gallop rhythm
- Decreased peripheral pulses and skin mottling in the extremities
- Decreased urine output and edema
- Diaphoresis
- Hepatomegaly
- Decreased activity
- Failure to thrive and feeding problems
- Diminished cardiac output

Tachycardia. **The heart attempts to compensate for the decrease in cardiac output (CO) by increasing either the heart rate (HR) or the stroke volume (SV) (CO = HR × SV).** Because the fetal myocardium has fewer contractile elements and is poorly innervated by the sympathetic nervous system, capacity to increase stroke volume is very limited. **Therefore increases in cardiac output are achieved mainly by increasing the heart rate.**

Cardiac Enlargement. Hypertrophy and dilation of the heart occur in response to the volume or pressure overload. This enlargement is evident on chest x-ray examination.

Gallop Rhythm. The gallop rhythm is an abnormal filling sound caused by dilation of the ventricles. It is heard as a triple rhythm on auscultation.

Decreased Peripheral Pulses/Mottling of the Extremities. Decreased cardiac output results in a compensatory redistribution of blood flow to vital tissues. **Peripheral tissue perfusion is decreased, which results in mottling of the skin and decreased pulses.**

Decreased Urine Output and Edema. **Decreased renal perfusion results in decreased glomerular filtration.** The body interprets this as a decrease in intravascular volume and begins to initiate compensatory mechanisms such as vasoconstriction and retention of fluid and sodium. **Neonates manifest this as weight gain and periorbital edema.**

Diaphoresis. Congestive heart failure leads to an increase in metabolic rate and increased activity of the autonomic nervous system, resulting in diaphoresis. This is representative of the increased workload of the heart in failure.

Hepatomegaly. The right ventricle in congestive heart failure is less compliant and does not adequately empty. This leads to elevated pressures in the right atrium, central venous system, and hepatic system. Hepatomegaly results from hepatic venous congestion.

Decreased Activity and Exercise Intolerance. **The decreased perfusion to peripheral tissues and the increased energy needed by the heart in failure leaves little energy for activities such as feeding and crying.** The infant in heart failure may sleep the majority of the time.

Failure to Thrive/Feeding Difficulties. Tachypnea compromises the infant's ability to feed. The basal metabolic rate increases in neonates with congestive heart failure. This necessitates a higher caloric intake (150 kcal or more).

Dysrhythmias. Abnormalities of the cardiac rhythm and murmurs are discussed individually later.

CARDIAC EXAMINATION

See "Specific Conditions" section.

LABORATORY DATA

Arterial Blood Gases. The $Paco_2$ in cardiac disease is often normal. It is usually increased if a primary pulmonary disease is present. Frequent monitoring of blood gases is unnecessary, but **the acid-base balance should be monitored closely.**

Four-Extremity Blood Pressure. **The measurement of blood pressure should be taken in both arms and both legs. A systolic pressure that is more than 10 mm Hg higher in the upper body compared with the lower body is abnormal** and suggests coarctation of the aorta, aortic arch hypoplasia, or interrupted aortic arch. However, this is a highly specific test with low sensitivity; the lack of systolic blood pressure gradient does not conclusively rule out aortic arch abnormalities.

Chest X-ray Examination. Frontal and lateral views (if possible) of the chest should be obtained. In neonates, the size of the heart may be difficult to determine because of the overlying thymus. Chest x-ray examination may be normal even in the presence of life-threatening CHD. However, the degree of pulmonary vascularity helps define the type of CHD present and is characterized as being increased, normal, or decreased. Likewise, the heart size should be evaluated and is described as being increased, normal, or decreased.

Electrocardiogram. Neonatal electrocardiogram (ECG) reflects the hemodynamic relationships that existed in utero. Many forms of CHD have minimal prenatal hemodynamic effects, and therefore the ECG is frequently "normal for age" despite significant structural defects (e.g., transposition of the great arteries, tetralogy of Fallot).

Echocardiogram. The echocardiogram is indispensable in the diagnosis of congenital heart disease.[4] Two-dimensional echocardiography, used to define cardiac anatomy, estimates pressures, measures gradients, and evaluates cardiac function[21] and, supplemented with Doppler and color Doppler, has become the primary diagnostic tool in pediatric cardiology. Noninvasive transthoracic echocardiogram is the most commonly used approach. **During the procedure, close monitoring is recommended with attention to vital signs, respiratory status, and temperature.** Recently, three-dimensional echocardiograms (3D Echos) that offer real-time three-dimensional imaging with 2 Dx-matrix probe and reconstructed 3D imaging using spatiotemporal image correlation (STIC) techniques[21] are being used.

Computed Tomography. More practitioners are finding 64-slice multidimensional computed tomography (64-MDCT) to be helpful in imaging some thoracic regions beyond the scope of echocardiograms, particularly after surgical revision. MDCT offers higher spatial resolution with shorter scan times.[31]

Magnetic Resonance Imaging. Magnetic resonance imaging (MRI) offers three-dimensional reconstruction and high-resolution images of the heart and great vessels. The MRI is of particular use in evaluating extracardiac vascular abnormalities, such as arch anomalies, vascular rings, and pulmonary arteriovenous anomalies. MRI provides high spatial resolution, excellent soft-tissue definition, a large field of view, and unrestricted demonstration of cardiovascular morphology; however, it does require sedation and a stable patient, and it is expensive.[13]

General Treatment Strategy

Optimal management of infants with heart disease requires specialized expertise. **Infants are monitored closely for hypoxia, hypoglycemia, acidosis, and congestive heart failure.**

The infant must be kept in an incubator or radiant heat warmer in which body temperature is maintained while color changes (pallor and increased cyanosis) may be observed. A cardiorespiratory monitor for continuous cardiac monitoring detects bradycardia, tachycardia, and dysrhythmias. Monitoring of oxygen saturations is helpful in determining adequacy of pulmonary blood flow and/or increased need for oxygen. **Respiratory effort is assessed** for tachypnea, shallow breathing, apnea, retractions, grunting, and nasal flaring. **Observe and document activity level such as feeding behavior, muscle tone, spontaneous movement, and seizure activity.**

MANAGEMENT OF CONGESTIVE HEART FAILURE

The medical management of congestive heart failure attempts to reverse the outlined process and helps the heart compensate with increased cardiac output.

Digoxin acts primarily as a positive inotropic (improves contractility) agent but decreases the heart rate and increases urine output (Box 24-3). Digoxin slows conduction at the atrioventricular (AV) node. This drug should be used with caution if acidosis, myocarditis, or obstructive lesions (e.g., tetralogy of Fallot, subvalvular pulmonary stenosis, asymmetric septal hypertrophy) are present. Diuretics such as furosemide (Table 24-4) help decrease total body water (which is increased as a result of congestive heart failure). In general, chronic fluid restriction and low-salt diets are not commonly used in newborns or infants with congestive heart failure.

Infants with congestive heart failure may be difficult to feed, and the process is often frustrating. They may have trouble sucking, swallowing, and breathing simultaneously. **They may have to rest frequently during a feeding, thus prolonging feeding times, and they may fall asleep exhausted before adequate caloric intake is achieved.** Because caloric requirements are higher in infants with CHD, the use of higher caloric formulas may be of benefit. Adequate nutrition must be ensured by the following:

- **Observing the infant's ability to nipple feed** (a soft, free-flowing [premature] nipple offers the least resistance to sucking and helps the infant conserve energy)
- **Providing adequate calories for growth** and, if necessary, **using alternative feeding methods** (i.e., gavage or continuous nasogastric drip) if the infant is sucking poorly

BOX 24-3 DIGOXIN DOSAGES AND COMMON SIDE EFFECTS

Digitalizing Schedule	
Preterm infant PO route: 20 mcg/kg total dose* Term infant PO route: 30 mcg/kg total dose*	Total dose is usually divided into three doses giving one half, then one fourth, then one fourth of the total dose q 8 hr. Check electrocardiogram rhythm strip for rate, PR interval, and dysrhythmias before each dose.
Maintenance Schedule	
Preterm infant PO route: 5-10 mcg/kg/day*	Total dose should be divided BID. Allow 12-24 hr between last digitalizing and first maintenance doses. It takes about 6 days to "digitalize" a patient with maintenance doses alone. The sign of digitalis effect is usually prolongation of the PR interval. The first sign of digitalis toxicity is usually vomiting, dysrhythmia, or bradycardia.
Term infant PO route: 5-10 mcg/kg/day	Drugs such as quinidine, amiodarone, and diuretics predispose to digoxin toxicity. The clearance of digoxin is directly related to renal function. Dosage must be reduced in patients with impaired renal function.

BID, Twice daily.
*Intravenous (IV) dose is 75% of oral (PO) dose.

TABLE 24-4 CARDIAC DRUGS

DRUG	ROUTE	DOSE	ONSET OF ACTION	COMMENTS
Atropine	IV	0.01-0.03 mg/kg/dose PRN (max 0.4 mg)	Seconds	May cause tachycardia, urinary retention, or hyperthermia
	PO	0.01-0.03 mg/kg/dose q 4-6 hr (max 0.4 mg)	Minutes	May cause tachycardia
	ETT	Give 2-3 times the IV dose followed by NS flush	Minutes	May cause tachycardia
Calcium chloride (10% solution)	IV	0.2-0.3 mL (20-30 mg)/kg/ dose q 10 min PRN (max 500 mg)	Minutes	Slow infusion; must be IV; potentiates digoxin, bradycardia
Calcium gluconate (10% solution)	IV	1-2 mL/kg/dose (100-200 mg/kg/ dose) q 10 min PRN (max 500 mg)	Minutes	Slow infusion (over 10-30 min); must be IV; potentiates digoxin, bradycardia/dysrhythmias
Captopril (Capoten)	PO	Younger than 2 months: Initial dose: 0.1-0.25 mg/kg/dose q 8-24 hr Titrate: up to 0.5 mg/kg/dose Older than 2 months: Initial dose: 0.3 mg/kg/day Titrate: up to 6 mg/kg/day in 1-4 divided doses	15 min +	Hypotension, tachycardia, increased BUN and serum creatinine, hypercalcemia

Data from Miller-Hoover SR: Pediatric and neonatal cardiovascular pharmacology, *Pediatr Nurs* 29(2):105, 2003.
Standard Concentrations: Each institution's concentration may vary; NOT to exceed maximum concentration per pharmacy reference manuals.
Neonatal Drug Guidelines Updated May 7, 2002.
BID, Twice daily; *BP,* blood pressure; *BUN,* blood urea nitrogen; *CNS,* central nervous system; *ETT,* endotracheal tube; *GI,* gastrointestinal; *IHSS,* idiopathic hypertrophic subaortic stenosis; *IV,* intravenous; *IM,* intramuscular; *KCl,* potassium chloride; *kg,* kilograms; *Maint.,* maintenance; *max,* maximum; *mcg,* micrograms; *mg,* milligrams; *min,* minutes; *NEC,* necrotizing enterocolitis; *NS,* normal saline; *PO,* per os; *PRN,* as needed; *q,* every; *QID,* four times a day; *TID,* three times a day.

Continued

TABLE 24-4 **CARDIAC DRUGS—cont'd**

DRUG	ROUTE	DOSE	ONSET OF ACTION	COMMENTS
Diazoxide (Hyperstat)	IV	5 mg/kg/dose q 30 min PRN	1-2 min	May cause hypotension or hypoglycemia
Dobutamine (Dobutrex)	IV	2-10 mcg/kg/min	Minutes	Do not use if IHSS or tetralogy of Fallot, may cause ventricular ectopy, tachycardia, or hypertension Incompatible with alkaline solutions
Dopamine (Intropin)	IV	5-10 mcg/kg/min	Minutes	Tachydysrhythmia, vasoconstriction, gangrene of extremities, anginal pain, and palpitations can occur; inactivated in alkaline solution
Epinephrine (1:10,000)	IV/ETT	0.1-0.3 mL/kg/dose (max 5 mL/dose) q 3-5 min PRN	Seconds	May cause tachycardia, dysrhythmias, or hypertension; not effective if acidosis is present
Esmolol (Brevibloc)	IV	*Loading dose:* 500 mcg/kg/min *Continuous infusion:* titrate 50-200 mcg/kg/min	Minutes	May cause bradycardia, hypotension, bronchoconstriction
Furosemide (Lasix)	IV PO	1-2 mg/kg/dose 1-4 mg/kg/dose	5-15 min 30-60 min	May cause metabolic alkalosis and hypokalemia; monitor electrolytes—may need KCl supplementation; renal calcification
Hydralazine (Apresoline)	IV PO	0.1-0.5 mg/kg q 3-6 hr 0.1-0.5 mg/kg q 6 hr; may increase to max of 2 mg/kg/dose q 6 hr	15-30 min Often days until titrated effect achieved	May cause lupus-like syndrome, tachycardia, or hypotension
Hydrochloro-thiazide (HydroDIURIL)	PO	1-2 mg/kg q 12 hr	1-2 hr	May cause electrolyte imbalance, may need KCl supplementation
Ibuprofen lysine (NeoProfen)	IV	10 mg/kg first dose; then 5 mg/kg second and third dose (q 24 hr)		Most effective in first 3 days of life Monitor urine output and creatinine levels; discontinue drug if dramatic decrease in urine output Significantly fewer adverse effects (compared with indomethacin) on renal and mesenteric blood flow; less oliguria and increase in serum creatinine levels
Indomethacin (Indocin)	IV	0.1-0.2 mg/kg/dose; may be repeated q 8 hr for a total of 3 doses		Less effective if administered after 7 days of age; probably will have no effect after 14 days Monitor urine output and creatinine levels; discontinue drug if dramatic decrease in urine output Contraindications: severe renal impairment, active bleeding in the CNS or GI tract, and NEC[10]
Isoproterenol (Isuprel)	IV	0.1-0.4 mcg/kg/min	30-60 seconds	May cause tachycardia/ventricular tachydysrhythmia; may also cause subendocardial ischemia
Lidocaine (Xylocaine)	IV	*IV bolus:* 1-3 mg/kg *IV drip:* 30-50 mcg/kg/min		May cause dysrhythmia, CNS agitation or depression
Milrinone (Primacor)	IV	*Loading:* 50 mcg/kg over 15 min *Maint.:* 0.25-0.75 mcg/kg/min		May cause ventricular dysrhythmias, ventricular fibrillation, or hypotension

TABLE 24-4 CARDIAC DRUGS—cont'd

DRUG	ROUTE	DOSE	ONSET OF ACTION	COMMENTS
Nitroprusside (Nipride)	IV	1-10 mcg/kg/min over 10 min to control BP; *chronic infusion:* 2 mcg/kg/min (protect from light; change solution q 4 hr)	Seconds	May cause hypotension and reflex tachycardia; may cause thiocyanate toxicity, especially if decreased renal function is present
Phentolamine (Regitine)	IV PO	1-20 mcg/kg/min 5 mg/kg/day QID	5-10 min	May cause hypotension; commonly used with an inotropic agent
Phenytoin (Dilantin)	IV	*Load:* 10-15 mg/kg over 5 min (slow infusion) *Maint.:* 3-5 mg/kg/day BID	5-10 min	May cause cardiac depression
	PO	3-5 mg/kg/day BID	2-4 hr	Therapeutic blood levels (5-20 mcg/mL)
Procainamide (Pronestyl)	IV	*Load:* 10-15 mg/kg/dose over 5 min (max 100 mg) *Maint.:* IV 30-80 mcg/kg/min	1-5 min	May cause hypotension or lupus-like syndrome
	IM	5-8 mg/kg q 6 hr	15-30 min	Same as for IV
Propranolol (Inderal)	IV	*Dysrhythmias:* 0.01-0.15 mg/kg/dose slow IV q 6-8 hr PRN (max single dose, 10 mg) *Hypercyanotic spell:* 0.15-0.25 mg/kg/dose slow IV push q 15 min (max dose 10 mg)	2-5 min	May severely decrease cardiac output
	PO	*Dysrhythmias:* 0.5-1 mg/kg/dose TID-QID (max daily dose 60 mg) *Hypercyanotic spell:* 1-2 mg/kg/dose QID	30-60 min	Same as for IV
Prostaglandin E_1 (Prostin VR)	IV	*Initial dose:* 0.05-0.1 mcg/kg/min cont. IV infusion *Maint.:* 0.01-0.05 mcg/kg/min cont. IV infusion	30 min	May cause apnea, fever, or hypotension
Spironolactone (Aldactone)	PO	1-2 mg/kg/day	3-5 days	Hyperkalemia, drowsiness, GI upset
Tolazoline	IV	*Test:* 1-2 mg/kg slow IV push *Maint.:* 1-2 mg/kg/hr	Minutes	May cause hypotension, GI or pulmonary hemorrhage
Adenosine	IV	30-250 mcg/kg		Slows the spontaneous heart rate and prolongs the PR interval; may cause transient complete heart block and hypotension; half-life is only 9.3 seconds so its effects quickly dissipate

Data from Miller-Hoover SR: Pediatric and neonatal cardiovascular pharmacology, *Pediatr Nurs* 29(2):105, 2003.
Standard Concentrations: Each institution's concentration may vary; NOT to exceed maximum concentration per pharmacy reference manuals.
Neonatal Drug Guidelines Updated May 7, 2002.
BID, Twice daily; *BP,* blood pressure; *BUN,* blood urea nitrogen; *CNS,* central nervous system; *ETT,* endotracheal tube; *GI,* gastrointestinal; *IHSS,* idiopathic hypertrophic subaortic stenosis; *IV,* intravenous; *IM,* intramuscular; *KCl,* potassium chloride; *kg,* kilograms; *Maint.,* maintenance; *max,* maximum; *mcg,* micrograms; *mg,* milligrams; *min,* minutes; *NEC,* necrotizing enterocolitis; *NS,* normal saline; *PO,* per os; *PRN,* as needed; *q,* every; *QID,* four times a day; *TID,* three times a day.

- **Anticipating the infant's hunger and offering feedings before the infant uses energy by crying**
- Positioning the infant in a semi-erect position for feeding
- Burping the infant after every half ounce consumed to help minimize vomiting
- **Weighing the infant daily** and checking for appropriate weight gain

Before discharge from the nursery, the infant should be in stable condition (e.g., feeding well and gaining weight appropriately).

An important fact for families to understand is that many infants gain weight very slowly because of their cardiac defects, regardless of the method of feeding used. The family of an infant in congestive heart failure needs support and teaching. **Explanation of the term *congestive heart failure* should be given early, because it is a frightening term for parents.** The term "heart failure" is often interpreted as "heart attack" or "cardiac arrest." Parents must understand that saying an infant is in heart failure does not imply that the infant's heart will stop beating. **A simple explanation describing heart failure as a condition in which the heart shows signs of being less able to pump sufficient blood to meet all the needs of the body helps decrease anxiety for the family.**

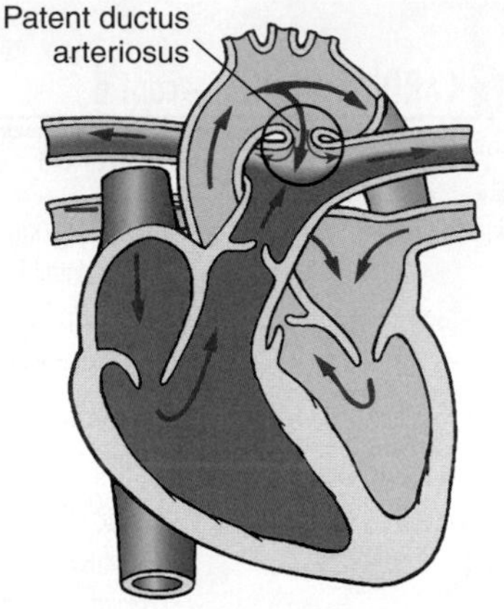

FIGURE 24-3 Patent ductus arteriosus. (Modified from Hockenberry MJ, Wilson D: *Wong's essentials of pediatric nursing,* ed 8, St Louis, 2009, Mosby.)

SPECIFIC CONDITIONS

Patent Ductus Arteriosus

PHYSIOLOGY

The ductus arteriosus is a normal pathway in the fetal circulatory system and allows blood from the right ventricle and pulmonary arterial system to flow into the descending aorta for ultimate delivery to the placenta (Figure 24-3). Functionally, the patent ductus arteriosus (PDA) closes within a few hours to several days after birth, but this closure is often delayed in premature infants. After birth, as a result of a decrease in the pressure of the pulmonary circulation and an increase in the pressure of the aorta, the blood flow through a PDA is predominantly from the aorta to the pulmonary artery (left-to-right shunt). The hemodynamic changes and the resultant clinical manifestations of a PDA depend on the magnitude of the pulmonary vascular resistance and the size of the ductal lumen.

Approximately 15% of infants with PDAs have additional cardiac defects (e.g., VSD, coarctation of the aorta, aortic stenosis, pulmonary stenosis). PDA can be associated with known syndromes, most commonly rubella.

DATA COLLECTION

History. Asphyxial insult or respiratory distress syndrome (RDS), inability to wean from a ventilator, and an increasing FIO_2 demand usually accompany PDA.

Physical Findings. Increased flow to the pulmonary circulation and volume overload of the left ventricle are the two major physiologic abnormalities in a PDA.

Cyanosis. Generally, cyanosis is not present in an isolated PDA, because the predominant shunt is from left to right.

Heart Sounds. Infants with a PDA may have an audible murmur as a result of the left-to-right shunting through the ductus during systole. **A grade I through III systolic murmur is best heard at the upper left sternal border with radiation to the left axilla and faintly to the back.** Although this murmur occasionally may spill into diastole, the classical continuous machinery-like murmur is an unusual occurrence in the newborn period. It is often helpful to briefly disconnect the newborn from the ventilator before auscultating. **There are cases of large PDAs in which no murmur is audible.**

Pulses. Because of the rapid upstroke and wide pulse pressure, the **peripheral pulses are bounding.** Pulses are hyperdynamic and easily palpated. **Assessment of the pulses should include palpation of palmar, plantar, and popliteal pulses.** The presence of an easily palpated pulse in these areas suggests the presence of an aortic run-off lesion, which is most commonly a PDA.

Congestive Heart Failure. Because of the volume overload of the left ventricle, the infant may show signs of congestive heart failure and pulmonary edema (see "Congestive Heart Failure" section).

Laboratory Data

Arterial Blood Gases. Arterial blood gas values are normal.

Chest X-ray Examination. Chest x-ray examination is normal in small shunts. Cardiomegaly is present with increased pulmonary vascularity in large shunts.

Electrocardiogram. The ECG may be normal, demonstrate left ventricular hypertrophy, or demonstrate combined ventricular hypertrophy.

Echocardiogram. Direct imaging is the preferred method both to diagnose patency and to determine the significance of the ductus arteriosus. An increased left atrial/aortic ratio suggests a moderate to large left-to-right shunt (i.e., PDA, VSD). **An echocardiogram should be performed before medical or surgical closure of the PDA to rule out a ductal-dependent lesion or other associated anomalies.** Color-flow Doppler mapping allows visualization of the PDA and aids in determining the size and direction of the shunt across the PDA (i.e., left to right, right to left, bidirectional).

Cardiac Catheterization. If the echocardiogram has eliminated a ductal-dependent lesion, cardiac catheterization is usually not necessary before treatment.

TREATMENT

Medical Management. Asymptomatic infants with PDAs generally do not require medical management or surgical ligation. These infants should be monitored for evidence of congestive heart failure, failure to thrive, increasing oxygen requirement, or other complications.

Symptomatic infants require ductal closure by either pharmacologic management with prostaglandin inhibitors such as indomethacin or ibuprofen lysine therapy (both are Food and Drug Administration [FDA]–approved cyclo-oxygenase [COX] inhibitors) or surgical ductal ligation. Medical management such as fluid restriction, watchful waiting, and ventilator support is rarely successful, especially in low-birth-weight infants. The current trend is to **treat early presymptomatic therapeutic PDA at 2 to 3 days of age after a confirmed echocardiogram.**[30] Although indomethacin was first reported in the 1970s and became first-line therapy for the treatment of PDA, ibuprofen lysine has been shown to be equally effective in closure rates and may be preferable because of its better toxicity profile.[25] Table 24-4 has indomethacin and ibuprofen lysine doses, contraindications, and side effects. **Urine output, as well as creatinine levels, should be continuously monitored with both medications. If urine output decreases dramatically, the drug should be discontinued.** Ibuprofen appears to have significantly fewer adverse effects on renal and mesenteric blood flow, as well as fewer issues with increased serum creatinine and oliguria.[34]

Surgical Treatment. Although surgical ligation of the ductus arteriosus through a lateral thoracotomy incision is a low-risk procedure when performed by an experienced surgical team, this should be reserved for those preterm infants who cannot tolerate or have failed pharmacologic intervention or when it is contraindicated. Questions have been raised about the long-term effects of surgical PDA closure in extremely-low-birth-weight infants and the relationship between ligation and bronchopulmonary dysplasia (BPD), severe retinopathy of prematurity (ROP), and neurosensory impairment.[14]

COMPLICATIONS AND RESIDUAL EFFECTS

Complications and residual effects, although rare, include recanalization, recurrent laryngeal or phrenic nerve palsies, and false aneurysms. The surgical mortality rate in the neonatal period is generally less than 1%.

PROGNOSIS AND FOLLOW-UP

Asymptomatic infants have an excellent prognosis, although close follow-up is necessary because if the ductus remains patent beyond infancy, repair is usually recommended. Symptomatic infants with PDA generally experience failure to thrive, continued congestive heart failure, increased oxygen requirements with resultant BPD, or pulmonary infections.

Ventricular Septal Defect

PHYSIOLOGY

VSD is the most common cause of congestive heart failure after the initial neonatal period. VSDs may involve various portions of the ventricular septum and are classified according to the anatomic position that they occupy when viewed from the right ventricle (Figure 24-4). Defects in the membranous septum are the most common type and have been found to close spontaneously 20% of the time.[12] In contrast, 65% of muscular VSDs close spontaneously.[12]

A VSD may occur as an isolated anomaly or may be part of a more complex cardiac lesion. Only isolated VSDs are discussed in this section. The effect of the VSD on the circulation depends on both the size of the VSD and the relative PVR. PVR is nearly systemic immediately after birth but rapidly falls to one-fourth to one-third systemic in the first several days of life.

In a small VSD, the left-to-right shunting at the ventricular level is minimal and the infants are asymptomatic.

Larger VSDs may have a moderate to large left-to-right shunt, resulting in congestive heart failure and pulmonary edema. Premature infants tend to have lower pulmonary vascular resistance at birth, allowing greater left-to-right shunting and therefore may be symptomatic. Infants with severe lung disease (e.g., RDS, BPD, pneumonia) may have elevated PVR and therefore minimal left-to-right shunting.

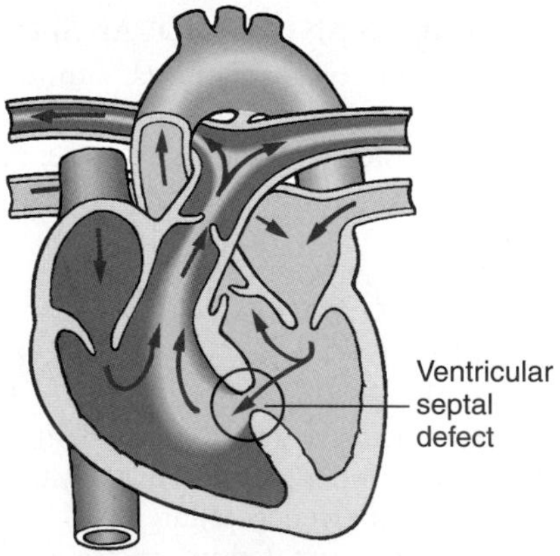

FIGURE 24-4 Ventricular septal defect. (Modified from Hockenberry MJ, Wilson D: *Wong's essentials of pediatric nursing*, ed 8, St Louis, 2009, Mosby.)

DATA COLLECTION

See Table 24-1 for infants at increased risk.

Physical Findings

Cyanosis. Infants with isolated VSDs are rarely cyanotic in the neonatal period.

Heart Sounds. Most infants with VSDs have a heart murmur. **The time when this murmur is first audible depends on the PVR and the size of the defect.** The murmur is typically a grade II to III/VI systolic murmur heard best at the lower left sternal border. A diastolic flow rumble at the apex indicates a large left-to-right shunt.

Congestive Heart Failure. Congestive heart failure is unusual in the newborn with an isolated VSD. When it occurs, however, it is a result of the volume overload of the left ventricle (see "Congestive Heart Failure" section).

Laboratory Data

Arterial Blood Gases. Arterial blood gas values are normal.

Chest X-ray Examination. A chest x-ray examination shows a normal to increased heart size with an increased pulmonary blood flow.

Electrocardiogram. The ECG in an infant with a VSD is usually normal but may demonstrate left or biventricular hypertrophy.

Echocardiogram. A two-dimensional echocardiogram can demonstrate the VSD in 90% of the cases. Doppler interrogation of the ventricular septum and color-flow mapping have greatly increased the accuracy of diagnosing even the smallest VSDs noninvasively. The use of color-flow studies is particularly advantageous in identifying the presence of multiple VSDs and the direction of blood flow across a VSD.

Cardiac Catheterization. A cardiac catheterization is diagnostic but not necessary in the neonatal period unless there is some question about the diagnosis or if surgery is being considered.

TREATMENT

Medical Management. Medical management of congestive heart failure associated with VSDs includes digoxin, diuretics, and caloric supplementation. Failure to thrive is an indication for surgical repair of the defect.

Surgical Treatment. Surgical treatment of a VSD consists of either suture closure or patching (using most commonly a synthetic material such as Dacron).

The surgical approach is through a median sternotomy incision. The defect is approached through the right atrium and tricuspid valve, thereby avoiding a right ventriculotomy.

If the infant is small (<2 kg) or if multiple muscular VSDs are present, it may be necessary to perform a palliative procedure called *pulmonary artery banding* to decrease pulmonary blood flow until the infant is older and can undergo debanding and closure of the VSDs. With improvements in surgical technique and technology, VSD closure can be performed safely and effectively in the younger pediatric population.[17]

COMPLICATIONS AND RESIDUAL EFFECTS

Complications or residual effects may include (1) a persistent shunt (residual VSD), (2) conduction abnormalities (right bundle-branch block and third-degree heart block), and (3) aortic or tricuspid insufficiency (<1%).

The mortality rate in infants is less than 5%, with higher mortality found in the neonatal period. Contraindications to primary VSD closure include the diagnosis of double-outlet right ventricle and multiple muscular VSDs. The combined risk of pulmonary banding plus later debanding and VSD closure is about 10%.

PROGNOSIS AND FOLLOW-UP

Depending on the anatomic type, approximately 50% of small VSDs may close spontaneously in the first months of life. If a large left-to-right shunt is persistent after 12 to 24 months of age, the infant is susceptible to the development of pulmonary vascular disease.

Coarctation of the Aorta

PHYSIOLOGY

Coarctation of the aorta is a localized constriction of the aorta that usually occurs at the junction of the transverse aortic arch and the descending aorta in the vicinity of the ductus arteriosus (Figure 24-5). However, coarctation can occur anywhere in the aorta from above the aortic valve to the abdominal aorta. The precise location of the coarctation and the presence or absence of associated anomalies affect the clinical presentation. Associated anomalies include PDA, VSD, and bicuspid aortic valve (50%). Coarctation is observed in approximately 10% of infants with Turner syndrome.

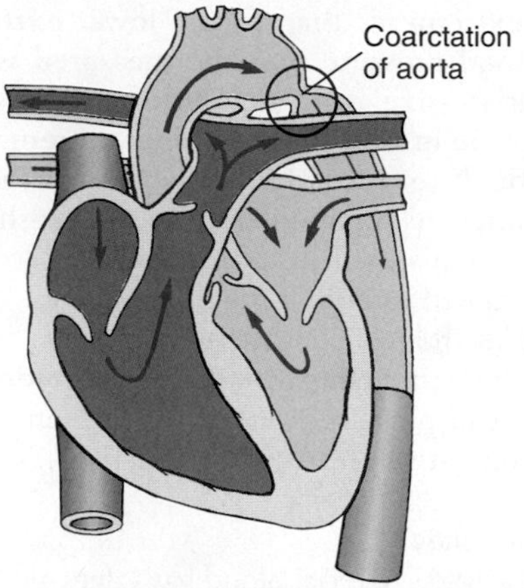

FIGURE 24-5 Coarctation of the aorta. (Modified from Hockenberry MJ, Wilson D: *Wong's essentials of pediatric nursing,* ed 8, St Louis, 2009, Mosby.)

DATA COLLECTION

Physical Findings. In utero, the majority of systemic blood flow to the lower body is via the ductus arteriosus. After ductal closure, the neonate with coarctation becomes critically ill because the left ventricle must suddenly generate adequate pressure to pump the entire cardiac output past a significant point of obstruction. **Newborns with critical coarctation of the aorta will then have signs and symptoms of congestive heart failure and low cardiac output. Severe coarctation of the aorta is a medical and surgical emergency.**

Cyanosis. Generally, cyanosis is not present in the newborn with isolated coarctation of the aorta.

Heart Sounds. A cardiac murmur generally is not found in an isolated, severe coarctation of the aorta. If other cardiac defects are present, however, a murmur may be heard. A soft grade I to II/VI systolic murmur may be present at the left sternal border, radiating to the left axilla and to the back. **A murmur heard only in the back is strongly suggestive of coarctation.** A gallop rhythm sometimes is present and is associated with congestive heart failure. The murmurs of associated anomalies, however, usually are dominant.

Pulses and Blood Pressure. The blood pressure proximal to the area of obstruction is higher than the blood pressure distal to the area of obstruction.

The most consistent physical finding in infants with critical coarctation of the aorta is a higher systolic blood pressure (>15 mm Hg) in the

upper extremities than in the lower extremities. This blood pressure must be measured with the appropriate-size cuff. In addition, pulses are easily palpable in one or both upper extremities but are difficult to palpate or are absent in the lower extremities. As mentioned earlier, pulses should be carefully evaluated in all extremities and blood pressures obtained in both arms and both legs.

Congestive Heart Failure. Congestive heart failure is a common finding in infants with severe coarctation and is the result of pressure overload on the left ventricle (see "Congestive Heart Failure" section).

Laboratory Data

Arterial Blood Gases. Arterial blood gas values are normal.

Chest X-ray Examination. Cardiomegaly may be seen on the x-ray film. Pulmonary vascularity is normal unless associated anomalies are present.

Electrocardiogram. Right ventricular hypertrophy is frequently present. Left ventricular hypertrophy or combined ventricular hypertrophy is rarely seen in the newborn period. The ECG may be normal.

Echocardiogram. The area of coarctation can often be visualized using two-dimensional techniques and color-flow mapping. However, cautious interpretation of the findings is suggested if a PDA is present.

Cardiac Catheterization. Cardiac catheterization can be diagnostic when performed before a surgical procedure to evaluate for other associated anomalies; however, it is rarely necessary.

TREATMENT

Medical Management. Congestive heart failure should be treated immediately and aggressively for stabilization before surgery. **Intractable congestive heart failure, acidosis, oliguria, and hypertension are indications for corrective surgery as soon as possible.** (See "General Treatment Strategy" discussion in "Congenital Heart Disease" section.) **Medical management consists of continuous intravenous infusion of prostaglandin E_1 (PGE_1) to keep the ductus arteriosus open, dopamine and/or dobutamine for inotropic support, and correction of metabolic acidosis, hypoglycemia, and anemia.** Since the introduction of PGE_1, emergency surgical repair is rarely necessary. Balloon angioplasty is rarely performed as a palliative emergency procedure.

Surgical Treatment. The two most common surgical procedures are resection of the coarctation with end-to-end anastomosis and the subclavian flap aortoplasty. With the former, the coarcted segment is resected and the ends of the aorta reanastomosed. With the latter, a longitudinal incision is made in the aorta across the coarctated site and continued to the end of the distally divided left subclavian artery. The left subclavian artery is used as a patch or flap to increase the diameter of the aorta. Both procedures are performed through a lateral thoracotomy incision and have been highly successful in relieving coarctation and providing for future growth of the aorta. Absorbable suture material often is used with the intention of decreasing the incidence of recoarctation from rigid suture lines.

COMPLICATIONS AND RESIDUAL EFFECTS

Complications and residual effects include (1) diminished or absent pulses in the left arm, (2) persistent hypertension, (3) Horner syndrome, (4) paraplegia (<0.5%), (5) mesenteric vasculitis, and (6) residual coarctation.

The overall operative mortality rate is as high as 20% in infancy. The high mortality rate is usually related to preoperative status and the presence of associated lesions.

PROGNOSIS AND FOLLOW-UP

Infants with mild coarctation require minimal care initially. If these patients are medically managed, close follow-up is mandatory, with repair likely at a later date.

Infants with severe coarctation require prompt medical and surgical treatment. If this therapy is instituted early, the prognosis generally is favorable. Untreated infants with severe coarctation often have a rapidly deteriorating clinical course with left intractable congestive heart failure, and the prognosis is guarded. After surgical repair, frequent follow-up is necessary to ensure adequate coarctation repair. Cardiac catheterization may be necessary several months to years after the surgical procedure is completed if recoarctation is suspected (20%). Balloon angioplasty can be performed if significant residual obstruction is found.

Critical Aortic Stenosis

PHYSIOLOGY

Obstruction of the left ventricular outlet may occur below the aortic valve, at the aortic valve, or above the aortic valve (subvalvular, valvular, or supravalvular aortic stenosis) (Figure 24-6). Valvular aortic

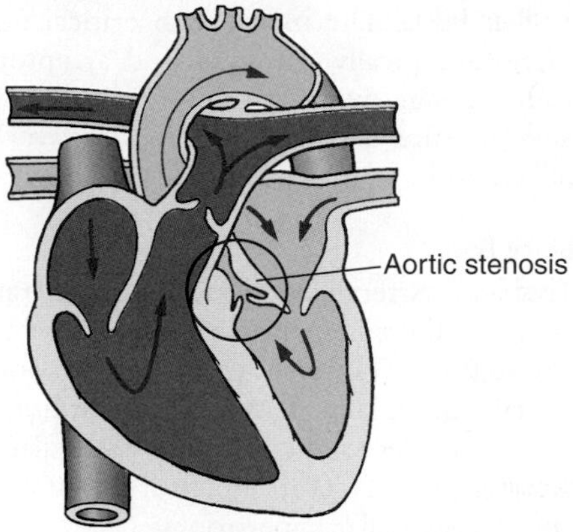

FIGURE 24-6 Aortic stenosis. (Modified from Hockenberry MJ, Wilson D: *Wong's essentials of pediatric nursing*, ed 8, St Louis, 2009, Mosby.)

stenosis is the most common type and is discussed here. A pressure gradient (the pressure difference from the left ventricle to the ascending aorta) of at least 60 mm Hg or more is indicative of significant aortic stenosis in the newborn.

DATA COLLECTION

Physical Findings. Although most infants with aortic stenosis are asymptomatic in the neonatal period, **a neonate with critical or severe aortic stenosis needs emergent treatment.** The infant with critical aortic stenosis has pale gray, cool skin with decreased perfusion and peripheral pulses.

Cyanosis. Cyanosis is generally not present in isolated valvular aortic stenosis.

Heart Sounds. A grade II to IV/VI harsh systolic murmur is typically heard in the upper right sternal border, radiating to the upper left sternal border and faintly to the neck. The intensity of the murmur is unrelated to the severity of the obstruction. An ejection click may be heard at the apex. A suprasternal notch thrill is sometimes palpable.

Congestive Heart Failure. Infants with critical aortic stenosis have congestive heart failure caused by a pressure overload of the left ventricle (see "Congestive Heart Failure" section).

Laboratory Data

Arterial Blood Gases. Arterial blood gas values are generally normal.

Chest X-ray Examination. A chest x-ray examination shows cardiomegaly with normal pulmonary vascularity.

Electrocardiogram. The ECG may be normal or demonstrate left ventricular hypertrophy. There is poor correlation between an electrocardiographic abnormality and the degree of aortic stenosis present.

Echocardiogram. The aortic valve is usually thickened and appears to close abnormally on an echocardiogram. Doppler interrogation can accurately estimate the systolic pressure gradient from the left ventricle to the ascending aorta and identify the level or levels of obstruction.

Cardiac Catheterization. Cardiac catheterization is diagnostic and may or may not be performed in cases of critical aortic stenosis. Some centers are performing balloon dilation of the aortic valve during the cardiac catheterization.

TREATMENT

Medical Management. Initial medical management includes treatment of low output state. **Positive end-expiratory pressure (PEEP) is helpful to overcome pulmonary venous desaturation from pulmonary edema. Inspired oxygen should be limited to FIO_2 of 0.5 to 0.6 unless severe hypoxemia is present.** Surgical intervention is necessary for critical aortic stenosis in the newborn (see "General Treatment Strategy" section). However, balloon dilatation of aortic valve stenosis in the cardiac catheterization laboratory has been a successful alternative to surgical intervention in selected newborns.

Surgical Treatment. Aortic valvotomy through a median sternotomy incision is the surgical procedure for correcting critical aortic stenosis in infants. This procedure can usually be accomplished in the newborn with inflow occlusion and circulatory arrest for 1 to 2 minutes. In older infants, cardiopulmonary bypass should be performed. The fused commissures of the valve are incised, permitting the leaflets to open freely during systole.

COMPLICATIONS AND RESIDUAL EFFECTS

Complications and residual effects include aortic insufficiency and residual aortic stenosis. The mortality rate in infancy ranges from 5% to 50%, with the highest risk involving the newborn with critical obstruction.

PROGNOSIS AND FOLLOW-UP

All patients with critical aortic stenosis will require lifelong follow-up. Further surgical or catheter intervention is frequently necessary.

Critical Pulmonary Stenosis with Intact Ventricular Septum

PHYSIOLOGY

In critical pulmonary stenosis with intact ventricular septum, the flow to the pulmonary artery from the right ventricle is obstructed. The obstruction may occur below the valve in the infundibular area, above the valve, or at the valve (subvalvular, valvular, or supravalvular). In valvular stenosis, the orifice of the pulmonary valve is markedly narrowed and the valvular tissue may assume the shape of a cone (Figure 24-7). The pulmonary artery distal to this area of stenosis may be dilated. Because the ventricular septum is intact, the right ventricle is subjected to a marked increase in pressure and becomes hypertrophied. A pressure gradient from the right ventricle to the pulmonary artery of 50 mm Hg or more is indicative of significant pulmonary stenosis in the newborn.

DATA COLLECTION

Physical Findings

Cyanosis. Cyanosis is generally not present in an isolated lesion but may occur in the presence of a right-to-left atrial shunt.

Heart Sounds. A harsh grade II to III/VI systolic murmur is heard in the upper left sternal border, radiating to both axillae and faintly to the back. Diastole is quiet. A murmur of tricuspid insufficiency (grade I/VI, soft, systolic murmur at the lower left sternal border) may be heard. An ejection click also may be heard at the left sternal border.

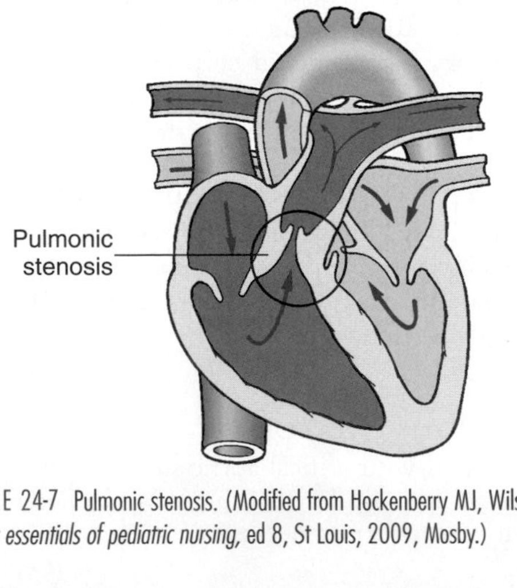

FIGURE 24-7 Pulmonic stenosis. (Modified from Hockenberry MJ, Wilson D: *Wong's essentials of pediatric nursing*, ed 8, St Louis, 2009, Mosby.)

Congestive Heart Failure. The infant with critical pulmonary stenosis typically has signs and symptoms of right-sided congestive heart failure resulting from excessive pressure overload (see "Congestive Heart Failure" section).

Laboratory Data

Arterial Blood Gases. Arterial blood gas values generally are normal unless there is an atrial right-to-left shunt.

Chest X-ray Examination. The chest x-ray examination may be normal but usually demonstrates cardiomegaly with normal or decreased pulmonary vascularity.

Electrocardiogram. The ECG may be normal or demonstrate right ventricular hypertrophy.

Echocardiogram. An abnormal pulmonary valve pattern on a two-dimensional echocardiogram is diagnostic. Doppler interrogation and color-flow mapping can accurately estimate the systolic pressure gradient from the right ventricle to the pulmonary artery and identify the level or levels of obstruction.

Cardiac Catheterization. Infants suspected of having critical pulmonary stenosis with an intact ventricular septum usually undergo cardiac catheterization as soon as possible. Catheter balloon valvotomy has become the treatment of choice for this defect. Successful balloon valvotomy is associated with excellent clinical results, and the need for repeat surgical procedures is quite low.

TREATMENT

Medical Management. PGE_1 has been used successfully to maintain the patency of the ductus arteriosus, thereby allowing adequate pulmonary blood flow until surgery or balloon dilation is performed. If balloon dilation has been successful, surgical intervention may be postponed or may not be necessary at all.

Surgical Treatment. The degree of pulmonary stenosis and the size of the pulmonary arteries determine surgical approach. If the right ventricle and pulmonary arteries are of adequate size, then pulmonary valvulotomy through a median sternotomy incision is the preferable procedure. This involves incising the pulmonary valve commissures, allowing the leaflets to open freely during systole. Like aortic valvulotomy, this procedure can often be performed under inflow occlusion.

COMPLICATIONS AND RESIDUAL EFFECTS

Complications and residual effects include pulmonary insufficiency and residual pulmonary stenosis.

The mortality rate for pulmonary valvulotomy is 17% in newborns.

If the right ventricle and pulmonary arteries are too small to allow antegrade flow, then a palliative procedure such as the Blalock-Taussig operation is performed. This procedure consists of bringing down the subclavian artery opposite the aortic arch and anastomosing it to the ipsilateral pulmonary artery or placing a Gore-Tex or Dacron tube graft (conduit) between the subclavian artery and the pulmonary artery.

Complications and residual side effects of Blalock-Taussig shunts include (1) diminished or absent pulses in the affected arm, (2) congestive heart failure from an overlarge shunt, and (3) inadequacy of the shunt. The mortality in this group is higher than in infants with adequate-size right ventricles and pulmonary arteries.

PROGNOSIS AND FOLLOW-UP

If a palliative shunt has been used, follow-up catheterization and surgical procedures should be anticipated either when the shunt becomes nonfunctional or when total repair is expected. If the lesion has been primarily corrected surgically in the neonatal period, repeated catheterization may be performed several months later to evaluate the residual obstruction if it is suspected. However, evaluation by echocardiogram may be sufficient without catheterization.

Atrioventricular Septal Defect, Endocardial Cushion Defect (Atrioventricular Canal)

PHYSIOLOGY

Nearly 70% of infants with complete atrioventricular canal have trisomy 21 (Down syndrome). The complete type of AV septal cushion defect is characterized by a large central hole in the endocardial cushion of the heart with free communication among all four chambers. The anterior leaflet of the mitral valve and the septal leaflet of the tricuspid valve both have clefts and are continuous with each other through the defect. Thus the AV valves are represented by a valve common to both sides of the heart (Figure 24-8).

These infants usually have a left-to-right shunt at both the atrial and ventricular levels. AV valve insufficiency also may be present. The symptomatology depends on the degree of shunting at the atrial and ventricular levels and the amount of AV valve insufficiency present.

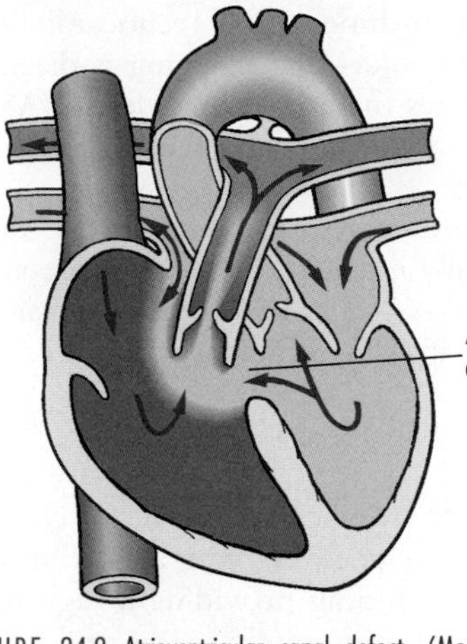

FIGURE 24-8 Atrioventricular canal defect. (Modified from Hockenberry MJ, Wilson D: *Wong's essentials of pediatric nursing,* ed 8, St Louis, 2009, Mosby.)

DATA COLLECTION

Physical Findings

Cyanosis. There may be some degree of cyanosis, particularly in the immediate neonatal period before the pulmonary vascular resistance has fallen.

Heart Sounds. Often there is **no murmur audible.** If AV valve insufficiency is present, a blowing, systolic, apical murmur with radiation to the left axilla or a VSD murmur is heard.

Congestive Heart Failure. Because of the large left-to-right shunt, which increases as pulmonary vascular resistance falls, these neonates typically present early in life with congestive heart failure. Congestive heart failure may be present because of volume overload of the ventricles as a result of AV valve insufficiency (see "Congestive Heart Failure" section).

Laboratory Data

Arterial Blood Gases. The $Paco_2$ may be elevated if there is severe AV valve insufficiency and pulmonary edema. The pH is usually normal. The Pao_2 usually is normal also.

Chest X-ray Examination. The heart size may be normal or increased. The pulmonary vascularity is generally increased.

Electrocardiogram. An ECG with a left axis deviation, counterclockwise loop in the frontal plane, and superior axis suggests AV septal defect.

Echocardiogram. A two-dimensional echocardiogram with Doppler and color-flow mapping is diagnostic and demonstrates the atrial septal defect (ASD), VSD, and common AV valve and the degree of AV valve insufficiency.

Cardiac Catheterization. Cardiac catheterization is diagnostic but generally not performed in the neonatal period in a typical AV septal defect. An echocardiographic diagnosis may be sufficient without cardiac catheterization.

TREATMENT

Medical Management. Medical treatment for congestive heart failure includes **digoxin and diuretics. Other measures including providing a high level of supplemental oxygen, nitric oxide, and maintaining a mild respiratory alkalosis.**

Surgical Treatment. If the infant does not respond to medical treatment and exhibits congestive heart failure, severe AV valve regurgitation, or pulmonary hypertension, surgical repair is necessary. The surgical procedure through a median sternotomy incision involves closing the ASD and VSD, separating the common leaflets of the mitral and tricuspid valves, and reconstructing the mitral valve.

COMPLICATIONS AND RESIDUAL EFFECTS

Complications and residual effects include (1) persistent shunt (residual ASD or VSD), (2) conduction abnormalities, (3) dysrhythmias and third-degree heart block, (4) mitral regurgitation, and (5) tricuspid regurgitation.

PROGNOSIS AND FOLLOW-UP

In the complete AV septal defect, congestive heart failure is a frequent problem and early surgical intervention generally is necessary. The prognosis after surgical repair in the neonatal period is guarded, with a generally favorable outcome if the surgery can be postponed until the infant is older than 6 months. The prognosis is also guarded if pulmonary hypertension persists after surgical intervention.

Ebstein's Anomaly

PHYSIOLOGY

Ebstein's anomaly is an uncommon but important anatomic heart defect when presenting in the neonatal period.[26] Anatomically, there is a downward displacement of the tricuspid valve into the body of the right ventricle. The resultant right ventricular cavity is smaller than normal and, because the elevated pulmonary vascular resistance is normally present in the newborn period, the cardiac output from the right ventricle to the pulmonary artery is decreased. This cardiac output generally increases as the pulmonary vascular resistance decreases after birth. Tricuspid insufficiency is present in varying degrees in the infant. There is a right-to-left shunt at the atrial level via the foramen ovale.

DATA COLLECTION

Physical Findings

Cyanosis. **Varying degrees of cyanosis are present,** depending on the amount of right-to-left shunting at the foramen ovale and the amount of blood that enters the pulmonary circulation by the right ventricle. In severe cases, the amount of pulmonary blood flow is markedly decreased, and these infants may be deeply cyanotic.

Heart Sounds. The second heart sound, S_2, is normal in the mildly affected infant, but the pulmonary component of S_2 may be diminished or inaudible in severely affected patients. A nonspecific systolic murmur is usually present and varies from a grade I/VI to a grade V/VI, representing tricuspid insufficiency. Diastolic murmurs, ejection clicks, and triple or quadruple rhythms are frequently heard.

Congestive Heart Failure. Newborns who are symptomatic usually have congestive heart failure resulting from volume overload of the left ventricle (see "Congestive Heart Failure" section).

Laboratory Data

Arterial Blood Gases. The Pao_2 may be normal to very low, depending on the amount of shunting at the atrial level. **Pao_2 values in the low 20s are not uncommon.**

Chest X-ray Examination. The chest x-ray examination shows cardiomegaly with decreased pulmonary vascularity. Massive cardiomegaly generally indicates severe tricuspid insufficiency.

Electrocardiogram. An ECG shows abnormal P waves and various degrees of heart block. The QRS complex generally demonstrates a right bundle-branch block pattern. **Wolff-Parkinson-White (WPW)** (preexcitation) syndrome frequently is present, and dysrhythmias are common.

Echocardiogram. A two-dimensional echocardiogram is diagnostic. Doppler interrogation and color-flow mapping are very useful in evaluating the amount of antegrade blood flow through the pulmonary valve, shunting at the arterial level, and the degree of tricuspid insufficiency present.

Cardiac Catheterization. There is an increased risk for dysrhythmias during catheterization. This procedure is not generally performed in the neonatal period unless a question about the differential diagnosis exists (to rule out pulmonary atresia).

TREATMENT

Medical Management. Medical management is aimed at **supporting the neonate through the initial period of transitional circulation.** Because of elevated pulmonary vascular resistance, pulmonary blood flow may be quite severely limited with profound hypoxemia and acidosis. **PGE_1 is used to maintain a patent ductus arteriosus. Other measures include providing a high level of supplemental oxygen and maintaining a mild respiratory alkalosis.** Both of these measures help decrease pulmonary vascular resistance and promote antegrade pulmonary blood flow. Recently, **oral sildenafil (Viagra) is being used in symptomatic neonates.** This pulmonary vasodilator reduces right ventricular afterload and helps improve forward flow of blood across the pulmonary valve.[1] **Ebstein's anomaly is often associated with WPW syndrome and supraventricular tachycardia.**

Surgical Treatment. Surgical treatment for Ebstein's anomaly is controversial and generally reserved for the severely symptomatic patient. The procedure, performed through a median sternotomy incision, involves repositioning the tricuspid valve and an anuloplasty to improve the competency of the valve. In addition, plication of the atrialized ventricle is performed. Replacing the tricuspid valve may be necessary.

COMPLICATIONS AND RESIDUAL EFFECTS

High mortality rate in neonates with Ebstein's anomaly is associated with pulmonary hypoplasia because of the massively enlarged right heart in utero that prevented pulmonary development.

Complications and residual effects include tricuspid insufficiency and dysrhythmias. The mortality in infancy is unknown because of insufficient data.

PROGNOSIS AND FOLLOW-UP

The prognosis for mild Ebstein's anomaly is generally favorable. Infants with severe Ebstein's anomaly generally improve as the pulmonary vascular resistance decreases and right ventricular output increases. Although surgery has been used successfully in the more severe forms of Ebstein's anomaly, the prognosis is less favorable in patients requiring surgical intervention.

The prognosis for neonates presenting with profound cyanosis caused by Ebstein's anomaly is quite grave.

Persistent Pulmonary Hypertension in the Newborn

PHYSIOLOGY

Infants with abnormally elevated PVR have persistent pulmonary hypertension of the newborn (PPHN) or persistent fetal circulation. These infants are generally hypoxic and acidotic but usually do not have severe pulmonary parenchymal disease or underlying cardiac disease. These infants have a right-to-left shunt at the ductal and atrial levels.

DATA COLLECTION

History. PPHN is usually associated with severe antepartum or peripartum conditions that involve hypoxia reflected by low Apgar scores. **These infants are generally term or late preterm and are symptomatic within the first hours after birth.** Associated findings may include polycythemia, hypoglycemia, or an anatomic abnormality such as congenital diaphragmatic hernia.

Physical Findings

Cyanosis. The milder cases of PPHN have **minimal transient tachypnea and cyanosis associated with stress (crying or feeding). Severe cases demonstrate marked cyanosis, tachypnea, acidosis, and decreased peripheral perfusion.**

Heart Sounds. A loud pulmonary component of S_2 and occasionally the systolic ejection murmur of tricuspid regurgitation (TR) are heard.

Congestive Heart Failure. Infants with PPHN may have congestive heart failure because of pressure overload of the right ventricle (see "Congestive Heart Failure" section).

Laboratory Data

Arterial Blood Gases. Arterial blood gas values demonstrate acidosis, hypoxia, and increased $Paco_2$. **If a blood gas measurement is obtained simultaneously from the right radial artery (preductal) and from the descending aorta with an umbilical artery**

catheter (UAC) (postductal), the right-to-left shunt at the ductal level can be documented. If blood gas measurements are repeated after intubation and pharmacologic intervention (see "Treatment" section), the degree of hypoxia is often reduced.

Pulse Oximetry. **Simultaneous preductal and postductal transcutaneous oxygen measurements may also be used.**

Chest X-ray Examination. The chest x-ray examination demonstrates mild to moderate cardiomegaly with normal pulmonary vascular markings. The lung fields may be clear.

Electrocardiogram. The ECG frequently is normal but may demonstrate right ventricular hypertrophy and signs of myocardial ischemia.

Echocardiogram. An echocardiogram helps evaluate cardiac structures and rule out cyanotic lesions. Evaluating the right ventricular and pulmonary artery pressures by Doppler interrogation and the degree of right-to-left shunting at the atrial and ductal levels is helpful.

Cardiac Catheterization. Cardiac catheterization usually is not performed.

TREATMENT

Medical Management. See Chapter 23.

d-Transposition of the Great Arteries

PHYSIOLOGY

d-Transposition of the great arteries (Figure 24-9) is one of the most common forms of serious heart

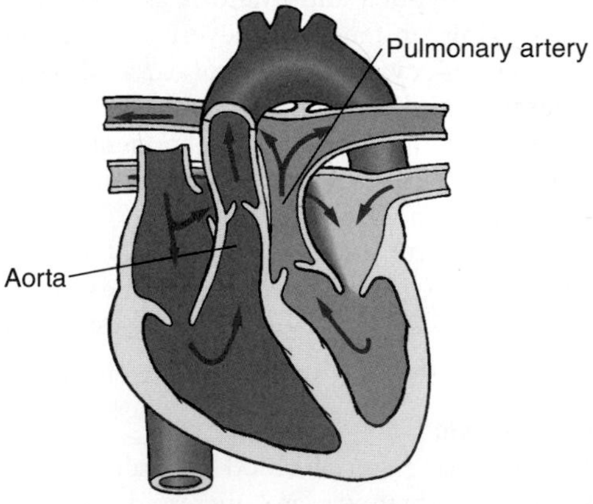

FIGURE 24-9 d-Transposition of the great arteries. (Modified from Hockenberry MJ, Wilson D: *Wong's essentials of pediatric nursing,* ed 8, St Louis, 2009, Mosby.)

disease. The aorta arises from the right ventricle, receives unoxygenated systemic venous blood, and returns this blood to the systemic arterial circulation. The pulmonary artery arises from the left ventricle, receives oxygenated pulmonary venous blood, and returns this blood to the pulmonary circulation. This creates a situation of "parallel circulations." The d-transposition anomaly can occur by itself or can be associated with other defects (e.g., PDA, ASD, VSD, pulmonary stenosis). Some patients with transposition have an associated ventricular septal defect, which allows for mixing between the parallel systemic and pulmonary circulations.

DATA COLLECTION

History. Transposition of the great arteries is more prevalent in males and is typically found in infants who are full term.

Physical Findings. The major physiologic abnormalities in d-transposition of the great arteries are an oxygen deficiency in the tissues and excessive workload of the right and left ventricles. **The only mixing of oxygenated and unoxygenated blood occurs in the presence of associated lesions** (e.g., patent foramen ovale, ASD, VSD, PDA, collateral circulation). The extent of the mixing depends on the number, size, and position of the anatomic communications, the pressure differential between the two systems, and changes in the systemic and pulmonary vascular resistances.

Cyanosis. These infants are usually **cyanotic within the first hours of life, leading to their early diagnosis. Cyanosis is present in varying degrees, depending on the amount of intracardiac mixing present.** Cyanosis may be mild if the mixing occurs through a significant VSD or PDA. Cyanosis is profound with intact ventricular septum or a closing PDA. **Oxygen therapy will be of limited benefit.** Only a certain amount of oxygenated blood can reach the systemic circulation, and administration of additional oxygen does not improve this situation. Enlargement of the interatrial communication by balloon septostomy (Rashkind procedure) during cardiac catheterization is commonly performed to establish adequate intercirculatory mixing for these infants.

After palliative procedures, the infant will continue to be cyanotic, especially in times of stress (crying, feeding, or exposure to cold temperatures). If the Pao_2, measured at rest in room

air, is not greater than 35 mm Hg or if persistent metabolic acidosis is present, inadequate intracardiac mixing should be suspected.

Heart Sounds. The aorta arises from the anterior (right) ventricle, and the closure of the aortic valve is easily heard. The S_2 is single with an increased intensity. Murmurs, if present, are usually those of associated lesions.

Congestive Heart Failure. The infant may show signs of congestive heart failure, but this is rare unless there is a large VSD or PDA present (see "Congestive Heart Failure" section).

Laboratory Data

Arterial Blood Gases. In neonates with transposition of the great arteries and an intact ventricular septum, **a very low Pa_{O_2} (15-20 torr) with normal Pa_{CO_2} and mild metabolic acidosis are often seen.**

Chest X-ray Examination. The chest x-ray examination may be normal or demonstrate either decreased or increased pulmonary vascularity. The cardiac silhouette may assume the shape of an "egg on a string." However, this finding is not diagnostic.

Electrocardiogram. The ECG may be normal or demonstrate right ventricular hypertrophy.

Echocardiogram. The echocardiogram is extremely useful in establishing the diagnosis and evaluating associated lesions in infants with transposition of the great arteries.

Cardiac Catheterization. Cardiac catheterization is diagnostic. A balloon septostomy is commonly performed to improve interatrial mixing.

TREATMENT

Medical Management. Serial venous and arterial pH measurements should be obtained to rule out the presence of a persistent metabolic acidosis that would suggest inadequate intracardiac mixing. Hyperventilation and treatment with sodium bicarbonate are important to promote alkalosis. PGE_1 infusion is used to maintain ductal patency.

Surgical Treatment. The arterial switch procedure in most centers is the treatment of choice for d-transposition of the great arteries. This procedure, through a median sternotomy incision, involves transection of the main pulmonary artery and the aorta above the respective valves. The pulmonary artery is anastomosed to the right ventricle, and the aorta is anastomosed to the left ventricle (the aortic valve becomes a functional pulmonary valve, and the pulmonary valve becomes a functional aortic valve). The coronary arteries are resected with a button of surrounding tissue and reanastomosed to the supravalvular area of the ascending aorta.

It is essential in performing this procedure that the left ventricular (LV) pressure is systemic. In infants with a VSD, the LV pressure tends to remain elevated; therefore this procedure may be postponed for several days or even months. However, once the LV pressure decreases below that of the right ventricle, the morbidity and mortality of surgery increase dramatically. Therefore infants with an intact ventricular septum require surgery within the first few days of life.

COMPLICATIONS AND RESIDUAL EFFECTS

Complications and residual effects of the arterial switch procedure include (1) dysrhythmias, (2) myocardial ischemia and infarction, and (3) aortic or pulmonary supravalvular stenosis.

PROGNOSIS AND FOLLOW-UP

Without treatment, 30% of these infants die within the first week of life, 50% die within the first month, 70% die within the first 6 months, and 90% die within the first year. With treatment, the mortality rate is reduced to approximately 5% or less.

Tetralogy of Fallot

PHYSIOLOGY

Tetralogy of Fallot is the most common cyanotic congenital heart defect. The four components of tetralogy of Fallot are VSD, overriding of the ascending aorta, obstruction of the right ventricular outflow tract, and right ventricular hypertrophy (Figure 24-10).

DATA COLLECTION

Physical Findings. Symptomatology in these infants relates to the degree of right ventricular outflow tract obstruction. Newborns who are symptomatic usually have severe right ventricular outflow tract obstruction.

Cyanosis. The predominant intracardiac shunt is right to left; therefore most infants with tetralogy of Fallot are cyanotic. However, if the right ventricular outflow obstruction is only mild or moderate, the intracardiac shunt is mainly left to right and the infant initially will not be cyanotic.

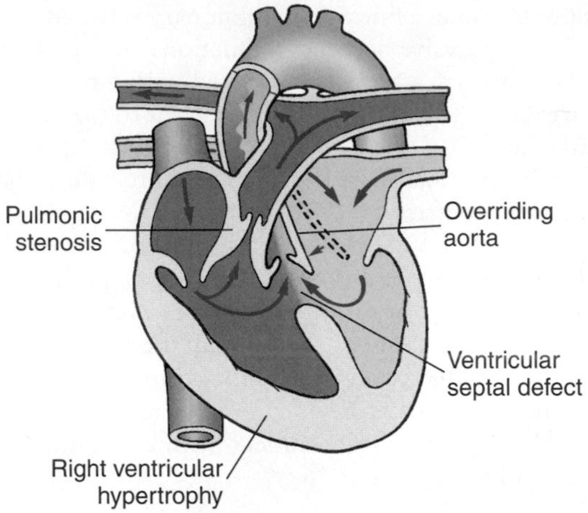

FIGURE 24-10 Tetralogy of Fallot. (Modified from Hockenberry MJ, Wilson D: *Wong's essentials of pediatric nursing,* ed 8, St Louis, 2009, Mosby.)

Infants with tetralogy of Fallot occasionally have hypercyanotic (or "tet") spells. These spells consist of cyanosis, irritability, pallor, tachypnea, flaccidity, and possible loss of consciousness. They may be the result of a transient increase in the obstruction of the right ventricular outflow tract (usually the muscular infundibular area) and **usually resolve with knee-chest positioning, oxygen, propranolol, or morphine.**

Heart Sounds. A grade II to IV/VI harsh systolic murmur at the mid to upper left sternal border is usually present but is diminished or absent during a hypercyanotic spell. The S_2 is usually loud and single (representing aortic closure).

Congestive Heart Failure. Congestive heart failure is uncommon in tetralogy of Fallot.

Laboratory Data

Arterial Blood Gases. The $PaCO_2$ and pH are normal. The PaO_2 is normal if the pulmonary stenosis is mild and there is little right-to-left shunting at the ventricular level. If the pulmonary stenosis, however, is more severe, the amount of right-to-left shunting increases and the PaO_2 falls.

Chest X-ray Examination. The classic chest x-ray examination in tetralogy of Fallot shows the shape of a boot with a normal-size heart. However, the classic chest x-ray pattern described is not common in the newborn. Pulmonary vascularity is either normal or decreased.

Electrocardiogram. The ECG demonstrates right ventricular hypertrophy.

Echocardiogram. The echocardiogram is suggestive when the overriding aorta can be demonstrated. Echocardiograms help identify the pulmonary valve to rule out pulmonary atresia. Doppler interrogation helps define the degree and level of pulmonary stenosis. Color-flow mapping identifies the VSD, as well as the direction of blood flow across the VSD.

Cardiac Catheterization. Cardiac catheterization is diagnostic and performed in the newborn when there is a question about the differential diagnosis (pulmonary atresia).

TREATMENT

Medical Management. Immediate medical management involves **establishing adequate pulmonary blood flow with PGE_1 infusion.** Digoxin is not routinely used because it may increase the amount of infundibular obstruction present. **Propranolol is the preferred drug for treating hypercyanotic spells, although morphine has been used successfully** (see "General Treatment Strategy" section).

Surgical Treatment. Total correction of tetralogy of Fallot involves intracardiac repair with patch closure of the large VSD and relief of the right ventricular outflow obstruction performed through a median sternotomy incision. Often a pericardial patch across the pulmonary valve annulus is necessary. Contraindications include small size of the infant, anomalous left anterior descending coronary artery, and hypoplastic pulmonary arteries.

Total surgical repair of tetralogy of Fallot is not usually carried out in the neonatal period. Surgery is usually performed electively within the first year of life.[15] More recently, repair at 3 to 6 months is recommended with successful outcomes.[11] If surgical intervention in infancy is warranted (i.e., the infant is severely hypoxic because of inadequate pulmonary blood flow), a systemic-to-pulmonary shunt is performed. The Blalock-Taussig operation is usually preferred (see description of the Blalock-Taussig operation on p. 697).

COMPLICATIONS AND RESIDUAL EFFECTS

Complications and residual effects include (1) diminished or absent pulses in the affected arm, (2) congestive heart failure from an overly large shunt, and (3) inadequate shunt. Mortality rate in infancy is 10%.

PROGNOSIS AND FOLLOW-UP

Surgery is recommended if the infant is symptomatic or refractory to medical care. Tetralogy of Fallot without surgery carries a grave prognosis. Long-term follow-up after corrective surgery has indicated impaired neurodevelopment, both in intellectual and behavioral functioning.[22]

Pulmonary Atresia with Intact Ventricular Septum

PHYSIOLOGY

Pulmonary atresia is characterized by complete agenesis of the pulmonary valve. This lesion produces severe signs or symptoms soon after birth and is not compatible with life unless there is an associated interatrial communication and an additional pathway of entry for blood into the pulmonary circulation (through a PDA or collateral blood flow). Because flow to the lungs may depend on a PDA, death may occur when this structure closes. The right ventricle is usually hypoplastic but may be normal or dilated, depending on the degree of tricuspid insufficiency present. The presence of sinusoidal connections between the right ventricle and the coronary arteries is associated with poorer long-term survival.[8]

DATA COLLECTION

Physical Findings

Cyanosis. **Cyanosis is always present in varying degrees,** depending on the amount of pulmonary blood flow from the PDA and degree of atrial right-to-left shunting.

Heart Sounds. The S_2 is single, and a soft systolic murmur is heard as a result of either the PDA or tricuspid insufficiency in about one half of the infants with pulmonary atresia.

Congestive Heart Failure. Congestive heart failure is usually present with moderate to severe tricuspid insufficiency (see "Congestive Heart Failure" section).

Laboratory Data

Arterial Blood Gases. The pH and $Paco_2$ are usually within normal range. **The Pao_2, however, usually is very low (20 to 30 torr), unless there is a large shunt at the ductal or bronchial collateral level.** In some cases, the amount of pulmonary blood flow is insufficient, and the **pH may be low, reflecting metabolic acidosis.**

Chest X-ray Examination. The heart appears enlarged on x-ray examination if tricuspid insufficiency is present. Pulmonary vascularity is either decreased or normal, depending on the amount of shunting through the PDA or collateral blood flow.

Electrocardiogram. The ECG is usually normal but may demonstrate left ventricular hypertrophy.

Echocardiogram. The two-dimensional echocardiogram with Doppler and color-flow mapping can identify absence of blood flow across the pulmonary valve and is diagnostic.

Cardiac Catheterization. Cardiac catheterization is diagnostic and may be performed if the diagnosis is suspected. A balloon atrial septostomy may be performed at the time of catheterization. Catheterization is also used to define the coronary artery anatomy before surgery.

TREATMENT

Medical Management. PGE_1 **is used to maintain patency of the ductus arteriosus until surgical intervention** (see "General Treatment Strategy" section).

Surgical Treatment. In most medical centers, a systemic-to-pulmonary shunt such as the Blalock-Taussig operation is performed through a lateral thoracotomy incision. However, some institutions are performing a pulmonary valvulotomy or a pulmonary outflow patch procedure in addition to a shunt. This establishes an open pathway through the atretic valve area between the pulmonary artery and the right ventricle. Antegrade blood flow through the right ventricle and pulmonary artery then promotes growth of these areas. The pulmonary valvotomy and pulmonary outflow patch procedures are performed through a median sternotomy incision.

COMPLICATIONS AND RESIDUAL EFFECTS

Complications and residual effects of the Blalock-Taussig operation include (1) diminished or absent pulses in the affected arm, (2) congestive heart failure from an overlarge shunt, and (3) inadequate shunt. The mortality rate in infants is 25% or higher.

PROGNOSIS AND FOLLOW-UP

Pulmonary atresia is fatal without surgical intervention. If a palliative shunt is performed, catheterization and further surgical procedures should be anticipated when the shunt becomes inadequate. If primary surgical correction is undertaken in the newborn period, catheterization should be anticipated to evaluate residual obstruction. Despite the development of newer surgical techniques, the prognosis in these infants is guarded.

Total Anomalous Pulmonary Venous Return

PHYSIOLOGY

Total anomalous pulmonary venous return (TAPVR) occurs when all pulmonary veins drain into the systemic venous system with complete mixing of pulmonary and systemic venous return. The presence of an ASD is necessary to sustain life (Figure 24-11). The four main varieties of TAPVR are as follows:

- Supracardiac (most common), in which the drainage is to the superior vena cava through the innominate vein
- Cardiac, in which the pulmonary veins drain into the coronary sinus or directly into the right atrium
- Infracardiac, in which the four veins join behind the heart, pass through the diaphragm, and connect to the portal venous system or a systemic vein
- Mixed

Each of the various types of anomalous drainage can occur with or without obstruction along the pulmonary venous pathway. The presence or absence of obstruction profoundly affects the clinical course.

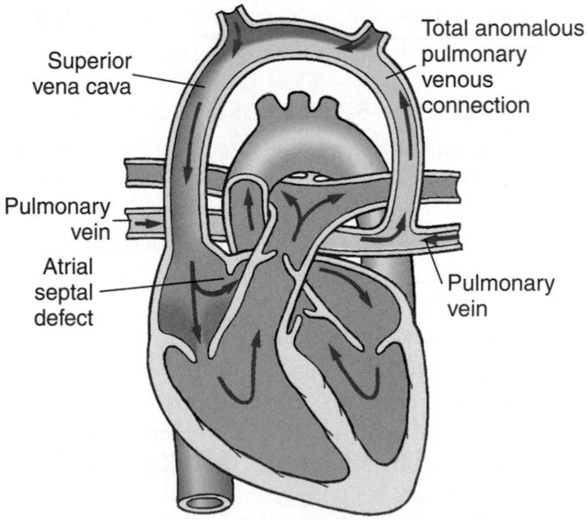

FIGURE 24-11 Total anomalous pulmonary venous return. (Modified from Hockenberry MJ, Wilson D: *Wong's essentials of pediatric nursing*, ed 8, St Louis, 2009, Mosby.)

DATA COLLECTION

Physical Findings

Cyanosis. Infants with obstructed or unobstructed TAPVR are frequently cyanotic. Because all pulmonary venous return (oxygenated blood) ultimately enters the right atrium (as opposed to the left atrium), **a right-to-left shunt at the atrial level is necessary to sustain life.**

Heart Sounds. Murmurs are rarely heard in infants with TAPVR and, when present, are nonspecific.

Congestive Heart Failure. Infants with **unobstructed TAPVR usually show signs of congestive heart failure** resulting from volume overload of the right ventricle. Infants with **obstructed TAPVR generally do not demonstrate evidence of congestive heart failure** but typically demonstrate pulmonary venous congestion (see "Congestive Heart Failure" section).

Laboratory Data

Arterial Blood Gases. The pH and $Paco_2$ are usually normal. The Pao_2 may be within the normal range if there is a large amount of pulmonary blood flow (always associated with severe congestive heart failure). If the pulmonary blood flow is limited, secondary to obstruction of blood flow, the Pao_2 may be low, but this is rare.

Chest X-ray Examination. If the TAPVR is obstructed, the chest x-ray examination will demonstrate pulmonary venous congestion without cardiomegaly. If the TAPVR is unobstructed, the chest x-ray examination will demonstrate a marked increase in pulmonary vascularity and cardiomegaly.

Electrocardiogram. An ECG may demonstrate right axis deviation, right ventricular hypertrophy, and right atrial enlargement.

Echocardiogram. An echocardiogram is diagnostic, but it is sometimes difficult to visualize the pulmonary veins by this method. The diagnosis of TAPVR is strongly suggested when an extra vascular structure is seen behind the small left atrium. With color-flow mapping, the right-to-left shunting across the atrial septum, as well as the anomalous venous return as it enters through the atrium, superior vena cava, or coronary sinus, can be visualized.

Cardiac Catheterization. Infants suspected of having TAPVR may undergo cardiac catheterization to define the type of TAPVR and presence or absence of obstruction. A Rashkind balloon septostomy may be performed at that time to improve intraatrial mixing.

TREATMENT

Medical Management. Obstructed TAPVR is a surgical emergency. Nonobstructed TAPVR may be medically treated temporarily (prostaglandin and ventilatory support), although surgery at the time of diagnosis is generally recommended (see "General Treatment Strategy" section).

Surgical Treatment. Surgical correction of TAPVR depends on the variety. Supracardiac and infracardiac varieties require surgical reimplantation of the common vein into the left atrium. Intracardiac TAPVR can usually be surgically repaired by realigning the atrial septum during closure of the ASD and directing the anomalous veins to the left atrial side. All repairs are performed through a median sternotomy incision.

COMPLICATIONS AND RESIDUAL EFFECTS

Complications and residual effects include pulmonary venous obstruction and dysrhythmias. The mortality rate varies from 5% to 25% in infancy, depending on thc anatomic type.

PROGNOSIS AND FOLLOW-UP

Infants with nonobstructed TAPVR generally do well if the lesion is recognized early and early corrective surgery is performed. The prognosis for obstructed TAPVR is less favorable despite early surgical intervention.

Tricuspid Atresia

PHYSIOLOGY

In tricuspid atresia, there is complete agenesis of the tricuspid valve with no direct communication between the right atrium and right ventricle. Systemic venous blood entering the right atrium is shunted through a patent foramen ovale or ASD into the left atrium. If a large VSD is present, the right ventricle and pulmonary arteries may be normal in size. If the ventricular septum is intact but a large PDA is present, the right ventricular cavity may be hypoplastic and the pulmonary arteries are usually slightly decreased or normal in size (Figure 24-12). About 30% of these infants will have transposition of the great arteries.

DATA COLLECTION

Physical Findings

Cyanosis. The degree of cyanosis varies. **Newborns will have marked cyanosis if the pulmonary blood flow is compromised.**

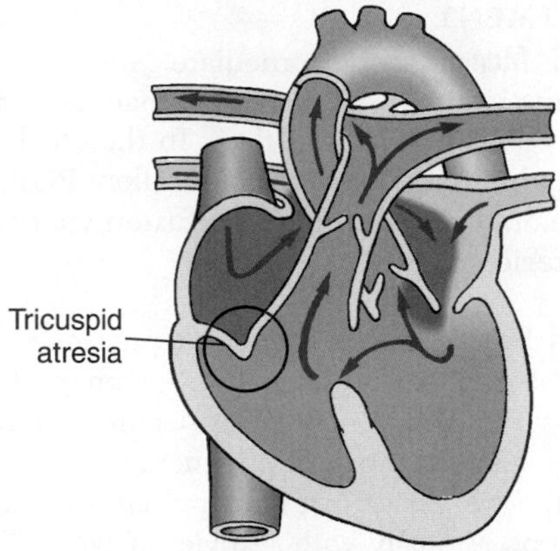

FIGURE 24-12 Tricuspid atresia. (Modified from Hockenberry MJ, Wilson D: *Wong's essentials of pediatric nursing,* ed 8, St Louis, 2009, Mosby.)

Heart Sounds. A single S_2 is present in infants with tricuspid atresia. Murmurs of associated shunts (VSD and PDA) may be present.

Congestive Heart Failure. Congestive heart failure may be present with a large shunt (PDA or VSD) (see "Congestive Heart Failure" section).

Laboratory Data

Arterial Blood Gases. The pH and $Paco_2$ usually are normal. The Pao_2 may vary from near normal if there is a large VSD or PDA to extremely low if there is limited shunting into the pulmonary system.

Chest X-ray Examination. A chest x-ray examination is nondiagnostic and may show a normal heart size or cardiomegaly. Pulmonary vascularity may be normal, decreased, or increased, depending on the degree of pulmonary blood flow.

Electrocardiogram. An ECG usually demonstrates left axis deviation with a counterclockwise loop, a superior axis in the frontal plane, and left ventricular electrical dominance.

Echocardiogram. Absence of the tricuspid valve and presence of a hypoplastic right ventricle are diagnostic of tricuspid atresia. Color-flow mapping can identify the right-to-left shunt at the atrial level and the presence of a VSD or PDA.

Cardiac Catheterization. An infant suspected of having tricuspid atresia usually undergoes cardiac catheterization and a balloon septostomy. A balloon septostomy is performed to improve intraatrial mixing.

TREATMENT

Medical Management. Immediate medical management is aimed primarily at maintaining adequate pulmonary blood flow. In the usual case of severely limited pulmonary blood flow, **PGE_1 infusion maintains pulmonary perfusion via the ductus arteriosus.**

Surgical Treatment. The preferred procedure in the neonatal period is a systemic-to-pulmonary shunt such as the Blalock-Taussig operation performed through a lateral thoracotomy incision.

Definitive "repair" of tricuspid atresia is accomplished occasionally with a single operation (Fontan procedure) or, more frequently, a staged procedure (Glenn followed by a Fontan). These operations involve anastomosis of the systemic venous return directly to the pulmonary artery. Any associated defects present are also repaired. Definitive repair is performed through a median sternotomy incision.

COMPLICATIONS AND RESIDUAL EFFECTS

Complications and residual effects include heart failure, pleural effusions, renal or liver failure, persistent shunts, conduit obstruction, dysrhythmia, and protein-losing enteropathy. The mortality rate in infancy is unknown, but in older children it is approximately 10% to 25%.

PROGNOSIS AND FOLLOW-UP

The prognosis for tricuspid atresia is guarded. The Fontan procedure may improve this prognosis.

Truncus Arteriosus

PHYSIOLOGY

Truncus arteriosus is characterized by one great artery arising from the left and right ventricles, overriding a VSD. This common artery has one valve and gives rise to (in order) the coronary arteries, the pulmonary arteries, and the brachiocephalic arteries (Figure 24-13). A coexisting VSD is present in more than 98% of cases. Truncus arteriosus is classified into three types, depending on the origins of the pulmonary arteries:

1. Type I—A short, main pulmonary artery arises from the common trunk that bifurcates into the right and left pulmonary arteries.
2. Type II—The right and left pulmonary arteries arise directly from the posterior surface of the common trunk.

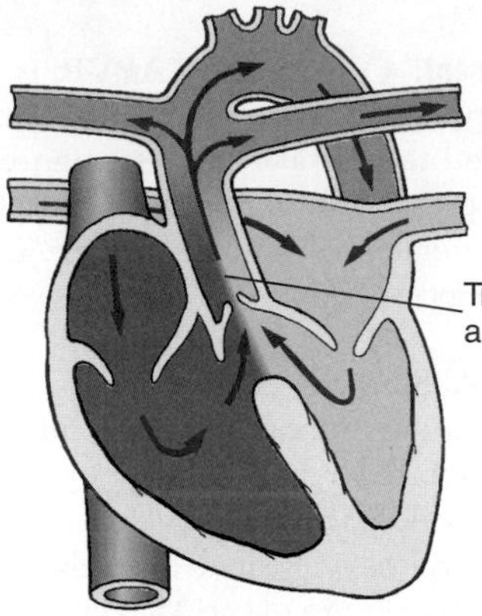

FIGURE 24-13 Truncus arteriosus. (Modified from Hockenberry MJ, Wilson D: *Wong's essentials of pediatric nursing,* ed 8, St Louis, 2009, Mosby.)

3. Type III—The right and left pulmonary arteries arise directly from the lateral walls of the common trunk.

The ductus arteriosus is absent in approximately 50% of infants with truncus arteriosus. Between 30% and 35% have a right aortic arch. Extracardiac anomalies are present in 20% to 40% of cases.

DATA COLLECTION

Physical Findings. In truncus arteriosus, the common trunk receives a mixture of unoxygenated blood from the right ventricle and oxygenated blood from the left ventricle. Blood flow to the lungs varies with the type of truncus but is usually increased and at systemic level pressure.

Cyanosis. Cyanosis may be present at birth but varies in intensity according to the amount of pulmonary blood flow. Minimal cyanosis indicates adequate pulmonary blood flow.

Heart Sounds. The first heart sound, S_1, is normal, but the S_2 is single and loud because of the single valve of the common trunk. A loud systolic ejection click is frequently heard.

A loud pansystolic murmur maximal at the lower left sternal border that radiates to the entire precordium is commonly heard. A mid-diastolic rumble may be present. If the truncal valve is insufficient, a blowing diastolic murmur may be heard. A wide pulse pressure also may be present.

Congestive Heart Failure. Congestive heart failure may be present shortly after birth or appear between 2 and 3 weeks of age. The presence of congestive heart failure depends on the amount of pulmonary blood flow. Persistently high pulmonary arteriolar resistance in the first few weeks of life decreases pulmonary blood flow, and congestive heart failure may not be present. However, if the truncal valve is severely abnormal, congestive heart failure may be present shortly after birth (see "Congestive Heart Failure" section).

Laboratory Data

Arterial Blood Gases. The pH and $Paco_2$ are usually normal. If there is no obstruction to pulmonary blood flow, the Pao_2 may be near normal (usually associated with severe congestive heart failure). If the pulmonary blood flow is restricted, the Pao_2 may be extremely low.

Chest X-ray Examination. Cardiomegaly, displayed pulmonary arteries, and increased vascular markings are typical findings on the chest x-ray examination.

Electrocardiogram. Combined ventricular hypertrophy is most often seen in an ECG. Left atrial enlargement is also commonly found.

Echocardiogram. A two-dimensional echocardiogram is helpful in establishing the diagnosis and in differentiating tetralogy of Fallot from truncus arteriosus. In addition, the echocardiogram is used to identify the number of truncal valve leaflets, the presence of truncal valve insufficiency, or stenosis.

Cardiac Catheterization. A cardiac catheterization is diagnostic and is usually performed on an infant suspected of having truncus arteriosus.

TREATMENT

Medical Management. **Medical management of these infants consists of stabilizing and treating congestive heart failure when present.** Calcium should be closely monitored because of the possibility of DiGeorge syndrome or 22q deletion syndrome.

Surgical Treatment. Repairing of truncus arteriosus is rare in the newborn period and is usually carried out at 6 weeks to 6 months of age. It consists of separating the pulmonary artery from the common trunk, closing the VSD with a patch, and inserting a right ventricular-to-pulmonary artery valved conduit. The use of homograft conduits for repair of truncus arteriosus has become more common. Total repair of truncus arteriosus is performed through a median sternotomy incision.

COMPLICATIONS AND RESIDUAL EFFECTS

Complications and side effects include pulmonary vascular disease, residual shunts, truncal valve insufficiency, and conduit obstruction. The mortality rate is 40% to 50% in infancy.

PROGNOSIS AND FOLLOW-UP

The natural history depends on the amount of pulmonary blood flow and the competency of the truncal valve. Without treatment, more than half of these infants die before 3 months of age. Survival past 1 year of age ranges from 15% to 30%. Truncus arteriosus is often associated with DiGeorge syndrome, which has a wide spectrum of clinical manifestations.

Hypoplastic Left Heart Syndrome

PHYSIOLOGY

Hypoplastic left heart syndrome represents a clinical spectrum that includes severe coarctation of the aorta, severe aortic valve stenosis or atresia, and severe mitral valve stenosis or atresia (Figure 24-14). The left ventricle and ascending aorta are hypoplastic. Coronary blood flow occurs in a retrograde fashion into the small ascending aorta through the PDA. The resultant poor myocardial perfusion leads to rapid decompensation.

DATA COLLECTION

Physical Findings

Cyanosis. These infants are usually **not truly cyanotic but, rather, have severe pallor and a grayish skin**

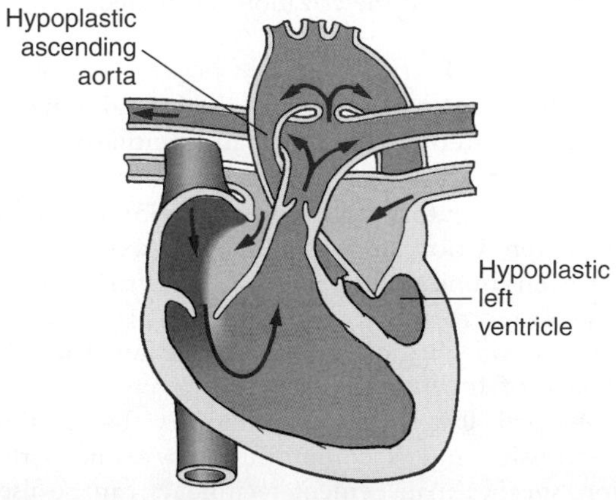

FIGURE 24-14 Hypoplastic left heart syndrome. (Modified from Hockenberry MJ, Wilson D: *Wong's essentials of pediatric nursing,* ed 8, St Louis, 2009, Mosby.)

color as a result of marked poor perfusion, vasoconstriction, and congestive heart failure.

Heart Sounds. A nonspecific systolic murmur is heard in approximately two thirds of infants with hypoplastic left heart syndrome.

Congestive Heart Failure. Congestive heart failure is present in all cases as a result of right ventricular volume and pressure overload (see "Congestive Heart Failure" section).

Laboratory Data

Arterial Blood Gases. **The arterial blood gas may represent the single best indicator of hemodynamic stability.** Low arterial saturation (75% to 80%) with normal pH indicates an acceptable balance of systemic and pulmonary blood flow with adequate peripheral perfusion. Elevated oxygen saturation (>90%) with acidosis represents significantly increased pulmonary and decreased systemic flow with probable myocardial dysfunction.

Chest X-ray Examination. Cardiomegaly with increased pulmonary vascularity and pulmonary edema is seen on the x-ray examination.

Electrocardiogram. An ECG frequently demonstrates right axis deviation and right ventricular hypertrophy. However, the ECG may be normal.

Echocardiogram. An echocardiogram is usually diagnostic with a small left ventricular cavity and ascending aorta, mitral and aortic valve atresia or hypoplasia, and a dilated right ventricle (RV).

Cardiac Catheterization. Cardiac catheterization carries a high risk in infants with hypoplastic left heart syndrome and is usually not necessary if the echocardiogram is diagnostic. If there is a question about the differential diagnosis, a heart catheterization is indicated.

TREATMENT

Medical Management. **Pharmacologic maintenance of ductal patency with PGE_1 and ventilatory support to increase pulmonary resistance is used.** A mild respiratory alkalosis (pH 7.35) is helpful. Hyperventilation and supplemental oxygen have not been found to be beneficial. Small to moderate doses of inotropes may be useful in the treatment of hypotension. **Surgical intervention offers the only chance of survival.**

Subatmospheric Oxygen. When pulmonary blood flow is excessive and is compromising systemic perfusion, specific management techniques can be used to increase PVR and thus create a balance between systemic and pulmonary perfusion. **This increase in PVR can be accomplished clinically by administration of inspired CO_2, permissive hypercapnia, hypoventilation, or administration of subatmospheric concentrations of inspired oxygen.** The administration of CO_2 or subatmospheric concentrations of oxygen is preferred because of the risk for atelectasis with hypoventilation or permissive hypercapnia. The choice between the two is based on institutional or caregiver preference.

Surgical Treatment. Recent advances in surgical treatment have made it possible to treat this lesion with a multistaged approach. The **Norwood procedure** is performed initially, consisting of enlargement of the atrial septal defect, ligation of the PDA, anastomosis of the pulmonary artery to the ascending aorta and the aortic arch, and creation of an aortopulmonary shunt (Blalock-Taussig shunt) to maintain pulmonary blood flow. In the second stage, the aortopulmonary shunt is removed and an anastomosis is made between the superior vena cava and the pulmonary artery; it is called a **bidirectional Glenn shunt** and is performed at 6 to 12 months of age. The final stage is the **Fontan procedure,** which connects the inferior vena cava to the pulmonary artery; this is generally done at 18 to 36 months of age. **Cardiac transplantation is an alternative surgical option.** In some centers, the Norwood procedure is performed as a bridge to transplantation, allowing the infant to survive until a donor heart is available.

Heart Transplantation in Infants

Approximately 10% of infants born with congenital heart disease have severe, complex lesions that preclude corrective surgery. For some of these infants, heart transplantation may offer the only chance of long-term survival. **Hypoplastic left heart syndrome is the most common indication for heart transplantation in early infancy.** Cardiomyopathies are another indication.

Heart transplantation in infancy is severely limited by donor availability. There is a scarcity of donor hearts in this age and size group, and 31% of infants younger than 6 months on transplant lists die waiting for donors.[2]

Dysrhythmias

When evaluating an infant with a dysrhythmia, it is essential to assess simultaneously the

electrophysiology and hemodynamic status. A neonate with poor perfusion and hypotension should first be treated for shock. A 12-lead ECG can then be done for definitive diagnosis of the type of dysrhythmia. When analyzing the ECG for the mechanism of dysrhythmia, a notation should be made in three main areas: (1) rate; (2) rhythm; and (3) QRS morphology.

PHYSIOLOGY

The development of the cardiac conduction system continues after birth with a steady increase in the sympathetic innervation of the heart. This accounts for the observed heart rate variability and the high frequency of benign dysrhythmias in the newborn. Premature ventricular beats (Figure 24-15), brief episodes of ectopic atrial rhythms, wandering atrial pacemakers (Figure 24-16), and even brief episodes of sinus arrest are all frequently seen in the newborn period. **The majority of these dysrhythmias do not require immediate treatment; however, if they persist, the presence of congenital heart disease, sepsis, drug toxicity, persistent hypoxia, adrenal insufficiency, disorders of electrolyte and acid-base balance, hypoglycemia, and hypocalcemia should be considered.**

All cardiac tissue is capable of generating a spontaneous depolarization. However, the sinoatrial (SA) node, atrioventricular (AV) node, and His-Purkinje system consist of specialized conductive tissue with rapid spontaneous depolarization. The SA node is the normal pacemaker of the heart because it has the fastest rate of spontaneous depolarization. If, however, the spontaneous depolarization of the SA node is delayed or slower than normal, an escape rhythm (Figure 24-16) is generated by either the AV node or His-Purkinje system (these rhythms are called *nodal escape* or *ventricular escape,* respectively). Dysrhythmias also can originate from an automatic "ectopic" pacemaker located anywhere in the heart. These **ectopic pacemakers become more active in the presence of hypoxia, acidosis, digoxin toxicity, abnormal sympathetic nervous system stimulation, increased wall tension (congestive heart**

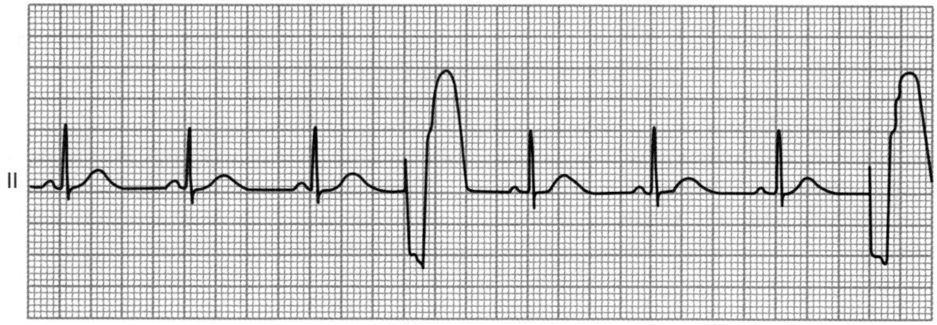

FIGURE 24-15 Premature ventricular beats.

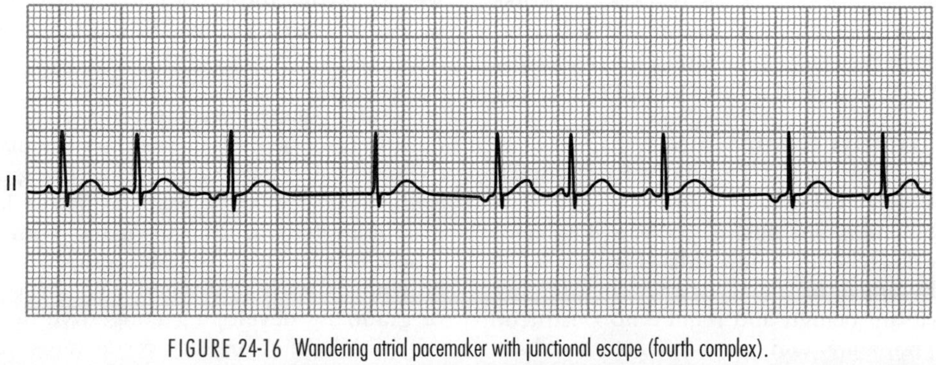

FIGURE 24-16 Wandering atrial pacemaker with junctional escape (fourth complex).

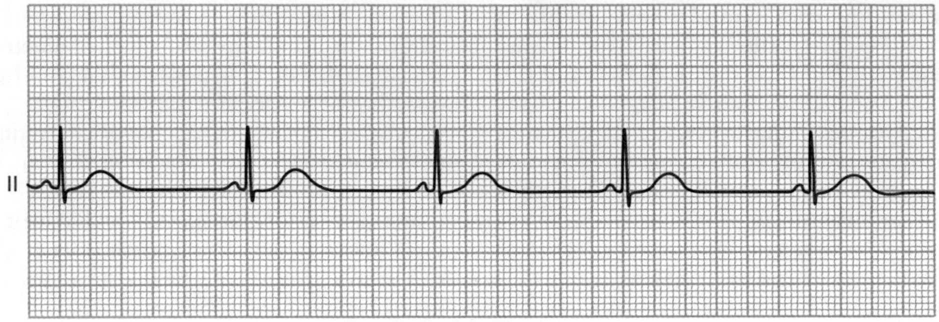

FIGURE 24-17 Sinus bradycardia.

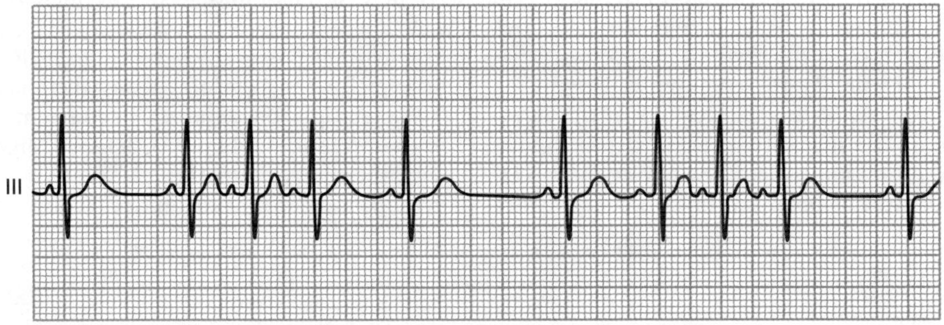

FIGURE 24-18 Sinus dysrhythmia.

failure), or altered electrolyte balance. Drug therapy for dysrhythmias is based on the ability of certain medications to alter the electrophysiologic properties of cardiac tissue. One class of antidysrhythmic drugs directly increases the automaticity of certain cardiac fibers. Examples of such drugs are quinidine, procainamide, lidocaine, and phenytoin (see Table 24-4). Other drugs directly or indirectly affect the autonomic nervous system activity. Propranolol is a beta-adrenergic blocker and works in this fashion. Digoxin exerts its chronotropic activity by altering the sympathetic and parasympathetic nervous system response within the heart.

BENIGN DYSRHYTHMIAS: SINUS BRADYCARDIA, SINUS TACHYCARDIA, AND SINUS DYSRHYTHMIA

Of normal premature infants, 35% to 40% have brief episodes of sinus bradycardia (Figure 24-17), sinus tachycardia, or sinus dysrhythmia (Figure 24-18) that are benign and require no treatment. Healthy premature and term infants may have heart rates that range from 90 to 200 beats/min. Sustained heart rates (>15 seconds) above or below this range should be evaluated with a 12-lead ECG and rhythm strip. These are important, because artifact created by the bedside monitors often makes accurate interpretations of dysrhythmias impossible.

SUPRAVENTRICULAR TACHYCARDIA

Supraventricular tachycardia (SVT) (Figure 24-19) is the most common tachydysrhythmia in the newborn period. SVT is the result of dual AV nodal pathways, rapid conduction through an accessory bundle (WPW syndrome), or the existence of an ectopic atrial pacemaker. SVT is occasionally associated with Ebstein's anomaly of the tricuspid valve, d-transposition of the great vessels, cardiomyopathy, or myocarditis. These lesions are present in 10% to 25% of infants with SVT and should be excluded with the appropriate evaluation. **Newborns with prolonged SVT have a history of gradually developing congestive heart failure with findings of anxiety, restlessness, tachypnea,**

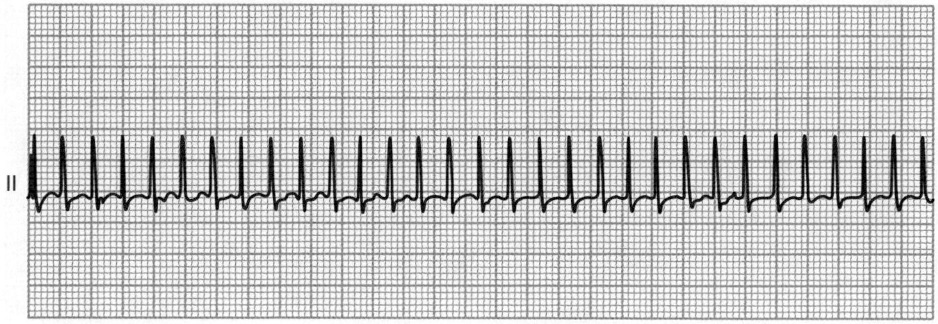

FIGURE 24-19 Supraventricular tachycardia.

and poor feeding. These symptoms develop after 12 to 24 hours of SVT. SVT often starts and ceases abruptly.

Criteria for SVT include (1) persistent ventricular rate over 200 to 220 beats/min, (2) a fixed and regular R-R interval, and (3) little variability in heart rate with various activities (e.g., crying, feeding, apnea).

Treatment. Various maneuvers may be used to attempt to convert the infant to normal sinus rhythm (NSR). Vagal maneuvers (unilateral carotid pressure, gagging, rectal stimulation) may be attempted but rarely work. Ocular compression should never be used. Stimulation of the diving reflex using an ice bag applied to the infant's face may be attempted. (Caution must be used in this procedure to ensure adequate ventilation for the infant.) **For infants without WPW syndrome, digoxin is the initial therapy. Parenteral digitalization usually abolishes this dysrhythmia within 12 hours. Propranolol is used as drug therapy for infants with SVT caused by WPW syndrome in the absence of congestive heart failure.** In premature infants, propranolol may cause apnea and hypoglycemia. **Adenosine, a purinergic agonist, is an especially effective antidysrhythmic drug for treatment of SVT. Adenosine slows the sinus rate and produces transient AV block, interrupting the SVT.** Overdrive atrial pacing has been successful in converting SVT to NSR. However, **direct-current (DC) cardioversion (1 to 2 watt-seconds/kg) is the most effective mode of treatment.** The defibrillator must always be in the synchronous mode. **If cardioversion is successful, maintenance drug therapy should be initiated.** Other antidysrhythmic drugs such as digoxin have been used to treat this disorder. Recently, however, it has been suggested that digoxin not be used in WPW syndrome and that this disorder be ruled out before digoxin is used. If not contraindicated, digoxin should be administered using standard doses (see Box 24-3).

Propranolol administered intravenously (IV) may be used if the patient is not in congestive heart failure, although it is very risky and not usually recommended. Beta-blocking agents may inhibit circulating catecholamines, which are needed for the maintenance of adequate cardiac output in the face of congestive heart failure. **Esmolol is another beta-blocking agent that can be administered IV for SVT (see Table 24-4).**

If the SVT fails to convert using the methods outlined previously, other drugs such as amiodarone, flecainide, or procainamide may be necessary. **After conversion to NSR, maintenance drug therapy should be continued for 6 to 12 months or longer. Relapses during the first 48 hours are common (70%) and should be anticipated.**

Fetal SVT is uncommon but, when present, can be associated with severe congestive heart failure and hydrops fetalis. Fetal SVT requires aggressive management, including conversion with maternally administered propranolol and digoxin. A favorable outcome usually can be expected for fetal SVT. Failure to control the fetal SVT in the presence of fetal hydrops is an indication for delivery.

ATRIAL FLUTTER AND FIBRILLATION

The presence of atrial flutter (Figure 24-20) is often suggestive of a serious organic heart disease (endocardial fibroelastosis, Ebstein's anomaly of the tricuspid valve, or complex heart defects). Atrial

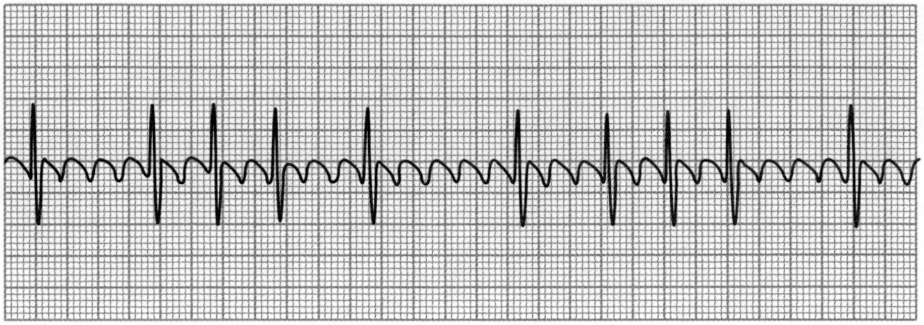

FIGURE 24-20 Atrial flutter.

flutter is diagnosed when (1) the atrial rate is greater than 220 beats/min; (2) the P waves are very regular; and (3) there is a characteristic sawtooth pattern, indicating a flutter wave. The ventricular rate will vary depending on the degree of AV block present. **Atrial fibrillation is extremely rare and almost always indicates a serious organic heart disease.** The prognosis for atrial flutter and fibrillation tends to be less favorable than that of SVT. These tachydysrhythmias have been reported to be more difficult to treat in utero, more likely to be associated with structural heart defects, and more likely to develop hydrops fetalis. Some cases of atrial flutter have been found in infants with an intracardiac catheter (in right atrium by echo) and/or those receiving broad-spectrum antimicrobials.[23]

Treatment. **The treatment of atrial flutter or fibrillation is DC cardioversion or overdrive atrial pacing followed by maintenance therapy with digoxin.**

VENTRICULAR TACHYCARDIA

Ventricular tachycardia is relatively rare and is usually seen with severe medical illnesses such as hypoxemia, shock, electrolyte disturbances, and digoxin toxicity.

Treatment. **Ventricular tachycardia is best treated with immediate DC cardioversion. Lidocaine may be used as a bolus (1 to 2 mg/kg IV) or as a continuous IV infusion of 20 to 30 mcg/kg/min. After conversion, maintenance therapy should be initiated using phenytoin, propranolol, lidocaine, procainamide, or amiodarone. Phenytoin, 2 to 4 mg/kg, may be effective if the dysrhythmia is the result of digoxin toxicity.**

COMPLETE ATRIOVENTRICULAR BLOCK

In complete heart block, the ventricular rate is slower than the atrial rate and there is no association between the ventricular and atrial rates. **Complete heart block can be seen in infants with myocarditis or endocardial fibroelastosis. There is a strong association between congenital heart block and maternal collagen diseases such as systemic lupus erythematosus (SLE).** Often these mothers have no signs or symptoms of lupus, but laboratory confirmation is often possible.

Treatment. **No treatment is necessary unless the ventricular rate falls below 55 beats/min or the infant becomes symptomatic, in which case a pacemaker is necessary. Isoproterenol may increase the ventricular rate until a pacemaker is placed.**

SICK SINUS SYNDROME

Sick sinus syndrome (SSS) is a broad term used to describe dysrhythmias resulting from abnormal sinus node function and includes a wide array of bradydysrhythmias, including sinus bradycardia, sinus pause/arrest, sinoatrial exit block, and slow escape rhythms, including junctional bradycardia. Although **most commonly acquired during surgical repair for CHD** (because of the proximity to the sinus node), **SSS can be congenital.** Mutations in the cardiac sodium channel gene *SCN5A* can result in congenital SSS.[37]

PARENT TEACHING

If the diagnosis of CHD is made prenatally by fetal echocardiography, parent education begins before the birth of the infant (see the Parent

Parent Teaching

KEY POINTS FOR PARENTS OF NEWBORNS WITH HEART DISEASE

- Refer to a pediatric facility experienced with infants with heart disease.
- Reassure and support family for understanding that "this is not their fault."
- Explain all tubes, monitors, and equipment to decrease anxiety.
- Help parents accept and understand their infant's diagnosis.
- Encourage parental bonding with their infant and participation in care.
- Detail home care, to include medications, signs and symptoms, when to call physician.
- Encourage normal activity.
- Explain the necessity of subacute bacterial endocarditis protection.
- Supply parents with resource information—booklets, brochures, Internet resources.

Teaching box above). Expectant parents should be referred to a pediatric facility experienced in providing complex medical and surgical care for infants with CHD. Arrangements should be made for parents to meet with key members of the medical and surgical team and tour the intensive care units. The period of diagnosis, hospitalization, and early caregiving at home is extremely stressful.

The diagnosis of CHD in their infant is a frightening experience and causes much distress to parents. When an infant is born with a heart defect, the parents may grieve over the loss of the healthy newborn they had anticipated and experience shock, denial, guilt, anger, despair, or confusion. **Therefore comprehensive teaching, reassurance, and support are essential for the well-being of both the infant and the family. Understanding the heart defect aids in decreasing anxiety as well as allowing parents to provide good care after discharge.**

Explain the infant's heart defect to the parents. **Draw or show a picture of the heart defect, explaining briefly and simply the normal circulation of the heart and how the circulation of their infant's heart differs from normal.** This explanation should be repeated often for parental understanding and retention. Careful explanation of all tubes, monitors, equipment, and procedures in the nursery also helps decrease parental anxiety.

Heart defects are not visible lesions. Most of these infants will appear quite normal and healthy. Thus it may be difficult for some parents to accept that anything is wrong with their infant. In addition, parents are under great emotional and sometimes physical stress (from labor and delivery), which decreases their ability to hear and retain explanations about the defect. Patience and repetition of explanations is important.

Some parents may be unable at first to respond to their newborn with a heart defect. **Health care providers should facilitate bonding and decrease the parent's fear of holding or caring for their infant by encouraging interaction with the infant and enabling parents to participate in their infant's care.** The parents' confidence in caring for their infant at home should be established in the nursery. **Parents must feel comfortable caring for their infant and have the opportunity to demonstrate their ability to do so before discharge from the hospital.**

Teaching home care of the infant before discharge should be detailed and include medications, signs to observe, and guidelines for care. It is critical that these be written instructions that can be referred to often. Parents should telephone the physician if the infant demonstrates (1) poor feeding for 1 to 2 days or sweating with feeds, (2) vomiting most of feedings for a 12- to 24-hour period, (3) fast or labored breathing for several hours, (4) decreased activity level, (5) weight loss or failure to gain weight, and (6) frequent respiratory illnesses.[28]

All medications should be explained in detail, including their purpose, action, and administration. Parents should be made aware of the potential adverse effects (side effects) of all of their infant's medications. Parents should be observed giving medications in the nursery before the infant is discharged.

Cyanotic heart disease is particularly disturbing to parents because their infant's skin color is "blue." Parents should be cautioned that their infant will appear blue, especially around the mouth, mucous membranes, hands, and feet, and the blueness will increase with activity such as crying, feeding, and bowel movements. Parents should notify the physician about any of the previously listed symptoms in addition to (1) greatly increased cyanosis, especially if associated with fast or labored breathing, (2) decreased movement in any or all of the extremities, (3) decreased responsiveness or eyes deviating to one side, and (4) seizure activity such as jerking motions or stiffness followed by the infant becoming floppy or limp.[28]

Many parents will develop a narrow, disease-oriented focus. **Emphasize to parents that their infant should be treated as normally as possible. There is no activity restriction for infants with heart disease, because infants "self-limit" according to their capacity.** It is difficult for parents with a firstborn infant with heart disease to differentiate "normal baby problems" from cardiac-related problems. For these parents, as well as other parents of children with cardiac defects, it is particularly important to have open communication among the family, primary care provider, and cardiologist. Parents should be encouraged to call these medical personnel as needed for support, answers to questions, and reassurance. **Support groups of parents whose children have heart defects provide information, empathy, and practical tips to parents dealing with medical or surgical interventions for their child's heart defect.**

Active participation in care helps alleviate some of the parents' stress. Parental participation enables opportunities for parents to practice under the guidance of professionals and enables professional assessment of parental abilities, individualizing care, and building on existing competencies. **Parents should be encouraged to provide comfort measures such as touch and to assist with diaper changes, positioning, and oral care, even during the critical phase of illness. During the postoperative and convalescent phase of hospitalization, parents should assume more of the infant's care, such as feeding, care of the incision, and medication administration. Before discharge, parents should be encouraged to room with and completely care for their infant,** with nursing assistance available as needed.

Normal Newborn Care and Maintenance

Emphasis on **infection prevention strategies,** such as handwashing before handling the infant, avoiding ill contacts, and avoiding large crowds, is especially important to teach parents. The trip home should occur in a **proper car seat** with perhaps a small blanket placed over the chest to ensure that the safety straps do not rub the wound. Standard pediatric immunizations are delayed until just after surgery. **Provide information about the infant's prognosis and follow-up care and anticipatory guidance about special growth and development considerations. Provide explicit instructions on when to call the health care provider.**

Infectious Endocarditis Protection

Infants with congenital heart disease are at increased risk for developing adverse outcomes associated with infectious endocarditis (IE), also known as *bacterial endocarditis (BE).* Recently, the guidelines for the prevention of IE have changed dramatically. The American Heart Association's Endocarditis Committee extensively reviewed published studies and found no conclusive evidence to link dental or gastrointestinal (GI) or genitourinary (GU) tract procedures with the development of IE in most patients with congenital heart defects.[6] **Antibiotic prophylaxis with dental procedures is recommended only for patients with cardiac conditions (e.g., prosthetic valves, previous endocarditis, cardiac transplant) associated with the highest risk for adverse outcomes from endocarditis. Antibiotic prophylaxis is also recommended for the following categories of CHD: (1) unrepaired cyanotic CHD; (2) completely repaired CHD with prosthetic material, such as conduits; and (3) repaired CHD with residual defects adjacent to prosthetic material.**[6] Parents are encouraged to speak with their pediatric cardiologist regarding any questions related to IE antibiotic prophylaxis.

Activity

Normal newborn activity is encouraged after discharge. Special precautions are indicated for handling. **Teach parents to avoid picking the infant up under the arms until the wound and underlying structures are healed.**

Supporting Ongoing Development

Infants are at risk for neurodevelopmental abnormalities for a number of reasons. The incidence of brain abnormalities is higher than in the general population. Review normal developmental milestones, provide pragmatic strategies to maximize infant development, and fully inform parents about their infant's increased risk for developmental delay. Referral to early intervention programs may be helpful.

Parenting an infant with CHD requires adaptation, coping, and evolution—from diagnosis to discharge from the hospital and through caretaking and parenting at home. **Parents need an outlet so that they feel free to share their thoughts and concerns in a nonjudgmental environment. Consultation with a mental health professional may enable the family to recognize and build on strengths that will help them cope with this enormous challenge.**

FUTURE RESEARCH

Improvements in the diagnosis and treatment of CHD have drastically reduced the morbidity and mortality associated with these defects. Future research lies in increasing knowledge about the genetic contributions to CHD. Genetic tests are available for many syndromes strongly associated with structural CHD (e.g., Noonan syndrome, pulmonary valve stenosis) and most chromosomal abnormalities associated with CHD (e.g., Down syndrome, complete atrioventricular septal defect [AVSD]).[37] There is a genetic test (fluorescent in situ hybridization [FISH]) for DiGeorge syndrome, which is often associated with interrupted aortic arch (IAA), tetralogy of Fallot (TOF), or truncus arteriosus. Further research also is being done on the development of surgical and technologic approaches for cardiac surgery of the fetus, as well as reduction of mortality associated with the pediatric cardiac surgery patient. Tissue engineering is also an emerging area of inquiry with the focus on bioengineering of pediatric heart valves and vascular tissue.

REFERENCES

1. Aggarwal S, Chintala K, Humes RA: Sildenafil use in a symptomatic neonate with severe Ebstein's anomaly of the tricuspid valve, *Am J Perinatol* 25(2):125, 2008.
2. Allen HD, Driscoll DJ, Shaddy RE, et al, editors: *Moss and Adams heart disease in infants, children, and adolescents: including the fetus and young adults*, ed 7, Philadelphia, 2008, Lippincott Williams & Wilkins.
3. American Heart Association: *Children with congenital or acquired heart disease*, Dallas, 2008, The Association. Accessed October 4, 2009, from www.americanheart.org.
4. Bakiler AR, Ozer EA, Kanik A, et al: Accuracy of prenatal diagnosis of congenital heart disease with fetal echocardiography, *Fetal Diagn Ther* 22:241, 2007.
5. Bentham J, Bhattacharya S: Genetic mechanisms controlling cardiovascular development, *Ann NY Acad Sci* 1123(1):10, 2008.
6. Bobhate P, Pinto R: Summary of the new guidelines for prevention of infective endocarditis: implication for developing countries, *Ann Ped Cardiology* 56:58, 2008.
7. Castanada A: Congenital heart disease: a surgical-historical perspective, *Ann Thorac Surg* 79(5):S2217, 2005.
8. Cloherty JP, Eichenwald EC, Stark AR: *Manual of neonatal care*, ed 5, Philadelphia, 2004, Lippincott Williams & Wilkins.
9. Dice JE, Bhatia J: Patent ductus arteriosus: an overview, *J Pediatr Pharmacol Ther* 12:138, 2007.
10. Donze A, Smith JR, Bryosky K: Safety and efficacy of ibuprofen versus indomethacin for the treatment of patent ductus arteriosus in the preterm infant: reviewing the evidence, *Neonatal Netw* 26(3):187, 2007.
11. Gaca AM, Jaggers JJ, Dudley LT, et al: Repair of congenital heart disease: a primer—part 2, *Radiology* 248:44, 2008.
12. Garne E: Atrial and ventricular septal defects: epidemiology and spontaneous closure, *J Matern Fetal Neonatal Med* 19(5):271, 2006.
13. Gutierrez FR, Ho M, Siegel MJ: Practical application of magnetic resonance in congenital heart disease, *Magn Reson Imaging Clin N Am* 16(3):403, 2008.
14. Kabra NS, Schmidt B, Roberts RS, et al: Neurosensory impairment after surgical closure of patent ductus arteriosus in extremely low birth weight infants: results of the trial of indomethacin prophylaxis in preterms, *J Pediatr* 150:229, 2007.
15. Karamlou T, McCrindle BW, Williams WG: Surgery insight: late complications following repair of tetralogy of Fallot and related surgical strategies for management, *Nat Clin Pract Cardiovasc Med* 3:611, 2006.
16. Kirk EP, Sunde M, Costa MW, et al: Mutations in cardiac T-box factor gene *TBX0* are associated with diverse cardiac pathologies, including defects of septation and valvulogenesis and cardiomyopathy, *Am J Hum Genet* 81(2):280, 2007.
17. Kohon B, Butler H, Kirshbom P, et al: Closure of symptomatic ventricular septal defects: how early is too early? *Pediatr Cardiol* 29(1):36, 2008.
18. Lee W, Comstock CH: Prenatal diagnosis of congenital heart disease: where are we now?, *Ultrasound Clinics* 1:2, 2006.
19. Lopez V, Keen CL, Lanoue L: Prenatal zinc deficiency: influence on heart morphology and distribution of key heart proteins in a rat model, *Biol Trace Elem Res* 122(3):238, 2008.
20. Mahle WT: Physical examination and pulse oximetry in newborn infants: out with the old, in with the new? *J Pediatr* 152:747, 2008.

21. Maulik D: Echocardiography in detection of fetal heart abnormalities, *J Matern Fetal Neonatal Med* 19:9, 2006.
22. Miller SP, McQuillen PS, Hamrick S, et al: Abnormal brain development in newborns with congenital heart disease, *N Engl J Med* 357:1928, 2007.
23. Obidi E, Touba P, Sharma J: Atrial flutter in a premature infant with a structurally normal heart, *J Matern Fetal Neonatal Med* 19:113, 2006.
24. O'Connor M, McDaniel N, Brady WJ: The pediatric electrocardiogram. III. Congenital heart disease and other cardiac syndromes, *Am J Emerg Med* 26(4):497, 2008.
25. Ohlsson A, Walia R, Shah S: Ibuprofen for the treatment of patent ductus arteriosus in preterm and/or low birth weight infants, *Cochrane Database Syst Rev* 1:CD003481, 2008.
26. Pashia SE: Ebstein's anomaly, *Neonatal Netw* 26(3):197, 2007.
27. Pierpont ME, Basson CT, Benson Jr DW, et al: Genetic basis for congenital heart defects: current knowledge, *Circulation* 115:3015, 2007.
28. Pye S, Green A: Parent education after newborn congenital heart surgery, *Adv Neonatal Care* 3:147, 2003.
29. Rao PS: Perinatal circulatory physiology: its influence on clinical manifestations of neonatal heart disease. I, *Neonatol Today* 3(2):6, 2008.
30. Sekar KC, Corff KE: Treatment of patent ductus arteriosus: indomethacin or ibuprofen? *J Perinatol* 28(suppl 1):S60, 2008.
31. Spevak PJ, Johnson PT, Fishman EK: Review of surgically corrected congenital heart defects: utility of 64-MDCT, *AJR Am J Roentgenol* 191(3):854, 2008.
32. Tanner K, Sabrine N, Wren C: Cardiovascular malformations among preterm infants, *Pediatrics* 116(6):1536, 2005.
33. Tomita H, Takamuro M, Soda W, et al: Increased serum high-sensitivity C-reactive protein is related to hypoxia and brain natriuretic peptide in congenital heart disease, *Pediatr Int* 50:436, 2008.
34. Turck CJ, Marsh W, Stevenson JG, et al: Pharmacoeconomics of surgical intervention versus cyclooxygenase inhibitors for the treatment of patent ductus arteriosus, *J Pediatr Pharmocol Ther* 12(3):183, 2007.
35. Wooley CF, Miller PJ: William Osler, Maude Abbott, Paul Dudley White, and Helen Taussig: The origins of congenital heart disease in North America, *Am Heart Hosp J* 6(1):51, 2008.
36. Wren C, Reinhardt Z, Khawaja K: Twenty-year trends in diagnosis of life-threatening neonatal cardiovascular malformations, *Arch Dis Child Fetal Neonatal Ed* 93(1):F33, 2008.
37. Zeigler VL: Congenital heart disease and genetics, *Crit Care Nurs Clin North Am* 20(2):159, 2008.

RESOURCES FOR PARENTS

American Heart Association: *Children with congenital or acquired heart disease*: www.americanheart.org.

Congenital Heart Defects.com, sponsored by Baby Hearts Press: www.congenitalheartdefects.com.

Congenital Heart Information Network: www.tchin.org.

Kids With Heart National Association for Children's Heart Disorders: www.kidswithheart.org.

Little Hearts, Inc, national nonprofit organization: www.littlehearts.org.

Pediheart Organization: www.pediheart.org.

25

NEONATAL NEPHROLOGY

MACKENZIE S. FROST, LUCY FASHAW, JACINTO A. HERNANDEZ, AND M. DOUGLAS JONES, JR.

In utero, the fetal kidney is not necessary for toxin removal or fluid and electrolyte homeostasis; that is primarily the placenta's function. By contributing to amniotic fluid, the fetal kidney instead has an essential role in the normal development of the fetus. After birth, as the infant adapts to the external milieu, the kidney gradually assumes its role as regulator of fluid and electrolyte homeostasis. At birth, renal function changes dramatically, complicating clinical assessment. Assessment is an even greater challenge in the premature infant.

The more complicated an organ is in its development, the more subject it is to maldevelopment. In this aspect, the kidney outranks most other organs. **Abnormalities of the genitourinary system constitute up to 30% of all anomalies diagnosed prenatally.**[116] Anomalies may cause problems during the neonatal period, but they may also not be clinically apparent until the infant is an older child or adult.

Neonatal renal disease is important not just during the neonatal period but also as it may affect adult renal pathology. Congenital renal dysplasias, renal obstructive disorders, and cystic diseases account for a substantial percentage of patients with end-stage renal failure. Furthermore, a growing body of data supports a link between prenatal and neonatal events and later hypertension in adolescents and adults.[21,89,109]

NORMAL DEVELOPMENT

Anatomic Development of the Kidney[115,116]

The mammalian embryo progressively develops three sets of excretory organs, all of which might be termed the "embryonic kidney." The pronephros and mesonephros regress in the human but induce the metanephros, the direct precursor of the adult kidney (Figure 25-1). The pronephros, a solid mass of cells along the nephrogenic cord, is located at the cervical level at approximately 3 weeks' gestation. Degeneration of the pronephros begins soon after its formation, and regression has completely occurred by week 5. The pronephros has no excretory function but plays an important role in the formation of the mesonephros. The primitive ureter of the pronephros forms the wolffian, or mesonephric, duct via fusion of the pronephric tubular buds. The mesonephric duct then induces the formation of the second kidney, the mesonephros, at approximately 4 weeks of gestation. The mesonephros develops from the nephrogenic cord and forms 40 pairs of thin-walled tubules and glomeruli with excretory function. Portions of the mesonephric duct system are retained in the male fetus and form the ducts of the epididymis, the ductus deferens, and the ejaculatory duct. The remainder of the mesonephric duct system in the male infant has degenerated by the 4th month of gestation as the metanephric kidney develops. In the female, near-complete degeneration has occurred by the 3rd month of gestation.

The metanephros appears at 4½ to 5 weeks' gestation. The metanephric kidney is the product of a series of inductive interactions between the metanephric mesenchyme and epithelial ureteric bud. Initially, the ureteric bud grows from the mesonephric duct into the mesenchymal portion of the urogenital ridge; concomitantly, the metanephric mesenchyme changes, becoming histologically distinct from the surrounding tissue. When the metanephric mesenchyme and ureteric bud make contact, a condensation of cells begins along the surface of the bud. These cells are the beginnings of pretubular aggregates that undergo mesenchymal-to-epithelial transformation to become the segmented nephron. The condensed mesenchyme is also thought to produce

Please note that the **PURPLE** type in each chapter is intended to make it easier to identify clinically applicable material.

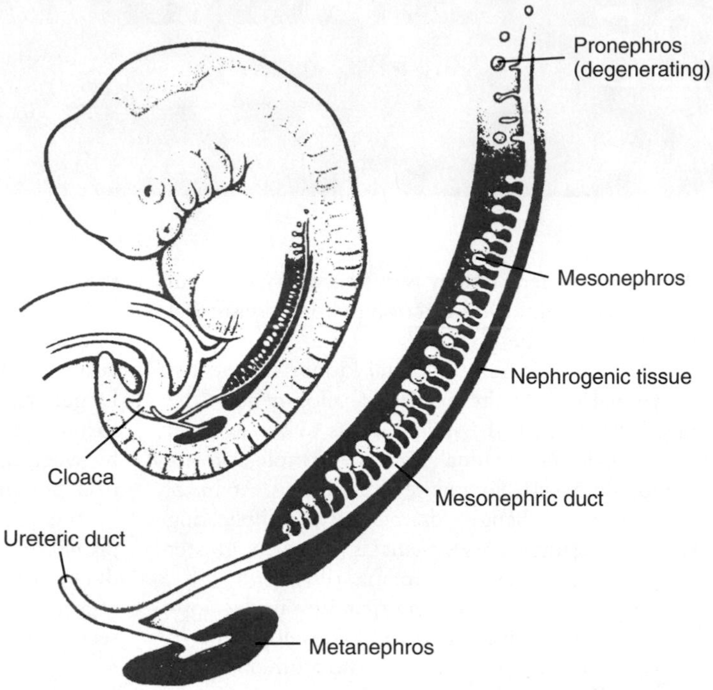

FIGURE 25-1 Schematic representation of overlapping stages in embryogenesis of human kidney. See text for detailed description. (From Holliday MA: Developmental abnormalities of the kidney in children, *Hosp Pract* 13:101, 1978.)

a number of stem cells, which remain undifferentiated and proliferative. These cells serve to maintain a supply of precursor cells until the completion of nephron development. Thus the epithelial portion of the adult kidney is derived from both the metanephric mesenchyme, via the stem cells ultimately responsible for individual nephron formation, and the ureteric bud, whose migration and division determine the pattern of formation of the urinary collecting system via its pretubular aggregates. The ureteric bud migrates to the most caudal end of the nephrogenic cord and finally to the lumbar region by week 8 of gestation. The ureteric bud also rotates 90 degrees medially along the longitudinal axis. Abnormalities in ascent or rotation can lead to pelvic kidneys, horseshoe kidneys, or crossed fused ectopia. Anomalies of the kidney often accompany anomalies of the ureter, as well as other portions of the urinary tract. **Congenital anomalies of the kidney and urinary tract (CAKUT) are a family of diseases with a diverse anatomic spectrum of kidney anomalies (agenesis, dysplasia, hypoplasia) and ureteropelvic anomalies (megaureter, agenesis, hydronephrosis, vesicoureteric reflux, posterior urethral valves, and ureteral duplications).**[48]

Nephrogenesis is the process of nephron formation via growth and differentiation of multiple cell types and leads to formation of the overall renal architecture. The process begins in the renal cortex closest to the medulla (juxtamedullary nephrons) and proceeds in a dichotomous branching centrifugal pattern with the outermost (superficial cortical) nephrons forming last. There are multiple phases of growth and structural reorganization following the interactions between the mesonephric mesenchyme and the ureteric bud. The formation of the collecting system is controlled by the branching pattern of the ureteral bud, and this occurs at the same time as the formation of functional nephron units. Four progressive phases of nephrogenesis occur during which the nephron proceeds through several intermediate forms. By the fourth stage, there is a definitive glomerulus with highly differentiated visceral and parietal epithelial cells. The vascular system development occurs in concert with nephron formation. The surrounding major vessels and spinal ganglia grow into the metanephros to complete the remaining cell types, and vessel architecture is similar to the newborn kidney by 15 weeks of gestation.

Physiologic Development and Clinical Assessment[5,21,38,59]

Although newborn kidneys are usually described as "immature," they are perfectly suited to their usual responsibilities. During the latter part of gestation, their primary role is maintenance of amniotic fluid volume. This requires a large volume of urine with a relatively high concentration of sodium. Thus **fetal urine output is on the order of 10 mL/kg/hr of sodium-rich urine.** Fetal fractional excretion of sodium (FENa) (i.e., the fraction of sodium in glomerular filtrate that appears in urine) is especially high, approximately 15%. This compares with less than 1% in a growing infant born after a full-term pregnancy.

The next major responsibility is during the first week of life. **Fetuses have a large amount of extracellular fluid (ECF).** ECF as a percentage of body weight progressively diminishes throughout gestation: (1) approximately 65% of body weight at 26 weeks of gestation; (2) 40% at full-term; and (3) 25% by 1 year of age. Most of the postnatal reduction occurs in the first week of life and is the primary reason that body weight may decrease by up to 10% in breast-fed term infants and even more in premature infants. The newborn kidney can handle this challenge without difficulty. Finally, in subsequent weeks, the kidney has no trouble retaining the electrolytes needed for growth and no trouble producing dilute urine to accommodate the large water load presented by breast milk. Growth itself is a powerful homeostatic ally. A substantial portion of carbohydrates, electrolytes, and nitrogenous wastes from protein absorbed from breast milk are never presented to the kidney for excretion. They are incorporated into the growing body.

Only when the neonatal kidney has to cope with unexpected derangements of water, electrolyte, or acid-base status secondary to premature birth or illness, especially illness accompanied by cessation of growth, does its relative lack of ability to concentrate urine, excrete extra sodium and potassium loads, conserve sodium (in preterm infants), and regulate acid-base status become problematic. In older children and adults, normal kidneys can correct for substantial errors in clinical judgment as to water and electrolyte administration or creation and correction of acid-base abnormalities. This is not so with neonatal kidneys, especially in smaller preterm infants.

With that in mind, it is helpful to review specific aspects of neonatal renal function.

Nephron Development[21,89]

The process of forming the adult complement of approximately 600,000 nephrons in each kidney is complete by 34 to 36 weeks gestational age (GA). Development proceeds in centrifugal fashion, with juxtamedullary nephrons developing first and superficial cortical nephrons last.[5] **In general, nephron development continues at approximately the same rate even if the infant is born prematurely.** In other words, development continues whether *in utero* or *ex utero.* For example, a premature infant born at 28 weeks of gestation will not complete nephrogenesis for another 6 to 8 weeks (Figure 25-2). Despite continued nephrogenesis, infants with intrauterine growth restriction and those born with extremely low birth weights may never achieve a normal number of nephrons. This has been termed ***congenital oligophrenia.*** Compromised renal function and elevated blood pressures have been reported on long-term follow-up of small preterm infants.

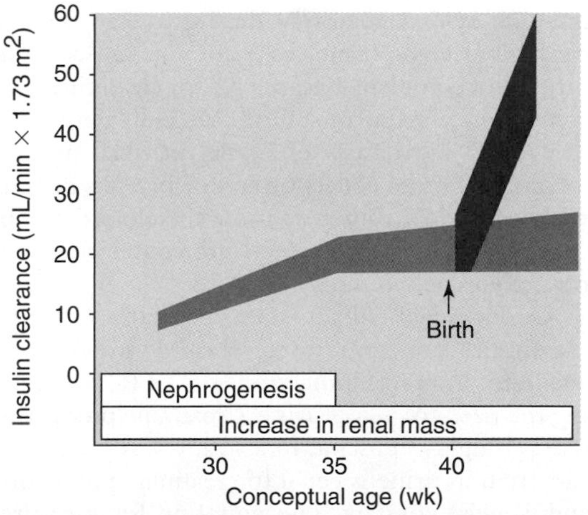

FIGURE 25-2 Correlation of glomerular filtration rate (GFR) as measured by insulin clearance and post-conceptual age. Note marked increase in GFR postnatally. However, this increase in GFR does not occur after 40 weeks unless birth occurs. If birth occurs before nephrogenesis is complete (usually at 35 weeks), this increase will not occur until 34 to 36 weeks postmenstrual age. (From Guignard JP: Neonatal nephrology. In Holliday MA, Barratt TM, Vernier RL, editors: *Pediatric nephrology,* ed 2, Baltimore, 1987, Williams & Wilkins.)

Glomerular Filtration Rate*

Glomerular filtration rate (GFR) is the rate at which filtrate of renal blood, or more precisely of renal plasma, appears in proximal renal tubules. **A primary physiologic limitation of the neonatal kidney, increasingly so with decreasing gestational age, is limited GFR.** For the fetus, the placenta serves to maintain fluid and electrolyte composition and clearance of metabolic wastes. Thus renal arterial blood flow is approximately 5% of fetal cardiac output as compared with 25% later on. After full-term birth, GFR doubles to triples in the first weeks of life (see Figure 25-2) and then further increases to adult levels between 1 and 2 years of life.

The situation is different in infants born before 34 to 36 weeks GA. For example, GFR is approximately 5 mL/min/1.73 m^2 or approximately 0.5 mL/kg/min (30 mL/kg/hr) in a 24-week infant. That increases little in absolute terms until 34 to 36 weeks of gestation (see Figure 25-2). Thereafter GFR increases rapidly, as it does in full-term infants although, as just mentioned, it may never reach normal adult values.

In clinical settings, GFR may be estimated using the clearance of creatinine. For this to be accurate, serum creatinine concentration must be constant, creatinine in the urine must represent creatinine in glomerular filtrate with no creatinine added or taken away during passage through renal tubules, and urine collection must be carefully timed and complete. Because serum creatinine concentrations change after birth, filtered creatinine is reabsorbed by tubules, especially in small preterm infants, and urine collection in newborns is difficult without bladder catheterization; therefore determination of creatinine clearance is uncommon in neonatal intensive care units (NICUs).

Under ideal steady-state conditions, serum creatinine concentrations should provide an accurate indirect indication of GFR, eliminating the need to collect urine. Creatinine production rate is roughly constant. In a steady state, creatinine excretion in urine is equal to creatinine production and likewise constant. **The equation for measurement of GFR with creatinine is as follows:**

$$\text{Serum creatinine concentration} = \frac{\text{Urinary creatinine excretion}}{\text{GFR}}$$

*References 5,6,21,59,89,96,107.

Serum creatinine concentration is thus equal to a constant divided by GFR. Therefore a true increase in creatinine concentration from 0.4 to 0.5 mg/dL, a 25% increase, indicates a reduction in GFR of 20%; the inverse of 1.25 is 0.80.

As mentioned, strict steady-state conditions are often absent in the neonatal period. **Nevertheless, serum creatinine concentration is useful as a general indicator of renal function.** In full-term infants, as GFR increases, creatinine concentration falls during the first week of life from 0.8 to 1.2 mg/dL, reflecting maternal creatinine concentrations, to neonatal levels of 0.2 to 0.3 mg/dL. The rate of decrease depends on hydration and clinical status. **Rising or stable serial serum creatinine concentrations or an isolated value exceeding 0.5 mg/dL after 1 week of age indicates renal dysfunction.**

In preterm infants, the steep increase in GFR does not occur until nephrogenesis is complete at 34 to 36 weeks postmenstrual age (PMA). Furthermore, filtered creatinine is reabsorbed along the tubule. This increases with decreasing gestational age and PMA. As a result, creatinine concentrations often rise in the first 24 to 48 hours and are then slow to fall. Gestational-age– and postnatal-age–based graphs are needed to identify abnormal values.[6,107] After the initial increase in creatinine concentration, concentration should slowly fall. A secondary rise indicates renal dysfunction.

Tubular Function[5,49]

Urine flow depends on both GFR and tubular reabsorption. **Fetal GFR is approximately 30 mL/kg/hr, yet fetal urine output is 10 mL/kg/hr. GFR in full-term infants is approximately 90 mL/kg/hr, yet urine output is 2 to 3 mL/kg/hr.** The difference is the activity of the renal tubule.

Oliguria is ordinarily defined as urine output of less than 1 mL/kg/hr. However, urine output may transiently decrease immediately after birth to less than 1 mL/kg/hr because tubular reabsorption of water increases because of an increase in fetal antidiuretic hormone (ADH) during labor. Nevertheless, 50% of full-term infants void by 12 hours, 92% by 24 hours, and 99% by 48 hours of life. Causes for prolonged failure to void include poor cardiac output or blood pressure, primary renal dysfunction, and obstruction to urine flow. After transient oliguria/anuria, urine flow rate increases as the newborn excretes his or her physiologically expanded fetal extracellular fluid volume as described earlier.

Proximal Tubular Function*

The proximal tubule is responsible for reabsorbing glucose, amino acids, and most of the bicarbonate, sodium chloride, and water in glomerular filtrate. In smaller preterm infants, tubular transport mechanisms are insufficient to prevent spillage of each of these in varying degrees.

Sodium[8,15,23,30,99]

Physiologic diuresis in the first week of life is accompanied by physiologic natriuresis. The kidney is then responsible for conserving sufficient dietary sodium for growth. This is a challenge for preterm infants (Figure 25-3). Thus **premature infants often require extra sodium intake to compensate for what amounts to obligatory sodium wastage.** Conversely, in the presence of a sodium load (e.g., from administration of large amounts of sodium chloride), the neonatal kidney cannot compensate with a rapid increase in FENa. The result is edema and possibly circulatory overload.

Potassium[5,41]

The kidney is an important site for regulation of potassium balance. In the adult, it is responsible for maintaining zero balance. In contrast, to sustain the neonate, the kidney must maintain positive potassium balance. In this context, it is less surprising that mechanisms for potassium excretion are underdeveloped at birth.

Serum potassium concentrations tend to be high in neonates (5.5 to 6 mEq/L).[59] The levels are not of pathologic significance and perhaps play a role in supporting growth. This serves to point out the importance of growth as a homeostatic mechanism. Some clinicians have the impression that nonoliguric hyperkalemia in small preterm infants is less common since routine institution of early parenteral protein administration.

*References 5,8,15,20,30,49,59,99.

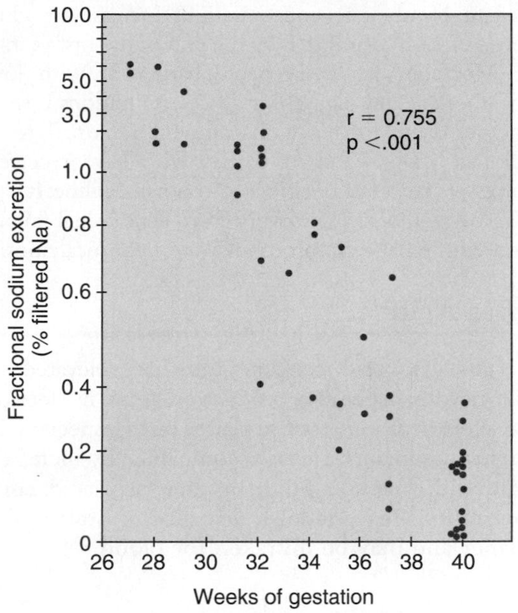

FIGURE 25-3 Decrease in fractional excretion of sodium occurs with increasing postconceptual age. *Na,* Sodium. (From Siegel S, Oh W: Renal function as a marker of human fetal maturation, *Acta Paediatr Scand* 65:481, 1976.)

Acid-Base Balance[5,59,84]

By adult standards, serum bicarbonate concentrations are low in full-term newborns (19-21 mEq/L) and even lower (16-20 mEq/L) in premature infants. Lower serum bicarbonate concentrations reflect limited ability to cope with the higher acid load from high protein intake and acid generated with formation of new bone. The capacity of the neonatal proximal tubule to reabsorb filtered bicarbonate is one-third that of an adult. Proximal tubular bicarbonate reabsorption is further compromised if ECF is over-expanded with crystalloid solutions; because proximal tubular sodium and bicarbonate reabsorption are closely linked, bicarbonate is wasted as sodium reabsorption decreases to rid the body of excess sodium chloride. The capacities of the collecting duct to secrete hydrogen ions and of the proximal tubule to make ammonia to buffer secreted hydrogen ion are also limited. The net result is limited capacity to correct metabolic acidosis. Limited ability to achieve minimal urine pH values is relative. If serum bicarbonate is low enough (e.g., 14 to 15 mEq/L), the kidney can completely reabsorb the smaller amount of filtered bicarbonate and achieve a urine pH of 5.

Serum bicarbonate concentrations increase to adult levels of 24 to 26 mEq/L by the end of the first year.

Metabolic acidemia (see Chapter 8) with low bicarbonate and high chloride concentrations is seen in premature infants with transient proximal renal tubular acidosis and in infants who have received excessive amounts of chloride in normal saline. It can also be seen during recovery from acute renal failure and with renal vein thrombosis and nephrocalcinosis.

Uric Acid[101]

Serum uric acid concentrations are elevated in the newborn because production from nucleotide breakdown is increased just after birth, especially in premature infants. This is accompanied by increased uric acid excretion. **High urinary uric acid concentrations leave reddish uric acid crystals in the diaper and may be mistaken for blood.**

CONGENITAL AND ACQUIRED RENAL ABNORMALITIES

Chromosomal Disorders[115,116]

Although lower urinary tract and renal anomalies are seldom the presenting feature of chromosomal disorders, they frequently form part of a multisystem malformation syndrome caused by chromosomal anomalies. Renal disorders seen with chromosomal disturbance include fused kidneys, duplication defects, renal agenesis or hypoplasia, hydronephrosis and hydroureter, renal dysplasia or cystic disease, hypospadias, micropenis, and cryptorchidism.

The overall pattern of malformation with individual chromosomal disorders is usually sufficient for diagnosis; however, variation can be seen from one individual to another, even for patients with aneuploidy. Although certain renal anomalies are characteristic of certain chromosomal disorders, no one renal malformation is unique to any particular chromosomal disorder.

Consequences of obstruction of the developing nephron unit include hydronephrosis, hydroureter, and cortical cysts. Severe obstruction leads to renal dysplasia or agenesis. Dysplasia and agenesis may also be secondary to developmental growth failure and may be unilateral or bilateral. In the case of the multicystic dysplastic kidney, there may be no evidence of obstruction, whereas in other cases, dysplasia may be secondary to lower tract dysfunction and obstruction. Typically, the dysplastic kidney does not keep up with somatic growth and gradually shrinks and disappears.

Acquired Disorders*

Three drugs commonly used in neonates may cause renal damage and dysfunction: furosemide, aminoglycosides, and nonsteroidal anti-inflammatory drugs (NSAIDs). GFR changes with gestational and postnatal age, making it difficult to relate toxicity to dosage.

Furosemide may cause electrolyte and acid-base disturbances, including hyponatremia, hypochloremia, hypokalemia, and metabolic alkalosis. It increases calcium excretion and may be associated with nephrocalcinosis and less commonly with nephrolithiasis, secondary hyperparathyroidism, and osteopenia. Although nephrocalcinosis can occur without furosemide, there is little doubt that furosemide increases the risk. Calcification and the additional complication of renal tubular acidosis may be ameliorated or reversed by promotion of calcium reabsorption by addition of a thiazide diuretic.[93,97] The long-term effects of nephrocalcinosis in preterm infants are not clear. **Ototoxicity is another complication of furosemide, especially when used in combination with aminoglycosides.**

Aminoglycosides have long been one of the commonest causes of drug-induced nephrotoxicity. Pharmacokinetic monitoring can achieve desired concentrations (peak 6 to 8 mcg/mL and trough <2 mcg/mL) and reduce risk. The neonate may be at less risk for nephrotoxicity from aminoglycosides than is the mature kidney. However, gentamicin-induced renal toxicity was recently confirmed in the neonatal kidney without any relationship to peak and trough serum levels. In fact, the long-term effects of neonatal aminoglycoside exposure on renal development have yet to be adequately evaluated. **Ototoxicity is the second main adverse effect of aminoglycosides and, in contrast to nephrotoxicity, is irreversible.**

The nephrotoxicity induced by aminoglycosides manifests clinically as nonoliguric renal failure, with a slow rise in serum creatinine and a hypo-osmolar urine developing after several days of treatment. The nephrotoxicity of the aminoglycosides is believed to be secondary to a small percentage of retained drug within the kidney's proximal epithelial cells. At low

*References 9-12,41,42,52,54,73,110.

or appropriate doses, tubular alterations can generate proteinuria, hypo-osmotic urine, and increases in blood urea nitrogen (BUN) and creatinine reflecting a decrease in GFR. At higher doses of aminoglycosides, tubular wasting of potassium, magnesium, and calcium, along with decreased water reabsorption, bicarbonate, and glucose concomitantly with tubular necrosis, can be seen.

Since the 1970s, premature infants with symptomatic patent ductus arteriosus (PDA) have been treated with indomethacin, a nonspecific prostaglandin inhibitor. Indomethacin, as well as other NSAIDs, has been shown to have various side effects including hemodynamic changes in cerebral, mesenteric, and renal circulations. **The renal side effects seen with indomethacin appear to be related to three phenomena, as follows:**

1. Intrauterine cyclooxygenase (COX) inhibition may induce renal dysplasia and dysgenesis and alter renal maturation by slowing glomerular maturation.
2. Oligohydramnios may be the end result of fetal indomethacin exposure with concomitant decline in renal blood flow and glomerular filtration.
3. Indomethacin given for closure of PDA may induce and exacerbate renal failure by changing the balance of cortical juxtamedullary nephron perfusion.

The fragile balance of vasoconstrictor (mediated by angiotensin II, endothelin) and vasodilatory (atrial natriuretic peptide, nitric oxide, prostaglandins, kallikrein-kinin) forces is now altered in favor of vasoconstriction and further reduction of the already low GFR.

For preterm infants and newborns, the administration of NSAIDs should be done with care and frequent monitoring of renal function, even though these changes often are reversible. When a change or decline in GFR is noted (e.g., plasma creatinine increase), then the administration of NSAIDs should be halted. **Indomethacin has been shown to have clinically important renal side effects including proteinuria, oliguria, renal failure, hyperkalemia, and hyponatremia.** Patients at higher risk include those with persistent patent ductus arteriosus, dehydration, and simultaneous administration of other nephrotoxic drugs. Unfortunately, the combined use of furosemide and indomethacin does not improve outcome. At this time, in the absence of large randomized and controlled trials, guidelines for NSAID administration must rely on animal studies. In addition, there are no studies on the effect of selective COX inhibitors on PDA closure.

The neonatal patient, particularly the low-birth-weight infant, is now exposed to an increased use of invasive procedures and broad-spectrum antimicrobial therapy and therefore is at a higher risk for systemic fungal sepsis. Agents for therapy include amphotericin B, which is associated with adverse effects, including infusion reactions with hemodynamic instability and nephrotoxicity with electrolyte disturbances.

Multiple studies have indicated that **maintenance of adequate fluid and electrolyte balance before amphotericin B administration may prevent nephrotoxicity.** In particular, two strategies, use of a liposomal amphotericin system and salt-loading before amphotericin B administration, are employed. To date, no definitive controlled data exist that show an ameliorated risk for liposomal amphotericin B. **Salt-loading, on the other hand, before amphotericin B therapy, of greater than 4 mEq/kg/day may reduce nephrotoxicity;** the exact mechanism by which sodium reduces the incidence and severity of amphotericin B–induced nephrotoxicity has not been shown. Suggestions have been made that amphotericin B–enhanced tubuloglomerular feedback is reversed by high sodium intake.

GENERAL DATA COLLECTION[38,55,66,109]

History

A complete family history of renal disease or syndromes that involve the kidneys is important. Prenatal exposures to maternal infection, drugs, toxin, or medication intake are risk factors. Paternal smoking and advanced age may also be associated with an increased risk for urinary tract anomalies.

The quantity of amniotic fluid is an indicator of fetal renal function since fetal urination is responsible for most of the amniotic fluid volume beginning in the second trimester of pregnancy. Normally, amniotic fluid volume increases during gestation, peaking at 34 weeks of gestation. **Severe fetal genitourinary abnormalities result in oligohydramnios (Table 25-1). Severe urinary concentrating defects (e.g., diabetes insipidus and Bartter syndrome) have been associated with polyhydramnios. Perinatal asphyxia is a risk factor for renal damage.**

TABLE 25-1 PERINATAL INDICATORS SUGGESTIVE OF ABNORMALITIES OF THE GENITOURINARY TRACT

FINDING	SUSPECTED ABNORMALITY
Oligohydramnios	Bilateral renal agenesis, polycystic kidney disease, or dysplasia Amnion nodosum
Polyhydramnios	Nephrogenic diabetes insipidus, trisomy 18 or 21, anencephaly, esophageal or duodenal obstruction, Klippel-Feil syndrome, Bartter syndrome
Enlarged placenta (>25% of infant birth weight)	Congenital nephrotic syndrome
Velamentous insertion of umbilical cord	Increased congenital anomalies
Asphyxia neonatorum	Renal failure
PHYSICAL EXAMINATION	
Hypertension	See text
SKIN	
Hemangioma	Hemangioma of kidney or bladder
Edema	Congenital nephrotic syndrome, hydrops fetalis
Adenoma sebaceum	Tuberous sclerosis—cystic kidneys
HEAD	
Encephalocele	Meckel's or Meckel-Gruber syndrome—polycystic kidney disease
Cleft lip and palate	Urinary tract anomalies
Macroglossia	Beckwith-Wiedemann syndrome—renal dysplasia Johanson-Blizzard syndrome—hydronephrosis, orofacial-digital syndrome—renal microcystic disease
EYES	
Phakoma (tubular sclerosis)	Angiomyolipoma of the kidney
Retinitis pigmentosa	Medullary cystic disease of the kidney
Cataracts	Cystic disease, Lowe syndrome, Wilms' tumor, congenital rubella
Aniridia	Wilms' tumor
EARS	
Low-set or malformed	Increased risk for renal abnormalities, Potter syndrome
Ear tags	Branchio-oto-renal (BOR) syndrome
Preauricular pits	
SKELETON	
Hemihypertrophy	Wilms' tumor
Spina bifida	Neurogenic bladder
Arthrogryposis	Oligohydramnios, Potter syndrome
Dysplastic nails	Nail patella syndrome

Modified from Retek AB: Genitourinary problems in children, *Hosp Pract* 11:133, 1976.
VATER, Vertebral defects, imperforate anus, tracheoesophageal fistula, and radial and renal dysplasia.

TABLE 25-1 PERINATAL INDICATORS SUGGESTIVE OF ABNORMALITIES OF THE GENITOURINARY TRACT—cont'd

FINDING	SUSPECTED ABNORMALITY
SKELETON—cont'd	
Vertebral anomalies	VATER syndrome—renal dysplasia
Polydactyly	Meckel's or Meckel-Gruber syndrome—polycystic kidney disease
ABDOMEN	
Absence of abdominal musculature	Prune-belly syndrome
Single umbilical artery	Increased congenital anomalies of the urinary tract
Umbilical discharge	Patent urachus
Abdominal mass	See Table 25-6
Hepatomegaly	Storage diseases—renal tubular dysfunction, Beckwith-Wiedemann syndrome, Zellweger syndrome
PULMONARY	
Spontaneous pneumothorax	Increase in renal anomalies
Pulmonary hypoplasia	Oligohydramnios
GENITOURINARY—MALE	
Undescended testes	Prune-belly syndrome, Noonan syndrome, Lawrence-Moon-Biedl syndrome
Congenital absence of vas deferens	Renal agenesis or ectopia
Hypospadias	Increase in renal anomalies
Abnormal urinary stream	Bladder dysfunction or urethral outlet obstruction
GENITOURINARY—FEMALE	
Enlarged clitoris	Adrenogenital syndrome
Cystic mass in urethral region	Ectopic ureterocele, paraurethral cyst Sarcoma botryoides
Bulging in vagina	Hydrometrocolpos
Abnormal urinary stream or dribbling	Bladder dysfunction, urethral obstruction
Common cloaca	Urinary tract abnormalities
URINALYSIS	See text
RECTAL	
Deficient anal sphincter tone	Neurogenic bladder dysfunction
Dilated prostatic urethra	Posterior urethral valves, prune-belly syndrome
Masses	Tumor
Anal atresia	VATER syndrome—renal dysplasia (see text)

Signs and Symptoms

Physical findings that are indicators of genitourinary tract abnormalities are outlined in Table 25-1.

Laboratory Data

IMAGING STUDIES[87,109,115]

Fetal ultrasound can provide (1) estimation of amniotic fluid volume, (2) information on the appearance and echogenicity of kidneys, and (3) evidence of renal and/or lower tract dilation. Prenatal ultrasonography can define anatomy but does not accurately predict function. Mild dilation does not necessarily mean obstruction. More severe dilation and reduced amniotic fluid volume are more likely to mean obstruction and compromised renal function. The more severe the dilation (>7 mm after 32 weeks of gestation), the more likely the infant will need either follow-up or even surgical intervention. The later in pregnancy that dilation is found, the more likely hydronephrosis will be confirmed postnatally.

Nuclear scans are most useful when abnormalities are severe (e.g., lack of renal perfusion). A **voiding cystourethrogram** evaluates the lower urinary tract and is typically reserved for more mature infants.

URINALYSIS

Specific Gravity. Specific gravity in term infants ranges from 1.001-1.005 to 1.015-1.020. **Specific gravity is useful as an indicator of urine osmolality and thus of the ability of the kidney to concentrate and dilute. However, it can be altered by the presence of glucose, protein, and urinary contrast agents.** In that case, osmolality must be measured directly and compared with serum osmolality.

Glucosuria. Trace quantities of glucose may be found occasionally in term infants and more frequently in premature infants. Even minor elevations of plasma glucose concentrations may cause glucosuria. Large glucose loads may cause osmotic diuresis.

Urinary pH. Urinary pH is typically around 6, although most neonates can achieve a urine pH of 5. Urine pH is frequently 7 or greater in premature infants with proximal renal bicarbonate wasting.

Hematuria.[19,76] **Hematuria is defined as more than 5 to 6 red blood cells per high-power field (hpf).** A positive dipstick test occurs with hemoglobinuria from hemolysis and with myoglobinuria from muscle breakdown, usually from asphyxia. Hematuria may occur if kidneys are damaged during delivery, especially with an enlarged kidney (e.g., cystic disease, obstruction). **Hematuria is common in perinatal asphyxia.** Other conditions associated with hematuria are renal vein thrombosis, urinary tract infections, sepsis, renal artery embolization (especially from umbilical artery catheters), renal necrosis, hypercalciuria, coagulopathies, and, rarely, congenital glomerulonephritis or nephrosis. Factitious hematuria may occur as a result of blood from circumcision, perineal irritation, and uterine bleeding caused by withdrawal from maternal hormones. If hematuria is persistent, it should be evaluated with urine culture, assessment of proteinuria and urine calcium excretion, assessment of GFR, and an anatomic evaluation of the kidneys.

Pyuria.[38] Pyuria is common in newborns, especially females. As many as 25 to 50 white blood cells (WBCs) per hpf may be observed in the first days of life. Pyuria may indicate infection, and a urine culture should be obtained if clinically indicated. However, pyuria also may indicate noninfectious renal injury.

Proteinuria.[77] A positive dipstick test for protein indicates the amino groups of proteins. Although convenient, dipstick testing is subject to limitations. Because albumin and low-molecular-weight proteins give positive results, dipstick testing cannot distinguish between glomerular and tubular proteinuria. An alkaline urine (pH of ≈8) may give a false-positive result. The test may also be confounded by prolonged immersion of the strip and by the presence of detergents, WBCs, or bacteria in the urine. If urine is concentrated, small amounts of protein can give a falsely elevated reading; conversely, if the urine is dilute, important amounts of protein will go undetected.

ACUTE RENAL FAILURE

Pathophysiology

Acute renal failure (ARF) in the newborn is a relatively common problem. Although the precise incidence and prevalence of acute renal failure in the NICU is unknown, several studies have shown an incidence between 6% and 24%.[3,4,103] ***ARF* is defined as the sudden deterioration of the kidney's baseline function and is usually characterized by an increase in** the blood concentration of creatinine and nitrogenous waste products, by a decrease in the GFR, and by the inability of the kidney to appropriately regulate fluid and electrolyte homeostasis.

After birth, the serum creatinine in the newborn is a reflection of maternal renal function and cannot be used as a measure of renal function in the newborn shortly after birth.[4,20,22,96] **In full-term healthy newborns, the serum creatinine declines to about 0.4 to 0.6 mg/dL at about 2 weeks of age.** In premature infants, this postnatal decline in serum creatinine is at a slower rate. As a general rule, **the more premature the infant, the higher the serum creatinine. Any rising serum creatinine from initial baseline or a serum creatinine greater than 1.5 mg/dL with normal maternal function should be investigated.**

A decline in urine output is a common clinical manifestation of ARF (e.g., prerenal failure, hypoxic-ischemic insults, or cortical necrosis), but **many forms of ARF are associated with normal urine output** (e.g., nephrotoxic renal insults).

Etiology

There are many different causes of renal failure in the newborn (Box 25-1). These causes are typically classified as prerenal, intrinsic renal disease including vascular insults, and obstructive uropathy. The preponderance of factors causing ARF in the newborn are prerenal in nature (e.g., hypoxia, hypovolemia, hypotension); primary intrinsic renal disease and obstructive uropathy are much less common.

In ***prerenal failure,*** renal function is decreased because of decreased renal perfusion and the kidney is intrinsically normal. **Renal hypoperfusion results from true volume contraction (e.g., hemorrhage, dehydration, third space losses) or from a decreased effective blood volume (e.g., congestive heart failure, cardiac tamponade).**

Timely correction of the underlying disturbance and restoration of normal perfusion will return renal function to normal. Alternatively, profound and prolonged hypoperfusion can lead to intrinsic kidney damage. However, the evolution of prerenal failure to intrinsic renal failure is not sudden, and a number of compensatory mechanisms work together to maintain renal perfusion when it is otherwise compromised.[4,55]

Acute tubular necrosis (ATN) can evolve from prerenal failure if the insult is severe and sufficient enough to result in vasoconstriction and patchy

BOX 25-1 ETIOLOGY OF ACUTE RENAL FAILURE IN NEWBORNS

Prerenal Failure

Decreased True Intravascular Volume

- Dehydration
- Gastrointestinal losses
- Salt-wasting renal or adrenal disease
- Central nephrogenic diabetes insipidus
- Third space losses (sepsis, traumatized tissue)

Decreased Effective Intravascular Blood Volume

- Congestive heart failure
- Pericarditis, cardiac tamponade

Intrinsic Renal Disease

Acute Tubular Necrosis

- Ischemic/hypoxic insults
- Drug induced
  - Aminoglycosides
  - Intravascular contrast
  - Nonsteroidal anti-inflammatory drugs
- Toxin mediated
  - Endogenous toxins
  - Rhabdomyolysis, hemoglobinuria
- Interstitial nephritis
  - Drug induced—antibiotics, anticonvulsants
  - Idiopathic
- Vascular lesions
  - Cortical necrosis
  - Renal artery thrombosis
  - Renal venous thrombosis
- Infectious causes
  - Sepsis
  - Pyelonephritis
- Obstructive uropathy
  - Obstruction in a solitary kidney
  - Bilateral ureteral obstruction
  - Urethral obstruction

Congenital Renal Diseases

- Dysplasia/hypoplasia
  - Cystic renal diseases
    - Autosomal recessive polycystic kidney disease
    - Autosomal dominant polycystic kidney disease
    - Cystic dysplasia

From Andreoli SP: Acute renal failure in the newborn, *Sem Perinatol* 28:112, 2004.

tubular necrosis. The prognosis of ATN is good, except when the severity of the insult leads to the development of cortical necrosis. The recovery of the renal function depends on the underlying events that precipitated the ischemic/hypoxic insult. The length of time before recovery is quite variable (few days to several weeks). **Return of renal function may be accompanied by a diuretic phase with excessive urine output. During this phase, close attention to fluid and electrolyte balance is very important to ensure adequate fluid management to promote recovery and prevent additional renal damage.**

In the newborn, some forms of renal failure may have a prenatal onset in congenital diseases, such as renal dysplasia with or without obstructive uropathy, and in genetic diseases, such as autosomal recessive polycystic kidney. **Acute renal failure in the newborn is also commonly acquired in the postnatal period because of hypoxic ischemic injury and toxic insults.** In fact, asphyxia is the most common cause of acute tubular necrosis in the term neonate (65%), both oliguric and nonoliguric.[82] In the premature infant, sepsis is the most common cause (35%). Patients with congenital heart disease appear to be especially vulnerable to tubular necrosis after cardiac catheterization and cardiac surgery. **Nephrotoxic ARF in newborns is commonly associated with the administration of aminoglycoside antibiotics, NSAIDs, intravascular contrast media, and amphotericin B.** Indomethacin therapy to promote closure of the patent ductus arteriosus in premature neonates is associated with renal dysfunction in approximately 40% of exposed infants. These alterations are usually reversible.[2,9,39,45] Nephrotoxic ARF from exposure to endogenous compounds such as hemoglobinuria or myoglobinuria is very rare in the newborn.

Renal artery thrombosis and renal venous thrombosis will result in renal failure if bilateral or if either occur in a solitary kidney. In addition to acute renal failure, infants may demonstrate hypertension, gross or microscopic hematuria, thrombocytopenia, and oliguria.

Diagnosis

The diagnosis of acute renal failure in the newborn is not an easy one since oliguria is not a consistent finding and serum creatinine is an unreliable predictor of glomerular filtration in neonates. However, **serum creatinine values consistently above the 99th percentile, prolonged oliguria, or failure to achieve a diuresis is clinically significant.**

The urine osmolality, urine sodium concentration, fractional excretion of sodium, and renal failure index have been proposed for use to help differentiate prerenal failure from ATN. This differentiation is based on the premise that the tubules are working appropriately in prerenal failure and therefore can conserve salt and water appropriately, whereas in ATN, the injured tubules cannot conserve sodium appropriately.[63,68,69,102] However and of importance, because the renal tubules in newborns and premature infants are relatively immature, the distinction between prerenal failure and ATN is not as clear-cut as we would like to see. **In the newborn, values suggestive of hypoperfusion are urine osmolality greater than 350 mOsm/L, urine sodium less than 20 to 30 mEq/L, and a fractional excretion of sodium of less than 2%. Alternatively, values suggestive of ATN are urine osmolality less than 350 mOsm/L, the urine sodium greater than 30 to 40 mEq/L, and the fractional excretion of sodium greater than 2.5%. Similarly, a urine creatinine–to–serum creatinine ratio of greater than 40 implies water conservation and a prerenal cause, whereas a ratio of less than 20 suggests intrinsic renal damage. These values vary greatly, according to gestational age and maturity. Some newborns, particularly premature infants, may have prerenal failure with urinary indices suggestive of ATN.**[17] Therefore it is important to recognize the limitations of these indices in assessing renal failure in the newborn period (Table 25-2).

A **renal ultrasound examination** should be performed in all neonates with suspected ARF to assess for possible urinary tract obstruction, renal vein thrombosis, and congenital renal abnormalities such as dysplasia, polycystic disease, and aplasia.[34]

Prevention

The prevention of ARF in the preterm and term infant is a complicated discussion. Nonetheless, the following are some recommendations:

- Minimization of perinatal asphyxia
- Avoidance of maternal and infant ACE-inhibitor use
- Aggressive management of hypoxemia, hypovolemia, hypotension, acidosis, and hypothermia
- Early detection and treatment of infections
- Careful attention to agents with vasoactive or nephrotoxic properties, which can exacerbate renal injury (e.g., diuretics, aminoglycosides, NSAIDs)

TABLE 25-2 ETIOLOGY OF ACUTE RENAL FAILURE IN THE NEONATE

	URINARY INDEXES OF ACUTE RENAL FAILURE				
	U_{na} (mEq/L)	FENa (%)	RFI	U/P_{cre}	U/P_{osm}
Pretubular	31.4 ± 19.5	0.95 ± 0.55	1.29 ± 0.82	29.2 ± 15.6	>1.3
Renal parenchymal (tubular) obstruction	63.4 ± 34.7	4.25 ± 2.2	11.6 ± 9.6	9.6 ± 3.6	>1

Data from Mathews OP, Jones AS, James E, et al: Neonatal renal failure: usefulness of diagnostic indices, *Pediatrics* 65:57, 1980.

Pretubular: Hypotension/sepsis, shock, hypovolemia/dehydration, hemorrhage, hypoproteinemia, cardiac failure, renal artery stenosis, hypoxemia, asphyxia, glomerulonephritis, mechanical ventilation, pressor agents.

Renal parenchymal (tubular): Acute tubular necrosis, corticomedullary necrosis, asphyxia neonatorum, pyelonephritis, interstitial nephritis, polycystic kidney disease, renal parenchymal/aplasia/hypoplasia, intrauterine infection, endogenous toxins (uric acid, hemoglobinuria, myoglobinuria), exogenous toxins (aminoglycosides, indomethacin, contrast media), renal vein thrombosis, disseminated intravascular coagulation, congenital nephrotic syndrome.

Obstruction: Ureteral obstruction, urethral obstruction.

Cre, Creatinine (mg/dL); *FENa,* fractional excretion of sodium; *Osm,* osmolarity (mOsm/L); *P,* plasma concentration; *RFI,* renal failure index ($U_{na} \times P/U$ creatinine); *U,* urine concentration.

Management/Treatment

Once the diagnosis of ARF has been established, management of its metabolic derangements needs to be initiated promptly and involves appropriate management of fluid balance, electrolyte status, acid-base balance, and nutrition, as well as initiation of renal replacement therapy when appropriate.[4,13,35]

WATER BALANCE

Prerenal causes require increasing perfusion of the kidney by fluid therapy and restoring cardiac output and blood pressure to normal. **A fluid challenge of 10 mL/kg of body weight of crystalloid for the small preterm infants and up to 20 mL/kg of body weight for the term infant should be attempted.** With no signs of congestive heart failure and continuing oliguria or anuria, **fluid administration continues now with the administration of colloid, 5% albumin,** in a similar amount. Central venous pressure (CVP) is an important, underutilized parameter in measuring the appropriateness of fluid therapy. Use of CVP is especially important in infants with capillary leak syndrome or third spacing of fluid postoperatively. These infants appear fluid overloaded but may be intravascularly depleted.

Diuretic therapy has some potential benefits (removal of fluid), but the conversion of oliguric to nonoliguric ARF has not been shown to alter the course of the acute renal failure. **When using diuretics in newborns with ARF, potential risks and benefits need to be considered. In fact, diuretics may cause dehydration and further exacerbation of the failure.** Mannitol (0.5 to 1.0 g/kg over several minutes) may increase intratubular urine flow and may limit cell damage. However, **in neonates (particularly premature infants), mannitol should be avoided because of its hyperosmolarity and increased risk for intraventricular hemorrhage (IVH).**

The use of "renal" dose dopamine to improve renal perfusion after an ischemic insult has become very common in intensive care units.[4,29,58,105] However, there is very little evidence that it decreases the need for dialysis or improves survival.

ELECTROLYTE AND ACID-BASE DISTURBANCES

Mild hyponatremia is very common in acute renal failure and usually is the result of fluid overload with dilutional hyponatremia. This level of hyponatremia responds very well to fluid restriction or water removal by dialytic therapy. **In severe cases (serum sodium <120 mEq/L), there is a greater risk for seizures and correction to a sodium level of approximately 125 mEq/L with hypertonic saline should be considered.**

Hyperkalemia is a common and potentially life-threatening complication. The risk for disturbances of the cardiac rhythm secondary to hyperkalemia increases with the presence of acidosis and hypocalcemia. **Severe hyperkalemia requires prompt therapy with sodium bicarbonate, intravenous glucose and insulin, and intravenous**

calcium gluconate.[4,67] Severe hyperkalemia in some cases of ARF is an indication for dialysis or hemofiltration.

Hypocalcemia and acidosis are very common in ARF. **Severe acidosis can be treated with intravenous or oral sodium bicarbonate, oral sodium citrate solutions, and/or dialysis therapy.** When considering treatment of acidosis, it is important to consider the serum ionized calcium level. **Correction of acidosis would decrease the amount of ionized calcium and may precipitate tetany and/or seizures.** Finally, hyperphosphatemia is a very common electrolyte abnormality noted during ARF. **Hyperphosphatemia should be treated with dietary phosphorus restriction and with oral calcium carbonate.**

In many instances, ARF is associated with marked catabolism, and malnutrition can develop rapidly, leading to delayed recovery from ARF. Prompt and proper nutrition is essential in the management of the newborn with ARF.

RENAL REPLACEMENT THERAPY

The purpose of acute renal replacement therapy is to remove endogenous and exogenous toxins and to maintain fluid, electrolyte, and acid-base balance until renal function returns. Indications for this type of therapy include fluid overload, severe acidosis, hyperkalemia with electrocardiogram (ECG) changes, symptomatic uremia, hyperuricemia, hyperammonemia, and drug overdose (e.g., theophylline, gentamicin, vancomycin). **Renal replacement therapy may be provided by peritoneal dialysis (PD), intermittent hemodialysis (HD), and hemofiltration (HF) or continuous renal replacement therapy (CRRT) with or without a dialysis circuit.** Despite the preferential use of hemofiltration by pediatric nephrologists for neonates and small infants with ARF, PD, and HD still remain important therapeutic modalities for ARF in neonates.[31,46,64]

CONTINUOUS RENAL REPLACEMENT THERAPY (HEMOFILTRATION)[33,36,65]

Over the past several years, renal replacement therapy with hemofiltration, including continuous venovenous hemofiltration (CVVH) or with the addition of a dialysis circuit to the hemofilter (continuous venovenous hemodiafiltration [CVVHD]), has become increasingly popular in the treatment of ARF (Figure 25-4). **The advantages of hemofiltration include that it can result in rapid fluid removal, does not require the patient to be hemodynamically stable, and is administered continuously, avoiding rapid solute and fluid shifts as occurs in hemodialysis.** The disadvantages include that hemofiltration may require constant heparinization.[90]

In recent years, improvements in the technologies of CRRT have made it more suitable for use in neonates.[26,32] For some centers, CRRT has become the standard of care for neonatal acute dialysis. CVVHD offers a great alternative, especially in the infant with labile hemodynamic status, in whom HD and PD are not feasible.[98,113]

HEMODIALYSIS

Hemodialysis (HD) has the advantage of rather quickly correcting metabolic abnormalities, and

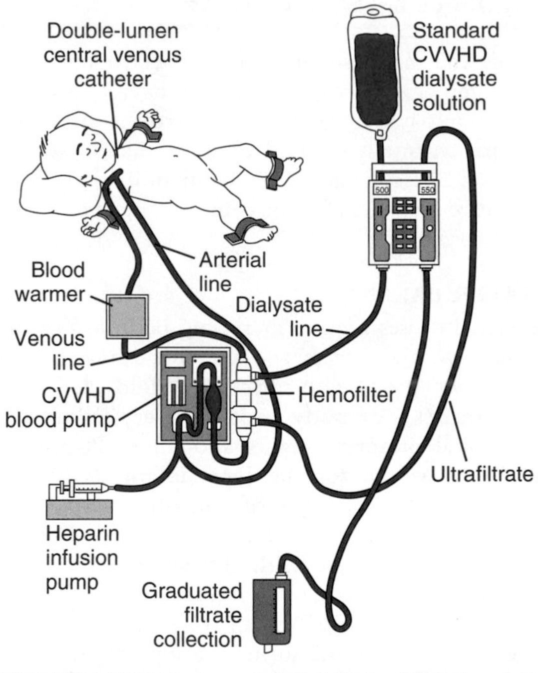

FIGURE 25-4 Continuous venovenous hemodiafiltration (CVVHD) in newborn. Blood access is provided by a central venous line. Blood is pumped through the system by a hemofiltration pump at a blood flow of 5 to 8 mL/kg/min (minimum 30 mL/min). A constant heparin infusion is maintained to keep an activated clotting time between 180 and 220 seconds. The amount of ultrafiltrate is regulated (according to the individualized needs) by using an infusion pump at filter outflow. A standard CVVHD dialysate solution is used unless severe metabolic acidosis develops. Before the blood is returned to the patient, it is passed through a blood warmer to prevent hypothermia.

hypervolemia can be corrected by ultrafiltration as well.[26] The disadvantages include the need for heparinization, the need for skilled nursing personnel, and the need for vascular access. Relative contraindications include hemodynamic instability or severe hemorrhage.

PERITONEAL DIALYSIS

Traditionally, acute peritoneal dialysis (PD) has been a major modality of therapy for ARF in the neonate when vascular access may be difficult to maintain.[46,47] Advantages of PD include that it is relatively easy to perform, it does not require heparinization, and the newborn does not need to be hemodynamically stable to undergo PD. The disadvantages include a slower correction and the potential for peritonitis.

As a renal replacement therapy, PD is useful for both the acute and chronic setting; therefore it remains the intervention of choice for the neonate with end-stage renal disease (Figure 25-5 and Table 25-3). The goal of long-term PD is ideally to permit normal growth and development up to the time of transplantation, if needed. Although technically challenging, long-term PD has been performed in very-low-birth-weight (VLBW) infants

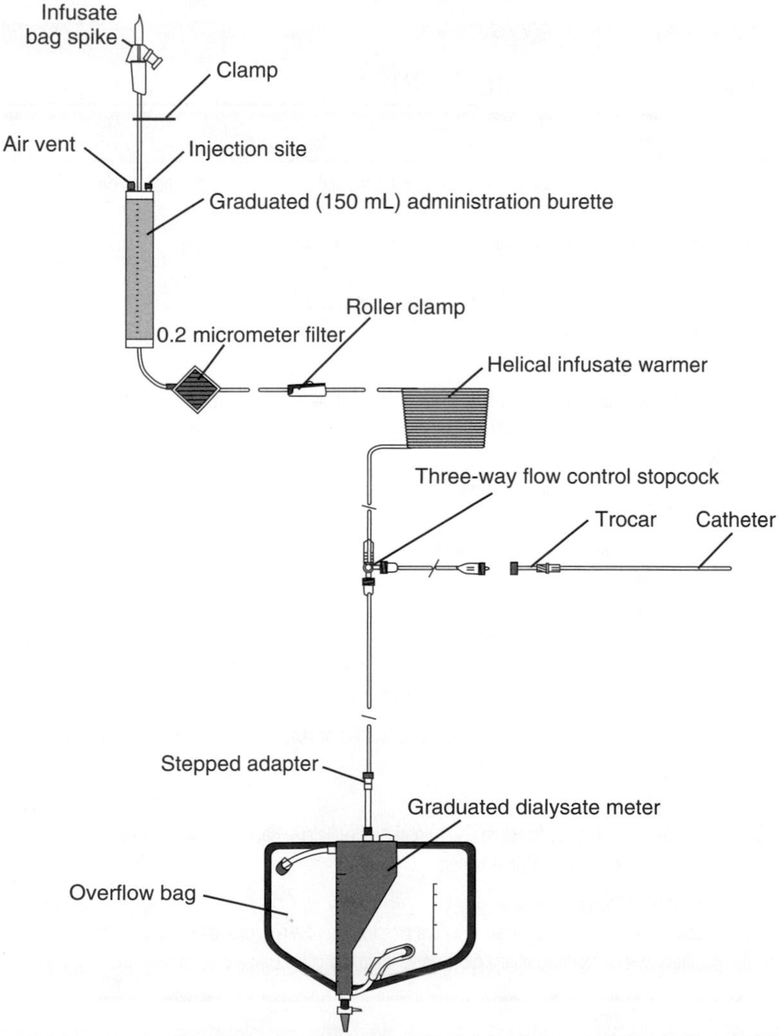

FIGURE 25-5 Example of a commercially available dialysis set for neonatal peritoneal dialysis. Graduated burette in this closed system allows easily varying amount of dialysate delivered. Helical coils allow dialysate to be warmed in same manner as in exchange transfusion. Graduated meter allows accurate measurement of outflow. (Courtesy Utah Medical Products, Midvale, Utah.)

with birth weight as low as 930 grams.[4,111] Currently, despite the fact that there has been a clear improvement in the availability of infant catheters and dialysis tubing, chronic dialysis remains extremely time consuming, challenging, and demanding for the infant, the family, and medical personnel. Ultimately, this is a home-based therapy ostensibly provided by parent(s). Although renal replacement therapy for infants has become a standard-of-care therapy, the final decision to begin chronic dialysis remains in the hands of both the parents and the multidisciplinary team. Mortality remains high for the infant group, with 20% to 50% dying within the first year of life.

Outcome and Prognosis

In the newborn infant, the prognosis and recovery from acute renal failure highly depends on the underlying etiology of the ARF.[3,7,32,56] Factors that are associated with mortality include multiorgan failure, hypotension, need for pressors, hemodynamic instability, and need for mechanical ventilation and dialysis.[28,35]

Newborns who have suffered substantial loss of nephrons as may occur in cortical necrosis, hypoxic/ischemic injury, and nephrotoxic injury are at significant risk for late development of chronic renal failure long after the initial insult.[80,114] Newborns

TABLE 25-3 NURSING CARE PLAN FOR PERITONEAL DIALYSIS IN THE NEONATE

PROBLEMS	NURSING ACTIONS
Potential peritonitis	1. Sterile technique to be used at all tubing connections and bag spikes; all connections clamped and taped. 2. Assess PD effluent with each drain for color, turbidity, and the presence of fibrin. 3. If turbidity exists: a. Obtain cell count, differential, and Gram stain and culture PD fluid b. Administer antibiotics as ordered 4. Occlusive dressing at catheter site.
Potential fluid overload or dehydration	1. Measure and record the exact amount of inflow and outflow of dialysate with each exchange. 2. Weigh neonate at regular intervals during drain to determine his or her real weight. 3. Assess fluid reabsorption: a. Peripheral and dependent edema b. Weight gain c. Failure to drain out all of dwell volume 4. Assess for dehydration: a. Weight loss b. Poor skin turgor and sunken eyes c. Hypotension 5. Notify physician of weight discrepancies or other symptoms.
Potential temperature maintenance problems	1. Warm all PD fluid to body temperature by blood warmer or heating pad immediately before inflow.
Inflow or outflow obstruction	1. Check for kinks in line. 2. Reposition patient, inflow and/or drain bags. 3. Plain radiograph of the abdomen to check position of catheter—should be toward pelvis. 4. Add heparin to dialysate if fibrin is present.
Potential respiratory compromise	1. Use smaller exchange volumes. 2. Position patient with HOB elevated to reduce pressure from the abdomen on the diaphragm. 3. If distress exists after drain, obtain chest x-ray film to rule out pneumonia or hydrothorax.

HOB, Head of bed; *PD,* peritoneal dialysis.

with ARF need lifelong monitoring of their renal function, blood pressure, and urinalysis. Typically, the late development of chronic renal failure will first become apparent with the development of hypertension, proteinuria, and eventually an elevated BUN and creatinine.[4]

HYPERTENSION*

Hypertension is a significant clinical problem in the neonate cared for in a NICU setting. The incidence of hypertension in healthy term infants appears to be quite low, and the majority of hypertensive infants have a definable etiology. Nearly universal blood pressure monitoring in nurseries with established normal blood pressure ranges enables more frequent diagnosis. A hypertensive infant may be quite ill, with symptoms similar to those of an infant with sepsis or heart or lung disease. If the infant is properly diagnosed and treated, the outcome is favorable.

*References 1,25,27,38,50,60,74,112,117.

Blood pressures (BPs) vary by gestational age, body weight, cuff size, and state of alertness. Normal values have been developed by body weight and postnatal age. BP increases by 1 to 2 mm Hg/day for the first 3 to 8 days after birth and by 1 mm Hg/week for 5 to 7 weeks. It reaches a steady value for the first year of life by 2 months of age. How the percentile ranking for an infant's BP will track into later childhood or adulthood is still unclear. Normal values for BPs in infants are shown in Table 25-4.

Etiology

The causes of hypertension can be seen in Box 25-2. All infants with hypertension must first be assumed to have a specific etiology.

Diagnosis

Accurate, reliable measurements of BP are critical to prevent falsely elevated (or depressed) values. Under study conditions, the best measurement of BP is the direct arterial measurement, usually through an umbilical artery catheter (UAC). Older

TABLE 25-4 BLOOD PRESSURE IN HEALTHY TERM NEWBORNS DURING THE FIRST 4 WEEKS OF LIFE

			MEASURED PRESSURES (mm Hg)		
AGE	n	STATE	SYSTOLIC	DIASTOLIC	MEAN
1 hour[62]	17		70	44	53
12 hours[62]	17		66	41	50
1 day[106]	46	Asleep	70 ± 9	42 ± 12	55 ± 11
		Awake	71 ± 9	43 ± 10	55 ± 9
3 days[106]	46	Asleep	75 ± 11	48 ± 10	59 ± 9
		Awake	77 ± 12	49 ± 10	63 ± 13
6 days[106]	46	Asleep	76 ± 10	46 ± 12	58 ± 12
		Awake	76 ± 10	49 ± 11	62 ± 12
2 weeks[118]	566		78 ± 10	50 ± 9	
3 weeks[118]	77		79 ± 8	49 ± 8	
4 weeks[118]	642		85 ± 10	46 ± 9	

Adapted from Tulassay T, Ramanathan R, Evans JR, et al: Renal vascular disease in the newborn. In Taeusch HW, Ballard RA, Gleason CA, editors: *Avery diseases of the newborn*, ed 8, Philadelphia, 2005, Saunders.

BOX 25-2 ETIOLOGY OF HYPERTENSION IN THE NEONATE

Vascular

- Renal artery stenosis
- Renal artery thrombosis
- Coarctation of the aorta
- Hypoplastic abdominal aorta
- Renal vein thrombosis
- Idiopathic arterial calcification

Renal

- Renal dysplasia or hypoplasia
- Polycystic kidney disease (autosomal dominant or recessive)
- Renal failure
- Obstructive uropathy
- Reflux nephropathy
- Pyelonephritis
- Glomerulonephritis

Tumors

- Wilms' tumor
- Neuroblastoma

Endocrine

- Adrenogenital syndrome
- Cushing disease
- Hyperaldosteronism
- Thyrotoxicosis

Other

- Closure of abdominal wall defects
- Fluid overload
- Genitourinary surgery
- Hypercalcemia
- Increased intracranial pressure
- Medications
    - Phenylephrine
    - Corticosteroids
    - Theophylline
    - Deoxycorticosterone
- Seizures
- Chronic lung disease/bronchopulmonary dysplasia

Data from Adelman RD: Neonatal hypertension. In Loggie JMH, Horan MJ, Hohn AR et al, editors: *NHLBI workshop on juvenile hypertension*, New York, 1983, Biomedical Information Corporation; Gulgnard JP: Neonatal nephrology. In Holliday MA, Barratt TM, Vernier RL, editors: *Pediatric nephrology*, ed 2, Baltimore, 1987, Williams & Wilkins.

techniques such as auscultation, palpation, and flush blood pressure measurements have been replaced by Doppler measurements and oscillometry. These latter two techniques correlate well with direct arterial measurements for systolic BP but not diastolic BP. **Cuff selection is also important, because cuffs that are too small give falsely high values. The cuff should completely encircle the extremity and be the largest cuff possible without impinging on the joints.** The position for measuring BP is always supine. BPs in extremities elevated above the level of the heart will be erroneously low; the converse is true of pressures taken below the level of the heart. BP can vary greatly with state of alertness and crying.

Frequently a sick infant will have a BP measured both directly through an arterial catheter and indirectly by oscillometry. Discrepancies between these measurements are often difficult to resolve. Oscillometric pressure may be inaccurate because of improper cuff size or equipment problems, or arterial blood pressure may be so low that oscillometry is difficult. Direct measurements may be inaccurate because of equipment malfunction, improper placement of the transducer in relation to the heart, or partial catheter occlusion.

Data Collection

HISTORY*

Many infants who develop hypertension have had a UAC. Although ultrasound imaging has shown that the incidence of associated aortic and/or renal artery thrombosis is high and therefore the potential for renal artery embolism as a cause for hypertension is likewise high, documented renal infarction is relatively uncommon. It is possible that embolism in some infants may be sufficient to cause hypertension but too small to be identified without, or even with, arteriography. It is also possible that in many such infants, the UAC was simply part of management rather than causative. **Hypertension is common in infants with severe bronchopulmonary dysplasia** for reasons that are unclear; this usually occurs long after a UAC has been removed, even after discharge.

*References 1,25,27,60,95,100,112.

SIGNS AND SYMPTOMS

An infant with blood pressures above the 95th percentile for similar gestational age and postconceptual age (PCA) (on three measurements 3 days in a row [unless severe, meaning more than 30% above expected for age]) should be considered hypertensive. In general, a term infant with blood pressures consistently exceeding 95 mm Hg systolic or 75 mm Hg diastolic should be considered hypertensive. In premature infants, the definition varies with gestational and postnatal age and is defined in reference to graphically displayed normal data.[25,112] **BP measurements should be taken in all extremities to rule out coarctation of the aorta.**

Severe hypertension may present as congestive heart failure with respiratory distress and hepatomegaly and with neurologic symptoms (seizures, tremor, and abnormalities in tone). Infants with mild and moderate hypertension are usually asymptomatic. In long-standing hypertension, funduscopic examination may show typical changes of hypertensive retinopathy.

LABORATORY DATA[25,91,112]

Diagnosis of hypertension requires full evaluation. This should include gray-scale **ultrasound examination** to evaluate renal anatomy and look for aortic and renal artery thrombi. Color-flow Doppler should be used to look for flow abnormalities. **Renal scintigraphy** can identify side-to-side differences in renal function. **Magnetic resonance angiography (MRA)** adds information about the anatomy of larger vessels, but MRA resolution is insufficient to identify disorders in small vessels. Classic contrast angiography is seldom performed in newborns.

Serum creatinine concentrations are usually normal. Urinalysis is also usually normal, but **hematuria and proteinuria also may be noted either as a sign of a cause of hypertension or as a result of hypertension.** Plasma renin activity, thyroid function studies, plasma and urinary steroids, and urinary catecholamines will be indicated in selected patients. **The effects of hypertension should be sought, including a cardiac evaluation and funduscopic examination by an ophthalmologist.**

Treatment[60,88,112]

There are no firm indications for treatment of hypertension in infancy. The long list of available antihypertensive medications has not been systematically studied. Therefore treatment relies on case-series data, older clinical trials, expert opinion, and personal experience.

There is general agreement that hypertension should be treated if systolic blood pressure exceeds 100 to 110 mm Hg, although rapid normalization of long-standing hypertension may be detrimental and must be avoided. A definable cause, such as urinary tract obstruction, abdominal tumor, or coarctation, should be treated surgically. Nephrectomy may be necessary in medically unmanageable, severe hypertension.

Medical management should begin with correction of salt or fluid overload if either exists. Drugs and dosages commonly used in the neonate are shown in Table 25-5. Captopril and enalapril are commonly used in NICUs and after discharge. They should be started with extreme caution if bilateral renal artery obstruction is suspected; dramatic, prolonged decreases in blood pressure with renal failure and neurologic abnormalities have been reported. Calcium channel blockers are also used. Within recommended dosing, they do not typically cause fluid retention or reflex tachycardia. For an acute hypertensive crisis, intravenous (IV) hydralazine, labetalol, nicardipine, and nitroprusside are used.

Prognosis[25,27,112]

Prognosis for these patients is excellent if BP is controlled medically or cured surgically. These infants have normal somatic growth and development. Antihypertensive medications are usually unnecessary after 1 to 2 years of follow-up. Poor renal growth may occur on the side of a renal artery lesion, and renal function scans tend to be persistently abnormal. Creatinine clearance is usually normal.

ABDOMINAL MASSES

Abdominal masses in neonates reflect a wide spectrum of pathologies, ranging from small lesions found incidentally to large ones occupying the entire peritoneal cavity; from unilocular cysts to complex solid ones; from lesions that can cause significant morbidity and mortality to

TABLE 25-5 ANTIHYPERTENSIVE MEDICATIONS FOR USE IN THE NEONATAL PERIOD*

MEDICATIONS	DOSE	SCHEDULE	ROUTE	COMMENTS
Propranolol	1-4 mg/kg/dose	BID-TID	PO	Contraindicated in heart failure, possibly in CLD/BPD, sedation
	0.025-1 mg/kg/dose	BID	IV	
Hydralazine	0.25-1.5 mg/kg/dose (max 4.5 mg/kg/dose)	BID-QID	PO	Tachycardia, sodium retention
	0.1-0.5 mg/kg/dose with a beta blocker 0.4-0.8 mg/kg/dose (sole agent)	q 6 hr	IV	
Captopril	0.1-2 mg/kg/dose	TID	PO	Leukopenia, rash, proteinuria, hyperkalemia, acute renal failure, seizures
Enalapril	0.1-0.3 mg/kg/dose	q 12-24 hr	PO	Hypotension
Enalaprilat	0.005-0.05 mg/kg/dose	q 12-24 hr	IV	Hypotension
Diazoxide	1-5 mg/kg/dose	q 4-24 hr	IV	Hyperglycemia, fluid retention, hyperuricemia
Sodium nitroprusside	0.5-10 mcg/kg/min	Continuous infusion	IV	Keep covered in foil, careful observation for infiltration of IV or varying rate of administration

BID, Twice a day; *CLD/BPD,* chronic lung disease/bronchopulmonary dysplasia; *IV,* intravenous; *kg,* kilogram; *mcg,* microgram; *mg,* milligram; *PO,* per os, orally; *QID,* four times a day; *TID,* three times a day.

*No reported experience in the newborn with nifedipine, clonidine, labetalol, or verapamil. Furosemide (Lasix) and thiazides are not antihypertensive medications but are used for volume overload.

entities that may be safely observed. This spectrum is further broadened by the variety of organs that can give rise to such masses.[14,16,24,38]

In the era of almost universal prenatal ultrasound, many such masses are identified, and some are even treated, before delivery. Others are discovered during the course of a thorough routine examination of the neonate. **Although most of these babies are otherwise healthy, the news is likely to disturb the new parents. It is incumbent upon the infant's physician to determine the nature of the mass in a timely, safe, and cost-effective manner.**[14,40,43]

Diagnosis

Slightly more than 50% of abdominal masses present during the newborn period are of renal origin.[61,71] The literature offers no consistent data on frequency of abdominal masses in infants, but there is general agreement about the urgent need to evaluate these infants quickly and thoroughly and to reach an accurate diagnosis before planning intervention.

PHYSICAL EXAMINATION

To examine the abdomen, the infant should be in the supine position. Inspection of the abdomen before manual exploration enables the examiner to note a mass that may be missed on a tense abdomen. The shape of the abdomen should be noted. The position of the umbilicus and the presence of any hernias should be assessed. Bimanual palpation using the flat surface of the fingers while supporting the infant's flank with the other hand permits the exploration of the abdomen during deep palpation. **Characteristics of the mass to note include location, size, shape, texture, mobility, and tenderness.** The mass should be categorized as solid, cystic, or air-filled; however, the differentiation between solid and cystic masses can be difficult on physical examination. Percussion may be used to outline the suspected area, and transillumination is sometimes helpful.

If gastric distention or intestinal obstruction is suspected, a nasogastric tube is inserted and air and fluid evacuated. If there is a question of urinary retention, the infant should be re-examined after placement of a urinary catheter or after inducing voiding with a Credé maneuver. Rectal examination, applied judiciously, may provide useful information, such as in a suspected intra-pelvic or intra-abdominal mass. Upon the recognition of an abdominal mass, findings of the entire physical examination should be reviewed in this light. Clues to the nature of the lesion may be external or distant to the mass.

LABORATORY DATA

Radiographic imaging is usually the next step. Plain films may provide a surprising amount of information, such as organomegaly and calcifications in a number of tumors or displacement of the intestines, as a subtle clue to the nature or even presence of a mass.

Additional information can be expected from **ultrasonography (US).** This modality, with ever-increasing image resolution, is an excellent screening tool. It is noninvasive, accessible for bedside studies, radiation-free, and painless and can provide detailed information on the location, nature, and vascularity of the mass and adjacent structures. When this diagnostic tool is incapable of differentiating dysplasia and hydronephrosis, **renal scintigraphy** is indicated to better assess renal function. Rarely a percutaneous nephrostogram is performed to determine whether cysts result from obstruction or dysplasia. A **voiding cystourethrogram** is the method of choice to diagnose vesicoureteral reflux. **Computed tomography (CT) or magnetic resonance imaging (MRI)** is occasionally indicated, especially in differentiating renal masses and extent of the disease.

DIFFERENTIAL DIAGNOSIS

The differential diagnosis in the infant with an abdominal mass is shown in Table 25-6. The workup of most abdominal masses requires only a thorough physical examination and few (goal-oriented) studies. Usually, the location of the mass is a very useful clue to the possible organ involved and the most likely diagnosis[14]:

1. ***Flank:*** The most common causes of flank masses are of renal origin, hydronephrosis or multicystic kidney. Other flank masses of importance are the solid tumors of the kidney, such as the benign congenital mesoblastic nephroma (the most common) and Wilms' tumor. Another group of flank masses are of juxtarenal origin: neuroblastoma, adrenal hemorrhage, various necrotic lesions, bronchogenic cyst, and infradiaphragmatic (extralobar) pulmonary sequestration. Renal vein thrombosis is an unusual cause of flank mass.
2. ***Right upper quadrant (RUQ):*** Most RUQ masses usually involve the liver and biliary tract. In fact, the typical presentation of the most common benign hepatic tumor, infantile hepatic hemangioma (hemangioendothelioma), is a palpable RUQ mass. Other masses include the

TABLE 25-6 NEONATAL ABDOMINAL MASSES

TYPE OF MASS	PERCENT OF TOTAL
RENAL MASSES	
Hydronephrosis	55
Multicystic dysplastic kidney	
Polycystic kidney disease	
Mesoblastic nephroma	
Renal ectopia	
Renal vein thrombosis	
Nephroblastomatosis	
Wilms' tumor	
GENITAL MASSES	
Hydrometrocolpos	15
Ovarian cyst	
GASTROINTESTINAL MASSES	
Duplication	15
Volvulus	
Complicated meconium ileus	
Mesenteric-omental cyst	
"Pseudocyst" proximal to atresia	
NONRENAL RETROPERITONEAL MASSES	
Adrenal hemorrhage	10
Neuroblastoma	
Teratoma	
HEPATOSPLENOBILIARY MASSES	
Hemangioendothelioma	5
Hepatoblastoma	
Hepatic cyst	
Splenic hematoma	
Choledochal cyst	
Hydrops of gallbladder	

From Kirks DR, Merten DF, Grossman H, et al: Diagnostic imaging of pediatric abdominal masses: an overview, *Radiol Clin North Am* 19:527, 1981.

benign mesenchymal hamartomas, the hepatoblastoma (the only significant primary hepatic malignancy in neonates), and the choledochal cyst.

3. ***Left upper quadrant (LUQ):*** Splenic cysts are very rarely diagnosed.
4. ***Mid-abdominal:*** Abdominal masses in the mid-abdomen usually involve the intestine. Duplications of the gastrointestinal (GI) tract occur anywhere from the esophagus to the anus and are either cystic (the most common) or tubular. Usually, they are present as an asymptomatic palpable mass but may also cause pain, intestinal obstruction, GI bleeding, or even volvulus.

   Other mid-abdominal masses may include intestinal lymphatic malformations, meconium diseases, mid-abdominal wall defects, and omphalomesenteric remnants. Failure of the vitelline duct to resorb completely may lead to a variety of related entities, including Meckel's diverticulum and omphalomesenteric sinus, cyst, or fistula.
5. ***Pelvic:*** A residual pelvic mass in a female infant after voiding may represent an enlarged vagina (hydrocolpos) or uterus (hydrometrocolpos). Such a mass should trigger a close look at the perineum and vaginal introitus. Other pelvic masses may represent ovarian masses, urachal cyst, and teratomas. Cystic ovarian tumors are more common than solid ones, and the majority are benign; however, every cystic ovarian mass needs to be investigated. Some malignancies have been reported.

INTRINSIC RENAL PARENCHYMAL ABNORMALITIES[79,81]

Renal abnormalities can be classified by the amount of tissue, differentiation of tissue, and position of the kidneys.

Congenital absence or agenesis of renal tissue can occur unilaterally or bilaterally. Unilateral renal agenesis is seen more frequently (1:1000 live births) and may manifest as a solitary kidney on examination with enlargement caused by compensatory hypertrophy. Unilateral agenesis has been associated with Turner, Poland, and VATER (***v***ertebral defects, imperforate ***a***nus, ***t***racheo***e***sophageal fistula, and ***r***adial and ***r***enal dysplasia) syndromes. Bilateral agenesis, also known as ***Potter disease,*** is seen rarely, with an incidence of 1 per 4000 births.

Hypoplasia is a deficiency in the amount of renal tissue expressed as an abnormally small kidney. Morphologically, the kidney is normal, and renal function is unaffected in the neonatal period. Later in life, patients can sometimes "outgrow" their renal function.

Signs and Symptoms

In unilateral agenesis, patients are often asymptomatic and are diagnosed inadvertently on ultrasound or based on the significant association with malformations of the lower genitourinary tract. There is no need for long-term follow-up if only a solitary kidney without additional involvement is found.

In bilateral agenesis, the majority of affected infants are male and small for gestational age, with a history of maternal oligohydramnios. The characteristic facial features accompanying Potter syndrome include wide-set eyes, parrot-beak nose, receding chin, and large, low-set ears with little cartilage. Other associated malformations include pulmonary hypoplasia, hydrocephalus, meningocele, multiple skeletal anomalies, and imperforate anus. Death usually occurs within hours to several days.

Differentiation of Tissue[79,85,86]

Abnormalities in renal tissue differentiation are most commonly expressed as dysplastic kidneys. Renal dysplasia is a failure of the metanephric tissue to mature appropriately, frequently because of obstruction of the urinary tract early in gestation. The result is a persistence of immature structures and very little normal functioning renal tissue.

Renal dysplasia may be seen in one or both kidneys and involving the entire kidney, segments of the kidney, or microscopic areas (foci) of a kidney. Dysplasia is most commonly expressed as cyst formation. Bilateral multicystic dysplastic kidneys (MCDKs) are nonfunctional and not compatible with life. Unilateral MCDK involvement is both the most common cystic lesion of the neonatal kidney and one of the most frequently palpated abdominal masses in the newborn. Unilateral MCDK shows no predilection for males or females or for involvement of right or left kidney. Usually the ureter is absent, atretic, or stenotic. No orifice is found in the bladder. The kidneys are extremely hypoplastic, enlarged, diffusely cystic with almost complete loss of the reniform configuration. The histopathologic landmark of MCDK is nests of cartilage and mesenchymal mantles surrounding primitive tubules. Renal function and structure may be normal in the remaining kidney of infants with unilateral dysplasia; however, frequently vesicorectal reflux or ureteropelvic junction (UPJ) obstruction is present in the contralateral kidney. Therefore a voiding cystourethrogram should be performed on every patient. In addition, hypertension is a potential complication (estimates of 20% have been made) of MCDK and requires treatment or long-term follow-up.

Renal dysplasia is usually sporadic, but some familial cases have been reported. A lack of blood flow on 99mTc DPTA nuclear renal scan confirms the diagnosis of dysplasia.

Treatment

Generally, these kidneys involute with time; therefore a conservative rather than surgical approach is recommended. The association between renal dysplasia and neoplasia has not been confirmed. However, removal of the kidney is sometimes indicated if its size prevents adequate nutrition.

POLYCYSTIC KIDNEY DISEASE[18,37,51,53,83]

Pathophysiology

Polycystic kidney disease (PKD) may present as one of two types in the infant: (1) autosomal recessive polycystic kidney disease (ARPKD); and (2) autosomal dominant polycystic kidney disease (ADPKD). Traditionally, ADPKD has not been associated with onset during the first year of life, but recent studies have confirmed both presentations in the infant and, conversely, ARPKD has been reported in the older child.

ARPKD manifests with varied severity, but it is always bilateral. The kidneys become enlarged with a proliferation of renal tubules and dilated collecting tubules. These are not true "cysts," and the kidney has a reniform shape. Various combinations of cystic renal disease and hepatic disease occur in ARPKD including dilation of collecting tubules in the kidney, congenital hepatic fibrosis because of ductal plate malformation, and nonobstructive dilation of intrahepatic bile ducts (Caroli disease). Autosomal dominant disease involves cyst formations in any portion of the nephron, Bowman's space, and liver. Of affected individuals, 50% have cysts in other visceral organs including the liver, pancreas, spleen, and lung. There is a strong association between ADPKD and cerebral artery aneurysms.

Data Collection

HISTORY

Criteria for making a definitive diagnosis for both diseases have been developed. Autosomal recessive disease includes infants with the following: (1) congenital hepatic fibrosis on liver biopsy or evidence of portal hypertension; (2) renal histologic studies consistent with collecting tubule ectasis; or (3) a sibling with the disease. Infants diagnosed with ARPKD have either a positive parental history or known liver cysts or berry aneurysm.

SIGNS AND SYMPTOMS

Both types of PKD can manifest initially with an abdominal mass. The infant may present with bilateral flank masses, hepatic enlargement, Potter facies caused by oligohydramnios, oliguria, acute renal failure, hypoplastic lungs, respiratory distress, and spontaneous pneumothorax. Hypertension is common in both types of the disease.

LABORATORY DATA

Differentiation of ADPKD versus ARPKD may be difficult, even with ultrasound, because radiographic studies are not consistently accurate in discerning differences. Indeed, retrospectively, it is not uncommon to find infants misclassified.

Treatment

Management consists of serial monitoring of blood pressure, renal function, and urine cultures. Neonates with either form of PKD need aggressive treatment of hypertension with captopril as the drug of choice, treatment of any urinary tract infection, and aggressive nutritional management.

HYDRONEPHROSIS[70,72,78]

Physiology

The collecting system of the kidney is composed of the ureter, pelvis, and calyces, all of which function as a system for removing urine from the kidney. **Hydronephrosis, one of the most common abdominal masses in the newborn, involves a dilation of the pelvis and calyces, most often as a result of congenital obstruction.** The impaired movement of urine from severe or chronic obstruction may lead to dysplastic and cystic changes that further impair kidney function if the obstruction occurs early in gestation.

The most common ureteral site of obstruction is at the ureteropelvic junction (UPJ). The infant presents with a ballooning of the renal pelvis. Obstruction at the ureterovesical junction (UVJ), also known as ***congenital megaureter*** in its primary form, occurs more often in the male infant. UVJ obstruction more frequently affects the left ureter. Posterior urethral valves (PUVs) in males are the major cause of urethral obstruction. This distal obstruction may result in bladder hypertrophy, hydroureter, and hydronephrosis if severe. Dysplastic changes can be seen if the obstruction occurs early in gestation. The neonate with PUV is at risk for developing an ascending infection and subsequent renal damage. Prune-belly syndrome, also known as ***Eagle-Barrett syndrome,*** is a less common cause of obstruction and dilation of the pelvis and calyces. There is a strong male predominance. This triad of anomalies includes (1) absence or hypoplasia of the abdominal wall muscles, (2) bilateral cryptorchidism, and (3) urinary tract abnormality. The loose, shriveled abdomen is responsible for the "prune belly" appearance, which diminishes with age and does not require surgical correction. Renal dysplasia is usually seen in prune-belly syndrome and may range from mild to severe involvement. The enlarged bladder may be seen in conjunction with a patent urachus draining urine. The prostatic urethra is usually hypoplastic.

Etiology

The etiology of most types of hydronephrosis remains unclear. Primary prune-belly syndrome may be a result of a mesenchymal developmental arrest. A variant of the syndrome also can be seen as a sequela of an intrauterine distention of the abdomen by an obstructed urinary system. The existence of this secondary cause of prune-belly syndrome is controversial. Another cause of calyceal dilation not associated with obstruction is vesicoureteral reflux, as discussed further in the "Urinary Tract Infection" section.

Infants may have few if any symptoms, and there are usually no physical findings unless a bladder or kidney is palpated on routine examination. These infants can present with a poor urinary stream and frequently with failure to thrive.

Treatment[70]

Mild to moderate unilateral obstruction does not require immediate treatment. Close follow-up is indicated for monitoring of kidney growth and obstruction as surgery may be a postnatal consideration; bilateral dilation with normal amounts of amniotic fluid is managed with close observation. Treatment of bilateral dilation with decreased amniotic fluid depends on the gestational age of the fetus.

A viable fetus with dilated collecting systems, initial normal amount of amniotic fluid, and evidence of decreasing amniotic fluid should be delivered early. Other conditions such as bilateral vesicoureteral reflux, prune-belly syndrome, and primary megaureter may present with dilated collecting systems and are not amenable to in utero surgery. Surgical intervention in utero is very controversial and center dependent, and the morbidity of this therapy is very high.

Complete obstruction at the UPJ is surgically corrected. For uterovesical obstructions, surgical correction involves excising the stenotic segment in the obstructed megaureter, as well as ureteric reimplantation, and is successful in the large majority of infants. Management of obstruction secondary to PUV depends on the age at presentation and infant's condition. After initial stabilization, relief of obstruction with a catheter provides quick decompression. Permanent repair consists of removal of the obstructing valves. The use of a vesicostomy versus a higher diversion is controversial.

RENAL VEIN THROMBOSIS[57,75,94]

Renal vein thrombosis (RVT) can be an acute life-threatening condition or insidious with the development of microhematuria and inflammation.

RVT is associated with conditions that cause circulatory collapse and decreased oxygenation within the kidney.

Etiology

Perinatal causes of neonatal RVT include maternal diabetes, toxemia, maternal thiazide therapy, polycythemia, placental insufficiency, birth asphyxia, prematurity, respiratory distress syndrome (RDS), and sepsis. Angiography has also been associated with RVT. Thrombosis most often occurs in the smaller renal veins rather than in the main renal vein.

Data Collection

SIGNS AND SYMPTOMS

The involved kidney may enlarge secondary to obstruction to blood flow and forms a palpable flank mass. Other clinical symptoms may include hematuria (60% of cases), anemia, oliguria, and thrombocytopenia (<75,000 platelets).

LABORATORY DATA

Positive blood on dipstick testing, urine output of less than 1 mL/kg/hr, and a low platelet count may indicate RVT.

Treatment

Management includes treatment of the underlying illness, treatment of sepsis if suspected, fluid therapy, and possibly dialysis in select cases. Heparin therapy remains controversial for RVT. Surgical excision of the thrombus is not usually indicated during the acute phase but may be appropriate at a later time. Rarely is nephrectomy necessary. Renal tubular dysfunction is often observed after recovery from RVT.

MISCELLANEOUS CAUSES OF ABDOMINAL MASS

Wilms' tumor, also known as *nephroblastoma,* is the most common intraabdominal tumor seen in children and occurs at a rate of 8 to 9 per 100,000 per year in the United States; two thirds of patients present in the first 3 to 6 months of life. The tumor is described as firm, smooth, and confluent with the kidney or attached to the organ. Both kidneys are involved in 10% of cases. This condition has an excellent prognosis with treatment. Surgical removal of the tumor is followed by irradiation for most patients and chemotherapy.

Neuroblastoma, on the other hand, is the most common malignant tumor in infancy. The primary site of the tumor may be any area of neural crest tissue, with the most common site identified in the adrenal gland. Presenting in the neonate as a palpable abdominal mass, this tumor may also cause urinary obstruction. Prognosis is related to the site of the primary tumor, histologic appearance of the tumor, staging of the disease, and age of the patient.

RENAL TUBULAR DISORDERS[5,104,108]

Although most of the renal tubular disorders are congenital, they rarely manifest clinically during the newborn period. However, in sick infants admitted to the intensive care unit, **these tubular abnormalities can lead to severe and frequently life-threatening electrolyte disorders.**

Etiology

With the advent of routine prenatal ultrasound, a number of newborns referred for evaluation of polyhydramnios and polyuria have been diagnosed with diabetes insipidus (central or nephrogenic) and Bartter syndrome. In addition, obstruction of the urinary tract, which is frequently diagnosed prenatally, is commonly associated with renal tubular acidosis (RTA), particularly the hyperkalemic type (type IV).

Data Collection

HISTORY/SIGNS AND SYMPTOMS

Infants with Fanconi syndrome and distal RTA most commonly present after the neonatal period with the complaint of failure to thrive. Frequently a history of previous admissions to the hospital for evaluation of sepsis or dehydration is obtained.

LABORATORY DATA

The diagnosis of Fanconi syndrome is confirmed by demonstration of a generalized dysfunction in the proximal tubule, evidenced by the presence of glycosuria, proteinuria (low-molecular-weight proteins), bicarbonaturia, phosphaturia, and uricosuria. Distal RTA is diagnosed by demonstrating a decreased urinary excretion of ammonium; if the result is a negative number (less than zero), then distal RTA is ruled out. A positive urine net charge (higher than zero) is consistent with RTA. However, because of the presence of other organic anions in the urine during the first 2 weeks of life, the validity of this test during the neonatal period has been questioned. Disorders of vitamin D metabolism or phosphate reabsorption (rickets) usually manifest by the end of the first year of life, after the child starts walking. Infants with diabetes insipidus typically present during the first 2 months of life with dehydration and a sepsis-like picture.

Complications

Thus, although most of the tubular disorders are not clinically evident at birth, the clinician should keep a high index of suspicion in those infants with prenatal diagnosis of urologic abnormalities or serious abnormalities in water and electrolyte metabolism. **Early evaluation and treatment of renal tubular disorders may prevent catastrophic complications** such as life-threatening episodes of dehydration and delayed growth and development.

URINARY TRACT INFECTION[44,105]

Urinary tract infections (UTIs) affect approximately 1% of full-term infants and 3% of premature infants. Male infants are affected 5 times more frequently than females. Vesicoureteral reflux is a common radiographic finding in infants. Primary reflux is seen in abnormalities of the vesicoureteral junction, ureteral duplication, and ureterocele. Secondary reflux is associated with infection, PUV, and neurogenic diseases.

Etiology

Abnormalities of the urinary tract are responsible for a large number of UTIs in the neonate. Whether the infection is ascending from the bladder or hematogenously spread is a matter of debate. **The high association of reflux with UTI makes determining the etiology of reflux a priority for planning appropriate treatment.** Reflux is graded on a four-point scale, with grade IV denoting massive hydronephrosis and hydroureter.

Maternal urinary infections also have been associated with neonatal UTIs. Symptomatic manifestations include abnormal weight loss during the first days of life, decreased feeding, dehydration, irritability, lethargy, cyanosis, jaundice, and septicemia. In some cases, the affected kidneys are palpable. Infected infants also may be asymptomatic.

Data Collection

LABORATORY DATA

Evaluation of a neonate with suspected UTI includes immediate urine and blood cultures and a complete blood count (CBC). The optimum method of obtaining urine for culture is **suprapubic aspiration of the bladder or catheterization.** Catheterization may not be recommended in the neonate because of possible urethral stricture formation in the male and frequent culture contamination in the female. **Urine obtained in a urine bag should not be used for cultures because it is easily contaminated. With diagnosis of UTI, radiographic evaluation should be undertaken to rule out anatomic abnormality.** This should include **ultrasound and voiding cystourethrogram (VCUG).** Grades of reflux are diagnosed by voiding cystourethrogram; thus sterile urine is necessary before a VCUG is undertaken. **Renal scintigraphy and CT scan** may be needed to evaluate renal scarring and damage.

Treatment

Pyuria (10 to 15 WBC per hpf) can be observed in the neonate normally. Treatment for UTI is indicated when an organism is cultured from the urine. Any growth in a urine specimen obtained by suprapubic aspiration should be considered to represent an infection if the procedure was cleanly done. Any aspiration of bowel contents must affect the interpretation of culture results. **Traditional antibiotic coverage consists of both ampicillin and an aminoglycoside.** The advent of third-generation cephalosporins has allowed for excellent gram-negative coverage without the nephrotoxicity of the aminoglycosides. ***Escherichia coli* is the organism**

most often implicated in neonatal UTIs, followed by *Klebsiella.* Sulfonamides are contraindicated in the neonate because of their potential to complicate hyperbilirubinemia.

Antibiotic therapy should continue for 10 to 14 days, with a follow-up urine culture 3 days after therapy is discontinued. Many practitioners recommend antibiotic prophylaxis until significant reflux or anatomic abnormality is ruled out.

NEUROGENIC BLADDER[92,105]

Neurogenic bladder is an anatomic interruption of the micturition reflex normally triggered by a full bladder. The bladder may be flaccid and unable to empty urine or spastic and hyperreflexive and unable to store urine. **Infants with lumbosacral spinal malformations commonly have a urinary tract dysfunction known as *neurogenic bladder.*** Lower motor neuron deficit causes bladder atony, and upper motor neuron deficit can cause spasticity.

Data Collection

SIGNS AND SYMPTOMS

Often there is a mixed presentation of symptoms. **The flaccid bladder requires aggressive intervention in the neonate. Diagnosis begins immediately at the bedside when the newborn has no apparent voiding stream or the urine flow rate falls below expectations without other explanations.** Further clarification of the diagnosis can be made by VCUG and by cystometric studies.

Treatment

Surgical intervention is indicated in the neonate with neurogenic bladder when there is severe reflux with renal damage present or recurrent UTI. The urologist creates a vesicostomy to allow the free flow of urine into diapers.

Complications

Early diagnosis and intervention for infants with neurogenic bladder can decrease the risks of the complications associated with this problem. Long-term complications of neurogenic bladder include UTI and vesicoureteral reflux leading to hydronephrosis, electrolyte imbalances, and permanent damage to the kidney.

PARENT TEACHING

Because many renal problems are secondary to abnormalities, parents should be assured that nothing they did or did not do caused the anomaly. Grief work over the loss of the perfect infant is necessary before attachment and care giving are possible (see Chapters 29 and 30). Genetic counseling enables parents to make informed choices about subsequent pregnancies (see Chapter 27).

Most infants with renal problems require accurate intake and output measurement. The importance and necessity of measuring intake and not overfeeding must be stressed to parents, as well as the necessity of saving and weighing diapers. Infants who are fluid restricted may be "difficult" for care providers and parents because they are fussy and irritable. Adherence to the prescribed formula or breast milk is very important to regulate sodium intake and fluid retention.

Long-term complications that parents may have to recognize or manage must be explained and written instructions given. Because abnormalities in renal function and anatomy may be sequelae of renal diseases, follow-up by a pediatric nephrologists or urologist for urinalysis, cultures, and other diagnostic tests is important. General health maintenance is also important, because growth failure may be a manifestation of ongoing or recurring renal problem.

The importance of administering antihypertensive medications must be stressed to parents. Because hypertension is often a silent condition, the need for continuation of medications must be thoroughly explained. Side effects of hypertensive medications such as sedation, tachycardia, and excessive weight gain, as well as the necessity of medical follow-up, also must be emphasized.

REFERENCES

1. Adelman RD: Neonatal hypertension. In Loggie JMH, Horan MJ, Hohn AR, et al, editors: *NHLBI workshop on juvenile hypertension,* New York, 1983, Biomedical Information Corporation.
2. Adelman RD, Wirth F, Rubio T: A controlled study of the nephrotoxicity of methicillin and gentamicin plus ampicillin in the neonate, *J Pediatr* 111:888, 1987.

3. Andreoli SP: Acute renal failure in the newborn, *Curr Opin Pediatr* 17:713, 2002.
4. Andreoli SP: Acute renal failure in the newborn, *Semin Perinatol* 28:112, 2004.
5. Arant BS: Renal and genitourinary diseases. In McMillan J, Feigen RD, DeAngelis CD, et al, editors: *Oski's pediatrics,* Philadelphia, 2006, Lippincott Williams & Wilkins.
6. Auron A, Mhanna MJ: Serum creatinine in very low birth weight infants during their first days of life, *J Perinatol* 26:755, 2006.
7. Basile DP, Donohoe D, Roethe K, et al: Renal ischemic injury results in permanent damage to peritubular capillaries and influences long-term function, *Am J Physiol* 281:F887, 2001.
8. Baum M: Developmental changes in proximal tubule NaCl transport, *Pediatr Nephrol* 23:185, 2008.
9. Brion LP, Campbell DE: Furosemide in indomethacin-treated infants: systematic review and meta-analysis, *Pediatr Nephrol* 13:212, 1999.
10. Brion LP, Campbell DE: Furosemide for symptomatic patent ductus arteriosus in indomethacin-treated infants, *Cochrane Database Syst Rev* 3:CD001148, 2001.
11. Brion LP, Primhak RA: Intravenous or enteral loop diuretics for preterm infants with (or developing) chronic lung disease, *Cochrane Database Syst Rev* 1:CD001453, 2002.
12. Brion LP, Soll RA: Diuretics for respiratory distress syndrome in preterm infants, *Cochrane Database Syst Rev* 3:CD001454, 2008.
13. Bunchman TE: Infant dialysis: the future is now, *J Pediatr* 136:1, 2000.
14. Chandler JC, Gauderer MWL: The neonate with an abdominal mass, *Pediatr Clin N Am* 51:979, 2004.
15. Chevalier RL: The moth and the aspen tree: sodium in early postnatal development, *Kidney Int* 59:1617, 2001.
16. Chevalier RL: Perinatal obstructive nephropathy, *Semin Perinatol* 28:124, 2004.
17. Choker G, Gouyon JB: Diagnosis of acute renal failure in very preterm infants, *Biol Neonate* 86:212, 2004.
18. Cole BR, Conley SB, Stapleton SB: and Southwest Pediatric Nephrology Study Group: Polycystic kidney disease presenting in the first year of life, *J Pediatr* 111:693, 1987.
19. Cruz C, Spitzer A: When you find protein or blood in the urine, *Contemp Pediatr* September, 1998.
20. Drukker A, Guignard JP: Renal aspects of the term and preterm infants: a selective update, *Curr Opin Pediatr* 14:175, 2002.
21. Drukker A, Mosig D, Guignard JP: The renal hemodynamics effect of aspirin in newborn and young adult rabbits, *Pediatr Nephrol* 16:113, 2001.
22. Engle WD: Evaluation of renal function in acute renal failure in the neonate, *Pediatr Clin North Am* 33:129, 1986.
23. Ertl T, Hadzsiev K, Vincze O, et al: Hyponatremia and sensorineural hearing loss in preterm infants, *Biol Neonate* 79:109, 2001.
24. Farmer DL: Urinary tract masses, *Semin Pediatr Surg* 9:109, 2000.
25. Flynn JT: Neonatal hypertension: diagnosis and management, *Pediatr Nephrol* 14:332, 2000.
26. Forni LG, Hilton PJ: Continuous hemofiltration in the treatment of acute renal failure, *N Engl J Med* 336:1303, 1997.
27. Friedman AL, Hustead VA: Hypertension in babies after discharge from a neonatal intensive care unit, *Pediatr Nephrol* 1:30, 1987.
28. Gallego N, Perez-Caballero C, Estepo R, et al: Prognosis of patients with acute renal failure without cardiomyopathy, *Arch Dis Childhood* 84:258, 2001.
29. Galley HF: Renal dose dopamine: will the message get through? *Lancet* 356:2112, 2000.
30. Gallini F, Maggio L, Romagnoli C, et al: Progression of renal function in preterm neonates with gestation age less than or equal to 32 wks, *Pediatr Nephrol* 15:119, 2000.
31. Geary DF: Initiation of renal replacement therapy in infancy. In Warady BA, Fine RN, Alexander SR, et al: *Pediatric dialysis,* Netherlands, 2004, Kluwer.
32. Goldstein SL, Currier H, Graf CD, et al: Outcome in children receiving continuous venous hemofiltration, *Pediatrics* 107:1309, 2001.
33. Gong WK, Tan TH, Foong PP, et al: Eighteen years in pediatric acute dialysis: analysis of predicted outcome, *Pediatr Nephrol* 16:212, 2001.
34. Gordon I, Barratt TM: Imaging the kidneys and urinary tract in the neonate with acute renal failure, *Pediatr Nephrol* 1:321, 1987.
35. Gouyon JB, Guignard JP: Management of acute renal failure in newborns, *Pediatr Nephrol* 14:1037, 2000.
36. Gregory M, Bunchman TE, Brophy PD: Continuous renal replacement therapies for children with acute renal failure and metabolic disorders. In Warady BA, Fine RN, Alexander SR, et al, editors: *Pediatric dialysis,* Netherlands, 2004, Kluwer.
37. Guay-Woodford L, Desmond R: Autosomal recessive polycystic kidney disease: the clinical experience in North America, *Pediatrics* 111:1072, 2003.
38. Guignard JP: Neonatal nephrology. In Holliday MA, Barratt TM, Vernier RL, editors: *Pediatric nephrology,* ed 2, Baltimore, 1987, Williams & Wilkins.
39. Guignard JP, Gouyan JB: Adverse effects of drugs on the immature kidney, *Biol Neonate* 53:243, 1988.
40. Gunn TR, Mora JD, Pease P: Antenatal diagnosis of urinary tract abnormalities by ultrasonography after 28 week gestation: incidence and outcome, *Am J Obstet Gynecol* 172:479, 1995.

41. Gurkan S, Estilo GK, Wei Y, et al: Potassium transport in the maturing kidney, *Pediatr Nephrol* 22:915, 2007.
42. Hein G, Richter D, Manz F, et al: Development of nephrocalcinosis in very low birth weight infants, *Pediatr Nephrol* 19:616, 2004.
43. Helin I, Persson PH: Prenatal diagnosis of urinary tract abnormalities by ultrasound, *Pediatrics* 78:879, 1986.
44. Hellstrom M, Jacobsson B, Jodal U, et al: Renal growth after neonatal urinary tract infection, *Pediatr Nephrol* 1:269, 1987.
45. Holler B, Omar SA, Farid MD, et al: Effects of fluid and electrolyte management on amphotericin B-induced nephrotoxicity among extremely low birth weight infants, *Pediatrics* 113:608, 2004.
46. Holmberg C, Ronnholm K: Maintenance peritoneal dialysis during infancy. In Warady BA, Fine RN, Alexander SR, et al, editors: *Pediatric dialysis*, Netherlands, 2004, Kluwer.
47. Hölttä T, Rönnholm K, Jalanko H, et al: Clinical outcomes of pediatric patients on peritoneal dialysis under adequacy control, *Pediatr Nephrol* 14:889, 2000.
48. Ichikawa I, Kuwayama F, Pope JCIV, et al: Paradigm shift from classic anatomic theories to contemporary cell biological views of CAKUT, *Kidney Int* 61:889, 2002.
49. Jones DP, Chesney RW: Tubular function. In Avner ED, Harmon WE, Niaudet P, editors: *Pediatric nephrology*, ed 5, Philadelphia, 2004, Lippincott Williams & Wilkins.
50. Jones JE, Jose PA: Neonatal blood pressure regulation, *Semin Perinatol* 28:141, 2004.
51. Kalia A, Brouhard BH, Travis LB, et al: Renal transplantation in the infant and young child, *Am J Dis Child* 143:47, 1988.
52. Kao LC, Warburton D, Cheng MH, et al: Effect of oral diuretics on pulmonary mechanics in infants with chronic bronchopulmonary dysplasia: results of a double-blind crossover sequential trial, *Pediatrics* 74:37, 1984.
53. Kaplan BS, Kaplan P, Ruchelli E: Inherited and congenital malformations of the kidneys in the neonatal period, *Clin Perinatol* 19:197, 1992.
54. Kapur G, Mattoo T, Aranda JV: Pharmacogenomics and renal drug disposition in the newborn, *Semin Perinatol* 28:132, 2004.
55. Karlowicz GM, Adelman RD: Nonoliguric and oliguric acute renal failure in asphyxiated neonates, *Pediatr Nephrol* 9:718, 1995.
56. Katz A, Bock GH, Mauer M: Improved growth velocity with intensive dialysis: consequence or coincidence, *Pediatr Nephrol* 14:710, 2000.
57. Keidan I, Lotan D, Gazit G, et al: Early neonatal renal venous thrombosis: long-term outcome, *Acta Paediatr* 83:1225, 1994.
58. Kellum JA, Decker JM: Use of dopamine in acute renal failure: a meta-analysis, *Crit Care Med* 29:1526, 2001.
59. Kelly LK, Seri I: Renal developmental physiology: relevance to clinical care, *NeoReviews* 9:e150, 2008.
60. Killian K: Hypertension in neonates: causes and treatments, *J Perinat Neonatal Nurs* 17:65, 2003.
61. Kirks DR, Merten DF, Grossman H, et al: Diagnostic imaging of pediatric abdominal masses: an overview, *Radiol Clin North Am* 19:527, 1981.
62. Kitterman JA, Phibbs RH, Tooley WH: Aortic blood pressure in normal newborn infants during the first 12 hours of life, *Pediatrics* 44:959, 1969.
63. Kleinman LI, Stewart CL, Kaskel FJ: Renal disease in the newborn. In Edelmann CM, editor: *Pediatric nephrology,* ed 2, Boston, 1992, Little, Brown.
64. Ledermann SE, Scanes ME, Fernando ON, et al: Long-term outcome of perinatal dialysis in infants, *J Pediatr* 136:24, 2000.
65. Lieberman K: Continuous arteriovenous hemofiltration in children, *Pediatr Nephrol* 1:330, 1987.
66. Lindemann R: Congenital renal tubular dysfunction associated with maternal sniffing of organic solvents, *Acta Pediatr Scand* 80:882, 1991.
67. Malone TA: Glucose and insulin versus cation-exchange resin for the treatment of hyperkalemia in very low birth weight infants, *J Pediatr* 118:121, 1991.
68. Mathew OP, Jones AS, James E, et al: Neonatal renal failure: usefulness of diagnostic indices, *Pediatrics* 65:57, 1980.
69. Matos V, Drukker A, Guignard JP: Spot urine samples for evaluating solute excretion in the first week of life, *Arch Dis Child Fetal Neonatal Ed* 80:F240, 1999.
70. McLean RH, Gearhart JP, Jeffs R: Neonatal obstructive uropathy, *Pediatr Nephrol* 2:48, 1988.
71. McVicar M, Margouleff D, Chandra M: Diagnosis and imaging of the fetal and neonatal abdominal mass: an integrated approach, *Adv Pediatr* 38:135, 1991.
72. Mesrobian HO: Urologic problems of the neonate: an update, *Clin Perinatol* 34:667, 2007.
73. Mingeot-Leclercq MP, Tulkens PM: Aminoglycosides: nephrotoxicity, *Antimicrob Agents Chemother* 43:1003, 1999.
74. Mirmiran M, Kok JHL: Circadian rhythms in early human development, *Early Hum Dev* 26:121, 1991.
75. Mocan H, Beattie TJ, Murphy AV: Renal vein thrombosis in infancy: long term follow-up, *Pediatr Nephrol* 5:45, 1991.
76. Moxey-Mims M: Hematuria and proteinuria. In Kher KK, Schnaper HW, Makker SP, editors: *Clinical pediatric nephrology,* ed 2, Abingdon, Oxon, United Kingdom, 2007, Informahealthcare.

77. Moxey-Mims M, Stapleton FB: Renal tubular disorders in the neonate, *Clin Perinatol* 19:159, 1992.
78. Murphy JI, Kaplan GW, Packer MG, et al: Prenatal diagnosis of severe urinary tract anomalies improves renal function and growth, *Child Nephrol Urol* 9:290, 1988.
79. Murugasu B, Cole BR, Hawkins EP, et al: Familial renal adysplasia, *Am J Kid Dis* 18:490, 1991.
80. Polito C, Papale MR, La Manna AL: Long-term prognosis of acute renal failure in the full term newborn, *Clin Pediatr* 37:381, 2001.
81. Pope JC, Brock JW, Adams MC, et al: How they begin and how they end: classic and new theories for the development and deterioration of congenital anomalies of the kidney and urinary tract, CAKUT, *J Am Soc Nephrol* 10:2018, 1999.
82. Portman RJ, Carter BS, Gaylord MS, et al: Predicting neonatal morbidity after perinatal asphyxia: a scoring system, *Am J Obstet Gynecol* 162:174, 1990.
83. Potter EL: Normal and abnormal development of the kidney, Chicago, 1972, Year Book.
84. Quigley R, Baum M: Neonatal acid base balance and disturbances, *Semin Perinatol* 28:97, 2004.
85. Rabelo E, Oliveira EA, Diniz JS, et al: Natural history of multicystic kidney conservatively managa prospective study, *Pediatr Nephrol* 19:1102, 2004.
86. Reznik VM, Kaplan GW, Murphy JL, et al: Follow-up of infants with bilateral renal disease detected in utero, *Am J Dis Child* 142:453, 1988.
87. Richards DS: Ultrasound for pregnancy dating, growth and diagnosis of fetal malformation. In Gabbe SG, Niebyl JR, Simpson JL, editors: *Obstetrics: normal and problem pregnancies*, ed 5, Philadelphia, 2007, Churchill Livingstone.
88. Robinson RF, Nahata MC, Batisky DL, et al: Pharmacologic treatment of chronic pediatric hypertension, *Pediatr Drugs* 7:27, 2005.
89. Rodríguez-Soriano J, Aguirre M, Oliveros R, et al: Long-term renal follow-up of extremely low birth weight infants, *Pediatr Nephrol* 20:579, 2005.
90. Ronco C, Brendolan A, Bragantini L, et al: Treatment of acute renal failure in newborns by continuous arteriovenous hemofiltration, *Kidney Int* 29:908, 1986.
91. Roth CG, Spottswood SE, Chan JCM, et al: Evaluation of the hypertensive infant: a rational approach to diagnosis, *Rad Clin N Am* 41:91, 2003.
92. Roussan MS: Neurogenic bladder dysfunction, *Med Times* 109:43, 1981.
93. Schell-Feith EA: Etiology of nephrocalcinosis in preterm neonates: association of nutritional intake and urinary parameters, *Kidney Int* 58:2102, 2000.
94. Schmidt B, Andrew M: Neonatal thrombosis: report of a Prospective Canadian and International Registry, *Pediatrics* 96:939, 1995.
95. Seeman T, John U, Blahova K, et al: Ambulatory blood pressure monitoring in children with unilateral MCDK, *Eur J Pediatr* 160:78, 2001.
96. Sertel H, Scopes J: Rates of creatinine clearance in babies less than one week of age, *Arch Dis Child* 48:717, 1973.
97. Shankaran S, Liang KC, Ilagen N, et al: Mineral excretion following furosemide compared with bumetanide therapy in premature infants, *Pediatr Nephrol* 9:159, 1995.
98. Shooter M, Watson M: The ethics of withholding and withdrawing dialysis therapy in infants, *Pediatr Nephrol* 14:347, 2000.
99. Siegel S, Oh W: Renal function as a marker of human fetal maturation, *Acta Paediatr Scand* 65:481, 1976.
100. Sitka U, Weiner TD, Berle K, et al: Investigation of the rhythmic function of heart rate, blood pressure, and temperature in neonates, *Eur J Pediatr* 153:117, 1994.
101. Sniderman S, Charlton VE: Routine postnatal care and observation. In Rudolph CD, Rudolph AM, editors: *Rudolph's pediatrics*, ed 21, New York, 2003, McGraw Hill.
102. Springate JE, Fildes RD, Feld LG: Assessment of renal function in newborn infants, *Pediatr Rev* 9:51, 1987.
103. Stapleton FB, Jones DP, Green RS: Acute renal failure in neonates: incidence, etiology and outcome, *Pediatr Nephrol* 1:314, 1987.
104. Sulyok E, Guigard JP: Relationship of urinary anion gap to urinary ammonium excretion in the neonate, *Biol Neonate* 57:98, 1990.
105. Swinford RD, Bonilla-Felix M, Cerda RD, et al: Neonatal nephrology. In Merenstein GB, Gardner SL, editors: *Handbook of neonatal intensive care*, ed 6, St Louis, 2006, Mosby.
106. Tan KL: Blood pressure in full-term healthy newborns, *Clin Pediatr* 26:21, 1987.
107. Thayyil S, Sheik S, Kempley ST, et al: A gestation- and postnatal age-based reference chart for assessing renal function in extremely premature infants, *J Perinatol* 28:226, 2008.
108. Vainio JS, Uvsitalo MS: A road to kidney tubules in the WNT pathway, *Pediatr Nephrol* 15:151, 2000.
109. Vanderhcydcn T, Kumar S, Fisk NM: Fetal renal impairment, *Semin Neonatol* 28:279, 2003.
110. Wahlig TM, Thompson TR, Sinaiko AR: Drug use in the newborn: effects on the kidney, *Clin Perinatol* 19:251, 1992.
111. Warady BA, Bunchman T: Dialysis therapy for children with acute renal failure: survey results, *Pediatr Nephrol* 15:61, 2000.
112. Watkinson M: Hypertension in the newborn baby, *Arch Dis Child Fetal Neonatal Ed* 86:F78, 2002.
113. Watson AR, Shooter M: The effects of withholding and withdrawing dialysis. In Warady BA, Fine

RN, Alexander SR, et al, editors: *Pediatric dialysis*, Netherlands, 2004, Kluwer.
114. Wood EG: Risk factors for mortality in infants and children on dialysis, *Am J Kid Dis* 37:573, 2001.
115. Woolf AS: Developmental anatomy and physiology. In Morgan SH, Grunfeld JP, editors: *Inherited disorders of the kidney,* Oxford, 1998, Oxford University Press.
116. Woolf AS, Winyard PJD: Molecular mechanisms of human embryogenesis: developmental pathogenesis of renal tract malformations, *Pediatr Dev Pathol* 5:108, 2002.
117. Wu J, Cornelissen G, Tarquini B: Circaseptan and circannual modulation of circadian rhythms in neonatal blood pressure and heart rate. In Hayes D, Pauly J, Reiter R, editors: *Chronobiology: its role in clinical medicine, general biology and agriculture,* New York, 1990, Wiley-Liss.
118. Zinner SH, Rosner B, Oh W, et al: Significance of blood pressure in infancy: familial aggregation and predictive effect on later blood pressure, *Hypertension* 7:411, 1985.

26 NEUROLOGIC DISORDERS

M. TERESE VERKLAN AND SUZANNE M. LOPEZ

The developing nervous system provides ongoing challenges for researchers and clinicians. Investigations continue in a wide variety of areas, yet basic mechanisms for a pathophysiologic understanding of common events such as neonatal seizures and intraventricular hemorrhages (IVHs) remain unclear.

Improved neonatal care in recent years has not significantly reduced neurologic sequelae. How much of this is a reflection of survival of sicker and more immature infants is difficult to assess. Primary neurologic disease and secondary neurologic complications from such common conditions as cardiopulmonary disease, metabolic derangements, shock, infection, and coagulopathy still represent major problems encountered in every intensive care nursery. Serious anomalies still appear with regularity, yet in small numbers.

This chapter deals with selected topics in neonatal neurology, including congenital malformations, trauma, seizures, hypoxic-ischemic encephalopathy, and IVH.

CONGENITAL MALFORMATIONS

Physiology, Etiologic Factors, and Clinical Features

Congenital malformations of the nervous system occur when the usual sequence of maturation and development is interrupted (Table 26-1).[39] Present at birth, the etiology is multifactorial and sometimes unclear. Although strictly destructive lesions (e.g., hydranencephaly resulting from bilateral carotid artery occlusion) are separate from primary failures of morphogenesis, both may be included in the broad category of congenital malformations. The distinction between the two types lies in an understanding of the causes.

Understanding congenital malformations requires an appreciation of the normal embryologic sequence.[39] The clinical and pathologic identification of normal and abnormal structures makes it possible to determine the timing of the insult or development failure. Once timing is established, an appropriate search for the cause can be made.

Neural Tube Defects

The incidence in the United States of neural tube defects (NTDs) is approximately 1 to 2 in 1000 births (see the Critical Findings box on p. 749).[41] Although the prevalence of NTDs has decreased, they are one of the most common congenital anomalies contributing to morbidity and mortality in neonates.[2] Changes in vertebral, vascular, meningeal, and dermal structures are typically found along with the defects. The more common types of NTDs include anencephaly, encephalocele, myelomeningocele, and occult spina bifida.[5] Genetic and environmental factors play a role in the development of NTDs. Familial incidence also plays a role; when one family member is affected, the risk increases by 2% to 3% in subsequent offspring and doubles if two or more family members are affected.[5] Cytogenic abnormalities are found in approximately 2% to 16% of neonates who have an isolated NTD.[35] Teratogen exposure has also been linked to NTDs.[39] A prepregnancy history of diabetes, specific drugs (especially anticonvulsants and sulfonamide drugs), and maternal hyperthermia secondary to using a hot tub or sauna have been identified as risk factors.[17] Recently, prepregnancy maternal obesity also has been linked to an increased risk.[64]

Please note that the **PURPLE** type in each chapter is intended to make it easier to identify clinically applicable material.

TABLE 26-1	CENTRAL NERVOUS SYSTEM DEVELOPMENT AND RELATED DEFECTS	
MATURATIONAL PROCESS	**TIME**	**ASSOCIATED DEFECTS**
Neural tube defects (dorsal induction, neurulation)	3-4 weeks	Craniorhachischisis Anencephaly Myeloschisis Encephalocele Myelomeningocele Arnold-Chiari malformation
Prosencephalic development[61]	2-3 months	Cyclopia Holoprosencephaly Arrhinencephaly Septo-optic dysplasia Agenesis of corpus callosum Agenesis of septum pellucidum
Proliferation	2-4 months	Microcephaly Megalencephaly Neurocutaneous syndromes (?)
Migration[61]	3-5 months	Schizencephaly Lissencephaly Pachygyria (macrogyria) Microgyria (polymicrogyria) Neuronal heterotopias
Neuronal organization and functional organization	6 months	Down syndrome (?) Mental retardation (?) Genetic epilepsy (?)
Myelination[61]	2nd trimester[61]	Anoxic/ischemic damage

Critical Findings

NEURAL TUBE DEFECTS

- As many as 50% or more of neural tube defects (NTDs) are preventable.
- Two thirds of American women fail to ingest an adequate amount of folic acid, and enriched grain products supply only one fourth of daily need.
- All women of childbearing age should consume **400 mcg** of folic acid daily even when not planning to become pregnant.
- **At increased risk:** women with a prior NTD pregnancy. For these women, the recommended dose of folic acid is **increased to 4 mg daily**. It should be taken at least 1 month before conception.
- **Sources:** Dietary supplements, enriched grain products, and consumption of foods with folic acid content (citrus fruit, beans, leafy greens).
- The Centers for Disease Control and Prevention (CDC,) the American Academy of Pediatrics (AAP), and the March of Dimes have all recommended an increase in the amount of folic acid used to fortify grain products from 140 mcg to 350 mcg per 100 g of grain.
- Inadequate education of women continues to be a problem.

The major environmental factor linked to NTDs is a dietary level of folic acid.[27] Folic acid supplements before and during pregnancy have been cited as substantially lowering the incidence of these NTDs. The U.S. Public Health Service issued a recommendation that women of childbearing years consume 400 mcg of folic acid each day to prevent NTDs. The American Academy of Pediatrics (AAP) also supports this recommendation.[9,16,27,39,41] Such an intake can be achieved by dietary supplementation of folate, adding folic acid to U.S. enriched grain products (e.g., bread, flour), and consuming foods containing folic acid (e.g., citrus fruit, beans, leafy greens). The Food and Drug Administration (FDA) required all enriched grain products to be fortified with folic acid by 1998.[6,16] In spite of this, it has been reported by the Centers for Disease Control and Prevention (CDC) that two thirds of American women fail to ingest an adequate amount of folic acid.[9] It has been argued that the amount of folic acid supplementation in grain products may be inadequate, supplying only about one fourth of daily need.[40] Noting the 26% decrease in the incidence of NTDs after the FDA required 140 mcg folic acid per 100 g of grain, the March of Dimes recommended an increase in the level of folic acid fortification.[37,62] Others, including the CDC and AAP, concur with this recommendation to increase the requirement to 350 mcg folic acid per 100 g of grain.[7]

A Cochrane review concluded that supplementation of folate provides "a strong protective effect against neural tube defects." Recommendations were made to increase availability of information about folate. Another recommendation was to advise women with a prior NTD pregnancy of the increased risk for future pregnancy and to provide them with folate supplementation.[34] For women with a prior NTD pregnancy, the recommended dosage of folic acid is increased to 4 mg daily, which should be taken for at least 1 month before conception.[6,16,20] Unfortunately, it has been reported that some health care providers in contact with women of childbearing age are not counseling them about the importance of folic acid consumption or the appropriate amount to take.[20] It should not be expected that an improved consumption of folic acid will totally prevent all NTDs because of etiologic factors such as the environment and genetics.

At the end of the first embryonic week, the primitive streak is present on the rostral surface of the embryo. A second streak, the notochordal process, develops alongside the primitive streak. The notochord is responsible for the induction of both the neural plate and the neurenteric canal. Cells proliferate along the lateral margin of the neural plate to form the neural folds around the central neural groove.[61]

Cells at the apex of the neural folds make up the neural crest. Schwann cells, pia-arachnoid cells, sensory ganglia, melanocytes, and various secretory cells arise from the neural crest. The neural folds meet and fuse with the rostral (anterior) and caudal (posterior) ends (neuropore), closing by approximately the end of the fourth embryonic week.[61]

Failure of development at this stage results in the defects of neurulation (or dorsal induction). The most severe of these defects is craniorachischisis, in which there is significant malformation of the brain (as in anencephaly), absence of the posterior skull, and an open spine along the full length of the spinal cord. Only a few affected embryos survive to early fetal stages.[61]

Anencephaly is similar to craniorachischisis without the spinal defect. There is essentially no normal brain tissue above the brainstem and thalami, and parts of those structures are malformed. Onset is thought to occur before 24 days' gestation. About one fourth of the fetuses survive into the neonatal period, but three fourths are stillborn. The majority of anencephalic infants die within the first week of life without intensive care.[61]

Myeloschisis involves the failure of the posterior neural tube to close. There is no well-defined sac protruding from the defect.[8]

Encephaloceles are caused by a limited failure of closure at the rostral (head) end of the neural tube. Extensions of meninges or brain tissue through the skull may occur on the ventral or rostral surface.[61]

Myelomeningoceles (or even the more limited meningoceles) are a limited form of myeloschisis with failure of closure at the caudal (tail) end of the neural tube. With meningocele, the meninges protrude through the vertebrae and are contained within a sack. The spinal cord and nerve roots are generally in normal position, which improves the outcomes for these children. Unfortunately, myelomeningoceles, the more common defect, result in protrusion of both meninges and spinal cord through the opening in the spinal column. Neurologic deficits occur below the level of the protrusion.[35,47,56] The Arnold-Chiari deformities usually are included here. These malformations, often seen with myelomeningoceles, involve structures of the brainstem and cerebellum. Generally, the cerebellar tonsils are pulled down through the foramen magnum, and the brainstem is elongated in later life. Hydrocephalus is common. Dilation of ventricles often occurs without increased head circumference or clinical symptoms of increased intracranial pressure in this group of infants; therefore serial computed tomography (CT) or ultrasonographic scans should be performed. Symptoms of brainstem involvement may be present. Open myelomeningoceles and anencephaly (any defect in which the spinal or cranial contents are "open" to the outside) are associated with an elevation of alpha fetoprotein (AFP) in the amniotic fluid. This is important in prenatal diagnosis.[61]

Segmentation Defects

After formation and closure of the neural tube, the development of the different regions of the brain begins to occur. Suprasegmental structures are formed. The division of the brain into hemispheres, formation of the ventricular system, and formation of the major gyral patterns are all part of this period of development. Major areas of the brain, including the cerebellum, basal ganglia, brainstem nuclei, thalamus, and hypothalamus, form at this time.[61] Defects of segmentation and cleavage occur during this phase of neural development. For unknown reasons, defects of segmentation and cleavage are far less common than defects of neurulation. Because these malformations involve abnormalities of ventral induction rather than dorsal induction (e.g., neurulation), the face, eyes, nose, mouth, and hair are also involved in the malformation. These features always should be investigated carefully for specific anomalies.

Holoprosencephaly is characterized by a single midline lateral ventricle, incomplete or absent interhemispheric fissure, absent olfactory system, midfacial clefts, and hypotelorism. The most severe form of holoprosencephaly is cyclopia (a single fused midline eye) and supraorbital nasal structure. At times, the nasal structure and eye are absent. An intermediate form is cebocephaly, which includes ocular hypotelorism (abnormally decreased space between the eyes) and a flat nose with single nostril.[61]

When any of these malformations are suspected or when features suggestive of them are seen, careful examination of the hair, eyes, ears, mouth, and nose may reveal other related anomalies.

Migration and Cortical Organizational Defects

A critical aspect of brain development has yet to be described. The remaining development of the brain takes over twice as long as previously described development and includes cellular proliferation, migration, organization, and myelination. Cells that later form the cerebral cortex begin in the germinal matrix (near the caudate nucleus around the lateral ventricles). These cells then migrate in a radial fashion to their final positions near the surface of the brain. Abnormalities of cellular migration result in collections of gray matter in unusual places (heterotopias), abnormal gyri and sulci, abnormal spaces in the brain, and frequent clinical signs of gray matter dysfunction. Frequently, these clinical problems are not apparent in the newborn period.

Microcephaly means "small brain" and is manifested as a head circumference measuring greater than two standard deviations below average for infants at that gestational age.[17] Microcephaly may be (1) genetic (dominant, recessive, sex-linked) or chromosomal (translocation [see Chapter 27]); (2) caused by teratogens (cocaine, alcohol); (3) caused by infection (rubella, cytomegalovirus); or (4) of unknown cause. Occasionally there is a paucity of germinal matrix cells or they fail to adequately migrate, resulting in a brain cortex with a decreased number of neuronal cells.[61]

In ***lissencephaly,*** the brain is smooth in appearance, having little or no gyri (convolutions). Although not generally present at birth, microcephaly usually occurs within the first year in type I lissencephaly. Appearance is marked by hollowing at both temples, a small jaw, and hypotonia. Neonatal seizures may be present, but seizures are more commonly present at 6 to 12 months of age. Another form of type I lissencephaly is Miller-Dieker syndrome, in which craniofacial deviations occur. In type II lissencephaly, macrocephaly is generally present at birth or develops soon afterward. Retinal, cerebellar, and muscular abnormalities always are present.[61]

Clinical features of lissencephaly include seizures, microcephaly, hypotonia, feeding problems, scarcity of movement, upturned nares, temporal hollows, small jaw, protruding and long upper lip, and abnormalities on the electroencephalogram (EEG). Later, mental retardation and severe spasticity may be noted and death may occur.[61]

Additional Defects

Cerebellar malformations are quite varied. Most often, at least a portion of the cerebellum is preserved, but total absence is possible. Hemispheric aplasia or vermal aplasia is seen, and familial forms have been reported. The ***Dandy-Walker cyst*** is another complex malformation involving the cerebellum in which the fourth ventricle is dilated into a cystic structure. The foramina of Magendie and Luschka are atretic, and hydrocephalus results. The cerebellum is small and displaced upward. Associated anomalies include heterotopias, agenesis of the corpus callosum, aqueductal stenosis, and syringomyelia. Causation is unknown. The differential diagnosis includes an arachnoid cyst of the posterior fossa. In the case of an arachnoid cyst, the fourth ventricle is not part of the malformation and is normal, although it may be displaced.[61]

Clinical features of the Dandy-Walker cyst include frequent progressive hydrocephalus, associated malformations that cause additional specific symptoms, possible absence of symptoms in the newborn period, enlargement of the occipital shelf and posterior part of the skull, and clinical symptoms of increased intracranial pressure.[61]

Craniosynostosis is the abnormally early closure (fusion) of the bones of the skull. Causation of this malformation is unknown. The premature closure of sutures may involve one or many sutures, with resulting deformity of the skull. Numerous terms are used to describe the shapes the skull assumes when craniosynostosis is present.[61]

Craniosynostosis should be suspected in the presence of microcephaly or misshapen head. Appropriate evaluation requires x-ray films of the skull and a CT scan to define which, if any, of the sutures are stenosed and what problems might exist with brain structure (pressure or malformation).[61]

Hydrocephalus may occur in many different situations from many separate causes. An inherited X-linked form exists. Intrauterine infection is another cause. Hydrocephalus may be associated with many of the malformations described previously. Hydrocephalus results when the normal flow of ventriculospinal fluid is obstructed. This may be the result of an atretic portion of the ventricular system, blockage from the outside, inflammation within the ventricular system causing a permanent blockage, or (very rarely) overproduction of ventriculospinal fluid.[35,61]

Data Collection

The diagnosis of malformations of the central nervous system (CNS) may be quite obvious (as in anencephaly) or more subtle. Careful examination of all newborns results in the identification of most malformations. At times, the diagnosis is suspected not on the basis of findings on examination but because of an accompanying sign, such as seizures.[5]

Two very important tests have become available in recent years that allow prenatal diagnosis of certain congenital malformations of the nervous system. Ultrasonographic examination (an abdominal ultrasound scan of the mother) provides an opportunity to identify certain malformations by viewing the fetus during development. Hydrocephalus, encephaloceles, myelomeningoceles, and anencephaly may be identified prenatally. Determination of AFP in the amniotic fluid and maternal serum allows the identification of anencephaly and open myelomeningoceles. A non-enclosed nervous system is associated with a significant rise in AFP in the amniotic fluid. Amniocentesis provides the amniotic fluid necessary for this determination. Testing of maternal serum for AFP also is an option and at some centers may be used along with ultrasonography for diagnosis, allowing amniocentesis to be omitted.[61] Clinical signs and symptoms have been described for each individual nervous system malformation presented earlier in this chapter.

Treatment

Limited treatment is available for congenital malformations of the nervous system. A variety of strategies are available for reducing secondary complications or providing earlier management to handle these complications more efficiently.

The greatest efforts and accomplishments have been made for infants with congenital malformations who might be expected to have productive lives. When secondary complications are managed appropriately, the majority of children with myelomeningoceles are ambulatory (total or partial) and continent of urine.[61]

Myelomeningocele generally is surgically repaired as soon as possible (within 24 to 48 hours).[5,35,47,61] Prevention of infection is paramount. In addition to sterile technique, prophylactic antibiotics have been shown to be beneficial.[61] **Trauma to the area should be avoided by keeping the infant in the prone position and maintaining sterile gauze moistened with warm, sterile normal saline.** Tape should be avoided.[5,35,44] Preventing fecal contamination is vital. Several authors recommend the use of a sterile, plastic drape fastened above the anus but below the lesion to keep fecal material isolated from the site.[35,44] **Latex precautions also should be initiated, because these infants have an increased propensity for developing sensitivity to latex.**[5]

In addition, spina bifida has been repaired in utero at early gestational age. Such repairs have risks for both mother and fetus but have resulted in reported significant drops in the number of infants developing hydrocephalus that would require a postnatal ventriculoperitoneal shunt.[15] Because of a lack of improved neurologic outcomes overall, a multicenter randomized controlled trial (RCT) is underway to compare intrauterine therapy to conventional postnatal care to better identify procedure-related benefits and risks.[15]

Some of the malformations are lethal very soon after birth (anencephaly), limiting management options for **comfort measures and family support.** When appropriate, genetic counseling should be requested. **For other malformations, treatment requires management of symptoms such as seizures, signs of increased intracranial pressure, and infection.** A consult to neurosurgery is indicated. Other helpful consults may include physical therapy, infectious diseases, urology, and orthopedics.[35] For hydrocephalus, shunting may become necessary. See Box 26-1, the Parent Teaching box on pp. 754-755, and Figure 26-1).[61]

The one situation in which microcephaly could be considered surgically treatable is total craniosynostosis. Generally, skull deformity is present in infants with craniosynostosis, and it is always wise

BOX 26-1 POSTOPERATIVE VENTRICULOPERITONEAL SHUNT CARE

- Positioning:
  - Place infant on unaffected side (may position on shunt side with "doughnut" over operative site once incision has healed). Keep head of bed flat (15 to 30 degrees) to prevent too-rapid fluid loss.
  - Support head carefully when moving infant.
  - Turn q 2 hr from unaffected side of head to back.
- Shunt site:
  - Use strict aseptic technique when changing dressing.
  - Pump shunt if and only as directed by neurosurgeon.
  - Observe for fluid leakage around pump.
- Observe and document all intake and output. Watch for symptoms of excessive drainage of CSF:
  - Sunken fontanel
  - Increased urine output
  - Increased sodium loss
- Observe, document, and report any seizure activity or paresis.
- Observe for signs of ileus:
  - Abdominal distention (serially measure abdominal girth)
  - Absence of bowel sounds
  - Loss of gastric content by emesis or through orogastric tube
- Perform range-of-motion exercises on all extremities.
- Observe and assess for symptoms of increased intracranial pressure (shunt failure):
  - Increasing head circumference (measure head daily)
  - Full or tense fontanel
  - Sutures palpably more separated
  - High-pitched, shrill cry
  - Irritability and/or sleeplessness
  - Vomiting
  - Poor feeding
  - Nystagmus
  - Sunset sign of eyes
  - Shiny scalp with distended vessels
  - Hypotonia and/or hypertonia
- Observe and assess for signs of infection:
  - Redness or drainage at shunt site
  - Hypothermia and/or hyperthermia
  - Lethargy and/or irritability
  - Poor feeding and/or poor weight gain
  - Pallor
- Parent teaching:
  - Demonstrate and receive return demonstration of drug administration.
  - Teach parents side effects of medications.
  - Document on NICU's routine discharge teaching checklist with routine care.

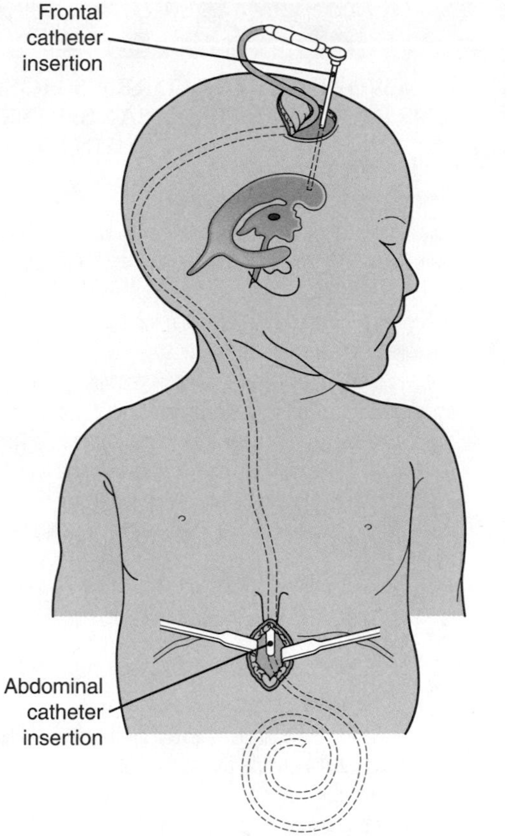

FIGURE 26-1 Ventricular peritoneal shunt. (From Rothrock LC: *Alexander's Care of the Patient in Surgery,* ed 13, St Louis, 2007, Mosby.)

to consider the presence of craniosynostosis in any infant with a small head. If present, total craniosynostosis should be treated surgically.[35]

The management of congenital hydrocephalus consists primarily of early shunting as soon after birth as possible. Fetal surgery for placement of a ventriculoamniotic shunt has been proposed, but an improvement in outcomes compared with surgery after birth is uncertain. In addition, hydrocephalus in a fetus is often associated with serious developmental abnormalities that may increase morbidity and mortality.[61]

In Volpe's series, outcome was variable and the procedures were not as reliable as hoped. It was not always possible to distinguish true hydrocephalus from ventriculomegaly without increased pressure. Shunting soon after birth often produces a far better outcome

Parent Teaching

WOLFSON CHILDREN'S HOSPITAL PARENT HANDOUT: NEWBORN VENTRICULOPERITONEAL SHUNT (FOR USE WITH VENTRICULOPERITONEAL SHUNT TEACHING CHECKLIST)

Purpose of Ventriculoperitoneal Shunt

- Ventricles are compartment-like spaces that are located in the normal brain. Spinal fluid forms daily in these ventricles. This clear fluid flows out over the brain and down around the spinal cord. Spinal fluid helps cushion the brain from injury, keeps the brain moist, and carries away waste products.
- Hydrocephalus is a condition in which an abnormally large amount of spinal fluid builds up in your baby's ventricles and usually is caused by a blockage in the spinal fluid path. Because the ventricles continue to make spinal fluid daily, a buildup of fluid occurs when it cannot escape. This excess fluid can cause pressure on the brain and result in permanent damage to the brain unless it is properly treated.
- The purpose and function of your baby's VP shunt is to allow the excess spinal fluid to drain through a tube from the ventricle into the abdomen, where it is absorbed.

Pathway of the Ventriculoperitoneal Shunt

- A small incision is made on the scalp, and the tube is passed through the skull and into the ventricle. Located under the skin, the tube passes behind the ear, down the side of the neck, and continues to the abdomen, where a second incision is made to put the end of the tube into the abdominal cavity. A third incision is sometimes needed in the neck area with some babies.
- The scalp incision will be hidden as your baby's hair grows. You will see and feel the shunt tubing (like a large vein under the skin), but it is barely noticeable after the baby gains weight.

Signs and Symptoms of Shunt Infection

- The shunt is at risk for infection because it is a foreign object located inside the body. You will have to watch for these signs of shunt infection and report them **immediately** to your doctor:
  - Temperature of 101° F or higher
  - Swelling, redness, or drainage along the pathway of the shunt tube
  - Lethargy or irritability (change in behavior)
  - Loss of appetite or poor feeding

Signs and Symptoms of Shunt Failure/Increased Intracranial Pressure

- The spinal fluid contains proteins and chemicals that may build up and block off the shunt. It is also possible for tissue within the brain or abdomen to block the shunt or for the shunt device itself to fail. This shunt failure (malfunction) means that the spinal fluid will once again build up and result in pressure on the brain and possible irreversible damage. Therefore it is very important for you to watch for the signs of increased pressure in the brain that occurs with shunt failure and report them to your doctor immediately:
  - Lethargy or sleepiness
  - Unusual irritability, fussiness, or excessive crying
  - Repeated vomiting
  - Poor feeding
  - Bulging soft spot when baby is sitting up quietly
  - Shrill, high-pitched cry
  - Eyes that look downward
  - Increase in spaces between the bones of the skull
  - Seizures/posturing

Reason and Importance of Prompt Treatment of Health Problems

- Prompt treatment of your baby's health problems (e.g., ear infections, skin infections) is important to prevent infections spreading to the shunt. It is also vital to seek medical care for signs of shunt infection or failure as noted.

Importance of Close Medical Follow-up

- Your baby will have to be followed up by a neurosurgeon and your pediatrician after being discharged. Bring the baby to every follow-up appointment so that your baby's head can be measured and physical condition can be evaluated. Your baby will also go to the Developmental Evaluation Clinic where a specialist in baby development can examine him or her. If development problems occur, this will ensure early diagnosis and treatment.

Care of the Shunt

- You can handle, cuddle, and play with your baby like any baby. Your baby also can sleep in any position after the initial postoperative period.

Courtesy Baptist Medical Center, Wolfson Children's Hospital, Jacksonville, Fla.

than would be assumed, with minimal motor deficit and only a mild to moderate deficit in intellect.[61]

Monitoring of pregnancies with fetal ultrasound allows the detection of congenital hydrocephalus. Induction of lung maturation with steroids has been suggested to allow a preterm delivery (with a smaller head) without excessive pulmonary complications. In this way, a permanent shunt can be placed sooner than with term delivery.[61]

Parent Teaching—cont'd

BAPTIST MEDICAL CENTER
WOLFSON CHILDREN'S HOSPITAL
JACKSONVILLE, FLORIDA

Wolfson Children's Hospital at Baptist Medical Center

VENTRICULOPERITONEAL (VP) SHUNT TEACHING CHECKLIST

GOAL/SKILL	NURSING (Date and Initials)	CARE GIVER #1	CARE GIVER #2	CARE GIVER #3
1. Verbalizes understanding of reason for VP shunt.	H - "An Introduction to Hydrocephalus" ☐			
2. Identifies the pathway of the VP shunt and the shunt's function.	H - "Ventriculoperitoneal Shunt" (Newborn) ☐ H - "Hydrocephalus and Shunts" (For infants with Cordis Shunts) ☐ H - "Your Valve System for Hydrocephalus" (For Cordis Valve System Shunts) ☐ H - "Just Like Any Other Little Beagle" ☐ V - "Just Like Any Other Little Beagle" ☐			
3. Lists signs and symptoms of shunt infection and emergent need to notify MD.				
4. Lists signs and symptoms of shunt failure and emergent need to notify MD.				
5. Discuss the reason and importance of prompt treatment of health problems.				
6. Verbalizes understanding of importance of close medical follow-up.				

SIGNATURE/INITIAL		TEACHING CODES	PARENT SIGNATURE(S)
		L - Lecture/Discussion D - Demonstration (or return demo) U - Verbalizes Understanding R - Reinforced Teaching V - Video H - Handout E - Equipment	 PATIENT LABEL

20-207 Rev 5/96

Complications

Many of the expected complications were dealt with previously in the sections describing the malformations and their associated problems. It is difficult to separate true complications from problems resulting from the malformation. For example, hydrocephalus develops in many infants with myelomeningocele and may be present at birth.[5,47] Other complications or associated problems of myelomeningocele include bowel and bladder incontinence, meningitis, urinary tract infections, and paralysis.[35]

Malformations carry with them altered anatomy and physiology that is reflected in abnormal function. Common general problems include seizures, mental retardation, sensorimotor abnormalities, disturbances in primary sensory function such as vision and hearing, orthopedic problems, and vegetative functions.[61]

The problems encountered are ordinarily explained on the basis of the malformation. Often midline defects in the brain (particularly at the base of the brain) have clinical problems involving the hypothalamus. Diabetes insipidus may be present.

To some extent, the anatomy predicts the types of problems. Involvement of the cortex causes seizures, retardation, and sensorimotor problems. White matter damage can cause spasticity. If the brainstem is involved in the malformation, apnea, deafness, sleep disturbance, oculomotor disturbances, and problems with sucking and swallowing may be seen. Spinal cord lesions cause quadriplegia or paraplegia. Genitourinary problems and, to a lesser extent, gastrointestinal problems also are seen.

Apnea and other brainstem findings may occur when the malformation involves the brainstem, as in Arnold-Chiari deformity, Dandy-Walker cyst, occipital encephalocele, and arachnoid cyst.

Pituitary-hypothalamic dysfunction may manifest itself in impaired temperature regulation, thyroid abnormalities, diabetes insipidus, and adrenal insufficiency.

Most of the complications occur after the newborn period, although causation is present at birth and includes seizures, retardation, spasticity, genitourinary problems, and orthopedic problems. In many circumstances, the problem is already present but functional expression, such as impaired ambulation, mental retardation, or deafness, is lacking. In the infant's follow-up examinations, careful attention must be given to problems likely to develop or intensify with age. When a specific malformation is identified, it is necessary to become familiar with the expected problems, not only to anticipate problems as they appear but also to lessen any secondary damage that might occur if they go unrecognized.

Parent Teaching

Parents of an infant born with congenital malformations are faced with a stressful event that may develop into a major life transition. Parents, especially mothers, report feelings of guilt and self-blame, although they may not initially share these feelings with hospital staff. After the birth of a malformed child, they go through stages of grief (see Chapters 29 and 30): shock or denial, anger, bargaining, depression, and acceptance. Some authors question whether full acceptance occurs for the family of the handicapped child because of return of grief and sorrow each time a developmental milestone is missed or the child experiences illness.[38,44]

Social support received from hospital personnel, family, and friends can help parents feel less stressed and more able to cope with the illness of their infant. **The ability of the staff to accurately anticipate and assess parental feelings and concerns can be invaluable when assisting families through this difficult time.** Parents should be encouraged to verbalize their feelings and fears in a supportive environment. Reassurances, when appropriate, should be provided (e.g., parents were not responsible for the congenital malformation; it is normal for the mother to experience [or at least report] more fears than her husband). **The ultimate goal of intervention is to reduce stress, assist families to confront fears, improve coping, and facilitate the bonding process.**[38]

Infants with congenital malformations present such a complex variety of problems that parent teaching and emotional support need to begin as early as possible. Often parents know from the time of birth or earlier that a major problem exists. In other circumstances, the anomaly is detected only after appropriate studies are performed.

When the infant is not viable, care should be directed at meeting the emotional needs of the family. **Every effort should be made to give family members positive experiences and memories by encouraging early parental holding of the infant and, whenever possible, participation with care** (see Chapter 30). Anticipatory counseling from social services and chaplain staff can help the family during grieving and with funeral arrangements. There are also questions about etiologic factors and genetics, and these questions should be dealt with according to the family's wishes (see Chapter 27).

If serious handicaps are anticipated and the infant is expected to survive, the parents should be encouraged to participate in the care of the infant from the beginning. Both adjustment and specific aspects of care within the circumstance will be enhanced and learning will be more effective if parents are supported. **A multidisciplinary team approach to parent education and support allows individualized hospital resources for specific needs of the patient and family.** In addition to medical, nursing, social service, and chaplain involvement, team members can be drawn from psychology, developmental specialists, physical therapy/occupational therapy, and other services based on specific needs and circumstances. **Parent teaching and support must be individualized according to the anomaly.** When available, support groups, integrative discharge planning, and specialized clinics can help with post-discharge care and parent education.

Parent teaching for the mothers and fathers of infants with congenital anomalies should (1) be started early, (2) involve the parents in the care of the infant, (3) use the resources of the hospital for specialized help, and (4) continue after the infant has gone home from the hospital.[38]

TABLE 26-2 ANATOMIC CLASSIFICATION OF BIRTH INJURIES

SITE OF INJURY	TYPE OF INJURY
Scalp	Caput succedaneum Subgaleal hemorrhage Cephalhematoma
Skull	Linea fracture Depressed fracture Occipital osteodiastasis
Intracranial	Epidural hematoma Subdural hematoma (laceration of flax, tentorium, or superficial veins) Subarachnoid hemorrhage Cerebral contusion Cerebellar contusion Intracerebellar hematoma
Spinal cord (cervical)	Vertebral artery injury Intraspinal hemorrhage Spinal cord transection or injury
Plexus injuries	Erb's palsy Klumpke's paralysis Total (mixed) brachial plexus injury Horner syndrome Diaphragmatic paralysis Lumbosacral plexus injury
Cranial and peripheral nerve injuries	Radial nerve palsy/nerve injuries Medial nerve palsy Sciatic nerve palsy Laryngeal nerve palsy Diaphragmatic paralysis Facial nerve palsy

BIRTH INJURIES

Physiology and Etiology

Birth injuries (birth traumas) are the direct result of difficulties encountered during the delivery process. These may be minor injuries without expected sequelae or the direct cause of death in the neonatal period. Classification of birth injuries usually is etiologic (predisposing factors or mechanisms of injury) or anatomic. An anatomic classification is used in this discussion to illustrate commonly encountered problems (Table 26-2).

The timing of birth injuries can be used to identify and describe causes. Etiologic classification of birth injuries includes uterine injury (antenatal), fetal monitoring procedures, abnormal or difficult presentations or methods of delivery, and multifactorial injuries. It should be recognized that the same injury might have multiple causations. Thus a cephalhematoma could be the result of forceps delivery, vacuum extraction, or routine vaginal delivery. A variety of specific predisposing factors increase the risk for birth injury, as follows:

- Macrosomia
- Cephalopelvic disproportion
- Dystocia
- Prematurity
- Prolonged or precipitous labor
- Breech presentation
- Forceps usage
- Rotation of fetus

- Version and extraction
- Handling after delivery

Multiple factors often are present. When multiple predisposing factors are present, a single underlying maternal disease often links them. A common example is that of a premature, macrosomic fetus with a diabetic mother in whom labor is not progressing properly.

The common factors that are present in deliveries complicated by birth injuries are as follows:

- **Unusual progress of labor**
- **Unusual size or shape of the fetus (large for gestational age or hydrocephalus)**
- **Problems encountered during delivery (dystocia or forceps application)**
- **Unusual or unexpected presentations (breech or unexpected twin)**

The maternal history must always be explored for the underlying disease process or conditions that might increase the risk for a birth injury.

Prevention

Most birth injuries may be preventable, at least in theory. Careful attention to risk factors and the appropriate planning of delivery should reduce the incidence of birth injuries to a minimum. Transabdominal ultrasonography facilitates predelivery awareness of macrosomia, hydrocephalus, and unusual presentations. Particular pregnancies then may be delivered by controlled elective cesarean section to avoid significant birth injury. Care must be taken to avoid substituting a procedure of greater risk. Often a small percentage of significant birth injuries cannot be anticipated until the specific circumstances are encountered during delivery. Emergency cesarean section may provide last-minute salvage, but in these circumstances, the injury truly may be unavoidable.

SPECIFIC BIRTH INJURIES

Injuries to the Scalp

The three commonly encountered forms of extracranial hemorrhage are caput succedaneum, subgaleal hemorrhage, and cephalhematoma and are distinguished not only in clinical manifestations but also in pathophysiology (see the Critical Findings box at right.[61] These three extracranial scalp injuries are included with neurologic birth injuries, not because they have associated neurologic problems but because the family or health care providers often raise the question of possible neurologic involvement.

Critical Findings

EXTRACRANIAL HEMORRHAGE

There are three common forms of extracranial hemorrhage but with different etiology and clinical assessment findings, as follows.

1. Caput succedaneum
   a. *Etiology:* Trauma to scalp (usually vertex vaginal delivery) results in hemorrhagic edema superficial to the aponeurosis of the scalp.
   b. *Findings:* Soft, pitting edema that crosses suture lines.
2. Cephalhematoma
   a. *Etiology:* Mechanical trauma; most common in primiparous women, with delivery using forceps or in vacuum-assisted deliveries.
   b. *Findings:* Firm, tense collection of blood confined by the sutures. Area often increases in size after delivery. No significant blood loss. Blood collects beneath the periosteum (subperiosteal).
   c. *Warning:* Associated with linear skull fracture in up to 25% of the cases.
3. Subgaleal hemorrhage
   a. *Etiology:* Forces that compress and then drag head through pelvic outlet.
   b. *Findings:* Firm swelling that crosses suture lines and is fluctuant to palpation. Blood collection is under the aponeurosis (connective tissue connecting the occipital and frontal muscles). Bleeding (swelling) may continue after birth and dissect along tissue planes into the neck.
   c. *Warning: Acute blood loss may occur.* Presenting symptom may be shock.
      Monitor VS for signs of shock:
         Elevated HR
         Decreasing BP
      Monitor baby for signs of shock:
         Pallor
         Delayed capillary refill time
         Diminished tone
         Respiratory distress
      Transfusion may be necessary: type and crossmatch.
      Serial Hct should be followed.
      Elevated bilirubin is a common complication as a by-product of broken-down red blood cells.

BP, Blood pressure; *Hct,* hematocrit; *HR,* heart rate; *VS,* vital signs.

PHYSIOLOGY AND ETIOLOGY

Caput succedaneum is caused by trauma to the scalp, usually during a routine vertex vaginal delivery. The caput is the result of hemorrhagic edema superficial to the periosteum of the scalp. Therefore spread of the edema is not restricted to suture lines and is soft and pitting because of its superficial location.[35,61]

Forces that compress and drag the head through the pelvic outlet are associated with ***subgaleal hemorrhage.*** Significant acute blood loss can occur with shock as the presenting symptom. Bleeding may continue after birth with enlargement of the accumulated blood and dissection of the blood along tissue planes into the neck. Such a hemorrhage carries the greatest potential for complications, but fortunately it is the least common form of birth injury to the scalp.[32,35,61]

Cephalhematoma is a subperiosteal collection of blood that is confined by the skull sutures. The incidence is 1% to 2% of all live births. The cause is nearly always mechanical trauma, and its occurrence is more common in primiparous women and in forceps or vacuum-assisted delivery. Males are generally more likely to be affected than females. It is associated with an underlying linear skull fracture in up to 25% of cases. The firm, tense collection of blood frequently increases in size after birth, but significant blood loss does not occur.[5,35,61]

DATA COLLECTION

With caput succedaneum, physical examination reveals soft, pitting edema that is diffuse and crosses suture lines. Laboratory tests are not needed.[35,61]

Because the subgaleal collection of blood is under the aponeurosis (connective tissue connecting the occipital and frontal muscles) and superficial to the periosteum, subgaleal hemorrhage crosses suture lines. It is firm but fluctuant to palpation. **Vital signs should be carefully monitored for symptoms of shock. Pallor, delayed capillary refill time, diminished tone, respiratory distress, elevated heart rate, or decreasing blood pressure should be observed for and treated promptly.** Transfusion may be necessary. **The hematocrit should be serially followed, and bilirubin levels should be determined during recovery.**[35,61]

Cephalhematomas may occur anywhere but are most commonly found in the parietal area on one side. Because the location of the blood is subperiosteal, the blood is confined by suture lines. Symptoms are normally absent. A skull fracture underlying the cephalhematoma is present in 10% to 25% of affected infants. X-ray examination of the skull defines the fracture. Rare complications include infection, osteomyelitis, hyperbilirubinemia, meningitis, and late-onset anemia.[35,61]

TREATMENT

Usually, no treatment is necessary for any of these three lesions. **In subgaleal hemorrhage, treatment of blood loss and shock may be necessary. During resolution, the breakdown of the blood may cause hyperbilirubinemia requiring treatment** (see Chapter 21).[35,61]

PARENT TEACHING

Parents of an infant with caput succedaneum should understand that the swelling is outside of the cavity of the brain and will usually reabsorb within 48 hours.[35] **Careful preparation of the parents for the acute side effects of subgaleal hemorrhage is important. Parents should be warned of the possibility of swelling and discoloration of the face, head, and neck.** The purpose of serial hematocrit and bilirubin checks should be explained. Parents can expect 2 to 3 weeks for the swelling to resolve.[35] Parents of an infant with a cephalhematoma should be instructed that the cephalohematoma may enlarge but that they should not be concerned unless localized changes occur, suggesting secondary infection (erythema, induration, or drainage). This lesion should not be drained and may be evident for 6 to 8 weeks and leave a small calcification after reabsorption of hemorrhage. The hemorrhage can be significant enough to cause hyperbilirubinemia or anemia. **Outpatient evaluation of bilirubin levels and hematocrit may be needed in some cases.**

Skull Fractures

Three forms of skull fracture should be identified and differentiated: linear fractures, depressed fractures, and occipital osteodiastasis.[35,61]

PHYSIOLOGY AND ETIOLOGY

Linear skull fracture (a nondepressed fracture) is the most common type of skull fracture. The result of compression of the skull during delivery, **a linear skull fracture most often has no associated injuries and causes no symptoms.** Bleeding may be seen extracranially (common) or intracranially (rare).

Intracranial bleeding causes symptoms referable to the bleeding rather than to the fracture itself.[35,61]

The typical depressed skull fracture is of the "ping-pong" type, an indentation without loss of bony continuity. When forceps are used during delivery, the direct cause of injury may result but is often without complications or sequelae. When neurologic signs are present, direct cerebral injury, intracranial bleeding, or free bone fragments should be suspected.[35,61]

DATA COLLECTION

A linear skull fracture usually produces no signs or symptoms unless intracranial bleeding has occurred. Skull x-ray films most frequently demonstrate a parietal fracture. A depressed skull fracture may be noted by presence of a visible depression or a palpable "ping-pong" fracture in the parietal or temporal area. No other signs and symptoms are present unless intracranial bleeding or focal irritation of the cortex causes them. **Evaluation with a skull x-ray examination or CT scan is necessary to delineate the fracture and to identify complications.**

TREATMENT

No treatment is necessary for a linear skull fracture. Treatment of a depressed skull fracture varies and centers on the mode of treatment and the necessity of treatment for fractures that create no neurologic symptoms. **If free bone fragments or clots are identified, neurosurgical intervention is necessary.** More conservative approaches are indicated when no complications are present. Noninvasive treatments such as vacuum extractors and breast pumps have been used with success to raise the depressed bone segment.[61]

COMPLICATIONS

With a linear skull fracture, the single complication to be aware of is a "growing" skull fracture. A dural tear may allow leptomeninges to extrude into the fracture site, setting up the possibility of a leptomeningeal cyst. As the cyst enlarges, the edges of the fracture may fail to fuse and even spread apart, giving the appearance of a "growing" fracture. Palpation and x-ray examination demonstrate the lesion. Surgical correction may be necessary to ensure healing and prevent further complications. With a depressed skull fracture, intracranial bleeding and direct cerebral injury with seizures or residual neurologic deficit are rare.

PARENT TEACHING

Parents should be instructed to have the fracture site monitored for several months to ensure that reunion of the bone has taken place. Patients will require no other aftercare unless neurosurgical intervention was necessary or complications developed.

Intracranial Birth Injuries

Three major forms of bleeding occur intracranially: epidural hematoma, subdural hemorrhage, and subarachnoid hemorrhage (see the Critical Findings box on p. 761). Added to these are cerebellar hemorrhages, cerebellar contusions, and cerebral contusions. Each has its own particular set of symptoms and signs and complications and sequelae. IVH usually is not related to trauma and is covered separately in this chapter.

PHYSIOLOGY AND ETIOLOGY

An ***epidural hematoma*** is pathophysiologically difficult to form in newborns because of a relatively thick dura. When present, it is almost always accompanied by a linear skull fracture across the middle meningeal artery.

Subdural hemorrhage is more common in term infants than in preterm infants and occurs from trauma tearing veins and venous sinuses. Although some assume its presence represents birth trauma, several authors indicate that this is not necessarily the case.[61,65] Subdural hemorrhage has been linked with maternal use of aspirin and also to maternal ingestion of phenobarbital.[61] Four major pathologic entities are defined: (1) laceration of the tentorium, (2) laceration of the falx, (3) laceration of the superficial cerebral vein, and (4) occipital osteodiastasis. Tentorial laceration causes a posterior fossa clot with compression of the brainstem. The straight sinus, Galen's vein, lateral sinus, and infratentorial veins may be involved. Laceration of the falx is caused by rupture of the inferior sagittal sinus. The laceration usually occurs at the junction of the tentorium and the falx, and the clot appears in the longitudinal cerebral fissure over the corpus callosum. Laceration of superficial cerebral veins causes subdural bleeding over the convexity of the brain. Subarachnoid bleeding or contusion of the brain also may be present.[36,61]

A subarachnoid hemorrhage is the most common type of neonatal intracranial hemorrhage. In term infants, trauma is the most common

Critical Findings

INTRACRANIAL BIRTH INJURIES

1. Epidural hematoma
   a. *Occurrence:* Rare.
   b. *Location:* Bleeding occurs into the epidural space. Blood is located between the inner area of skull bone and the periosteum.
   c. *Pathophysiology:* Most (not all) with history of traumatic labor or delivery.
   d. *Clinical findings:*
      Increased intracranial pressure (swollen fontanel).
      Seizures may occur.
   e. *Associated problems:* Almost always accompanied by a linear skull fracture.
2. Subdural hemorrhage
   a. *Occurrence:* More common in term infants than in preterm.
   b. *Location:* Bleeding is produced from tear of cerebral vein or sinus, which is often accompanied by a tear in the dura. Exact location of the hematoma depends on the location of the bleeding source.[61]
      Laceration of the tentorium
      Laceration of the falx
      Laceration of the superficial cerebral vein
      Occipital osteodiastasis
   c. *Pathophysiology:*
      Debate as to whether its presence indicates birth trauma. Volpe indicates that most cases result from trauma.[61]
      Linked to maternal use of aspirin and maternal ingestion of phenobarbital.
   d. *Clinical findings:*
      Neurologically abnormal at birth, if massive bleed:
      Seizures
      Stupor or coma
      Skew deviation of eyes
      Pupil changes: unequal pupils, poorly responsive pupils, fixed and dilated pupils
      Nuchal rigidity
      Apnea and bradycardia
      Signs of increased intracranial pressure
   e. *Associated problems:* Risk for herniation with lumbar puncture.
3. Subarachnoid hemorrhage
   a. *Occurrence:* Most common type of neonatal intracranial hemorrhage.
   b. *Location:* Blood is within the subarachnoid space but not because of extension from other areas. Small hemorrhages are more common than large ones. Source believed to be small vascular channels.[61]
   c. *Pathophysiology:*
      Term: Usually caused by trauma
      Preterm: Usually caused by hypoxia
   d. *Clinical findings:*
      Most common: Minimal or no symptoms
      Seizures (especially with term infants): "Well baby with seizures"
      Apnea (especially with preterm infants)
      For massive bleed (rare): Sudden and marked deterioration; death
      Associated problems:
         Usually none for infants without significant trauma or hypoxia.
         After major bleed:
            Hydrocephalus (most common sequela)
            Neurologic residual
            Death

cause, whereas in preterm infants, hypoxia is more often the cause. Small hemorrhages are more common than massive ones and usually result from venous bleeding. Underlying contusion may be present.[3,36,61]

Cerebral contusions are uncommon as an isolated event. Focal blunt trauma is necessary to produce a contusion. Pathologically, focal areas of hemorrhage and necrosis are seen. Shearing forces may cause slit-like tears in the white matter.

Cerebellar contusion and ***intracerebellar hemorrhage*** are uncommon events usually seen in association with occipital osteodiastasis and infratentorial subdural hemorrhage. These are catastrophic events, as described, and most often result in the death of the patient.

DATA COLLECTION

For epidural hemorrhage, the signs and symptoms may be diffuse (increased intracranial pressure with a bulging fontanel) and may include focal or lateralizing seizures, eye deviation, and hemisyndromes. **Laboratory tests should include x-ray examination to look for fractures and CT scanning to identify bleeding.**

Infants with subdural hemorrhage are neurologically abnormal at birth. **Tentorial lacerations and laceration of the falx tend to produce signs by pressure on the brainstem.** These signs include skew deviation of the eyes, apnea, coma, or unequal pupils. Nuchal rigidity and opisthotonos are signs of progressive herniation. Signs and symptoms of subdural hemorrhage from laceration of the superficial cerebral veins are variable. Small clots may produce no identifiable dysfunction. Typical signs are those of focal or lateralized cerebral dysfunction, although increased intracranial pressure may occur. **CT scans including views of the posterior fossa should be obtained immediately when a subdural hemorrhage is suspected. Lumbar puncture is not used as a diagnostic tool because of the risk for herniation.**[61]

With subarachnoid hemorrhage, underlying contusions may cause focal neurologic signs. Often no significant increase in intracranial pressure is found acutely. Irritability and a depressed level of consciousness may persist. **Seizures are common in term infants, whereas apnea is common in preterm infants.** Diagnosis generally is made with CT scan. If a lumbar puncture is performed, it is generally done for another reason (e.g., meningitis workup) and shows elevated red blood cells (RBCs) and protein.[3,36,61] For infants without serious injury from trauma or hypoxia, the prognosis is good.[61] Focal signs predominate in cerebral contusions.

TREATMENT

Surgical evacuation of epidural and subdural clots may be necessary as emergency procedures. Subdural taps may be useful in the symptomatic infant with subdural bleeding from laceration of superficial cerebral veins. **Many infants with intracranial bleeding may require treatment of seizures.**[36,61] In the presence of coagulation defects, prompt intervention may require platelets, vitamin K, or replacement therapy for deficient coagulation factors.[3,36,61]

COMPLICATIONS

The complications of epidural hemorrhage range from none to permanent neurologic deficits with or without seizure. Sequelae of subdural hemorrhage occur in 20% to 25% of affected infants. The most common sequelae are focal neurologic signs. Seizures and hydrocephalus are seen less often. Hydrocephalus is the major potential complication of subarachnoid hemorrhage and directly alters outcome.[61]

PARENT TEACHING

Because long-term outcome is variable and may be abnormal even in infants who appear normal at discharge from the nursery, parent teaching must be individualized. **Emphasize the need for appropriate follow-up and intervention.** Referral to available support groups is usually beneficial.

Spinal Cord Injuries

PHYSIOLOGY AND ETIOLOGY

Injuries to the spinal cord (usually the cervical portion) are seen most often in complicated breech deliveries. Before cesarean sections were routinely performed for breech delivery, fatal attempts to deliver vaginally often were associated with intraspinal hemorrhage. The breech presentation in conjunction with a hyperextended head is the most dangerous situation and is worsened by fetal depression. Traction, rotation, and torsion cause mechanical strain on the vertebral column. Cephalic deliveries are not entirely safe because of the difference in mechanical forces; a different clinical picture is seen with a higher-level lesion.[22,61]

DATA COLLECTION

Clinical manifestations depend on the severity and location of the injury. Clinical syndromes include stillbirth or rapid neonatal death, respiratory failure, and spinal shock syndrome. High cervical cord injuries are more likely to cause stillbirths or rapid death of the neonate. Lower lesions cause an acute cord syndrome. Common signs of spinal shock include flaccid extremities (may involve just the lower extremities if the cervical cord is spared), asensory level, diaphragmatic breathing, paralyzed abdominal movements, atonic anal sphincter, and distended bladder. **Useful laboratory tests include magnetic resonance imaging (MRI) or CT scan of the spine and somatosensory-evoked potentials to help determine the extent and site of the lesion.** The differential diagnosis includes dysraphism, neuromuscular disease, and cord tumors.[22,61]

COMPLICATIONS

After the acute phase, chronic lesions include cysts, vascular occlusions, adhesions, and necrosis of the spinal cord. Flaccid or spastic quadriplegia is expected. Some infants with spinal cord injuries are respirator dependent, and bowel and bladder problems continue.

PARENT TEACHING

Parents should understand fully the implications of severe injury to the spinal cord. Recovery is frequently minimal to nonexistent. Continued specialized care may be necessary, including ventilator therapy. The overwhelming implications for the family cannot be emphasized strongly enough.

An individualized multidisciplinary team approach to discharge planning is vital to parental confidence and a timely discharge. The problems of both patient and family are complex and not limited to medical concerns. A successful discharge is unlikely unless family emotional, financial, and educational concerns are addressed early in the planning process. The timely assessment of needs and involvement of supportive agencies allow resolution of problems well before the projected discharge date. Such assistance should include early family referral to available federal programs for financial aid (e.g., Supplemental Security Income [SSI]) and assistance with patient transportation to their multiple outpatient follow-up appointments. Early assessment of equipment needs and home nursing requirements is also of primary importance and should include a determination of the availability of these resources in the community, parent acceptance of their use, and whether the home can accommodate them (i.e., adequate electrical system and space).

Plexus Injuries

PHYSIOLOGY AND ETIOLOGY

Plexus injuries occur more commonly than cord injuries and result from lateral traction on the shoulder[55] (vertex deliveries) or the head (breech deliveries).[61] Risk factors include large infant, fetal depression, breech delivery, and a variety of obstetric factors.[13,35,61] Any factor resulting in a difficult vaginal delivery of the baby can increase the risk for injury (e.g., prolonged second stage of labor, placenta previa).[13,55] A study of 35,796 infants (54 with brachial plexus injury) concluded that brachial plexus injury is not predictable before delivery.[12] Some authors note the preventability of some risk factors.[61] Estimates of the incidence of brachial plexus injuries range from 0.5 to 2 per 1000 live births.[61] Extremely mild cases often have undetectable findings and may remain unidentified.

Pathologic changes range from edema and hemorrhage of the nerve sheath to actual avulsion of the nerve root from the spinal cord. Of the reported cases of plexus injuries, 90% involve the cervical nerve 5 (C5) to C7 nerve roots and are classified as ***Erb's palsy***.[22,61] In a small minority of cases, the C4 nerve root is also affected, causing diaphragmatic problems. The site of injury in Erb's palsy is Erb's point where C5 and C6 nerve roots join to form the upper trunk. ***Total brachial plexus palsy*** occurs in 8% to 9% of the cases and has findings referable to C5 to thoracic nerve 1 (T1) (and possibly C4). When T1 is involved, the sympathetic fibers become affected with an ipsilateral ***Horner syndrome*** (ptosis, anhidrosis, and miosis) and possible delay in pigmentation of the iris. Klumpke's palsy rarely occurs in the newborn period and involves only the distal upper extremity (hand), whereas the muscles in the proximal extremity are normal. When both distal and proximal weakness occur, it should be classified as total plexus palsy.[13,61]

DATA COLLECTION

Signs of brachial plexus palsies vary somewhat, most often because of the overlap of pure clinical syndromes. Shoulder and arm findings are characteristic of a true Erb's palsy. Involvement of the hand and fingers is seen in total forms or Klumpke's palsy. Table 26-3 lists the specific cord levels involved in various functions that might be addressed.

TABLE 26-3 BRACHIAL PLEXUS EXAMINATION: DISTINGUISHING FEATURES

PART EXAMINED	SPINAL LEVEL
Diaphragm movement (downward)	C4 (C3-5)
Deltoid muscle	C5
Spinatus muscle	C5
Biceps muscle	C5-6
Brachioradialis muscle	C5-6
Supinator of arm	C5-6
Biceps tendon reflex	C5-6
Wrist extensors	C6-7
Long extensor of the digits	C6-7
Triceps tendon reflex	C6-7
Wrist flexor	C7-8, T1
Finger flexors	C7-8, T1
Dilator of iris (sympathetic chain, Horner syndrome)	T1
Eyelid elevator (full elevation) (same as above)	T1
Moro reflex (shoulder abduction)	C5
Moro reflex (hand motion)	C8-T1
Palmar grasp	C8-T1

Evaluation of diaphragmatic function by x-ray examination is at times necessary. CT myelography or MRI may be necessary to identify nerve root avulsion, which generally should be suspected when recovery does not occur. Electromyography often shows abnormalities early in the course of the injury, suggesting that the process actually may have begun in the last weeks of pregnancy rather than at the time of delivery.[61]

Clinical syndromes of plexus injuries include Erb's palsy, total palsy, and Klumpke's palsy. Erb's palsy accounts for about 90% of plexus injuries.[22,61] It involves the upper part of the plexus, C5 to C7 and occasionally C4. The shoulder and upper arm are involved, and the biceps reflex is decreased. When C4 is involved, diaphragmatic dysfunction is present.

Total palsy occurs less frequently than Erb's palsy. Plexus involvement is diffuse (C5 to T1 and occasionally C4). The upper and lower arm and hand are involved. Horner syndrome (ptosis, anhidrosis, and miosis) exists when T1 is involved. The diaphragm is affected when C4 is involved. Biceps and triceps reflexes are decreased.[22,61]

Klumpke's palsy is rare in the neonatal period (see the preceding).[61] The lower part of the plexus, C8 to T1, is involved. The lower arm and hand also are involved. T1 involvement is associated with Horner syndrome. Triceps reflex is decreased.

TREATMENT

Treatment includes passive range-of-motion exercises followed by a gradual increase of activity to the affected limb. Treatment may include immobilization for 1 to 5 days to prevent contractures initially; finger and wrist splints also may be necessary.[61] For infants failing to achieve sufficient functional recovery by 3 months of age, surgical intervention is considered.[13,61]

COMPLICATIONS

Associated trauma may occur and should be carefully investigated. Common associated injuries include clavicular fracture, shoulder dislocation, cord injury, facial nerve injury, and humeral fracture. Full recovery of plexus function was seen in 88% to 92% of cases in the first year of life during the National Collaborative Perinatal Study.[61] Children who show no signs of improvement during the first 3 months after delivery should be referred to a clinic specializing in brachial plexus injury. Rarely, nerve graft surgery of the injured nerve root is necessary.

PARENT TEACHING

Parents should be taught passive range-of-motion exercises to encourage the infant's mobility and prevent contractures. Instructions should begin before discharge from the hospital. Usually a neonatal nurse or occupational or physical therapist gives the instructions.

Parents may equate the presence of a brachial plexus injury with poor obstetric care. This is often not the case. The awareness of early changes on electromyography should be used to help families understand that the factors causing injury to the plexus begin before the onset of labor.

Cranial and Peripheral Nerve Injuries

Median and sciatic nerve injuries usually are postnatal and result from brachial and radial artery punctures (median nerve) and inferior gluteal artery spasm (umbilical artery line drug instillation). Recovery is variable.

Median nerve palsy is manifested by decreased pincer grasp, decreased thumb strength, and the continuous fixed position of the fourth finger. ***Sciatic nerve palsy*** presents with decreased hip abduction and distal joint movement. Hip adduction, flexion, and rotation are normal, because the femoral and obturator nerves control them. ***Radial nerve damage*** usually is seen in conjunction with a humeral fracture. Prolonged labor is normally present. Congenital bands may also be causative. Recovery takes place over weeks to months. Radial nerve palsy is manifested by wrist drop (decreased finger and wrist extension) and normal grasp.

Laryngeal nerve palsy may be seen in conjunction with facial or diaphragmatic paralysis. If the paralysis is unilateral, a hoarse cry may be heard. Bilateral involvement causes breathing to be difficult and the vocal cords to remain closed in the midline. It is essential to rule out intrinsic brainstem disease. Often the presence of other brainstem-related abnormalities such as oculomotor problems, apnea, or facial palsy helps clarify this. Evoked potentials, both brainstem auditory and somatosensory, also may help rule out brainstem involvement.

Laryngeal nerve palsy is manifested by difficulty in swallowing (superior branch), difficulty in breathing (bilateral), and difficulty in vocalizing (recurrent branch). Also, the head is held high and fixed laterally with slight rotation. Severe cases may require tracheotomy and assisted feedings by gavage or gastrostomy tube.[61]

Diaphragmatic paralysis is most often seen in association with plexus injuries (80% to 90% have an associated plexus injury) and has the same cause. Some series involving unilateral paralysis have a mortality rate of 10% to 20%. Most patients recover fully in 6 to 12 months. Although fewer than 10% of patients have bilateral diaphragmatic paralysis, the mortality rate for these patients is almost 50%. Treatment has consisted of using rocking beds, electric pacing of the diaphragm, continuous positive airway pressure (CPAP), respirators, or plication. Because diaphragmatic paralysis may occur in other conditions such as a myotonic dystrophy, attention to the differential diagnosis is important, particularly when an associated brachial plexus problem is not present.[61]

Diaphragmatic paralysis is demonstrated by respiratory difficulty in the first few hours of life. X-ray film shows elevation of the hemidiaphragm with paradoxic movement that may disappear on positive end-expiratory pressure (PEEP) or CPAP.[22,61]

Facial palsy may be part of intrinsic brainstem disease (see previous discussion of laryngeal nerve palsy) or other conditions such as Möbius syndrome, myotonic dystrophy, or facial muscle agenesis. When it is traumatic in origin, facial palsy is thought to be caused by the position of the face on the sacral promontory at the exit of the nerve from the stylomastoid foramen.[61] Normally, both the upper (temporofacial) and lower (cervicofacial) branches are involved. Known complications (from lack of total resolution) include contractures and synkinesis. Cosmetic surgical procedures occasionally are necessary but often are delayed for years.

Facial palsy is seen on the left side in 75% of cases. Features include a widened palpebral fissure, flat nasolabial fold, and decreased facial expression. Most infants completely recover within 3 weeks, although some infants continue to have deficits months later.[61]

PARENT TEACHING

Infants with facial palsy may require the use of artificial tears if unable to completely close the eye on the involved side. Occasionally it may be necessary to tape the eye to prevent injury to the cornea. **Parents also should be taught to expect some drooling of formula from the corner of the mouth during feedings.**

Most infants with laryngeal nerve palsy recover in the first 6 to 12 months of life. **Symptoms initially require supplemental parent education and support. An infant's risk for aspiration necessitates careful feeding and appropriate response if choking occurs.** Additional education for gavage feedings, a tracheotomy, or an apnea monitor may be necessary for the parents of a few infants. The teaching requirements for the infant with diaphragmatic paralysis must also be tailored to meet the individual needs and circumstances of the infant and family involved.

NEONATAL SEIZURES

Seizures may be the most frequent and often the only clinical sign of central nervous system dysfunction in the neonate.[46,61] The occurrence of neonatal seizures typically prompts urgent medical attention. Seizures raise immediate concerns about the underlying cause of the brain disorder, associated clinical condition, the effect seizures may have on the developing brain, the need for anticonvulsant drugs, and the effect these drugs may have on the neonate with seizures.[46,61]

Although the exact incidence of neonatal seizures is difficult to ascertain, Volpe noted marked differences in incidence associated with variations in birth weight, ranging from 57.5 per 1000 infants weighing less than 1500 g to 2.8 per 1000 infants weighing 2500 to 3999 g at birth.[5,61] **Seizures occur more frequently during the neonatal period than at other periods of life.**[31]

Neonatal seizures increase the risk for impaired neurologic and developmental functioning in infancy and increase the risk for death.[22,45] Volpe notes that **multiple or extended neonatal seizure activity is associated with significantly poorer prognosis than when seizures are controlled.**[61] There is also a suspected predisposition to cognitive, behavioral, or epileptic complications later in life.[31,46]

Recognition of neonatal seizures with identification of etiology and prompt treatment is critical. Although not a disease entity, seizures are commonly related to significant disorders, which may require specific treatment. Untreated neonatal seizures may interfere with supportive therapies such as assisted ventilation and nutrition. Finally, **experimental data suggest that seizures themselves may result in brain injury.**[61]

Seizures result when an excessive synchronous electrical discharge of neurons within the CNS occurs (i.e., depolarization).[35,61] **Neonatal seizures are not a specific disease entity but, rather, a symptom.**[5,22] They may be associated with any disorder directly or indirectly affecting the CNS. Primary intracranial processes that may result in neonatal seizures include meningitis, intracranial hemorrhage (subdural, intraventricular, primary subarachnoid), encephalitis, and tumor.

However, **seizures also occur secondary to systemic or metabolic disturbances** including hypoglycemia, hypoxia-ischemia, hypocalcemia, hypomagnesemia, hyponatremia, and drug withdrawal.[4,35,61] A link between intrapartum fever and unexplained seizure activity in term infants also has been made in the literature. The presence of fever increased the likelihood of such seizure activity by four times the norm, even when the presence of infection was not found.[33]

Seizures are signs of malfunctioning neuronal systems. Seizures occur when the neurons within the central nervous system excessively depolarize (extreme simultaneous electrical discharge). Volpe notes that **a seizure is defined clinically as a paroxysmal alteration in neurologic function, that is, behavioral, motor, or autonomic function.**[61] These clinical signs may or may not be accompanied by abnormalities of the surface EEG. Clinical presentation of seizures is considerably different in the newborn period when compared with the well-organized seizure activity seen in older children and adults. The incomplete neurophysiologic development of a premature infant results in even less organized seizure activity than that seen with the term infant.[61]

TABLE 26-4 COMMON CAUSES OF NEONATAL SEIZURES

CLASSIFICATION	CAUSES
Acute metabolic conditions (Do blood gases, pH, HCO_3^-, Na, K, Ca, Mg, glucose, blood urea nitrogen [BUN])	Hypocalcemia Hypoglycemia; hyperglycemia Hypomagnesemia Pyridoxine dependency or deficiency Hyponatremia; hypernatremia
Inherited metabolic conditions (acidosis is common; assess urine amino acids, organic acids, NH_3, galactose)	Maple syrup urine disease Nonketotic hyperglycemia Hyperprolinemia Hyperglycinemia Galactosemia Urea cycle abnormalities Organic acidemias
Infections (12% of cases; assess cerebrospinal fluid [CSF]; culture blood, CSF; polymerase chain reaction assay in CSF; imaging)	Viral encephalitis; herpes or enterovirus infection Congenital infections Bacterial meningitis Sepsis Brain abscess Septic venous thrombosis
Intracranial hemorrhage (15% of cases; imaging; CSF examination)	Subdural hematoma Cerebral contusion Subarachnoid hemorrhage Epidural hemorrhage Intraventricular hemorrhage (premature)
Hypoxic ischemia (0-3 days) most common (60%)	
Congenital malformations	
Neonatal drug withdrawal (see Chapter 11) (e.g., opiates)	
Local anesthetic intoxication	
Kernicterus	
Specific nongenetic syndromes	
Benign familial neonatal seizures	
Idiopathic (in only 10%, no cause is found)	

Etiology and Data Collection

Neonatal seizures may be caused by a variety of acute and chronic stresses on the brain.[4,22,35,46,61] Table 26-4 lists the general groups of causes of neonatal seizures. The search for a cause proceeds in an orderly, methodical way. Most often, the known **history of perinatal problems narrows the differential diagnosis to one or two likely causes. Acute metabolic changes that are likely to cause seizures should be rapidly investigated first.** Blood glucose should be immediately checked both in the neonatal intensive care unit (NICU) (Accu-Chek with glucose meter reading) and in the laboratory, because hypoglycemia is a dangerous but very treatable cause of seizures (Table 26-5).[35,61]

Volpe[61] also listed **lumbar puncture as the other urgent laboratory test to be completed because bacterial meningitis is another dangerous but**

TABLE 26-5 DRUG THERAPY FOR NEONATAL SEIZURES

DRUG	DOSE	COMMENTS
Glucose	10% solution 2 mL/kg bolus intravenously (IV) if hypoglycemic.[61] *Maintenance:* as high as 8 mg/kg/min IV[61] (see Chapter 15).	Treat if hypoglycemic with glucose meter testing (e.g., Accu-Chek; One Touch II).[68]
Phenobarbital (drug of choice for neonatal seizures)	*Loading:* 20 mg/kg IV given slowly over 10-15 min; additional 5 mg/kg can be given 1 hour after dose to maximum of 40 mg/kg total for refractory seizures.[61,68,69]	*Therapeutic level:* 15-40 mcg/mL[69] (obtain levels any time); respiratory depressant; incompatible with other drugs in solution.
	Maintenance: 3-4 mg/kg/24 hr in 2 divided doses beginning no earlier than 12 hours after last loading dose.[61,69]	Maintain adequate oxygenation and ventilation.[61]
Fosphenytoin (Cerebyx) preferred over phenytoin* (added if seizures not controlled by phenobarbital alone)	Fosphenytoin dose is expressed in phenytoin equivalents (PE); fosphenytoin 1 mg PE = phenytoin 1 mg.[69] *Loading:* 15-20 mg PE/kg intramuscularly (IM) or intravenously† (IV) given slowly over minimum of 10 min. Flush IV with normal saline before and after.[69]	*Fosphenytoin advantages:* high water solubility; pH value closer to neutral; faster, safe rate of administration; safe to give IM; absence of tissue injury with IV infusion; easy to prepare in IV solution.[61] *Therapeutic level:* measure trough serum phenytoin (not fosphenytoin) 48 hr after IV loading dose; 10-20 mcg/mL desirable level.[69]
	Maintenance: 4-8 mg PE/kg/24 hr IM or IV slow push (see above for dilution); infuse no faster than 1.5 mg/kg/min. Flush IV before/after with normal saline (NS).[69] Maintenance should be initiated 24 hr after loading dose.[69] Term infants greater than 1 wk of age may need up to 8 mg PE/kg/dose every 8-12 hr.[69]	Monitor blood pressure closely during infusion; can be given with lorazepam or phenobarbital at terminal injection site.[69] Safety with newborns still not clearly established; use with caution in infants with hyperbilirubinemia.[61,69]
Phenytoin used instead of Cerebyx to control seizures that are not controlled by phenobarbital alone	*Loading:* 15-20 mg/kg IV infusion over at least 30 min (no more rapidly than 0.5 mg/kg/min). Flush with NS before and after giving.[69] ***Never give IM!*** Never give in central lines.[69] *Maintenance:* 4-8 mg/kg/24 hr‡ IV slow push (no more rapidly than 0.5 mg/kg/min) or by mouth (PO). Flush with NS before and after. Absorption erratic with PO route. No IM administration.[69] Term infants greater than 1 week of age may need up to 8 mg/kg/dose q 8-12 hr.[69]	*Phenytoin disadvantages:* incompatible with glucose and all other drugs; cannot be given IM (crystallizes in the muscle); rapid administration can result in bradycardia, dysrhythmias, hypotension.[69] The pH of IV solution is 12, which is very irritating to veins.[69] Extravasation may result in tissue necrosis.[61,69] *Therapeutic level:* measure trough level 48 hr after loading dose. Serum level 6-15 mcg/mL initially and 10-20 mcg/mL after the first few weeks.[69]
Pyridoxine (vitamin B_6) as indicated	50-100 mg IV push or IM.[61,69]	Used to diagnose and treat seizures resulting from pyridoxine (vitamin B_6 deficiency).[61,69] Monitor electroencephalogram (EEG) while giving.[69] Protect from light.[69] Diagnostic when seizures cease within minutes and the EEG normalizes within minutes or hours.[61]

*Appears to be preferred, although safety has not been clearly established.[61]
†Must be diluted in NS or D_5W to a concentration of 1.5 to 25 mg PE/mL for IV use.[69]
‡Volpe cited 3-4 mg/kg/24 hr IV in divided doses every 12 hr, starting 12 hr after loading dose.[61]

Continued

TABLE 26-5 DRUG THERAPY FOR NEONATAL SEIZURES—cont'd

DRUG	DOSE	COMMENTS
Lorazepam (Ativan) for seizures uncontrolled by phenobarbital and fosphenytoin (or phenytoin if used)[61]	0.05-0.1 mg/kg IV slow push over several min.[61,69]	Enters brain rapidly; onset of action in less than 5 min.[61] Monitor for respiratory depression.[61,69] Monitor IV site for phlebitis or extravasation.[69] Safer to use than diazepam (Valium), which is contraindicated for use in the newborn.[61]
ADDITIONAL THERAPY AS INDICATED:		
Calcium gluconate, 5% solution		
Magnesium sulfate, 50% solution		
IV antibiotics (bacterial infection) (see Chapter 22)		
Acyclovir (herpes) (see Chapter 22)		

*Appears to be preferred, although safety has not been clearly established.[61]
†Must be diluted in NS or D_5W to a concentration of 1.5 to 25 mg PE/mL for IV use.[69]
‡Volpe cited 3-4 mg/kg/24 hr IV in divided doses every 12 hr, starting 12 hr after loading dose.[61]

treatable cause of seizures. Sepsis should never be overlooked as a potential cause. The infectious agent (e.g., meningitis, encephalitis, empyema, abscess, septic thrombosis, ventriculitis) may directly affect the CNS. **Systemic infection may cause seizures** through the complication of shock, coagulopathy, impaired oxygenation, and multisystem organ failure. When the cerebrospinal fluid (CSF) is examined, not only should the changes associated with infection be identified but also evidence of bleeding (RBCs) or cell destruction (protein) may be found.[14,61]

Structural studies are routinely performed as part of the evaluation. At present, the most useful studies are **CT scans and cranial ultrasonographic examination,** which can document intracranial hemorrhage.[22,46,68]

The **infant's history should be carefully reviewed** to narrow the possible causes to the most likely ones. Physical examination may further narrow the differential diagnosis. Once the history and physical examination are completed, blood should be drawn for assessment of arterial blood gases, electrolytes, glucose, calcium, and magnesium.[22,35,46,61,68]

Appropriate cultures must be obtained. Usual culture sites or specimens include blood, urine, CSF, and pharyngeal or tracheal aspirate. The CSF should be examined for RBCs and white blood cells (WBCs), organisms (by Gram stain), protein, and sugar.[14,22,35,46,68]

Ultrasonographic examinations are particularly useful for identifying and following the clinical course of intraventricular bleeding and hydrocephalus. The infant is not exposed to radiation, either immediately or long-term. Complications, either immediate or long-term, have not been identified. The test may be repeated as often as needed and usually is performed at the bedside. CT scan or MRI also may be indicated.[61]

Clinical Seizure Types

Simultaneous EEG and video recording allow the accurate diagnosis of difficult-to-assess subtle behaviors, apneic and bradycardic spells, and the jerks and twitches commonly seen in preterm newborns.[41] Many have been surprised to find no correlation between events thought to be seizures and changes on the EEG.[61]

Seizures result from excessive simultaneous electrical discharge or depolarization of neurons.[22,48,61] They are a **manifestation of an underlying disorder rather than being an isolated disorder.** As a paroxysmal alteration of neurologic function, behavioral, motor, or autonomic clinical phenomena are associated with EEG seizure activity, and there are also clinical phenomena not consistently correlated with EEG seizure activity. An increasing body of literature indicates that epileptic phenomena can be formed at subcortical levels and are therefore not detectable by surface-recorded EEG.[61] The Critical Findings box on p. 769 lists classification types and usual EEG findings. It has been noted also that many neonatal

Critical Findings

TRADITIONAL CATEGORIZATION OF NEONATAL SEIZURES

CLASSIFICATION/TYPES	CLINICAL MANIFESTATIONS	DEFINITION/DESCRIPTION
Clonic • Focal clonic • Multifocal clonic	• Rhythmic jerks (1-3/sec) • Rate slows during seizure • + Electroencephalogram (EEG) seizure activity	• Focal: well-localized to a body part • Multifocal: several body parts jerking simultaneously or in migrating order
Tonic • Focal tonic • Generalized tonic	• Characterized by posturing • Focal: + EEG seizure activity • Generalized: usually no EEG seizure activity	• Focal: continued posturing of limb or a posturing (asymmetric) of trunk or neck • Generalized: extension of lower limbs with either upper limb extension (looks like decerebrate posturing) or upper limb flexion (looks like decorticate posturing)
Myoclonic • Focal myoclonic • Generalized myoclonic	• Faster jerking than in clonic seizures • Flexor muscles (limbs) involved • Focal: usually no EEG seizure activity • Generalized: + EEG seizure activity	• Focal: flexor jerking of upper limbs • Generalized: bilateral jerking of upper extremities; sometimes lower limbs are involved; often single or irregular jerks
Subtle (more common in the premature infant)	• Abnormal behavioral, autonomic, or motor activities that do not result from the other 3 seizure classifications • + EEG seizure activity with only some of the seizure activities	• Ocular: nystagmus, horizontal or vertical deviation of eyes, staring episodes, eyelid flutter or blinking • Facial: repetitive sucking, mouth movements, tongue protrusion, chewing, drooling • Limb: bicycling, swimming movements, "boxing" or "hooking" motions, stepping • Apnea: only 2% result from seizures • Autonomic or vasomotor changes

seizures identified by EEG are not correlated with motor and behavioral seizure activity—a phenomenon called *electroclinical dissociation*. The most immature infants are more prone to such seizures.[48,61]

Focal clonic and multifocal clonic seizures are the most likely to have true cortical origins. Eye blinking, a clonic manifestation, or nystagmus may be seen. Focal clonic seizures have been seen as an important manifestation of cerebral infarction in the neonate.[48,61] **Apnea with electrical seizure activity has been seen as an ictal manifestation but is more commonly seen in a full-term infant.** The majority of apneic episodes in the premature population are not epileptic in origin.[48,61]

The lack of ongoing monitoring of brain activity in most neonatal units makes accurate identification of seizures extremely difficult. The best correlation can be made by obtaining an EEG during periods of suspected seizure activity. The EEG may confirm clinical manifestations as true epileptic seizure activity. As discussed, however, there is evidence that epileptic discharges may be present without EEG detection.[48,61]

The traditional categorization of neonatal seizures is presented in the Critical Findings box above. The classification does not have the same significance as that of the International Classification of Seizures in older individuals. Some general observations may pertain, even with the confusion surrounding the accurate diagnosis of neonatal seizures. However, **seizures continue to be more difficult to recognize in neonates. Newborn jitteriness compounds this difficulty, so care must be taken to avoid mistaking this jitteriness for seizure activity (see the Critical Findings box on p. 770).**[46,61]

Episodes characterized as tonic and subtle are most likely to be seen in premature infants. Tonic episodes are quite commonly associated with IVH. Clonic and multifocal clonic seizures are more common in term infants. Myoclonic seizures often include a metabolic cause, such as nonketotic

Critical Findings

SEIZURES VERSUS JITTERINESS

CLINICAL OBSERVATIONS	SEIZURE	JITTERINESS
Ocular abnormalities (eye deviations or staring)	Yes	No
Gentle restraint of the involved body part halts the activity	No	Yes
Activity is easily elicited with stimulation (e.g., voice, motions)	No	Yes
Dominant movement is a slower clonic jerking having both fast and slow elements	Yes	No
Tremor in which the amplitude and rate of the alternating movements are equal	No	Yes
Autonomic changes are present (e.g., apnea, tachycardia, elevated blood pressure, pupil changes, increased salivation)	Yes	No

hyperglycemia or urea cycle disorder (see the Critical Findings box on p. 769 for a review).

Prevention

Many neonatal seizures can be successfully prevented through careful attention to possible metabolic changes expected on the basis of the infant's condition. Hypoglycemia, hypocalcemia, hypomagnesemia, and often hypoxia can be anticipated and controlled.

Seizures resulting from intracranial malformations, infections, or prenatal injury most often cannot be prevented. Inherited metabolic disorders may not be identified until after initial symptoms, which may include seizures, appear.[48]

Whether neonatal seizures can be prevented by pretreatment of the mother in high-risk situations contributing to neonatal seizures has not been adequately investigated. As progress in antenatal treatment of the fetus continues, this may become an area for further investigation.[61]

Treatment

The rational treatment of neonatal seizures involves a vigorous attempt to achieve four specific goals: acute treatment, correction, prevention, and minimization.

ACUTE TREATMENT

The first goal is acute treatment of prolonged or multiple seizures and status epilepticus. **Prolonged seizures and frequent, multiple seizures may result in metabolic changes and cardiorespiratory difficulties.** Seizures are associated with increased energy consumption by the neurons and may interfere with adequate oxygenation. The neonatal brain appears to be less sensitive to seizure-induced injury than the adult brain; however, repeated seizures may be detrimental to the developing nervous system.[23] **Although it may not always be possible, vigorous efforts should be made to control the seizure activity. When the administration of a single drug does not result in lasting control, a second or third should be tried.**[48,61,63]

The most common drugs used for the control of acute seizures and status epilepticus in the newborn are phenobarbital and phenytoin (see Table 26-5). In a randomized controlled study, these two drugs equally performed in controlling EEG-confirmed seizures; combined therapy was needed in over half of the infants, regardless of which drug was received first.[61] Both drugs are given in loading doses of 15 to 20 mg/kg.[48,63,69] In most infants, this load achieves a blood level within the therapeutic range.

Because both drugs are always given intravenously (IV) for this indication, the blood level is promptly achieved.[48,61,63,69] **When these antiepileptic drugs are unsuccessful in bringing the seizure(s) under control, alternative drugs, lorazepam or midazolam, may be used.**[63,69] Fosphenytoin (Cerebyx) has significantly decreased the adverse effects associated with phenytoin, but information is still limited regarding its safety and efficacy in neonates.[63,69] However, some important features of fosphenytoin differentiate it from phenytoin and should be appreciated if fosphenytoin is eventually approved for use in newborns. With fosphenytoin, potential is less for local toxicity such as phlebitis. An additional advantage of the use of fosphenytoin over phenytoin is the ability to administer fosphenytoin intramuscularly (IM) if no IV sites are available. A considerable advantage of fosphenytoin is that it can be infused safely at a much faster rate than that for phenytoin, but the safety of its use in newborns has not yet been proven.[61]

CORRECTION

The second goal is **correction of underlying remediable causes.** This goal is often more important than the first goal, because some seizures induced by metabolic abnormalities cannot be controlled with antiepileptic drugs until the metabolic derangement is corrected. It is especially inappropriate to treat a newborn with antiepileptic drugs before correctable causes have been excluded.

After blood has been drawn for glucose, calcium, magnesium, electrolytes, and blood gas determination, therapy may begin. **It is always proper to administer glucose. Inspired oxygen concentration may be raised temporarily if hypoxia is suspected.** In refractory seizure situations, the **IV administration of 50 to 100 mg pyridoxine** ideally should be performed under simultaneous EEG monitoring so that the true causes of pyridoxine dependency or deficiency can be detected.[48,61]

PREVENTION

Prevention of future seizures is the third goal (see Table 26-5). Seizure prophylaxis is a worthwhile goal for patients of all ages, but it is often not easily achieved in newborns. Often, despite the appropriate and vigorous administration of several antiepileptic drugs, seizures persist for several days, only to remit spontaneously and never return. **Despite this observation, attempts to provide adequate seizure prophylaxis seem justified.**

Phenobarbital remains the most studied and used drug for seizure control in the newborn.[46,48,61,63] Because the half-life of phenobarbital is long and may vary from 40 to 200 hours, serum concentration is monitored and it may not be necessary to give routine maintenance doses on a fixed schedule.[69]

Phenytoin also is used extensively in neonatal seizures.[48,61,63,69] Although it may be very useful in acute treatment, phenytoin often is quite difficult to use as a maintenance drug. The most frequently encountered problem is the extremely variable half-life in newborns. It is not predictable, and frequent blood level determinations are necessary to estimate a useful half-life for the individual infant.[61,63] This pharmacokinetic problem is dramatically compounded by oral administration in which the medication interacts with milk proteins and is absorbed erratically.[69] It is reasonable to avoid altogether the oral use of phenytoin in the newborn.

A second problem is the variability in binding of phenytoin to albumin in blood. Bilirubin competes for protein binding sites and results in an increase in free phenytoin levels.[69] The binding is affected by the amount of albumin, concurrent drugs, and other poorly understood factors. Because changes in binding alter the amount of drug available to enter the brain, there is often little control over the true unbound "level."[48,61,63]

Maintenance doses of phenobarbital (3 to 5 mg/kg) should be given after blood level determinations indicate that the level is dropping.[69] Phenytoin and fosphenytoin maintenance doses are difficult to predict. Frequent blood level assessments may be necessary.[48,61,63]

If unbound levels of phenytoin are available, these are often easier to use to ensure that a therapeutic range is maintained. Because the characteristic signs of phenytoin toxicity are cerebellar, they are ordinarily not recognized in the newborn. One must rely on the accurate determination of blood levels to safeguard against excessive administration. Maintenance doses for phenytoin range from 4 to 8 mg/kg IV every 24 hours for the neonate.[63,69] Phenytoin should be given slowly when pushed IV (never exceeding 0.5 mg/kg/min).[69]

Other antiepileptic agents such as carbamazepine and valproic acid are used less frequently. Fewer data about safety, effectiveness, and dosage are available than for phenobarbital, phenytoin, and lorazepam.[48,61,63]

MINIMIZATION

The fourth goal is minimization of the side effects of antiepileptic drug therapy. In the attempt to control seizures, the potential of antiepileptic drugs to produce side effects must not be ignored. **Drug-induced encephalopathy may mimic the clinical changes seen in hypoxic-ischemic encephalopathy (HIE) or numerous metabolic derangements.** The possibility that the pharmaceutical agent may be causing some of the findings being attributed to the underlying disorder always exists. Likewise, improvement in the underlying disorder may be masked by changes induced by the drug.

More significant side effects such as respiratory or cardiovascular depression produced by large doses of any of the drugs, hepatotoxic changes induced by valproic acid, or hyperbilirubinemia intensified by diazepam are rare but worthy of recognition.[61,63,69]

The issue of long-term side effects of the antiepileptic drugs is far from being settled. Virtually all of the drugs used have been shown in animal or tissue culture studies to have detrimental effects on the growth or development of the brain. The extent to which any of this information can be transferred to the human situation remains the subject of extensive investigation.[48,61,63]

Complications and Outcome

Studies to date have been unable to separate the effect of the seizure from the effect of the cause. Early hypocalcemia, not uncommonly found in stressed newborns, is an example of a relatively benign cause of neonatal seizures. These infants have an excellent chance of recovery without complications. For acute treatment, 1 to 2 mL/kg of a 10% solution of calcium gluconate (10 to 20 mg/kg of elemental calcium) should be diluted in an appropriate IV solution and infused IV over 10 to 30 minutes. The infant should be closely monitored by electrocardiogram (ECG) during infusion of IV calcium.[48,69] The infusion should be halted if the heart rate falls below 100 beats/min.[69]

Separate from any discussion of the direct effect of seizures on the developing brain is the question of whether seizures in the newborn period predispose to later seizures. Again, cause seems to be the most important factor. Those seizures caused by transient metabolic changes that do not cause other permanent neurologic dysfunction are themselves likely to be transient and not occur outside the neonatal period. Seizures caused by congenital anomalies or those accompanied by obvious permanent brain damage are likely to persist.

Important prognostic findings and signs can be grouped to provide a general guide to assess newborns with seizures. ***Factors favoring a good prognosis*** include transient metabolic causes (hypocalcemia, hypomagnesemia), normal neurologic examination, normal EEG findings, and benign familial neonatal seizures.

Factors favoring a poorer prognosis include the presence of a congenital malformation, seizures persisting for more than several days, presence of a major IVH with seizure activity, severely abnormal EEG findings (burst suppression, extremely low voltage, isoelectric), or major signs on neurologic examination (hemi-syndrome, multiple brainstem signs, and severe hypotonia with unresponsiveness).[48,61]

Parent Teaching

Lay terms such as "fit" or "spell" provide a hint of the fear that seizure activity can instill in parents. **Parent teaching should focus not only on providing pertinent information but also on correcting existing misinformation.** Parents may initially have difficulty believing that an infant is experiencing a seizure, because a neonatal seizure is difficult to recognize. It is also not unusual for parents to expect staff to insert items in the mouth, perform cardiopulmonary resuscitation (CPR), restrain or shake the infant, or institute other measures once they understand that the infant is having a seizure.

Parents may express an urgent and understandable need to know the cause and the long-term outcomes of the seizure activity. **Supply careful explanations of tests being performed and their purpose in identification of the cause of the seizure.** The long-term impact on the infant may be harder to predict for the parents, although the presence of certain factors can result in a poorer or better prognosis (see "Complications and Outcome" section). Close follow-up after discharge by both medical and developmental services is vital.

Once the parents are home with the infant, their ability to recognize seizures and appropriately intervene is crucial. Careful documentation of teaching and parent understanding will allow the nursing staff to build on previous knowledge and skills. Parent handouts should focus on the skills and goals listed on the teaching checklist (see the Parent Teaching box on p. 773). **Care should be taken to use short, easy-to-understand sentences and to explain all terminology that parents might find confusing** (e.g., what an EEG is). Without parent handouts, attempting to teach the volume of necessary information is more stressful on both the caregiver and the family. Handouts improve the parents' retention of new and complex material and are available for reference after discharge.

Parent Teaching

SEIZURE DISORDER FAMILY TEACHING CHECKLIST

BAPTIST MEDICAL CENTER
WOLFSON CHILDREN'S HOSPITAL
JACKSONVILLE, FLORIDA

Wolfson Children's Hospital at Baptist Medical Center

SEIZURE DISORDER FAMILY TEACHING CHECKLIST

GOAL/SKILL	PRESENTATION/ NURSE DEMONSTRATION DATE AND INITIAL	CARE GIVER/ PATIENT DEMONSTRATION DATE AND INITIAL	CARE GIVER/ PATIENT DEMONSTRATION DATE AND INITIAL	COMMENTS/ HANDOUTS DATE AND INITIAL
1. Verbalizes understanding of seizure pathophysiology.				Handouts given:
2. Describes signs that indicate a seizure.				
3. Lists important observations to make during a seizure.				"Seizure Recognition"
4. Describes care of a child during a seizure.				
5. Identifies child's a. medication, dosage and schedule b. side effects of anticonvulsants c. consequences of non-compliance d. correct administration of medication				Medication ______ Dosage ______ Schedule ______ Medication handout given ______
6. Verbalizes how to seek emergency assistance from home.				
7. Identifies resources for families with a child with a seizure disorder.				
VIDEOS FOR PARENTS (Date that care giver/ patient views)	______ "How Medications Work" ______ "Understanding Seizure Disorders"			

Courtesy Wolfson Children's Hospital, Jacksonville, Fla, 1996.

Providing parents with a form for documenting seizures is also helpful. Documentation can guide the parents in making appropriate observations during seizure activity (e.g., date, time, duration, seizure activities observed, color changes, behavior after seizure). Parents should practice using this form while the infant is in the hospital so that staff members can assist them with their assessments and documentation. **Parents should also administer the medications whenever possible during the infant's hospitalization to establish skills and reinforce their confidence.**

A multidisciplinary team approach to discharge planning is crucial for the provision of effective discharge teaching. This planning and parental education must be initiated early in the hospitalization for successful outcomes. After discharge, a multidisciplinary approach to follow-up is also necessary.

In summary, discharge from the hospital after the diagnosis and treatment of neonatal seizures is a period of both relief and increased anxiety for parents, other family members, and caregivers. **For infants with a good prognosis, efforts should be made to help family members look past the neonatal seizures and view their newborn as "healthy." For infants whose neurologic outcome will clearly not be normal, clinicians should stress the needs of the child with multiple handicaps.** The clinician should take the lead in providing the basis for this discussion and guidance in the normalization of the lives of these infants and children.

HYPOXIC-ISCHEMIC ENCEPHALOPATHY

Pathophysiology

A common cause of brain damage in newborns is HIE.[61] ***Hypoxemia* refers to a diminished amount of oxygen in the blood, and *ischemia* refers to a diminished amount of blood perfusing the brain.** Either of these may result in the lack of a sufficient oxygen supply to the brain. ***Asphyxia*** refers to the impairment of the exchange of respiratory gases, implying low oxygen and high carbon dioxide in the blood.[29,35,60,61] When comparing hypoxemia and ischemia, ischemia is more important. With ischemia, the brain lacks a supply of both oxygen and glucose, which increases likelihood of brain injury. During the perinatal period, hypoxia or ischemia (or a combination of them both) is usually the outcome of asphyxia.[29,60,61]

Injury to the brain is thought to occur at two time periods. The initial insult is caused by the hypoxemia and/or ischemia. Once cerebral circulation and oxygenation are restored, there is a resolution of the acute event and a return of cellular energy metabolism.[36,60] During the reperfusion, glutamate is cleared, lactate levels are reduced, and high energy phosphate levels are returned to normal.[61] **Eight to sixteen hours after this initial acute event, a second decrease in high energy phosphate levels can be seen** and reaches a nadir at approximately 24 to 48 hours.[60,61]

The ratio of phosphocreatine/inorganic phosphate decreases, nitric oxide vasodilates the cerebral circulation, and calcium shifts into the cell, disrupting the sodium-potassium-ATPase pump. Levels of glutamate, arachidonic acids, prostaglandins, and uric acid are increased. Adhesion molecules in platelets and leukocytes are activated by free radicals, promoting occlusion of the microvasculature. The reduced delivery of oxygen and glucose perpetuates the insult.[28,60,61] **As mitochondria become more dysfunctional, clinical deterioration including the presence of seizure activity becomes evident.** Animal research has shown that neuronal protein loss can be noted by 6 hours and is very evident by 18 hours.[58] **The period of time before the occurrence of the secondary energy failure is the targeted therapeutic window in which an intervention may ameliorate injury.** It has been demonstrated that the secondary energy collapse is the consequence of the hypoxic-ischemic event rather than the cause of it.[58,61]

Etiology

HIE occurs in 1 to 2 of every 1000 live term births, and 0.3 per 1000 demonstrate significant neurologic sequelae.[30,35,61] Approximately 20% of these outcomes can be associated with primarily antepartum events (e.g., hypotension of the mother, intrauterine growth restriction [IUGR], maternal diabetes).[60,61] When hypoxic-ischemic insults are linked primarily to intrapartum events (e.g., cord prolapse, abruptio placentae, traumatic delivery), they occur in 35% of the cases.[60,61] Primarily postnatal occurrences (e.g., cardiac failure with congestive heart disease, pulmonary failure) have a 10%

incidence.[60,61] Finally, 35% of HIE cases occur from a combination of both antepartum and intrapartum difficulties.[30,60,61]

In a publication by the AAP and the American College of Obstetricians and Gynecologists (ACOG), the authors note that new information indicates that **intrapartum hypoxia is usually not the only cause of neonatal encephalopathy or cerebral palsy (CP).**[1] The authors state that "less than a quarter of infants with neonatal encephalopathy have evidence of hypoxia or ischemia at birth, and, therefore it is inappropriate to label most newborns with encephalopathy as having hypoxic-ischemic neonatal encephalopathy."[1] Rather than occurring during labor and delivery, they state that the majority of cases of neonatal encephalopathy and CP can be linked to events that occur before the onset of labor. They also emphasize that HIE is just a single subset of neonatal encephalopathy and **define HIE as neonatal encephalopathy with hypoxia occurring in the intrapartum period with no evidence of any other abnormality.**[1] Because of limitation in our current ability to determine the actual timing of the insult, it is often hard to identify/quantitate the antepartum contribution separately from the intrapartum.

The AAP and ACOG task force established criteria to be used in defining an acute intrapartum event that is adequate to produce CP.[1] The task force listed four criteria that must all be present:

1. **Metabolic acidosis** in fetal cord arterial blood obtained at delivery (pH <7 and base deficit [BD] ≥12 mmol/L)
2. **Severe or moderate neonatal encephalopathy** with an early onset occurring in infants born at 34 weeks' gestation or less
3. **CP**, either spastic quadriplegia or dyskinetic type
4. **Other identifiable etiologies (trauma, infections, genetic or coagulation disorders) must be excluded**

The task force also cited criteria "that collectively suggest an intrapartum timing (within close proximity to labor and delivery (e.g., 0 to 48 hours) but are nonspecific to asphyxial insults"[3,60]:

1. "A sentinel (signal) hypoxic event occurring immediately before or during labor"[1]
2. "A sudden and sustained fetal bradycardia or the absence of fetal heart rate variability in the presence of persistent, late, or variable decelerations, usually after a hypoxic sentinel event when the pattern was previously normal"[1]
3. Apgar scores of 0 to 3 occurring later than 5 minutes after birth
4. Multisystem involvement with an onset within 72 hours of birth
5. The presence of evidence of acute nonfocal cerebral abnormality shown on early imaging study

Prevention

Prevention of HIE requires the avoidance of hypoxic-ischemic insults. Anticipation of risk factors in the antepartum period, monitoring of the fetus during the intrapartum period, and prompt intervention when needed are discussed in the literature.[61] Chorioamnionitis has been linked to the development of encephalopathy and CP in the term infant.[67] **After delivery, management includes maintaining adequate oxygenation and carbon dioxide levels and preserving adequate perfusion while avoiding fluctuations in blood pressure or systemic hypotension.**[35,60,61] **Serum glucose levels should be kept stable** (Volpe recommends 75 to 100 mg/dL[61]). Although neuronal injury may result from hypoglycemia, allowing marked hyperglycemia may result in hemorrhage or increase cerebral lactic acid levels.[61] **Promptly diagnose seizure activity and provide treatment.**[35,61] **Seizures have been linked to swift falls in glucose levels in the brain (secondary to heightened cerebral metabolic rate), lactic acid increases in the brain, apnea and hypoventilation (which worsens hypoxia and elevated CO_2 levels), and marked increases in arterial blood pressure (with resultant increased likelihood of IVH).** When seizure activity of infants is poorly controlled, the incidence of severe neurologic sequelae rises.[46,48,61,63]

Data Collection

HISTORY

Infants with intrapartum causes of HIE are symptomatic in the newborn period. These infants have fetal distress in utero, are depressed at birth, and have prolonged low Apgar scores. **Most have evidence of systemic organ damage: renal, cardiac, and sometimes pulmonary dysfunction is readily apparent, accompanying the neurologic features**

of HIE. Diagnosis of HIE depends on careful prenatal and perinatal history-taking and a thorough postnatal neurologic examination. Severe and persistent neurologic findings suggest an unfavorable prognosis. Risk for more severe neurologic sequelae increases when the duration of the neurologic abnormalities in the neonate lengthens. Conversely, when neurologic abnormalities depart by week 1 or 2, the prognosis is excellent.[60,61]

SIGNS AND SYMPTOMS

The neurologic findings vary by the stage of HIE (see the Critical Findings box below). Seizures occur within the initial 12 hours after birth and are almost always subtle seizure activity.[22,35,36,49,61] Generalized tonic seizures occur in the preterm, whereas multifocal clonic seizure activity occurs in the term infant (see the Critical Findings box on p. 769).[22,35,36,61]

LABORATORY DATA

Essential laboratory data to reflect liver, renal, or cardiopulmonary dysfunction include a complete blood count (CBC), sodium, potassium, calcium, phosphorus, magnesium, glucose, blood urea nitrogen (BUN) and creatinine, urinalysis, liver function studies, enzymes (aspartate transaminase [AST], serum creatine kinase), echocardiogram, blood gases, lumbar puncture with CSF analysis, and cultures of CSF and blood.[22,36,60,61] Acidosis, hypoxemia, and hypercarbia are frequent findings after asphyxia. Other parameters needing correction include a low blood sugar (hypoglycemia), hypocalcemia, hyponatremia, and, more rarely, hyperammonemia.[22,35,36,61]

One should sample the spinal fluid to assess bleeding and to rule out infectious possibilities. Chest radiograph is recommended. The infant should be monitored with an amplified EEG for seizures.[22,36] EEGs not only confirm or rule out the diagnosis of seizures but also may be used to identify the severity of hypoxic-ischemic brain injury and assess future prognosis.[35,61] In a term infant, a severely abnormal pattern such as burst suppression, very low amplitude, or isoelectric EEG suggests an ominous prognosis.[22,36,48,61]

Accurately performed ultrasonography may show periventricular increased echo densities, but most scans of the term neonate do not show such changes.[61] **MRI scans are most valuable in follow-up at 2 to 3 months, but early CT or MRI scans may demonstrate areas of cerebral edema or of ischemic injury.** Hyperdense areas are characteristic of hemorrhagic infarction on CT scans.[22,36,61] MRI is the diagnostic tool of choice for the neonate with hypoxic-ischemic injury.[61] Even conventional MRI can display abnormal findings as early as the first day. Diffusion-weighted MRI has a greater sensitivity and can display abnormal findings within hours of birth.[61]

Critical Findings

STAGES OF HYPOXIC-ISCHEMIC ENCEPHALOPATHY AND NEUROLOGIC ASSESSMENT

STAGE	NEUROLOGIC ASSESSMENT
Stage I: Mild encephalopathy	Hyperalert, with normal tone and activity, exaggerated response to stimulation, reactive pupils, no seizure activity
Stage II: Moderate encephalopathy	Hypotonic, weak suck, constricted but reactive pupils; periodic breathing or apnea Development of seizure activity or lethargy indicates deteriorated status
Stage III: Severe encephalopathy	Stupor or coma, absent reflexes, pupils nonreactive, no spontaneous activity, requires mechanical ventilation

Treatment

Treatment includes the broad principles of adequate ventilation, gas exchange, and perfusion; maintenance of normal glucose, calcium, and electrolyte levels; control of seizures; and prevention and control of brain swelling.[22,36,50,60]

Current clinical trials support possible benefits of "modest" hypothermia as a neuroprotective intervention for moderate hypoxic-ischemic encephalopathy. Although the exact mechanisms underlying the neuroprotective strategy of hypothermia is not totally elucidated, a Cochrane review has found it to be **beneficial in term neonates suffering from HIE.[24]** Because the long-term efficacy and safety issues have not been established, **hypothermia is considered to be an evolving therapy that should be used in NICUs that strictly follow the recommendations of the protocols used in**

the CoolCap and the National Institute of Child Health and Human Development (NICHD) trials.[21,54]

Eligibility criteria for neonatal cooling are listed in Box 26-2. The NICU must be well organized and prepared to screen the neonate and have equipment ready to initiate cooling within 6 hours after the initial insult because this is the window of opportunity. First, the baby is examined to determine if the eligibility criteria are met. Before or as the neonate is being screened, equipment can be assembled and the blanket is pre-cooled and placed at the bedside. The neonate is always admitted and/or transported in a warmed bed on servocontrol to ensure that a thorough physical and neurologic examination may be carried out. Care should be taken with provision of heat support since overheating is potentially very dangerous and has been shown to markedly add to the neurologic damage. After cooling, rewarming should be done gradually because rapid rewarming may cause vasodilatory shock and rebound seizures. **A total body-cooling hypothermia protocol is outlined in Box 26-3.**

Other new therapies under study include the use of free radical scavengers (e.g., allopurinol), magnesium sulfate, and excitotoxic amino acid antagonists.[19,57,61] The use of calcium channel blockers resulted in marginal benefits, and the risks of these drugs outweigh these benefits.[57]

Complications

A variety of sequelae may result from selective neuronal necrosis. Outcome depends on the degree of insult to the brain. When asphyxiated infants exhibit HIE, there is a 20% to 50% mortality rate within the newborn period. Sequelae include hyperactivity, attention deficits, spastic diplegia, motor difficulties, intellectual deficits, and impairments of vision.[35] Other complications include CP, mental retardation, deafness, epilepsy, and learning disabilities.[61]

Cooling reduces mortality without increasing major disability in survivors.[24] Selective head cooling has shown a significant reduction in major neurodevelopmental disability but not a significant decrease in mortality.[24] Total body cooling has demonstrated significant reductions in both mortality and major neurodevelopmental disability.[24,53] The benefits of cooling on survival and neurodevelopment outweigh short-term adverse effects. Adverse

BOX 26-2 CRITERIA FOR NEONATAL COOLING FOR HIE

Screening Inclusion Criteria

- Postmenstrual age ≥36 weeks
- Admitted ≤6 hours of age with a diagnosis of encephalopathy
- pH ≤7 or base deficit >16 mmol/L on cord blood or blood gas within first hour of life (for head cooling)
- pH 7.01-7.15 and base deficit 10-15.9 mmol/L in the first hour of life (for whole body cooling)
- If no blood gas available in the first hour, there also must be:
  - Evidence of an acute perinatal event, <u>or</u>
  - 10-minute Apgar score <5, <u>or</u>
  - Assisted ventilation (PPV or CPAP) initiated at birth and continued for a minimum of 10 minutes

Inclusion Criteria

- Seizure activity present
- Diagnosis of moderate or severe encephalopathy, which includes any one of the following:
  - Lethargy
  - Decreased tone (may have normal peripheral tone but have central hypotonia), abnormal tendon reflexes, myoclonus, weak suck, abnormal Moro reflex
  - Any evidence of seizures
  - Abnormal breathing
  - Moderate to severe EEG amplitude reduction (lower margin <5 microvolts and/or upper margin <10 microvolts) on a 20-minute aEEG or evidence of seizures

Exclusion Criteria

- >6 hours of age
- Severe intrauterine growth restriction (<1.8 kg)
- Major congenital anomaly
- Head trauma resulting in severe intracranial hemorrhage (head cooling)
- Prophylactic high-dose anticonvulsants (head cooling)
- Parents do not grant consent
- Inability to initiate cooling by 6 hours of age

Data from Gluckman PD, Wyatt JS, Azzopardi D, et al: Selective head cooling with mild systemic hypothermia after neonatal encephalopathy: multicentre randomised trial, *Lancet* 365:663, 2005; Higgins RD, Tonse NKR, Perlman J, et al: Hypothermia and perinatal asphyxia: executive summary of the National Institute of Child Health and Human Development workshop, *J Pediatr* 148:2, 170, 2006; and Shankaran S, Laptook AR, Ehrenkranz RA, et al: Whole-body hypothermia for neonates with hypoxic-ischemic encephalopathy, *N Engl J Med* 353:1574, 2005.

aEEG, Amplitude-integrated electroencephalogram; *CPAP,* continuous positive airway pressure; *EEG,* electroencephalogram; *HIE,* hypoxic-ischemic encephalopathy; *PPV,* positive pressure ventilation.

BOX 26-3 TOTAL BODY–COOLING HYPOTHERMIA PROTOCOL[21,24,54,60]

- Place the precooled blanket, covered with one regular hospital baby blanket, under the baby.
- Insert (nasally) an esophageal temperature probe to T6-9, or approximately 2 centimeters above the diaphragm.
- After an x-ray film confirms the probe's position, the radiant warmer is turned to manual control with the heater in the *off* position and the radiant warmer temperature probe is left in place.
- The cooling machine (Blanketrol II [or III]) is placed on auto control to maintain the esophageal temperature at 33.5° C (92.3° F) for 72 hours. Although some fluctuation is expected, it should be no more than 1° C higher or lower than the target (32.5° to 34.5° C or 90.5° to 94.1° F). If using the Blanketrol II, the water temperature in the blanket is better stabilized when two blankets are connected together, such that one blanket is under the neonate and the other is hung next to the radiant warmer.
- The set point, patient esophageal temperature, skin temperature, and water (blanket) temperature are recorded on a specific hypothermia flow sheet, while a standard nursing flow sheet documents axillary temperature, blood pressure, heart rate, and skin condition.
- Effects of cooling may include the following:
  - Decreased perfusion to the extremities (caused by cold stress) may affect reliability of pulse oximetry values.
  - Decrease in the resting heart rate, which may result in blood pressure fluctuations.
  - It may be necessary to adjust the temperature of the blood gas analyzer (to the baby's temperature) to increase accuracy of blood gas results.
- At exactly 72 hours of hypothermia, the cooling machine is turned to the warming mode. Auto control is increased by 0.5° C every hour for 6 hours until the set temperature is 36.5° C.
- The blanket is turned off, the esophageal probe is removed, and the heater on the radiant warmer is turned on with the servocontrol set to 0.5° C warmer than the neonate's skin temperature. The servocontrol set point is increased by 0.5° C each hour until the axillary or skin temperature reaches 36.5° C. Wide fluctuations in heart rate and blood pressure should be anticipated.
- As the neonate approaches discharge, a Whole Body Hypothermia Discharge Checklist is completed to ensure that a brain MRI, developmental evaluations, and follow-up appointments with the high-risk clinic and neurologist have been done.

effects of neonatal cooling are transient and minimal: (1) bradycardia, (2) hypotension, (3) thrombocytopenia, (4) coagulopathy, and (5) renal impairment. Overcooling (especially <28° C) is associated with added risks of dysrhythmias and bradycardia.

INTRAVENTRICULAR HEMORRHAGE

Physiology

The problem of bleeding into and around the ventricular system has received more attention in the past two decades than any other neurologic problem in neonates. In large measure, this relates to the **frequency with which the problem develops, generally estimated to be 15% in premature infants weighing 1500 g or less.**[22,36,61] The growth of routine cranial ultrasonographic examination in premature infants has resulted directly from the need to evaluate this common problem. With the advent of CT and ultrasonographic scanning, a large number of infants who were not otherwise suspected of having intraventricular bleeding are diagnosed on scans.

Although the bleeding is regularly spoken of as *intraventricular* and *intracranial hemorrhage,* these terms do not accurately reflect its causes. Highly vascularized areas, which have relatively fragile and poorly supported blood vessels, are the source of bleeding. **In a premature infant, the most common source of hemorrhage is the subependymal germinal matrix.**[26,43,61] The width of the matrix is 2.5 mm at 23 to 24 weeks but decreases to 1.4 mm at 32 weeks. By 36 weeks, almost complete involution has occurred. Volpe lists principal clinical features in a premature baby requiring a ventilator secondary to respiratory distress syndrome. **Approximately 90% of bleeding events occur in the first 72 hours of life, and at least one in two affected infants experiences hemorrhage in the first 24 hours.**[36,61]

The incidence of IVH in term infants is approximately 3.5%, making IVH both an uncommon and unanticipated diagnosis. **Approximately 50% of cases of IVH in the term newborn are caused by asphyxia or trauma with symptoms occurring within the first 2 days after delivery.** About 25% of these infants with IVH have no significant risk factors (e.g., delivery without occurrence of trauma or asphyxia, a neonatal history without complications before the hemorrhage). Symptoms in this group may appear as late as 3 to 4 weeks after delivery.[36,61]

In term infants, the choroid plexus of the lateral ventricles is the most common site in which bleeding originates.[3,22,36,61] **In premature infants, the germinal matrix, in the subependymal area adjacent to the caudate nucleus, is the primary**

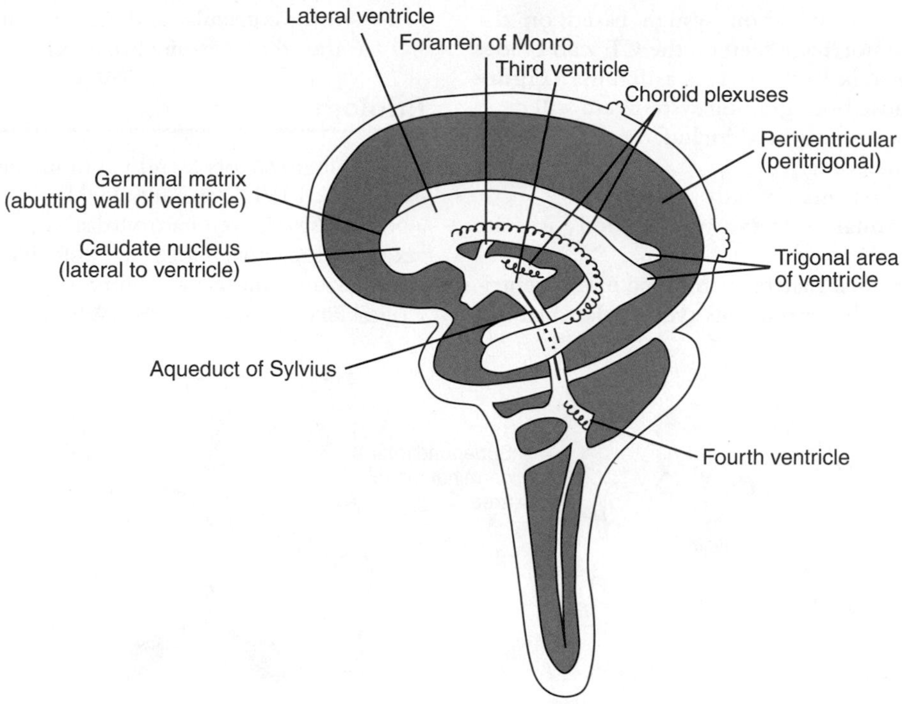

FIGURE 26-2 Central nervous system/ventricular system.

site of bleeding.[3,11,43,61] Both of these are areas of high arterial and capillary blood flow; in addition, they use an anatomically awkward venous drainage system, eventually draining into the internal cerebral vein (Figure 26-2).

The extent of bleeding generally predicts the likelihood of complications and sequelae. Bleeding may be confined to the germinal matrix or the choroid plexus, or it may enter the ventricular system. When filled under pressure, the ventricular system may dilate. Blood may also extravasate out into the brain parenchyma (more likely with germinal matrix bleeding than with choroid plexus bleeding).

Several classification schemes have been used, each trying to assess the degree of bleeding or amount of blood present. Ideally, a classification should relate to pathophysiology, treatment, or outcome; however, with present knowledge, this is not possible.

Volpe listed **three grades of germinal matrix IVH using ultrasonographic scanning to identify the presence and extent of blood in the germinal matrix and lateral ventricles (Table 26-6).** A "separate notation" is made for the existence of "periventricular hemorrhage infarction or of other parenchymal lesions." He clarified the use of this separate notation by noting that these abnormalities are not usually the result of simple "extension" of matrix or IVH hemorrhage into "normal brain parenchyma."[61] Others also use this classification system.[25]

TABLE 26-6 GRADING OF SEVERITY OF GERMINAL MATRIX—INTRAVENTRICULAR HEMORRHAGE BY ULTRASOUND SCAN

SEVERITY	DESCRIPTION
Grade I	Germinal matrix hemorrhage with no or minimal intraventricular hemorrhage (10% of ventricular area on parasagittal view)
Grade II	Intraventricular hemorrhage (10%-50% of ventricular area on parasagittal view)
Grade III	Intraventricular hemorrhage (greater than 50% of ventricular area on parasagittal view; usually distends lateral ventricle)
Separate notation	Periventricular echodensity (location and extent)

From Volpe JJ: *Neurology of the newborn,* ed 5, Philadelphia, 2008, Saunders.

An older classification system based on the extent of hemorrhage seen on the CT scan grades germinal matrix hemorrhages as follows (**Figure 26-3**). Because both grading systems are still cited in the literature, we have included each.

0—No bleeding

I—Germinal matrix only

II—Germinal matrix with blood in the ventricles

III—Germinal matrix with blood in the ventricles and hydrocephalus (ventricular dilation)

IV—Intraventricular and parenchymal bleeding (other than germinal matrix)

Etiology

The etiologic factors identified in infants who have experienced IVH are multiple.[11,45,59] These include asphyxia, severe respiratory distress, pneumothorax, hypoglycemia, shock, acidosis, blood transfusions, seizures, and rapid volume expansion (see the Critical Findings box on p. 781). What appears to be the

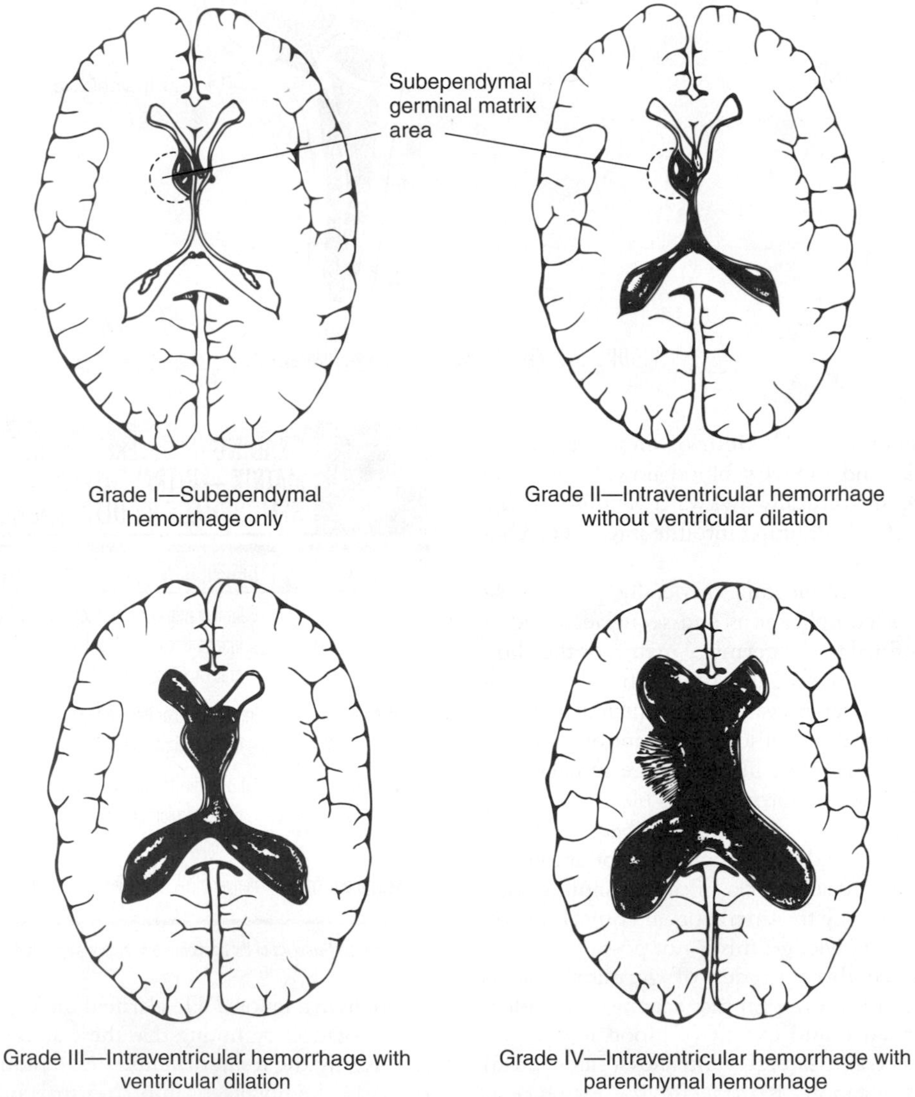

FIGURE 26-3 Periventricular-intraventricular hemorrhage, grades I to IV. (From Rozmus C: Periventricular-intraventricular hemorrhage in the newborn, *Matern Child Nurs* 17:79, 1992.)

common factor underlying the pathologic condition is a fluctuation/alteration in cerebral blood flow[61] that causes the numerous and thin-walled blood vessels in the germinal matrix to bleed.[22,36,61]

Critical Findings

FACTORS THAT PREDISPOSE THE PREMATURE INFANT TO INTRAVENTRICULAR HEMORRHAGE

Prematurity

- Birth weight less than 1500 g
- Less than 34 weeks' gestation

Asphyxia (see Chapters 4 and 8)

- Before, during, after birth

Respiratory (see Chapters 8 and 23)

- Idiopathic respiratory distress syndrome
- Hypoxia
- Positive pressure ventilation
- Pneumothorax
- Apnea

Cardiovascular (see Chapter 4)

- Rapid volume expansion
- Elevated venous pressure
- Elevated or lowered arterial pressure (shock; transfusions)

Hematologic (see Chapter 20)

- Hyperosmolarity
- Coagulation disorders
- Hyperviscosity

Metabolic (see Chapters 8, 14, and 15)

- Hypoglycemia/hyperglycemia
- Hypernatremia/hyponatremia
- Metabolic acidosis
- Rapid pH shifts

Miscellaneous

- Hypothermia (see Chapter 6)
- Acetylsalicylic acid ingestion by mother
- Neonatal pain (see Chapter 12)
- Neonatal environmental stressors (see Chapter 13)

Modified from Gardner S, Hagedorn M: Physiologic sequelae of prematurity: The nurse practitioner's role. VIII. Neurologic conditions, *J Pediatr Nurs* 6:265, 1992.

Intraventricular bleeding tends to occur in the first few hours or days of life. The profound physiologic changes normally seen after birth are coupled with the multiple problems (primarily cardiorespiratory) typically experienced by the premature infant, making intraventricular bleeding common. The degree to which the aggressive management of premature newborns has a role in the development of bleeding cannot be accurately assessed. Generally, although not exclusively, sicker infants both require more intervention and have a greater likelihood of bleeding. In a recent study of 3721 premature infants, the authors concluded that a significant reduction in the incidence of IVH would occur if "extremely premature infants, the vast majority of patients suffering from IVH, didn't have to be transferred postnatally to another hospital."[18]

Data Collection

Some infants, generally those who are term, have IVH associated with severe asphyxia. Premature infants often show one or more of the following: birth weight less than 1500 g, gestational age less than 34 weeks, shock, respiratory distress syndrome (RDS), need for blood transfusions, coagulopathy, hyperviscosity, hypoxia, and birth asphyxia.[22,36,61]

Because premature infants, particularly those weighing less than 1500 g, tend to have multiple problems, it is not surprising that the clinical presentation of germinal matrix hemorrhage may range from subtle (or even undetectable) to catastrophic.

Deterioration in clinical condition followed by apnea, flaccid quadriparesis, unresponsiveness, and death from circulatory collapse is a recognizable syndrome. **Common signs of germinal matrix hemorrhage include apnea, hypotension, drop in hematocrit, flaccidity, areflexia, full fontanel, tonic posturing, and oculomotor disturbances.**

When intracranial bleeding is suspected, appropriate studies of intracranial structures should be performed as soon as possible. **For periventricular-intraventricular hemorrhage, both ultrasonography and CT scanning are useful tools for defining the presence of bleeding and for following its evolution.** Ultrasonographic scanning is listed by Volpe as "the procedure of choice in the diagnosis of germinal matrix-IVH."[61] Because ultrasonography is the safer procedure and uses no radiation, it should be used for follow-up.

Treatment and Intervention

The primary treatment of IVH is supportive care. Ventilatory support, maintenance of oxygenation, regulation of acid-base balance, suppression of seizures, and treatment of any attendant coagulopathy are all extremely important in reducing mortality and morbidity. The role that successful management has in the amelioration or prevention of complications is unclear.

Many therapies have been proposed or used but remain unproven. Therapies are listed not to recommend their general clinical use but, rather, to suggest ways the problem has been approached.

When the hemorrhage is confined to the germinal matrix, little can be done, even from a theoretic standpoint.

Intraventricular fibrinolytics (streptokinase/urokinase) have been used to dissolve the clot and prevent hydrocephalus. After intraventricular blood clots were successfully dissolved by urokinase in the adult population with subsequent improved outcomes, several neonatal studies were completed. Initial favorable results were followed by two studies that showed no benefit from the use of fibrinolytic therapy.[61]

Care must be given to reduce the risk for continued bleeding, to maintain perfusion of the brain, and to reduce wide fluctuations in blood pressure, oxygenation, and pH.[22,35,36]

Medications to reduce intracranial pressure and treat secondary effects of the bleeding include furosemide, acetazolamide, and steroidal agents. Mannitol and glycerol also have been used.

Helpful pharmacologic preventive agents (glucocorticoids and possibly phenobarbital administered prenatally and indomethacin, vitamin E, and phenobarbital postnatally) show varying success in the literature. Antepartal prophylactic use of phenobarbital to prevent IVH or neurologic disabilities in the preterm infant is not supported by research.[10,63] Vitamin K administration to women before preterm delivery is not preventive of periventricular hemorrhage in the preterm neonate.[10] Postnatal prophylactic use of phenobarbital in preterm infants to prevent IVH results in a greater requirement for mechanical ventilation, and it is recommended that phenobarbital not be used for this purpose.[66]

Complications

The complications from IVH relate to the underlying causes and the extent of bleeding. Massive bleeding with dilation of the ventricular system is much more likely to cause an acute change in brain function, with increased intracranial pressure, brainstem abnormalities, and apnea. Milder degrees of hemorrhage may be asymptomatic or associated with seizurelike events, changes in muscle tone, or apnea.

When bleeding extends into the parenchyma, porencephaly may result from liquefactive necrosis or ischemia-induced encephalomalacia. Follow-up structural brain studies may show hypodense areas in which blood was present; later they may show areas of porencephaly.

The most common complication is posthemorrhagic hydrocephalus. The risk is directly related to the severity of the hemorrhage, with up to 10% of survivors of mild IVH and 65% to 100% of survivors of severe IVH showing progressive ventricular dilation.[5] Evidence of posthemorrhagic hydrocephalus should be investigated in all survivors of germinal matrix hemorrhage. CT scanning or ultrasonography to assess ventricular size should be used because clinical signs alone are not reliable.[5,22,61] CP, visual and hearing difficulties, problems with fine or gross motor control, seizures, and mental disabilities are other possible complications.[5,25,61]

With the hope of avoiding the necessity of placing a shunt, some attempts at control of the hydrocephalus have been made. Osmotic and diuretic agents, including furosemide, isosorbide, and acetazolamide, have been used to reduce the formation of CSF, although the practice has not gained widespread acceptance.

Outcome studies have been difficult to assess. Clearly, the sickest infants tend to do poorly. They also tend to have more complications, including CNS complications. There is a clear correlation between the grade of bleed and the likelihood of significant neurologic residua, but the correlation is far from perfect.[22,36,61] The influence of other factors on neurologic outcome may be more significant than that of the actual bleed itself. Hypoxia, hypoperfusion, and other conditions known to damage the developing nervous system cannot easily be separated as individual factors in outcome. Patients with grades I and II hemorrhages usually do as well as patients with no hemorrhage. Patients with grades III and IV hemorrhages most often have moderate to severe developmental disability.

Parent Teaching

Parents of an infant with IVH should be involved with their infant's care plan. The rationale for a minimal handling protocol needs to be explained. Encouraging parents to participate in setting "time out" and "touch me" times will facilitate their ability to visit and assist with care. **During visits, they should be encouraged to recognize signs of overstimulation and become knowledgeable about the appropriate interventions to take to calm the infant.**

The infant with IVH has varying degrees of problems.[5,11,61] Often the acute situation resolves without ongoing problems. In these cases, parents should understand the possible complications such as hydrocephalus that may occur in the short term. **Teaching the parents to measure head circumference and alerting them to the signs of increased intracranial pressure such as poor feeding, posturing, eye movement difficulties, full fontanel, and lethargy enable them to participate more fully in the medical follow-up** (see the Parent Teaching box on pp. 754–755). Up to 80% to 90% of infants with hydrocephalus need a shunt because of ventricular dilation.[4,5]

Parents must understand the risk for long-term neurologic sequelae. **Despite the difficulty of predicting sequelae with any degree of certainty, parents should understand that mental and motor handicaps, delays in the acquisition of milestones, seizures, and problems associated with hydrocephalus and potential shunt placement may occur.**[5,11,45,61] Specific preparation for these potential problems should begin in the nursery but will be increased during follow-up visits if the possibility for such problems seems greater. Prompt and appropriate referral to medical specialists and supportive services is important in both inpatient and outpatient settings. Parents may find support and information from national and state organizations (see the "Parent Resources for Neurologic Disorders" section).

REFERENCES

1. American Academy of Pediatrics and American College of Obstetricians and Gynecologists: *Neonatal encephalopathy and cerebral palsy: defining the pathogenesis and pathophysiology*, Washington, DC, 2003, The College.
2. Back S: Congenital malformations of the central nervous system. In Taeusch H, Ballard R, Gleason C, editors: *Avery's diseases of the newborn,* ed 8, Philadelphia, 2005, Saunders.
3. Barks JD, Donn SM: Intracranial hemorrhage. In Donn SM, editor: *Michigan manual of neonatal intensive care,* ed 3, Philadelphia, 2003, Hanley & Belfus.
4. Blackburn ST: *Maternal, fetal and neonatal physiology: a clinical perspective,* ed 3, Philadelphia, 2007, Saunders.
5. Blackburn ST, Ditzenberger GR: Neurologic system. In Kenner C, Lott JW, editors: *Comprehensive neonatal care: an interdisciplinary approach,* ed 4, Philadelphia, 2007, Saunders.
6. Bol KA, Collins JS, Kirby RS: National Birth Defects Prevention Network: Survival of infants with neural tube defects in the presence of folic acid fortification, *Pediatrics* 117:803, 2006.
7. Brent RL, Oakley GP, Mattison DR: The unnecessary epidemic of folic acid-preventable spina bifida and anencephaly, *Pediatrics* 106:825, 2000.
8. Bruner JP, Tulipan N, Reed G, et al: Intrauterine repair of spina bifida: preoperative predictors of shunt-dependent hydrocephalus, *Am J Obstet Gynecol* 190:1305, 2004.
9. Centers for Disease Control and Prevention (CDC): *Folic acid now frequently asked questions* (last review January 30, 2008). Accessed November 1, 2008, from www.cdc.gov/ncbddd/folicacid/faqs.htm.
10. Crowther CA, Henderson-Smart DJ: Vitamin K prior to preterm birth for preventing neonatal periventricular haemorrhage, *Cochrane Database of Syst Rev* 3: CD000229, 2008.
11. deVries L, Rennie JM: Preterm cerebral hemorrhage. In Rennie JM, Roberton NRC, editors: *Roberton's textbook of neonatology,* ed 4, Edinburgh, 2005, Elsevier Health Sciences.
12. Donnelly V, Foran A, Murphy J, et al: Neonatal brachial plexus palsy: an unpredictable injury, *Am J Obstet Gynecol* 187:1209, 2002.
13. Dunham EA: Obstetrical brachial plexus palsy, *Orthop Nurs* 22:106, 2003.
14. Edwards MS: Postnatal bacterial infections. In Fanaroff AA, Martin RJ, editors: *Neonatal-perinatal medicine: diseases of the fetus and infant,* ed 7, vol 2, St Louis, 2002, Mosby.
15. Fichter MA, Dornseifer U, Henke J, et al: Fetal spina bifida repair: current trends and prospects of intrauterine neurosurgery, *Fetal Diagn Ther* 24:318, 2008.

16. Geisel J: Folic acid and neural tube defects in pregnancy, *J Perinat Neonatal Nurs* 17:268, 2003.
17. Gleeson JG, Dobyns WB, Plawner L, et al: Congenital structural defects. In Swaiman KF, Ashwal S, Ferriero DM, editors: *Pediatric neurology: principles and practice,* ed 4, St Louis, 2006, Mosby.
18. Gleissner M, Jorch G, Avenarius S: Risk factors for intraventricular hemorrhage in a birth cohort of 3721 premature infants, *J Perinat Med* 28:104, 2000.
19. Gunes T, Ozturk MA, Koklu E, et al: Effect of allopurinol supplementation on nitric oxide levels in asphyxiated newborns, *Pediatr Neurol* 36(1):17, 2007.
20. Hauser KW, Lilly CM, Frias JL: Florida health care providers' knowledge of folic acid for the prevention of neural tube defects, *South Med J* 97:437, 2004.
21. Higgins RD, Tonse NKR, Perlman J, et al: Hypothermia and perinatal asphyxia: executive summary of the National Institute of Child Health and Human Development workshop, *J Pediatr* 148:2, 170, 2006.
22. Hill A: Neurological and neuromuscular disorders. In MacDonald MG, Mullett MD, Seshia MMK, editors: *Avery's Neonatology: pathophysiology and management of the newborn,* ed 6, Philadelphia, 2005, Lippincott Williams & Wilkins.
23. Holmes GL, Ben-Ari Y: The neurobiology and consequences of epilepsy in the developing brain, *Pediatr Res* 49:320, 2001.
24. Jacobs S, Hunt R, Tarnow-Mordi W, et al: Cooling for newborns with hypoxic ischaemic encephalopathy, *Cochrane Database Syst Rev* 4: CD003311, 2007.
25. Jones MW, Bass WT: Perinatal brain injury in the premature infant, *Neonatal Netw* 22:61, 2003.
26. Kirby CL: Posthemorrhagic hydrocephalus: a complication of intraventricular hemorrhage, *Neonatal Netw* 21:59, 2002.
27. Klusman A, Heinrich B, Stopler H, et al: A decreasing rate of neural tube defects following the recommendations for periconceptional folic acid supplementation, *Acta Paediatr* 94:1538, 2005.
28. Kumar A, Ramakrishna VK, Basu S, et al: Oxidative stress in perinatal asphyxia, *Pediatr Neurol* 38:3, 181, 2008.
29. Laptook AR: Hypoxic-ischemic-encephalopathy. In Lawson EE, Lehmann CU, Nogee LM, et al, editors: *eNeonatal Rev,* vol 2(5), 2008, p 1.
30. Lavery SV, Randall KS: Cerebral monitoring of the term infant, *Neonatal Netw* 27(5):329, 2008.
31. Levene M: The clinical conundrum of neonatal seizures, *Arch Dis Child Fetal Neonatal Ed* 86:F75, 2002.
32. Levene MI: Intracranial haemorrhage at term. In Rennie JM, Roberton NRC, editors: *Roberton's textbook of neonatology,* ed 4, Edinburgh, 2005, Elsevier Health Sciences.
33. Lieberman E, Eichenwald E, Mathur G, et al: Intrapartum fever and unexplained seizures in term infants, *Pediatrics* 106:983, 2000.
34. Lumley J, Watson L, Watson M, et al: Periconceptional supplementation with folate and/or multivitamins for preventing neural tube defects, *Cochrane Database Syst Rev* 3: CD001056, 2008.
35. Lynam L, Verklan MT: Neurologic disorders. In Verklan MT, Walden M, editors: *Core curriculum for neonatal intensive care nursing,* ed 4, Philadelphia, 2009, Saunders.
36. Madan A, Hamrick SEG, Ferriero DM: Central nervous system injury and neuroprotection. In Taeusch H, Ballard R, Gleason C, editors: *Avery's diseases of the newborn,* ed 8, Philadelphia, 2005, Saunders.
37. March of Dimes: *New folic acid seal helps women choose enriched grain foods to help prevent birth defect* (last review January 29, 2008). Accessed November 1, 2008, from www.marchofdimes.com/cgi-bin/.
38. Miller M, Elixhauser A, Zhan C: Patient safety events during pediatric hospitalizations, *Pediatrics* 111:1358, 2003.
39. Mitchell LE: Epidemiology of neural tube defects, *Am J Med Genet C Semin Med Genet* 135:88, 2005.
40. Molloy AM, Kirke PN, Troendle JF, et al: Maternal vitamin B_{12} status and risk of neural tube defects in a population with high neural tube defect prevalence and no folic acid fortification, *Pediatrics* 123:917, 2009.
41. Moore KL, Persaud TVN: The nervous system. In Moore KL, Persaud TVN, editors: *Before we are born: essentials of embryology and birth defects,* ed 7, Philadelphia, 2007, Saunders.
42. Reference deleted in proofs.
43. Papile L: Intracranial hemorrhage and vascular lesions. In Fanaroff AA, Martin RJ, Walsh MC, editors: *Fanaroff and Martin's neonatal-perinatal medicine: diseases of the fetus and infant,* ed 8, St Louis, 2005, Mosby.
44. Rathnau CH: The ABCs of genetics, *Central Lines* 17:21, 2001.
45. Rennie JM: Assessment of the neonatal nervous system. In Rennie JM, Roberton NRC, editors: *Roberton's textbook of neonatology,* ed 4, Edinburgh, 2005, Elsevier Health Sciences.
46. Rennie JM: Seizures in the newborn. In Rennie JM, Roberton NRC, editors: *Roberton's textbook of neonatology,* ed 4, Edinburgh, 2005, Elsevier Health Sciences.
47. Sarnat HB: Embryology and malformations of the central nervous system. In Fanaroff AA, Martin RJ, editors: *Neonatal-perinatal medicine: diseases of*

the fetus and infant, ed 7, vol 2, St Louis, 2002, Mosby.

48. Scher MS: Neonatal seizures. In Taeusch H, Ballard R, Gleason C, editors: *Avery's diseases of the newborn*, ed 8 Philadelphia, 2005, Saunders.
49. Shalak LF, Laptook AR, Velaphi SC, et al: Amplitude-integrated electroencephalography coupled with an early neurologic examination enhances prediction of term infants at risk for persistent encephalopathy, *Pediatrics* 111:351, 2003.
50. Shankaran S: The postnatal management of the asphyxiated term infant, *Clin Perinatol* 29:675, 2002.
51. Reference deleted in proofs.
52. Reference deleted in proofs.
53. Shankaran S, Pappas A, Laptook AR, et al: Outcomes of safety and effectiveness in a multicenter randomized, controlled trial of whole-body hypothermia for neonatal hypoxic-ischemic-encephalopathy, *Pediatrics* 122:e791, 2008.
54. Shaw PS, Ohlsson A, Perlman M: Hypothermia to treat neonatal hypoxic ischemic encephalopathy, *Arch Pediatr Adolesc Med* 161:951, 2007.
55. Smith SA, Ouvrier R: Peripheral neuropathies. In Swaiman KF, Ashwal S, Ferriero DM, editors: *Pediatric neurology: principles and practice*, ed 4, St Louis, 2006, Mosby.
56. Thompson DNP: Postnatal management and outcome for neural tube defects including spina bifida and encephalocoeles, *Prenat Diagn* 29:412, 2009.
57. Vannucci RC, Palmer C: Hypoxia-ischemia: neuropathology, pathogenesis, and management. In Fanaroff AA, Martin RJ, editors: *Neonatal-perinatal medicine: diseases of the fetus and infant*, ed 7, vol 2, St Louis, 2002, Mosby.
58. Vannucci RC, Towfighi J, Vannucci SJ: Secondary energy failure after cerebral hypoxia-ischemia in the immature rat, *J Cereb Blood Flow Metab* 24:1090, 2004.
59. Vergani P, Patane L, Doria P, et al: Risk factors for neonatal intraventricular haemorrhage in spontaneous prematurity at 32 weeks gestation or less, *Placenta* 21:402, 2000.
60. Verklan MT: The chilling details: hypoxic ischemic encephalopathy, *J Perinat Neonatal Nurs* 23:59, 2009.
61. Volpe JJ: *Neurology of the newborn*, ed 5, Philadelphia, 2008, Saunders.
62. Wald NJ: Folic acid and the prevention of neural-tube defects, *N Engl J Med* 350:101, 2004.
63. Ward RM, Lugo RA: Drug therapy in the newborn. In MacDonald MG, Mullett MD, Seshia MMK, editors: *Avery's neonatology: pathophysiology & management of the newborn*, ed 6, Philadelphia, 2005, Lippincott Williams & Wilkins.
64. Watkins ML, Rasmussen SA, Honein MA, et al: Maternal obesity and risk for birth defects, *Pediatrics* 111:1152, 2003.
65. Whitby EH, Griffiths PD, Rutter S, et al: Frequency and natural history of subdural haemorrhages in babies and relation of obstetric factors, *Lancet* 362:846, 2004.
66. Whitelaw A, Odd D: Postnatal phenobarbital for the prevention of intraventricular hemorrhage in preterm infants, *Cochrane Database Syst Rev* 3: CD001691 2008.
67. Willoughby RE, Nelson KB: Chorioamnionitis and brain injury, *Clin Perinatol* 29:603, 2002.
68. Yager JY, Vannucci RC: Seizures in neonates. In Fanaroff AA, Martin RJ, editors: *Neonatal-perinatal medicine: diseases of the fetus and infant*, ed 7, vol 2, St Louis, 2002, Mosby.
69. Young TE, Mangum B: *Neofax*, ed 21, Montvale, NJ, 2008, Thomson Reuters Publishing.

PARENT RESOURCES FOR NEUROLOGIC DISORDERS

The Hydrocephalus Association: 870 Market Street, Suite 705, San Francisco, CA 94102; Phone: (888) 598-3789 toll free; Phone: (415) 732-7040; Fax: (415) 732-7044; Website: www.hydroassoc.org;. E-mail: info@hydroassoc.org.

Support Center of New Jersey: 2516 Route 35, North Manasquan, NJ 08736; Phone: (732) 528-8080; Fax: (732) 528-4744; NJ only: (800) 372-6510; Website: www.familysupportnj.com.

National Organization for Rare Disorders (NORD): PO Box 1968, Danbury, CT 06813-1968; Phone: (800) 999-6673 (help line); Phone: (203) 744-0100; Fax: (203) 798-2291; Website: www.rarediseases.org; E-mail: orphan@rarediseases.org.

National Dissemination Center for Children with Disabilities (NICHCY): PO Box 1492, Washington, DC 20013; Phone: (800) 695-0285 (V/TTY); Fax: (202) 884-8441; Website: www.nichcy.org; E-mail: nichcy@aed.org.

Epilepsy Foundation of America: 4351 Garden City Drive, Landover, MD 20785-7223; Phone: (800) 332-1000 toll free; Website: www.epilepsyfoundation.org.

National Hydrocephalus Foundation: 12413 Centralia, Lakewood, CA 90715-1623; Phone: (888) 857-3434 toll free; Phone: (562) 402-3523; Fax: (562) 924-6666; Website: www.nhfonline.org;. E-mail: hydrobrat@earthlink.net.

Spina Bifida Association of America: 4590 MacArthur Blvd, NW, Suite 250, Washington, DC 20007-4226; Phone: (800) 621-3141 toll free; Phone: (202) 944-3285; Fax: (202) 944-3295; Website: www.sbaa.org; E-mail: sbaa@sbaa.org.

American Self-Help Group Clearing House: 100 East Hanover Avenue, Suite 202, Cedar Knolls, NJ 07927-2020; Phone: (800) 367-6274 toll free (NJ only); Phone: (973) 326-6789; Website: www.selfhelpgroups.org.

American Epilepsy Society: 342 North Main St., West Hartford, CT 06117; Phone: (860) 586-7505; Website: www.aesnet.org.

Medic Alert: 2323 Colorado Ave., Turlock, CA 95382; Phone: (888) 633-4298 toll free; Fax: (209) 669-2450; Website: www.medicalert.org.

27 GENETIC DISORDERS, MALFORMATIONS, AND INBORN ERRORS OF METABOLISM

ANNE MATTHEWS AND NATHANIEL H. ROBIN

A neonate born with a malformation, a genetic syndrome, or an acute metabolic disorder presents a management challenge for the neonatal intensive care unit (NICU) staff. If these conditions are not suspected and diagnosed in a critically ill neonate, an appropriate course of action might not be taken. Thus a specific diagnosis becomes imperative. An accurate diagnosis provides the staff with information about the cause of the condition, points the way toward appropriate treatment, and indicates the prognosis so that the most appropriate care of the infant can be initiated. Moreover, the broader issues of providing supportive care and counseling for the affected infant's family can be addressed.

Genetic evaluation is a complex process that requires expertise in differentiating normal variations from abnormal findings and knowledge of the principles of embryology and dysmorphology to provide an accurate diagnosis. Skills in obtaining detailed information of prenatal and family histories may be equally important.

The field of genomics and genetic medicine has witnessed an explosion of new knowledge, much of which has been generated by the efforts of the Human Genome Project.[13] Advances in understanding of the genetic basis of development and function, as well as the interaction of genes and the environment, continue to provide new insights into human health.

This chapter presents a concise overview of the major categories of genetic disorders and the appropriate techniques to establish specific diagnoses. For an excellent review and detailed explanation of concepts, terminology, and specific genetic mechanisms, refer to *Thompson and Thompson Genetics in Medicine.*[37] See Box 27-1 for a comprehensive list of terms.

GENETIC PRINCIPLES

Genes

A ***gene*** is a segment of a deoxyribonucleic acid (DNA) molecule that codes for the synthesis of a single polypeptide and contains the hereditary information needed for development or function. DNA, which allows the storing, duplicating, and processing of hereditary information, consists of two long strands twisted around each other to form a double helix. Each strand of DNA is composed of four nucleotides: guanine (G), adenine (A), thymine (T), and cytosine (C). The specific order of the nucleotides determines the precise information that will be encoded at that site. Genes can (1) regulate other genes by turning them "on" or "off," (2) specify the exact structure of proteins, which then control the activities of the cells, and (3) specify ribonucleic acid (RNA), which is necessary for protein synthesis.

Chromosomes

Genes are packed in linear order on chromosomes. ***Chromosomes*** are found in the nuclei of cells. In

Please note that the **PURPLE** type in each chapter is intended to make it easier to identify clinically applicable material.

BOX 27-1 **GLOSSARY**

Aerocentric chromosome A chromosome with the centromere near the end of the chromosome.
Allele One of a pair or series of alternate forms of a gene at the same locus.
Aneuploid Any chromosome number that is not an exact multiple of the haploid set.
Autosome A chromosome that is not a sex chromosome.
Centromere The primary constriction of a chromosome in which the long and the short arms meet.
Chromatid After replication of a chromosome, two subunits attached by the centromere can be seen; each is called a *chromatid,* and after separation, each becomes a chromosome of a daughter cell.
Chromosomes The microscopic structures in the cell nucleus composed of DNA and proteins that contain the genes.
Congenital Present at birth.
Dermatoglyphics The dermal ridge patterns on the digits, palms, and soles.
Diploid Two copies of all chromosomes; the number of chromosomes normally present in somatic cells. In humans, this is 46 and is sometimes symbolized as *2N.*
Dominant A gene (allele) that is expressed clinically in the heterozygous state. In a dominant disorder, the mutant allele overshadows the normal allele.
Dysmorphic Morphologic abnormality, often a minor physical finding that may or may not have any cosmetic or functional significance and is present in less than 4% of the newborn population.
Fluorescence in situ hybridization (FISH) Molecular cytogenetic method for detection of microdeletions of chromosomes.
Gamete Mature reproductive cell, the egg or the sperm, containing the haploid number of chromosomes.
Gene The functional unit of heredity.
Genotype A person's genetic constitution.
Haploid One copy of all chromosomes; the number of chromosomes present in the gamete; in humans this is 23 and can be symbolized as *N.*
Hemizygous The condition in which only one copy of a gene is normally present, so its effect is expressed because there is no counterpart gene present (e.g., the genes on the X or Y chromosome of the male).
Heterozygote An individual who has two different alleles at a given locus of two homologous chromosomes.
Homologous chromosomes Members of the same chromosome pair; normally they have the same number and arrangement of genes.
Homozygote An individual who has two identical alleles at a given locus of two homologous chromosomes.
Karyotype The standard pictorial arrangement of chromosome pairs, numbered according to centromere position and length.
Locus The position or place that a gene occupies on a chromosome.
Malformation A primary structural defect that results from a localized error of morphogenesis; abnormal development.
Metacentric chromosome Chromosome with the centromere in the center of the chromosome.
Monosomy Absence of one chromosome of one pair.
Mosaicism Presence in the same individual of two or more different chromosomal constitutions.
Mutation A heritable alteration in the genetic material.
Nondisjunction Failure of two homologous chromosomes to separate equally during cell division into two daughter cells, resulting in abnormal chromosome numbers in gametes or somatic cells.
Phenotype The observable expression of traits either physically or biochemically.
Recessive A gene (allele) that is expressed clinically in the homozygous state. In a recessive disorder, both genes at a given locus must be abnormal to manifest the disorder.
Sex chromosomes The X and Y chromosomes.
Syndrome Recognizable pattern of multiple malformations that occur together and have the same cause.
Transcription The process by which complementary messenger RNA is synthesized from a DNA template.
Translation The process whereby the amino acids in a given polypeptide are synthesized from the messenger RNA template.
Translocation Transfer of all or part of a chromosome to another location (i.e., on the same or another chromosome) after chromosome breakage.
Trisomy The presence of three homologous chromosomes rather than the normal two.
X-linked A gene located on an X chromosome.
Zygote A fertilized egg that develops into an embryo.

humans, normal somatic cells contain 46 chromosomes (diploid number), of which 44 are termed *autosomes* and 2 are *sex chromosomes.* Females have two X chromosomes (XX), and males have an X and a Y chromosome (XY). Gametes—eggs or sperm—contain 23 chromosomes (haploid number). In the zygote and somatic cells, chromosomes are paired (homologs). In each pair, one homolog is maternal and the other is paternal in origin. Each chromosomal pair has unique morphologic characteristics that allow it to be distinguished from other chromosomes, such as size, position of the centromere, and the unique banding pattern that is demonstrated by special staining techniques (Figure 27-1).[19] To pass

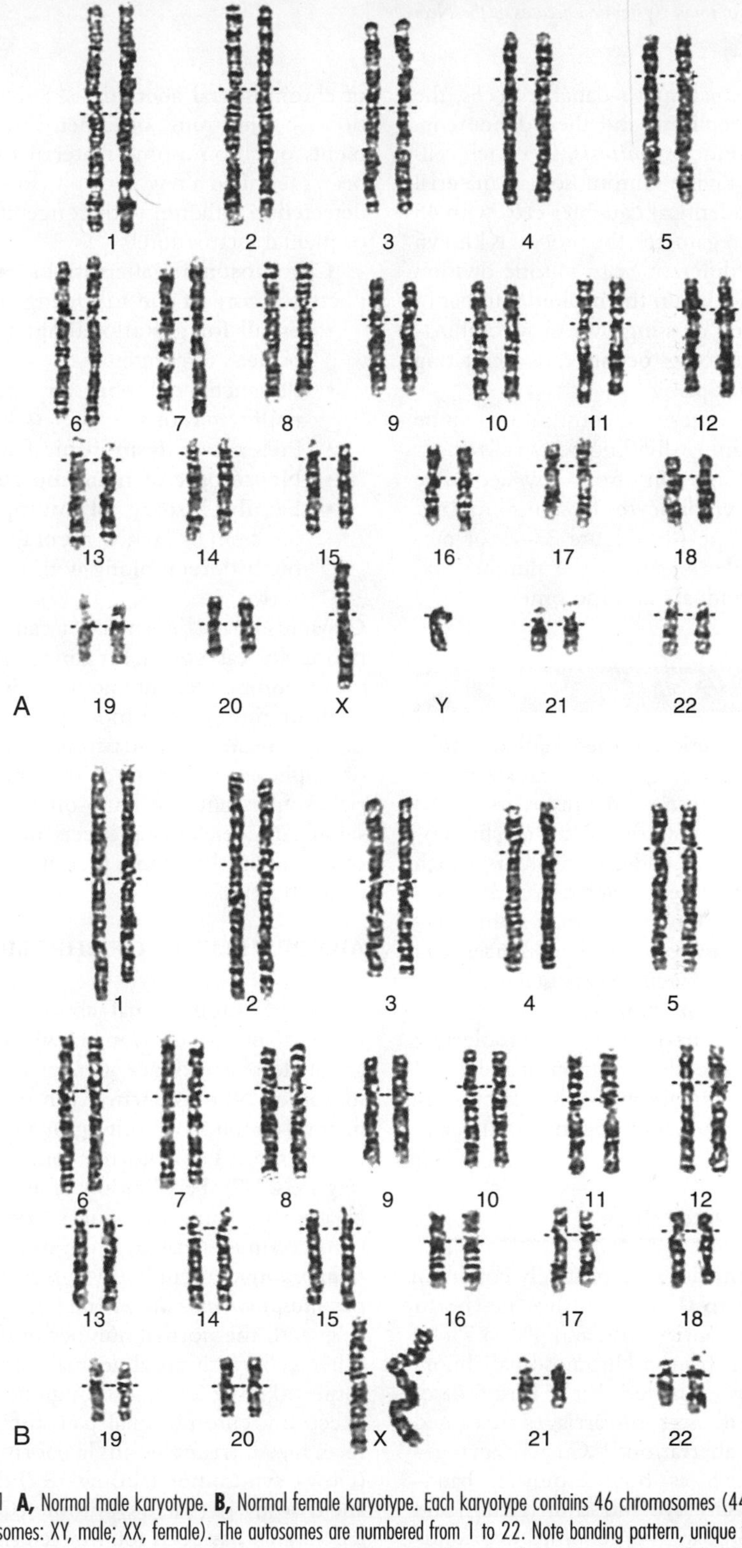

FIGURE 27-1 **A,** Normal male karyotype. **B,** Normal female karyotype. Each karyotype contains 46 chromosomes (44 autosomes and 2 sex chromosomes: XY, male; XX, female). The autosomes are numbered from 1 to 22. Note banding pattern, unique for each chromosomal pair. (Courtesy Dr. Loris McGavran, Ph.D., Cytogenics Laboratory at the University of Colorado at Denver and Health Sciences Center, Denver.)

on the genetic information to daughter cells, the chromosomes must replicate and then divide correctly. Somatic cells undergo ***mitosis,*** in which cells replicate and then divide chromosomal material into two genetically identical daughter cells with 46 chromosomes each. In gametes, the process is known as ***meiosis,*** which is different from mitotic division in that daughter cells contain the haploid number of chromosomes (23) and crossing over or recombination between two homologs occurs, thus facilitating genetic variation in offspring.[37]

An individual's chromosome constitution can be determined by examining dividing body cells under certain laboratory conditions from any accessible tissue such as blood lymphocytes or skin fibroblasts. The resulting karyotype (see Figure 27-1), or pictorial arrangement, demonstrates the number and structure of that individual's chromosomes.

ETIOLOGY

Malformations and genetic disorders caused wholly or partly by genetic factors can be categorized into four major areas: (1) chromosomal disorders caused by numeric or structural abnormalities of chromosomes; (2) single-gene or mendelian disorders, which are secondary to single-gene mutations; (3) complex or multifactorial disorders resulting from interaction of genes and environmental influences; and (4) abnormalities caused by environmental exposures of the fetus during development.

More recently, better understanding of molecular processes has allowed the identification of additional genetic mechanisms contributing to genetic disorders: germline mosaicism, genomic imprinting, and uniparental disomy.

Chromosomal Disorders

Chromosomal abnormalities are relatively common. Approximately 0.5% to 0.7% of all live newborns have a chromosomal abnormality, and 4% to 7% of perinatal deaths result from a chromosomal abnormality. Moreover, it is estimated that at least 50% of all recognized first-trimester miscarriages are caused by a chromosomal aberration.[18] Current cytogenetic techniques, such as high-resolution banding, fluorescence in situ hybridization (FISH), and microarray-based comparative genomic hybridization (array-CGH), have increased the detection rate of chromosomal aberrations. Submicroscopic deletions, duplications, or other abnormal rearrangements of chromosome material that may not have been identified a few years previously are now being detected in children with congenital malformations or mental retardation.

Chromosomal aberrations should be suspected in any of the following situations:

- **Small for gestational age** for weight, length, or head circumference
- Presence of one or more **congenital malformations**
- Presence of **dysmorphic features**
- **Neurologic or neuromuscular dysfunction**
- **Family history of multiple miscarriages** or siblings with **mental retardation or birth defects** along with one or more of the above

Chromosomal abnormalities can be classified into two major categories: (1) abnormalities of chromosome number (aneuploidy), in which there is an extra or missing chromosome; and (2) abnormalities of chromosome structure that result in the loss or duplication of part of the chromosomal material. Abnormalities of autosomes usually have more significant deleterious effects on the development of the infant than those seen with sex chromosome abnormalities.

ABNORMALITIES OF CHROMOSOME NUMBER

Numeric chromosomal abnormalities occur as a result of nondisjunction in which aberrant segregation leads to loss or gain of one or more chromosomes. Nondisjunction can occur during either meiosis or mitosis, resulting in an abnormal gamete (egg or sperm) or abnormal somatic cell, respectively (Figure 27-2). Fertilization of an aneuploid gamete by a normal gamete produces a zygote with an extra chromosome ***(trisomy)*** or missing chromosome ***(monosomy).*** Aneuploidy in somatic cells results in ***chromosomal mosaicism*** (i.e., the presence of some cells with the normal number of chromosomes and other cells with an abnormal number of chromosomes) (Figure 27-3). Although nondisjunction may affect any chromosomal pair, the most commonly recognized trisomies in liveborns are trisomy 21 (Down syndrome), trisomy 18 (Edward syndrome), and trisomy 13 (Patau syndrome). On the other hand, trisomy 16 has been found exclusively in spontaneous abortions.[18] The most common monosomy is

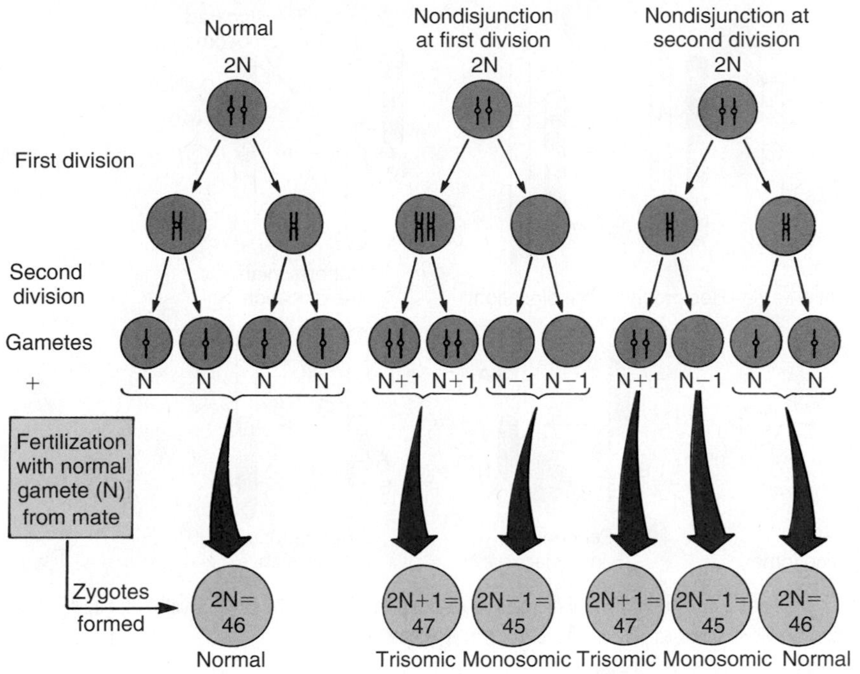

FIGURE 27-2 Nondisjunction. During formation of gametes, errors of nondisjunction can occur during either first or second meiotic division.

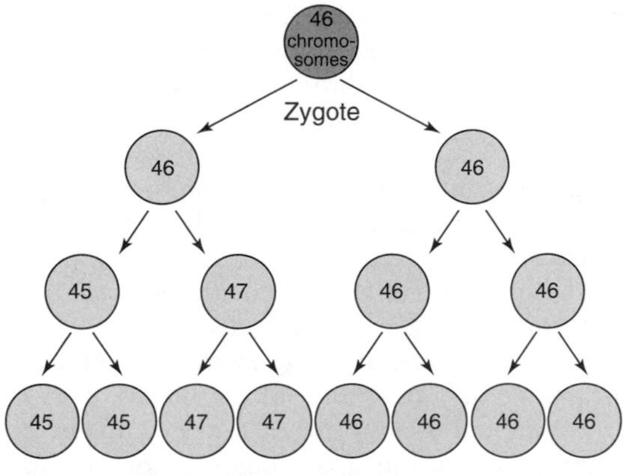

FIGURE 27-3 Mosaicism. Nondisjunction occurring after fertilization and zygote formation results in some cells containing the normal 46-chromosome complement and other cells having an abnormal number of chromosomes.

45,X, Turner syndrome. As a rule, numeric chromosomal abnormalities are associated with intrauterine growth restriction (IUGR), dysmorphic features, malformations, and mental retardation. Physical abnormalities may be milder or absent in the newborn with mosaicism.

ABNORMALITIES OF CHROMOSOME STRUCTURE

Structural abnormalities have been described in all chromosomes. These include deletions, translocations, duplications, and inversions (Figure 27-4). A ***deletion*** is a loss of chromosome material and results in partial monosomy for the chromosome involved. Loss of material from the end of a chromosome is known as a *terminal deletion,* as seen in 5p−, or cri du chat syndrome. An ***interstitial deletion*** involves a loss of chromosomal material that does not include the ends of the chromosome. A terminal deletion of both arms of a chromosome may result in reattachment of the remaining arms, leading to a formation of a ring chromosome. The presence of additional chromosome material results in ***duplication*** or partial trisomy of a chromosome. ***Translocation*** is the detachment of a chromosome segment from its normal location and its attachment to another chromosome. The translocation is balanced if the cell contains two complete copies of all chromosomal material, although in different order. In an unbalanced translocation, the rearrangement results in partial trisomy or monosomy.

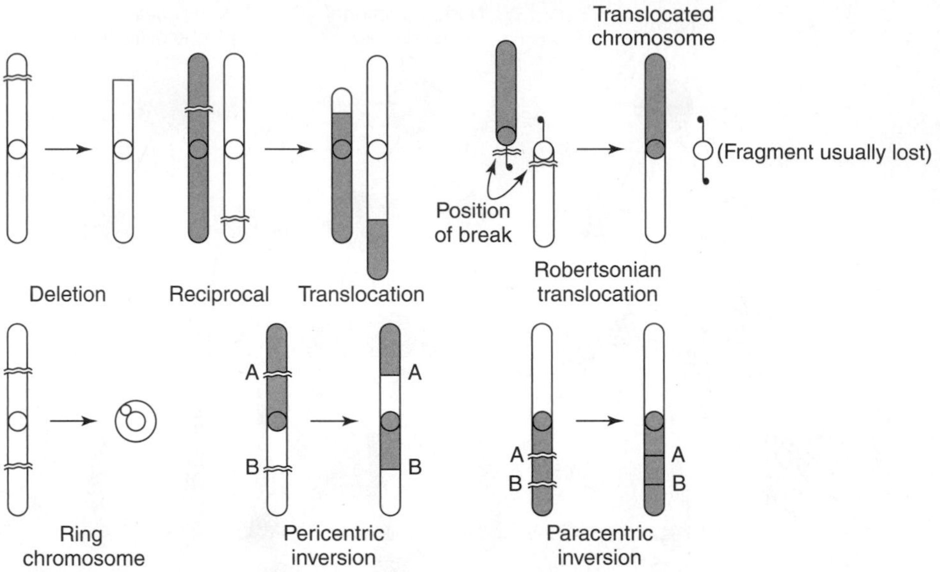

FIGURE 27-4 Schematic example of structural chromosomal abnormalities. (From Hathaway WE, Groothius J, Hay W, editors: *Current pediatric diagnosis and treatment*, ed 10, Norwalk, Conn, 1991, Appleton & Lange.)

Translocations can be reciprocal or robertsonian. A reciprocal translocation involves exchange of segments between two chromosomes (e.g., part of the short arm of chromosome 4 trades a place with a part of chromosome 10). Robertsonian translocations involve two acrocentric chromosomes fused at their centromeres. The most common robertsonian translocation is formed between chromosomes 14 and 21.[22]

Inversions are the result of a double break in a single chromosome and reinsertion of the chromosomal material that has been inverted. Inversions are either pericentric (including the centromere) or paracentric (without the centromere). The most common inversion is a small pericentric inversion of chromosome 9, which is considered to be a normal variant, found in approximately 1% of the general population.[37] All other inversions may produce gametes that result in an individual with an unbalanced rearrangement (i.e., having both a duplication and a deletion of some chromosome material, such as that seen in recombinant 8 syndrome).

MICRODELETIONS AND SYNDROMES

At times, structural chromosomal abnormalities are submicroscopic and therefore cannot be detected by conventional cytogenetic techniques. **FISH is a molecular cytogenetic method that facilitates the detection of microdeletions.** FISH uses segments of fluorescently labeled DNA called *probes,* constructed so that each probe can attach only to a specific segment of a chromosome, which then will be fluorescent during a microscopic visualization. In the case of a deletion of that chromosome segment, the probe cannot attach to the chromosome; thus the fluorescent segment is missing from the deleted segment of that chromosome.[45]

The most recent advance being used to detect very small submicroscopic deletions and duplications is ***comparative genomic hybridization*** (array-CGH).[15] This technology blends molecular techniques with cytogenetics and allows the genome to be scanned at a higher resolution than conventional techniques. DNA from a patient sample and DNA from a control sample are differentially labelled, mixed in equal proportions, and hybridized to DNA substrates fixed on an array platform (i.e., bacterial artificial chromosomes [BACs] or oligonucleotides [short segments of DNA usually 8-50 base pairs]). This technique can measure the difference between two different DNA samples in copy number (dosage) of a particular segment of DNA. Thus microscopic gains and losses from a patient sample can be quantified.[15]

Microdeletions result in phenotypic abnormalities. A number of well-recognized microdeletion syndromes may be suspected in the NICU. ***Prader-Willi syndrome,*** caused by an interstitial deletion of chromosome 15 (q11q13), usually manifests in a newborn as severe hypotonia, feeding difficulties, and micropenis or hypoplastic labia.[9] ***Williams syndrome*** is caused by an interstitial deletion or mutation of the elastin gene (ELN) on the long arm of chromosome 7 (7q11).[35] The condition is often first seen in an affected newborn in the postterm period; the infant is small for family size. There may be a congenital heart defect, in particular, supravalvular aortic stenosis or peripheral pulmonic stenosis; hypotonia; failure to thrive with gastroesophageal reflux; poor suck and swallow; and vomiting and irritability or colic. Infantile hypercalcemia is seen in approximately 20% of these infants. Subtle dysmorphic facial features may be noted in the newborn.[35]

One of the **most commonly seen microdeletion syndromes is velocardiofacial syndrome (VCFS),** which is characterized by cleft palate or velopharyngeal insufficiency, hypernasal speech, learning disabilities, conotruncal heart defects, and characteristic facies. VCFS actually represents one of a spectrum of clinical disorders all known to be caused by a deletion in chromosome 22q11 (del22q11). These include ***DiGeorge syndrome*** (DGS) (conotruncal heart defect, hypocalcemia, and thymic hypoplasia) and conotruncal anomaly face syndrome (CTAF) (conotruncal heart defects and typical facies). In addition, del22q11 has been found in 11% to 16% of cases of nonsyndromic congenital conotruncal heart disease and has been reported to present as apparently isolated neonatal hypocalcemia or learning problems.[14] Overall, del22q11 has an estimated incidence of 1 in 2000 to 4000 newborns. The availability of molecular cytogenetic testing by FISH has led to appreciation of both the high incidence of the del22q11, as well as the increasing variety of clinical presentations that can be seen even within a single family.[32]

In the newborn period, the characteristic facial features are seldom obvious. However, most affected individuals manifest some of these findings by early childhood. Most prominent is the nose, which is described as long, with a "built up nasal bridge, squared off nasal root, and bulbous nasal tip."[42] The eyes appear narrow and slitlike, the mala (cheeks) are flat, and the jaw is recessed. The ears usually are small and in some way abnormally formed. There may be an overt cleft of the secondary palate, a bifurcated uvula, a subtle submucosal cleft, or cleft lip with or without cleft palate. Other nonstructural palatal abnormalities can be seen, most commonly velopharyngeal insufficiency. In an older child or adult, this presents as hypernasal speech; in a newborn, one sees excessive nasal regurgitation. Congenital heart disease (CHD) is seen in 35% of del22q11 patients. The type of CHD is fairly specific and includes those lesions classified as "conotruncal heart defects" (truncus arteriosus, interrupted aortic arch, tetralogy of Fallot, left-sided aortic arch, vascular rings, and some types of ventricular septal defects [VSDs]). Perhaps the most consistent finding in patients of all age-groups is long, thin fingers and toes. Additional nonspecific findings include abundant scalp hair; hypospadias; renal abnormalities that can include renal agenesis; tortuous retinal vessels; ectopic/aberrant/unilateral absence of carotid and vertebral artery; microcephaly; and microdontia (there are 166 different findings to date).[42]

Developmental delay, learning disabilities, or mental retardation is common and quite variable. Behavioral and psychiatric problems are common but underappreciated findings in VCFS. These individuals have a characteristic personality, marked by a flattened affect and abnormal social interaction, ranging from being intermittently withdrawn to socially precocious. A host of other psychiatric diagnoses have been seen in patients with VCFS.

Both DiGeorge syndrome and VCFS have been recognized as being caused by deletions in 22q11. More than 95% of cases of DGS and VCFS are deleted. In a small number of patients with DGS, point mutations in TBX1 have been found when no deletion was identified.[50] There are a few cases of VCFS in which no 22q11 deletion or TBX1 mutation has been found. Thus obtaining family histories and examining parents for subtle features of the syndrome are important. In many cases, the infant has inherited the abnormality from a parent.

CLINICAL EXAMPLES OF CHROMOSOMAL ABNORMALITIES

Down Syndrome. Down syndrome has an incidence of approximately 1 in 600 live births. Approximately 95% of cases are caused by nondisjunction involving chromosome 21, 4% are caused by a translocation, and 1% are mosaic. Down syndrome may manifest

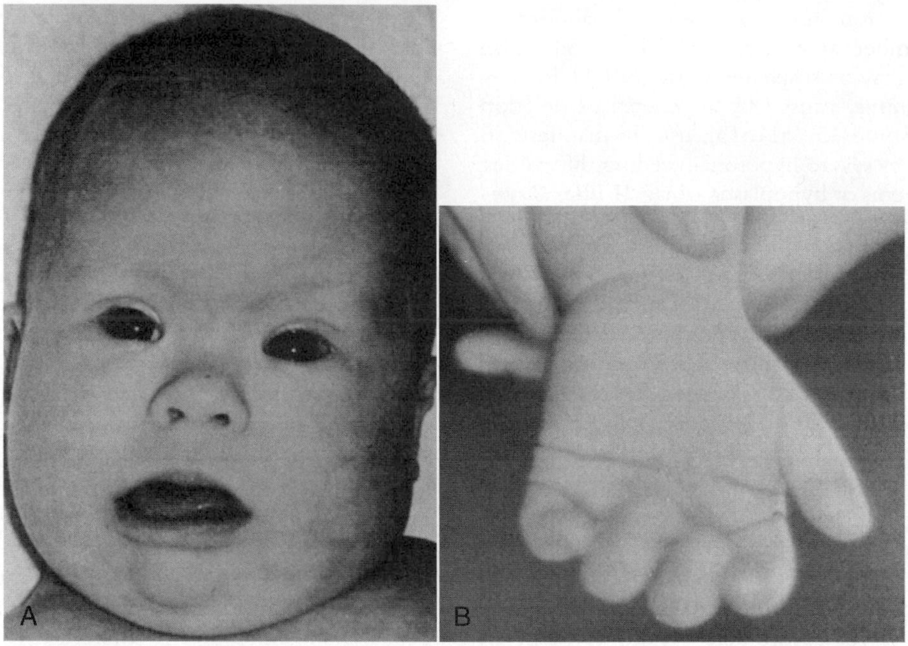

FIGURE 27-5 Infant with Down syndrome. ***A,*** Note midface hypoplasia, epicanthic folds, and depressed nasal bridge. ***B,*** Single palmar crease. (*A* from Cohen MM: *The child with multiple birth defects,* ed 2, New York, 1997, Raven Press. *B* courtesy Dr. Eva Sujansky, Genetic Services at The Children's Hospital, Denver, Colo.)

with marked hypotonia; a number of major malformations, most commonly congenital heart defects, duodenal atresia, and tracheoesophageal fistula; and a characteristic pattern of dysmorphic features. The classic phenotype seen in Down syndrome includes a flattened occiput, midfacial hypoplasia, depressed nasal bridge, upward-slanting palpebral fissures, epicanthic folds, grayish speckling of the iris (Brushfield spots), micrognathia, excess nuchal skin, single palmar creases (simian creases), single flexion creases and in-curving of the fifth fingers (clinodactyly), and increased distance between the first and second toes (Figure 27-5).

In full-term infants with the classic phenotype of Down syndrome, the clinical diagnosis is not difficult. However, it is imperative that cytogenetic studies be done to confirm the diagnosis and to differentiate a nondisjunctional trisomy from a translocation. This distinction has important implications for recurrence risks (see discussion in "Prevention" section). In premature infants, the classic facial phenotype is frequently missing, making clinical diagnosis more difficult. The presence of an atrioventricular (AV) canal or duodenal atresia with minor malformations, such as abnormal dermatoglyphics, should alert the clinician to the possibility of Down syndrome.

Trisomy 18. Trisomy 18 has an incidence of 1 in 6000 live births. The major phenotypic features include prenatal growth restriction, complex cardiac malformations, abnormal muscle tone, microcephaly, prominent occiput, short sternum, low-set and malformed ears, corneal opacities, micrognathia, peculiar hand posturing with the second and fifth digits overlapping the third and fourth, hypoplasia of fingernails, abnormal dermatoglyphics, prominent calcanei, and deep plantar furrows between the first and second toes (Figure 27-6). The prognosis is poor, and the majority of infants with trisomy 18 die within the first few months of life. Infants who have survived into childhood are profoundly retarded.

Trisomy 13. Trisomy 13 is seen in approximately 1 in 15,000 live births. Phenotypic features include prenatal and postnatal growth restriction, microcephaly,

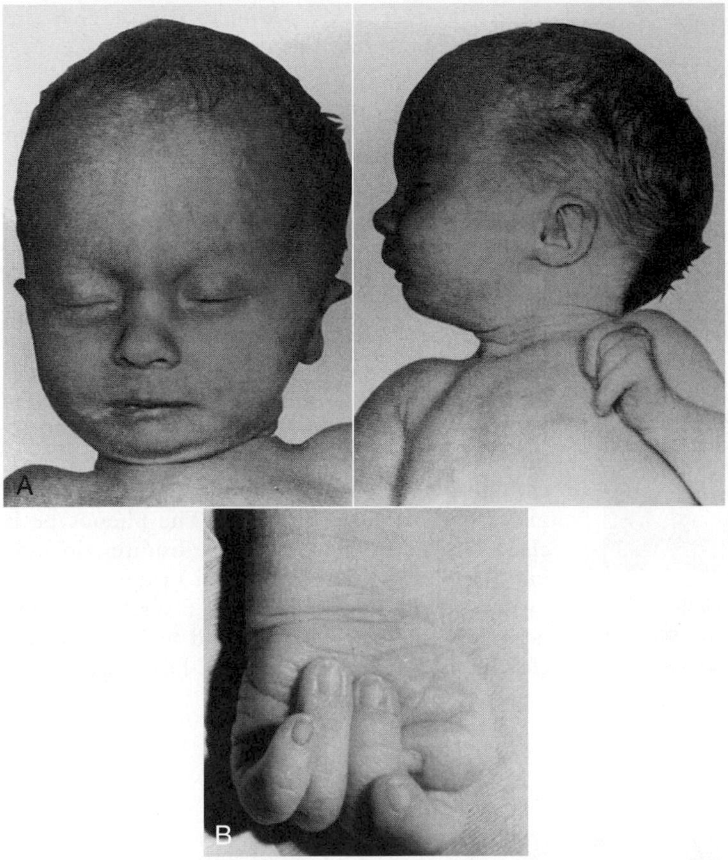

FIGURE 27-6 Infant with trisomy 18. ***A,*** Typical facies with small chin, abnormal pinna, and prominent occiput. ***B,*** Typical hand posturing with overlapping fingers. (From Paerregaard P, Mikkelsen M, Froland A, et al: Trisomy no. 17-18: report of two cases, *Acta Pathol Microbiol Scand* 67:479, 1966.)

sloping forehead, coloboma of the iris, microphthalmia or anophthalmia, low-set or malformed ears, cleft lip and palate, postaxial polydactyly, and abnormal palmar creases and dermatoglyphics (Figure 27-7). Internal abnormalities may include a number of central nervous system (CNS) malformations, such as holoprosencephaly, cardiac malformations, omphalocele, renal malformations, and urogenital abnormalities such as cryptorchidism in males and uterine malformations in females. The prognosis is extremely poor for these infants, with most dying within the first few months of life.

Turner Syndrome. The only monosomy to be seen in live births is that of Turner syndrome—females with a 45,X karyotype. In addition, it is the only numeric abnormality of the sex chromosome that may be identifiable at birth. Turner syndrome has an incidence of 1 in 5000 female births.[40] Clinical features that may be evident in the newborn period are a short, webbed neck or redundant skin on the back of the neck and marked lymphedema of the dorsum of the hands and feet (Figure 27-8). Congenital heart defects are seen in approximately half of the patients, with 30% having a coarctation of the aorta. Renal anomalies may also be present.[23] Prognosis is usually excellent but depends on the presence and severity of the congenital heart defect. Intelligence is normal; however, some females with Turner syndrome have been noted to have problems with spatial perception or fine motor abilities.[40]

Cri du Chat. Cri du chat, or "cat cry" syndrome, is the result of loss of the terminal end of the short arm of chromosome 5 (5p−). The name of the syndrome reflects the unusual catlike, weak cry these infants have in the neonatal period. These infants are usually small for gestational age, hypotonic, and microcephalic and may have ocular hypertelorism, epicanthic folds, downward slant of the palpebral

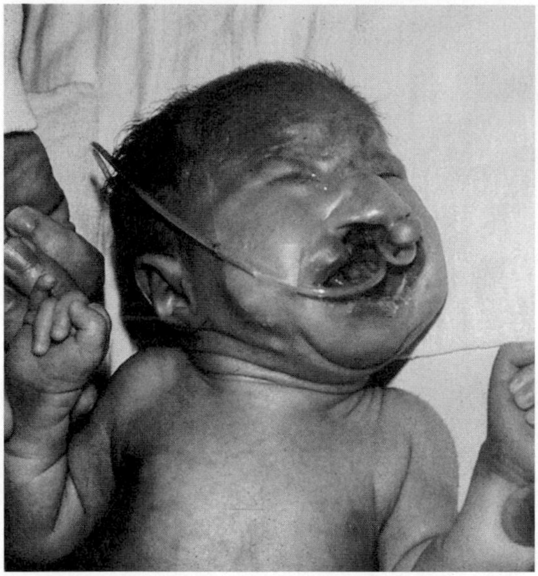

FIGURE 27-7 Infant with trisomy 13. Facial clefts and microcephaly; abnormal positioning of the hands. (From Hathaway WE, Groothuis J, Hay W, editors: *Current pediatric diagnoses and treatment*, ed 10, Norwalk, Conn, 1991, Appleton & Lange.)

fissures, low-set ears, and micrognathia. They are significantly mentally retarded.

San Luis Valley Syndrome. Recombinant 8 or the San Luis Valley syndrome, named for the area in which many of these individuals were first identified, is an example of an unbalanced pericentric inversion with both a duplication and a deletion of chromosome 8 material. The pericentric inversion of chromosome 8 found in a parent and other relatives of a child with recombinant 8 syndrome has no phenotypic consequence because it is a balanced rearrangement. However, a carrier is at risk for producing unbalanced gametes during meiosis. In recombinant 8 syndrome, there is a deletion of chromosomal material of the short arm of chromosome 8 and a duplication of chromosome material of the long arm of 8. The phenotype is characterized by unusual facial features, including a wide face, depressed nasal bridge, hypertelorism, down-slanting palpebral fissures, upturned nose, long philtrum, low-set and malformed ears, cleft lip or cleft palate, congenital heart disease, and renal abnormalities.[43]

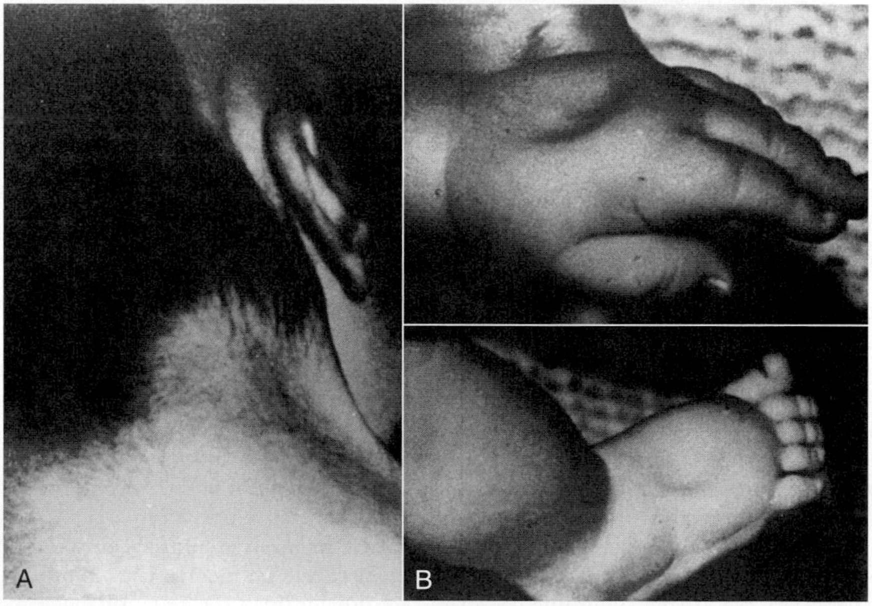

FIGURE 27-8 Female infant with Turner syndrome. ***A,*** Webbed neck with low posterior hairline. ***B,*** Lymphedema of the dorsal surfaces of the hands and feet. (From Knuppel R, Drukker JD, editors: *High risk pregnancy: a team approach*, Philadelphia, 1988, Saunders.)

PREVENTION

The identification of chromosomal abnormalities in the newborn is important, not only for management issues about the infant but also because of the recurrence risks the abnormality carries for the family. In general, numeric chromosomal abnormalities carry low recurrence risks (approximately 1% to 2%).[18] In the presence of structural abnormalities, recurrence risks depend on whether one of the parents carries a balanced rearrangement. If parental chromosomes are normal, the recurrence risk is minimal. However, if a parent carries a balanced chromosomal rearrangement, the recurrence risk is significantly increased. The exact risk figure varies with the nature of the specific chromosomal rearrangement and, in some cases, the sex of the carrier parent. In either situation, prenatal diagnosis for chromosome analysis is available for parents and families concerned about recurrence risk.

Single-Gene Disorders

McKusick's online catalog of mendelian inherited disorders currently lists more than 19,000 entries with approximately 6000 single-gene disorders with known patterns of inheritance.[38] Many of these disorders are singularly rare; however, collectively, they affect about 1% of the population. Single-gene disorders are the result of either a single or double dose of an abnormal gene. **Single-gene disorders are classified as autosomal dominant, autosomal recessive, X-linked dominant, and X-linked recessive.** Humans have two copies of each gene located at identical places (gene loci) on homologous chromosomes. In a single-gene disorder, an abnormal or mutated allele (an alternate form of a gene) is found on one or both members of a pair of chromosomes.[37] Individuals with identical alleles at a particular locus are homozygous for the gene. Individuals with different alleles are heterozygous for the gene. Because males have only one X chromosome and most genes located on the Y chromosome do not correspond to those located on the X, males are hemizygous for the genes on the X chromosome. Abnormal genes located on one of the 44 autosomes are the cause of autosomal disorders: **disease-causing genes located on the X chromosome are the cause of X-linked disorders.** Disorders are ***dominant*** when the phenotype is expressed in the presence of only one copy of the mutated gene. In ***recessive disorders,*** the phenotype is expressed only when both chromosomes carry the mutated gene.

AUTOSOMAL DOMINANT DISORDERS

Autosomal dominant disorders are ones in which the disorder is expressed in the heterozygous state. Major characteristics include the following: (1) multiple generations are affected (i.e., an infant would have an affected parent); (2) both males and females are affected, and both sexes can transmit the disorder to their offspring (i.e., male-to-male transmission can occur); (3) there is a 50% risk for each offspring to inherit the gene from an affected parent; and (4) individuals who do not have the gene cannot transmit the disorder to their offspring.

A negative family history does not rule out the presence of an autosomal dominant disorder. Possible explanations for a negative family history are the following: (1) the infant's disorder is a result of a new mutation; (2) a parent has a very mild expression of the disorder and may not have been previously diagnosed; (3) nonpaternity; (4) decreased penetrance (i.e., not all individuals with the gene have phenotypic abnormalities [skipped generation]); and (5) germline mosaicism for the mutation (see the "Nontraditional Inheritance" section).

Dominant disorders that may be seen in the NICU include skeletal dysplasias, such as ***achondroplasia*** (abnormality in the *FGFR3* gene), ***osteogenesis imperfecta*** (abnormality in *COL1A1* or *COL1A2*), ***Apert and Crouzon syndromes*** (abnormality in the *FGFR2* gene), ***Treacher Collins syndrome*** (abnormality in *Treacle* gene), and ectrodactyly (Figure 27-9).[1]

AUTOSOMAL RECESSIVE DISORDERS

Autosomal recessive disorders are expressed only in the homozygous state. Thus to be affected, an individual usually inherits an abnormal gene from each parent. The parent who is heterozygous for a disease-causing gene is usually phenotypically normal and is called a ***carrier.*** Major characteristics of autosomal recessive inheritance include (1) phenotypically normal parents, (2) affected siblings, (3) both males and females affected, (4) offspring of two carrier parents (25% risk for being affected), (5) unaffected siblings have a two-thirds chance of being carriers, and (6) possibly an increased incidence of consanguinity (mating between blood relatives).

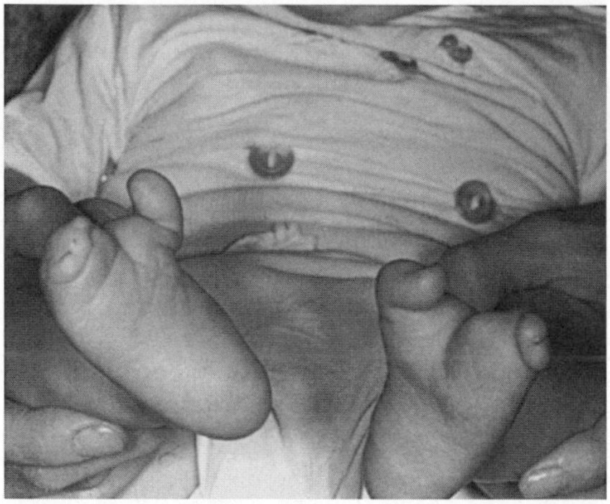

FIGURE 27-9 Ectrodactyly (lobster claw deformity) of the feet. (Courtesy Dr. Eva Sujansky, Genetic Services at The Children's Hospital, Denver, Colo.)

Autosomal recessive disorders that may be identified in the neonatal period include many of the metabolic disorders (e.g., ***phenylketonuria [PKU], galactosemia,*** and isovaleric acidemia) and some of the ***multiple-malformation syndromes*** (e.g., Meckel-Gruber syndrome), ***cystic fibrosis presenting with meconium ileus, Zellweger*** (cerebrohepatorenal) ***syndrome*** (Figure 27-10), and skeletal dysplasias such as achondrogenesis. The specific gene or biochemical defect for many of these disorders is now known.

X-LINKED DISORDERS

X-linked disorders are caused by an abnormal gene (or genes) located on the X chromosome. **Most X-linked disorders are recessive.** The X-linked recessive disorders are phenotypically expressed in hemizygous males; heterozygous females are generally phenotypically normal and are called ***carriers.***

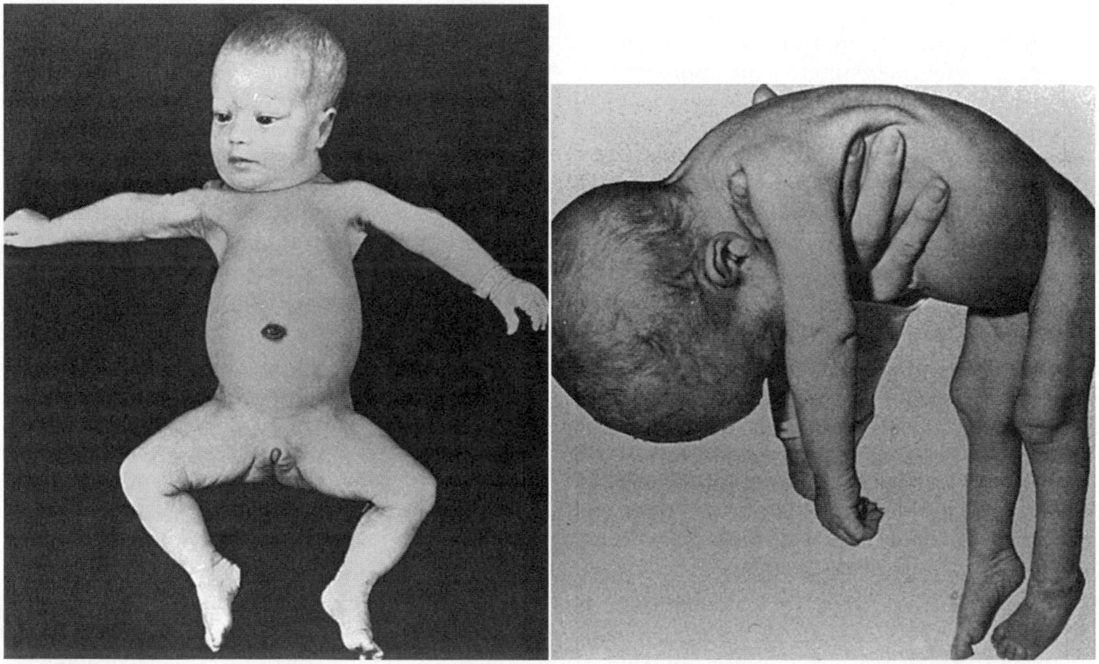

FIGURE 27-10 Infant with Zellweger syndrome, an autosomal recessive disorder. Note the high forehead, narrow facies, and extreme hypotonia. (*Left* from Jan JE, Hardwick DF, Lowry RB, et al: Cerebro-hepato-renal syndrome of Zellweger, *Am J Dis Child* 119:274, 1970. *Right* from Passarge E, McAdams AJ: Cerebro-hepato-renal syndrome: a newly recognized hereditary disorder of multiple congenital defects, including sudanophilic leukodystrophy, cirrhosis of the liver, and polycystic kidneys, *J Pediatr* 71:691, 1967.)

Affected fathers do not have affected sons (no male-to-male transmission); however, all daughters of affected males are carriers. A carrier female has a 50% chance of having an affected male offspring.

Occasionally, heterozygous females may be phenotypically affected, although usually less severely than males. If females are severely affected, other mechanisms, including homozygosity for the X-linked gene, may be responsible for the phenotype. **X-linked recessive disorders** that may be recognizable in the newborn period include **factor VIII and IX deficiency** (classic hemophilia A and B), X-linked hydrocephalus, and Opitz syndrome.

X-linked dominant disorders occur when the abnormal gene located on the X chromosome is expressed in both the hemizygous and heterozygous states. As in X-linked recessive conditions, there is no male-to-male transmission, because the affected male passes his Y chromosome and not his X chromosome to his sons; however, all of the daughters of an affected male will inherit his X chromosome and thus be affected. Each son and daughter of an affected female has a 50% risk for being affected; males usually are more severely affected than females. Only a few disorders are known to be **inherited as an X-linked dominant,** such as **incontinentia pigmenti, hypo-phosphatemia** (vitamin D–resistant rickets), and **ornithine transcarbamylase** (OTC) deficiency. Early diagnosis of OTC deficiency is important because, if untreated, it leads to neonatal hyperammonemia and death in affected males. In affected females, the clinical picture can be variable, ranging from an asymptomatic infant to one who presents in the first week of life with lethargy, vomiting, and protein avoidance, ending in seizures and coma.

Complex and Multifactorial Disorders

Complex, common non-mendelian disorders, often called ***multifactorial disorders,*** are the result of both environmental and genetic factors.[21] Most isolated single malformations, including congenital heart defects, neural tube defects, cleft lip and palate, pyloric stenosis, and club feet, are inherited in this manner. In addition, the more complex, common familial disorders, such as diabetes mellitus, coronary artery disease, affective disorders, and mild mental retardation, are the result of multifactorial inheritance. In contrast to single-gene inheritance, multifactorial disorders recur within families without a characteristic pedigree pattern and recurrence risks are based on empiric data.[37]

Multifactorial inheritance is explained as a liability model with a threshold effect.[21] The general population as a whole has an underlying genetic predisposition for multifactorial traits and disorders that follow a normal distribution curve; only in those individuals in whom the genetic predisposition exceeds the threshold will the malformation actually be expressed (Figure 27-11).

Major characteristics of complex/multifactorial inheritance include the following: (1) no consistent pedigree pattern exists between families (i.e., there may be only an isolated occurrence, or the disorder may be seen among siblings, in multiple generations, or scattered throughout the family); and (2) recurrence risks are not constant, as in single-gene disorders, but are influenced by a number of factors. These factors include the following:

- The number of family members affected (i.e., the more family members affected, the higher the recurrence risk becomes)
- The degree of relatedness to those affected (i.e., first-degree relatives are at higher recurrence risk than second- or third-degree relatives)
- The severity of the defect (i.e., the more severely affected an individual is, the higher the recurrence risk)

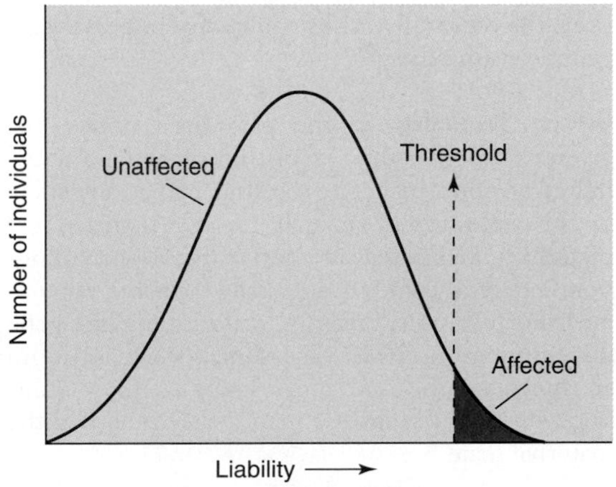

FIGURE 27-11 Multifactorial inheritance. Liability curve with a threshold beyond which the trait is expressed.

- The frequency of the disorder, which may vary with ethnic background (e.g., neural tube defects have a higher incidence among English and Irish populations)
- The gender of the individual (for disorders in which one gender is more commonly affected than the other [e.g., pyloric stenosis is more common in males]; if the less commonly affected gender has the defect, then the recurrence risk is higher)

With the increasing sophistication of ultrasound diagnosis during pregnancy, a number of these isolated malformations can now be diagnosed before delivery. Moreover, in the case of neural tube defects, it has been shown that folic acid supplements may decrease the incidence of spina bifida by as much as 70% in women of reproductive age.[34]

NONTRADITIONAL INHERITANCE

Germline Mosaicism. Spectacular growth in the field of molecular genetics and its technologies in only the past few years has enabled the clarification of the inheritance patterns of many genetic disorders and birth defects that were previously unknown or unclear. For example, the lethal form of osteogenesis imperfecta (OI) occurring in multiple offspring of unaffected parents was thought to be the result of autosomal recessive inheritance. However, improved molecular techniques have documented it to be the result of germline mosaicism; that is, the mutation occurs in the gonad of one of the parents, who then has some gametes with and others without the OI mutation. This distinction alters the recurrence risks and is very important for genetic counseling.[37]

Genomic Imprinting. In the past, little notice was given to whether the sex of the parent who transmitted an abnormal gene to offspring had any effect on the expression of genes. It is now recognized that maternally and paternally derived genes may function differently, and this is called *genomic imprinting.*[48] For example, offspring who inherit the gene for Huntington disease (autosomal dominant) from an affected father are more likely to have childhood onset of the disease than if they inherited the maternal gene.

Uniparental Disomy. Uniparental disomy is the result of inheriting both copies of a chromosome from one parent and none from the other.[48] It is assumed that for normal growth and development, a child must receive both maternal and paternal genes; if both copies of a gene originate only from one parent, the development is abnormal. Uniparental disomy has been seen in cystic fibrosis with short stature and in the Prader-Willi, Angelman, and Beckwith-Wiedemann syndromes. The parental origin of a child's chromosomes can be identified only by molecular analysis; routine chromosome analysis usually is not helpful.

The possibility of a nontraditional pattern of inheritance makes genetic counseling more complex than previously thought. Thus it is imperative that health care providers be aware of such complexities and refer families to a geneticist or genetic counselor for a more detailed discussion when appropriate.

INBORN ERRORS OF METABOLISM

Genetic disorders in which defects of single genes cause clinically significant blocks in metabolic pathways are known as *inborn errors of metabolism.* Recognition of disorders caused by inborn errors of metabolism has increased rapidly in recent years, and they are now recognized as important causes of disease in the newborn and pediatric age-group.[44] **Inborn errors of metabolism include defects of carbohydrate, amino acid, organic acid, and purine metabolism; disorders of fatty acid oxidation; lysosomal storage diseases; and disorders of peroxisomes.** Remember that inborn errors can present at any time and may affect almost any organ system. Specific disorders that should be considered in symptomatic newborns include galactosemia, OTC or carbamoyl-phosphate synthetase (CPS) deficiency, maple syrup urine disease, nonketotic hyperglycinemia, propionic and methylmalonic acidemias, isovaleric acidemia, and glutaric acidemia type II.[24]

Although the majority of infants are not found to have an inborn error of metabolism as the etiology of their illness, early recognition is imperative and may be considered a medical emergency if appropriate treatment is to be initiated. Many of these disorders can be treated effectively; if untreated, they are lethal in the newborn period. Moreover, without the appropriate diagnosis, parents would not be aware of recurrence risks in future offspring.

Inborn errors of metabolism should be included in the differential diagnosis for any critically ill newborn in the following instances: (1) suspicion of neonatal sepsis; (2) recurrent vomiting or altered consciousness; (3) clinical findings of hypoglycemia, seizures, parenchymal liver disease, unusual odor, hyperammonemia, or unexplained acidosis; or (4) a family history of a sibling affected with similar symptoms, mental retardation, or sudden infant death syndrome.[24]

In general, laboratory analysis depends on the presenting symptoms seen in the newborn. Laboratory studies that should be obtained before any treatment is begun are electrolytes, ammonia, glucose, urine pH, urine-reducing substances, and urine ketones. Clues to a possible inborn error are (1) hypoglycemia and ketonuria in the newborn, (2) acidosis with recurrent vomiting and hyperammonemia, and (3) acidosis that is difficult to correct and is out of proportion to the clinical state. If other underlying disorders are not readily apparent, additional laboratory tests that may be appropriate are serum and urine amino acids and urine organic acids.[44] Moreover, molecular (DNA) testing is available for several disorders.[27]

NEWBORN SCREENING

Inborn errors of metabolism, when unrecognized and untreated, may lead to severe consequences, including mental retardation and death in some instances. Thus the goal is to identify, treat, and prevent major sequelae whenever possible. Newborn screening accomplishes this goal for a growing number of disorders (Box 27-2). Screening criteria that should be met are relatively high frequency of the disorder, severity of symptomatology in untreated individuals, availability of treatment, simplicity of obtaining tissue for testing, and availability of a simple screening test with high sensitivity and specificity and reasonable cost. Recently, there have been major changes in the laboratory technologies available for newborn screening—specifically, the introduction of tandem mass spectrometry (MS/MS).[10] Using MS/MS technology, a single blood spot from a newborn can detect more than 50 inborn errors of metabolism.[36] Although many of the disorders detectable by MS/MS are rare, screening has been instituted in most states because screening remains inexpensive and a variety of disorders can be identified in a single assay. In most instances, additional testing adds approximately $25 to $60 to the cost of the newborn screen.[31]

BOX 27-2 A PARTIAL LIST OF DISORDERS THAT ARE SCREENED FOR IN NEWBORN SCREENING PROGRAMS

Defects Identifiable by Tandem Mass Spectrometry (MS/MS)

Amino Acid Disorders and Urea Cycle Disorders

Phenylketonuria
Homocystinuria
Hypermethioninemia
Argininosuccinic acidemia
Citrullinemia
Argininemia
Tyrosinemia types I and II

Organic Acid Disorders

Maple syrup urine disease
Isovaleric acidemia
Methylmalonic acidemia
Propionic acidemia
Glutaric acidemia type I
Isobutyryl-CoA dehydrogenase deficiency
3-Hydroxy-3-methylglutaryl-CoA lyase deficiency
2-Methylbutyryl-CoA dehydrogenase deficiency
3-Methylcrotonyl-CoA carboxylase deficiency

Fatty Acid Oxidation Disorders

Medium-chain acyl-CoA dehydrogenase deficiency
Short-chain acyl-CoA dehydrogenase deficiency
Very-long–chain acyl-CoA dehydrogenase deficiency
Long-chain hydroxyacyl-CoA dehydrogenase deficiency
Glutaric acidemia type II
Carnitine palmityl transferase deficiency type II
Carnitine/acylcarnitine translocase deficiency
Multiple CoA carboxylase deficiency
Trifunctional protein deficiency

Disorders Screened by Other Methodologies

Congenital adrenal hyperplasia
Galactosemia
Sickle cell disease and hemoglobinopathies
Hypothyroidism (congenital)

Data from the National Newborn Screening and Genetics Resource Center; website: http://genes-r-us.uthscsa.edu.

MS/MS has been used for many years to measure metabolites in blood and urine. However, the technology has been applied recently to newborn screening programs. A mass spectrometer is an instrument that separates and quantifies ions based on their mass/charge ratios (m/z). In MS/MS, there are two spectrometers in a series. After sample preparation from the dried blood spot, the process of tandem mass is automated and the analysis is computerized. The process takes only a few seconds, and an entire screen takes less than 2 minutes.[31] The MS/MS system is capable of handling a high volume of samples; thus it is an excellent technology for use in newborn screening. Currently the false-positive rate is 0.3% for all disorders.[52]

Screening for metabolic disorders is mandated by individual states, and all states require screening for phenylketonuria (PKU), hypothyroidism, congenital adrenal hyperplasia, sickle cell disease, s-beta thalassemia, and galactosemia.[36] However, the American Academy of Pediatrics (AAP) and the American College of Medical Genetics have recommended that all states screen for a core panel of 29 treatable disorders and an additional 25 conditions that may be detected by screening.[3] The additional disorders most often screened for include amnio acid disorders (homocystinuria, maple syrup urine disease), organic acids (glutaric, methylmalonic, and propionic acidemias), disorders of fatty acid metabolism (medium-chain and very-long–chain acyl-CoA dehydrogenase deficiency), hemoglobinopathies, and others such as biotinidase deficiency, congenital adrenal hyperplasia, and cystic fibrosis.[3]

Each state decides individually what will be included in its newborn screening program. Although some states require all of the tests on their list to be mandatory, other states offer a supplemental program in addition to the mandated program, often called *expanded newborn screening.* Testing for disorders listed on the mandated program is necessary, and only parents objecting on religious grounds may decline the mandated screen (e.g., Ohio Revised Code 3701.501). In those states offering a supplemental program, parents can choose whether or not to screen their child for the disorders listed. The program is optional, and no extra blood or additional tissue is necessary.[26] In most situations, parents are asked to sign a participation form to opt-in to the supplemental program. With more than 30 states now using MS/MS in their newborn screening process,[36] state legislators are constantly changing and updating their screening practices. It behooves the clinician to periodically check with the state newborn screening program for updates. The National Newborn Screening and Genetics Resource Center (NNSGRC) provides up-to-date information.

Any screening test may give both false-positive and false-negative results; this includes those identified by MS/MS. **Thus a positive screen result must be followed by a confirmatory diagnostic test.**[3] Moreover, if there is clinical suspicion of a particular disorder in spite of a negative screening result, further diagnostic testing is warranted. **In addition to confirming positive screens, clinicians may have to deal with the concern for increased parental anxiety based on false-positive screens.** Waisbren et al found in a prospective interview study of 254 mothers and 153 fathers that stress levels of parents whose infants had false-positive screening results were significantly higher than those with normal results.[46] Thus for clinicians in the NICU setting, being cognizant of the potential for an increased number of positive newborn screening results is important for the care of the neonate, as well as for parent teaching. (For an in-depth review of those disorders that may be part of the newborn screening program, refer to the AAP's newborn screening recommendations.)[3]

Newborn Hearing Screening. Newborn hearing screening tests are now available that have high sensitivity when administered properly.[4] Hearing loss is present in approximately 1 to 2 per 1000 infants. Research has demonstrated that there are both genetic and nongenetic causes of deafness. Sixty percent of prelingual deafness has a recognizable genetic etiology, and of these, the most common cause of autosomal recessively inherited nonsyndromic hearing loss results from mutations in the connexin 26 *(Cx26)* gene, a member of the connexin family of gap junction proteins.[51] Commercial DNA–based screening tests are now available to detect common genetic forms of deafness including *Cx26* and mitochondrial deafness.[5] The AAP has recommended that all newborns be screened for hearing loss before the age of 3 months.[2] The American College of Medical Genetics has recommended, in addition to screening and subsequent confirmation of hearing loss by diagnostic tests, that protocols be developed to ensure that appropriate genetic counseling be provided if diagnostic testing includes genetic testing.[5] This would provide families with accurate information about causes and recurrence risks for parents, siblings, and other family members.

ABNORMALITIES RESULTING FROM ENVIRONMENTAL EXPOSURES

Environmental exposures may have adverse (teratogenic) effects on fetal development, resulting in malformations and functional neurodevelopmental abnormalities in infants and children. The four major prerequisites needed for teratogenic action are as follows[20]:

1. The agent must have the **potential to be teratogenic.** Few conclusive data are available about the teratogenicity of most chemicals and drugs in humans. Animal studies provide most of the currently available data on the teratogenicity of agents; however, not all are always applicable to human situations. To prove that an agent is teratogenic, a causal relationship between the exposure and presence of a malformation must be documented; just the history of an exposure to an agent is not sufficient. Although very few agents have been documented to be teratogenic in humans, a few stand out, such as alcohol, cocaine, anticonvulsants, and isotretinoin (Accutane) (Figure 27-12).
2. The **timing of the exposure** during pregnancy is of major importance. For the agent to adversely affect the fetus, it must be present during organogenesis or histogenesis. Exposures occurring within the first 2 weeks after conception, before cell differentiation, will cause no damage or result in fetal wastage. Exposures occurring from 2 to 12 weeks of gestation (period of organogenesis) may result in major malformations. After completion of development of the major organ systems, harmful exposures usually do not result in malformations but can be responsible for organ dysfunction. However, some agents may morphologically disrupt previously intact organs.[11] On the other hand, it has been shown that if the harmful exposure to an agent such as alcohol has been discontinued, the damage is less severe than if the exposure continues throughout the pregnancy.
3. **Dosage of the teratogen is related to the severity of the teratogenic effect;** the higher the dose, the more severe the effect and the higher the frequency of affected fetuses.
4. Finally, **genetic makeup or genetic susceptibility of the mother and fetus** may affect the metabolism, as well as tissue sensitivity to the teratogen.

Teratogenic agents may be divided into four categories: (1) infectious agents, (2) chemical agents (drugs and environmental agents), (3) radiation, and (4) maternal factors. Chapter 2 provides excellent overviews of most of these exposures.

Traditionally, only maternal exposures to teratogens have been implicated in malformations. There has been a concern that some paternal exposures also may be teratogenic. Theoretically, a teratogen excreted in the semen could be introduced into the fetal environment and potentially be teratogenic to the developing fetus.[12]

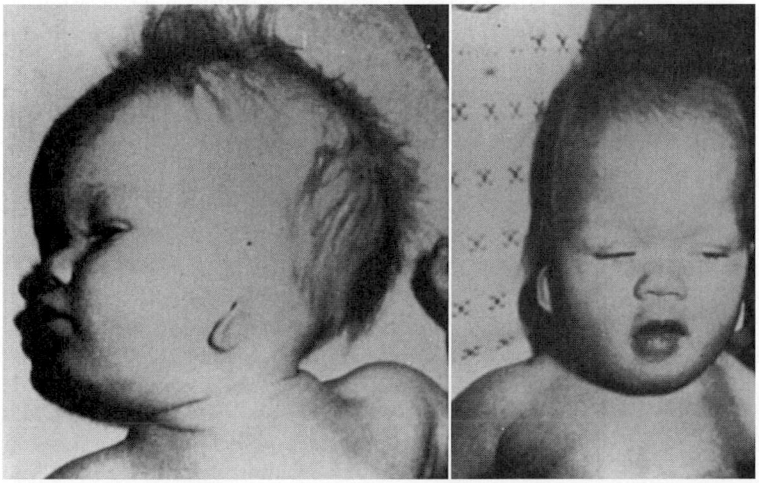

FIGURE 27-12 Infant exposed to Accutane in utero. Note dysmorphic face and auricles with atretic ear canal. (Courtesy Dr. Eva Sujansky, Genetic Services at The Children's Hospital, Denver, Colo.)

Teratogenic exposures should be considered in the differential diagnosis of congenital malformations and CNS dysfunction if one can document fetal exposure and the phenotype is compatible with the known effects of the suspected teratogen. The recognition of exposures is important for genetic counseling; if they can be avoided during subsequent pregnancies, recurrence risk is not increased. Frequently there is phenotypic overlap between the fetal abnormalities caused by specific teratogens and other syndromes. The family should be referred to a genetics clinic to rule out chromosomal, single-gene, and sporadic syndromes with overlapping phenotypes.

DATA COLLECTION

A genetic evaluation consists of the same components found in any medical evaluation; however, the emphasis may be different. Moreover, to make an accurate diagnosis and assessment, medical information about extended family members may have to be obtained. An excellent overview of the evaluation of the neonate with single or multiple congenital anomalies is published by the American College of Medical Genetics and available at their website.[5]

History

Prenatal and perinatal histories, from a genetic standpoint, should elicit information about potential teratogenic exposures including maternal disease and acute illness. Fetal growth and behavior (e.g., fetal movement, swallowing) provide important clues for the assessment of fetal neuromuscular function. Thus information about fetal position, movement, and amount of amniotic fluid should be obtained. Perinatal history should include the duration of gestation, anthropometric birth measurements including head circumference, and information about perinatal adaptation. In a newborn with abnormal CNS functioning, it may be difficult to differentiate between primary maldevelopment and dysfunction caused by perinatal complications. An abnormal newborn with a genetic disorder may present with signs suggestive of birth asphyxia (i.e., hypoxia, acidosis, hypotonia, seizures). Moreover, because many a priori abnormal newborns have an increased frequency of perinatal complications, a documented birth injury does not rule out the presence of a genetic cause.

Family history may be extremely helpful in clarifying the causes and risk for recurrence. The information obtained from the parents may have to be complemented by physical examination of the parents and other family members and review of the medical records. This may be necessary because parents may not be aware that different defects in family members may be an expression of the same disorder. For example, an autosomal dominant gene may cause mild hypoplasia of thumbs in one family member and complete absence of thumb and radii in another.

A three-generation pedigree also should be obtained that includes health information about parents, siblings, grandparents, aunts, uncles, and cousins. Specifically, information about miscarriages, stillbirths, childhood deaths, relatives born with congenital malformations and birth defects, mental retardation, and other disorders that "run in the family" should be obtained.[6] Information about ethnic background and consanguinity also should be collected.

Physical Examination

A physical examination should enable the examiner to detect major and minor malformations (dysmorphic features). *Minor malformations* are defined as structural variations found in less than 4% of the general population and that have no significant medical or cosmetic effect. This is in contrast to structural variations that are found in more than 4% of the newborn population and represent a normal variation, such as a mongolian spot and capillary hemangioma on the forehead. Minor malformations may provide important clues to the identification of a specific syndrome. **None of the minor malformations as an isolated finding are clinically significant; however, a combination or pattern of minor malformations may indicate a specific disorder.** For example, dysmorphic features such as up-slanted eyes, epicanthic folds, hypertelorism (Figure 27-13), and abnormal dermatoglyphic pattern (Figure 27-14) in an infant with a congenital heart defect are suggestive of Down syndrome. **Minor malformations also may alert the clinician to the presence of major malformations.** For example, preauricular ear tags are associated with an increased frequency of inner ear malformations and hearing impairment. In addition, **the greater the**

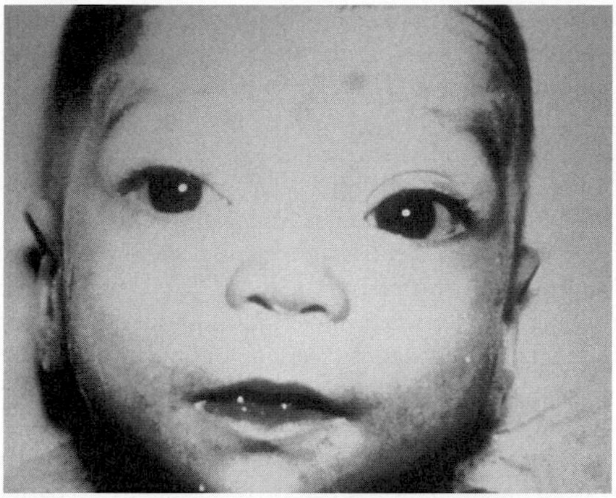

FIGURE 27-13 Dysmorphic feature of hypertelorism. Note wide-spaced eyes. (From Gilbert-Barness E, Kapur RP, Oligny LL et al: *Potter's pathology of the fetus, infant, and child,* ed 2, St Louis, 2007, Mosby.)

number of minor malformations an infant has, the higher the chance of finding one or more major malformations.[28]

If minor malformations are identified, the parents of the infant should be examined. Presence of the same minor malformation in one of the parents may indicate a benign familial feature. Alternatively, finding the same dysmorphic features in other family members may represent an inherited genetic disorder. A mild syndactyly between the second and third toes is frequently an isolated, inherited finding without clinical significance. However, syndactyly associated with craniosynostosis may represent an autosomal dominant disorder with variable expression and significant clinical sequelae.

If an infant looks dysmorphic, documentation of specific features should be recorded. Actual measurements compared with age-related norms should be used to measure body proportions, length of extremities, and such facial features as distance between eyes, length of eye fissures, size of ears, and length of philtrum. Description of the other features, such as the shape of the neck (webbed) or the chest size (widely spaced nipples), or a specific description of any skin lesions including size, shape, location, and color (hyperpigmented or hypopigmented) may provide important clues for a specific diagnosis. **Dermatoglyphic analysis**—the analysis of the dermal ridges on the digits, palms, and soles—may prove useful for determining the timing of a fetal insult.[49] Development of ridges begins during the thirteenth week of gestation and is complete by the nineteenth week. Thus many chromosomal and genetic disorders have disruptions of the dermal ridge patterns. For example, an infant with Down syndrome may have a single palmar crease (simian crease), a single flexion crease of the fifth digit, and an open field pattern (tibial arch) on the hallucal area of the foot.[49] Moreover, specific descriptors or, even more useful, photographs, should be used to describe dysmorphic findings.

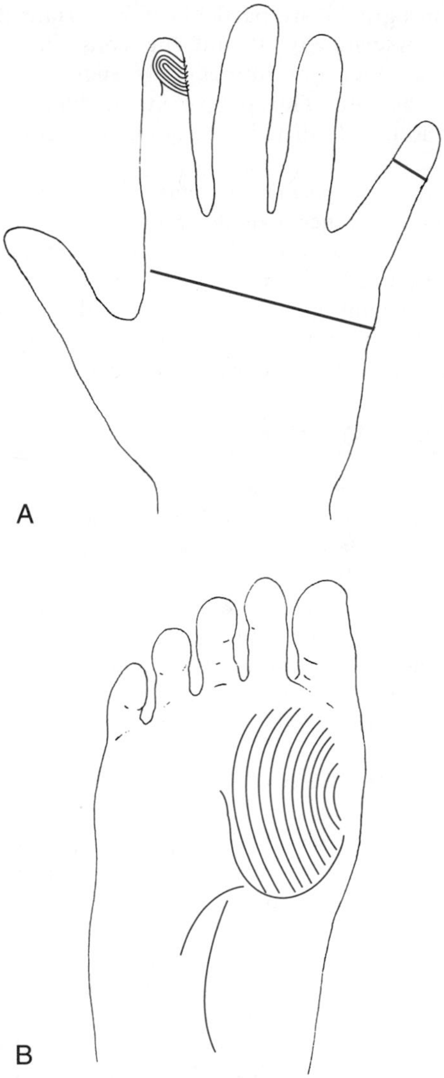

FIGURE 27-14 Dermatoglyphics commonly seen in infants with Down syndrome. ***A,*** Ulnar loop on the second digit, single flexion crease on the fifth digit, and single palmar crease (simian line). ***B,*** Tibial arch pattern on hallucal area of foot.

Photographs are particularly important if the infant is critically ill and the constellation of findings does not immediately suggest a specific syndrome. Thus the patient's findings may be more accurately shared with other clinicians in the future.

Smith's Recognizable Patterns of Human Malformation[23] and other texts document a large number of syndromes, some of which are quite rare and may not be immediately recognized by neonatal staff. It may be helpful and important to **consult a clinician who is familiar with dysmorphology and syndromology to help establish a diagnosis.**

Laboratory Data

When a genetic disorder is suspected, a number of diagnostic studies may be useful in delineating a diagnosis, including chromosome analysis, CGH array, molecular DNA testing, biochemical studies to rule out inborn errors of metabolism, radiographs, organ imaging, and when appropriate, autopsy. Not all of these studies are routinely used in all patients, but selection of studies is based on clinical suspicion of a particular disorder.

CHROMOSOME ANALYSIS

Routinely, results of chromosome analysis may not be available for several weeks. However, if results of chromosome analysis are urgently needed for clinical management, chromosome analysis from bone marrow can be available within a few hours and preliminary results from blood lymphocyte culture can be obtained in 48 hours. Indications for chromosome analysis have been listed previously. **However, chromosome analysis should be obtained in all critically ill infants for whom there is no plausible explanation for their grave clinical course, before death occurs.** For postmortem examination, chromosomes also may be obtained from any tissue—in particular, intracardiac blood, thymus, skin, and gonad. Under sterile conditions, these tissues should be obtained as soon as possible after the infant's demise. Tissue should be transported to the laboratory in a tissue culture medium or sterile saline solution, not in formalin.

MOLECULAR DNA ANALYSIS

There is a growing list of disorders for which the gene has been identified, and thus molecular diagnostic tests are commercially available. Although the Genetic Alliance, an international coalition comprising more than 600 advocacy, research, and health care organizations, lists 830 genetic conditions at their website *(www.geneticalliance.org),* not all those disorders are amenable to DNA testing. Moreover, often a clinical diagnosis of a recognized syndrome does not require additional diagnostic testing.[5] However, if the diagnosis is not clear, if there is a need to confirm a diagnosis for management issues, or if additional information about a clinically recognized disorder is needed for family planning and genetic counseling, then DNA testing may be extremely helpful.[5]

Whenever the health care professional has a reasonable suspicion of a specific diagnosis based on clinical phenotype, it is reasonable to suggest molecular testing if it is available to confirm the diagnosis and provide appropriate genetic counseling. However, the clinician must remember that mutational analysis is complex and, although it can confirm a diagnosis when the test result is positive, a negative result may not determine conclusively that the neonate is not affected.[1] Some disorders (listed with their gene symbol or chromosomal locus) that might be seen in the neonate for which molecular gene testing is available are listed in Table 27-1.

BIOCHEMICAL STUDIES

A critically ill neonate who has a condition suggestive of an inborn error of metabolism or who has no specific diagnosis should have blood and urine sent for appropriate biochemical studies (specified in the "Inborn Errors of Metabolism" section). If such studies have not been obtained, postmortem tissue such as liver should be obtained and frozen for later biochemical analysis. **Care providers should request detailed instructions from a laboratory specializing in testing for inherited metabolic disorders about which tissue is appropriate and how it should be obtained, stored, and shipped to the laboratory.**

RADIOGRAPHS

X-ray examination should be obtained if a skeletal dysplasia or other skeletal abnormality is suspected or if the differential diagnosis includes a genetic syndrome that has skeletal defects as part of the phenotype. Moreover, if a localized skeletal defect is found, a skeletal survey should be obtained to identify other possible skeletal defects.

TABLE 27-1 PARTIAL LIST OF DISORDERS SEEN IN THE NEWBORN PERIOD WHERE DNA MOLECULAR TESTING IS AVAILABLE CLINICALLY

SYNDROME	GENE	CHROMOSOMAL LOCATION
Apert and Crouzon	*FGFR2*	10q26
Achondroplasia and thanatophoric dysplasia	*FGFR3*	4p16
Cystic fibrosis	*CFTR*	7q31
Congenital myotonic dystrophy	*DMPK*	19q13
Miller-Dieker	Microdeletion	17p13.3
Osteogenesis imperfecta	*COL1A1* or *COL1A2*	17q21.3-q22
Pfeiffer	*FGFR1*	10q26
Prader-Willi and Angelman	Uniparental disomy, imprinting, deletion	15q11.3-q13
Smith-Lemli-Opitz	*DHCR7*	11q12-q13
Treacher Collins	Treacle (*TCOF1*)	5q32-q33
Velocardiofacial/DiGeorge	Microdeletion	22q11
Waardenburg type 1	*PAX3*	2q35
Waardenburg type 2	*MITF*	3p14.1-p12.3
Williams	*ELN* (elastin)	7q11.2
Wolf-Hirschhorn	Microdeletion	4p16.3

ORGAN IMAGING

Organ imaging by **ultrasonography, magnetic resonance imaging (MRI), and computed tomography (CT) scan should be used to rule out structural abnormalities of major organs** such as the brain, heart, and kidneys. Malformations may be suspected on the basis of clinical symptoms such as anuria or on the basis of known nonrandom associations of certain birth defects, such as the vertebral/anal/tracheoesopageal fistula/renal/radial (VATER) association. In addition, some dysmorphic features are associated with major malformations, and one must rule out these features. For example, there is an increased incidence of underlying midline brain defects associated with some facial dysmorphic features.

AUTOPSY

In the event of a neonate's death, an autopsy may provide crucial information for the establishment of a correct diagnosis. As outlined, chromosome analysis, biochemical studies, x-ray examination, and photographs all should be included. **In the absence of a specific, confirmed diagnosis, the family should be strongly encouraged to consent to an autopsy, and a tissue sample should be frozen for further testing.** Without this valuable information, subsequent genetic counseling of the parents, including clarification of the causes and recurrence risks, becomes impossible.

TREATMENT AND INTERVENTION

For most genetic disorders and malformations, there are no "cures" and only **symptomatic treatment is available; that is, conventional medical and surgical interventions are instituted, although the basic genetic defect is not corrected.** Surgical intervention for specific malformations will depend on the malformation, its cause, and prognosis. For example, surgical repair of a cleft lip and palate usually has an excellent outcome, although the underlying genetic cause has not been altered. In other instances, the diagnosis may provide direction and guidance to the health care professionals and family as to the appropriate course of action. An infant born with a hypoplastic left side of the heart may be considered a candidate for a heart transplant. However, if the cardiac malformation is the result of a chromosomal abnormality with an extremely poor prognosis, such as trisomy 13, the management of that infant may be palliative rather than corrective.

With the diagnosis of a metabolic disorder, treatment may be one of a nutritional or pharmacologic approach, such as the restriction of phenylalanine in an infant with PKU or the replacement of a deficient hormone, such as thyroid supplements in hypothyroidism. For some conditions, such as OI, the best approach may be educating the parents on specific techniques of holding and caring for an infant to prevent further fractures. In some disorders, organ or tissue transplantation may be appropriate. Bone marrow transplantation has been found to be effective in treating select genetic disorders, including lysosomal storage disorders[39] and beta thalassemia.[33] Because specific treatment leading to a cure is not available for most genetic disorders, the use of genetic counseling and available reproductive alternatives, such as prenatal diagnosis, in vitro fertilization, preimplantation diagnosis, and artificial insemination by donor, are acceptable alternatives for some families.

THE HUMAN GENOME PROJECT

The year 2000 marked the announcement that the vast majority of the human genome had been sequenced.[13] This international effort, funded in part by the National Institutes of Health (NIH), began in 1990 with the development of genetic and physical maps of the human genome and completed its initial goals in 2000 with a draft of the sequencing of the 3 billion base pairs of the human genome. Defining the sequence of the human genome is only the beginning of the application of that knowledge to current and future research opportunities that will provide avenues for innovative therapies. New powerful technologies for understanding gene expression are being applied to designing drugs that will moderate disease pathways. Collins et al have noted that "microarray technologies have catapulted many laboratories from studying the expression of one or two genes in a month to studying the expression of tens of thousands of genes in a day."[13] The field of genomics is also providing opportunities to predict responsiveness to drug therapies, because reactions to drugs often are based on individual genetic variations. With the identification of common gene variants involved in drug action or metabolism, health care professionals might be able to predict an infant's response—good or bad—to a particular drug regimen.[13]

With the numerous advances in molecular genetics, it is predicted that many genetic disorders and malformations may be amenable to treatment in utero or after birth. In utero correction of such birth defects as urinary tract malformations, myelomeningocele, and diaphragmatic hernia has been successful.[7,16,17] In 1990, the first human trial of gene therapy was undertaken at the NIH. The treatment was somatic gene replacement in a 4-year-old child with adenosine deaminase deficiency, a rare inherited disorder that destroys the immune system.[29] Successful efforts using improved gene therapy techniques continue with this disorder.[8] Since that time, a number of gene therapy trials for other genetic disorders have been done. Although the arena of gene therapy in general has been somewhat disappointing, the results have led to new areas of research and experimentation with new promising techniques.[41] The development of safer and more effective vectors based on technologies spearheaded by the Human Genome Project should provide significant improvements in gene therapy, such as that seen in an application of gene therapy with hemophilia B.[25]

PARENT TEACHING

The birth of any infant with a malformation or genetic disorder is a devastating event for any family. The neonatal staff find themselves on the front lines helping families deal with the infant's problems and providing the best environment for both the critically ill newborn and his or her family. In general, the most difficult factor for most parents and families to deal with is the unknown. Thus once again, the need for an accurate diagnosis becomes paramount (see the Parent Teaching box on p. 809). Moreover, even when the diagnosis carries a very poor prognosis, parents would prefer having the information so they can realistically anticipate and prepare for what is to come.[47] Currently, many parents obtain information

Parent Teaching

- Genetic diagnosis is essential not only for management of the neonate's condition but also for counseling.
- Genetic counseling assists parents and care providers in addressing management issues such as cause and diagnosis, prognosis, treatment and interventions, short-term and long-term care, and follow-up.
- Genetic counseling assists parents in decisions about future pregnancies or the use of assistive reproductive technologies.

about their infant's malformation or genetic disorder through prenatal diagnosis and have already begun the process of anticipatory grief by the time the infant is admitted to the NICU. Parental feelings of disbelief, shock, anger, or despair may have already been replaced with a "sense of relief" about confirmation of the abnormalities and a need to deal with the situation at hand.[30]

Chapter 30 provides an excellent review of the grief and mourning process that parents will experience when their anticipated "perfect baby" is born with a malformation or genetic disorder.

From a genetic counseling standpoint, a number of principles should be incorporated into the plan of care for the neonate and his or her family. First—and it cannot be overstated—an accurate diagnosis is essential if genetic counseling is to be provided. Even with what appears to be an isolated malformation, a genetics consultation may be appropriate to rule out other causes, such as single-gene disorders or chromosomal abnormalities. After establishing the diagnosis, one can realistically address the prognosis, treatment, and other management issues with the family. Finally, at the appropriate time for the family, recurrence risks and options for future pregnancies can be addressed.

Certainly, the busy and stressful environment of the NICU is not the most conducive atmosphere for obtaining and providing detailed information. **However, it is very appropriate for the geneticist to make an initial contact with the family in the NICU, where basic information about the pregnancy and perinatal and family histories can be obtained that will aid in diagnosis and defining the cause.** Diagnosis and management then can be addressed by the neonatal staff and geneticist. Later, at a time appropriate for the family, such issues as recurrence risks can be addressed. Eventually the family should receive a written summary of all the issues discussed for their own documentation.

The genetic evaluation is a complex and multifaceted process that cannot be done in isolation; it requires a team approach. The geneticist can assist the neonatal intensive care staff in determining the diagnosis, cause, and prognosis so that appropriate management of the infant can be implemented and aid in future counseling of the families they serve. The neonatal staff should use the genetics team as a resource for consultation and assistance in providing infants and families with the most appropriate and complete health care available.

REFERENCES

1. American Academy of Pediatrics: Molecular genetic testing in pediatric practice: a subject review, *Pediatrics* 106:1494, 2000.
2. American Academy of Pediatrics: Newborn and infant hearing loss: principles and guidelines for early detection and intervention programs, *Pediatrics* 120:898, 2006.
3. American Academy of Pediatrics: Newborn screening expands: recommendations for pediatricians and medical homes—implications for the system, *Pediatrics* 121(1):192, 2008.
4. American College of Medical Genetics: Newborn screening: toward a uniform screening panel and system, *Genet Med* 8:15, 2006.
5. American College of Medical Genetics: *Evaluation of the newborn with single or multiple congenital anomalies: a clinical guideline,* Accessed October 26, 2009, from www.acmg.net.
6. Bennett RL: The family medical history, *Prim Care Clin Office Pract* 31:479, 2004.
7. Bruner JP, Tulipan N, Paschall RL, et al: Fetal surgery for myelomeningocele and the incidence of shunt-dependent hydrocephalus, *JAMA* 282:1819, 1999.
8. Calazzana-Calvo M, Hacein-Bey S, de Saint Basile G: Gene therapy of human severe combined immunodeficiency (SCID)-X1 disease, *Science* 288:669, 2000.
9. Cassidy SB, McCandless S: Prader Willi syndrome. In Cassidy SB, Allanson JE, editors: *Management of genetic syndromes,* ed 2 Hoboken, NJ, 2004, Wiley-Liss.
10. Chace DH, Kalas TA, Naylor EW: Use of tandem mass spectrometry for multianalyte screening of dried blood specimens from newborns, *Clin Chem* 49:1797, 2003.
11. Clayton-Smith J, Donnai D: Human malformations. In Rimoin DL, Connor JM, Pyeritz RE, et al: *Emery and Rimoin's principles and practice of medical genetics,* ed 5, New York, 2006, Churchill Livingstone.

12. Colie CF: Male mediated teratogenesis, *Reprod Toxicol* 7:3, 1993.
13. Collins FS, Green ED, Guttmarcher AE, et al: A vision for the future of genomics research, *Nature* 422(6934):835, 2003.
14. Driscoll DA, Salvin J, Sellinger B, et al: Prevalence of 22q11 microdeletions in DiGeorge and velocardiofacial syndromes: implications for genetic counseling and prenatal diagnosis, *J Med Genet* 30:813, 1993.
15. Edelmann L, Hirschhorn K: Clinical utility of array CGH for the detection of chromosomal imbalances associated with mental retardation and multiple congenital anomalies, *Ann NY Acad Sci* 1151:157, 2009.
16. Flake AW: Fetal therapy: medical and surgical approaches. In Creasy RK, Resnick R, editors: *Maternal and fetal medicine,* ed 4, Philadelphia, 1998, Saunders.
17. Flake AW, Crombleholme TM, Johnson MP, et al: Treatment of severe congenital diaphragmatic hernia by fetal tracheal occlusion: clinical experience with fifteen cases, *Am J Obstet Gynecol* 183:1059, 2000.
18. Gardner RJM, Sutherland GR: *Chromosome abnormalities and genetic counseling,* ed 3, New York, 2003, Oxford University Press.
19. Gersen SL, Keagle MB: *Principles of clinical cytogenetics,* ed 2, Totowa, NJ, 2005, Humana Press.
20. Hanson JW: Human teratogens. In Rimoin DL, Connor JM, Pyeritz RE, et al: *Emery and Rimoin's principles and practice of medical genetics,* ed 5, New York, 2006, Churchill Livingstone.
21. Harper PS: *Practical genetic counseling,* ed 6, Oxford, England, 2004, Hodder Arnold.
22. Hay WW, Levin MJ, Deterding RR, et al: *Current pediatric diagnosis and treatment,* ed 19, Norwalk, Conn, 2008, McGraw Hill.
23. Jones KL, editor: *Smith's recognizable patterns of human malformation*, ed 6 Philadelphia, 2005, Saunders.
24. Kamboj M: Clinical approach to the diagnosis of inborn errors of metabolism, *Pediatr Clin North Am* 55(5):1113, viii, 2008.
25. Kay MA, Manno CS, Ragni MV: Evidence for gene transfer and expression of factor IX in haemophilia B patients treated with an AAV vector, *Nat Genet* 24:257, 2000.
26. Lamb DL: *Current parent experiences with the Ohio Newborn Screening program since the implementation of the supplemental newborn screening program, dissertation*, Cleveland, Ohio, 2004, Case Western Reserve University.
27. Levy HL, Albers S: Genetic screening of newborns, *Annu Rev Genom Hum Genet* 1:139, 2000.
28. Marden AM, Smith DW, McDonald MN: Congenital anomalies in the newborn infant, including minor variations, *J Pediatr* 64:357, 1964.
29. Marwick C: Two more cell infusions on schedule for gene replacement therapy patient, *JAMA* 265:2311, 1991.
30. Matthews AL: Known fetal malformations during pregnancy: a human experience of loss, *Birth Defects Orig Artic Ser* 26:168, 1990.
31. McCandless SE: A primer on expanded newborn screening by tandem mass spectrometry, *Prim Care Clin Office Pract* 31:583, 2004.
32. McDonald-McGinn DM, Tonnesen MK, Laufer-Cahana A, et al: Phenotype of the 22q11.2 deletion in individuals identified through an affected relative: cast a wide FISHing net!, *Genet Med* 3:23, 2001.
33. Michlitsch JG, Walters MC: Recent advances in bone marrow transplantation in hemoglobinopathies, *Curr Mol Med* 8(7):675, 2008.
34. Mitchell LE: Epidemiology of neural tube defects, *Am J Med Genet C Semin Med Genet* 135:88, 2005.
35. Morris CA: *Williams syndrome,* University of Washington. Accessed October 26, 2009, from www.geneclinics.org.
36. National Newborn Screening and Genetics Resource Center: website. Accessed December 20, 2008, from http://genes-r-us.uthscsa.edu/resources/newborn/msmstests.htm.
37. Nussbaum RL, McInnes RP, Willard HF: *Thompson and Thompson genetics in medicine,* ed 7, Philadelphia, 2007, Saunders.
38. Online Mendelian Inheritance in Man, OMIM (TM). McKusick-Nathans Institute for Genetic Medicine, *Johns Hopkins University (Baltimore, Md) and National Center for Biotechnology Information*, National Library of Medicine (Bethesda, Md), 2009. Accessed October 26, 2009, from www.ncbi.nlm.nih.gov/omim/.
39. Pastores GM, Barnett NL: Current and emerging therapies for the lysosomal storage disorders, *Expert Opin Emerg Drugs* 10(4):891, 2005.
40. Robinson A, Bender B, Linden M, et al: Sex chromosome aneuploidy: the Denver prospective study, *Birth Defects Orig Art Ser* 26:59, 1990.
41. Schuchman EH, Desnick RJ: Strategies for the treatment of genetic disease. In Rimoin DL, Connor JM, Pyeritz RE, editors: *Emery and Rimoin's principles and practice of medical genetics,* ed 5 New York, 2006, Churchill Livingstone.
42. Sprintzen RJ: Velo-cardio-facial syndrome. In Cassidy SB, Allanson JE: *Management of genetic syndromes,* ed 2, Hoboken, NJ, 2004, Wiley-Liss.
43. Sujansky E, Smith AC, Prescott KE, et al: Natural history of recombinant syndrome, *Am J Med Genet* 47:512, 1993.
44. Thomas JA, Van Hove JLK: Inborn errors of metabolism. In Hay WW, Levin MJ, Deterding RR, et al: *Current pediatric diagnosis and treatment,* ed 19 Norwalk, Conn, 2008, McGraw Hill.

45. Tkachuk DC, Pinkel D, Kuo WL, et al: Clinical applications of fluorescence in situ hybridization, *Genet Anal Tech Appl* 7:49, 1991.
46. Waisbren SE, Albers S, Amato S, et al: Effect of expanded newborn screening for biochemical genetic disorders on child outcomes and parental stress, *JAMA* 290:2564, 2003.
47. Walker AP: Genetic counseling. In Rimoin DL, Connor JM, Pyeritz RE, et al: *Emery and Rimoin's principles and practice of medical genetics,* ed 5 New York, 2006, Churchill Livingstone.
48. Walter J, Paulsen M: Imprinting and disease, *Semin Cell Dev Biol* 14:101, 2003.
49. Wertelecy W: Dermatoglyphics. In Stevenson RE, Hall JG, editors: *Human malformations and related anomalies,* ed 3 New York, 2006, Oxford University Press.
50. Yagi H, Furutani Y, Hamada H, et al: Role of TBX1 in human del 22q.11 syndrome, *Lancet* 362:1366, 2003.
51. Zelante L, Gasparini P, Estivill X, et al: Connexin 26 mutations associated with the most common form of non-syndromic neurosensory autosomal recessive deafness (DFNB1) in Mediterraneans, *Hum Mol Genet* 6:1605, 1997.
52. Zythovicz TH, Fitzgerald EF, Marsden D, et al: Tandem mass spectrometric analysis for amino, organic and fatty acid disorders in newborn dried blood spots: a two-year summary from the New England Newborn Screening Program, *Clin Chem* 47:1945, 2001.

RESOURCE MATERIALS

OMIM: (www.ncbi.nlm.nih.gov/).

Online Mendelian Inheritance of Man database is a catalog of genetic disorders and human genes. It is overseen by its originator, Dr. Victor A. McKusick, and maintained by the National Center for Biotechnology Information (NCBI). The database contains information about known inherited disorders, including information about the genes responsible for the disorder, a clinical synopsis, and references.

Gene Reviews and Gene Tests: (www.genereviews.org).

Gene Reviews and Gene Tests is an online database developed and maintained by the University of Washington. Gene Reviews lists over 466 genetic disorders that have information authored by experts for a particular disorder. A wealth of information is presented including (1) major clinical features of the disorder, (2) what is known about the genetics and inheritance, and (3) suggestions about a differential diagnosis for the findings. Each entry has an extensive reference list and information about support groups and is updated on a regular basis. The site also includes an international directory of laboratories for genetic testing (both clinical and research) and a listing of international genetics and prenatal diagnosis clinics. Educational materials are available about genetics, genetic disorders, and genetic testing including an illustrated glossary.

Genetic Alliance: (www.geneticalliance.org).

The Genetic Alliance is a coalition of hundreds of genetic advocacy organizations health professionals, clinics, hospitals, and companies. Type in a disorder and be transported to that support group's website for information about the disorder and resources for people with the disorder.

Genetics Home Reference: (http://ghr.nlm.nih.gov/).

The *Genetics Home Reference* is the National Library of Medicine's website for consumer information about genetic conditions and the genes or chromosomes responsible for those conditions. Summaries are provided about hundreds of genetic disorders. Each summary also contains information and web links to other resource materials.

28 NEONATAL SURGERY

HAROLD N. LOVVORN III, JOSHUA BRIAN GLENN, ANNETTE S. PACETTI, AND BRIAN S. CARTER

Congenital malformations may be found in up to 3% of all newborns and are an important cause of morbidity, early infant death, and chronic disability. Although overall infant mortality has declined, the mortality attributable to birth defects has increased, and up to 22% of neonatal deaths have been attributed to congenital malformations.[12] In the past decade, improvements in prenatal imaging and perinatology have allowed earlier diagnosis and intervention for surgically correctable malformations. Because of the complexity of accurate prenatal imaging and diagnosis, many anomalous conditions continue to escape early detection and present to the neonatology and surgical teams with advanced developmental consequences. The care of a neonate with a major congenital malformation therefore may be resource intensive and costly. In a study of one regional neonatal intensive care unit (NICU), newborns with major congenital malformations accounted for 27% of NICU referrals, 32% of total NICU days, and 40% of NICU costs. Moreover, surgery was more frequent in newborns with major malformations, and one third required ongoing medical support at the time of discharge.[47] Early diagnosis, comprehensive neonatal care, and a multidisciplinary approach are necessary to ensure an optimal outcome for both parent and child.

This chapter briefly describes the embryology, clinical history, diagnostic evaluation, and therapeutic intervention of common neonatal surgical conditions.

DIAPHRAGMATIC HERNIA

Physiology and Etiology

Congenital diaphragmatic hernia (CDH) is a defect in closure of the diaphragm that occurs in 1 in 4000 live births. A posterolateral defect, or Bochdalek diaphragmatic hernia (Figure 28-1), accounts for nearly 95% of all CDHs and may be left-sided (95%) or right-sided (5%). Much less common is the Morgagni diaphragmatic hernia (Figure 28-2), which results from a failure of anteromedial closure and resides in a substernal location. Several theories have been proposed to explain the mechanism for how this maldevelopment of the diaphragm occurs, but currently the most widely accepted theory is failure of the pleuroperitoneal canal to close completely during the 8th week of gestation. If a patent pleuroperitoneal canal persists through the 11th week of gestation, a period when the intestine returns from its normal herniation into the umbilical cord, the stomach, bowel, and spleen may be forced into the chest. Resultant compression of the developing lung leads to a variable extent of pulmonary hypoplasia.

Despite many studies in both animal models and infants over the past four decades, the causes of the pathophysiologic changes that occur in the underdeveloped lung are not well understood. Recognition of the associated abnormal physiologic mechanisms has failed to define these alterations as cause or effect for the malfunctioning lung. In addition to alveolar hypoplasia, a concomitant abnormal development of the pulmonary vasculature is a major contributor to the clinical challenges in managing CDH and its inherent risk for pulmonary hypertension.[67,83] Postnatal blood flow through these hypoplastic lungs is compromised by both a reduced total number of pulmonary arterioles and an increased muscularization of the arteriolar bed. As a result, pulmonary vasculature capacitance is reduced and responsiveness to signals for smooth muscle relaxation may be lost. Persistent pulmonary hypertension after birth maintains patency of and blood flow through natural fetal shunts (the foramen ovale and the ductus arteriosus). Resultant pulmonary hypoperfusion and systemic hypoxemia may be extreme and are often recalcitrant to conventional therapy and irreversible.

Please note that the **PURPLE** type in each chapter is intended to make it easier to identify clinically applicable material.

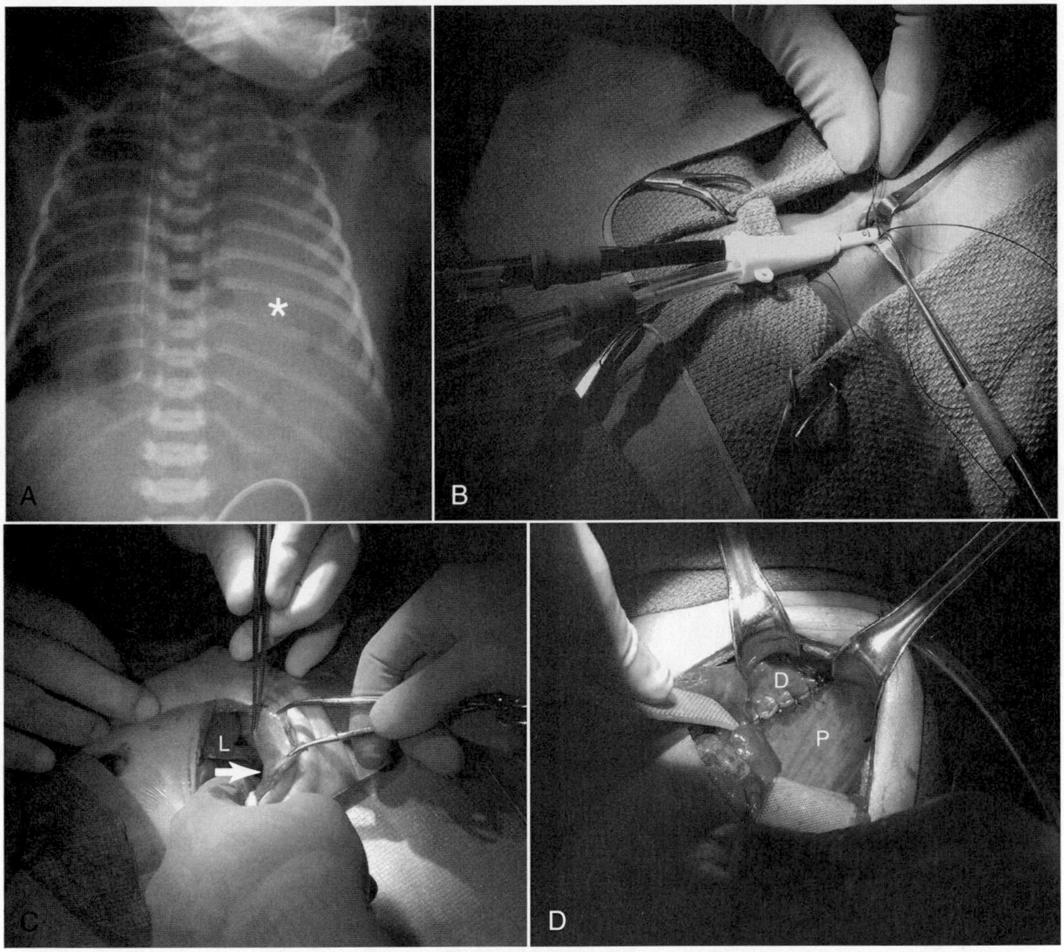

FIGURE 28-1 Newborn with left congenital diaphragmatic hernia (CDH), or Bochdalek diaphragmatic hernia. **A,** Chest radiograph shows liver herniation *(asterisk)* into the left chest. Note displacement of heart to right and minimally aerated lung on left. **B,** Dual-lumen venovenous cannulation via right internal jugular vein for extracorporeal life support (ECLS). **C,** Four days later, baby had stabilized on ECLS, so repair was performed in neonatal intensive care unit (NICU) on ECLS. Note left lobe of liver *(L)* herniating beneath a diminutive anterior leaflet of the left diaphragm (in forceps). Left lobe of liver is between forceps and surgeon's index finger. **D,** Defect required a biosynthetic patch (P; D, anterior leaflet of diaphragm). (Courtesy Dr. H. Lovvorn, Vanderbilt University Medical Center.)

Data Collection

HISTORY

Technologic advances in ultrasonography have facilitated earlier and more accurate ***antenatal diagnosis*** of diaphragmatic hernias, permitting planning of intervention and counseling of parents, as appropriate. The mother may then be transferred to deliver in a high-risk perinatal center with the appropriate level of neonatal and surgical support on standby, which is clearly less morbid than transferring the ill newborn with CDH. Although in utero surgical techniques to promote lung growth and passive reduction of the herniated abdominal contents seemed promising initially, as of this writing, a moratorium remains in place on this approach in the United States because a demonstrable survival benefit has not been shown, largely because of advances made in postnatal care of CDH.[86] Some fetal surgery centers, particularly European, continue to explore minimally invasive

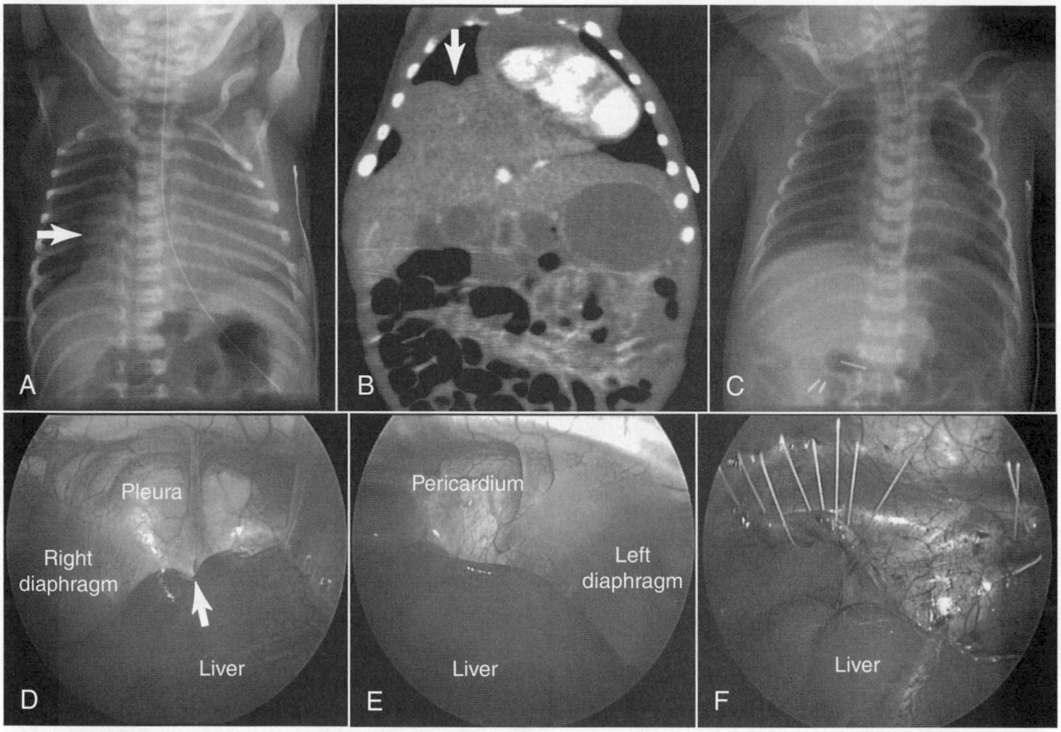

FIGURE 28-2 Newborn with anterior Morgagni diaphragmatic hernia. **A**, Chest radiograph. **B**, Computed tomography (CT) scan. *Arrows* on **A** and **B** show liver herniation. **C**, Postoperative chest radiograph shows complete reduction of liver and correction of hernia. **D** through **F**, Laparoscopic technique to repair large anterior defect: right and left diaphragms are sutured to abdominal wall anteriorly; sutures are passed through the entire wall of abdomen, and knots are secured below skin level. *Arrow* shows groove in liver corresponding with CT scan image. (Courtesy Dr. H. Lovvorn, Vanderbilt University Medical Center.)

means to promote lung growth in utero and thereby reduce the herniated abdominal contents. The Achilles' heel of fetal intervention, however, is the risk of preterm labor and the consequent morbidity of prematurity, risks which collectively must be weighed against a term delivery but with profound compromise in lung development.

SIGNS AND SYMPTOMS

Respiratory distress may develop immediately after birth or after an initial period of relative stability. If significant pulmonary hypoplasia is present and fetal circulation persists, the newborn may become rapidly symptomatic, heralded by profound hypoxic respiratory failure and circulatory shock. **Because much of the bowel is herniated into the chest, the abdomen appears scaphoid and the anteroposterior diameter of the chest may enlarge as the bowel distends with air. Breath sounds are diminished or absent on the affected side, and the mediastinum may be displaced toward the contralateral side.** Associated anomalies of the cardiovascular system may include patent ductus arteriosus, aortic coarctation, and hypoplastic left heart syndrome and require echocardiographic evaluation. Other associated anomalies requiring evaluation include central nervous system (CNS) malformations, genitourinary anomalies, esophageal atresia, omphalocele, cleft palate, and cardiovascular defects.[72]

LABORATORY DATA

Mixed respiratory and metabolic acidemia is present on blood gas evaluation. A chest radiograph is obtained and shows bowel herniated into the ipsilateral thoracic space with contralateral displacement of the heart. An echocardiogram is necessary to assess cardiac function, degree of pulmonary hypertension, and presence of significant congenital cardiac anomalies. Nonrotation of the intestine is an understood feature of CDH and does not require specific evaluation as a newborn.

Treatment

PREOPERATIVE CARE (STABILIZATION)

As soon as a diaphragmatic hernia is suspected, an orogastric tube should be placed to prevent further distention of the stomach and bowel and to alleviate compression of the lung. The newborn with CDH commonly requires endotracheal intubation and mechanical ventilation to maintain adequate gas exchange. Because cardiac function may also be compromised, a combination of inotropic and vasopressor medications such as dopamine, dobutamine, and milrinone may be needed. The earlier the infant becomes symptomatic, the more severe the respiratory compromise and the poorer the prognosis may be. **Pulmonary hypertension and lung hypoplasia are the major determinants of early outcome.**

A significant number of CDH newborns may have such severe pulmonary hypertension refractory to conventional or alternative (e.g., high-frequency oscillation or jet) ventilation that extracorporeal life support (ECLS; venovenous and venoarterial) may be required to establish effective gas exchange and end-organ perfusion. **The overriding principle in stabilizing CDH newborns is to reduce barotrauma and oxygen toxicity that result in chronic lung disease. Strategies now emphasize gentle ventilation and permissive hypercapnia, so long as arterial pH does not drift significantly low (<7.25).**[8]

OPERATIVE INTERVENTION

Surgical repair does not alter early outcome. Therefore the baby's condition should be stabilized and efforts directed toward the management of the associated pulmonary hypoplasia and hypertension. Early repair within the first 72 hours of life is indicated only in infants with little or no pulmonary dysfunction. If severe pulmonary insufficiency is present, medical therapies of conventional or high-frequency mechanical ventilation, inhaled nitric oxide, or ECLS are instituted. If these modalities are successful in stabilizing the baby, **surgical repair is generally performed between 4 and 14 days of life.**[67,87] If ECLS has been needed to stabilize the newborn with CDH, some centers advocate herniorrhaphy while on bypass, whereas other centers recommend repair after decannulation (see Figure 28-1).

Most commonly through a subcostal transabdominal approach, the surgeon reduces the stomach, intestine, and spleen from the chest to the abdominal cavity and repairs the diaphragmatic defect. If the defect is large, a prosthetic patch may be required to complete closure of the hernia. Closure of the abdominal wound may be difficult too because of underdeveloped abdominal wall musculature and loss of abdominal domain. In these circumstances, if abdominal closure is not possible or may result in abdominal hypertension, simple skin closure or prosthetic silo placement may be necessary to cover the abdominal contents, leaving a large ventral hernia for future repair when the abdominal domain is adequate and the baby is more stable. Chest tube placement depends on risk for bleeding, which may be significant if repair is performed on ECLS (because of anticoagulation during extracorporeal membrane oxygenation therapy), or if risk of pneumothorax is anticipated. Minimally invasive techniques to repair CDH may also be used in newborns (see Figure 28-2) but may not be well tolerated in the most fragile neonates. Appropriate patient selection is of prime importance.[28] Thoracoscopic and laparoscopic techniques to repair CDH have been described and may be better suited for infants who present out of the newborn period and without physiologically significant pulmonary hypoplasia or hypertension.

POSTOPERATIVE CARE

The principal postoperative concern remains effective ventilation and oxygenation while imparting the least amount of barotrauma and toxicity. If conventional mechanical ventilation fails, **high-frequency oscillation and inhaled nitric oxide** are employed.[49,56] **ECLS** is reserved in this setting as a salvage therapy for babies who revert back to fetal circulation and who do not respond to these less invasive modalities.

Complications and Prognosis

The survival rate for newborns with CDH and who require mechanical ventilation in the first 18 to 24 hours of life is approximately 64%. If an infant with a diaphragmatic hernia does not present with respiratory distress in the first 24 hours of life, survival approaches 100%. As improvements in gentle ventilation strategies have emerged, a gradual, albeit small, increase in survival has been realized.[49,56,72,83] **The primary early pathophysiologic consequence of CDH is pulmonary hypertension. Late complications include chronic lung disease, recurrent diaphragmatic hernia, gastroesophageal reflux, growth restriction, and neurodevelopmental delay.**[4,25] Basic and clinical research continue in an effort to identify improved therapies for the complex pulmonary dysfunction associated with congenital diaphragmatic hernia.

ESOPHAGEAL ATRESIA AND TRACHEOESOPHAGEAL FISTULA

Physiology and Etiology

Esophageal atresia (EA) occurs between 1 in 3000 and 1 in 4500 live births and represents **a spectrum of anomalies** that arise early in gestation (3 to 6 weeks) when the trachea normally buds from the primitive foregut. Failure in the normal development of the esophagus and in complete separation of the trachea from the esophagus gives rise to EA and distal tracheoesophageal fistula (TEF) in 85% of cases, isolated EA in 8%, TEF without EA in 5%, and EA with proximal or proximal and distal fistulas in 2%. Etiologies for this collection of defects remain unclear, but it is suspected that genetic alterations in and environmental insults on rapidly proliferating foregut stem cells during this critical period of organogenesis account for such diverse yet predictable esophageal malformations. Aberrations at the cellular level in muscle fibers of the distal esophagus may help explain the nearly universal symptoms of dysmotility and gastroesophageal reflux after operative repair.[46] Because other developing organs are vulnerable to the same insults in this critical period of gestation, **associated anomalies are common** (50% to 70%), particularly vertebral, anorectal, cardiac, genitourinary, limb, and gastrointestinal (e.g., duodenal atresia).[80] In 11% to 33% of infants with EA and distal TEF, concurrent and severe tracheomalacia is present. Although EA, with or without TEF, has not been associated with a single gene defect, a high incidence has been observed in children with trisomy 21, or Down syndrome.[12,24]

Data Collection

HISTORY

Maternal **polyhydramnios** may suggest esophageal atresia or other conditions in which the fetus does not swallow amniotic fluid normally.

SIGNS AND SYMPTOMS

Babies with esophageal atresia are identified soon after birth because of excessive oropharyngeal secretions and inability to swallow saliva or feedings. Upon feeding, these babies quickly cough and regurgitate undigested formula. When attempting to pass an orogastric tube, obstruction is typically encountered between 8 and 12 cm from the lips, and the diagnosis of EA is established. If a distal TEF is also present, air passes into the stomach and bowel and is present on plain abdominal radiographs. **Respiratory distress** may arise if oropharyngeal secretions are aspirated or gastric secretions reflux through the TEF and into the lungs, which may incite profound chemical **pneumonitis.** Symptoms of an "H"-type fistula in the absence of esophageal atresia are less obvious and require a high index of suspicion. **Coughing and choking with feedings or recurrent pneumonia over the first months of life suggests the presence of an occult, often "H"-type, TEF.** (See the Critical Findings box below.)

PHYSICAL EXAMINATION

Once esophageal atresia has been established, the infant should be carefully examined to exclude other anomalies of the **VACTERL** association, a variable sequence of anomalies affecting the Vertebrae,

Critical Findings

ESOPHAGEAL ATRESIA AND TRACHEOESOPHAGEAL FISTULA

The following are critical assessment findings for esophageal atresia and tracheoesophageal fistula:
- Excessive secretions
- Feeding intolerance
- Inability to pass orogastric tube
- Abdominal distention
- Other findings associated with VACTERL

VACTERL, Vertebrae, Anus, Cardiac system, Trachea, Esophagus, Renal tract, Limbs.

Anus, Cardiac system, Trachea, Esophagus, Renal (urinary) tract, and Limbs.[18,41] Imperforate anus may be obvious or obscure if a perineal fistula allows passage of meconium stool. Echocardiography permits both the identification of significant cardiac anomalies and the presence of a right-sided or left-sided aortic arch, which have important implications in the operative approach.

LABORATORY DATA

After **obstruction is met with passing of an orogastric tube,** a plain radiograph of the chest and abdomen should be obtained. The orogastric tube is **often coiled in the blind proximal esophageal pouch,** typically visualized at the second or third thoracic vertebra and above the carina. The stomach and intestines may contain luminal air if a distal TEF is present. If no distal fistula exists, the abdomen on radiograph will appear gasless. In the rare setting of EA, distal TEF, and duodenal atresia, the abdominal gas pattern may show the classic "double bubble" sign, as gas fills the stomach and proximal duodenum only.

Treatment

PREOPERATIVE CARE

Once the diagnosis of EA is established, an orogastric tube is placed in the upper esophageal pouch and set to low continuous suction to prevent aspiration of oral secretions. While awaiting operation, the neonate should be kept in a supine position with the head of the bed elevated about 30 degrees and antacid and antireflux medication should be considered to minimize gastroesophageal reflux and the consequent risk of acid-induced pneumonitis. Operative repair, in general, is not an emergency procedure. Patients first should be evaluated thoroughly for other associated anomalies by physical examination, echocardiography to delineate the anatomy of the heart and great vessels, abdominal ultrasound of the kidneys and genitourinary tract, and plain radiographs of the spine and limbs. Newborns with cyanotic congenital heart disease may require a palliative cardiac procedure before reconstruction of the esophagus.

If babies with EA and distal TEF are born prematurely and have respiratory distress syndrome (i.e., "stiff," noncompliant lungs), a significant portion of mechanical tidal volumes, delivered under positive pressure, may be shunted preferentially through the fistula and into the stomach. As a result, effective ventilation is lost and critical gastric distention ensues, further restricting diaphragmatic excursion. **Emergent ligation of the TEF with gastrostomy tube insertion** is necessary in such instances to restore effective ventilation.

OPERATIVE INTERVENTION

The type of esophageal malformation dictates the surgical approach. Surgical repair of EA with or without TEF is generally not an emergency but should be carried out as soon as the patient is stable. If the infant is in otherwise good health and the gap between esophageal elements is not too large, **primary anastomosis** is indicated through a right thoracotomy and retropleural approach. To reduce the pain and potential morbidities associated with a thoracotomy, some surgeons recommend repair thoracoscopically (Figure 28-3).

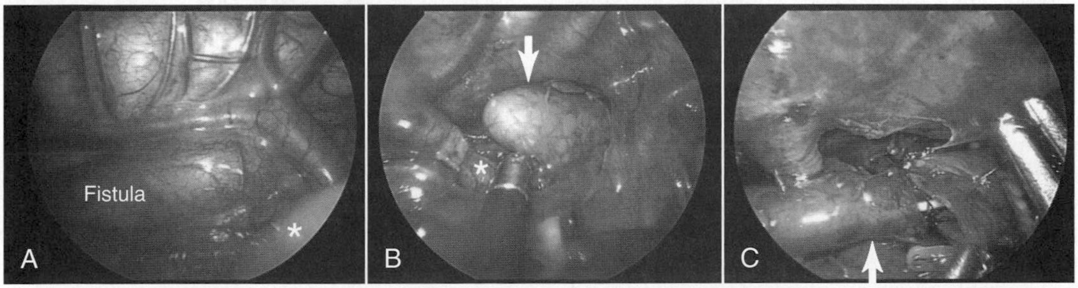

FIGURE 28-3 Thoracoscopic repair of esophageal atresia with distal tracheoesophageal fistula (TEF) in a newborn. **A,** View of TEF, which is distended from ventilation. Azygous vein is obscuring connection to trachea. **B,** After division of azygous vein, one can visualize the fistulous connection *(arrow)* of the distal esophagus to the posterior trachea. Upper atretic pouch has been mobilized and is being elevated with instrument. **C,** Suturing of upper esophagus to distal esophagus *(arrow)*. Replogle tube has been advanced through anastomosis after approximation of posterior row initially. For perspective of small working space, 3-mm and 5-mm instruments are used for this procedure. (Courtesy Dr. H. Lovvorn, Vanderbilt University Medical Center.)

Unfortunately, in isolated EA, the gap distance is generally too long to allow early primary repair. If the gap length is considered too great, with or without TEF, or if the child is too ill, a **delayed or staged repair** is planned. An early gastrostomy is placed for decompression and feeding, and the TEF, if present, is divided to prevent reflux into the tracheobronchial tree. After a variable period of time to allow **resolution of pneumonitis or maximum growth of the distal esophagus,** a second operation completes the repair. To promote lengthening and growth of the distal esophagus in cases of isolated EA, bougienage or balloon dilation may be performed via a mature gastrostomy tract.

POSTOPERATIVE CARE

Postoperative care includes appropriate pain control and pulmonary care, total parenteral nutrition (TPN), and a brief course of systemic antibiotics. **Tracheal and esophageal suction catheters should not come in contact with the newly repaired esophagus and trachea, because suture line disruption may cause a leak or recurrent fistula,** both potentially catastrophic complications. Antibiotic therapy is continued for 48 to 72 hours. A chest tube and/or retropleural drain is placed to control an anastomotic leak should it occur. Before initiating oral feedings, an esophagram is usually obtained within 7 to 10 days of repair to verify complete **anastomotic healing and absence of leak.** All EA babies have some degree of **esophageal dysmotility and gastroesophageal reflux (GER) after repair. Elevating the head of the bed 30 to 45 degrees, administering histamine H2 antagonists or proton pump inhibitors, and slow feeding may help control reflux symptoms.**

If delayed or staged repair is planned, secretions must be controlled. Suction catheters placed in the upper pouch are maintained to reduce the risk of aspiration. In rare cases, reconstruction using the native esophagus is not possible. In these circumstances, **esophageal replacement** using gastric or colon transposition is necessary. If the infant is not a candidate for early operation because of a lethal chromosomal defect or severe congenital heart disease, cervical esophagostomy and gastrostomy are performed to palliate the infant and esophageal replacement is performed later, as indicated.

Complications and Prognosis

Postoperative complications include anastomotic leak and/or stricture and esophageal dysmotility. **Anastomotic leaks** may occur in up to 20% of patients and generally are treated conservatively with chest tube drainage, parenteral nutrition, antibiotics, and tincture of time. The vast majority of leaks close without operative intervention but tend to heal with some degree of stricture, commonly amenable to dilation. **Strictures** often are associated with or exacerbated by GER and also may be treated successfully by esophageal dilation. If **GER** is complicated by stricture and is refractory to maximal medical therapy, a fundoplication procedure rarely may be necessary. Some degree of esophageal dysmotility usually exists because of poor peristalsis in the distal esophagus. The child may adapt to a poorly functioning esophagus by altering his or her feeding habits. However, in infancy, gastrostomy feeding may be necessary to prevent vomiting and aspiration.

With modern neonatal care and surgical techniques, long-term survival after repair of EA and TEF is excellent.[21] **Prognosis** depends largely on two factors: (1) the presence and type of cardiac anomalies, and (2) the presence of prematurity and respiratory distress syndrome. A useful system to predict survival is the Spitz classification, which stratifies infant survival by birth weight and major cardiac anomaly[74]:

- I: Birth weight equal to or greater than 1500 g, no major congenital heart disease (CHD), survival is greater than 97%
- II: Birth weight less than 1500 g or major CHD, survival is 59%
- III: Birth weight less than 1500 g and major CHD, survival is 22%

CONGENITAL CHEST MASSES

Physiology and Etiology

The most common congenital chest masses requiring surgical intervention in the newborn period are **congenital pulmonary airway malformations (CPAMs, also known as *cystic adenomatoid malformations*), pulmonary sequestrations (both intralobar and extralobar types), bronchogenic cysts, and congenital lobar emphysema.** Each of these malformations may exist alone or in combination with other anomalies.[7,44]

CPAM lesions are believed to arise from focal interruption in coordinated pulmonary progenitor cell growth, resulting in abnormal development of pulmonary tissues and structural distortion.

Histologically, CPAM is associated with increased cell proliferation and decreased apoptosis when compared with normal lung tissue. The CPAM lesion receives its blood supply from the pulmonary system but does not communicate with normally formed bronchial structures.

Anomalous development of the foregut is the accepted underlying etiology of both the bronchogenic cyst and pulmonary sequestration. Bronchogenic cysts are lined by ciliated columnar and/or cuboidal epithelium. The surrounding tissues resemble those of the normal bronchus and are generally, although not exclusively, located within the mediastinum along the tracheobronchial tree. Extralobar sequestrations are masses of primitive pulmonary parenchyma with no bronchial connection and are supplied by the systemic, not pulmonary, vasculature. Congenital lobar emphysema presents in the newborn period as a fluid-filled over-distended lobe that, under positive-pressure ventilation, may trap air and generate tension physiology. In many cases, though not all, congenital lobar emphysema is associated with the absence or hypoplasia of cartilaginous rings of the major and segmental bronchi. These structurally underdeveloped bronchi are prone to collapse on expiration, thereby trapping air.

Data Collection

HISTORY/SIGNS AND SYMPTOMS

Although rare, congenital lung malformations may lead to considerable morbidity, such as infection, hemorrhage, respiratory failure, and pulmonary hypoplasia, and may even prove lethal. Some lesions may escape **prenatal detection** and so appear later in development. Failure to recognize a malformation may lead to inappropriate intervention. For example, placement of a chest tube to manage suspected tension pneumothorax in a baby with congenital lobar emphysema may lead to lung injury and loss of tidal volume through the thoracostomy tube instead of into the remaining healthy lung.

Congenital Pulmonary Airway Malformation. CPAMs are usually detected prenatally and are nicely characterized on ultrasound but, if not, may be further delineated by fetal magnetic resonance imaging (MRI), as indicated.[42,81] In utero, these lesions may cause a variety of problems, from pulmonary hypoplasia (both ipsilateral and contralateral) to non-immune **hydrops fetalis** with congestive heart failure.

Polyhydramnios may also be present if the lesion compresses the esophagus and compromises fetal swallowing of amniotic fluid. Fetal intervention may be indicated if the gestation has not yet reached 34 weeks, in which case premature delivery might be planned. Large, fluid-filled cystic lesions may be amenable to thoracoamniotic shunt placement while in utero to relieve compression of intrathoracic structures and to restore hemodynamic status. Solid CPAM lesions arising early in gestation and causing similar complications have been resected in fetuses with promising results. If these lesions do not manifest with in utero pathophysiology (yet are of sufficient size), the neonate may develop **respiratory distress** shortly after birth. This process is responsible for the cystic appearance on radiographs. Babies may have mediastinal shift and a large air space, easily confused with a pneumothorax or diaphragmatic hernia. Sonography may be helpful to delineate a solid or cystic mass and should establish the diagnosis. CPAM may result in recurrent infections because mucociliary clearance is poor. Rarely, malignancy may arise in a CPAM in the form of pulmonary blastoma, rhabdomyosarcoma, or bronchoalveolar carcinoma.[42]

Pulmonary Sequestration. Pulmonary sequestration accounts for fewer than 10% of all congenital lung malformations and mostly occurs in the **lower lobes.**[7,44] A sequestration represents a mass of disorganized bronchopulmonary tissue without a normal bronchial communication and may have either a pulmonary or systemic vascular supply. The abnormal sequestered lung may be intralobar or extralobar and is classified according to pleural coverage, either within the pleural investment of the whole lung itself (intralobar) or outside of this normal pleural lining (extralobar). Sequestrations rarely may have some sort of communication with the foregut. Infants with an intralobar sequestration not detected prenatally may present outside of the newborn period and often with recurrent respiratory problems, such as **chronic cough,** or with **recurrent pneumonias,** either in the lesion or in the surrounding normal but compressed lung tissue. Plain radiographs may show simple consolidation. Anomalies associated with extralobar sequestration include diaphragmatic hernia and eventration and may share a similar dysregulated embryologic event, as approximately 95% of extralobar lesions are left-sided. Extralobar lesions may reside either above or below the left diaphragm. Older children may have exercise intolerance if a large systemic arteriovenous shunt exists. Systemic arterial flow through the lesion may produce a murmur and may lead to congestive cardiac failure. Squamous cell carcinoma, adenocarcinoma, and rhabdomyosarcoma may rarely arise in the sequestration.

Bronchogenic Cyst. Bronchogenic cysts may be considered a foregut duplication and arise from an abnormal budding of the ventral foregut. Approximately 85% are mediastinal and 15% are intrapulmonary. Bronchogenic cysts may be filled with air or fluid and may show air-fluid levels on plain radiographs.[77] As a result, bronchogenic cysts may become infected or simply grow over time and so may behave as a space-occupying and compressive lesion. Many cysts are asymptomatic or have vague symptoms and are discovered on routine chest radiographs. Infection, hemorrhage, and, in rare cases, late malignancy may occur. Associated respiratory symptoms include **stridor or wheezing.** Chronic air trapping may lead to emphysema, atelectasis, or both. Dysphagia, chest pain, and epigastric discomfort may also occur.

Congenital Lobar Emphysema. Although generally not discovered *in utero,* congenital lobar emphysema typically manifests in neonates as **hyperinflation** of one or more lung lobes. Causes include intrinsic absence or abnormality (bronchomalacia) of cartilaginous rings or external compression of a segmental bronchus by a large pulmonary artery.[44,65] Hyperinflation of a pulmonary lobe develops after birth as inspired air enters the affected lobe but cannot exit, because the positive pressure of expiration collapses the poorly structured airway. **Congenital lobar emphysema most commonly involves the upper lobes.** The left upper lobe is involved in roughly 41% of patients, the right middle lobe in 34%, and the right upper lobe in 21%. Involvement of the lower lobes is rare, occurring in fewer than 5% of patients. Neonates may present with mild to moderate **respiratory distress.** Mediastinal shift may develop with progressive air trapping, and decreased breath sounds are noted on the involved side. Infants who have a milder form of lobar emphysema will present with nonspecific findings, including cough, wheezing, respiratory distress, and cyanosis. Older children may present with recurrent chest infections. On plain radiographs obtained in neonates, the affected lobe may be hyperlucent or slightly opacified if alveoli remain fluid-filled. Associated cardiac anomalies may occur in as many as 10% of patients.

LABORATORY DATA

Routine chest radiograph is the initial evaluation tool in distinguishing congenital chest masses and is the principle study to establish the diagnosis of diaphragmatic hernia and congenital lobar emphysema in newborns. Sonography and/or **computed tomography (CT) scan of the chest** are useful means to evaluate CPAM, sequestrations and bronchogenic cysts, and lobar emphysema in older infants and children. The differential diagnosis of a hyperlucent hemithorax with mediastinal shift on chest x-ray in the newborn includes tension pneumothorax, cystic CPAM, diaphragmatic hernia with air-filled stomach or intestine in the chest, and congenital lobar emphysema.

Treatment

Surgical resection of these congenital chest masses is curative. Some small, asymptomatic lesions of sequestration or CPAM may be followed expectantly, as reports of spontaneous regression may be found in the literature. However, most lesions may be removed with little morbidity in an effort to minimize long-term complications of the various lesions. Operative approach to these lesions may be either via thoracotomy or thoracoscopy, depending on the suitability of the baby and the skill of the surgeon (Figures 28-4 and 28-5).

Special consideration to resection of the pulmonary lobe involved with congenital lobar emphysema should be given (Figure 28-6). Extreme caution must be followed upon induction of general anesthesia and endotracheal intubation with positive-pressure ventilation. Because of the collapsible airway and the propensity for air-trapping in congenital lobar emphysema, rapid development of tension physiology may ensue, compromising the well-being of the baby and necessitating emergent decompressive thoracotomy. Such pathophysiology is possible in any neonate with congenital lobar emphysema and requiring positive-pressure ventilation.

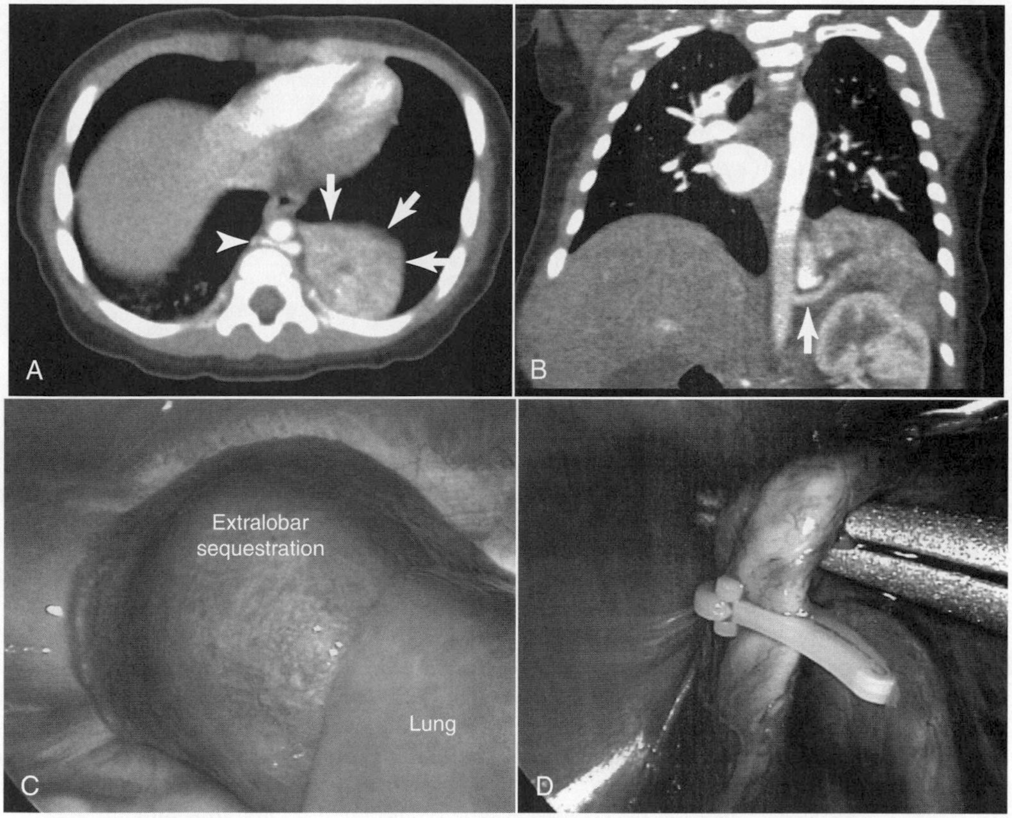

FIGURE 28-4 Thoracoscopic resection of a left-sided extralobar pulmonary sequestration (ELPS) in a newborn. **A** and **B**, Computed tomography (CT) scan shows ELPS at base of left chest (*arrows* in **A**). Note large vein coursing behind aorta in **A** *(arrowhead)* and large artery supplying lesion directly from aorta in **B** *(arrow)*. **C**, Thoracoscopic view of ELPS (looking toward diaphragm). **D**, Clipping of large artery and vein. Lesion is then removed through one of the port sites. (Courtesy Dr. H. Lovvorn, Vanderbilt University Medical Center.)

MALROTATION AND VOLVULUS

Physiology and Etiology

In the 4th week of gestation, the midgut exists as a straight tube deriving its blood supply from the superior mesenteric artery (SMA). The proximal limb of primitive intestine, representing the future duodenum, jejunum, and proximal ileum, lies in the midline and anterior to the SMA. The distal limb, destined to become the terminal ileum, ascending colon, and transverse colon, lies posterior to the SMA. During the 6th week of gestation, these segments of bowel, known collectively as the ***midgut,*** can lengthen rapidly by herniating through the incompletely closed abdominal wall and into the umbilical stalk. While lengthening outside of the coelomic cavity, the midgut undergoes a 270° counterclockwise rotation around the SMA axis. On return to the abdominal cavity, the duodenojejunal junction comes to rest in the left upper quadrant and becomes fixed in this location by the ligament of Treitz. At the end of the 11th week of gestation, midgut rotation is completed and the cecum now resides anterior and to the right of the SMA and is fixed in the right lower quadrant. Because of the counterclockwise nature of this intestinal rotation, the ascending colon and transverse colon lie to the right of the SMA. The hindgut (splenic flexure of the colon to the rectum) then fixes in the left hemiabdomen and derives its blood supply largely from the inferior mesenteric artery (IMA).

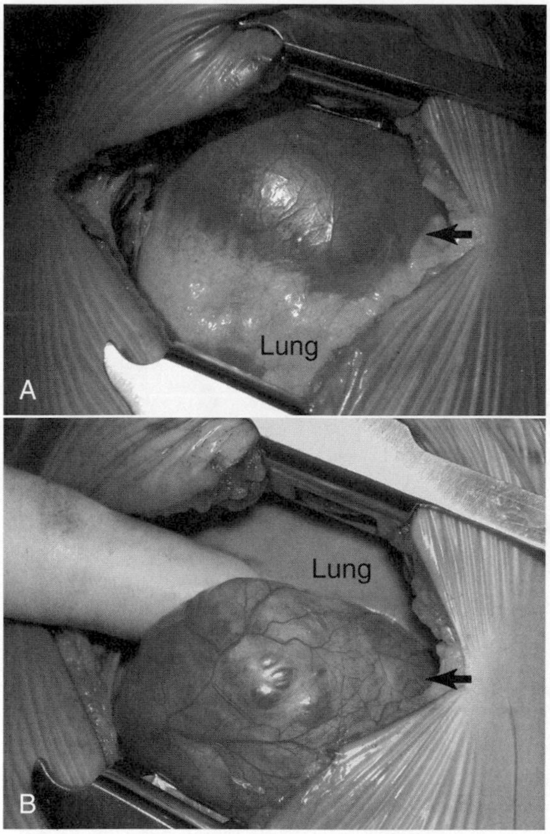

FIGURE 28-5 Thoracotomy in a newborn for congenital pulmonary airway malformation (CPAM). Views of anterior **(A)** and undersurface **(B)** of cystic lesion *(arrows)*. (Courtesy Dr. H. Lovvorn, Vanderbilt University Medical Center.)

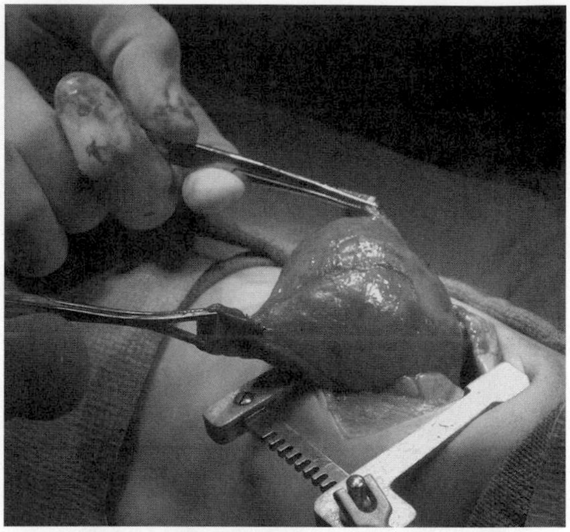

FIGURE 28-6 Thoracotomy in a newborn for congenital lobar emphysema. Note overdistended nature of emphysematous lobe compared with normal lobe just peering out from inferior aspect of wound. (Courtesy Dr. H. Lovvorn, Vanderbilt University Medical Center.)

Failure of this rotation and fixation results in the clinical condition termed *malrotation,* which covers a wide spectrum of rotational anomalies. Complete nonrotation is characterized by the entire small bowel existing on the right side of the abdomen and the colon principally to the left. Partial malrotation involves the improper fixation of a single segment. Complete malrotation is thought to occur from a lax umbilical ring allowing the gut to return en masse to the abdomen. Because proper rotation does not occur, the root of the mesentery is not anchored in the left upper quadrant and the superior mesenteric artery and vein loosely suspend the entire bowel without fixation. This unfixed, narrow mesenteric pedicle predisposes the midgut and its tenuous blood supply to twisting or **volvulus.** If volvulus occurs, the blood supply to the midgut may be compromised, leading rapidly to ischemia and bowel infarction. The majority of patients with midgut malrotation are diagnosed in the first month of life but may be seen with decreasing frequency in the older child or, rarely, the adult.[50,88]

By definition, malrotation also exists in several anomalies, including gastroschisis, omphalocele, and congenital diaphragmatic hernia, because the midgut is trapped and cannot rotate and fix properly in these conditions.

Data Collection

HISTORY

Malrotation may manifest in the newborn simply as a proximal mechanical bowel obstruction caused by abnormal attachments, or Ladd's bands, between the cecum and porta hepatis. These babies typically show some degree of **feeding intolerance** early on with or without bilious emesis. A more worrisome presentation of malrotation may arise should the bowel volvulize around its unfixed, narrow vascular pedicle. These babies present with an acute, high-grade proximal bowel obstruction. In a neonate who develops **midgut volvulus,** the first few days of life usually are unremarkable but then the baby develops **acute feeding intolerance and bilious emesis** in the absence

Critical Findings

MALROTATION AND VOLVULUS

The following are critical assessment findings for malrotation and volvulus:

- Lethargy
- Bilious emesis
- Abdominal distention
- Abdominal radiograph suggestive of intestinal obstruction
- Acidosis, leukocytosis, and shock, suggestive of volvulus

of abdominal distention. If diagnosis is delayed, intestinal ischemia sets in and **the symptoms may progress rapidly to an acute abdomen and profound shock as a result of gangrenous bowel. Abdominal wall erythema and distention are usually present in advanced stages of intestinal ischemia and are ominous findings.**[50,78]

SIGNS AND SYMPTOMS

The symptoms of nonvolvulized malrotation mimic those of duodenal stenosis or atresia, proximal jejunal atresia, or other conditions resulting in proximal intestinal obstruction. These babies develop **feeding intolerance** followed by **bilious emesis** and typically have a **scaphoid abdomen** on examination. **Midgut volvulus presents with a more sudden onset of signs, suggesting acute proximal intestinal obstruction.** If diagnosis is delayed, signs of intestinal ischemia become evident and include abdominal distention, lethargy, hypovolemic shock, and anuria. **The presence of bloody emesis or stools suggests intestinal ischemia with mucosal injury or necrosis.** In this setting, rapid diagnosis and prompt surgical intervention are essential to avoid extensive bowel loss or death. (See the Critical Findings box above.)

LABORATORY DATA

Plain abdominal radiographs may show a dilated stomach and proximal duodenum or, rarely, pneumoperitoneum in the presence of advanced intestinal necrosis. However, **the definitive study is an upper gastrointestinal (UGI) series,** which shows both abnormal rotation of the duodenum (malrotation) and partial obstruction (from Ladd's bands) or complete obstruction with a bird's beak suggesting midgut volvulus. A contrast enema may show an abnormal location of the cecum but is not diagnostic alone of malrotation and provides no information about the presence or absence of midgut volvulus.[75] Laboratory data are generally unremarkable unless bowel ischemia is present, as suggested by leukocytosis, anemia, and metabolic acidosis.

Treatment

PREOPERATIVE CARE

Although distinguishing between symptomatic malrotation with obstruction (Ladd's bands) and volvulus in its early stages may be difficult, these conditions should be managed similarly. **Gastric decompression, fluid resuscitation, correction of electrolyte and acid-base abnormalities, and parenteral antibiotics are instituted in the preoperative period. Emergent abdominal exploration should be considered in any infant with suspected or confirmed volvulus, because the bowel will be irreparably damaged in as little as 4 hours.** In this setting, prompt surgical intervention with continued intraoperative resuscitation is indicated to maximize the chances for bowel salvage and survival.

OPERATIVE INTERVENTION

Operative correction of malrotation without midgut volvulus includes division of Ladd's bands (to relieve duodenal obstruction), correction of the malrotation (by placement of the small bowel in the right of the abdominal cavity and the colon on the left), broadening the base of the mesentery by dividing its peritoneum, and appendectomy (the appendix and cecum will reside in the left upper quadrant). This procedure is best performed via laparotomy, and a laparoscopic approach has limited utility in the newborn.[9] The long-term results of the laparoscopic approach remain to be elucidated.[50] Cases of nonrotation in the older child may be amenable to laparoscopic techniques.

If volvulus is present, the bowel is detorsed and allowed to reperfuse (Figure 28-7). Necrotic segments of bowel are resected and stomas created as indicated. In select instances, substantial resection may result in short bowel syndrome. In these cases, marginal intestine may be left in place rather than removed and a planned reoperation performed within 24 to 36 hours to reevaluate the need for additional bowel resection. The objective of a **second-look laparotomy** is to allow continued resuscitation and marginally viable intestine the necessary time to recover. Bowel that

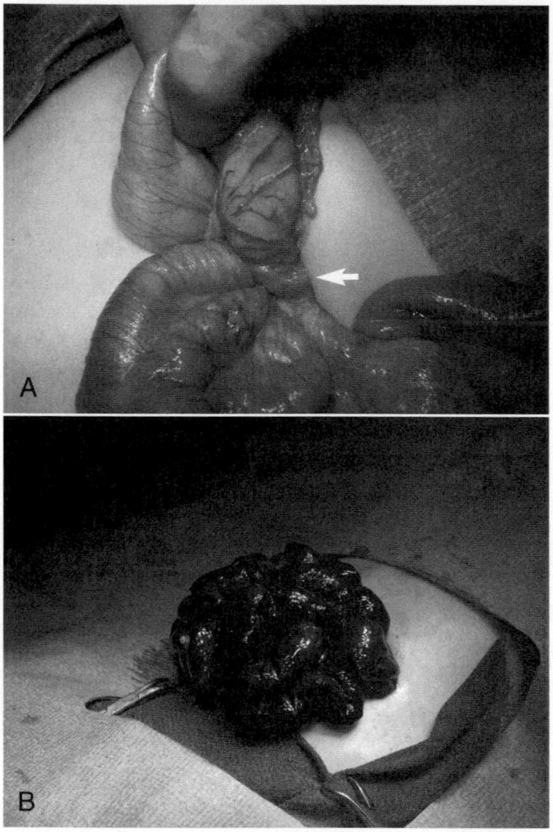

FIGURE 28-7 Two extremes of malrotation with midgut volvulus in newborns. **A**, Volvulus that presented before intestinal ischemia set in. *Arrow* shows 720° volvulus. Bowel is entirely viable. **B**, Delayed presentation of midgut volvulus with complete necrosis of intestine, a non-survivable injury. (Courtesy Dr. H. Lovvorn, Vanderbilt University Medical Center.)

is not salvageable will become more obviously non-viable but should not have perforated in this short period. This approach is designed to minimize the amount of total intestine resected.

Complications and Prognosis

Proximal obstruction related to Ladd's bands is corrected by the Ladd's procedure, and recurrent obstruction is rare. **The risk for subsequent volvulus is greatly reduced with Ladd's procedure but is not entirely eliminated.** Adhesive small bowel obstruction may occur later in life at the same rare incidence as after any other laparotomy.

The immediate postoperative care consists of nasogastric decompression and intravenous (IV) fluid therapy until the return of gastrointestinal function (4 to 6 days).[23] Conversely, the outcome after malrotation with midgut volvulus is predicated on the degree of intestinal resection.[48,50] Midgut volvulus is a leading cause of **short bowel syndrome** in infants and may render the infant dependent on TPN if extensive intestinal necrosis has occurred.

INTESTINAL ATRESIA

Physiology and Etiology

Any segment of the bowel may be narrowed **(stenosis)** or become discontinuous **(atresia).** Duodenal atresia is the most commonly involved bowel segment, followed by ileum, jejunum, colon, and stomach.[17]

Duodenal atresia results from failure of vacuolization (5th to 6th week of gestation) and recanalization (8th to 10th week of gestation). A vascular accident or segmental volvulus occurring later in utero is thought to give rise to jejunal, ileal, or colonic atresia.[47,66] Because duodenal atresia results from an early in utero event, a high incidence (30%) of anomalies may be associated and include trisomy 21, congenital heart disease, and VACTERL association.[24,27,61] Conversely, **intestinal atresia** occurs later in gestation and so is rarely associated with significant anomalies. Atresias are classified as membranes, fibrous cords, gap defect including mesentery, and "apple-peel" atresia.[84]

Data Collection

HISTORY AND PHYSICAL EXAMINATION

Commonly, a history of maternal **polyhydramnios** may be provided and the affected neonate may appear **small for gestational age (SGA).** The more proximal the site of intestinal atresia, the more likely the history of maternal polyhydramnios. Newborns with a proximal atresia (duodenum or jejunum) present with **early feeding intolerance and emesis and a scaphoid abdomen. Bilious emesis is present when the obstruction is distal to the ampulla of Vater, as is the case in approximately 85% of duodenal atresias. However, in 15% of cases, duodenal atresia occurs proximal to the ampulla of Vater and therefore the baby does not show bile-stained emesis or gastric aspirates.**

Critical Findings

INTESTINAL ATRESIA

The following are critical assessment findings for intestinal atresia:

- Maternal polyhydramnios
- Emesis (nonbilious vs. bilious depending on location of atresia)
- Abdominal radiograph suggestive of intestinal obstruction
- Abdominal radiograph with "double bubble" suggestive of duodenal atresia

The more distal the site of atresia and obstruction, the more likely that the infant will manifest significant **abdominal distention.** Babies with a distal intestinal atresia (ileum or colon) show typical features of a distal intestinal obstruction and develop abdominal distention often with visible intestinal loops.[66] If the atresia occurs early in gestation, the infant fails to pass meconium and only mucus is passed after birth. (See the Critical Findings box above.)

LABORATORY DATA

Initial evaluation of suspected duodenal atresia begins with a **plain abdominal radiograph** (flat and left lateral decubitus views), which classically shows a dilated, air-filled stomach and proximal duodenum in a pattern called the ***"double bubble" sign.*** A contrast study is not indicated unless air is present in the distal bowel, in which case malrotation with midgut volvulus cannot be excluded.

Abdominal radiographs that show **multiple distended loops of bowel** suggest a distal intestinal obstruction. In the setting of atresia of the small intestine or colon, abdominal radiographic images demonstrate dilation of intestinal segments proximal to the site of obstruction with absence of air in the distal bowel. For intestinal atresia distal to the duodenum, a **contrast enema** is generally performed and typically shows a **microcolon or unused colon** and no reflux of the contrast agent into the proximal bowel is observed.

Treatment

PREOPERATIVE CARE

Preoperative care includes orogastric tube decompression to reduce the risk of vomiting and aspiration, fluid resuscitation, and correction of electrolyte abnormalities. Preoperative **antibiotics** will be initiated.

OPERATIVE INTERVENTION

All forms of intestinal atresia require surgical correction to restore gastrointestinal tract continuity. Duodenal atresia is repaired through a diamond-shaped end-to-end anastomosis of the proximal and distal duodenum, and care must be exercised to prevent injury to the bile and pancreatic ducts. Repair of duodenal atresia may be performed either through a standard transverse right upper quadrant incision or laparoscopically (Figure 28-8). Other intestinal atresias are generally repaired by a standard end-to-end anastomosis. The size disparity between the dilated proximal loop and the decompressed distal loop may require that the proximal bowel be tapered or partially resected or the distal bowel may be cut obliquely to allow anastomosis (Figure 28-9). If these methods are not possible because of size discrepancy, then the segments just proximal and distal to the atresia may be brought out as stomas and intestinal anastomosis delayed to allow reduction in size of the dilated proximal segment and growth of the distal segment. When the caliber of the bowel becomes more comparable in size, anastomosis is performed.

POSTOPERATIVE CARE

Postoperatively, an orogastric tube remains in place to decompress the stomach until bowel function begins. Stomas must be protected from desiccation by covering with petrolatum gauze or a stoma appliance. Proximal ostomies have high output because of a lack of absorptive capacity and therefore require replacement of both fluid and electrolyte losses. The proximal output may be re-fed into a distal mucous fistula if present, but this technique may be challenging because of problems intubating the distal stoma and securing the feeding catheter to permit infusion. All infants endure a significant period of **bowel dysfunction** after surgery, and therefore temporary central venous access should be established to permit TPN support.[61,66,68] Furthermore, infants with intestinal atresia should undergo **screening for cystic fibrosis (CF),** which may contribute to both the development of the anomaly and ongoing bowel dysfunction.[11]

Complications and Prognosis

The overall prognosis for these patients is excellent unless severe associated anomalies are present. **Prolonged bowel dysfunction** is the primary complication after

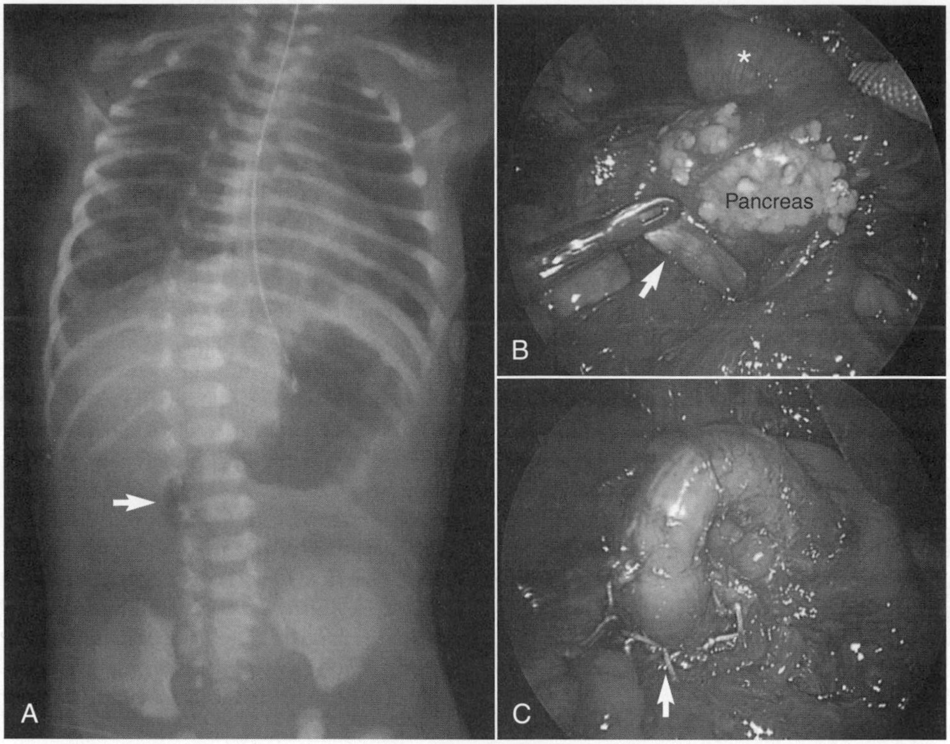

FIGURE 28-8 Duodenal atresia in a newborn. **A**, Abdominal radiograph shows classic "double bubble" sign. Orogastric tube is in stomach, and *arrow* shows air-filled proximal duodenum. **B**, Laparoscopic view of duodenal atresia. *Asterisk* depicts proximal dilated duodenum (compressed by instrument), and *arrow* shows small distal duodenum being elevated by a 3-mm bowel grasper. **C**, Completed anastomosis *(arrow)*. (Courtesy Dr. H. Lovvorn, Vanderbilt University Medical Center.)

surgical correction of intestinal atresia. In select cases, tapering of dilated bowel segments is attempted to enhance the recovery of bowel function.[61,73] Some infants fail to recover sufficient bowel function and require long-term parenteral nutritional support, either because of dysmotility or inadequate bowel length resulting from long segment atresia. Fortunately, the majority of patients have no long-term problems after postoperative recovery and return of bowel function.

NECROTIZING ENTEROCOLITIS

Physiology and Etiology

Necrotizing enterocolitis (NEC) is an inflammatory condition of the bowel of uncertain cause and occurs at a rate of 1 in 1000 live births and in 5% of infants born weighing less than 1500 grams (very low birth weight [VLBW]). NEC is fatal in 17% of all cases, in 20% of VLBW infants who develop the disease, and in as many as 40% to 50% of infants with a birth weight less than 1000 grams. NEC is primarily a disease of **premature infants,** although approximately 5% of cases occur in term babies. Despite intensive study, major advances in newborn intensive care, and improved survival of the VLBW preterm infant in the past two decades, the incidence of and mortality associated with NEC have changed little. In fact, the increase in survival of VLBW preterm infants has increased the size of the population at risk.

Perinatal stressors, an immature intestinal barrier, intestinal ischemia, bacterial colonization of the gut, and nutritional substrate in the gut lumen have all been implicated as contributing factors in the development of NEC. Other conditions that result in mucosal injury also have been linked to NEC: hypoxia; polycythemia; hyperosmolar feedings; gastrointestinal infection (bacterial or viral); and severe cardiopulmonary disease. Current research using

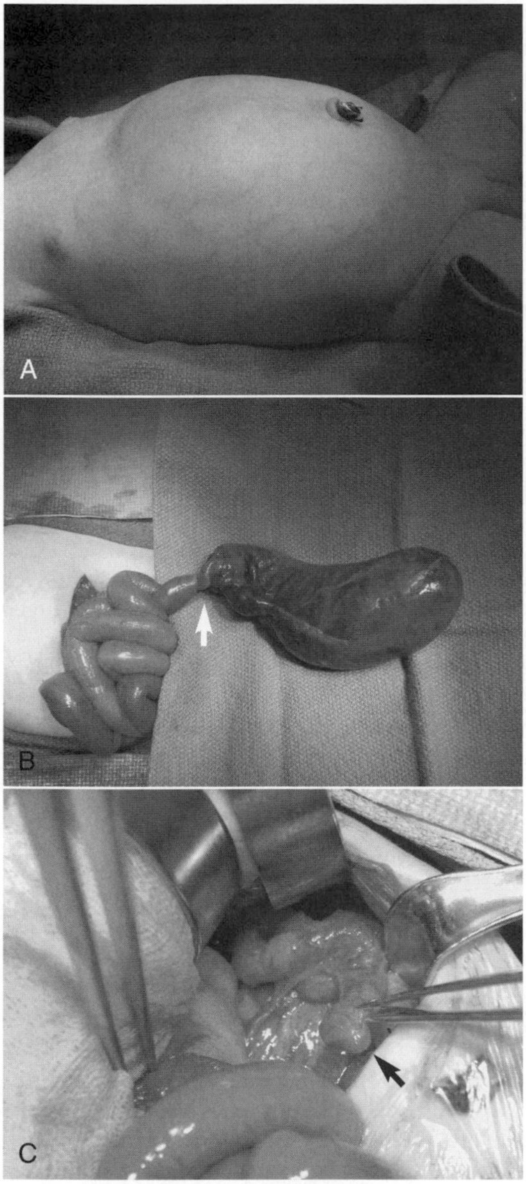

FIGURE 28-9 Newborn with colon atresia. **A**, Markedly distended abdomen. **B**, Atretic colon that has volvulized. *Arrow* shows twist, and note ischemic nature of volvulized colon. **C**, Distal microcolon elevated by forceps *(arrow)*. (Courtesy Dr. H. Lovvorn, Vanderbilt University Medical Center.)

animal models implicates up-regulation of multiple inflammatory mediators in the injured intestinal epithelia affected by NEC, and the presence of certain anti-inflammatory mediators may be cytoprotective.[14,29,37,63]

Critical Findings

NECROTIZING ENTEROCOLITIS

The following are critical assessment findings for necrotizing enterocolitis:

- Feeding intolerance
- Abdominal distention
- Bloody or Hemoccult-positive stools
- Thrombocytopenia, leukocytosis, leukopenia, and metabolic acidosis
- Pneumatosis intestinalis on abdominal radiograph
- Free air on abdominal radiograph in the presence of perforated viscus

Inflammation and ischemia initially involve the intestinal mucosa, but as the disease progresses, the muscular and subserosal layers of the bowel become involved. The intestinal wall becomes hemorrhagic and attenuated, with evidence of intramural gas **(pneumatosis)**. Histologically, the intestine shows features of acute and chronic inflammation with areas of coagulative necrosis. The ileocecal region is most commonly involved (50%), followed by disease limited to the colon (25%), or both large and small intestines (25%). Up to 15% of infants will develop pan-intestinal necrosis, or NEC-totalis, which is a non-survivable insult. Further, NEC is a significant risk factor for developing short bowel syndrome chronically if less than 40 cm of small bowel remains in the absence of the ileocecal valve or if, in its presence, less than 20 cm of bowel remains.[2,85]

Data Collection

HISTORY/SIGNS AND SYMPTOMS

The onset of NEC is heralded by the development of feeding intolerance, abdominal distention, and bloody stools in a premature infant receiving enteral feedings. A history of perinatal hypoxia, respiratory distress, congenital heart disease, or indomethacin administration for patent ductus arteriosus (PDA) closure often is elicited. As the disease progresses, the infant develops signs and symptoms of septic shock (lethargy, respiratory distress, temperature instability, hypotension, apnea, and oliguria). Examination reveals a distended and tender abdomen that may demonstrate erythema, induration, and pitting edema in severe cases. (See the Critical Findings box above.)

LABORATORY DATA

CBC and serum electrolyte evaluations typically reveal thrombocytopenia, leukocytosis or leukopenia, and metabolic acidosis. **Blood gas analysis** reveals that metabolic acidemia and lactate levels are elevated. **C-reactive protein (CRP) levels** are increasingly obtained and appear to be a good marker of onset, persistence, and resolution of NEC.[62] **Stool tests** may be positive for occult blood and reducing substances in more than 50% of cases. The diagnostic test of choice is the **flat plate (prone) plain abdominal radiograph and a left lateral decubitus abdominal radiograph.** Plain radiographs are carefully reviewed for the characteristic finding of **pneumatosis intestinalis,** or intramural bowel gas. The radiograph should be assessed for free air **(pneumoperitoneum),** which would suggest intestinal perforation. Other findings may include dilated bowel, **portal venous gas,** ascites, or a fixed bowel loop that does not change on repeated studies. Recently, ultrasound has been introduced in the diagnostic and prognostic evaluation of NEC.[71]

Treatment

PREOPERATIVE CARE

The only absolute and immediate indication for surgical intervention is intestinal perforation, which may be detected radiographically by the finding of **pneumoperitoneum. In a clinically stable infant without findings of perforation, medical management consisting of bowel rest, gastric decompression, fluid resuscitation, broad-spectrum antibiotic therapy, and TPN is indicated.** The infant is monitored carefully (serial abdominal examinations and radiographs every 8 hours) for signs of **intestinal gangrene.** More than half of infants respond to medical management, but up to 30% of infants treated medically may develop an **intestinal stricture** requiring surgical management.

A subset of infants continue to deteriorate despite maximum medical therapy, suggesting intestinal gangrene without intestinal perforation. Presence of intestinal gangrene should be considered in infants with persistent thrombocytopenia, leukopenia, hyperkalemia, refractory shock and acidemia, erythema of the abdominal wall, or a fixed, dilated intestinal loop on plain abdominal radiograph.[82]

OPERATIVE INTERVENTION

The principle of surgical management is to **resect all necrotic bowel while preserving as much of the intestinal length as possible.** In cases of extensive bowel involvement, only necrotic segments of intestine are removed and reoperation at 12 to 24 hours may be planned (a second look). After bowel resection, proximal and distal ostomies are created and the abdomen is thoroughly irrigated to reduce bacterial and fecal contamination. In severely premature infants weighing less than 1000 grams, **primary peritoneal drainage (PPD)** to decompress the abdomen after intestinal perforation may be performed in the NICU as an alternative to laparotomy. PPD and laparotomy may have comparable survival rates, but it is interesting to note that infants treated with PPD have substantial improvement in residual bowel length, which may be in part because up to one third of these patients do not require further operative therapy.[19] Nevertheless, laparotomy provides more definitive therapy and further aids in establishing the extent of diseased bowel, which, if NEC-totalis is discovered, may reduce futile care. In most cases, PPD should be considered a temporizing means, or "bridge to laparotomy," to allow complete resuscitation before definitive surgery (Figure 28-10).[10]

POSTOPERATIVE CARE

After laparotomy, supportive care (fluids, TPN, antibiotics) and bowel rest are continued for 10 to 14 days.[26] At 2 weeks postoperatively, low-osmolar elemental feedings may be started and advanced as tolerated. A stoma closure procedure is planned for 6 to 8 weeks after the initial surgery. All infants should undergo a preoperative contrast enema before ostomy closure to make certain the intestine and colon distal to the ostomy have not strictured.

Complications and Prognosis

Stomal prolapse or retraction, wound infection, intraabdominal abscess, and intestinal obstruction are early complications. Recurrent NEC is uncommon but may occur in approximately 5% of infants treated medically or surgically. **The most significant late complication is that of inadequate intestinal length (short bowel syndrome)** and the need for long-term parenteral nutrition. Preservation of the ileocecal valve is critically important to slowing intestinal transit and thereby limiting sequelae of short bowel syndrome. Babies at highest risk for short bowel syndrome have the ileocecal valve but less than 20 cm of small intestine or have no ileocecal valve and less than 40 cm of small bowel. **Survival in infants weighing more than 1000 g**

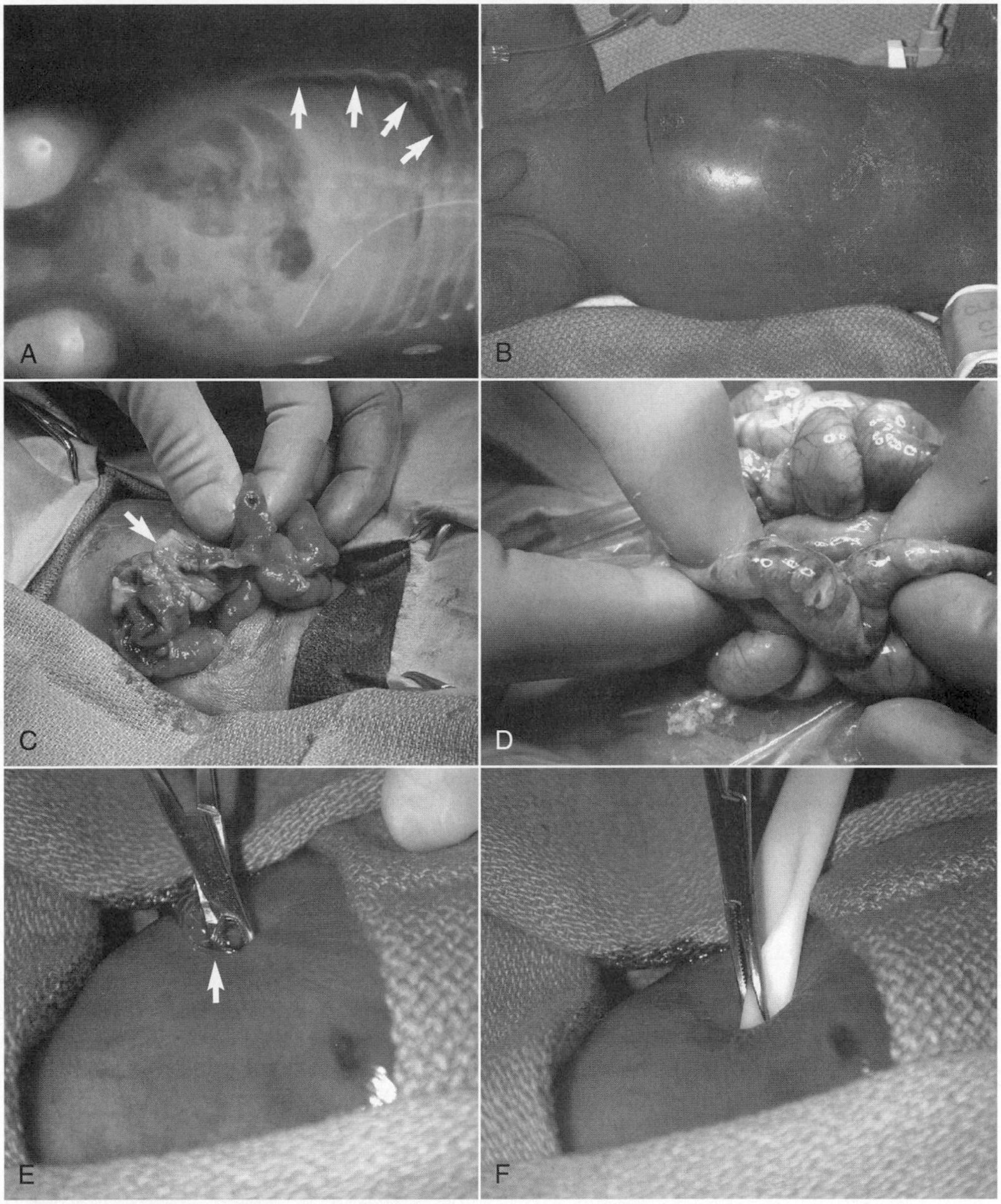

FIGURE 28-10 Several different examples of necrotizing enterocolitis (NEC) in extremely-low-birth-weight (ELBW) infants. **A**, Pneumoperitoneum on abdominal radiograph *(arrows)*. **B**, Same baby; note abdominal distention and discoloration. **C**, Findings of NEC at laparotomy: perforation is shown between surgeon's fingers. *Arrow* shows segment of gangrenous bowel. Bowel toward surgeon's middle finger is normal. **D**, Example of pneumatosis intestinalis; this baby had pan-intestinal necrosis. **E** and **F**, Placement of peritoneal drain in the neonatal intensive care unit (NICU). *Arrow* shows release of pneumoperitoneum (bubbles). (Courtesy Dr. H. Lovvorn, Vanderbilt University Medical Center.)

has improved from 50% to 80% over the past two decades. Severely premature infants weighing less than 1000 g still have a mortality rate in excess of 50%.[34,45]

MECONIUM ILEUS

Physiology and Etiology

Meconium ileus is an intestinal obstruction caused by **hyperviscous** secretions from the intestinal glands coupled with a lack of pancreatic enzymes necessary to help digest intestinal secretions and contents. The result is tenacious, viscous meconium that creates a sticky plug obstructing the lumen of bowel. The obstruction generally occurs within the terminal ileum, mimicking ileal atresia. More than 90% of infants with meconium ileus have **cystic fibrosis (CF),** a three-base-pair deletion on chromosome 7. This autosomal recessive gene defect results in alteration of the chloride channel transporter and therefore fluid flow across the apical surface of epithelial cells. Meconium ileus occurs in 10% to 25% of patients with CF; 20% of mothers have polyhydramnios. A family history of CF is present in 10% to 30% of cases.

This ileus associated with CF and retained meconium is in contrast to the **meconium plug syndrome (MPS),** which manifests as a failure to pass stool with obstruction in the colon and is not specific to CF. MPS is generally recognized as immaturity of the ganglion cells and generally is benign.[40] Rectal dilation and/or contrast enema usually results in passage of the meconium plug(s), and recurrence is uncommon; however, significant obstruction can develop with rare incidences of perforation. MPS, again in contrast to meconium ileus, is associated with Hirschsprung's disease in 15% of cases.

Data Collection

SIGNS AND SYMPTOMS

Meconium ileus is classified as **simple** (obstruction and obturation) or **complicated** (volvulus, intestinal atresia, perforation, meconium peritonitis). Uncomplicated meconium ileus presents as distal ileal obstruction caused by inspissated meconium (pellets) and proximal intestinal dilation. The onset of symptoms associated with simple meconium ileus begins 24 to 48 hours after birth. **Bilious emesis, progressive abdominal distention, and the failure to pass meconium suggest intestinal obstruction. The differential diagnosis in addition to meconium ileus includes ileal atresia, meconium plug, and Hirschsprung's disease.** Physical examination shows a patent anus that may express a small amount of gray meconium. Examination of the abdomen reveals moderate distention with a characteristic doughlike sensation on palpation because of the thickened meconium contained in the dilated bowel. Complicated meconium ileus often manifests more abruptly and progresses more quickly. Symptoms include abdominal distention within 24 hours of birth, respiratory distress (especially if a postnatal perforation has occurred), and an edematous, erythematous abdomen.[64] (See the Critical Findings box below).

LABORATORY DATA

Abdominal radiograph demonstrates a **"soap bubble"** appearance of the bowel caused by trapped gas within the meconium and also shows large, dilated (with air) loops of bowel with few air-fluid levels because of the viscous nature of the meconium. **A contrast enema shows a microcolon and pellets of inspissated meconium at the site of distal obstruction.** If in utero perforation has occurred, microcalcifications may also be present on plain abdominal radiographs.

Treatment

PREOPERATIVE CARE

If meconium ileus is suspected, **orogastric decompression, IV hydration, and electrolyte replacement** are instituted. Once the infant is appropriately hydrated, a diluted Gastrografin or Cysto-CONRAY enema should be attempted.[55] **Note: The infant**

> **Critical Findings**
>
> **MECONIUM ILEUS**
>
> The following are critical assessment findings for meconium ileus:
> - Abdominal distention
> - Bilious emesis
> - "Soap bubble" appearance of the bowel on abdominal radiograph
> - Microcolon on barium enema

should be adequately hydrated before the enema because of the hyperosmolarity of the Gastrografin or Cysto-CONRAY. Intra-colonic instillation of these water-soluble agents draws fluid into the bowel lumen, diluting the viscous meconium and facilitating passage. If the Gastrografin enema results in incomplete evacuation, it may be repeated over the next several days. However, if the Gastrografin enema fails to result in passage of meconium, complicated meconium ileus or ileal atresia may be present and operative intervention is indicated.[39,55]

OPERATIVE INTERVENTION

The goal of operative treatment is to relieve intestinal obstruction. For uncomplicated meconium ileus, several operative approaches are described to eliminate the obstructing inspissated meconium. Techniques include the following:

- Enterotomy with extraction of the tenacious meconium and irrigation of the bowel with saline solution or 2% *N*-acetylcysteine (Mucomyst)
- Resection of the affected segment with anastomosis
- Formation of chimney ostomies just proximal to the obstruction (Bishop-Koop procedure: bowel is divided to create an ostomy of the distal ileum for continued irrigations, and an internal anastomosis of the proximal to distal ileum is fashioned to maintain intestinal continuity)

More commonly now, a T-tube enterostomy may be created, in which a soft, small-caliber tube is securely placed within the bowel lumen and delivered through a separate wound in the abdominal wall (Figure 28-11). This tube, like the chimney ostomy, allows continued postoperative irrigations with normal saline or diluted Mucomyst to complete or maintain passage of intestinal contents. If complicated meconium ileus is identified, the obstructed segment is resected and ostomies are performed to permit postoperative irrigation. Ostomy closure usually is performed 4 to 6 weeks later.

POSTOPERATIVE CARE

Postoperatively, nasogastric tube decompression, nutritional support with TPN, and irrigation of the rectum or ostomies with saline solution or *N*-acetylcysteine (Mucomyst) are instituted. Once gastrointestinal function returns, feedings

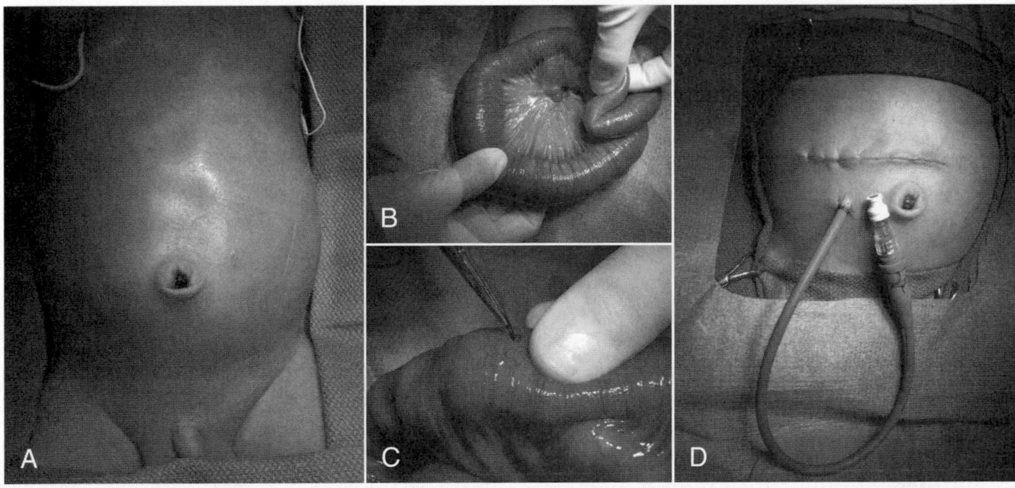

FIGURE 28-11 Newborn with meconium ileus as presenting feature of cystic fibrosis. **A**, Abdominal distention and visible intestinal loops on physical examination. **B**, Equal pressure is being applied to the bowel by both hands of the surgeon. Note how noncompressible the bowel in the right hand is secondary to the inspissated meconium. **C**, Note viscosity of meconium being teased out of the bowel lumen. **D**, After irrigation with Mucomyst and evacuation of the meconium, a tube enterostomy is placed for continued irrigation in the weeks after surgery. Once the baby's bowel is completely cleared of meconium and a full diet is tolerated, the tube may be removed. (Courtesy Dr. H. Lovvorn, Vanderbilt University Medical Center.)

using protein hydrolysate or elemental formula and pancreatic enzyme supplements are started. The diagnosis of cystic fibrosis is confirmed with genetic testing and sweat chloride testing.

Complications and Prognosis

One-year survival for infants with simple or complicated meconium ileus is favorable (>90%), but long-term survival is limited primarily because of the pulmonary complications of cystic fibrosis.[53,54] **Late gastrointestinal complications of CF** include distal intestinal obstruction syndrome (meconium ileus equivalent), appendicitis, intussusception, rectal prolapse, intestinal stricture, pancreatitis, and cholestatic liver disease.[53]

HIRSCHSPRUNG'S DISEASE

Physiology and Etiology

Hirschsprung's disease is a congenital intestinal disorder caused by a lack of ganglion cells in the bowel wall that prevents effective peristalsis. During development, neural crest cells (the progenitor or stem cells of the enteric nervous system) migrate along the intestinal tube to populate the entire gut in a craniocaudal fashion, with the distal colon, rectum, and sphincter being the last to be colonized. These progenitor cells divide, differentiate, and proliferate to form the enteric nervous system, of which the ganglion cells are a critical component. Arrest of migration, proliferation, and differentiation results in the **aganglionosis** found in Hirschsprung's disease, a well-recognized cause of distal intestinal obstruction in the newborn. At the site of arrest, a transition from normal to abnormal innervation is present and all intestine distal to this site will be aganglionic and therefore dysfunctional. The result is a functional obstruction that mimics mechanical intestinal obstruction. In brief, the pathophysiologic consequence of the absence of ganglion cells is loss of the ability of the involved rectum and colon to relax, and therefore the fecal stream cannot be passed effectively through this region and beyond. Rectosigmoid aganglionosis is most common (85%), with the remainder of patients developing variable lengths of more proximal colonic and, rarely, small intestine disease. Total colonic aganglionosis occurs in roughly 10% of cases.

Hirschsprung's disease occurs in 1 in 5000 live births, with a 4:1 male-to-female predominance. The majority of cases are sporadic (80% to 90%), but familial occurrences are well recognized and multiple genetic alterations have been identified in affected pedigrees. Associated anomalies are rare in sporadic cases but may be seen in as many as 25% of the familial cases. Babies born with Down syndrome also carry a higher incidence of Hirschsprung's disease (2%) than the population at large, and between 5% and 10% of Hirschsprung's patients will have Down syndrome.

Approximately 15% of Hirschsprung's neonates will present with meconium plug syndrome (MPS), an obstruction of the colon by inspissated meconium. However, in general, MPS is associated with immature ganglion development and is not indicative of the more serious Hirschsprung's disease.

Data Collection

SIGNS AND SYMPTOMS

Ninety-eight percent of normal infants pass meconium in the first 24 to 48 hours of life. Failure to pass meconium early, feeding intolerance, and abdominal distention suggest a diagnosis of Hirschsprung's disease. In some babies with a short segment of aganglionic bowel, spontaneous evacuation of stool may be noted and the infant may appear otherwise healthy. If **vomiting, abdominal distention, and constipation** (or paradoxic diarrhea resulting from watery stool escaping around the obstipated stool) continue, further investigation is indicated. Hirschsprung's disease may rarely escape detection during the newborn period, and in **older children,** a history of refractory and chronic obstipation may be the only symptom. Approximately 5% to 10% of affected infants will present with a picture of **enterocolitis (toxic megacolon),** characterized by fever, vomiting, abdominal distention/tenderness, foul-smelling diarrhea, and septic shock. The infant may rapidly deteriorate, with a 50% risk of death if the colon is not rapidly decompressed, either by transanal soft rubber tube irrigations or emergency colostomy. Fortunately, in most cases of Hirschsprung's disease, the infant is only mildly ill, allowing time for definitive diagnostic studies before surgical correction is undertaken.[15] (See the Critical Findings box on p. 833.)

Critical Findings

HIRSCHSPRUNG'S DISEASE

The following are critical assessment findings for Hirschsprung's disease:

- Failure to pass meconium within 48 hours of birth
- Feeding intolerance
- Abdominal distention
- Enterocolitis (fever, abdominal distention, foul-smelling diarrhea, sepsis)
- Transition zone on barium enema
- Absent ganglion cells and nerve hypertrophy on rectal biopsy

LABORATORY DATA

The diagnostic evaluation begins with a **contrast enema.** Surgical dogma states that the first enema should be a contrast enema. This study typically shows a contracted or spastic rectosigmoid colon, with contrast material entering the proximal dilated bowel. The area between the contracted and dilated bowel is called the ***transition zone.*** If the contrast enema is equivocal, an abdominal x-ray film should be obtained on the next day to evaluate extent of retained contrast material. Significant contrast material retained within the distal colon and rectum suggests the presence of Hirschsprung's disease. **Definitive diagnosis is made by performing a bedside suction rectal biopsy,** a well-tolerated procedure in neonates that does not require any analgesics or sedatives. On histology, the biopsy shows an absence of ganglion cells and a presence of hypertrophic nerve trunks within the submucosal and intermyenteric plexus. Conversely, if ganglion cells are observed on histologic examination, a diagnosis of Hirschsprung's disease is excluded.

Treatment

PREOPERATIVE CARE

In infants with Hirschsprung's-associated enterocolitis, **orogastric tube decompression, IV fluid resuscitation, broad-spectrum antibiotics, and correction of acid-base deficits and electrolyte abnormalities are promptly initiated.** Infants who are less ill with symptoms of obstruction are placed on nothing-by-mouth (NPO) status, and IV antibiotic therapy and orogastric decompression are instituted, permitting time to complete the diagnostic evaluation. Once the diagnostic evaluation is completed, transanal **rectal irrigations,** not enemas, are performed twice daily until surgery. Babies should have return to normal bowel function with these irrigations and may be fed enterally (so long as rectal irrigations continue) until definitive surgery.

OPERATIVE INTERVENTION

In the presence of profound enterocolitis, an emergency colostomy may be indicated. If necessary, **a colostomy** is performed at a site of normal bowel (ganglion cells present), as confirmed by a frozen section histologic examination. In select cases, the neonate will be too ill so operative time is minimized by the creation of a right-sided colostomy, because most affected babies have more distal colonic involvement. If the neonate presents with milder symptoms, one of several surgical options may be selected: (1) primary laparoscopically assisted endorectal pull-through (Figure 28-12), (2) primary transanal pull-through, or (3) **staged reconstruction** (temporary colostomy, followed by a pull-through in 3 to 6 months).[70] In all cases, multiple intestinal seromuscular biopsies are performed at the time of operation until the normally innervated bowel is identified. A coloanal anastomosis or colostomy is performed at the site of bowel that was proven normal by histologic examination. If the anastomosis or colostomy site is absent of ganglion cells, the neonate will remain symptomatic—the bowel will not function normally because of aganglionosis.

Several factors influence the decision to perform a **primary pull-through** procedure in neonates.[70] The neonate should be of sufficient gestational age and size (>2 kg), have rectosigmoid disease as demonstrated by contrast enema, not have significant proximal bowel distention, and not have evidence of advanced enterocolitis. Neonates who do not meet these criteria should be treated in a staged manner, with an immediate colostomy and a pull-through procedure delayed until later in infancy.[30,76]

POSTOPERATIVE CARE

The recovery period is generally straightforward, and supportive care is provided until the return of bowel function. For babies treated initially with colostomy, postoperative care includes teaching the parents about stoma maintenance and hygiene (Box 28-1). The **pull-through procedure** entails resecting abnormal aganglionic bowel and bringing ganglionic bowel to the anus. Several variations of the pull-through

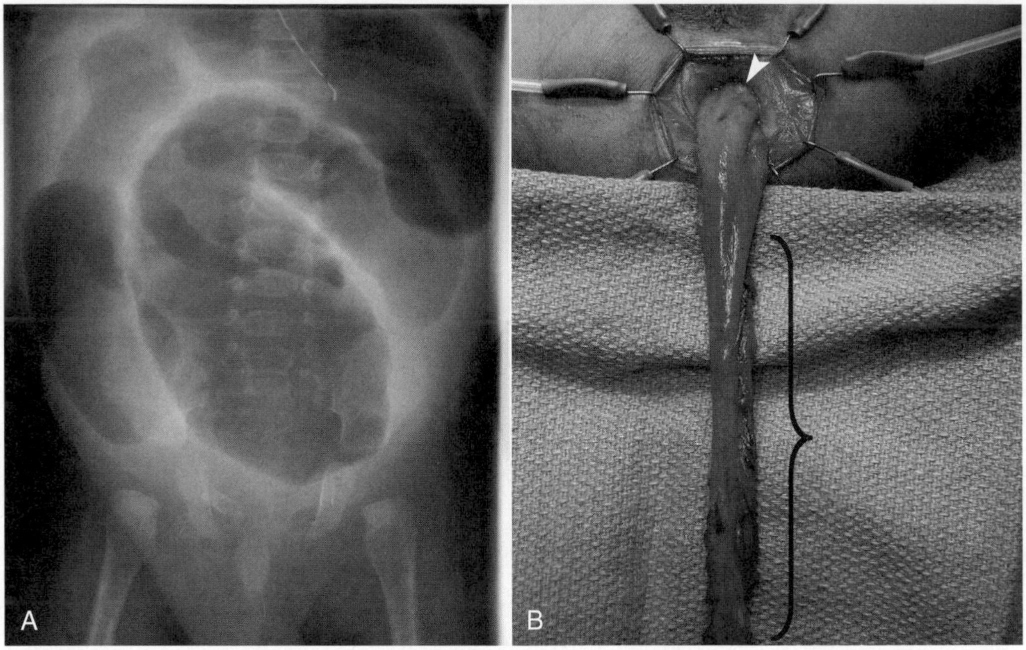

FIGURE 28-12 Newborn with Hirschsprung's disease. **A,** Plain abdominal radiograph shows distal intestinal obstruction 2 days after birth in a neonate who has failed to pass meconium. Note absence of gas in rectum/pelvis. **B,** After laparoscopic mobilization and transanal mucosectomy, the diseased bowel may be delivered through the anus. The *bracket* denotes the contracted, aganglionic bowel. *Arrowhead* shows biopsy performed laparoscopically that confirms region of ganglionated bowel. Coloanal anastomosis was performed at this level. (Courtesy Dr. H. Lovvorn, Vanderbilt University Medical Center.)

operation have been described; each has unique advantages and disadvantages, but in general, the results are similar regarding long-term stooling patterns. For neonates having a primary laparoscopically assisted endorectal pull-through, **first stool is usually passed within 24 hours of the procedure, at which time breast milk or Pedialyte may be introduced.** Feeds may be advanced to goal (according to tolerance) over the next 24 to 48 hours.

Complications and Prognosis

Early complications of the pull-through operation include inadequate blood supply to the coloanal anastomosis, anastomotic stricture, anastomotic dehiscence, and cuff abscess. Later complications include Hirschsprung's-associated enterocolitis, perianal excoriation, and recurrent **constipation.**[51] The infant usually thrives postoperatively and grows normally. It is not uncommon for the infant to have frequent stools during the immediate postoperative period, which gradually normalize to a lesser frequency. However, some children, despite a technically satisfactory operation, will experience recurrent constipation requiring some form of bowel management program with or without placement of a colostomy tube for antegrade enemas.[89]

ANORECTAL MALFORMATIONS

Physiology and Etiology

Anorectal malformations (ARMs) encompass a broad spectrum of hindgut anomalies, from isolated **imperforate anus** in boys and girls, which may include fistulous communications between the urogenital tract and rectum, to complicated **persistent cloaca** in females. Although the development of the cloaca and its subsequent septation into urogenital and anorectal tracts is not well understood, each organ system is recognizable as a separate entity by the 7th week of gestation. Therefore persistent cloaca in females arises from

BOX 28-1

INSTRUCTIONS FOR OSTOMY CARE

Supplies for Pouch Changes

Dry washcloths
Warm, wet washcloths or adhesive remover
Mild soap
Pattern or guide
Barrier wipes/Stomahesive powder (if skin is reddened or irritated)
Pouch
Stomahesive paste
Clamp or rubber band
Scissors
Optional: gauze pads, dry paper towel, cotton balls, or toilet paper

Directions

1. Gather supplies. (It is helpful to keep all supplies together in one place.)
2. Wash hands.
3. Trace pattern on the paper side of the pouch (wafer). The opening should fit closely around the stoma but not tightly or on top of the stoma.
4. Cut an opening in the wafer; use scissors to cut along the lines you traced on the wafer paper. (Cut several wafer patterns and pouches at once to save time when changing pouches.)
5. Gently remove the old wafer/pouch using adhesive remover or warm, wet washcloths.
6. Clean skin with a warm, soapy washcloth. Rinse well with warm water. (Do not use soaps that contain lotions or oils.)
7. If skin is reddened or irritated, apply a light dusting of Stomahesive powder and seal with barrier wipes. (The barrier wipes contain a skin sealer that protects the skin from stool and from tearing when the pouch is removed.)
8. Apply a small, thin line of Stomahesive paste around the stoma or around the opening cut in the wafer. (Stomahesive paste acts as caulking or filler, smoothing creases, dips, or scars, and helps prevent liquid from seeping under the wafer.)
9. Apply the wafer to the skin. Press around the stoma to ensure a good seal.
10. Hold your hand over the pouch for 1 minute to warm the wafer so it will stick to the skin.
11. If stool is liquid, you can place a gauze pad, for example, in the pouch to absorb liquid.
12. Place clamp or rubber band at the end of the pouch.

Helpful Hints

1. Always change a leaking pouch immediately. Do not use tape to seal a leak. As a rule, empty the pouch when it is ⅓ to ½ full. A full pouch can be heavy enough to fall off.
2. When emptying the pouch, turn the bottom of the pouch inside out before emptying; this makes it easier to clean the bottom of the pouch before applying rubber band or clamp.
3. You can squirt water into a pouch to clean it after emptying, but it is not necessary. You can also insert a ½-capful of mouthwash or an ostomy deodorizer into the pouch after emptying to control odors.
4. Never leave home without extra supplies (including a wafer/pouch that is already cut and ready for application) and clothing. Because checked baggage can be lost or stolen, always keep an extra supply in your "carry-on" luggage. Do not leave supplies in the car when the weather is either hot or freezing unless they are in a well-insulated bag, because extreme temperature will ruin pouches.
5. Use one-piece outfits to keep the infant's hands away from the pouch. Use empty paper towel or toilet paper rolls to help keep the infant's legs out of the way when emptying or changing the ostomy bag. Slit the roll up the side and wrap it around the infant's legs.

Special thanks to Elliott Douglass, RN, BSN, CWOCN, Wound, Ostomy, and Continence Nurse, Monroe Carell, Jr. Children's Hospital at Vanderbilt.

an arrest in development of the gut and its complete separation from urogenital tract between the 4th and 6th week of gestation. **Cloacal exstrophy** arises if disruption of the cloacal membrane occurs before the urorectal septum has separated the urinary bladder from the hindgut. Disruption of the cloacal membrane after septation results in exstrophy of the bladder only. Any insult occurring at this critical period of organogenesis places a number of organ systems at risk and accounts for the fact that 60% of infants with a persistent cloaca will have concomitant anomalies.[32]

Imperforate anus is the most common ARM, occurring in 1 in 5000 live births, and predominantly affects males (58%) more than females (42%). **Imperforate anus is characterized as low, intermediate, or high.** NOTE: **The higher the defect, the more likely the presence of other associated malformations.** A *high imperforate anus* is defined as the end of the rectum terminating above the levator ani muscles. Conversely, in *low imperforate anus,* the rectum descends below the levator complex. A fistulous connection to the perineum or urogenital tract is almost always present. In high lesions, the rectal fistula enters the membranous urethra in the male or, rarely, the vagina in the female. In low lesions, the rectal fistula empties on the perineum of both boys and girls or the posterior fourchette of the introitus, the most common site in girls.[59] Congenital **VACTERL** anomalies and trisomy 21 are common and require evaluation. Moreover, a high incidence of spinal dysraphism is observed with anorectal malformation; imaging of the spine is indicated.[79]

Data Collection

SIGNS AND SYMPTOMS

Most anorectal malformations are apparent on physical examination but may be missed if a careful inspection of the buttocks and anus is not performed. **Once the diagnosis is made, a fistula should be sought.** In low lesions, a thin membrane may be over the anal orifice or a fistula may be along the perineum and scrotal raphe of boys. In girls, the fistula most commonly terminates in the vestibule or fourchette of the introitus. If meconium passes in the urine or from the vagina, a high lesion is present. If the condition remains unrecognized, the infant develops signs and symptoms of distal intestinal obstruction. Down syndrome babies with an ARM usually (95%) have a high type variant of rectal atresia without genitourinary tract communication. (See the Critical Findings box below.)

Critical Findings

IMPERFORATE ANUS

The following are critical assessment findings for imperforate anus:

- Absence of anus or presence of anteriorly displaced perineal fistula
- Signs and symptoms of obstruction if diagnosis not made
- Perineal ultrasound study will identify the level of defect in the absence of a perineal fistula

LABORATORY DATA

A plain **abdominal radiograph** may show features of distal intestinal obstruction without rectal gas, but it will not reliably show the distal termination of the rectum. **Perineal ultrasonography** may be used to establish the termination of the rectum and its distance from the skin—data that may help operative planning. In boys with imperforate anus without a perineal fistula, a contrast study of the urethra should delineate a rectourethral fistula, if present. In girls without a perineal or vestibular fistula, **contrast genitogram** may help define the anatomic relationships of a persistent cloaca. A perineal fistula visible on physical examination does not usually warrant imaging of ARM. However, because of the possibility for VACTERL association, echocardiography and abdominal sonography of the genitourinary tract are indicated, as is a plain radiograph of the spine and limbs.

Treatment

PREOPERATIVE CARE

The infant should be kept on NPO status while evaluation of ARM is underway, and an orogastric tube should be placed to exclude esophageal atresia and to decompress the stomach. If a fistula is present on the perineum or at the fourchette, an early anoplasty may be performed, assuming the baby has no associated cardiac anomaly and is otherwise deemed to be a suitable candidate for a general anesthetic. If early repair is contraindicated, then the fistula tract may be dilated twice daily to promote elimination of fecal contents until the baby is a more suitable candidate for surgery. If no fistula is visualized and a high lesion or cloaca is present, a divided colostomy is performed and staged reconstruction is planned for later in infancy.

OPERATIVE INTERVENTION

For **low imperforate anus,** early reconstruction is performed either in the newborn period or in the first months of life if the infant can produce stools adequately through the fistulous tract with dilations. After **colostomy for high imperforate anus,** a formal repair is undertaken when the child is 3 to 6 months of age. Approached through a posterior sagittal incision (buttock), the fistula is separated from the urethra in boys or vagina in girls and the rectum is mobilized to lie within the center of the sphincter mechanism. The levator muscles

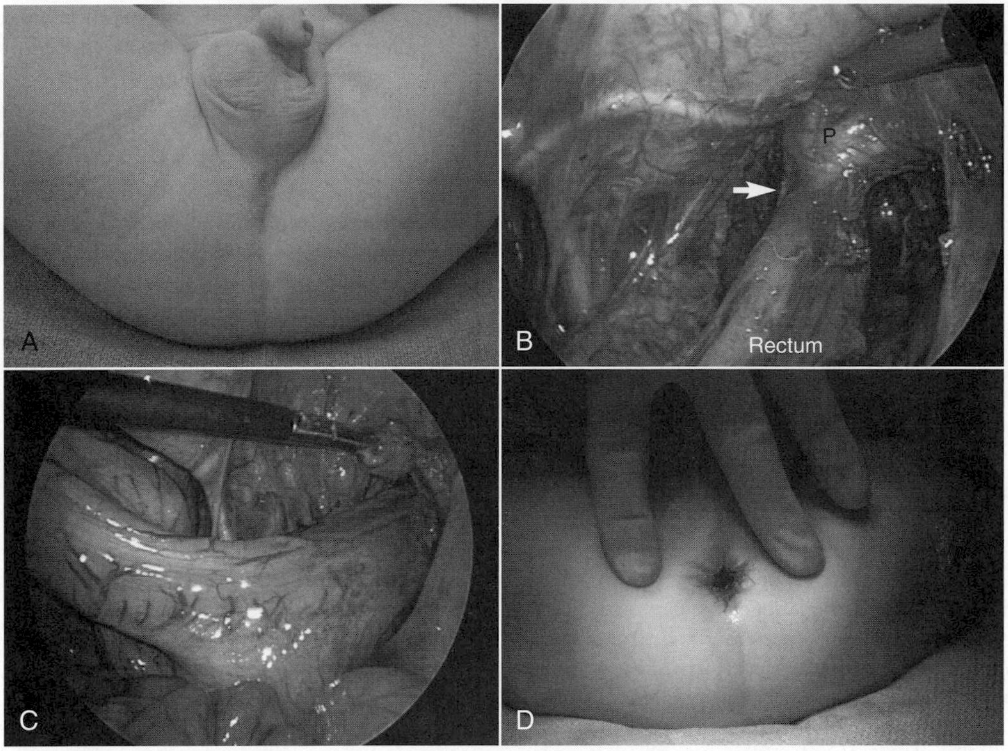

FIGURE 28-13 Male neonate with an anorectal malformation and rectourethral fistula. **A**, Flat perineum without cutaneous fistula. **B**, Laparoscopic view of pelvic structures after dissection. *Arrow* shows rectourethral fistula at level of prostate *(P)*. **C**, Fistula has been divided and ligated (held by 5-mm grasper), and rectum has been delivered through the center of the sphincter complex for colocutaneous anastomosis. **D**, Neoanus. (Courtesy Dr. H. Lovvorn, Vanderbilt University Medical Center.)

and sphincter are closed anteriorly and posteriorly around the rectum, which is then anastomosed to the perineal skin in a procedure known as a ***posterior sagittal anorectoplasty*** (*PSARP,* or *Peña procedure*).[60] Alternatively, to minimize wound complications and postoperative pain, a laparoscopic-assisted anorectoplasty may be performed (Figure 28-13). A Foley catheter should always be placed in boys at time of the definitive repair to assist in separation of the rectum from the urethra and to facilitate bladder drainage in the postoperative period; this catheter will be in place typically for 7 to 14 days after PSARP.

POSTOPERATIVE CARE

After anorectoplasty, simple skin care is all that is necessary, and a program of anal dilation is instituted 10 to 14 days postoperatively and will continue for 4 to 6 months. **After a colostomy, stoma care and teaching are begun with the parents.** Colostomy closure will be performed within 6 to 8 weeks of PSARP, assuming the neoanus is of adequate size and not strictured.

Complications and Prognosis

Mechanical complications of the stoma (prolapse, stenosis, and skin breakdown) may arise but generally do not require revision and should be temporized until stomal closure.[58] **Urinary tract infection (UTI)** or **hyperchloremic metabolic acidosis** may result from the fistulous connection of the rectum to the urinary tract. Antibiotic prophylaxis is instituted, and select infants may require bicarbonate supplement until the fistula is divided.

Constipation is the primary long-term problem after correction of low imperforate anus. Stricture of the anoplasty should always be considered and may be treated with anal dilation or, rarely, revision anoplasty.

High imperforate anus is most often complicated by **incontinence** and frequent soiling. Long-term results are influenced by the degree of sphincter muscle development and innervation. Approximately 25% of infants have good continence, 50% have fair continence, and 25% have poor results. Bowel programs and strategies have been developed to permit some degree of social continence so that permanent colostomy can be avoided.

OMPHALOCELE AND GASTROSCHISIS

Physiology and Etiology

Omphalocele and gastroschisis are distinct defects of the abdominal wall at or near the umbilicus.[6,43] **Omphalocele is characterized by the persistent herniation of the abdominal viscera through the umbilical ring, and the herniated contents are covered by the normal components of the umbilical cord: the peritoneum, Wharton's jelly, and amnion.** Omphalocele, also known as ***exomphalos,*** is a defect in abdominal wall development that may result from failure of embryonic enfolding as early as the 4th to 7th week of gestation or from failure of closure of the exocoelomic space, which is usually completed by the 12th week of gestation. **As many as 50% of neonates presenting with omphalocele will have an underlying chromosomal abnormality, most often trisomies 12 and 18 but also trisomy 21. Congenital heart lesions are seen in as many as 50% of affected infants.** Congenital syndromes involving an omphalocele are potentially lethal, usually as a result of the associated abnormalities. Cloacal exstrophy, occurring in 1 in 200,000 pregnancies, and the constellation of defects known as *pentalogy of Cantrell* likely represent the earliest of embryonic failures in the development of this spectrum of anomalies including omphalocele.

Gastroschisis is a full-thickness defect of the abdominal wall that occurs most commonly to the right of the umbilicus and exposes the extruded bowel to the amniotic fluid. It has been hypothesized that this defect results from a weakening of the anterior abdominal wall caused by a vascular accident involving the right omphalomesenteric artery, which takes over perfusion of the anterior abdominal wall during the 7th week of gestation. Gastroschisis occurs 3 to 4 times more frequently than omphalocele and is rising in developed countries for unknown reasons. This increasing incidence seems to be occurring in younger mothers, most frequently in those younger than 20 years, although no clear epidemiology has been correlated with this finding. **Gastroschisis typically is not associated with major congenital anomalies or syndromes, although 20% or more of affected infants have a concomitant intestinal atresia.**[33] This atresia is likely secondary to either the initial vascular accident thought to initiate the defect or compromise of the affected bowel segment arising from a constricting fascial defect.

Nonrotation of the intestine, by definition, is uniformly present in all incidences of these two conditions.

Data Collection

HISTORY

Abdominal wall defects are readily diagnosed by **antenatal ultrasonography,** which is helpful in planning future delivery and therapy.[13] Spontaneous or induced vaginal delivery should be considered in most cases of gastroschisis, because risk of bowel injury during delivery is minimal.[1,20,36] Babies with an omphalocele may also be delivered vaginally, but liver herniation or associated anomalies may dictate cesarean section.

In cases of gastroschisis, severe serositis resulting from exposure of the bowel to amniotic fluid makes closure more difficult and delays the return of bowel function. **Early delivery may be recommended for certain fetuses who have gastroschisis if sonographic evidence reveals progressive bowel distention and thickening, suggesting intestinal obstruction or severe serositis.** In cases of omphalocele, prenatal sonography should thoroughly evaluate the fetus for other potential anomalies and may be supplemented by fetal MRI.

SIGNS AND SYMPTOMS

Both anomalies present as a mass of abdominal contents extruding through an anterior abdominal wall defect. **Eviscerated bowel without a peritoneal covering characterizes gastroschisis, whereas an omphalocele is defined by a peritoneal covering of herniated bowel and often a segment of liver.** Gastroschisis defects are most commonly to the right of the midline and are found adjacent to the umbilical stalk, whereas omphalocele occurs through a central defect at the base of the umbilical cord.

Critical Findings

OMPHALOCELE AND GASTROSCHISIS

The following are critical assessment findings for omphalocele and gastroschisis:

- Typically detected on antenatal ultrasound examination
- Eviscerated bowel without peritoneal covering in gastroschisis
- Eviscerated bowel with peritoneal covering in omphalocele
- Diagnosis of omphalocele necessitates search for other associated anomalies

In contradistinction to gastroschisis, omphalocele carries a high incidence of significant associated anomalies, with cardiac and urinary tract malformations being most prevalent. Omphalocele also is a feature of several recognizable syndromes, including Beckwith-Wiedemann, prune belly, cloacal exstrophy, and pentalogy of Cantrell. Chromosomal defects are also identified with greater frequency in cases of omphalocele than gastroschisis and include trisomies 13, 18, and 21. Most babies with an omphalocele will deliver at term. Gastroschisis, in contrast, is associated with few anomalies outside of the gastrointestinal tract. Malrotation is understood to exist with gastroschisis, and so the most common associated anomaly is intestinal stenosis or atresia (10% to 15%), a rare finding in omphalocele. **Babies with gastroschisis are more commonly preterm and SGA.** (See the Critical Findings box above.)

LABORATORY DATA

In a neonate with **omphalocele,** a careful search for associated anomalies is performed before closure is attempted. **Echocardiography and an x-ray examination of the chest and spine** are performed to rule out cardiac, chest wall, diaphragmatic, and spinal anomalies. **Abdominal sonography** is obtained to evaluate integrity of the urinary tract. Newborns with gastroschisis do not require routine imaging of the heart and kidneys unless otherwise indicated.

Treatment

PREOPERATIVE CARE

Initial management of gastroschisis includes preservation of body heat and fluid, orogastric decompression, protection of the intestine, and prophylaxis against infection. Covering the exposed viscera minimizes heat and fluid loss. Wrapping the intestines in warm, saline-soaked gauze covered with a plastic wrap or placing the infant's torso into an impermeable, clear plastic bowel bag is generally employed. Both methods decrease evaporative losses; the bowel bag further allows continuous visual monitoring of the bowel. **With either method, it is imperative that the bowel be positioned to prevent constriction of the blood supply at the fascial level.**

Intravenous fluids and broad-spectrum antibiotics should be instituted early. To prevent bowel distention, **an orogastric tube is placed to low continuous suction.** In omphalocele, because the abdominal contents are covered naturally, less evaporative fluid and heat loss is encountered.

OPERATIVE INTERVENTION

Rarely, an infant with omphalocele may be too ill to undergo operation, may have other lethal malformations, or may have a "giant omphalocele," defined as the sac containing a significant portion of the liver (Figure 28-14). Under these circumstances, the newborn is given palliative care with a daily application of a desiccant or silver sulfadine to the abdominal sac. The result is eschar formation and subsequent epithelialization in 10 to 20 weeks. A large ventral hernia will remain, and if the patient survives, repair may be performed later in infancy. **For cases of omphalocele without liver herniation or significant associated anomalies, the sac may be removed and primary fascial closure accomplished shortly after birth;** alternatively, at a minimum, simple skin closure may be performed, with ventral hernia repair scheduled for later in infancy once the abdominal domain has been restored. Some cases of omphalocele will require biosynthetic fascial substitutes to accomplish visceral coverage.

For babies born with gastroschisis, **primary surgical repair** entails reduction of the herniated abdominal contents into the peritoneal cavity without increasing abdominal pressure to a point that ventilation, venous return, and intestinal blood supply are compromised. If the amount of eviscerated abdominal contents is small or moderate, primary repair is simple and safe. Before closure of gastroschisis, the surgeon searches carefully for associated atresia but may or may not attempt to restore intestinal continuity during the initial operation.

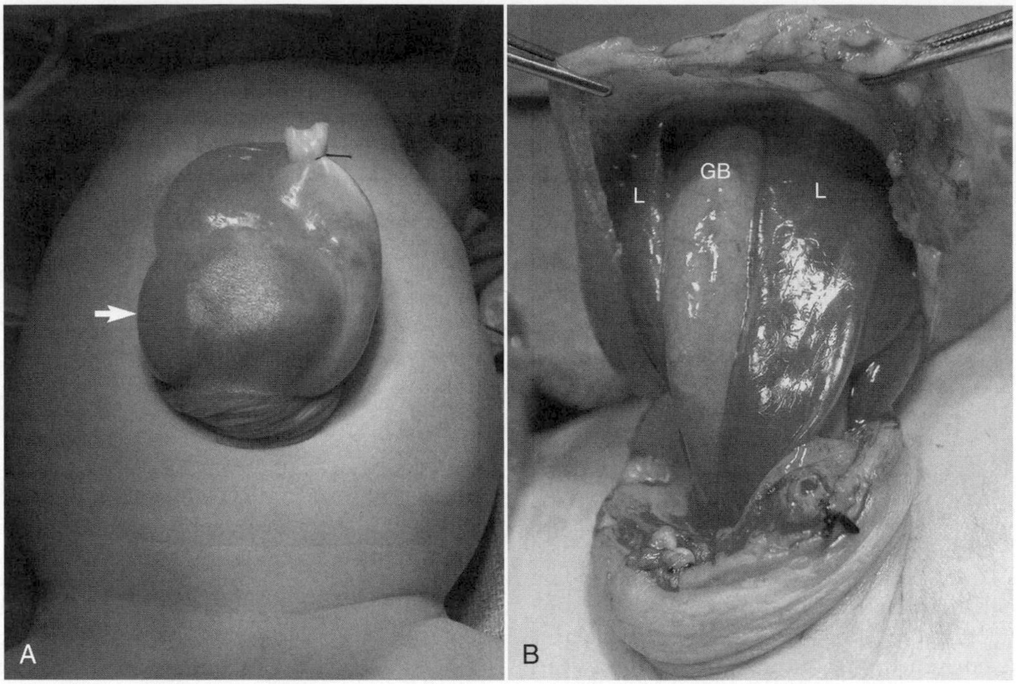

FIGURE 28-14 Neonate with omphalocele. **A,** *Arrow* shows liver contained within omphalocele sac. **B,** Dissection of sac contents. Liver is adherent to lining of sac. (*L,* Liver; *GB,* gallbladder.) Fascial defect was closed primarily. (Courtesy Dr. H. Lovvorn, Vanderbilt University Medical Center.)

If atresia is identified but inflammation and matting of the intestine will not permit safe anastomosis, the atretic bowel may be placed within a silo or returned to the abdomen primarily; re-exploration may be planned for 4 to 6 weeks later to allow the thickened, edematous bowel wall to normalize, facilitating anastomosis or enterostomy. If atresia is found but the bowel is not inflamed or matted, intestinal continuity may be restored at the initial operation or an ostomy created, with plans for delayed reconstitution 4 to 6 weeks later.

In select cases, the fascial defect may have to be enlarged to allow replacement of the herniated organs into the abdomen because of the small size of the fascial ring, loss of abdominal domain, and the amount of intestinal herniation. The inability to perform primary closure necessitates placement of a **Silastic silo** or patch to permit staged reduction (Figure 28-15). Over the ensuing 2 to 7 days, the herniated viscera are gradually returned to the abdomen on a daily basis by gravity (baby remains supine) and by applying gentle and constant pressure to the silo at the bedside (umbilical tape is tied sequentially along the silo until the intestine has reached the fascial level). Once all of the silo contents have been successfully reduced, the infant is returned to the operating room for removal of the silo and closure of the fascia.[69] While a silo is in place, most neonates will remain on antibiotics.

Complications and Prognosis

Bowel injury, respiratory compromise, and diminished venous return caused by abdominal hypertension may complicate recovery after primary fascial closure of abdominal wall defects. In this setting, the infant is returned to the operating room for placement of a silo. Rarely, a silo may become infected or separate from the fascia, complicating closure by this method.

Recovery of bowel function is uniformly delayed, especially in those with gastroschisis caused by exposure of the bowel to amniotic fluid and in those with intestinal problems (atresias, stenosis, perforation, necrosis, or volvulus).[5] A central venous catheter should be placed at the

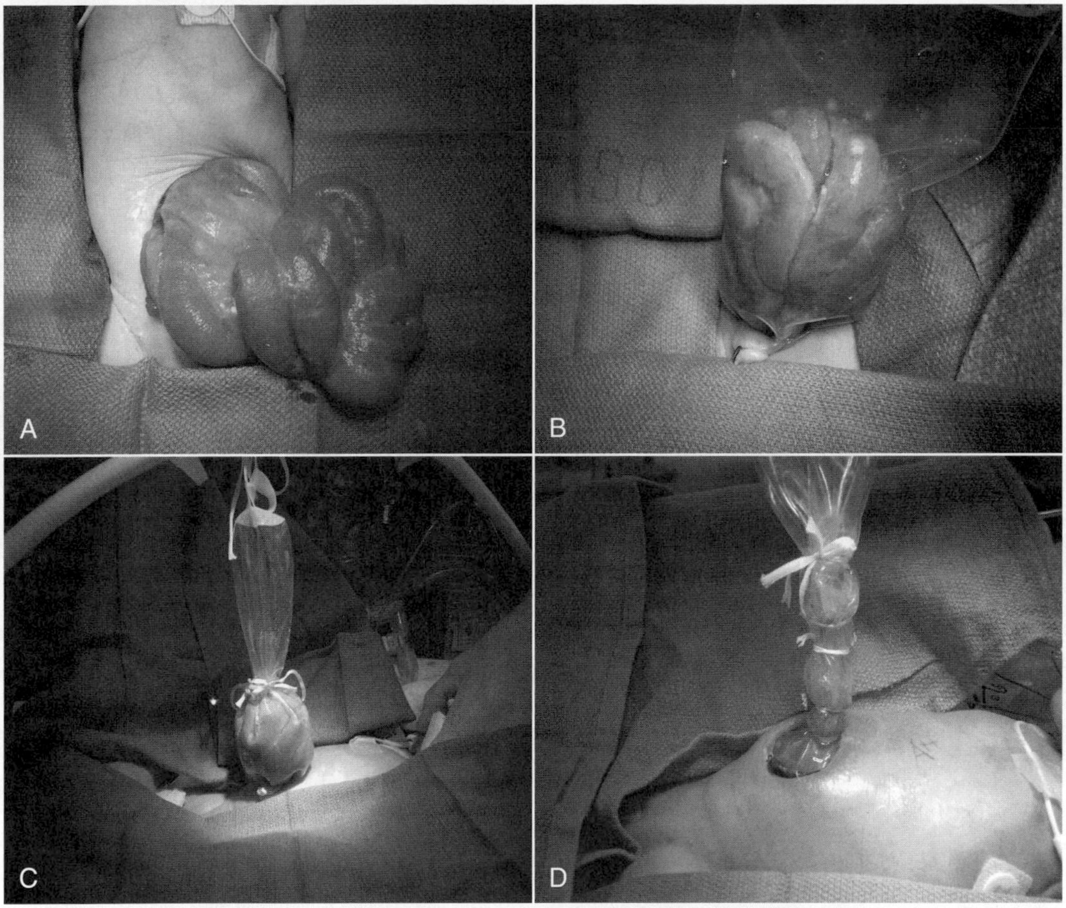

FIGURE 28-15 Neonate with gastroschisis. **A** and **B**, Note edema, thickening, and matting of bowel. Also, note scaphoid appearance of abdomen (loss of domain). As a result, bowel was placed in a Silastic silo. **C**, Postoperative day 1 after placement of silo. Note how the edema has largely drained from the bowel wall (gravity) and how much of the silo contents has reduced spontaneously. The first umbilical tape is placed to prevent bowel from rising in the silo. **D**, Postoperative day 5 (an umbilical tape is applied each day in the nursery) and the bowel has fully returned to the abdomen. The fascia is now ready for closure. (Courtesy Dr. H. Lovvorn, Vanderbilt University Medical Center.)

time of initial surgery for **long-term TPN support.** Intestinal stricture, incisional hernia, and adhesive bowel obstruction are possible short-term and long-term complications. The principle long-term morbidity associated with gastroschisis is short bowel syndrome. Morbidity for omphalocele is principally secondary to any associated anomalies and the challenges of abdominal closure. Otherwise, prognosis for both types of abdominal wall defects should be good.

NEONATAL TUMORS

Neonatal tumors are discovered in every 12,500 to 25,000 live births and account for 2% of all childhood malignancies.[52] The majority of affected neonates present with a mass at birth (or by day 28 of life), which may or may not have been identified on prenatal screening. The two most frequently encountered neonatal tumors are ***teratoma*** (principally sacrococcygeal [Figure 28-16] but also cervical

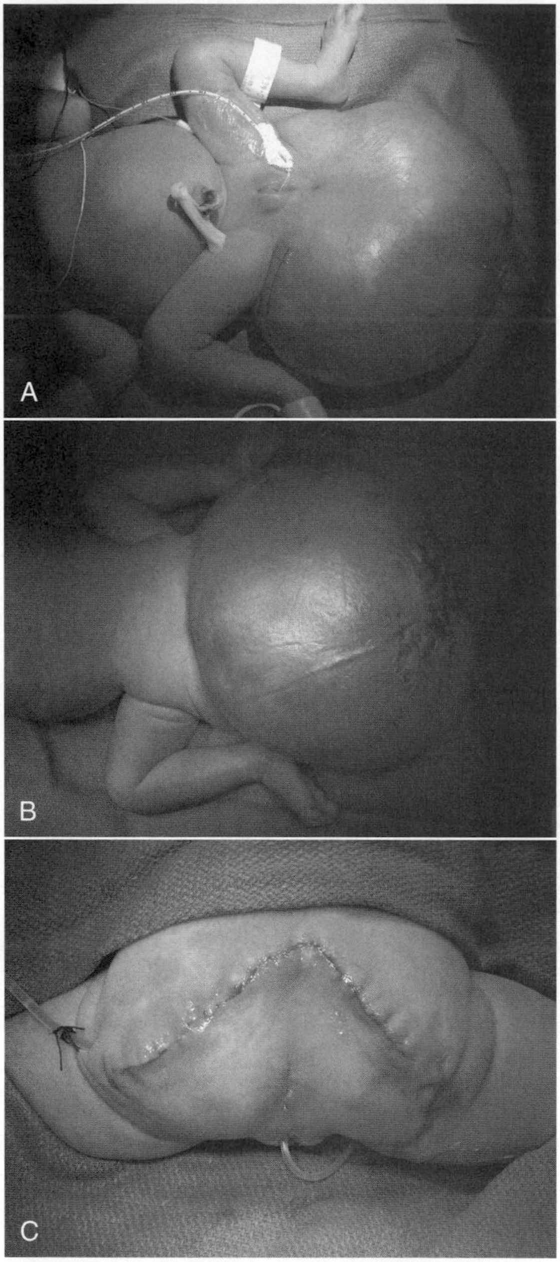

FIGURE 28-16 Female neonate with a huge sacrococcygeal teratoma. **A**, Anterior view. Note anal opening in anterior and just caudal to introitus. **B**, Posterior view. **C**, Immediately after resection. Incision will soften over time. (Courtesy Dr. H. Lovvorn, Vanderbilt University Medical Center.)

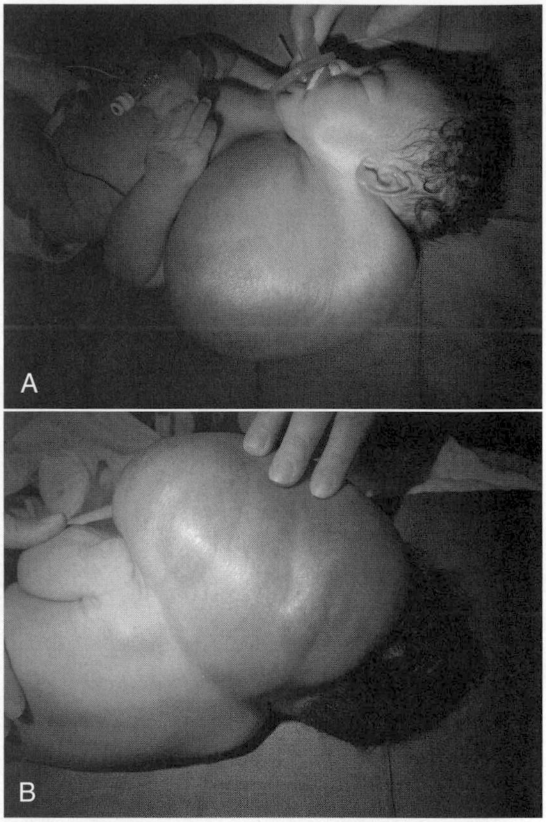

FIGURE 28-17 Huge cervical cystic hygroma. Teratomas show a similar appearance but tend to be more midline than hygromas. **A**, Anterior view. **B**, Posterior view. (Courtesy Dr. H. Lovvorn, Vanderbilt University Medical Center.)

[Figure 28-17]) and ***neuroblastoma.*** Soft tissue sarcomas, infantile myofibromatosis, renal tumors (benign mesoblastic nephroma and malignant Wilms' tumor), hepatoblastoma, and central nervous system tumors follow in frequency. Malignant tumors rarely arise in the newborn; however, some benign tumors encountered at birth may acquire malignant features later in infancy.

Nevertheless, although a neonatal tumor may be histologically benign, these tumors may be life threatening because of size, location, arteriovenous shunts, or rupture with hemorrhage. Some tumors show invasive or infiltrative characteristics, yet these may not have metastatic potential. Furthermore, screening programs have identified potentially malignant tumors earlier in development, such as for neuroblastoma in Japan, but have as yet failed to improve overall survival. Some neonatal tumors even show the potential for spontaneous regression. Taken together, neonatal tumors represent a protean mix of diseases that have a low malignant potential yet the biologic behavior may not be entirely predictable.

The etiology of solid malignancies in infants and children is an area of great interest. Many of these "congenital" tumors are classified as embryonal tumors because of retained features of embryonic development within the organ in which each tumor arises. Carcinomas, typical of adulthood, are virtually nonexistent in neonates. Under the microscope, many of these tumors show a recapitulation of cell types found in early embryonic development of the particular organ, but terminal differentiation of the progenitor cells has not been completed and so no functional tissue architecture is appreciated. Associated anomalies may be found in 15% of neonates with congenital tumors, and genetic defects are also relatively common.

Routine ***prenatal ultrasonography*** has contributed to an increasing diagnosis of fetal and neonatal tumors. It is interesting to note that several fetal tumors, particularly neuroblastoma, have a unique property to undergo spontaneous regression and involution by 12 months of age. As a result, the natural history of any given adrenal tumor and optimal management remain unclear. The Children's Oncology Group has an ongoing study to determine the natural history of adrenal masses in newborns or infants, presumed to be neuroblastoma. Patients are being enrolled into an "expectant management" arm, which should shed light on the natural history of these lesions.

Commonly, fetuses harboring an embryonal or germ cell tumor will be identified on antenatal screening. Some tumors—in particular, sacrococcygeal teratomas—may be so large as to cause dystocia or may present a significant risk for rupture during delivery, and either scenario could be disastrous. Further, a cervical teratoma or cystic hygroma may cause airway obstruction at birth. Fetuses with these occasionally huge cervical tumors should be delivered by cesarean section, bronchoscoped, and intubated before clamping of the umbilical cord, referred to as an ***EXIT procedure*** (**EX**-utero **I**ntra-partum **T**herapy). The tumor then may be resected electively once the extent of the disease and any associated anomalies have been fully evaluated.[35]

Most neonatal tumors are benign or of low malignant potential and tend to behave more favorably than the same type of tumor in older children. Neuroblastoma, for example, generally presents as stage I disease in 90% of infants younger than 1 year and is amenable to observation, if small, or complete resection. Hepatoblastomas presenting in the newborn period also tend to behave more favorably than when presenting later in infancy. Despite a collective rarity, presentation of malignant tumors in the newborn period does occur, and much work remains to identify determinants of tumorigenesis and pathogenesis.

MINIMALLY INVASIVE SURGERY

Laparoscopic or minimally invasive techniques are beginning to supplant many surgical procedures previously performed by laparotomy or thoracotomy. Laparoscopic procedures have been associated with decreased postoperative pain, earlier return to gastrointestinal function, shorter hospital stays, fewer wound complications, and improved cosmetic results, when compared with the corresponding open procedures.[31]

Laparoscopic techniques have been applied to many of the neonatal procedures described in this chapter. Indeed, laparoscopic Nissen fundoplication for gastroesophageal reflux disease (GERD) and laparoscopic-assisted pull-through procedures for Hirschsprung's disease are being performed routinely in the neonate and show shorter time to postoperative feeding, decreased hospital stay, and superior cosmesis. For example, thoracoscopic repair of esophageal atresia with tracheoesophageal fistula is beginning to be advocated as an equally effective approach, and supporters claim improved pain management and musculoskeletal benefits. Laparoscopic repair of duodenal atresia is also being performed with good results. Both thoracoscopic and laparoscopic techniques are being used increasingly to repair Bochdalek and Morgagni diaphragmatic hernias with good outcomes in neonates who do not require ECLS. Laparoscopic-assisted endorectal pull-through for Hirschsprung's disease and for anorectoplasty to correct ARM is becoming more and more a part of the neonatal surgeon's armamentarium.[70] However, pathophysiologic effects of pneumoperitoneum or iatrogenic pneumothorax are only recently being analyzed. Adverse consequences include the following[38]:

- Reduced intraoperative arterial saturation
- Increased carbon dioxide (CO_2) retention (CO_2 is used for abdominal insufflation, and diaphragmatic excursion may be compromised because of increased abdominal pressure)
- Oliguria or even anuria for up to 4 hours postoperatively

- Hypothermia
- Need for extended postoperative intubation if procedures exceed 100 minutes, which they often may

As experience increases and technical refinements are seen with improved optical systems and smaller instruments, a broader application of laparoscopy inevitably will occur in the neonatal patient population.

PARENT TEACHING

Preoperative

The advent of ever-increasing mechanisms of **prenatal diagnosis** allows parents to begin adjusting to the presence of certain malformations—some minor and others potentially lethal—before birth.[3] Research shows that parents experience various stages of grief, including shock, denial, anger, and sadness, when faced with such news. Although the intensity of the negative emotions associated with the initial diagnosis may lessen by the time of delivery, resolution of these emotions should not be expected. Expressions of fear, anxiety, and guilt are likely to remain for some time.[57]

Because parents' fears and fantasies about their infant's surgical diagnosis are frequently worse than reality, they should see their infant as soon as possible after birth and before surgery. Pictures of the infant should be taken before surgery and should include views with and without the defect if possible. Whenever time and patient condition allow, parents should be encouraged to hold their infant and pictures should be taken of the family with their newborn. In the event of a neonate's death, these pictures may be very valuable to the family. In the event neonatal transport from the birth hospital to a referral center is required, the transport team should do everything possible to ensure that the mother, who may be in the early recovery phase from her delivery, sees her infant before departure.[16]

The planned operative procedure and its expected results, as well as risks and alternatives, are discussed with the parents, ensuring that all questions and concerns are addressed. An informed consent for surgery is signed and witnessed. The **bedside nurse should be present when the physician meets with the family to discuss the operation, because the nurse is often the most consistent individual hearing explanations from the neonatologist, surgeon, and anesthesiologist and must answer questions, interpret information, and reassure an anxious family when these teams leave.** The nurse has a further important role in reassuring parents about postoperative analgesia and sedation for there infant. **Preoperative teaching can involve educating parents in recognizing pain cues in their baby, and they should be encouraged to discuss their concerns if they perceive their baby is experiencing discomfort. Care providers' sensitivity to the neonate's pain and advocating for pain relief are comforting for parents** (see Chapter 12).

Parents often fear what the infant will look like on return from surgery. Providing written material with simple drawings of the defects and operative procedure may help prevent postoperative surprises. Seeing another patient who has had a similar procedure and has the postoperative equipment that has been described (e.g., colostomy, orogastric tube, chest tube) may be helpful to the family as well.[57] The nursing staff must be careful, however, to protect the privacy of other patients and should get parental consent before visiting another infant for this purpose.

Intraoperative

Accompanying the infant to the preoperative area and seeing the infant as soon as possible after surgery are comforting to the parents. Progress reports of the surgery, if possible, are helpful for the anxious family members. After the operation, the pediatric surgeon should immediately see the parents to explain the procedure and any unexpected problems that occurred during the operation. It should be clear to both the family and the surgeon where this important communication will take place, and privacy should be protected during the interchange.

Postoperative

After surgery, the nurse should help parents focus on their infant rather than the surrounding intensive care environment. Although the nursing staff should identify the monitors, equipment, dressings, and foreign bodies on the baby and in the room and should explain the purpose of each to the family, encouraging parents

to comfort their baby will be of greatest benefit to their postoperative child (and to them). Early involvement in caregiving helps the parents feel as though they are essential to their child's recovery. Even in the immediate postoperative period, a parent can quietly sit and hold the infant's hand or take an axillary temperature. After most surgical procedures, mothers should be encouraged to express breast milk and may benefit from a lactation nurse consultation. Feeding issues may often remain a potential barrier to maternal confidence and maternal-infant interaction and warrant education and assistance during the postoperative period long before NICU discharge.[22]

If an infant is to be discharged home with an ostomy, parents begin to participate in stoma care as early as possible. Consultation with an enterostomal therapy nurse is of further benefit. Parents begin by learning to cleanse the skin around the ostomy or to prepare the appliance and peristomal salves. Gradually, parents will learn to increase their responsibilities of caregiving as their infant improves. Frequent practice improves proficiency and empowers parents for taking their infant home. Delay until a few days before discharge does not give parents adequate time for practice and familiarity for home care and does not serve the infant or family well. The same is true for infants who are discharged with other types of complicated care, such as home TPN or feedings through a gastrostomy tube and/or via a continuous feeding pump. Parent teaching includes the possibility of late postoperative complications and recognition of problems that may develop and a plan of action for dealing with them.

The importance of follow-up care is emphasized to the parents. It may be helpful for parents to talk with a "graduate" parent who had an infant with similar problems. Contact information about available resources, such as visiting nurses, graduate parents, and parent support groups is provided to parents before discharge. A concise history of hospitalization and the discharge plan are made available to all post-hospitalization health care providers, and a copy is provided to parents at the time of discharge. Encouraging parents to keep a copy of this discharge summary in their diaper bag increases the chances they will have it available should they be required to take their medically complex and vulnerable infant emergently to the hospital.

REFERENCES

1. Abdel-Latif NS, Bolisetty S, Abeywardana S, et al: Mode of delivery and neonatal survival of infants with gastroschisis in Australia and New Zealand, *J Pediatr Surg* 43:1685, 2008.
2. Adzick NS, Nance ML: Pediatric surgery, *N Engl J Med* 342:1651, 2000.
3. Aite L, Zaccara A, Nahom A, et al: Mother's adaptation to antenatal diagnosis of surgically correctable anomalies, *Early Hum Dev* 82:649, 2006.
4. American Academy of Pediatrics, Section on Surgery and the Committee on Fetus and Newborn: Postdischarge follow-up of infants with congenital diaphragmatic hernia, *Pediatrics* 121:627, 2008.
5. Arnold MA, Chang DC, Nabaweesi R, et al: Risk stratification of 4344 patients with gastroschisis into simple and complex categories, *J Pediatr Surg* 42:1520, 2007.
6. Aspelund G, Langer JC: Abdominal wall defects, *Curr Pediatr* 16:192, 2006.
7. Azizkhan RG, Crombleholme TM: Congenital cystic lung disease: contemporary antenatal and postnatal management, *Pediatr Surg Int* 24:643, 2008.
8. Bagolan P, Casaccia G, Crescenzi F, et al: Impact of a current treatment protocol on outcome of high-risk congenital diaphragmatic hernia, *J Pediatr Surg* 39:313, 2004.
9. Bax NM, van der Zee DC: Laparoscopic treatment of intestinal malrotation in children, *Surg Endosc* 12:1314, 1998.
10. Blakely ML, Gupta H, Lally KP: Surgical management of necrotizing enterocolitis and isolated intestinal perforation in premature neonates, *Semin Perinatol* 32:122, 2008.
11. Casaccia G, Trucchi A, Nahom A, et al: The impact of cystic fibrosis on neonatal intestinal obstruction: the need for prenatal/neonatal screening, *Pediatr Surg Int* 19:75, 2003.
12. Centers for Disease Control and Prevention: Trends in infant mortality attributable to birth defects: United States, 1980-1995, *MMWR Morb Mortal Wkly Rep* 47:773, 1998.
13. Chen CP, Liu FF, Jan SW, et al: Prenatal diagnosis and perinatal aspects of abdominal wall defects, *Am J Perinatol* 13:355, 1996.
14. Chokshi NK, Guner Y, Henri RF: The role of IL-10 in experimental necrotizing enterocolitis, *J Am Coll Surg* 207:S14, 2008 (abstract).
15. Coran AG, Teitelbaum DH: Recent advances in the management of Hirschsprung's disease, *Am J Surg* 180:382, 2000.
16. Cornette L: Transporting the sick neonate, *Curr Paediatr* 14:20, 2004.
17. DallaVecchia LK, Grosfeld JL, West KW, et al: Intestinal atresia and stenosis: a 25-year experience with 277 cases, *Arch Surg* 133:490, 1998.
18. de Jong EM, Felix JF, Deurloo JA, et al: Non-VACTERL-type anomalies are frequent in patients

with esophageal atresia/tracheo-esophageal fistula and full or partial VACTERL association, *Birth Defects Res A Clin Mol Teratol* 82:92, 2008.
19. Dimmitt RA, Meier AH, Skarsgard ED, et al: Salvage laparotomy for failure of peritoneal drainage in necrotizing enterocolitis in infants with extremely low birth weight, *J Pediatr Surg* 35:856, 2000.
20. Drewitt M, Michailidis GD, Burge D: The perinatal management of gastroschisis, *Early Hum Dev* 82:305, 2006.
21. Engum SA, Grosfeld JL, West KW, et al: Analysis of morbidity and mortality in 227 cases of esophageal atresia or tracheoesophageal fistula over two decades, *Arch Surg* 130:502, 1995.
22. Faugli A, Emblem R, Veenstra M, et al: Does esophageal atresia influence the mother-infant interaction?, *J Pediatr Surg* 43:1796, 2008.
23. Feitz R, Vos A: Malrotation: the postoperative period, *J Pediatr Surg* 32:1322, 1997.
24. Freeman SB, Torfs CP, Romitti PA, et al: Congenital gastrointestinal defects in Down syndrome: a report from the Atlanta and National Down Syndrome Projects, *Clin Genet* 75(2):180, 2009. Epub ahead of print: November 17, 2008.
25. Friedman S, Chen C, Chapman JS, et al: Neurodevelopmental outcomes of congenital diaphragmatic hernia survivors followed in a multidisciplinary clinic at ages 1 and 3, *J Pediatr Surg* 43:1035, 2008.
26. Gibbins S, Maddalena P, Golec L: Evidenced-based care for the infant with necrotizing enterocolitis, *Newborn Infant Nurs Rev* 8:144, 2008.
27. Grosfeld JL, Rescorla FJ: Duodenal atresia and stenosis: reassessment of treatment and outcome based on antenatal diagnosis, pathologic variance, and long-term follow-up, *World J Surg* 17:301, 1993.
28. Guner YS, Chokshi N, Aranda A, et al: Thoracoscopic repair of neonatal diaphragmatic hernia, *J Laparoendosc Adv Surg Tech* 18:875, 2008. Bottom of Form.
29. Guner YS, Chokshi N, Petrosyan M, et al: Necrotizing enterocolitis—bench to bedside: novel and emerging strategies, *Semin Pediatr Surg* 17:255, 2008.
30. Haricharan RN, Georgeson KE: Hirschsprung disease, *Semin Pediatr Surg* 17:266, 2008.
31. Harres AE: Minimally invasive neonatal surgery, *J Perinat Neonatal Nurs* 21:39, 2007.
32. Hendren WH: Cloaca, the most severe degree of imperforate anus: experience with 195 cases, *Ann Surg* 228:331, 1998.
33. Henrich K, Huemmer HP, Reingruber B, et al: Gastroschisis and omphalocele: treatments and long-term outcomes, *Pediatr Surg Int* 24:167, 2008.
34. Henry MCW, Moss RL: Neonatal necrotizing enterocolitis, *Semin Pediatr Surg* 17:98, 2008.
35. Hirose S, Farmer DL, Lee H, et al: The ex utero intrapartum treatment procedure: looking back at the EXIT, *J Pediatr Surg* 39:375, 2004.
36. How HY, Harris BJ, Pietrantoni M, et al: Is vaginal delivery preferable to elective cesarean delivery in fetuses with a known ventral wall defect? *Am J Obstet Gynecol* 182:1527, 2000.
37. Hunter JH, Williams M, Petrosyan M, et al: *Lactobacillus* species abrogates pathogen induced experimental necrotizing enterocolitis by attenuating inducible nitric oxide synthase production, *J Am Coll Surg* 207:S54, 2008 (abstract).
38. Kalfa N, Ecochard A, Patte C, et al: Tolerance of laparoscopy and thoracoscopy in neonates, *Pediatrics* 115:785, 2005.
39. Kao SC, Franken EA Jr: Nonoperative treatment of simple meconium ileus: a survey of the Society for Pediatric Radiology, *Pediatr Radiol* 25:97, 1995.
40. Keckler SJ, St. Peter SD, Spilde TL, et al: Current significance of meconium plug syndrome, *J Pediatr Surg* 43:896, 2008.
41. Keckler SJ, St. Peter SD, Valusek PA, et al: VACTERL anomalies in patients with esophageal atresia: an updated delineation of the spectrum and review of the literature, *Pediatr Surg Int* 23:309, 2007.
42. Lakhoo K: Management of congenital cystic adenomatous malformations of the lung, *Arch Dis Child Fetal Neonatal Ed* 94:F73, 2009.
43. Langer JC: Gastroschisis and omphalocele, *Semin Pediatr Surg* 5:124, 1996.
44. Langston C: New concepts in the pathology of congenital lung malformations, *Sem Pediatr Surg* 12:17, 2003.
45. Lemons JA, Bauer CR, Oh W, et al: Very low birth weight outcomes of the National Institute of Child Health and Human Development Neonatal Research Network, January 1995 through December 1996, *Pediatrics* 107:e1, 2001.
46. Li K, Zheng S, Xiao X, et al: The structural characteristics and expression of neuropeptides in the esophagus of patients with congenital esophageal atresia and tracheoesophageal fistula, *J Pediatr Surg* 42:1433, 2007.
47. Lindower J, Atherton H, Kotagal U: Outcomes and resource utilization for newborns with major congenital malformations: the initial NICU admission, *J Perinatol* 19:212, 1999.
48. Messineo A, MacMillan JH, Palder SB, et al: Clinical factors affecting mortality in children with malrotation of the intestine, *J Pediatr Surg* 27:1343, 1992.
49. Migliazza L, Bellan C, Alberti D, et al: Retrospective study of 111 cases of congenital diaphragmatic hernia treated with early high-frequency oscillatory ventilation and presurgical stabilization, *J Pediatr Surg* 42:1526, 2007.
50. Millar AJW, Rode H, Cywes S: Malrotation and volvulus in infancy and childhood, *Semin Pediatr Surg* 12:229, 2003.
51. Mills JLA, Konkin DE, Milner R, et al: Long-term bowel function and quality of life in children with Hirschsprung's disease, *J Pediatr Surg* 43:899, 2008.
52. Moore SW, Satge D, Sasco AJ, et al: The epidemiology of neonatal tumors, *Pediatr Surg Int* 19:509, 2003.
53. Munck A, Gérardin M, Alberti C, et al: Clinical outcome of cystic fibrosis presenting with or without

meconium ileus: a matched cohort study, *J Pediatr Surg* 41:1556, 2006.

54. Mushtaq I, Wright VM, Drake DP, et al: Meconium ileus secondary to cystic fibrosis: the East London experience, *Pediatr Surg Int* 13:365, 1998.
55. Navarro OM, Daneman A, Miller SF: Contrast enema depiction of small-bowel volvulus in complicated neonatal bowel obstruction, *Pediatr Radiol* 34:1020, 2004.
56. Ng GYT, Derry C, Marston L, et al: Reduction in ventilator-induced lung injury improves outcome in congenital diaphragmatic hernia? *Pediatr Surg Int* 24:145, 2008.
57. Nisell M, Ojmyr-Joelsson M, Frenckner B, et al: How a family is affected when a child is born with anorectal malformation: interviews with three patients and their parents, *J Pediatr Nurs* 18:423, 2003.
58. Patwardhan N, Kiely EM, Drake DP, et al: Colostomy for anorectal anomalies: high incidence of complications, *J Pediatr Surg* 36:795, 2001.
59. Peña A: Anorectal malformations, *Semin Pediatr Surg* 4:35, 1995.
60. Peña A, Hong A: Advances in the management of anorectal malformations, *Am J Surg* 180:370, 2000.
61. Piper HG, Alesbury J, Waterford SD, et al: Intestinal atresias: factors affecting clinical outcomes, *J Pediatr Surg* 43:1244, 2008.
62. Pourcyrous M, Korones SB, Yang W, et al: C-reactive protein in the diagnosis, management, and prognosis of neonatal necrotizing enterocolitis, *Pediatrics* 116:1064, 2005.
63. Radulescu A, Yu X, Chen Y, et al: HB-EGF knockout mice have increased susceptibility to necrotizing enterocolitis, *J Am Coll Surg* 207:S54, 2008 (abstract).
64. Rescorla FJ, Grosfeld JL: Contemporary management of meconium ileus, *World J Surg* 17:318, 1993.
65. Riedlinger WFJ, Vargas SO, Jennings RW, et al: Bronchial atresia is common to extralobar sequestration, intralobar sequestration, congenital cystic adenomatoid malformation, and lobar emphysema, *Pediatr Dev Path* 9:361, 2006.
66. Robb A, Lander A: Duodenal and small intestinal atresias and stenosis, *Surgery (Oxford)* 25:287, 2007.
67. Roessingh AS, de Buys AT, Dinh-Xuan: Congenital diaphragmatic hernia: current status and review of the literature, *Eur J Pediatr* 168:393, 2009. Epub ahead of print: December 23, 2008.
68. Sato S, Nishijima E, Muraji T, et al: Jejunoileal atresia: a 27-year experience, *J Pediatr Surg* 33:1633, 1998.
69. Sauter ER, Falterman KW, Arensman RM: Is primary repair of gastroschisis and omphalocele always the best operation? *Am Surg* 57:142, 1991.
70. Shinall MC Jr, Koehler E, Shyr Y, et al: Comparing cost and complications of primary and staged surgical repair of neonatally diagnosed Hirschsprung's disease, *J Pediatr Surg* 43:2220, 2008.
71. Silva CT, Daneman A, Navarro OM, et al: Correlation of sonographic findings and outcome in necrotizing enterocolitis, *Pediatr Radiol* 37:274, 2007.
72. Skari H, Bjornland K, Haugen G, et al: Congenital diaphragmatic hernia: a meta-analysis of mortality factors, *J Pediatr Surg* 35:1187, 2000.
73. Spigland N, Yazbeck S: Complications associated with surgical treatment of congenital intrinsic duodenal obstruction, *J Pediatr Surg* 25:1127, 1990.
74. Spitz L, Kiely EM, Morecroft JA, et al: Oesophageal atresia: at-risk groups for the 1990s, *J Pediatr Surg* 29:723, 1994.
75. Strouse PJ: Disorders of intestinal rotation and fixation (malrotation), *Pediatr Radiol* 34:837, 2004.
76. Teitelbaum DH, Cilley RE, Sherman NJ, et al: A decade of experience with the primary pull-through for Hirschsprung disease in the newborn period: a multicenter analysis of outcomes, *Ann Surg* 232:372, 2000.
77. Tireli GA, Özbey H, Temiz A, et al: Bronchogenic cysts: a rare congenital cystic malformation of the lung, *Surg Today* 34:573, 2004.
78. Torres AM, Ziegler MM: Malrotation of the intestine, *World J Surg* 17:326, 1993.
79. Torres R, Levitt MA, Tovilla JM, et al: Anorectal malformations and Down's syndrome, *J Pediatr Surg* 33:194, 1998.
80. Tovar JA: The neural crest in pediatric surgery, *J Pediatr Surg* 42:915, 2007.
81. Tran H, Fink MA, Cramer J, et al: Congenital cystic adenomatoid malformation: monitoring the antenatal and short-term neonatal outcome, *Aust N Z J Obstet Gynaecol* 48:462, 2008.
82. Ververidis M, Kiely EM, Spitz L, et al: The clinical significance of thrombocytopenia in neonates with necrotizing enterocolitis, *J Pediatr Surg* 36:799, 2001.
83. Waag K-L, Loff S, Zahn K, et al: Congenital diaphragmatic hernia: a modern day approach, *Semin Pediatr Surg* 17:244, 2008.
84. Waldhausen JH, Sawin RS: Improved long-term outcome for patients with jejunoileal apple peel atresia, *J Pediatr Surg* 32:1307, 1997.
85. Walesa PW, de Silva N, Kim JH, et al: Neonatal short bowel syndrome: a cohort study, *J Pediatr Surg* 40:755, 2005.
86. Walsh DS, Adzick NS: Fetal surgical intervention, *Am J Perinatol* 17:277, 2000.
87. Weber TR, Kountzman B, Dillon PA, et al: Improved survival in congenital diaphragmatic hernia with evolving therapeutic strategies, *Arch Surg* 133:498, 1998.
88. Williams H: Green for danger: intestinal malrotation and volvulus, *Arch Dis Child Educ Pract Ed* 92:ep87, 2007.
89. Yanchar NL, Soucy P: Long-term outcome after Hirschsprung's disease: patients' perspectives, *J Pediatr Surg* 34:1152, 1999.

29 FAMILIES IN CRISIS: THEORETICAL AND PRACTICAL CONSIDERATIONS

ROBERTA SIEGEL, SANDRA L. GARDNER, AND LORRAINE A. DICKEY

The technical advances that have characterized newborn care have resulted in marked decrease in mortality and morbidity in the high-risk infant. These developments have been accompanied by a heightened appreciation of the psychologic strain and emotional stresses encountered by the family of the sick neonate.[6,22,116,122,132] Realization of the need for a family-centered approach to perinatal care has emerged out of an enhanced understanding of individual and family functioning and their adaptation to stress.[9,10,70,84] It has become essential for perinatal health care teams to address the psychologic needs of families who are experiencing the painful crisis of the birth of a sick newborn.[122,182] This chapter discusses the complex psychosocial needs of families during this stressful period and offers concrete suggestions for intervention.

NORMAL ATTACHMENT

Emotional investment in the infant begins not at birth but during the pregnancy. The terms ***attachment*** and ***bonding***[101] are used to describe this process of relating between parents and their infant. Attachment behavior is characterized by the same qualities used to describe love: care, responsibility, and knowledge. Attachment is an individualized process, not an automatic one.[22,146]

The infant's need for the parent is absolute, but the parent's need for the infant is only relative. The neonate is totally dependent, both physically and emotionally, on the caregivers. Recognition of this unique relationship is evidenced cross-culturally by immediate and prolonged contact with no evidence of separation.[93,146] In most animal species, the mother engages in species-specific behaviors[101] that enable her to become acquainted with and claim the newborn. Interference during this critical period results in rejection by the animal mother and death of the young. In a recent study, adult rats whose mothers engaged in more species-specific behaviors (e.g., licking, grooming) showed significantly decreased levels of stress hormones.[119] Recent studies have shown a relationship between stressful environments, the health of the fetus, and caregiving ability (see Chapter 13). Parental attachment and appropriate caregiving behaviors are crucial for the infant's physical, psychologic, and emotional health and survival. Ultimately, this influence will affect the infant's well-being as an adult and a potential parent for a subsequent generation.

Critical and Sensitive Period

In the period immediately after birth, both mother and infant are physiologically and psychologically ready for reciprocal interaction.[101] Physiologically,

Please note that the **PURPLE** type in each chapter is intended to make it easier to identify clinically applicable material.

even though labor and birth are tiring, most mothers feel "high" and have an incredible surge of energy after birth. Psychologically, the family is ready to meet and interact with the long-awaited newcomer. Physiologically, the first hour of life is a time of alertness for the newborn. Before the sleep phase, the newborn is alert, makes eye-to-eye contact, fixes and follows, begins to search unassisted for the maternal nipple, and begins to feed. At birth, all five senses are operational and the infant is ready to cue and shape the environment (see Chapters 5 and 13).

This period of mutual readiness has been compared with the critical period in animals. This human "maternal sensitive period"[101] is the time immediately after birth in which the attachment process is initiated. Called the optimal but not the sole period for attachment to develop, the human critical period represents a reciprocal readiness for acquaintance. Positive effects of early and extended contact, rather than initial separation, have shown significant differences in caregiving behaviors that persist over time.

Sustained and early contact between parents and infant completes the process of labor and birth and gives the family the opportunity for interaction. The presence of the infant enables the parents to begin knowing the reality and individuality of their infant. Early parent-infant contact facilitates parent-infant attachment and contributes to the regulation of the newborn's physiology and behavior.[22,119,122,146] Early skin-to-skin contact between mothers and their infants results in significant benefits: (1) better breast feeding, (2) maintenance of infant body temperature, (3) higher blood glucose, (4) lower respiratory rate, (5) more affectionate maternal behavior, and (6) less infant crying.[139] Unnecessary "routines" and procedures that interfere with initial contact should be deferred until the initial acquaintance process is completed (see Chapter 5).

Failure to establish immediate contact because of medically indicated interventions necessary to sustain life does not promote attachment, but neither does it undermine the entire process of attachment.[42] Unlike animals, human mothers do not automatically reject their infant if they cannot interact immediately. Interference or failure to interact during the critical period does not condemn the resilient and adaptable human parent to rejection of or maladaptation to the infant.

Crisis Event: Pregnancy and Parenthood

Pregnancy, birth, and parenthood are almost universally defined as a life crisis.[93,146] Parenting is a major adjustment of the prepregnancy roles, lifestyle, and relationships. Because previous ideas and coping styles may not be helpful, life crisis situations challenge the individual with the potential for growth as new responses and solutions are used for problem solving. Periods of upheaval, change, and vulnerability provide a time of openness, receptiveness, and readiness for help from significant others (including professionals).

Influences on Parenting

Opportunities to experience parenting and observe others parent within a social setting are essential learning experiences for the development of parenting behaviors. The ability to parent is influenced by a multitude of factors that occur before, during, and after the birth of the infant. Previous life events, including degree of life stress/patterns of coping,[117,182,190] genetic endowment, being parented,[60,65,146] previous pregnancies,[97,116] anxiety and distress about parenting role,* and interpersonal relationships,[27,60,125,146] affect the experience of pregnancy and parenthood. The events of the current pregnancy,† their significance to the parent, and the availability of support and assistance influence parenting ability.‡

After birth, infant characteristics (e.g., responsiveness/vulnerability/severity of illness),[46,65,85] appearance,[22,52,114,134] parental feelings of loyalty and hope, the behavior of health professionals,§ separation from the infant,‖ an inability to protect their newborn from pain,[94,134,150] and hospital practices¶ may positively or negatively influence parents. Not only the occurrence of these events but also their meaning to the individual and the type of assistance received influence parenting abilities.

*References 43,53,65,81,82,85,125,134,146,182.
†References 27,76,101,115,122,146.
‡ References 89,122,125,134,146,182.
§References 43,53,63,81,82,101,112,114,125,132,135,190.
‖References 42,52,119,122,135,146,150.
¶References 22,42,43,62,65,76,85,89,99,112,122,132,146,192.

Cultural practices influence maternal and paternal attachment behaviors.* Studies indicate that cultural differences influence (1) parental emotional responses and perceptions of their infant's illness and disability, (2) parental utilization of services, and (3) parental interaction with health care providers.[25] Research demonstrates that how parents interact with their newborn varies based on their culture (e.g., Japanese mothers look at their babies more than Brazilian mothers do, who touch and interact more with them).[109] A recent study of Thai mothers in the neonatal intensive care unit (NICU) showed that the most frequent maternal behavior was touching (from infant's extremities to trunk), followed by inspection (of the infant's appearance and recognition of family traits), verbalization (e.g., to the infant and the nurse), and facial expression (e.g., smiling/crying/flat).[184] Viewing parental attachment behavior through the cultural eyes of the health care provider may result in negative assessments and labels about parent-infant attachment.[184] Differences in parent-infant interaction behaviors reflect cultural differences; therefore health care professionals' observations of these behaviors must be evaluated within the context of the family's culture.†

Steps of Attachment

Klaus and Kennell[101] have proposed nine steps in the process of attachment.

STEP 1: PLANNING THE PREGNANCY

Planning the pregnancy is the initial step of investment and commitment[146] in the life-altering prospect of parenthood. Pregnancies are planned in one of two ways: consciously or unconsciously. Who planned the pregnancy and why this particular time has been chosen are important indicators of the investment of each individual in the decision and in the pregnancy.

Carrying a pregnancy is not assurance that the baby is wanted. Although it may be a legal option, abortion may not be a cultural, moral, financial, or ethical option for the individual woman. Attachment of the mother (or father) to the infant is not ensured merely by the mother remaining pregnant, giving birth, and keeping the infant.

*References 25,85,93,117,134,141,155,163,164,171.

†References 11,93,114,134,141,155,163,164,171,184.

STEP 2: CONFIRMING THE PREGNANCY

Confirming the pregnancy occurs after the first and often subtle signs of pregnancy appear. Pregnancy confirmation begins the psychologic acceptance of the pregnancy. Delaying confirmation enables the fact of pregnancy to be denied and may influence progression to the acceptance stage.

STEP 3: ACCEPTING THE PREGNANCY

Accepting the pregnancy usually begins early in the pregnancy and is characterized by the emotional changes of primary narcissism, introversion, and passivity. Because the expectant mother is less interested in the outside world and more interested in her own inner world, the mother can become attuned to her own needs. Although she was previously engaged in active, extroverted behaviors, during the pregnancy she may contentedly participate in quieter, more introspective activities.

At this early stage of pregnancy, the fetus is not perceived by the woman as separate from herself but as an extension of her body. The psychologic changes of pregnancy have survival significance in that caring for herself ensures caring for the fetus as an integral part of herself.[117,146]

During the early months of pregnancy, the man and woman realize that parenting will require a major adjustment of prepregnancy roles, lifestyle, and relationships. The adaptation of parenthood is characterized by upheaval and change, losses and gains. Bombarded with phenomenal lifelong changes, the future parents experience the normal feeling of ambivalence.

STEP 4: FETAL MOVEMENT

Fetal movement, felt by the mother between 16 and 32 weeks of gestation, is the beginning of the acceptance of the fetus as an individual. Fetal movement is the first concrete evidence to the mother of the existence of another person within her. Hearing the baby's heartbeat, seeing the ultrasound images,[137] or experiencing an amniocentesis also confirms the reality of the fetus.[146] Fetal movement is such a significant event that often a pregnancy that began as unplanned and unwanted becomes wanted.

Perception of the first fetal movement is a happy event. When asked "How did you feel when the baby first moved?" most women respond in a happy tone and with a smile. Use of a negative tone or negative words to describe fetal movement is a concern because the individual (fetus) may already be perceived as an intruder.

STEP 5: ACCEPTING THE FETUS

Accepting the fetus as an individual begins with fetal movement. The fetus asserts individuality in controlling the movement; the mother can neither start nor stop these movements. With the realization of the concrete evidence of the presence of another person, parents begin the psychologic acceptance and personification of the fetus as a separate individual. Love for the fetus as a separate individual occurs as the parents invest a personality in the fetus and establish a relationship with that personality. Fantasies about how the baby looks, its sex, and the wish for a perfect, healthy infant are common.

Outwardly, preparations are made for the acceptance of an infant into the home; baby clothes and furniture are purchased, and a room is prepared. The fetus may be referred to by a nickname or a term of endearment. The baby's name may be chosen. Choosing a name is a highly personal and significant event. The meaning of the name and who chooses it illustrate the power holder and decision maker within the family. Prenatal questions such as the following may be asked after the birth to elicit information: "Do you have a nickname for the baby?" "Do you have a name picked out for the baby?" "Who picked it out?"

Whether the newborn meets parental expectations for "the right sex" may be crucially important for the parents to attach to the infant. "Do you have a sex preference for the baby?" may be asked before or after the birth to uncover this information. Often parents with a strong sex preference have chosen no names for a baby of the "wrong" gender. "It doesn't matter as long as it's healthy" is often heard and may indicate no conscious gender preference. However, unconsciously, the parents may have a strong gender preference as evidenced by a predominance of dreams about one gender. If dreams are equally divided between male and female children, there may indeed be no gender preference at the unconscious level.

Most parents are fearful of producing a defective child. This fear is experienced as dreams about dead, deformed, or damaged fetuses and babies or dreams with a central theme of destruction. These unconscious contents often are experienced as frightening nightmares that may be imbued with magical ideas such as "If I think (or talk about) it, it will come true." Both before and after birth, it is reassuring for parents to know that this is a common and scary phenomenon, that they aren't "crazy," and that the fears are not magical.

Parental expectations of the newborn are established before birth in the personification and relationship with the unseen, unheard fetus. After birth, the developmental task of parenthood is a working out of the discrepancy between the wished-for and the actual infant.[179] Before attachment to the actual infant can proceed, the fantasized child must be mourned.

STEP 6: LABOR AND BIRTH

Labor is a physiologic, maturational, and psychologic crisis for the family. Birth is the culmination of pregnancy and the reward for the work of labor. Parents' attitudes about the labor and birth experiences affect their reactions to the infant.[42] Newton and Newton[148] found mothers more likely to be pleased with their infant at first sight if the mothers were relaxed, calm, and cooperative; had rapport with the attendants; and received personalized, solicitous care. More recent research shows that continuous physical and emotional support during labor significantly improves birth outcomes for the mother (e.g., shortens labor duration, reduces the need for pain medication and operative vaginal and cesarean section birth) and the newborn (e.g., better Apgar scores, better/longer breast feeding, fewer NICU admissions, fewer complications of obstetric [OB] interventions because fewer OB interventions used). In addition to better physiologic outcomes, improved psychologic outcomes include (1) increase in maternal-infant attachment behaviors, (2) better confidence and ability to cope with labor, (3) better maternal satisfaction and personal control during labor, (4) enhanced maternal self-esteem, (5) positive attitudes toward mothering and family relationships, and (6) easier mothering (i.e., sees baby as less fussy).[75,167]

Paternal participation in labor and birth is an important issue. Many years ago, health care professionals saw no benefit to the presence of the father and even wished to exclude him because of imagined "horribles" such as increased infection rate, malpractice suits, and disruption of routines. Birth is a powerfully emotional experience; those who attend birth are more attached to the infant than those who do not attend.[101,122] Benefits attributed to a father's participation at labor and birth include use of less analgesia, a more supportive environment, and a deepened relationship[10] between parents and between parents and their infant.[122,158] Inclusion of the father in perinatal events may "hook" him for inclusion in parenting activities.[43,122] Rather than just a financial provider, fathering may be perceived as a psychologic necessity for both fathers and children.

Parental behaviors at birth indicate involvement and investment in the infant[71]:

- How does the mother or father look? At the sound of the infant's cry, parents smile and breathe a sigh of relief at this first breath of life. Support, joy, and happiness are positive feelings shared by couples at birth.
- What does the mother or father say? By speaking in a positive tone with words of affection and endearment, the parents relate to each other and to the new infant.
- What does the mother or father do? When offered the infant, both parents will reach out to take the infant. Spontaneously, parents engage in eye-to-eye contact and touch and explore the infant. Affectionate behaviors such as kissing, fondling, cuddling, and claiming characterize positive parental reactions.

A positive, self-affirming birth experience for the mother enhances her feelings of empowerment and self-esteem and thus her self-concept as a woman and mother.[75,146,167] A birth experience that does not meet parental expectations may have a negative effect on the self-concept of the mother, her perception of her ability to parent, and her relationship with the infant.[42] In fact, "so intricately are mother and infant entwined in a symbiotic relationship, that what is psychically positive for the mother is positive for the infant. What is psychically negative for the mother will affect the infant."[146] Labor and delivery that have been difficult or prolonged may influence the parents' overprotection, resentment, or antagonism toward the infant.[1]

So powerful is the labor and birth experience that women may be unable to proceed with parenting until psychic closure of the experience has occurred. Even women who experience a normal labor and birth process should recount the experience to others. Maternal perception of the events is obvious in tone and content of the recounting. ***Missing pieces***[1] is the term used to describe the aspects of labor and birth that are forgotten or unavailable to recall. Long labor, short labor, or medicated labor can cause missing pieces in the mother's memory of the birth. Labor that did not meet expectations because of difficulty, cesarean section, use of forceps, or episiotomy could also affect the mother.[1] To proceed with parenting, these women should be encouraged to fill in their knowledge gaps by asking questions or looking at pictures or films of the birth to reconstruct the situation.

STEP 7: SEEING

Seeing and touching are the species-specific ways in which humans attach to their young.[101] In a recent study, immediate attachment was facilitated by (1) positive maternal feelings toward the infant; (2) mother able to see infant immediately after birth; and (3) immediate contact between mother and infant.[22] Delayed attachment may occur when the infant is premature because he or she does not conform to parental expectations of a full-term baby.[22,42,184]

Eye contact between parents and their infant in the initial period after birth may be a positive release of parental feelings of warmth, closeness, and caring. As parents see and inspect the newborn, they begin claiming their infant—"He has my eyes"; "She has your nose"—and begin "letting go" of the prenatally fantasized child. Characteristics of each parent and the family are identified in the infant, and the newborn is claimed as a member of the family.[184]

The term ***en face position*** is used to describe the mother's (father's) eyes and the infant's eyes positioned in the same vertical plane.[101] This positioning enables the parent and the infant to look directly into each other's eyes, to focus, and to regard each other (Figure 29-1).

The newborn infant is an active participant in the acquaintance process, as he or she cues the mother with eye-to-eye contact. Even minutes-old newborns see and show a preference for the human face (within 7 to 12 inches from their face). The newborn can visually follow the parent's face and voice and signal the parent with facial expressions, movement, and vocalization, including a distress cry when separated from body contact with mother (see Chapter 13).

Deterrents to the infant's full participation include removal to the nursery, medication (from analgesia), and eye prophylaxis. Unless medically indicated (necessary for physical survival), newborns should remain with their parents after birth.[122] Because eye prophylaxis irritates and interferes with vision, the "routine" instillation immediately after birth (in the delivery room) can be delayed until after the initial acquaintance process is completed.

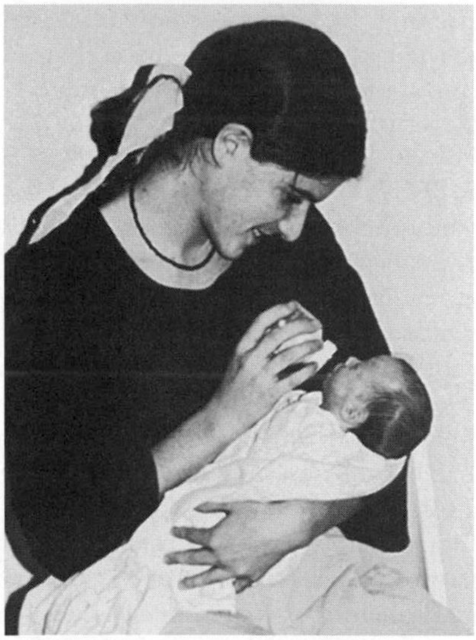

FIGURE 29-1 *En face position:* infant is held in close contact (mother's body touching infant's); mother is looking at infant *en face;* bottle is perpendicular to mouth; milk is in tip of nipple. (From Klaus MH, Kennel JH: *Parent-infant bonding,* ed 2, St Louis, 1982, Mosby.)

STEP 8: TOUCHING

Touching is important to the adult as a means of tactile and sensory knowledge of the infant. To the neonate, the stimulus *hunger*[1,2] is satisfied by the parents' touch and ministrations.

In exploring the infant, parents systematically use fingertip contact with the infant's extremities. Gradually, there is progression to palm contact with the infant's trunk (Figure 29-2). With the healthy term infant, this progression occurs within minutes of the first contact. After gaining confidence and preliminary knowledge, the parent will enfold the infant close to the parent's ventrum (a cuddling position).

With the preterm infant, this characteristic progression may take hours, days, or several visits (see Figure 29-2). Fear of harming the small, fragile preterm infant prevents parents from feeling at ease in touching him or her.[184] Until the parents feel confident that their actions will not harm the infant, they may be reticent to use palm contact with the trunk (vital organs). Not only the use of nurturing maternal touch but also the vulnerability of the premature

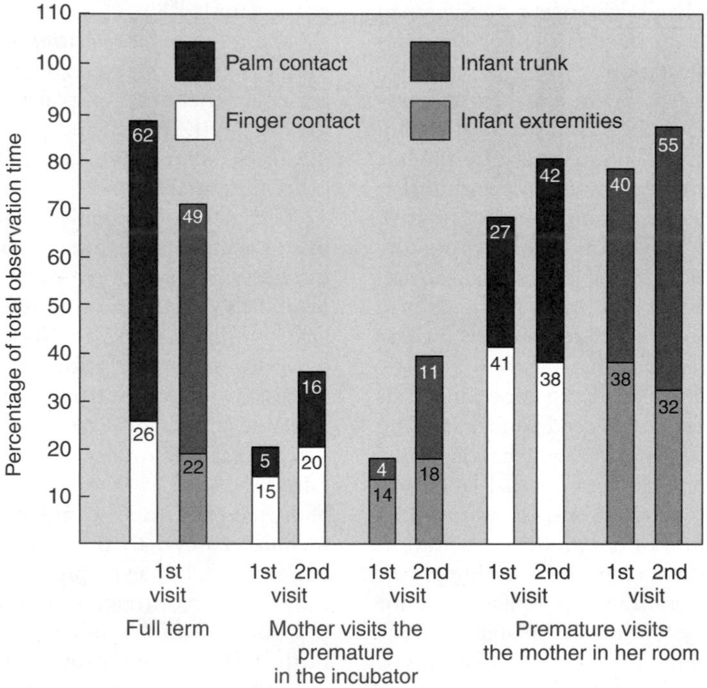

FIGURE 29-2 Fingertip and palm contact on trunk or extremities in three groups of mothers: (1) 12 mothers of term infants at their first visit, (2) 9 mothers who visited their premature infants in incubators in the NICU, and (3) 14 mothers whose premature infants were brought to their maternity rooms and placed in their beds. (From Klaus MH, Kennel JH: *Parent-infant bonding,* ed 2, St Louis, 1982, Mosby.)

infant affect how touch is perceived by the infant. A recent study showed that nurturing maternal touch was associated with more secure attachment in robust preterms and with less secure attachment in the most vulnerable infants.

Holding and cuddling the infant are significantly different from touching and exploring. The amount of holding influences mother-infant interaction with preterm infants.[107] Mothers who have only seen and touched their infant still experience "empty arms." The species-specific behavior of touch is not completely satisfied until the parent can hold the infant. Most mothers have a preference for holding their infants on the left. Explanations for this preference include hand dominance, importance of maternal heart beat, left breast sensitivity, and advantages in monitoring the infant. A more recent hypothesis proposes that maternal affective signals (both visual and auditory) are given to the infant's free left ear and processed by the more advanced right cerebral hemisphere.[175]

STEP 9: CAREGIVING

The final step of attachment, caregiving, is important for psychic closure of the task of bonding. A meta-synthesis of nine qualitative studies found two simultaneous processes necessary in the transition to motherhood: (1) engagement, a commitment to mothering that involves active attachment to the infant, experiencing the infant's presence, and involvement in caregiving for the infant; and (2) growth and transformation, which characterize the change of a woman into the new "self" of a mother.[146] Men also make the transition to fatherhood in the early postpartal period. A recent qualitative study of first-time fathers indicates that those who wanted to be highly involved in the care of their baby reported not feeling supported by the health care provider/hospital policies to engage in paternal and parental behaviors that favor involvement with their infant.[43] Fathers experienced more negative (63%) than positive (37%) interactions with nurses during the postpartum period.[43] Another study showed that 50% of new parents are worried about their ability to competently parent, the change in their relationship, and whether loneliness and boredom would be experienced by the mother who would be at home with the infant.[125] In assisting parental transition, nurses and all health care professionals should support, intervene, and utilize all encounters with both new parents as "teaching moments and opportunities."[43,121]

The relationship between the primary caregiver and the infant is reciprocal. In the caregiving relationship, both care provider and infant give to and receive from each other.[63,146] The physical and emotional needs of the helpless infant are satisfied by parental caregiving behaviors such as feeding, soothing, grooming, and playing. Based on the infant's ability to perceive and receive these ministrations, the infant responds to the care provider. Parental expectations of newborn responses include quieting, sucking, clinging and cuddling, looking, smiling, and vocalizing. The parent's capability to soothe and satisfy the infant provides emotional satisfaction and positive feedback about the parent's competency.

Personal needs for comfort, maintenance of homeostasis, and relief from painful experiences are infant expectations of the relationship with the care provider. Care-eliciting behaviors (e.g., crying, visual following, smiling) are neonatal cues used to signal the care provider that attention is needed. Relief from discomfort enables the infant to respond positively to the care provider. The infant experiences the world through the caregiver and quickly learns that the environment is either nurturing and loving or hostile and nonresponsive. Consistent, predictable nurturing and caregiving enable the infant to develop a sense of trust in the caregiver, the world, and the self (see Chapter 13).

Care by parents is the ideal neonatal care situation, because the infant learns and reacts to one set of cues or caregiving behaviors. Cared for by one or two people, the infant can regulate his physiologic behavioral processes (i.e., autonomic, neuroendocrine, behavioral, electrophysiologic) and develop synchrony with the parents.[112,122,146] Single caregiving improves the establishment of biorhythms of the neonate for sleep-wake cycles, feeding, and visual attentiveness. Multiple caregivers confuse the infant, increase distress with feeding, cause irritability, and upset visual attention. Care by parents provides for mutual cuing and acquaintance and a natural setting for observation of parent-infant interaction.[89,112,122,132]

PSYCHOLOGIC ADJUSTMENTS TO A SICK NEWBORN

The birth of a sick newborn with its consequent family disruption represents to the perinatal health care team a unique crisis, a dangerous opportunity[2] within which to practice preventive health care.[182,192] For the involved individual and family, this stressful event results in a period of psychologic disorganization during which their usual problem-solving mechanisms may not be adequate to cope with the events presented to them.[31] In addition to confronting this situational crisis, the individual or family must master the normal developmental process of parenthood.

Parental behavior and responses are determined not only by preexisting personality factors, social and cultural variables, and interactions with significant others[116] but also by the immediate situation in which the parents are placed.[42,122] In one recent study, six major sources of parental stress in the NICU were identified:

- Preexisting and concurrent personal and family factors
- Prenatal and perinatal experiences
- Infant illness, treatments, and appearance*
- Concerns about the infant's outcome
- Loss of the parental role†
- Health care providers‡

Situational factors can have an important bearing on the family's ability to cope with the crisis and thus affect the overall outcome (Box 29-1).

Families are psychologically vulnerable after the birth of a sick infant. During this period of temporary disorganization, there is a heightened receptivity to accepting help and being responsive to change, because the family is struggling for a way to cope with the crisis. Significant potentialities exist for individual and family emotional growth and development.[22,30,53,85] The perinatal health team has an opportunity to influence how the individual and family adapt to the crisis.§ By providing appropriate supportive interventions coupled with enlightened policies and attitudes that reflect family-centered principles (Box 29-2), the team can positively influence the family's coping, thus enhancing the likelihood for a successful resolution of the crisis and ultimately a healthy parent-child relationship. ||

Studies show a discrepancy between nurses' knowledge about the necessity of and their current practice of family-centered care.[157] Current practice of family-centered care scored significantly lower than scores representing necessity: Nurses do not consistently practice what they know to be necessary! NICU nurses scored significantly lower on the necessity scale than did pediatric and pediatric intensive care unit (PICU) nurses; nurses with fewer than 10 years of practice scored higher on the necessary and current use of family-centered principles than did nurses with more practice experience.[157] Organizational barriers to implementation include (1) the design of the health care system; (2) the lack of emotional support, guidance, and direction for the staff; (3) the lack of recognition, confidence, and support for nursing autonomy and skills to perform family-centered care; and (4) beliefs that dealing with families is stressful, interferes with care of the infant, and is "not part of my job."[5,37,53,157]

Family-centered care principles stress that parents are the most important persons in their infant's life, that they have expertise in caring for the infant, and that their values and beliefs should be central during NICU care.[70,84,89] Family-centered care demands a change from task-oriented, health care provider–centered care to a collaborative, relationship-based model of family

*References 22,42,52,65,114,134.

†References 22,42,53,85,89,114,134,146,192.

‡References 53,76,81,82,85,114.

§References 22,53,65,81,82,85,132,192.

||References 22,42,53,65,76,85,89,112,116,122,135,138,182.

BOX 29-1 SITUATIONAL FACTORS AFFECTING PARENTAL COPING*

1. The behaviors and attitudes of the hospital staff (physicians, nurses, and allied health professionals)
2. The sensitivity used in the process of separation and transfer of the infant to the intensive care unit or, in some cases, the referral hospital
3. The flexibility of hospital policy concerning parental and sibling involvement and visitation in the nursery
4. The instruction of parents in their infant's individual behaviors and characteristics (thus facilitating appropriate parent-child interaction and reciprocity) (see Chapter 13)
5. The staff's comprehension and appreciation of the psychosocial functioning of families and the family's responses and adaptation to stress and crisis
6. The employment of emotionally supportive intervention programs for parents within the nursery setting
7. The development of appropriate discharge planning to provide adequate follow-up care to the infant and family

* References 22,26,53,63,64,70,76,80,85,116,135,150,190.

BOX 29-2 PRINCIPLES OF FAMILY-CENTERED NEONATAL CARE

1. Family-centered neonatal care should be based on open and honest communication between parents and professionals on medical and ethical issues.
2. To work with professionals in making informed treatment choices, parents must have available to them the same facts and interpretation of those facts as the professionals, including medical information presented in meaningful formats, information about uncertainties surrounding treatments, information from parents whose children have been in similar medical situations, and access to the chart and rounds discussions.
3. In medical situations involving very high mortality and morbidity, great suffering, and/or significant medical controversy, fully informed parents should have the right to make decisions about aggressive treatment for their infants.
4. Expectant parents should be offered information about adverse pregnancy outcomes and be given the opportunity to state in advance their treatment preferences if their infant is born extremely prematurely and/or critically ill.
5. Parents and professionals must work together to acknowledge and alleviate the pain of infants in the neonatal intensive care unit (NICU).
6. Parents and professionals must work together to ensure an appropriate environment for infants in the NICU.
7. Parents and professionals must work together to ensure the safety and efficacy of neonatal treatments.
8. Parents and professionals must work together to develop nursery policies and programs that promote parenting skills and encourage maximum involvement of families with their hospitalized infants.
9. Parents and professionals must work together to promote meaningful long-term follow-up for all high-risk NICU survivors.
10. Parents and professionals must acknowledge that critically ill newborns can be harmed by overtreatment, as well as undertreatment, and must insist that laws and treatment policies be based on compassion. Parents and professionals must work together to promote awareness of the needs of NICU survivors with disabilities to ensure adequate support for them and their families. Parents and professionals must work together to decrease disability through universal prenatal care.

Modified from Harrison H: The principles for family-centered neonatal care, *Pediatrics* 92:643, 1993.

advocacy and empowerment.[53,70,89,112,127] Roles for families in family-centered care include (1) advocate for their infant, (2) peer support to other families, (3) participant in hospital committees, (4) collaboration with and education of clinicians, and (5) change-agent in health care settings.[48] Box 29-3 contains key components of family-centered care desired by families; they are remarkably similar to the "Principles of Family-Centered Neonatal Care" in Box 29-2. A web-based tool, the "Family-Centered Care Map" (available at *www.wickedstickz.com/samples/fcc/index.htm*), has been developed and studied.[49] This tool is based on 63 potentially better practices (PBPs) and is a joint effort of three NICUs (and their families), Vermont Oxford Network's Neonatal Intensive Care Quality Improvement Collaborative, and the Institute for Family-Centered Care. Use of the "Family-Centered Care Map" results in (1) improved growth for extremely-low-birth-weight (ELBW) preterms, (2) decreased length of stay for ELBW preterms by 13 days, and (3) better implementation of family-centered care principles.[91]

BOX 29-3 WHAT FAMILIES WANT IN FAMILY-CENTERED CARE[90]

- To be consistently and respectfully involved in decisions about the health care of their family member and their family members to be involved in ways they choose
- Health care providers to listen to the family's observations and incorporate their preferences about treatment into the plan of care
- Useful and understandable information from health care providers
- Personal connection—a relationship with health care providers; need personal connection and to be able to trust those providing care
- Patient comfort and pain control; important to family (and patient's) perception of the hospital experience
- Information and support for handling transitions in health care

Fenwick's research reports that mothers perceive their relationship with NICU nurses as either facilitating or inhibiting their ability to mother their preterms in the NICU. Actions that facilitate mothering are family-centered. Facilitative nursing actions include fostering the relationship between mother and infant by (1) assisting mothers to gain intimate knowledge and caregiving opportunities, (2) acknowledging the importance of the dyadic mother-infant and father-infant relationship, (3) recognizing that the mother is the infant's primary caregiver, (4) enhancing mother-infant interaction opportunities, and (5) collaborating with parents and relinquishing control to parents.[53,112]

Inhibitive nursing actions prevent and prohibit mothers and fathers from physical closeness and intimacy with their premature infants. Inhibitive nursing action (1) promotes patriarchal, authoritarian style of care delivery; (2) focuses on "protecting" the infant (from the parents); (3) maintains the nurse as the "expert" who retains control by directing and "allowing" parent involvement; and (4) dismisses parental worries, concerns, rights, and skills.[53] In the presence of inhibitive nursing actions, mothers are left with the feeling of "struggling to mother" in the NICU.[53] Mothers who are alienated and disaffected by these encounters feel angry, frustrated, distressed, inadequate, unsure, and anxious.[53] These feelings may result in (1) an inability to resume the relationship with the infant that has been interrupted by the stay in the NICU, (2) a delay in the mothering process, (3) feelings of depression or anxiety, and (4) affected perceptions of how they see themselves as mothers.[53] Maternal strategies to deal with highly tense NICU relationships include guarding and speaking out about the situation. Guarding strategies include (1) withholding their feelings about inhibitive nursing actions and smoothing over the relationship with the nurse(s), (2) withdrawing from the nursery, and (3) blaming oneself to justify the nurse's actions.[53] Mothers who spoke up did so only after tolerating a number of incidents, and often it was the father who complained. The consequences for speaking out may include (1) earning a reputation with the staff as a "troublemaker," (2) recrimination in the form of sanctions and punitive actions that result in a "struggle to mother," or (3) becoming a disenfranchised mother.[53]

As discussed, attachment is a complex developmental process. Many interrelated factors influence parental behavior and attachment toward the infant.[22] These include the infant, gender of the infant, social class, birth order, parental attitudes and expectations, events of the newborn period and post-discharge period, and level of family functioning.* Very important in any neonatal illness and subsequent hospitalization is the disruption and stress that is frequently created in the nuclear family system. It has been demonstrated that the family's functioning and its adaptation to stress have important effects on the family's relationship with the infant and the infant's later development. A crucial task of the perinatal health care team is to intervene in such a way as to assist families in using the unfortunate event of the birth of their sick infant to maximize their growth, adaptation, and reorganization during this period.*

To assist parents through the difficult experience of having a sick infant, it is helpful to identify the psychologic tasks and emotional reactions they experience. This section describes the six psychologic issues facing families; it discusses the clinical and behavioral indicators that parents are struggling with and then suggests interventions that the perinatal health care team can employ to help families. It is extremely important to remember that these are generalizations and that each family or person must be approached individually.[146] In addition, in assessing families' reactions, it is critical to look at how they cope over time. Initially, there may be a tremendous amount of upset, disruption, and upheaval within the individual or family system that eventually may lead to improved functioning and a sense of growth and mastery. The key is how the individuals or families reorganize, how able they are to return to a state of equilibrium, the coping strategies they are able to develop, and whether they are adaptive or maladaptive. Attachment and parenthood are complex, interactional developmental processes that must evolve and unfold over time.

Kaplan and Mason[97] describe four psychologic tasks with which parents of premature infants must deal:

1. Anticipatory grieving and withdrawal from the relationship established during pregnancy
2. Parental acknowledgment of feelings of guilt and failure
3. Resumption of the relationship with the infant that had been previously disrupted
4. Preparation to take the infant home

Two additional tasks are also significant:

5. Crisis events related to labor and delivery
6. Adaptation to the intensive care environment[53]

In general, these six psychologic tasks can be applied to any parent's reaction to a sick infant, with additional specific issues arising, depending on whether the infant was premature or born with a congenital anomaly.

*References 42,53,76,85,99,116,122,182.

*References 22,42,53,65,76,85,89,116,122,134,150,182,192.

Labor and Delivery

The first psychologic task involves working through the crisis events surrounding the labor and delivery. Medical problems occurring at any point during the pregnancy or delivery that threaten the health or survival of the fetus or mother can result in the parents delaying their planning and making an emotional investment in the fetus or infant. Parents may psychologically withdraw from the pregnancy as a way of protecting themselves. The parents of an infant born prematurely often do not have the necessary psychologic and physical time to prepare. This deprivation of time may interfere with the parents' ability to complete the final steps of attachment described earlier. Parents who have been concentrating on themselves in a healthy, narcissistic way may not yet be ready to transfer their investment to the infant, because they have been prematurely thrust into the role of parents.[85,122] There is an overwhelming sense of losing control of the events of the labor and delivery and their timing. Parents' wishes to retain the pregnancy can influence their attitude about the delivery and the infant.

On the other hand, some parents react in the opposite way: They may wish to be rid of the pregnancy as a way of dealing with their ambivalent feelings about the infant or their fear of the unknown and the uncertainty facing them. Many mothers of premature infants feel that their infants are alien[22,53,85]; they do not feel that the infant is really theirs, making it easier to have feelings of rejection toward the infant. In addition to feeling insufficient and inadequate about their ability to deliver an infant at term, they feel empty inside, as if something is missing. This seems to occur because the mother who has been predominantly concerned about herself, her body, and the fetus growing inside is not ready to transfer that emotional investment outside of herself. With a premature birth, there is usually a heightened sense of emergency and concern about the health and survival of the infant and, at times, the mother, who herself may have suffered complications.

In the case of a full-term infant born with a problem despite a problem-free pregnancy, there is a sense of overwhelming shock and disappointment.[150] Parents immediately sense the problem; as their apprehension mounts, they frequently imagine and fantasize the worst. Parents of a newborn with a malformation normally experience lowered self-esteem and view this event as an affront to their reproductive capabilities. The mother specifically views it as a failure of her feminine role. Parents often feel that they have failed and that the infant symbolically represents their own defectiveness. Parents not only fear for the infant, they fear for themselves and what this infant may mean to their future. The reaction of the parents is based on the specific psychologic, social, and cultural meaning of the defect to the parents and the manner in which the problem is discussed and handled with the parents by the health care team.[101]

The emotional reactions and feelings that parents have at and after the delivery of a sick infant range from shock, fright, and panic to anxiety and helplessness.[122,150] Parents may be so overwhelmed by the events that initially they may block any observable emotional response or affect. Staff interventions at this time are extremely important, because they lay the foundations for subsequent interactions between parents and health professionals. Early comments and influential statements during this critical time can have lasting impressions in the minds of parents. This is also an emotionally difficult time for physicians and nurses, because they too are struggling with their own feelings of inadequacy, failure, and helplessness. Unconsciously, in an attempt to deal with their own feelings, staff may withdraw from parents and not be emotionally available to help. This is a normal response but one that needs to be guarded against, because it only perpetuates a breakdown in relationships and communication with parents that are greatly needed at this time. Many helpful interventions can be employed that are sensitive and supportive and that facilitate the emerging relationship between the parents and their infant.

EARLY COMMUNICATION

In the labor and delivery phase, early communication with both parents is essential. Parents normally are apprehensive and extremely sensitive to explicit or implicit cues, such as actual statements by the staff, the atmosphere, looks, or a tone of voice that may indicate how things are progressing. Because of the emphasis on prepared childbirth, parents are extremely sophisticated in their knowledge of labor and delivery practices and immediately sense some deviation from what they expected. Prompt, direct explanations presented in a calm manner are important and reassuring to parents. This explanation of the process of what is or will be happening can be effective, because it helps organize the parents at a time when they are extremely vulnerable and feeling out of control.

Although it is normal for the staff to be guarded, members of the health care team should tell the parents the known facts and what actually is being done for their infant without giving any diagnosis, prognosis, or forecast for the future course of the infant. Avoiding or not talking to parents only accelerates parental anxiety and adds to their growing fantasies or distortions. It has been well established and documented that parents' fantasies about their infant's problems are usually worse than the reality. Parents often report that when they actually saw their infant, they were relieved because they had imagined that the infant would appear worse.

SUPPORT OF STAFF

It is also important that one of the staff members stays with the parents through labor, delivery, and recovery to offer continuous support and reassure the parents that communication will continue as soon as more information is known. This, again, is an uncomfortable time for the staff, because they may feel helpless and therefore may avoid parents or revert to performing more technical activities. Some parents may need someone to be with them, not only to talk to them but also, more important, to listen. On the other hand, some parents may not be able to talk or verbalize their concerns or fears. Others may wish to be alone with each other or any other significant person in their life. Because of the varying responses and needs of people, it is extremely important to be sensitive to individual differences in approaching parents.

Parents have expressed their desire to be together when given "bad news."[70,172] As much as possible, talking to both parents at the same time is helpful when discussing the infant's condition. This decreases their distortions and misconceptions, increases the communication and support between parents, and prevents either parent from feeling excluded. The assumption is commonly made that the father is in a better emotional state to hear about the infant; this misconception leads health professionals to mistakenly exclude or "spare" the mother, which only postpones her ability to begin to cope with the reality of her infant's condition. Sparing the mother may cause the parents to be in different stages of their understanding of the infant's medical condition and in different emotional states. Because emotional support between parents is so critical, the staff should avoid sparing, because it can add to the parents' difficulty in being attuned to each other's needs and creates more opportunities for the parents to be out of synchrony with each other. Both mothers and fathers of critically ill newborns generally find each other to be the greatest source of support in the first 2 weeks of NICU hospitalization.[122,190]

SEEING THE INFANT

The question usually arises about the value of the parents seeing their infant, especially if the infant is very small, not likely to survive, or profoundly malformed. Generally, it is assumed that it is psychologically better for parents to have had the opportunity to see their infant, but this must be individualized for each family and newborn. Seeing the infant helps facilitate attachment,[22,122,184] decrease exaggerated fantasies, decrease withdrawal from the infant, and enhance the parents' ability to grasp the reality of the situation. Because of the need to respect individual differences in people, the best approach is to give parents the opportunity to decide whether they together or individually want to see the infant. The opportunity to see and touch the infant in the delivery room or before transport may reduce stressful feelings verbalized by parents who see their infant for the first time in the NICU.

Ultimately this decision should be made by the parents with the support of the health care team. It is not uncommon to find a well-meaning family member, physician, nurse, or social worker advising the parents or making the decision himself or herself and concluding it would be in the parents' best interests not to see the infant. The following arguments are given: "It's better not to get attached." or "It would make them cry or upset them to see the anomaly." or "They could not handle it." or "They would lose control." This decision is for the parents, not the professional, to make.

Some parents may know unequivocally what they want to do; others may be ambivalent or indecisive. It is the role of the professional to give the parents assistance (information and support) in making the decision. The parents may need time to think about it or may have to discuss their fear and ambivalence first, before being able to decide. They may need some factual information and preparation from the professional, such as the appearance of the infant and a description of the equipment. They may need assurance that someone will stay with them. Although time often is a factor and a decision must be made quickly, it is important to move at the parents' pace. The professional should still follow as much as possible the principle of facilitating the parents in seeing the infant. If this is not possible for medical reasons related to the mother's condition, a self-developing or digital picture can be taken. If it is medically possible for the parents to touch or hold the infant, the parents should be offered that opportunity. Touching or holding not only facilitates attachment[22,107,122,184] but also can provide parents with an emotional experience that is sustaining and reassuring, helping them proceed through a critical time of separation.

The parents are very sensitive to the staff's attitude toward the infant as reflected by their comments and the manner in which the staff handle the infant. If the infant is regarded with respect and treated as important, the parent is given the feeling that the infant is seen as valued and worthwhile. This is especially important for parents of an infant with a congenital anomaly; the parents could wonder if their infant is viewed as "damaged goods" by society. In describing the infant to the parent, present a balanced picture of both the normal and abnormal aspects of the infant. In discussing the infant with the parents, staff should refer to the infant by name, if they have named the infant; this helps personalize the infant and establish the infant's unique identity.

CAREGIVING

To reinforce the caregiving needs of parents, discuss with them their plans to feed their infant. Support and encouragement should be given whether the parents have decided on breast feeding or bottle feeding. In most situations, breast feeding a sick infant may be possible. Many mothers can pump their breasts for milk that eventually will be given to the infant. There are many psychologic and physiologic reasons why breast feeding or pumping may be beneficial for mothers and infants alike (see Chapter 18). The breast-feeding or pumping experience helps the mother feel close to her infant and helps her feel that she has some control over what is happening to her infant; she can uniquely contribute to her infant's care in a way no one else can. Fathers, too, can participate in this activity by their support and interest in the actual breast feeding or the pumping and milk-collection activities. Many mothers can pump and eventually put the infant to breast, but others cannot because of emotional stresses, the condition of the infant, the length of time until the infant can feed, and the waning interest of the mother. Regardless of eventual success, the mother should be encouraged to try if she has an interest; then she can feel that she made an attempt to relate to her infant in this way. If a mother does not plan to breast feed or pump or if she tries but does not continue, she should not be made to feel guilty or that she failed in her role. She is already vulnerable to these feelings, having had an infant born with problems.

After the delivery, when the mother is taken to her room without a healthy infant, she usually experiences a void, as though an amputation has occurred.[65,101] She and those around her are beginning to grieve. The interventions of the staff should be flexible and sensitive to the individual needs of the family. Empathy, responsiveness, and an ability to listen to the parents are important at this time.[122]

Encouraging parents to verbalize and express their feelings and concerns (at their own pace), although difficult to do at times, is useful to the parents. Listening is as important to parents as giving them information.[76] Avoiding their grief gives the mother and father the impression that they are "bad parents" for having feelings of sadness, anger, guilt, or loss; this only increases their level of guilt and isolation. Prescribing tranquilizers also gives the message that is it not permissible to talk about what has happened to them and their infant. Tranquilizers only increase the feelings of unreality that normally are experienced. This stifles the parents' coping mechanisms at a time when the parents should begin to come to terms with what has happened.

Room assignments are a very personal matter, and the mother should be given a choice of where she will stay. Some mothers want to stay in a regular maternity unit; for others, this is too painful and they want to be in a separate area. Flexible visiting guidelines[36,62,122] for the father and other significant persons are essential so they can support one another through a difficult, uncertain period.

In talking to parents, bear in mind that the parents do not remember much of what has been said; it is very difficult for them to assimilate all that has happened, both cognitively and emotionally. It is important for the staff to move at the parents' own pace. If the infant has been transferred or the chances for survival are limited, the mother should be discharged or given a pass to visit the infant as soon as possible. It is also important to acknowledge to the mother (and father) that they are parents and that they did give birth to a baby. They need the congratulatory cards, gifts, and attention that they would have received normally.

Anticipatory Grieving

After labor and delivery, parents are struggling with the second psychologic task of anticipatory grieving and withdrawal from the relationship established during pregnancy. This task requires that parents acknowledge that their infant's life is endangered or that the newborn might die. Events surrounding the labor, delivery, and postpartum period may have indicated to the parents that their infant's chances for survival are diminished. If this has occurred, parents can then become involved in anticipatory grieving and withdrawal from the relationship established during pregnancy. Studies have shown that the decision to transfer an infant to a NICU alone is likely to initiate an anticipatory grief reaction.[42,150]

Parents also may experience feelings of grief and sadness over the loss of the expected, idealized child that they had wished for during the pregnancy. For some parents, attaching to a critically ill or malformed infant may be too overwhelming; parents may withdraw from the infant in an attempt to protect themselves from their feelings of hurt, disappointment, and guilt.[22,59,85] Some parents may feel ambivalent[85] about the infant; they may feel they could not love or cope with an infant who might die or who would have significant physical or mental problems. Feeling uncertain about whether they want the infant to survive can cause feelings of guilt that may cause the parents to withdraw from the infant as a way of avoiding confronting these difficult, painful feelings.

During this period, parents may find themselves in a very stressful position; they are faced with the task of balancing the painful realities of confronting a possible loss against their hopes of the intact survival of their infant.[70] The emotional withdrawal and grieving that parents experience is normal during the critical time that the infant's life is endangered or when parents are faced with the possibility that their infant may have a life-long problem. This withdrawal becomes pathologic only if it continues beyond the time the infant demonstrates definite signs (to the parents) of improvement and survival. In the case of a newborn with a permanent developmental or physical disability, parents who cannot grieve their idealized infant may maintain this withdrawal, which might lead to attachment difficulties and subsequent cognitive and emotional consequences for the infant.[179]

PARENTAL RESPONSES

Parents exhibit many emotional responses and behaviors that indicate they are struggling with the anticipatory grieving and withdrawal. Some parents are very sad, depressed, and teary, and others may be highly anxious, at times bordering on panic states; others react by having a flat affect, withdrawing, and appearing apathetic. Some parents may exhibit very angry, hostile, confrontational behavior as a way of dealing with their distress. Others may deny the situation by optimistically feeling that "everything will be OK."

Parents who typically are verbal may ask questions reflecting their concerns about their infant's survival; this is especially true after the infant has received medical attention and decisions are being made about treatment, including transfer to a NICU. The questions they ask physicians and nurses may include "Will he make it?" "What do you think his chances are?" "He'll be OK, won't he?" "Have you seen other babies with this problem?" "Do other babies make it?" and "How long will he be in the hospital?" Parents struggling with their fears may resist seeing, touching, or visiting the infant. If they do visit the infant in the NICU, they may remain distant by having little or no eye contact with the infant, refusing to touch, standing far from the warmer or incubator, and asking few or no questions of the staff. Parents may be reluctant to name the infant; when they do refer to the infant, they say "it," "she," "he," or "the baby." If the infant has been given a special or treasured family name, they may be reluctant to use it.

A common phenomenon occurs when parents, being protective of each other, discourage each other's involvement with the infant. This is especially true at the time of transport, when the transport nurse may suggest to the father or family members that the infant be shown to the mother before leaving. Many fathers are afraid this will increase the emotional attachment to the infant and thus the feelings of disappointment and loss if the infant should die. The father is usually very apprehensive about how to handle the mother's feelings of grief in addition to his own. This type of behavior also is true with regard to medical information; it is not uncommon for one parent to request that all communication go through him or her. The response is "My spouse is too upset or anxious and couldn't handle hearing any bad news." Many times it is actually the parent making the request who is most anxious and who is dealing with this anxiety by projecting it onto the other partner. Work and child-care responsibilities, transportation difficulties, and financial limitations are all legitimate reasons that parents may be unable to have frequent contact with their infant. However, these factors also may serve as unconscious ways to maintain distance from the infant.

Keep in mind that withdrawal and grieving are part of a necessary and natural process.[22] For parents to develop an attachment to and accept the reality of their infant's condition, they must experience their feelings of grief, sadness, anger, guilt, and disappointment over the loss of the expected infant.[179] This grieving serves to free the parents' emotional energy so that they can interact with and become attuned to their infant. Grieving enhances the parents' availability to the infant. This availability aids in their feeling competent to handle their infant. The goal, then, of the perinatal health care team's interventions is to help the family realize that their feelings are natural and normal and will be accepted.[22] Parents need permission to have their feelings. It is essential to acknowledge to parents that it is normal to be afraid of attaching to an infant who might die or have a handicap. Giving permission diminishes the guilt that the parents may feel about their behavior being abnormal or about being bad parents because they are afraid. Simple statements such as "Many parents tell us they are afraid of getting close to their baby" or "It's scary to attach when you think the baby may die" are helpful.

Sometimes it is useful for parents to verbalize their actual fears. They may fear their infant dying, being retarded, or being paralyzed. Once their fears are clarified in their minds and either confirmed or refuted by the medical staff, it is usually easier for parents to begin to accept their infant's diagnosis and prognosis and begin relating to the infant. Social workers can provide valuable emotional support to families in helping them deal with their realistic and unrealistic concerns.

COMMUNICATING MEDICAL INFORMATION

The role of the health care professionals in communicating medical information is important. There are many schools of thought about how to approach parents, ranging from being extremely cautious and pessimistic ("paint the bleakest picture") to being encouraging and optimistic ("give parents hope"). Although the approach should be individualized for each family, some professionals feel a balanced approach is the most beneficial. In a recent study, parents stated that information should be accurate, current, and comprehensive but not unduly pessimistic.[76] Parents need a realistic assessment of the situation that is honest and direct. Acknowledge the infant's condition and possible problems, but do not inundate parents with every potential problem that can arise.

Parents who hear "brain damage," "retarded," or "the baby will die" are not likely to forget these statements. These statements can linger in the minds of parents and adversely influence how they relate to their newborn.[80] They may believe that some day "brain damage will show up" or that the infant is susceptible and frail and needs to be treated cautiously for fear of a life-threatening condition. These children may become victims of the ***vulnerable child syndrome,***[4,56,80,154] a condition in which a child is overprotected by his or her parents and treated as if he or she had a medical problem or is in danger of death when neither is any longer the case. Parents who are told their newborn may die may have trouble attaching or becoming emotionally invested. When talking to parents, physicians and nurses should be judicious and careful in making statements of a sensitive nature. Definitive statements should be used only when appropriate and necessary. The long-term emotional implications of such statements should be weighed.

There are several other guidelines in communicating medical information to parents. As discussed, parents' perceptions of their infant's condition are extremely important, remain in parents' minds, and can affect their relationship with the infant. Parents easily misperceive information given to them. They may believe that a patent ductus arteriosus (PDA) indicates open-heart surgery and therefore worry that their infant has a heart condition. Or perhaps they think a bilirubin problem means their infant has liver disease. Therefore in beginning any discussion with parents, it is essential to determine and address their perceptions. A staff member might say, "Could you tell me what you understand about your baby's condition?" This will give the physician or nurse the opportunity to correct any misinformation or misconceptions and to hear about the parents' concerns. The perceived morbidity of the baby is a source of stress for both mothers and fathers. Parents' perceptions of the severity of their infant's illness are complex, change over time, and are affected by parental anxiety, infant size, amount and type of equipment and treatments, and amount and type of information received from health care providers.[80] A team member might specifically ask about the parents' concerns or worries: "Could you tell me what concerns you have about your baby?" Asking this can make communication between the perinatal health care team and parents more meaningful and helpful; unless the team deals with the parents' anxiety, discussions become one-sided lectures and benefit only the professional. Discussions should be a dialog between parent and professional.

During the course of a discussion and again at the end, it is useful to determine parents' interpretations of what has been said and modify and clarify as needed. The staff should avoid overloading a parent with lengthy explanations that are too technical. It is more productive to move at a pace that the parent can assimilate the information presented; it is not necessary to describe the entire course of respiratory distress syndrome or bronchopulmonary dysplasia. It is always preferable to use simple language that is understandable to a layperson. For some parents, the use of statistics is helpful; for others, it is not. Statistics can be confusing, because they do not apply to the individual case and can be misinterpreted easily. When asked about the frequency of brain damage with a grade III intraventricular hemorrhage, a team member might say, "A majority of these babies have some neurologic problem, but some do not." Vivid modifiers such as "This is the worst case of sepsis we have ever had" or "Your baby is the sickest baby in the nursery" are of no real benefit to the parents and only accelerate their fantasies and anxieties. Finally, if a referring physician and the nursery team are both communicating with the parents, it is essential to coordinate the particular approach. It is very confusing to parents and decreases their trust level for one to be pessimistic and the other optimistic.

CULTURALLY COMPETENT CARE AND COMMUNICATION

Providing culturally sensitive care in a growing multicultural and diverse society is essential and needs to be a constant pursuit in providing perinatal health care to childbearing families and those families who have an infant in the NICU.[92] It is important for the health care team to understand the values, beliefs, customs, and behaviors of the particular group(s) they serve. Culture influences beliefs about what causes illness and how that illness should be treated. The perinatal health care team needs to address cultural, linguistic, and spiritual competencies to provide family-centered care.[57,114] The National Perinatal Association has published an extensive resource guide that reviews specific cultural practices and beliefs of several ethnocultural and religious groups.[171] Another excellent resource that discusses health and illness in different populations is *Cultural Diversity in Health and Illness.*[180]

In the perinatal setting, some common areas that often emerge center around language, folk practices or traditional beliefs, and nonverbal communication.

Use of Language. If a language or educational barrier is encountered, a qualified interpreter who is bilingual and bicultural should be utilized[92] (Box 29-4). This is especially important in obtaining informed consent. A child or children should not be used as interpreters because they may have inadequate language skills and may be embarrassed by the topics being discussed. Interpreters should be familiar with medical information and terminology. A housekeeper or admissions clerk may be bilingual but have no understanding of the medical issues. Often information that is translated, even by a certified translator, is not understood by families if they are not literate. Some undocumented immigrants may have only a second-grade education and may be illiterate in their own native language (and embarrassed about disclosing this to the medical team). However, illiteracy does not mean the family is not intelligent. Some very intelligent parents can comprehend complex information if explained in a relevant manner.

Use of pictures augments what is being explained. Providing a list of common medical terms and educational materials in the native language of the parents is a useful tool. At times, despite numerous discussions about the infant's medical condition, the family may appear unable to comprehend what they have been told. Consider that even if the health care provider and family share the same language, the words may have different meanings depending on core cultural beliefs and values and the families' previous experiences.[13] What is considered an abnormality in our Western culture may not be in another culture.

BOX 29-4 GUIDELINES FOR THE EFFECTIVE CHOICE OF INTERPRETERS IN CLINICAL SETTINGS

Interpreter Choice

- Unless thoroughly fluent in patient's language, always use trained interpreter.
- Avoid strangers from waiting room or untrained staff as interpreters because of potential problems with accuracy, confidentiality, and medical terminology.
- Children should be interpreters of last resort because of problems with disruption of social roles, sensitive issues, and accuracy.
- Adult relatives or friends brought specifically to translate are acceptable alternatives when trained interpreters are not available, but there may be problems with accuracy, confidentiality, medical terms, and disrupted social roles.
- Always ask patient whether designated interpreter is acceptable.

Interpreter Use

- Clinician, interpreter, and patient or parent should be positioned in equilateral triangle so important nonverbal cues can be appreciated.
- Speak to and maintain eye contact with patient/parent, not interpreter.
- Ask interpreter to translate as literally as possible.
- If mistranslation or misunderstanding is suspected, return to issue later using different wording.
- Emphasize key instructions and explanations by repetition.
- Use visual aids (charts and diagrams) whenever possible.
- To verify quality and comprehension of translation, have patient/parent repeat information through back translation.

At End of Medical Visit

- Interpreter should write lists of instructions for patient or parent, particularly for prescriptions and other therapeutic interventions.
- Indicate to pharmacists that prescription instructions should be printed in the family's language.
- Interpreter should always accompany patient/parent to schedule follow-up appointments with receptionist.

Reprinted from Flores G: Culture and the patient-physician relationship: achieving cultural competency in health care, *J Pediatr* 136:14-23, 2000. Includes information from Perez-Stable, Pachter, and Putsch.

Folk Practices and Traditional Beliefs. Many cultures have their own set of beliefs and traditions about health, illness, and treatment. Many cultures believe that there is a balance between hot and cold forces in nature that are essential for health and harmony. These concepts, which are very prevalent in Latin and Asian cultures, are unrelated to temperature. Pregnancy is seen as "hot," as are vitamins and iron, and should be treated with "cold" products to regulate a proper balance in the system and avoid medical problems. To treat imbalance, one must know what conditions are viewed as hot and cold. There is no general agreement as to what is a hot or cold disease or food. The classification may vary from person to person, so it is imperative to understand the nature of the situation or problem from the perspective of the family.[180] Many of the following beliefs, however, are commonly accepted causes for illness, birth defects, or anomalies:

- *Mal ojo:* A type of magical occurrence caused by a look; the "evil eye" heats up the infant's blood, resulting in fever, crying, diarrhea, vomiting, and aches and pains. This is often treated by a curandero (a folk healer), a healing ceremony, or placing an amulet (azabache) or leather strap for protection on the infant.
- *Coraje:* Anger or frustration believed to sour breast milk, as well as affect an infant's intrauterine development. It is treated by wearing a good-luck charm in the bra and having a healing ceremony.[57]
- *Mollera caida:* Fallen fontanel is believed to occur when the breast or bottle is removed too quickly. It is believed the soft palate sinks in, causing feeding and swallowing difficulties. Treatment is performed by pushing up the soft palate with the thumb, pulling the hair, and sucking the fontanel.[54]
- *Susto:* A disease or illness resulting from fright. It is treated by relaxation and a cleansing ceremony or other specific actions to counter the susto.
- *Lunar or solar eclipse:* A cleft palate, some respiratory ailments, and birthmarks are often associated with an eclipse. It is treated by the pregnant woman wearing a red undergarment or a coin or key over the belly.

Traditional folk healers are multidimensional. In African cultures, they are diviners, herbalists, faith healers, and voodoo practitioners, as well as traditional midwives and birth attendants. Hispanic cultures use a wide range of curanderos (santeros in the Puerto Rican community) who range from massage therapists to faith healers and herbalists. Asians rely on medicinal plants or herbology, acupuncture, and moxibustion (heated pulverized wormwood applied to the skin), which restores the proper balance of yin and yang believed to be most helpful during the period of labor and delivery.[180]

In many cultures, decisions are made by a group of elders, removing the responsibility entirely from a new mother and father. Many societies view the whole family as more important than a single individual. Decisions about life and death may be deferred to the elders or the entire family. Ignoring this social structure can result in problems of mistrust and decreased cooperation and communication.

Nonverbal Communication. One must be aware of body language and nonverbal communication and its meaning. Eye contact with the doctor or nurse or authority figures is regarded as disrespectful in some cultures. Loud vocalization also may be considered disrespectful. Rather than openly contradicting a person of authority, a parent will nod as if to communicate agreement but never follow through. Often the parent is viewed as noncompliant. In most societies, touch and space are regulated by rules and social orders. What is acceptable in one group may be forbidden in another; therefore respect personal boundaries and space issues. For example, Southeast Asians typically do not like to be patted on the top of their head or shoulder because this is where the soul resides. In American Indian and Alaska Native populations, note taking is a taboo. Indian history has been passed down by means of verbal storytelling, and note taking is perceived as insensitive.[180]

Becoming culturally competent health care providers is an ongoing developmental process. One should be aware of the dimensions and complexities in caring for individuals from diverse cultural backgrounds. It is important to understand the family's core cultural dynamics, the meaning of the infant's illness, and the social context within which these life events are occurring. Specific customs, traditions, and taboos of each individual group are available in resource materials.[171,180]

COMMUNICATING MEDICAL INFORMATION: NEW RESEARCH

The principles of family-centered neonatal care clearly promote a certain approach. The first four principles concern communication, medical information, fully informed parental decision making, and parental advance directives (see Box 29-2). Recently, researchers have confirmed that information given to parents in the NICU is often communicated in euphemisms, vague statements, and half-truths and shields parents from uncertainties and controversies of NICU care.[70] Professional attitudes that may interfere with open, honest communication include (1) assuming that parents are too emotional to assimilate information and make a rational decision, (2) assuming that information about complications and poor outcomes may disrupt attachment to the neonate, (3) assuming that parental guilt and psychologic harm will ensue from decision making (despite research to the contrary), and (4) cultural and language differences.[70] A recent multicenter qualitative study of parental values in decision making about delivery-room resuscitation for their extremely preterm infants found that (1) all parents wanted to participate in decision making (although few parents recalled discussing options for delivery room resuscitation; even fewer recalled being offered "comfort care," even though this was documented in the chart), (2) parents did not report that physician predictions of morbidity and mortality were central to their decision making, and (3) religion, spirituality, and hope were the guiding values for most parents in making their decision.[23]

Many parents desire and can handle complete, specific, honest, detailed, unbiased, and meaningful information—the same facts and interpretation of those facts as the staff—delivered in a humane and respectful manner.[70] More recent research substantiates the parents' wishes. Parents express "remarkably uniform and unambiguous requests . . . to receive early, honest and detailed information in a comprehensible and sympathetic manner and to be together when given bad news."[156,p. 434] Prenatal consultation has been found to be useful by 80% of mothers in one study.[156] These researchers concluded that "in our population of educated mothers, most mothers prefer to be told exact statistics, rather than generalizations, concerning major neonatal morbidities."[156] Another group of researchers uses actuarial data for counseling parents about infants at the limits of viability and for morbidity counseling.[147] Accuracy of prenatal and postnatal counseling of parents is of concern, because information affects practice management and influences parental decision making.[104,147]

Individuals vary in their desire to be informed and involved in decision making. Individuals also vary in the manner in which they assimilate information. Some parents may want extensive information about their situation, whereas others may not. Some parents may not wish to be decision makers and should be able to delegate decision making to a physician of their choice.[70] However, physicians have an ethical and legal obligation[7,8] to give parents the facts from which to make an informed choice about their neonate's condition, illnesses, outcomes, and the risks and benefits of various interventions. Proactive risk management strategies include effective communication,[58] because legal action in the form of civil malpractice suits (60%) and criminal action may result from poor communication between parents and physicians. Because language and cultural barriers in medical settings are increasing, federal and state governments have established a number of laws ands standards to ensure that providers and health care organizations provide culturally and linguistically appropriate care.[86]

Poor understanding by parents may be the result of poor communication techniques, contradictory messages, poor parental health, inexperience with medical terminology, denial, language barriers, inability to ask questions, or lack of opportunity to review the information.[104] In one study, parents claimed that a neonatologist had never spoken to them, but, in fact, the conversation did occur and had been recorded.[105] In this study, parents were given a tape recording of their initial conversation with the neonatologist and any subsequent conversations of importance. The audiotape proved useful: 96% of the mothers and 68% of the fathers listened to the tape again an average of 2.5 and 1.8 times, respectively. Eighty-five percent of parents who listened to the tape had forgotten elements of the conversation, and two mothers did not recall that the conversation had ever occurred. Taped conversations were found helpful by 99% of parents and grandparents, 76% of nurses, and 36% of neonatologists. Forty percent of the physicians were not happy about having their conversations taped; "legal implications" was the most frequent reason given. As pointed out in the study, the "legal implications" work both ways; taping encourages precise, organized, clear, and humane communication of information while providing an "alibi" if a legal complication arises. A recent randomized, single-blind trial found that mothers in the audiotaped conversation group had enhanced recall about their infant's diagnosis, treatment, and outcome (for up to 4 months) when compared with the group without audiotapes (6 of the 98 mothers did not recall the conversation with the neonatologist).[102]

Research has documented that postpartum women have transient deficits in cognitive function, particularly in attention and memory function.[50] Because verbal communication may be poorly remembered, augmentation with written instructions is recommended.[9,50] In addition to relistening to an audiotape, if parents are given written information, such as an evidence-based table of the likely outcomes of babies at different gestations, they can look at it again to review it. Such an evidence-based table for infants from 23 to 28 weeks' gestational age has been presented in the literature for use with parents.[105] This table contains information about mortality statistics, need for assisted ventilation, prolonged use of oxygen, length of stay, use of phototherapy, PDA needing treatment, outcomes of brain scans, and long-term neurodevelopmental outcome. A NICU staff member can create a table for parents by using their most recent data.[103] With the advent of computerized databases (e.g., the Vermont Oxford Data Base) that compare statistics from multiple NICUs and a large cohort of infants, parents can be provided with statistical information from multiple NICUs to compare with the outcomes from the NICU in which their baby is hospitalized. Parents may need assistance in interpreting statistics and making them meaningful to their individual situation. Again, some parents may want and need this type of information, whereas others may not. All communication needs to be culturally and linguistically appropriate.

Ongoing research on the *outcome of gestation table (OGT)* has documented views of parents, nurses, and physicians.[103] The majority of parents and nurses interviewed favored the table; they agreed that the information was frightening but important for parents to know. Parents wanted to keep a copy, and nurses wanted a copy in the medical record. Parents also thought that the information was easy to understand, the table did not contain "too much" information, and although it was frightening, they still would rather have the information. The majority of physicians thought that the table was easy to understand but had "too much" information, and they were ambivalent about using it in their practice. Parents, nurses, and physicians all agreed that the table and its information were not misleading. Twenty-one percent of doctors disagreed about including a copy of the table in the medical record so that other health care providers would know what had been said to the parents. This finding was surprising to the researchers, who thought that inclusion of the table in the medical record would promote consistency in information given to the parents by different members of the perinatal team.

The Neonatal Research Network of the National Institute of Child and Human Development (NICHD) has developed a simple web-based tool (see "Websites for Parents of Premature Infants" at the end of this chapter) to enable clinicians (and parents) to utilize multiple factors, not just gestational age, in making decisions about intensive care for extremely preterm infants.[187] A prospective study of 22 to 25 weeks' gestation preterms (n = 4446) in the NICHD cohort found that the likelihood of favorable outcome of NICU care was best estimated with consideration of gestational age in addition to sex, use of antenatal steroids, single/multiple birth, and birth weight. Calculation of the risk-to-benefit ratio of use of NICU care for the extremely preterm infant provides both care providers and parents with information that is "less arbitrary, more individualized, more transparent and better justified"[187] for informed decision making than use of gestational age alone.[187]

The principles of family-centered neonatal care (see Box 29-2) also advocate full and free access to lay and medical literature pertaining to the neonate's condition, proposed treatments, and probable outcomes.[70] Recently, a multicenter study was conducted to create a family-centered care map to enhance the ability of the health care team to work with families to coordinate and deliver care in a holistic manner to meet the developmental, physical, and psychosocial needs of NICU patients and their families. This study led to the development of an innovative web-based resource to assist individual care providers and family advisors to provide comprehensive family-centered care to infants and families.[49] Medical literature, articles, books, and videos (in English and Spanish) should be available in the NICU or in the hospital library for the parents' use. A video such as *You Are Not Alone* (see "Resource Materials for Parents" at the end of this chapter) is available to help parents understand the impact on the family of long-term handicaps and to support them in making informed decisions. Access to the Internet has proven to be a source of medical information (some accurate; some inaccurate) for families, as well as professionals.

Users report they can receive information, support, relationships, and comfort from their online activities and connections. Although there are many benefits, less is known about the quality of information received and the potential for harm from online communication. Parents may be more comfortable seeking medical advice from anonymous people in cyberspace rather than consulting their own health care providers. When recommending the Internet as a resource, professionals should be aware of its benefits, as well as shortcomings.[45,111]

Acknowledgment of Guilt Feelings

The third psychologic task parents are dealing with simultaneously with anticipatory grieving and withdrawal is confronting and recognizing their feelings of failure and guilt in not delivering a healthy infant. Most parents struggling with feelings of inadequacy and guilt are likely to search for answers to the causes of their infant's situation. The mother may focus on concrete things, such as not eating well, the flu, intercourse, birth control pills, or an unwanted pregnancy. The father also may be concerned about his role in not helping his wife enough, placing too many demands on her, an argument he provoked that precipitated labor, or another family member with the same chromosomal abnormality. Parents search for reasons because they need to find a cause for such an event happening to them. It is harder for them to feel out of control and helpless than to feel guilty. Some parents place responsibility on themselves; however, others shift the blame to others in their external world, such as their spouse, extended family, doctor, nurses, or God. Often both parents are concerned with the disappointment that they have caused the other. They may withdraw from each other at a time when they both need acceptance and support.

Realistic answers from the medical team are helpful for some parents in diminishing guilt feelings; in other parents, the guilt may be so deeply integrated in their thinking that it is less easily overcome. For example, some parents may focus on irrational, unrealistic factors, such as "This is my punishment for not being a good wife or daughter" or "This is my punishment for running away from home when I was 15." It seems that the more irrational the parent's thinking, the harder it is to assuage and resolve the guilt. Many feelings of guilt and failure are normal and expected; the feelings are a problem when the parent does not respond to the infant's progress, because the infant may continue to represent the parent's failure.

PARENTAL RESPONSES

Parents demonstrate many behaviors that indicate they are struggling with guilt and failure. Some parents directly verbalize these feelings and attempt to obtain helpful answers from the staff. Less obvious are the parents who are markedly depressed and remain so despite any improvement in the infant. These parents demonstrate the classic signs of depression, such as apathy, loss of interest in appearance and self, withdrawal, and loss of self-esteem. They exhibit an overwhelming sense of helplessness, because they feel responsible for causing their infant's problem and are helpless to remedy the situation. Their guilt feelings cause them to be very self-deprecating and angry, a state that often results in depression. Other parents struggling with guilt are highly anxious about their ability to handle their infant; they feel they have harmed their infant and cannot tolerate facing that infant. Another manifestation of guilt is hostility and anger that is usually directed toward others, such as the spouse, the staff, or God. Instead of focusing their anger on themselves like a depressed parent, they direct it outward to rid themselves of their feelings of responsibility, projecting the guilt feelings onto others in their life. They may be angry at the physicians, nurses, or social workers for not making their infant healthy (if the infant is premature) or perfect (if the infant has a congenital defect). They may be hostile toward the social worker for not being able to help them with their financial problems. Unconsciously, they are trying to make the staff feel as guilty, helpless, and responsible as they do.

FACILITATING ADAPTATION

To intervene with parents, it is useful to help the parents become aware of and acknowledge their feelings of failure and guilt. By verbalizing their feelings, they can begin to identify the source of the guilt feelings, which may not always be clear to them. The staff can then intervene with appropriate information to modify and clarify the perceptions that may be the source of some of the parents' guilt feelings. Many parents directly ask about the causes of their infant's problem, and the medical team should provide them with appropriate information. Other parents are not as direct and verbal; they need to have the subject introduced. A staff member might ask, "Have you wondered why this has happened?" or "Many parents find themselves feeling responsible for their baby's problem, as if they failed. Have you had these feelings?" As parents begin to talk about their feelings, they often can test reality and discover the irrationality in their thinking. However, some parents continue to feel guilty even though they have been told they are not to blame. Guilt feelings are very complex and may take a long time to resolve; for some, they may never be completely resolved but at least the intensity of the feelings may diminish. If a child recovers from the illness, guilt can be more easily relinquished. If the child has a chronic problem, the parent is daily confronted with feelings of responsibility. The more irrational the source of the guilt, the harder it is to dispel. Because this persistent guilt can cause problems in the parents' relationship with each other and with the child, a referral to a perinatal social worker or other mental health professional may be indicated.

To facilitate support between parents, it is useful to ask whether they have shared their feelings of guilt and failure with each other. Often a spouse may assume that one is angry at or disappointed with the other. Discussing this may bring a tremendous sense of relief and reassurance. However, if the parents are blaming each other and relationship problems develop, a referral to a perinatal social worker or counselor is appropriate.

In some cases, there may be realistic reasons (either intentional or unintentional) why the parent may feel guilty about the infant's problem. Parental drug or alcohol abuse, domestic violence, an accident, or an inherited genetic problem may be a real reason. In these cases, the staff must acknowledge to the parent that there is a causal relationship and then give the parents support by allowing them to talk about their feelings. If causes were not intentional, it is helpful to acknowledge that fact; if they were, it is important to be nonjudgmental. A judging attitude only reinforces the feelings (e.g., guilt, concern, uncertainty)[166,173] parents are already experiencing and further alienates them from the infant and staff. The parents need help with the problem that initially led to the impairment of the fetus. When this type of psychosocial problem arises, the involvement of a perinatal social worker or other mental health professional is essential.

POSTPARTUM MOOD DISORDERS

The postpartum period has been viewed as a time of increased risk for the development of mood disturbances in women (and men). The symptoms may be transient and relatively mild (baby blues) or may be associated with significant impairment of functioning (e.g., postpartum depression and psychosis). Women with a history of mood disorders and those

BOX 29-5 SIGNIFICANT PREDICTORS OF POSTPARTUM MOOD DISORDERS

- History of previous depression
- Present depression and anxiety disorders
- Low self-esteem
- Negative, stressful life events
- Marital discord
- Poor social support
- Difficult infant temperament
- Child-care stresses
- History of endocrine dysfunction
- Maternity blues
- Single marital status
- Adolescent pregnancy
- Unplanned/unwanted pregnancy
- Low socioeconomic status

Data from Beck C: Recognizing and screening for postpartum depression in mothers of NICU infants, *Adv Neonatal Care* 3:37, 2003; O'Hara M, Gorman L: Can postpartum depression be predicted? *Prim Psychiatry* 11:42, 2004.

who experience depression during pregnancy are at greatest risk.[113] Box 29-5 lists significant predictors of postpartum mood disorders. Evidence suggests that mothers of premature infants or infants with problems and those with multiple births experience a higher rate of postpartum depression (PPD) than women who deliver a single full-term infant.[17,133]

PPDs usually are divided into three categories: (1) postpartum blues, (2) nonpsychotic postpartum depression, and (3) postpartum psychosis, although these disorders do exist along a continuum.[18]

Postpartum Blues

Postpartum blues (baby blues) affects approximately 50% to 80% of new mothers. Symptoms may include mood swings, sleep and appetite disturbances with periods of feeling anxious, irritability, and tearfulness interspersed with times of feeling well. Symptoms often begin within a few days of delivery and persist up to several days. Postpartum blues is time-limited and relatively benign. The symptoms worsen by the 5th or 7th day and tend to resolve by the 12th postpartum day. The occurrence of the "baby blues" does not necessarily indicate psychopathology; however, if the symptoms persist longer than 2 weeks, a further evaluation is needed because approximately 20% of women develop postpartum major depression.[6]

Postpartum Depression

Postpartum depression is relatively common. Several controlled studies reveal that between 12% and 20% of women experience a postpartum depressive episode and this rate is as high as 26% in adolescent mothers.[6,151,185] Most women begin to experience depressive symptoms within the first month after delivery, although some have reported symptoms during the pregnancy. Signs and symptoms include a depressed mood, lack of interest or pleasure in usual activities, guilt, impaired concentration, appetite disturbance, low self-esteem, feelings of hopelessness and worthlessness, and suicidal ideation.[12,18]

Postpartum Psychosis

Postpartum psychosis is a rare but extremely serious mental illness occurring in 1 to 2 per 1000 deliveries. It generally occurs within the first 2 to 3 weeks after delivery and requires immediate attention. The symptoms are crying, irritability, restlessness, sleep disturbances, delusions, hallucinations, and bizarre, irrational behavior. For example, a woman may view the baby as the devil, claim the infant is dead, or accuse the hospital staff of switching babies. There are significant risks of infanticide or suicide.

The causes of postpartum disorders are multifactorial. Pregnancy is a complex biologic process that takes place within a psychologic and social context. Some of the determinates are the psychologic makeup of the mother, hormonal changes associated with pregnancy,[51,126,160] genetics, socioeconomic issues, stress, the temperament and health of the baby, marital instability, ambivalence toward the pregnancy, and the emotional support system of the new mother.[6,149] When the features listed in the Critical Findings box on p. 871 occur in mothers with a sick infant, it may be hard to differentiate a normal reaction to an adverse situation, a grief reaction, from signs of PPD.

In general, postpartum disorders are often overlooked and not appreciated, thereby putting the mother at risk for the development of recurrent depression, which has been associated with deleterious effects on the cognitive, emotional, and social development of the infant.[1,17,18,113] Given the inherent stresses and emotional impact the birth of a sick infant(s) has on the mother and her family, it is recommended that universal screening for PPD be a part of every family assessment in the NICU. "Routine assessment will normalize the process, enhance awareness and increase the health care providers' comfort level and competency."[17]

Assessment Tools

Several assessment tools are designed to identify women with a substantial increased risk for PPD. Ideally it is recommended these assessment tools be administered at each trimester of pregnancy and periodically after delivery to assess a woman's risk status.[77] In the literature is an extensive discussion of the various assessment tools, checklists, and their reliability and predictability of PPD.[14,16,133] Although there are many tools, three seem to be used extensively: (1) the Postpartum Depression Screening Scale (PDSS)[17]; (2) the Postpartum Depression Predictors Inventory—Revised (PDPI-Revised) (Table 29-1) (these tools are also available in Spanish)[16,20,21] based on a meta-analysis of 84 studies published to identify significant risk factors of PPD[15]; and (3) the Edinburgh Postnatal Depression Scale (EPDS) (Table 29-2).[40,41]

The two scales, PDSS and PDPI-Revised, have different uses. The PDSS is a 35-item self-report Likert scale that assesses seven areas: (1) sleeping/eating difficulties, (2) anxiety/insecurity, (3) emotionality, (4) mental confusion, (5) loss of self, (6) shame or guilt, and (7) thoughts of self-harm.[17,19] The scale measures depressive symptomatology. The total score ranges from 13 to 175. If a mother's score is 80 or above, this is a positive screen for PPD and a referral for mental health follow-up is indicated. The mother completes the PDSS herself, and then it is scored. The tool is used only after delivery.

The PDPI-Revised is an inventory that (1) assesses a woman's risk status for developing PPD, (2) can be used during pregnancy and after delivery, and (3) should complement a clinician's professional judgment. It consists of 13 risk factors and is designed for a clinician and the woman to discuss each risk factor that might put her at risk for developing postpartum depression. There is no total score; rather, it is a tool providing detailed information on symptoms.

With some modifications as reported by a study in Australia, the PDPI-Revised has been used as a checklist that the woman administers herself. The information from the checklist was then used to initiate discussions by midwives and nurses with women about their postpartum depression.[69]

The EPDS is a 10-item screening questionnaire that (1) is completed by mothers (and fathers) and then scored by clinicians, (2) is useful as an inventory to identify parents at risk to initiate an open discussion about PPD, (3) requires minimal training to administer, and (4) is completed in less than 10 minutes. The EPDS is a reliable and valid measure of depression or anxiety disorders in fathers during the perinatal period[124] and can be used by pediatricians in the outpatient setting to help identify and assist mothers at risk.[35,73] The EPDS can be used at 6 to 8 weeks after delivery and is easy to score. The items are ordered and weighted to reflect severity of symptoms. A recent study found that the self-administered EPDS and the directed interview EPDS are equal in their ability to screen for postpartum depression and either technique should be used to screen for PPD.[96] A score of 12+ indicates the likelihood of depression but not its severity, although with this score, further assessment and possible intervention are recommended. If the woman or man scores positive on item 10, thoughts of harming oneself, immediate intervention is necessary.[14]

Many studies have demonstrated that mothers of sick or premature infants are at greater risk for psychologic distress than are mothers of full-term infants. These studies have looked at depressive symptoms in mothers during the hospitalization and after discharge. The goal of these studies, by using assessment tools, have been to identify (and ultimately treat) women at risk for depression,

Text continued on p. 877

Critical Findings

ADDITIONAL FEATURES OF POSTPARTUM MOOD DISORDERS

- Overconcern for the baby or excessive anxiety over the infant's health
- Guilt, inadequacy, worthlessness, especially feeling like a failure at motherhood
- Fear of losing control or "going crazy"
- Lack of interest in the baby
- Fear of harming the baby
- Obsession

TABLE 29-1 POSTPARTUM DEPRESSION PREDICTORS INVENTORY (PDPI)-REVISED AND GUIDE QUESTIONS FOR ITS USE

DURING PREGNANCY	CHECK ONE	
MARITAL STATUS		
1. Single	○	
2. Married/cohabiting	○	
3. Separated	○	
4. Divorced	○	
5. Widowed	○	
6. Partnered	○	
SOCIOECONOMIC STATUS		
Low	○	
Middle	○	
High	○	
SELF-ESTEEM	***YES***	***NO***
Do you feel good about yourself as a person?	○	○
Do you feel worthwhile?	○	○
Do you feel you have a number of good qualities as a person?	○	○
PRENATAL DEPRESSION		
1. Have you felt depressed during your pregnancy?	○	○
If yes, when and how long have you been feeling this way?		
If yes, how mild or severe do you consider your depression?		
PRENATAL ANXIETY		
Have you been feeling anxious during your pregnancy?	○	○
If yes, how long have you been feeling this way?		
UNPLANNED/UNWANTED PREGNANCY		
Was the pregnancy planned?	○	○
Is the pregnancy unwanted?	○	○
HISTORY OF PREVIOUS DEPRESSION		
1. Before this pregnancy, have you ever been depressed?	○	○
If yes, when did you experience this depression?		
If yes, have you been under a physician's care for this past depression?	○	○
If yes, did the physician prescribe any medication for your depression?	○	○
SOCIAL SUPPORT		
1. Do you feel you receive adequate emotional support from your partner?	○	○
2. Do you feel you receive adequate instrumental support from your partner (e.g., help with household chores or baby sitting)?	○	○
3. Do you feel you can rely on your partner when you need help?	○	○
4. Do you feel you can confide in your partner?	○	○
(Repeat same questions for family and again for friends)		

From Beck C: Revision of the postpartum depression predictors inventory, *J Obstet Gynecol Neonatal Nurs* 31:394, 2002.

Continued

TABLE 29-1 POSTPARTUM DEPRESSION PREDICTORS INVENTORY (PDPI)-REVISED AND GUIDE QUESTIONS FOR ITS USE—cont'd

DURING STATUS	CHECK ONE	
MARITAL SATISFACTION	***YES***	***NO***
1. Are you satisfied with your marriage (or living arrangement)?	○	○
2. Are you currently experiencing any marital problems?	○	○
3. Are things going well between you and your partner?	○	○
LIFE STRESS		
1. Are you currently experiencing any stressful events in your life such as:		
Financial problems	○	○
Marital problems	○	○
Death in the family	○	○
Serious illness in the family	○	○
Moving	○	○
Unemployment	○	○
Job change		
After delivery, add the following items:		
CHILD CARE STRESS		
1. Is your infant experiencing any health problems?	○	○
2. Are you having problems with your baby feeding?	○	○
3. Are you having problems with your baby sleeping?	○	○
INFANT TEMPERAMENT		
1. Do you consider your baby irritable or fussy?	○	○
2. Does your baby cry a lot?	○	○
3. Is your baby difficult to console or soothe?	○	○
MATERNITY BLUES		
1. Did you experience a brief period of tearfulness and mood swings during the first week after delivery?	○	○
COMMENTS		
______________________________		
______________________________		
______________________________		
______________________________		

TABLE 29-2 **EDINBURGH POSTNATAL DEPRESSION SCALE**

HEALTH VISITOR **NUMBER**

Today's date ______________________________ Baby's age ______________________________

Baby's date of birth ______________________________ Birth weight ______________________________

Triplets/twins/single ______________________________ Male/female ______________________________

How are you feeling?

As you have recently had a baby, we would like to know how you are feeling now. Please underline the answer that comes closest to how you have felt in the past 7 days, not just how you feel today.

Here is an example already completed:

I have felt happy:

Yes, most of the time
Yes, some of the time
Not very often
No, never

This means: "I have felt happy some of the time" during the past week.

Please complete the other questions in the same way.

In the past 7 days

1. I have been able to laugh and see the funny side of things:
   As much as I always could
   Not quite so much now
   Definitely not so much now
   Not at all
2. I have looked forward with enjoyment to things:
   As much as I ever did
   Rather less than I used to
   Definitely less than I used to
   Hardly at all
3. I have blamed myself unnecessarily when things went wrong:
   Yes, most of the time
   Yes, some of the time
   Not very often
   No, never
4. I have felt worried and anxious for no good reason:
   No, not at all
   Hardly ever
   Yes, sometimes
   Yes, very often
5. I have felt scared or panicky for no very good reason:
   Yes, quite a lot
   Yes, sometimes
   No, not much
   No, not at all

TABLE 29-2 EDINBURGH POSTNATAL DEPRESSION SCALE—cont'd

HEALTH VISITOR	NUMBER

In the past 7 days

6. Things have been getting on top of me:
   Yes, most of the time I haven't been able to cope at all
   Yes, sometimes I haven't been coping as well as usual
   No, most of the time I have coped quite well
   No, I have been coping as well as ever
7. I have been so unhappy that I have had difficulty sleeping:
   Yes, most of the time
   Yes, some of the time
   Not very often
   No, not at all
8. I have felt sad or miserable:
   Yes, most of the time
   Yes, some of the time
   Not very often
   No, not at all
9. I have been so unhappy that I have been crying:
   Yes, most of the time
   Yes, quite often
   Only occasionally
   No, never
10. The thought of harming myself has occurred to me:
    Yes, quite often
    Sometimes
    Hardly ever
    Never

EDINBURGH POSTNATAL DEPRESSION SCALE: SCORING SHEET

1. I have been able to laugh and see the funny side of things:	
As much as I always could	0
Not quite so much now	1
Definitely not so much now	2
Not at all	3
2. I have looked forward with enjoyment to things:	
As much as I ever did	0
Rather less than I used to	1
Definitely less than I used to	2
Hardly at all	3
3. I have blamed myself unnecessarily when things went wrong:	
Yes, most of the time	3
Yes, some of the time	2
Not very often	1
No, never	0

Continued

TABLE 29-2 EDINBURGH POSTNATAL DEPRESSION SCALE—cont'd

HEALTH VISITOR	NUMBER
4. I have felt worried and anxious for no good reason:	
No, not at all	0
Hardly ever	1
Yes, sometimes	2
Yes, very often	3
5. I have felt scared or panicky for no very good reason:	
Yes, quite a lot	3
Yes, sometimes	2
No, not much	1
No, not at all	0
6. Things have been getting on top of me:	
Yes, most of the time I haven't been able to cope at all	3
Yes, sometimes I haven't been coping as well as usual	2
No, most of the time I have coped quite well	1
No, I have been coping as well as ever	0
7. I have been so unhappy that I have had difficulty sleeping:	
Yes, most of the time	3
Yes, some of the time	2
Not very often	1
No, not at all	0
8. I have felt sad or miserable:	
Yes, most of the time	3
Yes, some of the time	2
Not very often	1
No, not at all	0
9. I have been so unhappy that I have been crying:	
Yes, most of the time	3
Yes, quite often	2
Only occasionally	1
No, never	0
10. The thought of harming myself has occurred to me:	
Yes, quite often	3
Sometimes	2
Hardly ever	1
Never	0

thereby decreasing the negative effect on infant development. General themes emerge from these studies.[17,18,133] Social support was consistently identified as extremely important both during the hospitalization and after discharge when the mother has full responsibility for the infant(s) for the first time. Increased stress at discharge, the isolation, and being disconnected from the NICU support network contribute to the risk for PPD. Therefore social support is necessary and can serve as a buffer to the effects of depression. Logsdon and Usui's work supported what other studies have found—that closeness to one's partner, social support, and self-esteem are important predictors of PPD regardless of ethnic diversity.[120] Stress and uncertainty surrounding the birth of a sick newborn increase the need for support. Support provided by the health care team to a mother's adaptation to the NICU environment, information communicated about the infant and his or her treatment, and accurate knowledge of infant development (at the time of discharge) can influence a mother's risk for PPD.[189] All of these factors indicate the need for enhanced family-centered care in the NICU and after discharge.

Mothers whose infants have chronic complications and who present long-term management challenges are more likely to experience more severe depressive symptoms.[133] In addition, the role of the hospital environment coupled with the appearance of the infant seems to contribute to maternal symptoms. In a study done in Japan, it was found that close emotional support of the father was much more significant than the existence of other modes of peripheral support.[144] This same study concluded that active intervention for PPD is necessary for the mother to be emotionally available to attach to the infant and cope with the infant's hospitalization and subsequent issues related to discharge. Most investigators believe that chronic exposure to maternal depression has long-term negative effects on a child's emotional, psychologic, and cognitive development.[113]

Treatment and Intervention

PPD and its symptoms present themselves along a continuum. Interventions should be guided by the severity of symptoms and the degree of impairment of the individual. Because PPD is a complex biologic and psychologic phenomenon, a comprehensive approach is needed including reassurance and support, psychoeducation, individual or group psychotherapy, and psychopharmacology.[55,78,79,142]

In childbirth classes, PPD should be addressed with anticipatory guidance discussing risk factors and early symptoms. Information brochures with resources should be available. Support groups often prepare mothers (and fathers) for the reality of parenthood and provide anticipatory guidance and counseling, skill building, validation, and acknowledgment of the concerns and frustrations of caring for a new infant. There are often support groups specifically for PPD available in one's local community and at the statewide level. Referral to national organizations such as *Postpartum Support International* and *Depression After Delivery* enable mothers and fathers to access many additional resources (see "Resource Materials for Parents" at the end of this chapter). Other interventions include visiting nurse services, nurse home visitors, parenting classes, referrals to child-care resources, and mutual aid hotlines. A recent meta-analysis found that *any* psychosocial or psychologic intervention (compared with routine postpartum care) reduced symptoms of depression as well as the likelihood of continued postpartum depression within the first year after giving birth.[44]

Many psychotherapy modalities[149,169] are recommended to mothers. Couples therapy may be part of the treatment plan if there is marital discord; however, even when there are no particular difficulties in the relationship, including the father can be useful in providing information and support for the mother. Suggestions for increased help around the home can be of tremendous value, allowing the mother to obtain adequate rest and care for herself. If the symptoms are very severe, psychiatric day treatment or inpatient hospitalization may be necessary. (In England, there are mother/baby inpatient units.) In cases in which the infant's life is in danger, protective services may have to be involved.

The use of medications (selective serotonin reuptake inhibitors, mood stabilizers, antidepressants, and antipsychotics) may be necessary. The use of hormonal manipulation has been investigated.[149] Referral to a clinician who is familiar with PPD is recommended.

The issue of breast feeding when considering psychotropic medications needs to be addressed.[28] Parents should be provided necessary information about the effects of these medications on the neonate so that the risks and benefits can be considered on an individual basis. All psychotropic medications enter the breast milk, so careful evaluation with the health care team needs to be undertaken (see Table 18-4).

ADAPTATION TO THE INTENSIVE CARE ENVIRONMENT

The fourth psychologic task involves adaptation to the intensive care environment.[53,65] All of the reactions of guilt, anxiety, fear, anger, and disappointment become heightened when parents attempt to adapt to this unfamiliar environment. They must learn a new language, establish trust in new relationships, and adapt to their role in this setting.[53,127] The intense and sometimes chaotic appearance of a high-risk nursery makes it a frightening experience that serves to increase parental feelings of helplessness and anxiety. Parents should gain a sense of security in this environment before initiating a caregiving role with their infant. There may be cultural and linguistic adaptations and geographic obstacles for families who live in small, rural communities and must travel to large, unfamiliar cities and adapt to large hospitals. Locating the hospital and finding accommodations and meals can become overwhelming to parents who have undergone much emotional turmoil. Meeting the infant's care provider, the competent physician and nurse, can sometimes evoke a mixture of positive and negative feelings. Parents may be reassured and grateful for care being given, but their feelings of uselessness, helplessness, and inadequacy can be reinforced.[150] The sophistication of the highly technical care and heroic measures provided to achieve survival for their infant may be met with both awe and uncertainty.[122] Family disruption is exaggerated by distance, especially if the infant was transported and the father must decide whether he is most needed with the infant, the infant's mother, or perhaps other children at home. Decisions must be made about work responsibilities, as well as child care. The financial concerns related to providing intensive care become an added stress on families and often are compounded by the travel expenditures necessary to visit the infant.

Parental Responses

In comparing the psychosocial adjustments of parents in the NICU, both parents may experience increased levels of emotional distress.[47] Mothers have been found to be more anxious, hostile, and depressed than fathers, with poorer adjustments related to work, sexual relations, social environment, and psychologic distress.[47] Mothers and fathers experience the NICU stay differently; mothers found the entire NICU experience and its aftermath more stressful than fathers.[47,85] It is important to include both mothers and fathers in assessments and interventions and to avoid overlooking the father's needs because he may be less accessible.[47,85,122] Fathers need communication, empathy, and support for the stressful experience of the NICU in a similar fashion as for mothers.[83]

A number of nonverbal and verbal signs indicate that parents are struggling to gain a sense of security in the NICU. Some parents appear frightened, overwhelmed, nervous, and withdrawn, asking few questions or being reluctant to call or visit. Others may be highly anxious and unable to focus on their infant and may instead concentrate on other activities or infants in the nursery. Some parents may ask many questions and become very interested in the technical aspects of their infant's treatment, such as respirator settings and laboratory values, in an attempt to understand and cope with their infant's illness.[46,122] Some parents, uneasy with entrusting their infant to strangers, may initially feel a need to remain at his or her side, maintaining a vigil. Some may wish to read the infant's chart or attempt to read material on their infant's particular condition. Others may become angry or upset at minor differences in the infant's care or the nursery policies, such as a respiratory setting being off a point or discrepancies in enforcing visitation guidelines.[53,62]

Research into the mother's needs in the NICU have found that the mother's priority is to safeguard her infant.[81,82] Mothers perceive that if they advocate for their own needs (e.g., to mother or care for the infant) in the NICU, they will be labeled as "difficult" or "demanding." Maternal needs in the NICU include information and interaction with their infant, emotional safety, and a supportive NICU environment in which to meet their needs (Table 29-3).[81,129] When these needs are thwarted, mothers feel helpless, powerless, and emotionally vulnerable and are less able to interact with their infant. A major barrier to implementing family-centered care is the mother's fear about how her needs, feelings, and actions affect the care of her baby. Family-centered care empowers mothers and fathers through collaboration with health care providers.

For families, the relationship with health care providers progresses through three stages: naïve trust, disenchantment, and guarded alliance.[127,129] Naïve trust, the belief that the family will be informed and involved in decision making, becomes disenchantment when unmet expectations, distrust, and anger result in the belief that the sick family member needs to be protected. A guarded alliance develops when families become more able to navigate the health care system and are involved, in control, and participate in the care of their sick member. Helpful interventions include (1) meeting individual family's needs,

TABLE 29-3 MATERNAL NEEDS IN THE NEONATAL INTENSIVE CARE UNIT

MATERNAL NEED	RECOMMENDATIONS FOR NICU STAFF
Empowering information	Give information about maternal situation in NICU (e.g., feelings, importance of her role as mother of the baby). Give information on how a preterm baby differs from a term baby and how to read/respond to her individual baby's cues/behaviors. Facilitate opportunities for parents to provide direct care for their infant. Understand parental need for modeling and role-modeling on preterm care tasks (e.g., feeding, bathing). Understand parental need for supportive appraisal—give positive feedback and reinforcement of maternal/paternal caregiving (e.g., feeding, diapering) and infant's responses to parental caregiving.
Continuity of care	Understand difficulty or impossibility of mother to negotiate actions with multitudes of caregivers. Use primary nursing for continuity of physical and emotional care for mothers, as well as infants.
Vigilant watching over	Understand maternal observations and actions to safeguard their infant and prevent injury or harm. Understand that mothers fear being seen as "difficult" by the staff, that voicing their concerns would jeopardize their baby's care. Understand mothers' perceptions that the nurse-to-patient ratio/acuity influences her behavior (i.e., mother is hesitant to advocate for her own needs for information, caregiving opportunities, and support). Mothers would shift their priority from interaction with the infant to safeguarding the infant from danger by delaying/rescheduling the activity with the infant. As a result, mothers often become disappointed and frustrated that a meaningful moment with their infant was denied.
Expert knowledge	Understand that, initially, nurses and other health care providers are seen as "experts" in care of the infant. With increasing confidence and caregiving, mothers become "expert" in knowing their own infant and what works best and are truly the "constant" in the multiple caregiving system of the NICU. Understand that mothers receive conflicting messages from health care providers about respect, acknowledgment, and value of growing maternal expertise.
Emotional safety in the NICU	Understand feelings of extreme emotional vulnerability/exposure experienced by mothers in the NICU. Empathy, emotional warmth, and understanding in interactions with nurses and other health care professionals provide mothers with emotional safety. Feelings of emotional vulnerability were engendered when (1) nurses' actions covertly communicated that the mother was a "bother" or an "intruder,"[129] (2) the mother focused energy on controlling her emotions and behaving so the nurse would approve, (3) the mother attempted to negotiate with the staff for access to her own infant, (4) health care providers were not empathetic about maternal worries, concerns, separation, and distress about their infant and need for frequent information,[129] and (5) there were breaches of confidentiality.

Modified from Hurst I: Mothers' strategies to meet their needs in the newborn intensive care nursery, *J Perinat Neonatal Nurs* 15:65, 2001; Hurst I: Vigilant watching over: mothers' actions to safeguard their premature babies in the newborn intensive care nursery, *J Perinat Neonatal Nurs* 15:39, 2001.

(2) providing a welcoming NICU environment, (3) personalizing the infant, (4) teaching parents to interpret their infant's cues and behaviors, (5) fulfilling the continuing need for information, and (6) forming partnerships with families in all aspects of decision making and caregiving,[127] including giving them the option to be present during procedures and participate in pain relief for their infant.[72,94,129,130]

Facilitating Adaptation

Many interventions can be employed to familiarize and orient families.[65,174] First, the obstetrician, transport team, or any other professional who has initial contact with parents can give them preparatory information and a description of intensive care. A booklet or video[65] in the native language of the parent that includes basic information and illustrative pictures is extremely useful and should include a discussion of the type of care being provided, normal feelings and reactions parents experience, financial information, a glossary of terms, breast-feeding information, available accommodations and meals, calling and visitation policies, the discharge policy, and a city map. Both at the time of transfer and later in the nursery, a self-developing picture or picture from a digital camera can be taken of the infant for the parents. If the infant is being transported, information should be given as to the general length of time of transport and by whom and when the parents will be contacted after the infant has been admitted and evaluated. A personal phone call from the staff with an introduction, information about the infant and unit, and an inquiry about parental visitation plans is useful. Parents feel less anxious when they have an orientation and a name to whom to relate. The staff can then be prepared to be available when the parents arrive.

Certainly, the first visit to the NICU is stressful, and members of the team should welcome the parents and stay with them to explain the equipment and procedures, answer questions, review the infant's course, give emotional support, and generally orient the parents to this new experience. Mothers who have not previously seen their baby report more stress in seeing their baby first in the NICU. Seeing the infant is stressful and may evoke shock, fear, guilt, and helplessness.[135] Be attentive to the mother's physical need; comfortable chairs and perhaps a wheelchair if the mother has had a cesarean section are helpful. The message needs to be conveyed that parents are welcome, that their presence makes a difference, and that they will be partners in the care of their infant.[127] Because many parents are uncertain about what questions to ask, it may be necessary at times to help parents construct questions (e.g., "Do you understand why we start IVs in the head?" or "Do you know what blood gases, hood oxygen, and CPAP are?") and repeat explanations using simple, nontechnical language. Relating to the parent's affect or emotional state seems to establish a rapport with the family and helps them feel that the staff is empathetic and understanding. If parents sense the staff's genuine concern and interest in them and their infant, it is easier for them to leave their infant in the staff's care.[129,135,150,179,191] A team member might say, "You look frightened or scared," or "This can be an overwhelming situation," or "You look like you want to cry." Facilitating the parents' relationship with the infant* is essential and can be done by offering the parents the opportunity to touch or stroke their infant, hold the infant if possible, or at least remove eye patches. Pointing out some of the unique personal characteristics of the infant is helpful. A staff member might say, "Your baby is very active," or "He responds well to touch," or "She seems to prefer lying on her side."

Families coming from out of town should be provided with a list of inexpensive housing and restaurants located near the hospital. In many cities, national and local businesses have established nearby homes run by local volunteer organizations for housing parents on a temporary basis. The homes have several sleeping rooms in addition to kitchen and laundry facilities and provide parents with a comfortable, homelike atmosphere at a nominal charge. A natural support system generally emerges among the parents using the home. A list of apartments, hotels, and boarding rooms reasonably priced and rented by the day or week also can be made available. Social workers often can secure food, parking, and cab vouchers to give to families to decrease some of the financial stresses.

Parents usually are concerned with the cost of their infant's hospitalization. Some parents feel that if they cannot pay, their child will receive less attention. Parents should be reassured that their infant's care will not depend on their ability to pay. However, they should be referred to the appropriate funding agencies, such as the Handicapped Children's Program

*References 122,129,179,182,190.

or Health Care Programs for Children with Special Needs, Social Security Disability, Title 19 Medicaid, and state child health insurance programs that provide financial assistance.

Because communication is critical, regular conferences between the family and staff (physicians, nurses, and social workers) should be instituted to give consistent medical information and emotional support; this is especially helpful with both extremely critical and long-term infants. Medical interpreters should be made available if parents do not speak English; the same principle applies for deaf parents. Parents should be given the names of the physicians and nurses taking care of their infant and the personnel's specific role in providing both care to the infant and communication to the family. If the physicians and nurses have a rotation system, this also should be explained from the beginning. At the end of a rotation, the transition can be facilitated by the oncoming physician's participation in even a brief conference with the outgoing physician, primary nurse, and parents.[68]

Primary nursing, especially for long-term infants, can be very helpful in providing for continuity of care.[68] The primary nurse has been identified by parents as the primary source and facilitator of information to parents and between parents and other health care providers and as the link between parents and infant. In a study of maternal values, mothers associated nurses with the human quality of the NICU, a wealth of knowledge about technology, and valuing the personal characteristics of the infants.[159] In the same study, mothers identified the most desirable attributes of care providers: (1) technical skill/competency, (2) caring about or "really liking" babies, (3) communication abilities, and (4) patience.[159]

Protection of patient privacy and confidentiality is an ethical and legal (state and federal) obligation. Compliance to protect patient privacy, secure private patient information, and protect patient confidentiality is mandatory (in the United States) under the Health Insurance Portability and Accountability Act (HIPAA96). Violations of patient privacy include (1) overheard conversations; (2) failure to identify a telephone caller; (3) failure to obtain written consent to communicate patient information by fax, e-mail, or any other written/electronic format; and (4) leaving patient charts open/accessible to others.[176] HIPAA violations may result in financial penalties ($100 to $250,000) and/or imprisonment. Parental access to the medical record is a legal right (HIPAA96) that cannot be denied by professionals or the hospital. However, institutions must have a specific policy to deal with parent requests for access to the medical record. Many institutions require the presence of a professional to answer questions and interpret medical language for parents as they read the chart. The principles of family-centered neonatal care advocate not only parental access to the complete medical record but also documentation by parents of their own observations in the medical record.[70] All of these activities must be in compliance with the HIPAA regulations.[29,176]

For out-of-town families, the telephone plays a major role in staff-parent communication. The establishment of a telephone calling schedule with families and a toll-free number, if available, can be useful. If the family lives out of town and cannot visit frequently, the local or referring physician can supplement the communication. This physician often knows the family and can talk with them in person. The physician, of course, should communicate regularly with the nursery team to obtain the current medical information and present a consistent approach to the family.

Resumption of the Relationship with the Infant

The fifth psychologic task entails the parents' reestablishment of a relationship with their infant and initiating their caregiving role, a process that usually begins when the infant's improvement revives previous hopes after a disappointing experience. Certain medical events may signal to the parents that it is safe to risk a relationship with the infant. These events may be a regular weight gain, changes in feeding patterns or methods, elimination of life support equipment or use of an incubator, the infant crying for the first time or becoming more active and responsive, or the infant's transfer from the NICU to a level II nursery. The parents may begin to read baby books or pamphlets about their infant's condition, buy clothes, set up the baby's room, send out birth announcements, or name the baby. If the infant has a congenital defect, the parents may become involved with genetic counseling and other parents whose infants have similar deficits.[123]

Parents must begin to shift their level of involvement and activity from that of passive participants to that of active primary caregivers.* This shift

*References 112,122,129,131,132,146,184.

includes the parents gaining confidence in their ability to care for their infant. The family who has been disrupted must reestablish themselves and recover from the crisis in an environment that is sensitive and supportive to this essential task.* The transfer of care from staff to parent is influenced by (1) the stability or lability of the infant's condition, (2) the physical health of the mother, (3) the level of parental support, and (4) the staff expectations.[122,150]

Several formalized intervention programs have been developed and tested for efficacy in assisting parents of NICU infants in relating to and parenting these vulnerable infants. An early educational-behavioral intervention program for NICU parents (Creating Opportunities for Parent Empowerment [COPE]) was developed and tested in a randomized controlled trial with 260 families.[131,132] Mothers in the COPE program had significantly less stress in the NICU, more positive interactions with their infants, and less depression and anxiety at 2 months corrected infant age when compared with the control mothers. Other study outcomes included (1) stronger parental beliefs about their role, (2) parents more able to read their preterm's cues and behaviors, and (3) shorter length of both NICU and hospital stays (by 4 days and 8 days for very-low-birth-weight [VLBW] preterms) when compared with the control group.[132] Another randomized study of an early intervention program found that parents who participated had a reduction in parenting stress after birth of their preterm infant.[95] The March of Dimes initiative to encourage family-centered care (NICU Family Support [NFS] Program) has been studied at 8 NFS sites by interviewing parents, NICU staff, and administrators. Findings include (1) culture change within the NICU resulting in increased family support, (2) enhanced overall quality of NICU care, (3) less stressed, more informed, and confident parents, and (4) increased receptivity of staff to the concept of family-centered care and its benefits.[38]

Involvement in caregiving lessens the parents' feelings of helplessness and frustration and facilitates their identification with their role as parents.† Alteration in their parental role is particularly stressful for mothers in the NICU.[22,76,80,134] The sense of parenthood for both mothers and fathers depends on expectations of the parental role, the infant's state of health, and the environment/professional attitudes in the NICU.[85,122] A study by Jackson[85] found that internalization of the parent role with a premature infant occurs over time and often involves initial feelings of alienation and responsibility that change to more confidence (at 3 to 6 months) and familiarity (at 18 months) with the parenting role. For weeks after birth, both parents experience alienation: (1) mothers felt ambivalence about their relationship with the baby and their new role as parent—a concern for the baby's welfare and a need to participate in and control the infant's care; and (2) fathers shared concern for the baby, felt unprepared for the birth, and were confident in delegating the baby's care to the NICU staff.[85] In this qualitative study, neither parent felt ready for the preterm infant's discharge to home. Taking on total responsibility for the baby's care resulted in both parents feeling insecure, fearful, and worried about the baby and the father taking on more responsibility for infant care. By 6 months of age, both parents had developed more confidence in the care and parenting of their preterm; by 18 months, parents had developed a feeling of relationship with their child.[85] For mothers of the smallest and sickest infants, concerns and worry about the infant remained even at 6 months.[85] Beginning as early as possible in the NICU, health care providers should encourage and facilitate parent participation in their infant's care.* Parents can provide skin care for their infant, learn to read and respond to infant cues, help turn the infant even if a respirator is attached, diaper the infant, and possibly feed the infant. If the parents are separated by distance, they can send family pictures that can be posted at the infant's bed; periodic pictures of the infant taken by the staff can be sent back to the family. Parents can send clothing, mobiles, simple toys, and even cassette tapes so that the infant can hear the parents' voices. Some mothers who are pumping send frozen breast milk (see Chapter 18). All of these reminders help the nursery staff to be aware of the real family that is genuinely interested. These personal attempts made by parents that help them feel they are important to their infant's development should be encouraged. Sometimes foster grandparents or volunteers can hold, feed, and talk to infants whose parents cannot visit frequently.

*References 22,42,63,70,80,112,122,131,132,146,150,184,190.
†References 42,76,112,122,129,131,132,146,182,184.

*References 42,80,122,129,132,182.

Kangaroo care (see Chapter 13), skin-to-skin contact between mother/father and infant by placing the infant in a vertical position between the mother's/father's breasts, has positive maternal/paternal, as well as neonatal, responses. Use of kangaroo care activates the maternal processes of a search for meaning and mastery of the experience of preterm birth, a recovery of self-esteem, maternal confidence, and enhancement in the parenting of a high-risk neonate.[26,80,88,100] Successive sessions of kangaroo care ease the pain and emotional suffering as mothers deal with loss and letting go and develop competence and confidence. Paternal attachment is also facilitated by fathers holding their infants and engaging in skin-to-skin contact.[122] A study by Sullivan[181] indicates that the earlier fathers hold their babies, the sooner they report feelings of love and warmth. The infant may become a reality to the father when he can hold his infant.[122,181] In the same study,[181] fathers reported delaying attachment until they were certain of the infant's survival.

The use of "graduate parents," parents who have had an infant in the NICU and who have successfully dealt with and resolved the crisis of the birth of their infant, can be extremely valuable.[70,80,122] They provide support to parents by sharing common feelings, reactions, and experiences about having a hospitalized infant. Graduate parents can provide support and practical assistance for mothers interested in breast feeding, parents who take their infant home on oxygen, or parents whose infant requires special medical care such as a shunt, tracheostomy, colostomy, or gavage feedings. Organized graduate parent groups in large tertiary settings have become a very popular means of providing support,[33,65,80-82] but locating one parent or couple to talk with parents in a small community can be just as helpful. Parent classes and Internet resources[80] also can be offered on a variety of topics such as breast feeding, infant development, premature infant development, sibling and family reactions, discharge, cardiopulmonary resuscitation, coping with the hospitalization, and special medical needs. These classes provide specific, didactic information combined with group discussions that are mutually supportive in nature. Social workers, nurses, and other related health care professionals (e.g., respiratory, occupational, and physical therapists) facilitate the group; graduate parents also participate as a resource.

A third type of support is counseling sessions. The purpose of these sessions is to discuss and deal with common issues among parents arising from the hospitalization of their infant and the effects on their marriage and family life. This type of session also has been helpful for parents whose infant has died. The sessions are usually short term and are conducted by the perinatal social worker and another staff member such as a physician, nurse, or chaplain. The focus of the group is not to give specific medical information but, rather, to provide parents with an opportunity to verbalize their feelings about their infant's hospitalization and receive emotional support.

Recently, telemedicine technologies have been used in the NICU to enhance medical, informational, and emotional support for families during and after hospitalization. Baby CareLink[61] is a telemedicine program that incorporates video conferencing and Internet technologies to enhance interactions among families, NICU staff, and community health care providers. The link contains information for families about relevant issues during and after hospitalization. The video conferencing module enables distance learning by the family in their home during the NICU stay and remote monitoring after discharge. A recent survey found that families using this technology were more satisfied with the unit's physical environment and visitation policy, possibly because of the ability to facilitate visitation via teleconferencing when family members could not be present in the NICU.[61] Websites for parents of premature infants, children, and adults in the family are available so that parents can support each other, discuss common problems, and share solutions; caution should be used, however, when recommending the Internet (see "Resource Materials for Parents" at the end of this chapter).

Visiting in the Neonatal Intensive Care Unit

VISITING GUIDELINES

Besides their spouse or significant other, parents identify their families and friends as the main source of support through the crisis of having a sick neonate.[129,190] Prohibiting visiting by family and friends or limiting visitors to "two at a time" can isolate parents from a major source of support. NICU visiting policies should be used as guidelines, rather than rules, to facilitate visiting and caregiving by parents and families.* Care providers should use good judgment and discretion about visitation while understanding and respecting the parents' need to be "in charge" of their infant (e.g., make decisions for their infant).† Lack of perceived control by parents is associated with increased anxiety, hostility, depression, and poorer adjustment.[53,122,129,182] A sense of parental control in the NICU is enhanced by parental decision making.‡ Parents should designate their infant's "guest list"—that is, other family and friends who can visit and perform caregiving activities in their absence.[129]

NICU visiting policies vary within the United States[36] and among European countries. Two thirds of surveyed nurseries "allow" parents to visit during medical rounds, whereas visiting during nurse report was more restricted.[36] When parental visits were restricted, confidentiality was cited as the determinant of the visiting policy.[36] In this same survey, 39% of parents "sometimes" or "often" complained about restricted visitation.[36] A discrepancy exists between parental requests and visitation practices in many NICUs. NICU staff should be open-minded and flexible in determining the policy on visitation during rounds, report, and emergencies.[10,62,70] Many parents are interested in being included in medical rounds to actively participate in the care, discussion, and decision making about their infant.[10,62,70] A recent qualitative study of 18 NICU parents included in interdisciplinary teaching rounds in a tertiary children's hospital found that parents (1) had a positive experience and were "comfortable" being included, (2) preferred rounds in which nurses were included and lay terminology was used, and (3) welcomed the ability to communicate, understand the plan, and participate with the team in decision making about their infant's care.[110] If parents and the NICU staff agree to parental participation in rounds, patient confidentiality can be maintained by moving rounds away from the bedside, speaking quietly, and inviting parents to participate in only their infant's care planning/medical rounds[10,62,70] in this or a separate meeting. Parents may be visitors to the hospital and NICU, but they are not "visitors" to their newborn; parents and family are the constants in the life of a child, whereas health care providers are only temporary "visitors" in the life of the child.*

Parents may be more comfortable in the NICU if they are accompanied by a family member or friend.[190] A study showed that black teenage mothers establish a relationship with their infant by visiting regularly and learning how to care for him or her.[135] The research states that when these young women bring a friend or family member with them to the NICU, they are more comfortable parenting and caregiving for their infants. Parental visiting patterns may be categorized by care providers as visiting "too much"[62] or "too little."[63] Financial constraints (e.g., transportation and child-care costs, loss of work time), chaotic social situations, or poor physical and mental maternal health may contribute to fewer visits.[80] Parents may fear that the infant will not survive, may feel helpless, or may not think their visits are important for their sick baby. Parents should be taught by example how important their presence and caregiving are to their baby's survival and recovery. In addition, parents need to be taught to interpret their infant's cues and behaviors (see Chapter 13). Maximizing every parental visit by scheduling care by parents† (e.g., bathing the baby, breast feeding, kangaroo care, nipple feeding) communicates the importance of parent care and enables them "to be an expert on how to care for your baby by the time the baby is ready to go home."

SIBLING RELATIONSHIPS

The inclusion of other children in the events surrounding the birth of a sick newborn is important. From a sibling's viewpoint, the anticipated birth of a new infant is a stressful time of noticeable physical and psychologic changes within the family. In preparation for the impending birth, the child is told that the mother will be going to the hospital for a few days and will return with a baby brother or sister. With the birth of a premature or ill infant, the mother may go to the hospital unexpectedly, stay a long time, and not return home with the anticipated playmate. Instead of a celebration of the expected happy event, parents are grieving the loss of the normal newborn and facing the current crisis of their sick infant.

*References 3,62,80,122,129,140.

† References 53,76,122,129,138,159.

‡ References 53,70,122,129,138,159,192.

*References 3,26,89,112,129,140.

†References 53,112,129,132,159,190.

Parents are often unsure about what to tell the other children and whether the children should see the infant. The siblings themselves may feel left out, rejected, or worried that they, too, may get sick. They may feel they are to blame and that their jealous feelings about their new rival may have caused this tragedy. Confused by their parents' distress, the other children may speculate that it is related to them and their "bad" behaviors. They may be disappointed and angry that they did not get the "playmate" they had wanted. Because parents are unsure about how to manage these issues, it is often helpful for the staff to introduce the topic.

Because children will make up an explanation for the infant's illness, it is better to have it based on accurate information. Before explaining the infant's condition to siblings, elicit their ideas and perceptions about "what is the matter." Any fears, fantasies, misconceptions, or accurate information is thus used to begin the explanation of "where the baby is." Explanations must be tailored to the individual child's cognitive and developmental level. The child should be told that the infant is sick but in a way that is different from his or her illnesses; the infant's illness is not "catching," and it is not like any of the illnesses that the child has experienced. To allay the siblings' fears about medical personnel, they should also be told that the nurses and physicians are trying to help the infant "get better." Because children between 2 and 6 years of age are involved in magical thinking, they should be told that they are not to blame and that they did not cause the infant's problem. If the infant is premature, a team member might say to the child, "The baby came out too early or too soon; he needed more time to grow inside." If the infant has spina bifida, a staff member might say, "The baby's spine did not grow right, so he may have trouble lifting his legs or walking."

A child of 3 years of age or younger usually does not understand much about the coming infant. More important to this age-group is the separation from parents who are frequently at the hospital. To ameliorate the separation, child-care arrangements should be structured so that the child is cared for by familiar people in a familiar environment. The best care arrangement is with a familiar person in the child's own home; second best would be a familiar person in the caregiver's home; and third best, an unfamiliar person in the child's own home. The least favorable, of course, is an unfamiliar person in an unfamiliar setting. Many hospitals have a child-care facility run by volunteers that allows the child the opportunity to go to the hospital to "see where Mommy and Daddy are going" yet allows the parents the chance to see their infant without having to care for their older child or children. Parents may also choose to include the young child in all or selected visits.

Children ages 3 years and older have more interest in babies and a better grasp of the physical meaning of life. Sometimes a picture of the baby or a look into the nursery through the windows is helpful to the other children. Many children benefit from visits to the nursery to see their brother or sister. The natural curiosity of the child about "what is going on" in the family is answered when the child actually sees the baby. Behavior problems such as bed-wetting, sleeping and eating difficulties, and difficult separations from parents may be prevented or reduced by the reassurance of a visit that decreases the sibling's worry about the baby.[1] Sibling visitation must be individualized for every family.

SIBLING VISITS

The decision to include siblings in the NICU depends to a great extent on the views, beliefs, and attitudes of the hospital staff. Generally, the staff's concerns about and resistance to sibling visitation focus on a fear of an increase in nosocomial infection, disruption of unit routine and order, and potential harm to young children from exposure to the NICU environment. Infection control is the responsibility of parents and professionals. Parents must be educated about the dangers of infection and instructed on how to screen their children for symptoms such as fever, cough, or diarrhea. Professional staff must inquire about the health of visiting siblings, including their exposure to communicable diseases. Both parents and children must wash their hands before entering the nursery; small stools allowing children to reach the sink are helpful. Cover gowns are no longer used by parents, siblings, or professionals. With vigilance, no increased bacterial colonization and no increased incidence of infection occur with sibling visits.[178]

Because sibling visitation may be beneficial, each NICU must evaluate the center's situation and consider instituting a sibling visitation policy.[62] The following general principles may be used in developing this policy:

- Communication and coordination between staff and family are necessary to promote successful sibling visitation.
- Children must be prepared, according to their age and development, for what they will see, hear, and feel in the NICU. Language should be simple and honest; pictures of the infant or other infants can be helpful.
- Parents and staff screen the visiting sibling for signs of illness that would exclude the child from visiting.
- Parents and child must scrub their hands thoroughly
- The initial visit should be held at a relatively quiet time in the nursery when a care provider can stay with the family. If the infant can be moved to a private room or family room area, this is preferable.

At the bedside, the child is introduced to the infant and seated on a chair or stool at eye level with the infant. The care provider then again explains the equipment the child sees and any of the infant's "interesting" behaviors such as crying because of hunger, sucking on a pacifier, or eyes open "looking at you." Children may even be included in age-appropriate caregiving tasks. Choosing clothes, handling diapers and blankets, holding the bottle, and touching and talking to the infant are all ways "to help." The child may bring a present to the infant such as a simple toy, music box, or handmade picture or photograph of the family. After a visit, both parents and staff should be available to talk about the visit or answer any questions. Some children, however, will not discuss the visit or ask questions until some later time. A method for enabling children to express their feelings in a nonverbal way is through play or books. A child who receives a book about physicians and hospitals or a "doctor" or "nurse" doll may "play out" feelings about the brother or sister and the hospital experience.

Creating a comfortable environment in which children feel free to ask questions is essential when siblings visit. Every question deserves an answer, even "I don't know," when appropriate. Children are often quite unrestrained in their remarks and questions. Comments such as "He's sure ugly!" or "Will he die?" or "Why is she tied up (restrained)?" are common. These may be embarrassing to parents who hesitate to make the same remarks or ask the same questions. If the infant is hospitalized for a long time, the other children may lose interest or even wish it were all over. This response may upset parents who themselves may be struggling with the same feelings. The longer the infant is hospitalized, the greater the pressure on time and financial resources. Family routines are disrupted by continuing hospitalization, and the disruption may strain family relationships.

Staff and parent response to sibling visitation has been positive in hospitals in which the policy has been implemented. Such a policy may facilitate family integrity and promotes mutual support during the stressful time of hospitalization. Another advantage of visitation is that the older siblings do not endure repeated separations caused by parental visits to the hospital but are included as important and special family members. The presence of siblings in a nursery can be a rewarding experience for family and staff alike and perhaps is the ideal example of providing safe yet comprehensive family-centered care.

Although a flexible sibling visitation policy is viewed as the best possible situation, some alternatives such as coloring books and children's books should be considered (see "Resource Materials for Parents" at the end of this chapter). Staff should be sensitive to the needs of the siblings and understand that the parents must deal with both time and financial constraints.

Psychosocial Conferences

Psychosocial conferences for staff members to discuss the dynamics of family functioning and the effect of a seriously ill newborn on the family can be quite useful. These conferences, usually led by perinatal social workers or other mental health professionals, can give staff the opportunity to discuss and better understand their own feelings and reactions to families, infants, and the many stresses related to working in a NICU. In addition, weekly rounds with the entire multidisciplinary team (physicians, nurses, home health nurse coordinator, social workers, case managers, and financial counselors) are an effective vehicle to discuss and develop medical discharge and psychosocial care plans about each infant and family. The involvement of perinatal social workers to assess and evaluate the psychosocial functioning of families, provide support and counseling services, and coordinate the discharge planning and follow-up care for the infant and family is essential. Social workers should evaluate all high-risk cases in addition to providing support in complicated medical conditions, including the death of the infant (Box 29-6). Programs

BOX 29-6 HIGH-RISK FACTORS INDICATING NEED FOR SOCIAL WORK INTERVENTION

1. Teenage pregnancy (ages 11 to 18 years)[22]
2. Single parent
3. Substance abuse[22]
4. Psychiatric history that interferes with appropriate functioning (including postpartum depression), especially as related to parenting abilities
5. Mother or father with a history of being physically or sexually abused or early deprivation by own family, or history of having abused or neglected own children
6. Battered women/domestic violence
7. Mental retardation, borderline intelligence, or significant physical handicaps
8. History of loss with previous pregnancy or loss of child because of stillbirth, birth defect, prematurity, abortion, custody case, or death
9. Rejection of or ambivalence about current pregnancy as manifested by requests for termination of pregnancy, attempted abortion, or relinquishment
10. No prenatal care with previous or current pregnancies
11. Pregnancy exacerbating extreme depression, anxiety, or suicidal thoughts
12. Stressful home or personal situation because of marital or financial problems or lack of support
13. Long-term hospitalization during pregnancy requiring intervention in helping family adjust by arranging for younger children at home or for financial assistance
14. Other children with physical or mental handicaps
15. Attachment difficulties with the infant
16. Prior history with social services
17. Inadequate housing and living arrangements and homelessness[186]
18. Inadequate food and other essentials[183]
19. Incarceration of mother/father[183]
20. Military families[177]
21. Undocumented immigrants

should be implemented for staff members to increase their competency and comfort level in identifying and intervening with psychosocial issues.[67,168]

Domestic Violence

Domestic violence is recognized as a serious risk factor for adverse pregnancy outcomes.[11] Studies have shown that injuries resulting from physical abuse are associated with low birth weight, preterm birth, and intrauterine growth restriction.[24,118,143,145] There is also an association of physical abuse with antepartum hemorrhage and perinatal death.[87] Perinatal violence and stress are significant risk factors for preterm birth in the teen population.[39,170] Abused women have reported a greater prevalence of substance abuse (alcohol, tobacco, and drugs), poor nutrition, and demographic risk resulting in a poor birth outcome. Late prenatal care and single marital status are predictors of decreased birth weight.[98]

Because domestic violence is so prevalent with serious negative effects on the entire family system, protocols and procedures (that are compliant with the policies of the setting [i.e., hospital, outpatient clinic, emergency room] and the reporting laws of the state) should be in place. Legal definitions of domestic violence vary by state. The health care team needs to be educated to recognize the signs and behaviors that may indicate domestic violence (and child abuse). The American College of Obstetricians and Gynecologists has guidelines for screening and advocates routine screening for all women. For a discussion about the benefits and risks of routine screening, refer to the U.S. Preventive Services Task Force recommendation statement.[188]

Because abuse is so pervasive and too serious to remain unidentified, health care providers should routinely ask all women patients about domestic violence (although men also can be victims).[128] Battering beginning during pregnancy is a very common phenomenon. Many assessment tools[32,74] (Boxes 29-7 and 29-8) are available that can be tailored to the practice setting. A recent article revealed that an anonymous computer-assisted self-interview offered an alternative approach to screening of women who are hesitant to disclose abuse directly to health care providers.[162] Another study conducted by the same investigators provided evidence that the great majority of pregnant women are not offended when screened for domestic violence and may increase their disclosure if they are told about state reporting mandates that preclude mandatory reporting for adults.[161]

Once a potentially abusive situation has been identified, culturally and ethnically sensitive interventions should be initiated. Interventions vary depending on the disclosures made by the mother or father (or partner) and the needs identified. Recommendations for interventions include the following: (1) discuss options with the victim, (2) help identify a safety plan, (3) make appropriate referrals, (4) comply with state statutes about reporting responsibility, (5) document assessments and interventions, and (6) refer for treatment and aftercare (essential). Because of the complexity of issues generated by domestic violence, a multidisciplinary team approach is recommended.

BOX 29-7 ASSESSMENT CHECKLIST FOR VICTIMS OF DOMESTIC VIOLENCE

Domestic Violence

Interview victim separately from spouse or boyfriend.

Risk Factors (Check Those That Apply)

_____ Financial problems, unemployment
_____ Divorce or separation, especially during pregnancy
_____ Drug or alcohol abuse by victim or perpetrator
_____ Victim or perpetrator physically abused as a child
_____ Overly protective or controlling perpetrator (refuses to leave room during examination or treatment)
_____ Suicide attempts by victim or perpetrator

Signs of Physical Abuse (Check Those That Apply)

_____ Self-induced or attempted abortions, multiple therapeutic abortions, miscarriages
_____ Abdominal or pelvic injuries, back or spine injuries (no fall or motor vehicle accident)
_____ Injuries to face, neck, throat, chest, breasts
_____ Injuries during pregnancy
_____ Increased drug or alcohol abuse during pregnancy
_____ Multiple injuries in various stages of healing
_____ Injury inconsistent with history
_____ Delay between injury and medical treatment
_____ Woman minimizes frequency or seriousness of injuries
_____ Repeated emergency department visits with multiple somatic complaints or with injuries of increasing severity
_____ Sexual assault by partner
_____ Suicide attempt
_____ Single car accident
_____ Fractures in various stages of healing
_____ Burns (cigarette, friction, splash, chemical)
_____ Head injuries
_____ Low self-esteem, sense of apprehension or hopelessness, depression by victim (laughing inappropriately, crying, no eye contact, angry, defensive)
_____ HOMICIDAL RISK: Presence of gun in home; perpetrator threatened to kill victim, or she believes he may kill her; overly jealous perpetrator; violent behavior by perpetrator toward nonfamily members; use of alcohol or drugs by perpetrator; increasing severity of injuries; perpetrator has killed pets; objectifies victim (calls names, body parts, animals)

From Haack D: *Suggested protocols for victims of spousal and elder abuse: a task force reference document for Colorado hospitals* (p. 6, Appendix B), Denver, 1992, Colorado Department of Health.

Transfer Back to the Referring Hospital

Transfer of the infant from a tertiary center back to the referring or local community hospital for convalescent care and discharge is a frequent occurrence. This can help facilitate the relationship between the infant and parents, because the infant will be more accessible. Parents generally view the transfer as positive if the hospital is closer to home and if they feel comfortable with the level of care provided. Transfer is stressful, and there is always an adjustment period any time a transfer occurs.[108] Parents must adapt to different personalities of medical personnel and different procedures and visiting policies. Preparing the parents for the transfer, orienting them to the new hospital, and talking to the staff of the referral hospital about the infant and the parents are important to help ease the transition.[108]

Preparation to Take the Infant Home

The sixth psychologic task for parents concerns preparations for taking the infant home. Parents must understand their infant's individual needs and personality characteristics and must feel a sense of competency in relating to their infant. Discharge is an anxiety-provoking event and ushers in the "crisis" of homecoming, which parents must face and master.[46,80,85,122,182] The unsuccessful resolution of the previously discussed five psychologic tasks can contribute to maladaptive parenting and a poor outcome for the infant, including the possibilities of attachment difficulties, overprotectiveness, failure to thrive, vulnerable child syndrome,[101] emotional deprivation, and battering.[34,101] To achieve a positive parent-child relationship after the hospitalization and through the transitional period that ensues, provision of appropriate follow-up support through the home adjustment period is crucial.[101,122,182]

Several behaviors demonstrate that parents are trying to understand the infant's care in preparation for discharge. First, parents may ask questions verbalizing a variety of concerns. For a premature infant, they might ask, "Do I need an apnea monitor at home?" or "Can the baby have visitors?" or "Do I have to wash my hands when handling the baby?" For an infant with a congenital defect such as spina bifida, the parents might ask, "Can I lay the baby on his back?" or "Can I bathe him?" or "Do I have to

BOX 29-8

ABUSE ASSESSMENT

For Pregnant Patients

These questions may help you when assessing female patients for abuse. For some women, answering "sometimes" to abuse questions is easier than "yes" or "no."

1. Do you know where you could go or who could help you if you were abused or worried about abuse?
   ______ Yes ______ No
   ______ If yes, where ______________________________
   ____
2. Are you in a relationship with a man who physically hurts you?
   ______ Yes ______ No ______ Sometimes
3. Does he threaten you with abuse?
   ______ Yes ______ No ______ Sometimes
4. Has the man you are with hit, slapped, kicked, or otherwise physically hurt you?
   ______ Yes ______ No ______ Sometimes
5. If yes, has he hit you since you've been pregnant?
   ______ Yes ______ No ______ Not Applicable
6. If yes, did the abuse increase since you've been pregnant?
   ______ Yes ______ No ______ Not Applicable
7. Have you ever received medical treatment for any abuse injuries?
   ______ Yes ______ No ______ Not Applicable
8. If you've been abused—remembering the last time he hurt you—mark the places on a body map where he hit you.
9. Were you pregnant at the time?
   ______ Yes ______ No ______ Not Applicable

When assessing for abuse, some women may be uncomfortable with the topic and may exhibit some of the behaviors below. For some women, these behaviors may be suggestive of abuse and disclosure of battering may follow at a later date.

Actions Suggestive of Abuse

1.	Laughing or "tittering"	Yes	No
2.	No eye contact (not applicable in some cultures)	Yes	No
3.	Crying	Yes	No
4.	Sighing	Yes	No
5.	Minimizing statements	Yes	No
6.	Searching/engaging eye contact (fear)	Yes	No
7.	Anxious body language (standing to leave, dropped shoulders, depressed)	Yes	No
8.	Anger, defensiveness	Yes	No
9.	Comments about emotional abuse	Yes	No
10.	Comments about a "friend" who is abused	Yes	No

From Haack D: *Suggested protocols for victims of spousal and elder abuse: a task force reference document for Colorado hospitals* (p. 11, Appendix E), Denver, 1992, Colorado Department of Health.

pump the shunt?" For an infant with a heart defect, the staff might be asked, "Do I need oxygen?" or "Do I have to handle him differently?" or "What about going to higher altitudes?" or "Is my baby at risk for sudden infant death syndrome (SIDS)?" All of these questions on the part of parents are typical and normal and represent the parents' working through their fears and anxieties.

On the other hand, parents who are highly anxious,[46] extremely overprotective, or very indifferent should be a concern to the health care personnel. The inability to deal with the task of taking the infant home may indicate some unresolved feelings related to the previous psychologic tasks. Although most parents whose infants have been in a NICU do admit to initially treating their infant differently until they "got to know their child," a group of parents who are excessively overprotective does exist. This type of behavior often stems from parents who are struggling with intense feelings of guilt and failure. These parents either protect their baby from everything because they feel so responsible for having caused the infant's initial problem or they demonstrate an indifference or lack of concern for the infant and the infant's welfare. Such parents may have an ambivalent attachment to their infant, who may continue to represent the threat of death or the parents' personal failure. This group of parents should be considered high risk for potential parent-child relationship difficulties and should be evaluated to determine an appropriate intervention.

At discharge, there are infants whose medical conditions are still fragile, and there is a substantial indication that these infants may not be normal and may have long-term problems. These infants may be temperamentally difficult to manage, and parents understandably treat them differently. These parents and infants need additional support and appropriate intervention (see Chapter 31).

The perinatal health care team can employ many interventions to assist parents with discharge and through the transitional period that follows (see Chapter 31). In the hospital, adequate teaching of caregiving skills that enable the parent to develop a sense of mastery and competence is of paramount importance. In addition to tasks of care, parents should participate in planning and providing developmentally appropriate care and be able to read and respond to their infant's cues (see Chapter 13). Maternal concerns about the infant's care center on elimination, feeding/weight gain, the infant's health (breathing, development, or ongoing medical problems),[80] and preparation of medications. If parents do not feel comfortable with their infant, their anxiety can cause adverse interactions with him or her. The parent needs to know the infant's mannerisms and behaviors; otherwise the parent may feel exhausted and resentful and then guilty. Teaching caregiving skills often can be facilitated in an environment that is less intense and crisis oriented than the NICU. Whenever possible, an infant should be transferred to a setting that is more conducive to the parents' initiation of the primary caregiving role, such as a special care or transitional nursery, a level II unit, or a general pediatric ward. Care by parents before discharge enables parents to assume full responsibility for their infant's care, tests the reality of caregiving, helps them learn caregiving activities and their infant's behavioral patterns, and confirms their readiness for independent parenting and the infant's readiness for discharge.[66,80,132,146]

Adequate discharge planning and follow-up arrangements should include general pediatric care, home health care, nurse home visitors, and parenting classes, especially for young or psychosocially high-risk parents.[106] Recent studies document positive effects of home visitation programs.[106,146,152,153] Referrals to county social service departments should be made for single mothers who are eligible for Temporary Assistance to Needy Families; Women, Infants, and Children (WIC) Program; Title 19 Medicaid; and state child health insurance programs. For infants with special problems (e.g., spina bifida, cerebral palsy, Down syndrome), referrals should be made for special programs that provide services for the infants and support groups for parents. Parents whose infants have special medical needs (e.g., gavage feedings, tracheostomy or colostomy care, oxygen, or ventilators) should be evaluated by the medical and nursing teams to determine helpful community resources (e.g., equipment, supplies, respite,[136,165] emergency care) and to make appropriate referrals. Home nursing care and homemaker services sometimes are covered by medical insurance and may be necessary to provide actual nursing activities and to relieve parents from the emotional burden inherent in caring for an infant with medical problems. For infants who are developmentally and physically disabled, developmental intervention programs and follow-up programs provided by many hospitals that have NICUs are extremely valuable. These infants are eligible for Part C of the Individuals with Disabilities Education Act (IDEA). Locating babysitters who will care for a child with special problems can be an overwhelming task for parents; cultivating a resource list for parents and suggesting that parents exchange services with each other also can be helpful. Graduate parents, neonatal nurses, or respite care organizations can provide a useful service to parents in this situation. Last, parents should be referred to appropriate funding agencies (e.g., Health Care Programs for Children with Special Needs, Title 19 Medicaid, state child health insurance programs, Social Security Disability) that provide financial assistance.

REFERENCES

1. Affonso D: Missing pieces: a study of post-partum feelings, *Birth Fam J* 4:159, 1977.
2. Aguilera D, Messick J: *Crisis intervention theory and methodology,* ed 3, St Louis, 1978, Mosby.
3. Ahmann E, Abraham M, Johnson B: *Changing the concept of families as visitors: supporting family presence and participation,* Bethesda, Md, 2003, Institute for Family-Centered Care.
4. Allen E, Manuel J, Legault C, et al: Perception of child vulnerability among mothers of former premature infants, *Pediatrics* 113:267, 2004.
5. Altimier L: Healing environments: for patients and providers, *Newborn Infant Nurs Rev* 4:89, 2004.
6. Altshuler LL, Cohen LS, Moline ML, et al: The expert consensus guideline series: treatment of depression in women, *Postgrad Med* (Spec No.): 1, 2001.
7. American Academy of Pediatrics: The initiation or withdrawal of treatment for high-risk newborns, *Pediatrics* 96:362, 1995.

8. American Academy of Pediatrics and American College of Obstetricians and Gynecologists: Perinatal care at the threshold of viability, *Pediatrics* 96:974, 1995.
9. American Academy of Pediatrics and American College of Obstetricians and Gynecologists: *Guidelines for perinatal care,* ed 6, Elk Grove, Ill, 2007, The Academy.
10. American Academy of Pediatrics, Committee on Hospital Care and Institute for Family-Centered Care: Family-centered care and the pediatrician's role, *Pediatrics* 112:691, 2003.
11. American Academy of Pediatrics, Committee on Pediatric Workforce: Ensuring culturally effective pediatric care: implications for education and health policy, *Pediatrics* 114:1677, 2004.
12. American Psychological Association: *Diagnostic and statistical manual of mental disorders,* ed 4, Washington, DC, 2000, The Association.
13. Ammon K: How to survive and thrive in a multicultural setting, *Natl Assoc Perinat Soc Work Forum* 22:2, 2002.
14. Baker L: Screening for postpartum depression, *Natl Assoc Perinat Soc Work Forum* 22:1, 2002.
15. Beck C: Postpartum depression: a metasynthesis, *Qual Health Res* 12:453, 2002.
16. Beck C: Revision of the postpartum depression predictors inventory, *J Obstet Gynecol Neonatal Nurs* 31:394, 2002.
17. Beck C: Recognizing and screening for postpartum depression in mothers of NICU infants, *Adv Neonatal Care* 3:37, 2003.
18. Beck CT: Postpartum depression: it isn't just the blues, *Am J Nurs* 106:40, 2006.
19. Beck CT, Gable RK: *Postpartum depression screening scale manual,* Los Angeles, 2002, Western Psychological Services.
20. Beck CT, Grable RK: Screening performance of the postpartum depression screening scale—Spanish version, *J Transcult Nurs* 16:331, 2005.
21. Beck CT, Records K, Rice M: Further development of the postpartum depression predictors inventory—revised, *J Obstet Gynecol Neonatal Nurs* 35:735, 2006.
22. Bialoskurski M, Cox C, Hayes J: The nature of attachment in a neonatal intensive care unit, *J Perinat Neonat Nurs* 13:66, 1999.
23. Boss RD, Holton N, Sulpar LJ, et al: Values parents apply to decision-making regarding delivery room resuscitation for high-risk newborns, *Pediatrics* 122:583, 2008.
24. Boy A, Salihu HM: Intimate partner violence and birth outcomes: a systematic review, *Int J Fertil Womens Med* 49:159, 2004.
25. Bracht M, Kandankery A, Nodwell S, et al: Cultural differences and parental responses to the preterm infant at risk: strategies for supporting families, *Neonatal Netw* 21:31, 2002.
26. Browne J: Early relationship environments: physiology of skin-to-skin contact for parents and their preterm infants, *Clin Perinat* 31:287, 2004.
27. Buist A, Morse C, Durkin S: Men's adjustment to fatherhood: implications for obstetric health care, *J Obstet Gynecol Neonatal Nurs* 32:172, 2003.
28. Burt V, Suri R, Altshuler L, et al: The use of psychotropic medications during breastfeeding, *Am J Psychiatry* 7:1001, 2001.
29. Calloway SD, Venegas LM: The new HIPAA law on privacy and confidentiality, *Nurs Adm Q* 26:40, 2002.
30. Caplan G: Patterns of parental response to the crisis of premature birth, *Psychiatry* 23:365, 1960.
31. Caplan G, Mason EA, Kaplan DM: Four studies of crisis in parents of prematures: 1965, *Community Ment Health J* 1:149, 2000.
32. Carroll JC, Reid AJ, Biringer A, et al: Effectiveness of the Antenatal Psychosocial Health Assessment (ALPHA) form in detecting psychosocial concerns: a randomized controlled trial, *Can Med Assoc J* 173:253, 2005.
33. Carvajal S: A parent support group in the NICU, *Central Lines* 18:4, 2002.
34. Catlin A: Child abuse prevention: still something to think about, *Central Lines* 19:6, 2003.
35. Chaudron LH, Szilagyi PG, Kitzman HJ, et al: Detection of postpartum depressive symptoms by screening at well-child visits, *Pediatrics* 113:551, 2004.
36. Chernick L, Cockrell T, Frech C, et al: Current staff attitudes regarding parental visitation within NICUs, *Pediatr Res* 47:391c, 2000.
37. Clark A, Carter P: Why do nurses see families as "trouble?" *Clin Nurse Spec* 16:40, 2002.
38. Cooper LG, Gooding JS, Gallagher J, et al: Impact of a family-centered care initiative on NICU care, staff and families, *J Perinatol* 27(suppl 2):S32, 2007.
39. Coverington D, Justason B, Wright L: Severity, manifestations, and consequences of violence among pregnant adolescents, *J Adolesc Health* 28:55, 2001.
40. Cox, JL, Holden JM: *Perinatal mental health: a guide to the Edinburgh Postnatal Depression Scale,* London, 2003, Gaskell.
41. Cox JL, Holden JM, Sagovsky R: Detection of postnatal depression: development of the 10-item Edinburgh Postnatal Depression Scale, *Br J Psychiatry* 150:782, 1987.
42. Damato E: Prenatal attachment and other correlates of postnatal maternal attachment to twins, *Adv Neonatal Care* 4:274, 2004.
43. De Montigny F, Lacharite C: Father's perceptions of the immediate postpartal period, *J Obstet Gynecol Neonatal Nurs* 33:328, 2004.

44. Dennis CL, Hodnett E: Psychosocial and psychological interventions for treating postpartum depression, *Cochrane Database Syst Rev* 4:CD006116, 2007.
45. Dhillon AS, Albersheim SG, Alsaad S, et al: Internet use and perceptions of information reliability by parents in a neonatal intensive care unit, *J Perinatol* 23:420, 2003.
46. Docherty S, Miles M, Holditch-Davis D: Worry about child health in mothers of medically fragile infants, *Adv Neonatal Care* 2:84, 2002.
47. Doering L, Dracup K, Moser D: Comparison of psychosocial adjustment of mothers and fathers of high-risk infants in the NICU, *J Perinatol* 19:132, 1999.
48. Dokken D, Ahmann E: The many roles of family members in "Family-Centered Care"—Part I, *Pediatr Nurs* 32:562, 2006.
49. Dunn MS, Reilly MC, Johnston AM, et al: Development and dissemination of potentially better practices for the provision of family-centered care in neonatology: the family-centered care map, *Pediatrics* 118:S95, 2006.
50. Eidelman A, Hoffman N, Kaitz M: Cognitive deficits in women after childbirth, *Obstet Gynecol* 81:764, 1993.
51. Epperson N: Postpartum mood changes: are hormones to blame?, *Zero to Three* 6:17, 2002.
52. Feldman R, Weller A, Leckman J, et al: The nature of the mother's tie to her infant: maternal bonding under conditions of proximity, separation and potential loss, *J Psychol Psychiatry* 40:929, 1999.
53. Fenwick J, Barclay L, Schmied V: Struggling to mother: a consequence of inhibitive nursing interactions in the neonatal nursery, *J Perinat Neonatal Nurs* 15:49, 2001.
54. Flores G: Culture and the patient-physician relationship: achieving cultural competency in health care, *J Pediatr* 136:14, 2000.
55. Gjerdingen D, Katon W, Rich DE: Stepped care treatment of postpartum depression: a primary care–based management model, *Womens Health Issues* 18:44, 2008.
56. Gleason TR, Evans ME: Perceived vulnerability: a comparison of parents and children, *J Child Health Care* 8:279, 2004.
57. Glick C: Smoothing the waters for compassionate health care: transcultural proficiency, *Natl Assoc Perinat Soc Work Forum* 24:1, 2004.
58. Gottfried AW, Gaiter JL: *Infant stress under intensive care*, Baltimore, 1985, University Park Press.
59. Grant P, Siegel R: *Families in crisis: birth of a sick infant.* Presented at the Perinatal Section Meeting of the American Academy of Pediatrics, Scottsdale, Ariz, April, 1978.
60. Gray J, Cutler C, Dean J, et al: Perinatal assessment of mother-baby interaction. In Helfer B, Kempe CH, editors: *Child abuse and neglect: the family and the community,* Cambridge, Mass, 1976, Ballinger Publishing.
61. Gray J, Pompilio G, Pursley D, et al: Baby CareLink: improving NICU care with telemedicine technologies, *Pediatr Res* 47:400a, 2000.
62. Griffin T: Visitation patterns: the parents who visit "too much, *Neonatal Netw* 17:67, 1998.
63. Griffin T: Visitation patterns: the parents who visit "too little, *Neonatal Netw* 18:75, 1999.
64. Griffin T: Facing challenges to family-centered care. I. Conflicts over visitation, *Pediatr Nurs* 29:135, 2003.
65. Griffin T: Facing challenges to family-centered care. II. Anger in the clinical setting, *Pediatr Nurs* 29:212, 2003.
66. Griffin T, Abraham M: Transition to home from the newborn intensive care unit: applying the principles of family-centered care to the discharge process, *J Perinat Neonatal Nurs* 20:243, 2006.
67. Gunn J, Hegarty K, Nagle C, et al: Putting women-centered care into practice: a new (ANEW) approach to psychosocial risk assessment during pregnancy, *Birth* 33:46, 2006.
68. Hack M: Continuity of neonatal care, *Lancet* 361:1809, 2003.
69. Hanna B, Jarman H, Savage S, et al: The early detection of postpartum depression: midwives and nurses trial a checklist, *J Obstet Gynecol Neonatal Nurs* 33:191, 2004.
70. Harrison H: The principles for family-centered neonatal care, *Pediatrics* 92:643, 1993.
71. Helfer B, Kempe CH: *Child abuse and neglect: the family and the community*, Cambridge, Mass, 1976, Ballinger.
72. Henderson DP, Knapp JF: Report of the National Consensus Conference on Family Presence During Pediatric Cardiopulmonary Resuscitation and Procedures, *J Emerg Nurs* 32:23, 2006.
73. Heneghan A, Mercer MB, DeLeone N: Will mothers discuss parenting stress and depressive symptoms with their child's pediatrician? *Pediatrics* 113:460, 2004.
74. Higgins LP, Hawkins JW: Screening for abuse during pregnancy: implementing a multisite program, *MCN Am J Matern Child Nurs* 30:109, 2005.
75. Hodnett E, Gates S, Hofmeyr GJ, et al: Continuous support for women during childbirth, *Cochrane Database Syst Rev* 3: CD003766, 2007.
76. Holditch-Davis D, Miles M: Mothers' stories about their experiences in the NICU, *Neonatal Netw* 19:13, 2000.
77. Horowitz JA: Community-based postpartum depression screening within the first month after delivery, *Contemp Nurse* 21:85, 2006.
78. Horowitz JA, Goodman J: Identifying and treating postpartum depression, *J Obstet Gynecol Neonatal Nurs* 34:264, 2005.
79. Howard M, Battle CL, Pearlstein T, et al: A psychiatric mother-baby day hospital for pregnant and postpartum women, *Arch Womens Ment Health* 9:213, 2006.
80. Hummel P: Parenting in the high-risk infant, *Newborn Infant Nurs Rev* 3:88, 2003.

81. Hurst I: Mothers' strategies to meet their needs in the newborn intensive care nursery, *J Perinat Neonatal Nurs* 15:65, 2001.
82. Hurst I: Vigilant watching over: mothers' actions to safeguard their premature babies in the newborn intensive care nursery, *J Perinat Neonatal Nurs* 15:39, 2001.
83. Hynan MT: Supporting fathers during stressful times in the nursery: an evidence-based review, *Newborn Infant Nurs Rev* 5:87, 2005.
84. Institute for Family-Centered Care: *Rationale for family-centered care*, Bethesda, Md, 2002, The Institute.
85. Jackson K, Ternestedt B, Schollin J: From alienation to familiarity: experiences of mothers and fathers of preterm infants, *J Adv Nurs* 43:120, 2003.
86. Jacobs E, Chen AH, Karliner L, et al: Legal and regulatory obligations to provide culturally and linguistically appropriate emergency department services, *Clin Ped Emerg Med* 5:58, 2004.
87. Janseen P, Holt V, Sugg N, et al: Intimate partner violence and adverse pregnancy outcomes: a population-based study, *Am J Obstet Gynecol* 188:1341, 2003.
88. Johnson AN: The maternal experience of kangaroo holding, *J Obstet Gynecol Neonatal Nurs* 36:568, 2007.
89. Johnson B, Abraham M, Parrish R: Designing the neonatal intensive care unit for optimal family involvement, *Clin Perinatol* 31:353, 2004.
90. Johnson B, Crocker L: *Privileged presence: personal stories of connections in health care,* Boulder, Colo, 2006, Bull Publishing.
91. Johnston AM, Bullock CE, Graham JE, et al: Implementation and case-study results of potentially better practices for family-centered care: the family-centered care map, *Pediatrics* 118:S108, 2006.
92. Joint Commission on Accreditation of Healthcare Organizations: *Joint Commission standards that support the provision of culturally and linguistically appropriate services*, 2006. Accessed November 2, 2009, from www.jointcommission.org.
93. Jordan B: *Birth in four cultures,* St Albans, Vt, 1978, Eden Press.
94. Joseph RA, Mackley AB, Davis CG, et al: Stress in fathers of surgical neonatal intensive care unit babies, *Adv Neonatal Care* 7:321, 2007.
95. Kaaresen PI, Ronning JA, Ulvund SE, et al: A randomized, controlled trial of the effectiveness of an early intervention program in reducing parenting stress after preterm birth, *Pediatrics* 118:e9, 2006.
96. Kaminsky LM, Carlo J, Meunch MV, et al: Screening for postpartum depression with the Edinburgh Postnatal Depression Scale in an indigent population: does a directed interview improve detection rates compared with a standard self-completed questionnaire? *J Matern Fetal Neonatal Med* 21:321, 2008.
97. Kaplan DM, Mason EA: Maternal reactions to premature birth viewed as an emotional disorder, *Am J Orthopsych* 30:539, 1960.
98. Kearny M, Munro B, Kelly U, et al: Health behaviors as mediators for the effect of partner abuse on infant birth weight, *Nurs Res* 53:36, 2004.
99. Klaus MH, Jerauld R, Kreger NC, et al: Maternal attachment: importance of the first postpartum days, *N Engl J Med* 286:460, 1972.
100. Klaus MH, Kennell JH: Mothers separated from their newborn infants, *Pediatr Clin North Am* 17:1015, 1970.
101. Klaus MH, Kennell JH: *Parent-infant bonding,* ed 2, St Louis, 1982, Mosby.
102. Koh THHG, Butow PN, Coory M, et al: Provision of taped conversations with neonatologists to mothers of babies in intensive care: randomised controlled trial, *BMJ* 334:28, 2007.
103. Koh THHG, Casey A, Harrison H: Use of an outcome by gestation table for extremely premature babies: a cross-sectional survey of the views of parents, neonatal nurses and perinatologists, *J Perinatol* 20:504, 2000.
104. Koh THHG, Harrison H, Morley C: Gestation versus outcome table for parents of extremely premature infants, *J Perinatol* 19:452, 1999.
105. Koh THHG, Jarvis C: Promoting effective communication in neonatal intensive care units by audiotaping doctor-parent conversations, *Int J Clin Pract* 52:27, 1998.
106. Koniak-Griffin D, Anderson N, Brecht M, et al: Public health nursing care for adolescent mothers: impact on infant health and selected maternal outcomes at one year postbirth, *J Adolesc Health* 30:44, 2002.
107. Korja R, Mauna J, Kirjavainen J, et al: Mother-infant interaction is influenced by the amount of holding in preterm infants, *Early Hum Dev* 84:257, 2008.
108. Kuhnly J, Freston M: Back transport: exploration of parents' feelings regarding the transition, *Neonatal Netw* 14:69, 1995.
109. Kussano C, Maehara S: Japanese and Brazilian maternal bonding behavior towards preterm infants: a comparative study, *J Neonat Nurs* 4:23, 1998.
110. Latta LC, Dick R, Parry C, et al: Parental responses to involvement in rounds on a pediatric inpatient unit at a teaching hospital: a qualitative study, *Acad Med* 83:292, 2008.
111. Lavitt M: Perinatal clients and the Internet: quality of online support and potential for harm, *Natl Assoc Perinat Soc Work Forum* 21:8, 2001.
112. Lawhon G: Facilitation of parenting the premature infant within the newborn intensive care unit, *J Perinat Neonatal Nurs* 16:71, 2002.
113. Lee DT, Chung TK: Postnatal depression: an update, *Best Pract Res Clin Obstet Gynaecol* 21:183, 2007.
114. Lee S, Lee KA, Rankin SH, et al: Acculturation and stress in Chinese-American parents of infants cared for in the intensive care unit, *Adv Neonatal Care* 5:315, 2005.

115. Leonard L: Prenatal behavior of multiples: implications for families and nurses, *J Obstet Gynecol Neonatal Nurs* 31:248, 2002.
116. Leung J, Spear M, Locke R, et al: Developmental changes in family reactions during their infant's prolonged hospitalization in the NICU, *Pediatr Res* 45:207a, 1999.
117. Lindgren K: A comparison of pregnancy health practices of women in inner-city and small urban communities, *J Obstet Gynecol Neonatal Nurs* 32:313, 2003.
118. Lipsky S, Holt V, Easterling T, et al: Impact of police reported intimate partner violence during pregnancy on birth outcome, *Obstet Gynecol* 102:557, 2003.
119. Liu D, Diorio J, Tannenbaum B, et al: Maternal care, hippocampal glucocorticoid receptors, and hypothalamic-pituitary-adrenal responses to stress, *Science* 277:1659, 1997.
120. Logsdon MC, Usui W: Psychosocial predictors of postpartum depression in diverse groups of women, *West J Nurs Res* 23:563, 2001.
121. London F: How to prepare families for discharge in the limited time available, *Pediatr Nurs* 30:212, 2004.
122. Lundqvist P, Jakobsson L: Swedish men's experiences of becoming fathers to their preterm infants, *Neonatal Netw* 22:25, 2003.
123. Masser-Frye D: Birth defects, genetics, and genetic counseling, *Natl Assoc Perinat Soc Work Forum* 21:1, 2001.
124. Matthey S, Barnett B, Kavanagh D, et al: Validation of the Edinburgh Postnatal Depression Scale for men and comparison of item endorsement with their partners, *J Affect Disord* 64:175, 2001.
125. Matthey S, Morgan M, Healey L, et al: Postpartum issues for expectant mothers and fathers, *J Obstet Gynecol Neonatal Nurs* 31:428, 2002.
126. Mayes L: Parental preoccupation and perinatal mental health, *Zero to Three* 6:4, 2002.
127. McAllister M, Dionne K: Partnering with parents: establishing effective long-term relationships with parents in the NICU, *Neonatal Netw* 25:329, 2006.
128. McFadden T: Understanding domestic violence, *Natl Assoc Perinat Soc Workers Forum* 24:1, 2004.
129. McGrath J: Building relationships with families in the NICU: exploring the guarded alliance, *J Perinat Neonatal Nurs* 15:74, 2001.
130. McGrath J: Family presence during procedures: breathing life into policy and everyday practice, *Newborn Infant Nurs Rev* 6:243, 2006.
131. Melynk B, Alpert-Gillis L, Feinstein N, et al: Creating opportunities for parent empowerment: program effects on the mental health/coping outcomes of critically ill young children and their mothers, *Pediatrics* 113:e597, 2004.
132. Melynk BM, Feinstein NF, Alpert-Gillis L, et al: Reducing premature infants' length of stay and improving parents' mental health outcomes with the Creating Opportunities for Parent Empowerment (COPE) neonatal intensive care unit program: a randomized controlled trial, *Pediatrics* 118:e1414, 2006.
133. Mew A, Holditch-Davis D, Belyea M, et al: Correlates of depressive symptoms in mothers of preterm infants, *Neonatal Netw* 22:51, 2003.
134. Miles M, Burchinal P, Holditch-Davis D, et al: Perceptions of stress, worry, and support in black and white mothers of hospitalized, medically fragile infants, *J Pediatr Nurs* 17:82, 2002.
135. Miles M, Wilson S, Docherty S: African American mothers' responses to hospitalization of an infant with serious health problems, *Neonatal Netw* 18:17, 1999.
136. Miller S: Respite care for children who have complex healthcare needs, *Pediatric Nurs* 29:80, 2002.
137. Mitchell L: Women's experience of unexpected ultrasound findings, *J Midwifery Womens Health* 49:228, 2004.
138. Montalvo N, Vila B: Parent's grand rounds speech on neonatal intensive care unit experience, *J Perinatol* 19:525, 1999.
139. Moore ER, Anderson GC, Bergman N: Early skin-to-skin contact for mothers and their healthy newborn infants, *Cochrane Database Syst Rev* 3: CD003519, 2007.
140. Moore K, Coker K, DuBuisson A, et al: Implementing potentially better practices for improving family-centered care in neonatal intensive care units: success and challenges, *Pediatrics* 11:e437, 2003.
141. Moore M, Moos M: *Cultural competence in the care of the childbearing families*, New York, 2003, March of Dimes Birth Defects Foundation.
142. Moses-Kolko EL, Roth EK: Antepartum and postpartum depression: healthy mom, healthy baby, *J Am Med Womens Assoc* 59:181, 2004.
143. Murphy C, Sehei B, Myhr T, et al: Abuse: a risk factor for low birth weight? A systemic review and meta-analysis, *Can Med Assoc J* 164:1567, 2001.
144. Nagata M, Yukiyo N, Hisanori S, et al: Depression in the early postpartum period and attachment to children: in mothers of NICU infants, *Infant Child Dev* 13:93, 2004.
145. Neggers Y, Goldenberg R, Cliver S, et al: Effects of domestic violence on preterm birth and lower birth weight, *Act Obstet Gynecol Scand* 83:455, 2004.
146. Nelson A: Transition to motherhood, *J Obstet Gynecol Neonatal Nurs* 32:465, 2003.
147. Neufeld M, Woodrum D, Tarczy-Hornoch P: Prenatal and postnatal counseling for parents of infants at the limits of viability, *Pediatr Res* 47:420A, 2000.

148. Newton N, Newton M: Mothers' reaction to their newborn babies, *JAMA* 181:206, 1962.
149. Nonacs R, Cohen L: Postpartum mood disorders: diagnosis and treatment guidelines, *J Clin Psychiatry* 59:34, 1998.
150. Nystrom K, Axelsson K: Mother's experience of being separated for their newborns, *J Obstet Gynecol Neonatal Nurs* 31:275, 2002.
151. O'Hara MW, Swain AM: Rates and risk of postpartum depression: a meta-analysis, *Int Rev Psychiatry* 8:37, 1996.
152. Olds D, Kitzman H, Cole R, et al: Effects of nurse home-visiting on maternal life course and child development: age 6 follow-up results of a randomized trial, *Pediatrics* 114:1550, 2004.
153. Olds D, Robinson J, Pettitt L, et al: Effects of home visits by paraprofessionals and by nurses: age 4 follow-up results of a randomized trial, *Pediatrics* 114:1560, 2004.
154. Olexa M: A longitudinal and concurrent examination of the vulnerable child syndrome: impact of maternal and child socio-emotional and behavioral status, *Dissertation Abstracts International* 62:3401, 2002.
155. Ottani P: Embracing global similarities: a framework for cross-cultural obstetric care, *J Obstet Gynecol Neonatal Nurs* 31:33, 2002.
156. Paul D, Epps S, Leef K, et al: Prenatal consultation with a neonatologist prior to preterm delivery, *J Perinatol* 21:431, 2001.
157. Petersen M, Cohen J, Parsons V: Family-centered care: "Do we practice what we preach?", *J Obstet Gynecol Neonatal Nurs* 33:421, 2004.
158. Phillips C, Anzalone J: *Fathering: participation in labor and birth*, ed 2, St Louis, 1982, Mosby.
159. Raines D: Values of mothers of LBW infants in the NICU, *Neonatal Netw* 17:41, 1998.
160. Rapkin A, Mikacich J, Moatakef-Imani B: Reproductive mood disorders, *Prim Psychiatry* 10:31, 2003.
161. Renker PR, Tonkin P: Women's views of prenatal violence screening: acceptability and confidentiality issues, *Obstet Gynecol* 107:348, 2006.
162. Renker PR, Tonkin P: Postpartum women's evaluations of an audio/video computer-assisted perinatal violence screen, *Comput Inform Nurs* 25:139, 2007.
163. Roberts K: Providing culturally sensitive care to the childbearing Islamic family, *Adv Neonatal Care* 2:222, 2002.
164. Roberts K: Providing culturally sensitive care to the childbearing Islamic family: Part II, *Adv Neonatal Care* 3:250, 2003.
165. Rollins J: Respite care and caring communities, *Pediatr Nurs* 29:80, 2003.
166. Sandelowski M, Barroso J: Motherhood in the context of maternal HIV infection, *Res Nurs Health* 26:470, 2003.
167. Sauls D: Effects of labor support on mothers, babies, and birth outcomes, *J Obstet Gynecol Neonatal Nurs* 31:733, 2002.
168. Schoening AM, Greenwood JL, McNichols JA, et al: Effect of an intimate partner violence educational program on the attitudes of nurses, *J Obstet Gynecol Neonatal Nurs* 33:572, 2004.
169. Segre L, Stuart S, O'Hara M: Interpersonal psychotherapy for antenatal and postpartum depression, *Prim Psychiatry* 11:52, 2004.
170. Shadigian EM, Bauer ST: Screening for partner violence during pregnancy, *Int J Gynaecol Obstet* 84:273, 2004.
171. Shah M: *Transcultural aspects of perinatal health care: a resource guide*, Washington, DC, 2004, National Perinatal Association.
172. Sharp M, Strauss R, Lorch S: Communicating medical bad news: parents' experiences and preferences, *J Pediatr* 121:539, 1992.
173. Shieh C, Kravitz M: Maternal-fetal attachment in pregnant women who use illicit drugs, *J Obstet Gynecol Neonatal Nurs* 31:156, 2003.
174. Siegel R: A family-centered program of neonatal intensive care, *Health Soc Work* 7:50, 1982.
175. Sieratzki J, Woll B: Why do mothers cradle babies on their left?, *Lancet* 347:1746, 1996.
176. Simon J: Communicating patient information in the HIPAA era: the good news and the bad news, *Adv Neonatal Care* 2:60, 2002.
177. Solbeck S: Working with military families: a perinatal perspective, *Natl Assoc Perinat Soc Work Forum* 22:4, 2002.
178. Solheim K, Spellacy C: Sibling visitation: effects on newborn infection rates, *J Obstet Gynecol Neonatal Nurs* 17:43, 1988.
179. Solnit AJ, Stark MH: Mourning and the birth of a defective child, *Psychoanal Study Child* 16:523, 1961.
180. Spector R: *Cultural diversity in health and illness*, Upper Saddle River, NJ, 2004, Pearson Prentice Hall.
181. Sullivan J: Development of father-infant attachment in fathers of preterm infants, *Neonatal Netw* 18:33, 1999.
182. Thomas K, Renaud M, DePaul D: Use of the Parenting Stress Index in mothers of preterm infants, *Adv Neonatal Care* 4:33, 2004.
183. Thureen P, Deacon J, Hernandez J, et al: *Assessment and care of the well newborn*, ed 2, Philadelphia, 2005, Saunders.
184. Tilokskulchai F, Phatthanasiriwethin S, Vichitsukon K, et al: Attachment behaviors in mothers of premature infants: a descriptive study in Thai mothers, *J Perinat Neonatal Nurs* 16:69, 2002.
185. Troutman B, Cutrona C: Nonpsychotic postpartum depression among adolescent mothers, *J Abnorm Psychol* 99:69, 1990.

186. Tuten M, Jones HE, Svikis DS: Comparing homeless and domiciled pregnant substance dependent women on psychosocial characteristics and treatment outcomes, *Drug Alcohol Depend* 69:95, 2003.

187. Tyson J, Parikh N, Langer J, et al, for the National Institute of Child Health and Human Development Neonatal Research Unit: Intensive care for extreme prematurity: moving beyond gestational age, *New Engl J Med* 358:1672, 2008.

188. U.S. Preventive Services Task Force: Screening for family and intimate partner violence: recommendation statement, *Ann Intern Med* 140:382, 2004. Website: http://ahrq.gov/clinic/3rduspstf/famviolence/famviolrs.htm.

189. Veddovi M, Kenny DT, Gibson J, et al: The relationship between depressive symptoms following premature birth, mothers' coping style, and knowledge of infant development, *J Reprod Infant Psychol* 19:313, 2001.

190. Weiss S, Chen J: Factors influencing maternal mental health and family functioning during the low birthweight infant's first year of life, *J Pediatr Nurs* 17:114, 2002.

191. Weiss S, Seed M: Precursors of mental health problems for low birth weight children: the salience of family environment during the first year of life, *Child Psychiatry Hum Dev* 33:3, 2002.

192. Whitfield M: Psychosocial effects of intensive care on infants and families after discharge, *Semin Neonatol* 8:185, 2003.

RESOURCE MATERIALS FOR CULTURAL COMPETENCY

Andrews M, Boyle J: *Transcultural concepts in nursing care*, ed 4, Philadelphia, 2003, Lippincott Williams & Wilkins.

Colorado Children's Healthcare Access Program: *Cross-cultural health care curriculum (syllabus)*, Available at http://www.cchap.org/cchc-syllabus/.

D'Avanzo CE: *Mosby's pocket guide to cultural health assessment*, ed 4, St Louis, 2008, Mosby. Available at www.nursingconsult.com/public/book/view/title.

Flores G, Laws B, Mayo SJ, et al: Errors in medical interpretation and their potential clinical consequences in pediatric encounters, *Pediatrics* 111(a):6, 2003.

Galanti G: *Caring for patients from different cultures*, ed 3, Philadelphia, 2004, University of Pennsylvania Press.

Lipson J, Dibble S, Menarck D, editors: *Culture and nursing care: a pocket guide*, San Francisco, 1998, UCSF Nursing Press.

Ngo-Metzger Q, Massagli MP, Clarridge BR, et al: Linguistic and cultural barriers to care, *J Gen Intern Med* 18:44, 2003.

Shah M: *Transcultural aspects of perinatal health care: a resource guide*, Washington, DC, 2004, National Perinatal Association.

U.S. Department of Health and Human Services, Office of Minority Health: *Cultural competency*. Available at www.omhrc.gov/templates/browse.aspx?lvl=1&lvlid=3.

Wiener ES, Rivera MI: Bridging language barriers: how to work with an interpreter, *Clin Pediatr Emerg Med* 5:93, 2004.

RESOURCE MATERIALS FOR PARENTS

Baby CareLink system: www.babycarelink.com.

Colorado Collective for Medical Health Care Decisions: *You are not alone (film)*, Denver, Colo, 1999, Nickel's Worth Publications. NICKELWRTH@aol.com.

D'Apolito K, McGrath J, O'Brien A: Infant and family-centered developmental care guidelines. In *National Association of Neonatal Nurses Practice Guidelines*, ed 3, des Plaines, Ill, 2000, The Association.

Davis D, Stein M: *Parenting your premature baby and child: the emotional journey*, Golden, Colo, 2004, Fulcrum Books.

Garcia-Prats J, Hornfischer S: *What to do when your baby is premature*, New York, 2000, Three Rivers Press.

Gracey K: A parent's guide for advocacy and involvement, *Adv Neonatal Care* 2:170, 2002.

Harrison H, Kositsky A: *The premature baby book: a parent's guide to coping and caring in the first years*, New York, 1990, St Martin's Press.

Institute for Family-Centered Care: *Parents on rounds*, Bethesda, Md, 2001, The Institute (video).

Johnson B: Institute for Family-Centered Care, 7900 Wisconsin Ave., Suite 405, Bethesda, MD 20814.

Johnson B, Crocker L: *Privileged presence: personal stories of connections in health care*, Boulder, Colo, 2006, Bull Publishing.

Johnson J, Johnson M, Hatcher D: *Special beginnings*, Omaha, Neb, 1994, Centering Corp.

Kahn R, Green R, Little G: *Dreams and dilemmas: parents and the practice of neonatal care*, Trustees of Dartmouth College and Richard Kahn (video), 1998.

Klein A, Ganon J: *Caring for your premature baby: a complete resource for parents*, New York, 1998, Harper Perennial.

Lafferty L, Flood B: *Born early: a premature baby's story for children*, Grand Junction, Colo, 1994, Songbird Publishing.

Linden D, Paroli E, Doron M: *Preemies: the essential guide for parents of premature babies*, New York, 2000, Pocket Books.

Madden S: *The preemie parents' companion: the essential guide to caring for your premature baby in the hospital, at home, and through the first years*, Boston, 2000, Harvard Common Press.

March of Dimes: Parent Care Kit: *(Parent—you and your baby in the NICU; Baby—a keepsake journal; NICU—a guide and glossary. Videos: First days: parenting in the NICU; When baby comes early: a parent's guide to prematurity)*, New York, 2002, March of Dimes Foundation. Website: http://www.marchofdimes.com.

March of Dimes: *Online parent support*. Website: www.marchofdimes.com/share.

Parlakian R, Lerner C: *Early arrival: finding the magic of everyday moments with your baby in the neonatal intensive care unit (NICU),* Washington, DC, 2006, Zero to Three. Available at wwwjjpi.com.

Rector L: *Supporting siblings and their families during intensive baby care,* Baltimore, Md, 2007, Paul H. Brookes Publishing.

Smith T: *Miracle birth stories of very premature babies: little thumbs up!,* Westport, Conn, 1999, Bergin & Garvey.

Society of Pediatric Nurses and American Nurses Association: *Family-centered care: putting it into action,* The SPN/ANA Guide to Family-Centered Care. Washington, DC, 2003, American Nurses Publishing.

Tracy A, Maroney D: *Your premature baby and child: helpful answers and advice for parents,* New York, 1999, Berkley Books.

Woodwell W: *Coming to term: a father's story of birth, loss, and survival,* Jackson, Miss, 2001, University Press of Mississippi.

Zaichkin J: *Newborn intensive care: what every parent needs to know,* ed 3, Petaluma, Calif, 2009, NICU Inc.

WEBSITES FOR PARENTS OF PREMATURE INFANTS

National Institute of Child Health and Human Development (NICHD) Neonatal Research Network: *Extremely preterm birth outcome data tool.* Available at www.nichd.nih.gov/about/org/cdbpm/pp/prog_epbo/.

Parent-to-parent support and discussion: *Preemie child—for parents of preemie survivors of school-age, adolescents, and adults.* Available at www.comeunity.com. *Preemie list—parents of preterm babies, infants and young children;* Preemie-L: *Homepage*—www.comeunity.com/prematurewww.preemie-l.org/*Resources for Parents of Preemies.*

RESOURCE MATERIALS FOR POSTPARTUM DEPRESSION

BOOKS

Beyond the blues: prenatal & postpartum depression: a treatment manual by Shoshana S. Bennett, Ph.D. and Pec Indman, Ed.D., MFT. A helpful book that can be purchased at a bookstore or online at: www.beyondtheblues.com.

I'm listening: a guide to supporting postpartum families by Jane Honikman. A guidebook to help organize postpartum parent support networks in the community. Can be purchased through Postpartum Support International.

Misconceptions: truth, lies, and the unexpected on the journey to motherhood by Naomi Wolf. This is a good book with a resource guide in the back.

Step by step by Jane Honikman. Ms. Honikman shares her own personal experience with PPD. Can be purchased through Postpartum Support International.

WEB RESOURCES

Depression after delivery (D.A.D.): www.depressionafterdelivery.com. Depression After Delivery, Inc., 91 East Somerset Street, Raritan, NJ 08869. Information Request Line: 1-800-944-4773 (4PPD).

PSI: Postpartum Support International: www.postpartum.net. Postpartum Support International, 927 North Kellogg Avenue, Santa Barbara, CA 93111.

Symptoms of Depression.com: www.symptoms-of-depression.com.

The Online PPD Support Group: www.ppdsupportpage.com.

30 GRIEF AND PERINATAL LOSS

SANDRA L. GARDNER AND LORRAINE A. DICKEY

As a life passage, pregnancy and birth are associated with hopes and expectations and joy and happiness for the future. Even though pregnancy and birth constitute a developmental crisis and major life change, expectant parents believe the gains of a healthy, happy child and family life offset any losses. Unfortunately, not all perinatal events have a happy ending. When pregnancy fails to produce a normal, healthy infant, it is a tragedy for the parents whose expectations of childbearing have not been fulfilled. Perinatal loss also affects their friends, family, and professional care providers.

Perinatal loss may be the first time a young adult has had the experience of coping with the illness or death of a loved one. Perinatal loss is especially significant because it (1) is sudden and unexpected, (2) is the most difficult loss to resolve[18]; (3) interrupts the significant developmental stage of pregnancy and the situational crisis of pregnancy[18]; (4) is the loss of a child who did not have the opportunity to live a full life[36,101]; (5) prevents progression into the next developmental stage of parenting that has been anticipated and rehearsed (at least in fantasy) during the pregnancy[64]; and (6) represents a narcissistic loss, a loss of self, for the parents.[96,119,120] Perinatal loss also often means interpersonal exclusion from the activities of childbearing friends and siblings.

Unfortunately, loss and grief often are thought of only in relation to death. However, as final and irreversible as death is, it is just one form of separation and loss. Although less obvious, other loss situations may have an equally crucial effect. Loss comes in many forms, and during the perinatal period, may occur without necessarily resulting in death. Circumstances of perinatal loss are parallel and, at the same time, different, because they all entail grief and mourning and yet each has unique dimensions and characteristics. The process of grief, its stages, and its symptoms are reviewed as a framework for understanding one's own feelings and those of others experiencing a loss. A desire to help and an idea of what is helpful and what is not helpful are essential for effective intervention by professionals.

THE GRIEF PROCESS

Grief, the characteristic response to the loss of a valued object, is not an intellectual and rational response.[38] Rather, it is personally experienced as the deep emotion of sadness and sorrow. To the individual, grief feels overwhelming, irrational, out of control, "crazy," and all-consuming. Mourning occurs in phases over time. After acknowledgment that the loved object no longer exists, gradual withdrawal of emotion and feeling occurs, so that eventual psychologic investment in a new relationship is possible.

A recent literature review of the theoretical perspectives of parental grief from the United States and United Kingdom reveals a change from a traditional to a "newer" model of grief in the Anglo-American culture.[29] Traditional models of grief emphasize the severing of bonds with the deceased, whereas "newer" understandings of parental grief emphasize parents retaining a relationship with their dead child. After reviewing nursing, medical, and social science publications and choosing relevant ones, Davies states: "…the concept of continuous bonds challenges the dominant assumption that resolution of grief is achieved through severing bonds with the deceased."[29] Parents wish to know

Please note that the **PURPLE** type in each chapter is intended to make it easier to identify clinically applicable material.

that their child's birth and death have meaning and purpose and that their child "mattered" and will be remembered by them and by others who have been "touched" and "changed" by him or her.[19]

For grief to occur, the object must have been valued by the individual so that its loss is perceived as significant and meaningful. Because, prenatally, there is an investment of love in the fetus or newborn, the neonate is a valued object. To the extent that prenatal attachment has occurred, grief should be expected and felt at the loss of the fetus or newborn. Therefore loss at birth is a significant loss of a valued (although as yet only fantasized) person.

Loss, whether real or imagined, actual or possible, is traumatic. The individual is no longer self-confident or confident about the surroundings, because both have been altered. Mourning and grief are forms of separation reactions. Fears of separation and abandonment are the universal fears of childhood regardless of age or developmental stage. Perhaps loss of a significant other awakens these childhood fears and reminds us of the basic "insecurity of all our attachments."[68]

Life changes are stressful to the individual because they threaten to disrupt continuity and a state of equilibrium.[88] Significant changes in the family configuration, such as accession of a new member, are normally a stressful occasion for family members. Perinatal complication or loss is even more of a stressful event for which the family has little or no preparation. The result of a crisis may be personal growth, maintaining the status quo, regression, or mental illness.[18,89] Often outcome depends on the type of help received during the crisis.

Decreasing the element of surprise through preparation for the situation to be encountered may modulate the effect of the event. Anticipatory grief[61,79,100] functions both to prepare and to protect the individual from the pain of impending loss. Prenatal diagnostic procedures, such as ultrasonography,[75] amniocentesis, and fetoscopy, can now detect a variety of severe or lethal birth defects. When there is forewarning that the pregnancy or newborn is not healthy, the parents may begin a process of anticipatory grief and psychologically prepare for the loss of their baby while hoping for his or her survival.[7]

Parental withdrawal from the relationship established during pregnancy accompanies the intense emotions of anticipatory grief. Detachment protects and defends the parent from further painful feelings associated with the investment of self in a doomed relationship. If anticipatory grief proceeds, the parent may detach to the point of being unable to reattach to the infant if he or she survives. In this situation, the infant survives but the relationship with the parents may be significantly impaired. Maintaining even a remote hope that the fetus or newborn will survive protects the parents from the full experience of grief and total detachment from the baby.

The degree of parental anticipatory grief is correlated with positive feelings about the pregnancy and the mode of delivery but not with the severity of the infant's illness. The greater the parental investment and the higher the expectations for the pregnancy, the more anticipatory grief is associated with the development of a perinatal complication. The relative severity of the medical problem is not associated with the degree of anticipatory grief.

PERINATAL SITUATIONS IN WHICH GRIEF IS EXPECTED

Loss is a fact of life, not just of death. Every stage of development requires a loss of the privileges of the preceding stage and movement into the unknown of the next stage. Any life event involving change or loss is accompanied by grief work, including moving, divorce, separation, death of a spouse or family member, injury or illness, retirement, job change, menopause, and even success.[88] The concept of loss is even applicable to the physiologic and psychologic events of normal pregnancy and birth. Certainly, when pregnancy fails to produce a live, healthy infant, a perinatal loss situation exists (Box 30-1). These perinatal losses, including stillbirth, loss of the perfect child, and neonatal death, are discussed in detail in this chapter.

Stillbirth

Stillbirth is the demise of a viable fetus that occurs after fetal movement when the fetus is invested by the parents with a personality and individuality. Because stillbirth occurs later in pregnancy than most abortions, there are increased parental expectations about the baby and the birth process. Selective abortions for genetic indications often are performed in the second trimester of pregnancy and involve the death of a wanted child. Even though parents understand the validity of the reason for terminating the pregnancy, sadness, guilt, and self-doubt often accom-

BOX 30-1 PERINATAL SITUATIONS IN WHICH GRIEF REACTION IS EXPECTED

1. Pregnancy
2. Birth
   - A. Normal
   - B. Cesarean section
   - C. Forceps
   - D. Episiotomy
   - E. Medicated
   - F. Prolonged or short labor
   - G. Place of birth
3. Postpartum (see Chapter 29)
   - A. "Postpartum blues"
   - B. Depression
   - C. Psychosis
4. Abortion
   - A. Spontaneous[13,82,83,109]
   - B. Therapeutic[13,98]
   - C. Elective
   - D. Selective
   - E. Selective reduction (for multiple gestation)[66,82,83]
5. Stillbirth
6. Loss of the perfect child
   - A. Premature
   - B. Deformed baby or baby with anomaly[40]
   - C. Sick newborn[78]
   - D. "Wrong" sex
7. Neonatal death
8. Relinquishment

pany the decision to abort. The anxieties related to termination procedures, which may include labor and birth, and the feelings of helplessness, isolation, and depression should be acknowledged and handled as in a stillbirth.

Fetal demise in utero happens either prenatally or in the intrapartum period. For 50% of stillbirths, death was sudden, without warning, and occurred from unexplainable causes. The majority of women whose fetus has died in utero spontaneously begin labor within 2 weeks of fetal demise. Carrying the dead fetus while waiting for spontaneous labor or induction is sad and difficult for the woman and her entire family. Feelings such as helplessness, disbelief, and powerlessness characterize this period. There is often an almost uncontrollable urge to flee and escape the unpleasant situation.

For the family who experiences an intrapartum demise, the joyous expectations of labor and birth suddenly change to fear, anxiety, and dread that the "worst" could have possibly happened to them. The suddenness of fetal demise in labor and birth affects both parents and professionals with feelings of shock, denial, and anxiety. Whether the loss is an early or late fetal loss, the woman and her family maintain hope by believing that the professional has made a mistake and that the fetus is still alive.[99] The onset (or continuation) of labor is approached with both hope and dread: hope that the infant may be born alive and dread that the infant's death will soon be a stark reality.

The discomfort of labor and birth is particularly difficult for the woman whose fetus has died, because her work will not be rewarded with a healthy infant. However, oversolicitous use of drugs at birth is not recommended, because they relegate the experience to unreality and give it a dreamlike quality.[128] Keeping parents together through this crisis is important for mutual support and sharing of the birth.[97] The deadening (and deafening) silence of a stillbirth forces the reality of the infant's death on both the parents and the professionals present at birth.[97]

In the past, at the birth of a stillborn, the mother was heavily sedated or anesthetized and the neonate was hidden and whisked away immediately. These women were often left with fears and fantasies: "Was the baby normal?" "What was the sex?" "What did the baby look like?" Seeing, touching, and holding the infant promote completion of the attachment cycle, confirm the reality of the stillbirth for both parents, and enable grief to begin.[10,99,128]

Because it is easier to grieve the reality of a situation than a mystical and dreamlike fantasy, contact with the stillborn enables parents to grieve the infant's reality rather than endure their most frightening fantasies about him or her.

After confirming the reality of the infant's death, a search for the cause, characterized by the universal question "Why did the baby die?" begins. Either or both parents may blame themselves or feel guilty about real or imagined acts of omission or commission. An autopsy may determine the cause of death, but most often the cause is unknown, even after an autopsy. However, an autopsy may be useful in reducing parental guilt and uncertainty about future pregnancies, as well as in aiding the recovery from the loss.[72,128] The "empty tragedy" of stillbirth forces the mother to deal with both the inner loss of the fetus and the outer loss of the expected newborn. Fathers experience stillbirth as a "waste of life," are especially appreciative of the tokens of remembrance from the baby, and need help in expressing their grief.[97]

Loss of the Perfect Child

Even though pregnancy ends in the birth of a live newborn, the pregnancy outcome may not be what the parents had anticipated. Birth of an infant who does not meet parental expectations represents the realization of the parents' worst fears: a damaged child. Newborns who are preterm, have an anomaly, are sick, or are the "wrong" gender or who ultimately die represent the loss of the fantasized perfect child.

After the birth of such a infant, parental reactions include grief and mourning for the loss of the loved object (the perfect child) while adapting to the reality and investing love in the defective baby.[42,106] This reaction is analogous to parental mourning at the death of a child.[106] However, unlike the finality of death, birth of a living, defective baby entails a persistent, constant reminder of the feelings of loss and grief because of parental investment of time, attention, and care for either a short time (preterm or sick newborn) or a lifetime (physically or mentally afflicted child).[91,106]

The psychic work involved in coping with the reality of the imperfect child and the inner feelings of loss is slow and emotionally painful.[40,91] The process is gradual and proceeds at an individual pace that cannot be hurried but can be facilitated and supported. Detachment from and mourning the loss of their fantasized child is necessary before parents are able to attach to the actual child.

Birth of an imperfect infant represents multiple losses for parents. A primary narcissistic injury, a threat to the female's self-concept as a woman and mother and the male's self-concept as a man and a father, occurs when a less-than-perfect infant is born.[27,28,40,58] Because the child is an extension of both parents, a less-than-perfect (i.e., deformed) child is equated with the perceived less-than-perfect part of the parental self. In the mind of the parent, the imagined inadequate self has failed and caused the birth of the damaged baby.[58]

Prematurity

Every woman expects to deliver a normal, healthy infant at term. Therefore the onset of premature labor is both physiologically and psychologically unexpected. Premature birth is a crisis and an emergency situation characterized by an increased concern for the survival of the newborn and often the mother. Premature labor and birth are accompanied by feelings of helplessness, isolation, failure, emptiness, and no control.[58,106] The negative and dangerous atmosphere surrounding the premature birth experience may influence the relationship with the premature infant, who also may be perceived as dangerous and negative.

Normal adaptations to pregnancy are abruptly terminated by the birth of a premature infant.[58] Prenatal fantasies about the infant and the new roles of mother and father are interrupted by a premature birth. This forces parents who are "not ready to not be pregnant" to grieve the loss of a term infant and imposes premature parenting on individuals not yet ready for the experience.

As discussed in Chapter 29, anticipatory grief is one of the normal psychologic tasks accompanying premature birth. Anticipatory grief may be decreased by early contact between parents and neonate and, conversely, increased by separation of parents from preterm newborn.[58] Prolonging anticipatory grief with failure to progress through the other tasks results in altered relationships with the parents if the preterm infant survives.

Deformed Infants or Infants with an Anomaly

In approximately 2 of every 100 births,[58] an infant is born with a birth defect. Because society values physical beauty, intelligence, and success, the birth of a physically or mentally defective baby is seen as a catastrophe in our culture.[127]

Recent medical advances now make it possible to identify potential fetal problems in utero. As parents receive the information antenatally, they begin the process of anticipatory grief. They experience feelings of shock, anger, guilt, and hope. At the birth of their baby, there usually is the confirmation of the anomaly, and parents must deal with the reality of the situation. Whether anticipated or not, however, the birth of a baby with a congenital defect is accompanied by ambivalent feelings for all concerned (parents, relatives, friends, and professionals). The first reactions to the reality of the situation are feelings of disbelief and shock. Feelings of shame, revulsion, and embarrassment at creating a damaged and devalued child are common.[104] Guilt, self-blame, and a search for a cause or reason for the tragedy are intermixed with feelings of anger.

The severity of loss and feelings of disappointment heavily burden the parents, a burden they may believe that no one else has experienced.[58] Their loneliness and isolation may be intensified by their self-imposed withdrawal from others. Unlike the birth of a healthy infant, the birth of a sick baby or one with an anomaly is not celebrated by society with announcements, visits, and gifts from friends and family. The negative responses of society's representatives (family, friends, acquaintances, and professionals) may increase the parents' negative feelings for a defective child.[127]

The extent of the infant's anomaly cannot be used as a criterion for the degree of parental grief reaction, although a gross, visible anomaly may elicit more emotional reaction than a hidden or minor one.[58] A seemingly "minor" anomaly as defined by the professional may represent a severe impairment to individual parents. The professional, who has had more contact with infants with a wide range of anomalies, views the individual infant's anomaly in a different context than that typical for the parents, who may have limited or no experience with a deformed child or adult. The professional also views the infant's defect from a less personal, more objective, and less narcissistic position than the new parents.

When the newborn is sick, the degree of mourning and parental feelings of grief and loss are not equated with the severity of the neonate's illness.[7,105] Even seemingly minor illnesses such as jaundice or respiratory difficulty requiring phototherapy or minimal oxygen supplementation are associated with parental concern for survival and feelings of grief and loss.[78] These feelings are often not acknowledged by the parents or professional care providers because of the non-serious medical nature of the condition. In the mind of the care provider, self-limiting and treatable conditions are compared with more serious and often fatal neonatal illnesses. The care provider feels relieved about the "minor" nature of the neonate's condition and conveys this to the parents—"This is an easy condition to remedy. You don't have anything to worry about. The baby will go home in a few days."

Thus only the medical aspects of the newborn's illness are dealt with, whereas parental feelings remain unspoken and unresolved.[16] In an altruistic attempt to reassure and comfort the family about the newborn's complete recovery, the professional unwittingly may discount the parents' real feelings. If the care provider is not concerned, parents may feel that they, too, should not be concerned and thus distrust and discount their own feelings.

Neonatal Deaths

The reactions accompanying neonatal illnesses are similar to the grief reactions experienced by parents whose infant dies.[7,123] Failure to acknowledge (even minor) neonatal illness as a loss situation and to work through the associated grief prevents parents from detaching from the image of the perfect child and taking on the sick newborn as a person to love. This may result in an aberrant parent-infant attachment. The liveborn infant who is critically ill or has a severe anomaly will be the focus of a "painful time of waiting"[10] for the family. They must deal with the uncertainty of whether their child will live and be healthy, live and continue to need extensive medical or special care, or die.

More deaths occur in the first 24 hours of life than in any other period of life. Yet death of a newborn is not the expected outcome of pregnancy. The majority of neonatal losses are caused by prematurity (80% to 90%) and congenital anomalies that are incompatible with life (15% to 20%). Regardless of the cause of death, even infants who live only a short time are mourned by their parents.[56] Prenatal attachment and investment of love in the newborn result in a classic grief reaction at the newborn's death.

Even a short period of life between birth and death gives parents an opportunity to know and take care of their infant.[108] Completion of the attachment process enables parents to psychically begin the next process of detachment. Attachment to the baby's reality encourages detachment from that reality rather than from the parents' most dreaded fears and fantasies about their infant. Parental contact with the child before death enables them to share life for a brief time.

In the case of multiple births, when one infant or more dies and the others live, parents simultaneously grieve the loss of the dead infant while attaching to the survivor.[60,82,83,110] In many situations of multiple birth, the surviving infant or infants are in an intensive care nursery. The diametrically opposite feelings of love and attachment and grief and detachment, as well as the anxiety associated with the care and well-being of the surviving infant, are emotionally draining for new parents. The process of grief may slow the parents' ability to become intimately involved with their surviving infant(s).[83,84,124] They may have ambivalent feelings toward the infant(s) who survives or toward the infant(s) who dies. With the loss of one infant of a multiple birth, there is less support for the grieving parents because the frequent response is that they should be thankful for the survival of one (or more) of their infants. Research shows that the death of a twin (or higher-order multiple) is as great a loss for a mother as the death of a singleton.[82,83,110] Helpful interventions include (1) acknowledging the uniqueness of every baby; (2) viewing, holding, and photographing the babies together—living and dead; (3) private time with each deceased infant; and (4) similar mementos and keepsakes from each infant, deceased and living, given to the parents.[82-84]

Generally, death of a newborn occurs despite everything done to prevent it. This provides parents with some measure of comfort in knowing that they did everything possible. Yet when the neonate is so severely ill or deformed that a decision about initiating or continuing life support is necessary, the parents have an extra burden. The situation may involve conflicts between physicians, nurses, and family wishes, causing significant personal anguish. As part of the federal Baby Doe regulations, most hospitals now have ethics committees that address the medical, legal, and ethical controversies (see Chapter 32). The decision-making process may be collaborative, parent initiated, directive, or nondirective.[82] Regardless of who makes this decision, it is primarily the parents who will live with the ramifications of that decision. When parents are involved in the decision-making process, they wonder if theirs was the right decision regardless of the decision. Whether the baby lives or dies, they wonder how a different decision would have changed their lives.

STAGES OF GRIEF

The experience of grief is a staged process that occurs over time. To detach both externally and internally from the lost loved object, emotional investment is withdrawn so that it may be invested in new love relationships.[61] Each stage of grief represents a psychologic defense mechanism used to help the individual adapt slowly to the crisis. This slow adaptation is purposeful, because it prevents the individual psyche from being overwhelmed by the pain and anguish of loss.[81]

Although the stage of grief is recognizable, the process of grief is dynamic and fluid rather than static and rigid. Parents, families, and professionals progress cyclically through the stages of grief rather than in an orderly progression from beginning to end. However, each person experiences the process of grief uniquely and at an individual rate. Knowledge of each stage is necessary to assess where an individual family member, the family as a unit, and the staff are in their grief process. This information is then used to support individuals when they are in their particular stage of grief. Rather than attempting to maneuver grieving individuals from stage to stage, contributing to their defense, or stripping individuals of their defenses, knowledgeable professionals are prepared to understand and honor the individual's grieving process. Regardless of the type of perinatal loss, the experience of that loss through staged grief work closely parallels the grief stages described by Elisabeth Kübler-Ross.[59]

The feelings of disbelief and rejection of the news are reflected in the responses "No! This couldn't happen to me!" "It isn't true! They've made a mistake!" This immediate response protects the individual from the shocking reality of loss by postponing the full effect of reality until the psyche can handle it.[99] By holding on to the fantasy of a positive outcome (e.g., the loss of the heartbeat is only temporary or the dead infant belongs to someone else), facing the awful truth and the grief associated with it is delayed at least temporarily.[99]

The initial stage of grief is characterized by overwhelming feelings of being stunned and surprised. This is often seen as emotional numbness, flat affect, or immobility.[128] Emotional detachment is often expressed as an inability to cope or respond with activities of daily living, an inability to remember what others have said, and a tendency to repeat the same question.[31,36] For the tragedy to be handled in manageable pieces without overwhelming the individual, the mind may acknowledge the event only intellectually and there is a corresponding lack of emotional reaction,[128] or the event may be compartmentalized so that only a part of the situation rather than the whole becomes the focal point of attention.

Anger is the result of a gradually developing awareness of the situation's reality. As the significance of their perinatal loss begins to dawn on them, parents (and significant others) experience the diffuse emotions of anxiety and anger.[58] With the full effect of their loss comes more focused feelings of bitterness, resentment, blame, rage, and envy of those with normal pregnancy outcomes.[59]

Social prohibitions against the expression of anger, especially for women, encourage this powerful emotion to be turned inward toward the self. Anger directed inward results in depression and a deepening sense of guilt. "Why?" and "What did I do wrong or not do right to have caused this to happen?" are the hallmarks of the self-examination and self-blame that accompany perinatal loss.[58,128] Answers are often irrational and have no cause-and-effect relationship with the reality of the circumstances. Irrational, feared causes include sexual intercourse (common worry of both men and women), career (of the mother) outside the home, superstitions, dietary habits, or lifting heavy objects.[128] Ideas of punishment (for past wrongs, for negative or ambivalent feelings, or for an unwanted pregnancy)[8] are often thought to be the reason for the failed outcome. The search for a reason to answer the question "Why me?" requires correct information to dispel unrealistic fantasies of causation. However, the question does not require a literal answer (often no concrete answer exists) but is merely a wish for a change in the situation.[8]

Anger directed outward is usually expressed as overt hostility to those in the immediate environment (family, children, care providers, and infant)[128] or toward God.[81] Fathers exhibit more anger than mothers do.[44] Blame and anger may be destructive forces in the relationships among family members and prevent these relationships from being a source of comfort and support. Venting of angry feelings toward professional care providers protects these family relationships for more positive interactions. Anger moves the grieving process along, but persistence of anger may prevent grief work from progressing to subsequent stages.

Bargaining may occur concomitantly with denial and shock as an attempt to prevent or at least delay the loss. Bargaining usually occurs with whoever the parents (family or staff) believe the Supreme Being is. The "Yes, but" of this stage is a form of "conditional acceptance" while still attempting to make the reality other than what it is.[8,59] With the defective infant, bargaining may take the form of shopping for a physician or searching for the magic cure.[127]

The onset of depression and withdrawal marks the stage of a greater level of acceptance of the tragedy. With the true realization of the effect of the loss, the individual acknowledges that indeed there is a reason to be sad. The predominant feelings of this stage are overwhelming sorrow and sadness[72] evidenced by tearfulness, crying, and weeping.[99] Feelings of helplessness, worthlessness, and powerlessness contribute to the sense that life is empty and futile. Withdrawal may be evidenced by requests to be left alone, by decreased or complete cessation of visits to the infant, and by silence.[59] The degree of withdrawal may be indicative of the depth of depression and the extent to which there is guilt and self-blame.[99]

Acceptance is the resolution stage of the grief process that is heralded by resumption of usual daily activities and a noticeable decrease in preoccupation with the image of the lost infant.[61] This stage usually is not witnessed by the perinatal professionals. The acceptance stage is characterized by emotional detachment of life's meaning from the lost relationship and reestablishing it independent of the lost object.[59,68] The lost relationship is seen in a new light—as giving meaning to the present.[68] The aggrieved person relinquishes that part of himself or herself that was defined in the lost relationship and establishes a new identity that is emotionally free to attach in another relationship.

For the family of a deformed child, acceptance is not an all-or-nothing proposition but, rather, a daily adaptation and coping with the child and the defect.[103] For the family, periods of frustration and sorrow alternate with periods of delight and enjoyment of the child. Because of the chronic sorrow experienced throughout the life of a defective child, the final stage of resolution of the family's grief is possible only after the child's death.[79,127]

The acceptance stage represents the ability to remember both the joys and sorrows of the lost relationship without undue discomfort.[38] With gradual integration of the loss, there are progressively fewer attacks of acute, all-consuming pain.[68] When recalling the lost infant, there are fewer feelings of devastation and more a feeling of sadness. The ability to "celebrate the loss" also identifies grief resolution. Celebration of the loss does not mean recall without sadness and sorrow but with an ability to find some meaning, some good, and some positive aspects in the situation (e.g., "At least we had our child for a time, even though it was a short time").

SYMPTOMS OF GRIEF

Although each person copes with grief in individual ways, there are expected reactions to loss situations. Knowledge of the differences and commonalities of the grief experience enables care providers to understand their own reactions, as well as to share their thoughts and feelings with the grieving family. The professional care provider must learn to "hear" what the family says about how and where each member is in the process of grief resolution. Often the "message" is not a direct reference to the loss or one's feelings but, rather, nonverbal communication. The professional must learn to recognize that individuals often communicate more by what they do and what they omit than by what they say.

The signs and symptoms of acute grief have been well described and include both somatic and behavioral manifestations of the emotional experience of the loss (see the Critical Findings box below). The behavior of the bereaved is characterized as ambivalent.[68] In certain perinatal situations, parents simultaneously hope that the infant will live and wish for the infant to die; they want to love and care for the infant and at the same time wish to reject him or her.[58] These feelings are frightening and socially unacceptable and therefore often remain unspoken.

Often the intensity of grief is greater when the relationship with and feelings about the lost person are ambivalent.[68] Even with the most positive of pregnancy outcomes, taking a newborn into the family results in ambivalent feelings for all family members. The degree of disruption that a perinatal loss brings to the family is equated with the severity of grief, especially because reproduction and a healthy perinatal outcome are highly valued in our society.[68]

Critical Findings

SIGNS AND SYMPTOMS OF GRIEF

1. Somatic (physiologic)
   a. Gastrointestinal system
      - Anorexia and weight loss
      - Overeating
      - Nausea or vomiting
      - Abdominal pains or feelings of emptiness
      - Diarrhea or constipation
   b. Respiratory system
      - Sighing respirations
      - Choking or coughing
      - Shortness of breath
      - Hyperventilation
   c. Cardiovascular system
      - Cardiac palpitations or "fluttering" in chest
      - "Heavy" feeling in chest
   d. Neuromuscular system
      - Headaches
      - Vertigo
      - Syncope
      - Brissaud's disease (tics)
      - Muscular weakness or loss of strength
2. Behavioral (psychologic)
   a. Feelings of:
      - Guilt
      - Sadness
      - Anger and hostility
      - Emptiness and apathy
      - Helplessness
      - Pain, desperation, and pessimism
      - Shame
      - Loneliness
   b. Preoccupation with image of the lost infant
      - Daydreams and fantasies
      - Nightmares
      - Longing
   c. Disturbed interpersonal relationships
      - Increased irritability and restlessness
      - Decreased sexual interest and drive
      - Withdrawal
   d. Crying
   e. Inability to return to normal activities
      - Fatigue and exhaustion or aimless overactivity
      - Insomnia or oversleeping
      - Short attention span
      - Slow speech, movement, and thought process
      - Loss of concentration and motivation

Data from Colgrove M: *How to survive the loss of a love,* New York, 1976, Lion Publishing; Lindemann E: Symptomatology and management of acute grief, *Am J Psychiatry* 101:144, 1944; Marris P: *Loss and change,* New York, 1974, Pantheon Books.

MALE-FEMALE DIFFERENCES

Although members of both genders have the same grief reactions, women express more symptoms (crying, sadness, anger, guilt, and use of medications)[34,50,51,70,93] than men. This difference in symptomatology does not represent a different experience of grief but merely a different expression of it. Understanding these differences and the reasons for them is crucial for care providers working with parents at the time of perinatal loss. Explaining these differences to parents is also crucial so that diverse grief responses do not become divisive in the relationship.[34,93]

The father's degree of investment in the pregnancy, impending parenthood, and the circumstances of birth all affect his feelings of loss. Because the father's body does not directly experience the changes of pregnancy, the pregnancy initially may be less of a reality to him than to the pregnant woman. This lag in the physiologic reality contributes to a lag in the psychologic investment of the father in the baby. The father's lag in psychologic investment often contributes to incongruent grieving, a difference in mother's and father's grief reactions. Fathers often comment that the infant became real when he felt the fetus move in the mother or at first sight of the new infant. Fathers who form an early attachment to the child feel sadness, disappointment, and often anger at being denied the expected son or daughter.[44,55,70,71,97] Conversely, fathers who have been normally ambivalent or overtly negative about the pregnancy may feel guilt and responsibility for the failed outcome.

Participation of the father in the events of labor and birth also influences his attachment and ultimately his feelings of loss. Exclusion decreases his involvement in these life-crisis events, whereas inclusion has many advantages for the mother, infant, and self (see Chapter 29). If the infant is ill, the father may initially have more and closer contact than the mother.[7] In the birth place, the father may see, touch, or hold the infant before the mother does. The father observes the initial resuscitation and stabilization and may accompany the infant to the nursery and on transport to a regional center. Often the father receives the first information and support about the infant's condition and returns to the hospitalized mother with the news. This early, prolonged contact coupled with the father's increased responsibility often contributes to the development of a closer and earlier bond between father and infant than between mother and infant. The initial lag in prenatal investment may be offset after birth by concentrated contact between the father and the baby, so that a loss is highly significant to the father.

Societal expectations about masculinity and femininity markedly influence the expression of grief. Society's message to men starts early in life: "Big boys don't cry" and "Don't cry, you'll be a sissy" (i.e., girl). The preferred male image in our society is the autonomous, independent achiever who is always strong and in control, even in the face of disaster.[44,45] In keeping with this image, the father may feel that he must make all the decisions and have all information filtered through him to protect the mother. However, this altruistic gesture prevents full disclosure to and involvement of the mother. Assuming the role of strong protector also involves a heavy price for the father in suppression of his own feelings and delay of his own grief work.[34,71,93] The role of "tower of strength" often engenders feelings of resentment from the mother. Although he attempts to live up to his (and society's) expectations of himself, the woman views his apparent lack of feelings and emotions, especially crying, as "He doesn't care." A recent study showed that distress experienced by the mother but not by her partner resulted in longer-term marital dissatisfaction for the mother.

Many men have difficulty dealing with irrational behaviors, as well as with the normal ambiguity and conflict of life. This difficulty makes the emotional response of grief and its accompanying ambivalent feelings and conflicts produce discomfort and anxiety in many men. The expression of appropriate human emotions becomes threatening and makes them feel vulnerable. To decrease the anxiety associated with grief and its expression, men often deal with feelings by denying them, increasing their workload, grieving internally, or withdrawing from the situation and refusing to discuss it.[70,93]

The father's attitude and ability to communicate about the loss may help or impede the mother's grief work.[100] Lack of communication between a couple may contribute to intense mourning, psychiatric disturbances, and severe family disruption.[56,93,118] Synchrony of grieving between the mother and the father is important in an ultimate healthy resolution for the family.[22,93] If the father denies and suppresses his own feelings of loss and grief, he may react to the normal signs and symptoms of grief in his partner as if they were abnormal. Often the father can resolve his grief faster than the mother, and he may become impatient with her continual "dwelling" on the loss. Sometimes fearing the woman's prolonged grief, the man decides to "spare her" from his feelings and does not discuss them with her. Instead of being comforting as intended, failure to share grief leads to isolation and alienation within the relationship.[58,93]

In some situations, the man may experience intense emotions several months after the death, not unlike those his partner experienced at the time of the crisis. Because these intense emotions occur so long after the crisis, he may not even associate them with the death.[31,58] A recent study found that at 30 months after the death of a baby, fathers were more distressed than the mothers, who were the more distressed initially after the death.[118]

TIMING OF GRIEF RESOLUTION

Parents

Emotional recovery from the pain of perinatal loss occurs with time. There is no complete agreement on the length of time necessary for the individual to resolve grief. Indeed, a specific timetable for mourning may be impossible to establish.[8] However, some general time frames are available for the duration of a normal grief reaction.

Acute grief reactions are the most intense during the first 4 to 6 weeks after the loss,[61,68,81] with some improvement noted 6 to 10 weeks later. Normal grief reactions may be expected to last from 6 months to 1 year[6,38,58,81] or 2 years.[68] Indeed, significant losses of a spouse or child may never be completely resolved[29,96,119]: "I'll never get over it."

One parameter for differentiating normal from pathologic grief has been the length of time for grief to be resolved. Grief work may still be categorized as normal even if it lasts longer than 1 year, especially if the person is working through unresolved grief from the past. Grief work is normally energy draining. Dealing with more than one grief or loss situation compounds the intensity of mourning and may prolong the grief reaction. Because perinatal loss represents more than the loss of the newborn (loss of the perfect child, loss of plans for the future, and loss of self-esteem), feelings of sadness and depression may still be evident for a year or longer.[58,70,118,128]

Sorrow and grief may even last a lifetime. For families of defective children, "chronic sorrow"[31,49,79,91,106] is experienced as long as the child lives. These parents live with the constant reminder of what is not and what the child will never be and can never do. The grief of death is final—parents do the work and go on; chronic sorrow is grieving on a daily basis. Expecting the parents to adjust to or accept their child's defect without any elements of lingering sadness is unrealistic. Although hampered by small sample sizes, research on the gender differences in chronic sorrow show more chronic sorrow in mothers than in fathers.[49,67] Chronic sorrow is a justifiable reaction to the daily stresses and coping necessary when a child is defective. The final stage of grief resolution is possible only with the finality of the death of the child.

Even when grief has been resolved, anniversary grief reactions are normal. Feelings of sadness, crying, and normal grieving behaviors may be reactivated at certain times. These anniversary reactions may not be limited to the infant's date of death but also may be felt on the expected date of delivery, on the actual birthday, or on seeing an infant of the same age and gender as the lost infant. Holidays may also reactivate grieving behaviors, especially those that bring together family and friends and recall memories of joy and happiness.

Staff

Those sharing a crisis (complication, illness, or death) often become closely attached, so that the loss is felt not only by the family but also by the professional care providers.* Repeatedly dealing with death and deformity increases the professional's exposure to personal feelings of grief and loss. This may be perceived either as a threat or a personal opportunity for growth.[37]

The critical variable in the ability to face or assist others in handling loss is the manner in which the care providers have been able to resolve their own personal losses. Unless the care providers can cope with personal feelings of loss and grief, they may not be able to give of the "self" to others. Care given without genuine involvement and responsiveness to the family's feelings does not facilitate and may actually impede the mourning process. Professionals who can deal honestly with their own feelings will be able to help others cope with theirs.[21,83]

*References 21,32,83,92,93,96.

Helping parents deal with their grief may be difficult for professionals because of their attitudes and feelings about perinatal loss. For professionals trained to preserve life, loss of the best pregnancy outcome or death itself represents both a personal and professional failure.[58] When success is equated with life, the failure of death (or loss) is associated with feelings of guilt, anger, depression, and hostility.[128] Just when professionals are expected to be supportive and therapeutic, they may be overwhelmed with their own feelings. Professionally, the care providers may feel helpless when all efforts inevitably result in no change in the outcome.

The feelings and stages of grief experienced by the family are the same ones felt by the staff who are attached to the parents and their newborn. Many professionals working in perinatal care are of childbearing age, so identifying with the parents and their plight is relatively easy. Because the sick, deformed, or dead infant could easily be that of the staff, they share with the parents the special stress of the loss of a child. The care provider often experiences the same fantasies of blame as the parents: "What did I do (or not do) to cause this?"

Repetitive contact with loss situations and death exposes the staff to recurring feelings of frustration, guilt, self-doubt, depression, anger, classic grief reactions, helplessness, sadness, hopelessness, loneliness, and covert relief.[32] Such uncomfortable feelings often lead to behaviors of avoidance and withdrawal as a means of self-protection; this has been called "compassion fatigue."[21,83,96] Adequate medical care may be given, but psychologic care of the family may be neglected.[64] The involved primary care providers may decrease their attachment to both parents and infant when an unfavorable outcome is inevitable. Withdrawing emotional support and involvement may spare the professional but only adds to parental feelings of isolation, inadequacy, and worthlessness. Professionals who have risked family attachment and shared grief work may be more cautious in future involvements to protect themselves from the pain of loss.

Asynchrony and individual differences in handling grief reactions also may cause problems among the professional staff. Constant exposure to perinatal loss may desensitize some individuals until they are blasé or even callous about the crisis, whereas the grief reactions of others parallel the family's reaction. Some staff members may have reached the stage of acceptance, whereas others who cannot let the infant go persist in the idea of a magical cure, a characteristic of denial. The rationale of prolonging the child's life may in reality be prolonging death, and inevitably one needs to accept death's finality.

Staff members cannot offer support to families experiencing loss unless they receive support in dealing with their own grief reactions.[21,37,39] Those who receive support learn about their feelings and how to handle them and so have no need to displace their pain to others. The three most effective ways that neonatal intensive care unit (NICU) nurses have identified to manage their stress after a neonate's death are (1) discussing with co-workers, (2) supporting and comforting the grieving family, and (3) talking with their own families.[32] Various formats are available for meeting staff needs, such as mutual support of colleagues or group sessions involving peer counseling on a long-term or short-term basis.[21,32,39,58,92] Group meetings provide a vehicle for support and for sharing information and feelings among staff members.[21,32,39,58,92] Facilitated by an objective person with expertise in group process and the concepts of grief, such meetings have the goal of helping the staff deal with their reactions so they will be better equipped to help the parents. Group sessions also serve to decrease stress, increase job satisfaction, and ultimately help prevent burnout. Staff members are encouraged to retain their humanity when an environment is created in which emotions are valued and their healthy expression facilitated, both at the time of loss and in its resolution.[53,92]

Sharing grief work with a family gives the care provider a chance for personal growth, to review past personal losses, and to evaluate the adequacy of their resolution. Helping others with loss or grief provides the professional with the opportunity to contemplate present and future losses, including one's own mortality. By working with those who have suffered a significant loss or death, a health care provider may gain a deeper perspective about life.

INTERVENTIONS

Those in a crisis feel an openness to help and assistance from others, so that those in the crisis emerge either stronger or weaker, depending on the help they receive.[17,89] This increased openness also makes those in a crisis more vulnerable to the reactions of others—to their facial expression, tone of voice, and choice of words. Helpful professional interventions provide psychologic assistance during a highly vulnerable period of personal development. The goals of intervention are to maintain the pre-crisis level of functioning and to improve coping and problem-solving skills beyond the pre-crisis level (i.e., to facilitate personal growth). Effective intervention is characterized by helping grief work get started, by supporting those who are grieving adaptively, and by intervening with individuals who display maladaptive reactions.[22,35]

For professionals, understanding parental perspectives of the experience of death of a newborn should enable provision of more sensitive and evidence-based care for grieving families. The results of two recent research studies give some insight into what is helpful and what is not helpful for grieving families. The first study was a systematic review of 61 studies and more than 6000 parents who suffered neonatal death.[43] This study found that parents valued emotional support, grief education, and attention to mother/baby. Non-helpful and distressing behaviors from health care providers included avoidance, thoughtlessness, insensitivity, and poor staff communication.[43] Another study conducted semi-structured interviews with mothers/fathers (n = 19) a mean of 1.9 years after death of their infant. This exploratory study found a low level of grief, effective coping, and factors important to parents in end-of-life care for their infant.[14] Review of the data from this study in Table 30-1 instructs health care professionals in helpful and non-helpful interventions during the stressful experience of a dying infant.[19] Because 76% of the dying infants were in the NICU or pediatric intensive care unit (PICU) and 42% of the families had hospice/palliative care team involvement,[14] perhaps the low level of grief and the positive adaptation by this small group of parents were because of the sensitive, helpful interventions of their health care providers.

TABLE 30-1 PARENTAL PERCEPTIONS OF GRIEF AND IMPORTANT FACTORS AT THE TIME OF INFANT DEATH: RESEARCH BASIS[14]

STUDY FINDINGS	COMMENTS
1. Parents scored significantly lower than other parents who had lost a child and other adults with grief experience.	1. Lower levels of grief were measured by the Revised Grief Experience Inventory (RGEI), a 22-item Likert scale.
2. Study investigators viewed parents as positively adapting after loss of their infant.	2. Mean scores were 33.16 (out of a highest possible score of 36) on the Post-Death Adaptation Score, a 10-item scale rated by professionals.
3. Seven important aspects of care:	3. Identified by parents:
A. Honesty	A. Parents expect professionals to be honest in giving information about the infant/condition to them. Parental anger results when (parental) perception is that honest information was not given.
B. Empowered decision making	B. Parents want to be involved in medical decision making, especially about withdrawing life support. Parents who had been involved were glad they had been part of the decision process and felt supported by the medical team. Parents felt anger and abandonment when the decision to withdraw support was not believed to be respected by professionals.
C. Parental care	C. Parents needed care as much as their baby; when staff were insensitive to their needs, parents felt upset.
D. Environment	D. Parents appreciated comforts of sleep/family rooms as well as private, quiet areas where the infant died with family/parents. People present at the death were more important than the place of death. Parents expressed fear when left at home with their dying infant; parents wished they had held the infant longer.
E. Faith/trust in nursing care	E. Parents had greater trust in nurses than other providers; most had positive experiences with their infant's nurses. Parents appreciated nurses personalizing and respecting the infant (using baby's name) as well as providing for the infant's comfort and opportunities for parental care of their baby. Negative experiences included mistakes in care and unprofessional behavior.

Continued

TABLE 30-1 PARENTAL PERCEPTIONS OF GRIEF AND IMPORTANT FACTORS AT THE TIME OF INFANT DEATH: RESEARCH BASIS[14]—cont'd

STUDY FINDINGS	COMMENTS
F. Physicians bearing witness	F. Parents thought it important that the physician be with them throughout the process, including being present at the time of the infant's death. Parents perceived the absence of the physician at the time of the child's death as negative, especially if they had been told that the physician would be there for them. Parents found it meaningful when the physician and other medical staff had contact with them after they had gone home.
G. Support from other hospital care providers	G. Parents appreciated support that they received from chaplains, social workers, and palliative care and child life workers. Parents also appreciated support and help from these providers in dealing with siblings.
4. Seven coping strategies:	4. Identified by parents:
A. Family support	A. Parents relied on family support to cope with the death, appreciated family presence at the hospital/home when the infant died, and found it helpful to talk to extended family about their infant. When extended family members were not supportive and avoided talking about the infant, parents were distressed.
B. Keeping the memory alive	B. All parents showed researchers mementoes of their dead infant and emphasized the importance of bringing things home (i.e., photos; plaster castings of hands/feet; blanket/clothes) from the hospital that had been used/belonged to the infant who died. Parents especially appreciated tangible reminders (i.e., garden/tree) and rituals to remember their infant.
C. Spirituality/faith	C. All families were comforted by their religious beliefs and found meaning and purpose in their infant's life and death. No families reported negative spiritual experience or abandonment of their religious beliefs.
D. Altruism	D. Many parents wanted and did "give back" to the hospitals that had cared for them and their dying infants. These altruistic acts took the form of monetary and equipment donations, volunteering, and becoming resource families to other parents with sick children.
E. Refocusing on life	E. Presence of other children in the family assisted parents continuing to focus on life and the daily requirements of their surviving children. All parents acknowledged that having another child would never replace the infant who died.
F. Validation of decision	F. Parents were comforted by autopsy results that validated that they had made the correct decision for their infant. Parents also appreciated when physicians communicated to them their support of the parents' decision.
G. Bereavement support groups	G. Bereavement support groups resulted in positive experiences for most families, especially in being able to talk freely about their dead infant with others who understood and were not uncomfortable. However, some parents did not feel validated in their grief/loss of an infant by other parents in the group whose children were "older" when they died.

Non-helpful Interventions

Caring for pregnant women and their infants is supposed to be a "happy" job. Birthing and caring for infants are supposed to be times of joy and celebration. Because no one expects death or loss to occur in maternity or nursery areas, when it does, both staff and families are shocked. To protect themselves from the reality of the situation or to "spare" the family, professionals may engage in interventions that do not help themselves or their patients. Such interventions may be meant altruistically but do not have the characteristics of effective intervention.

Maintaining the state of denial arrests grief work by preventing or delaying the acceptance of the reality of the loss situation. Progress toward resolution is not begun until the stage of disbelief is relinquished. Using drugs, not talking or crying about the loss, and using distraction all contribute to maladaptive reactions by maintaining the state of denial.

The use of tranquilizers, sedatives, and other drugs does not help the recipient but, rather, benefits the giver. Excessive use of these medications prolongs the denial stage by making the feelings and emotions foggy and dreamlike.[56] The energy needed to begin the grief work is dissipated by the effect of the medications. Avoiding the reality of the situation becomes easier when mind-altering drugs make the tragedy even more unbelievable.

Not talking about the loss is a powerful way of denying that it ever existed.[83,93] The inability of professionals to acknowledge that the loss has occurred and that the family is in pain maintains denial and repression.[16] Not discussing the loss prevents parents from learning the facts and facing their reality. Because a fantasy will be created to substitute for the unknown, the fantasy of what happened and why will be worse than the reality. By receiving truthful, honest communication, parents are not left to spend energy dealing with frightening fantasies.

Professional avoidance and unwillingness to talk with parents after a loss communicate other powerful messages that impede grief work. If the loss is not important enough to discuss, then perhaps it is not important at all. Not talking about the loss serves to reduce it and communicates to the parents, "I don't care; therefore neither should you." Avoidance of the topic or a hurried, businesslike or social communication that skirts the issue tells the parent that grief work is dangerous, that grief emotions are dangerous, and that others are afraid of grief and those experiencing it. In essence, not discussing the loss gives a clear nonverbal message to not grieve.

An inability to cry in response to a significant loss is not helpful and impedes grief work. The prohibition against crying may have been learned early in life or may be the result of unresolved grief work. Parents may feel the need to be strong for each other, their family, or the staff and thus do not cry. Sometimes role reversal occurs, so that the grieving person feels the need to support others rather than be the recipient of support. Often the significance of parental loss is neither recognized nor acknowledged by the professional for fear that he or she will cry. Rather than talking about the loss as a technique to facilitate tears, no one says anything so no one will cry, and no one's grief progresses through the grief stages.

Distraction is another way of denying the loss or its significance. Professionals, a spouse, or other family members try to distract parents from the feelings and emotions of acute grief by engaging in light, social conversation or by keeping them busy with work or recreation. Dealing only with the physical care and not the need for psychologic care after birth is a form of distraction used by care providers.[47] Parents are preoccupied with their shattered expectations of the past and the stark reality of the present, and they are not interested in distractions.

After an unfavorable perinatal outcome, the couple are often confused about their status: "Am I a mother or father…or not?" This experience has been called the "ambivalent transition into motherhood."[65] Failure to acknowledge the newly acquired role of mother or father (even if the fetus or newborn dies) discounts the parent's psychologic investment in the pregnancy, fetus, and newborn. Quickly removing the infant from the maternity or nursery areas or removing all the baby items from the home negates the infant's existence.[58] This is not helpful for grief resolution and prevents parents from making choices and decisions and thus maintaining control over the reality of the situation.

Isolation of the grieving family prevents the development of dependent relationships with others who might potentially provide support and comfort. Without others, parents cannot share their grief and may thus increase their feelings of guilt, anger, blame, and lack of self-worth at their failed pregnancy. Those directly experiencing a perinatal loss may be isolated from the rest of society, including their families, who do not view loss of a pregnancy or neonate as significant.[10,58,93] Empathy with the parents' definition of the loss as important is necessary for society to be supportive. The goal of recent research, professional literature, and education has been to sensitize the care provider to the effect of perinatal loss. Only recently have books specifically about perinatal loss become available to inform and assist parents.

To decrease contact with the grieving mother, the staff may neglect her or perform cursory physical care, or there may be overconcern for providing physical care.[71] Assigning a room at the end of the hall, not going into the room, delaying answering requests, and placing the mother on another floor are ways of avoiding families. Use of private rooms and room assignments off the maternity floor may be helpful but may allow staff to remove the unpleasant and uncomfortable situation. Early discharge to a supportive environment may be helpful but, without plans for follow-up, may merely be a way to remove the constant, painful reminder.

Keeping the childbearing couple together throughout the perinatal events facilitates a shared experience of the reality of the situation. Separation of the mother and father or of the couple from friends, family, and other children is not helpful. Exclusion of family members from the experience also excludes them from providing support for the mother and the couple. Relaxed visiting policies and as much contact as possible between the hospitalized mother and the father (and other family members) are important.[20,83]

Prohibiting contact between the parents and the infant allows fearful fantasies of the truth that are always more frightening than the reality of the situation. Delayed contact prolongs the state of disbelief and denial.[22] Restrictive visiting policies in the nursery, institutionalizing an infant without looking at all alternatives, or any other policy that separates parents from their infant does not facilitate grief. Especially in the case of a deformed, stillborn, or dead infant, the message of delayed or no contact is that the infant is too horrible and too unacceptable to be seen or touched. Because parental egos are so symbiotically attached to their offspring, an unacceptable child is equated with an unacceptable and unworthy self. The fantasy that the damaged or dead child is representative of the damaged and defective self is borne out in the behavior and separation policies of the care providers.

In an attempt to offer the grieving family comfort, friends, relatives, and even professionals often make comments that are non-supportive and nonhelpful[58,83]:

- "Well, you're young. You can have more babies."
- "Just have another baby right away."
- "Well, at least you have others at home."
- "It's better to lose her now when she's a baby than when she's 4 years old."
- "He never would have been totally normal anyway."
- "He was born dead. You didn't get a chance to know or get attached to him anyway."
- "It's God's will."

Clichés and platitudes such as these do not help because of the message they give about the parents and the infant.[99] These comments at best reduce and at worst negate the effect of prenatal attachment to the fetus. The importance of psychologic investment and attachment by the parents to this fetus or newborn is said to be basically unimportant and essentially nonexistent.[58] Because infants are viewed as an extension of the parent's self, "by a not very subtle process of identification, the parents see a part of themselves in the baby, and nobody likes to be told that part of them is better off dead."[99] Also, comforting parents whose infant has died with the information that the child was not perfect and never would have been normal and healthy reinforces their belief that they are as defective and unsatisfactory as their dead child.[58]

Such comments also convey a message about the importance of an individual life. Essentially, they say that one fetus or newborn is fairly interchangeable with another. They negate the importance of and indeed the existence of the infant for the parents, siblings, family, and society. The life of the individual is devalued, because he or she is easily replaced by "another baby." Comparing one infant's illness or deformity with another's is not helpful for parents whose own infant's deformity is certainly more important than any other infant's problem.

The power of words to help during grief is outweighed only by their power to not help. Because parents are increasingly open during a perinatal crisis, they are sensitive not only to what is said and how it is said but also to the nonverbal message. Giving premature or false reassurance may be more for relief of the professionals than for the parents.[17] Comments such as "It's okay" and "Everything will be all right" must be genuine and timed appropriately for the parent. Telling parents that they have a child with Down syndrome and then saying "But everything will be all right" is hardly helpful. Giving reassurance that subsequent pregnancies and infants will be all right or unaffected is not helpful before the parents are ready to think about and project into the future.

The basic terminology accompanying perinatal grief situations may be upsetting to parents. Instead of *dead,* professionals often substitute less frightening and less final words. The use of *loss* when *death* is appropriate may be misinterpreted (especially by children). The terms *lose, loss,* and *lost* connote misplacing, so that comments such as "I'm sorry you lost your baby" may be responded to by "I didn't lose (misplace) my baby. My child died." Medical professionals skirt the use of the words *dead, died,* and *die.* Care providers are taught as students to use the word *expired* when referring to a patient who has died. Meant to soften the effect of *dead,* the word *expired* may have its own effect, as a mother whose infant son died wrote in a poem: "The baby expired they said, as if you were a credit card."[113]

Other situations that do not facilitate grief work include dealing with multiple losses or stresses and ambivalence or mental illness.[128] The reaction to the loss of a significant relationship is intensified in the context of multiple losses, stresses, and problems.[83,128] Because perinatal losses represent not only a loss of the wished-for perfect child but also a threat to the parental self, self-concept, and self-worth, they represent situations of multiple loss.[119,120]

Helpful Interventions

Professionals have an opportunity to make a significant difference in the outcome after the crisis of perinatal loss for the individual, the couple, and the family. A care provider who is knowledgeable about the grief process and comfortable in sharing another's grief is equipped to assist the family and its members toward a long-term healthy adjustment rather than a dysfunctional and pathologic adjustment. Interventions that are helpful for family members also assist staff members in their own grief work.

Factors that influence an individual's personal experience of grief (and ultimately appropriate interventions) are outlined in Box 30-2. Care for the grieving is individualized through assessing these factors, planning, and continually evaluating the individual.[34,35,83,96] Eliciting such personal information may not be as difficult as it first seems. Those in crisis often spontaneously share crucial data with little prompting. The importance of active listening to questions and comments or a more formalized therapeutic interview process may provide the needed encouragement and permission to begin communication.

BOX 30-2 FACTORS TO EVALUATE IN INDIVIDUALIZING GRIEF INTERVENTIONS

1. Previous losses
   a. Type
      - Separation
      - Divorce
      - Death
      - Spontaneous abortion (miscarriage)
      - Elective or selective abortion
      - Period of infertility
      - Relinquishment of child
      - Perinatal loss
   b. Timing in the life cycle
      - Distant
      - Recent
   c. Coping styles (of each individual and the family as a unit)
   d. Grief work
      - Resolved
      - Unresolved
2. Prenatal attachment
   a. Degree of psychologic investment in relationship with fetus or newborn
   b. Decision making about pregnancy and infant
      - Planned or unplanned
      - Wanted or unwanted
   c. Meaning of pregnancy and infant to individual and family
   d. Parental expectation about childbearing
3. Nature of the current loss
   a. Timing
      - Sudden and expected
      - Anticipatory grief
   b. Definition and meaning of the event (death, deformity) to individual members of the family
   c. Multiple losses
      - Self
      - Perfect child
   d. Nature and severity
      - Of loss
      - Of defect
4. Cultural influences (also see Chapter 29)
   a. On experience and the expression of grief
   b. Societal expectations dictate acceptable and unacceptable behaviors of mourning
5. Strengths (individual and family)
   a. Support system (family, friends, religious, community, or social agencies) mobilized when necessary
   b. Stable relationships: couple supportive of each other
   c. Financial stability
   d. Coping abilities: can evaluate, plan for, and adjust to novel situations
   e. Good health
   f. Receptive and intelligent
   g. Realistic expectations about childbearing and childrearing

A history of previous losses and their type and timing in the life cycle are important data for the care provider dealing with the current loss. Past experiences with a crisis or loss influence an individual's behavioral and coping style with current problems.[121] Experiencing a previous perinatal loss affects a subsequent pregnancy.[24,95] These pregnancies are characterized by guarded emotions, marking the progress of the pregnancy and seeking out or avoiding various behaviors.[23-26,121] A previous perinatal loss may compound the individual's reaction to a current loss. Dealing with problems alone, receiving help and support from others, and withdrawing altogether are possible ways of coping with the loss.

The degree of attachment and the meaning of the pregnancy and impending parenthood to the family define expectations and influence reactions if an optimal outcome does not occur. The experience of grief depends on whether the loss situation was sudden and unexpected or if there was forewarning about a problem or complication. The definition and meaning of the crisis (e.g., the nature and severity of a deformity, the finality of death, or the chronic sorrow of a defective infant) reflect the individual's and family's value system and previous crisis experience. The process of grief is affected by the event itself, the previous and current coping mechanisms, and the family's definition of the event. Consideration of all of these factors is crucial in instituting appropriate intervention.

Cultural practices among families and professionals often differ (see Chapter 29).[94] For example, in some cultures, it may not be acceptable to see or hold your baby (as in some Native American cultures). In the Muslim culture, the family is the primary system of support and it is rare to see a Muslim family emote publicly. It is critical for health care practitioners to recognize cultural and religious differences to minimize misinterpretations and conflicts with families. With increasing immigration, practitioners must be able to respond with a more ethnic-sensitive approach.[20,35,63,77,104] It is essential to be creative and flexible, thus respecting families' cultural and religious belief systems.[2,117,125] Studies show that cultural differences influence (1) parental emotional response to and perception of their infant's illness and disability, (2) parental utilization of services, (3) parental interactions with health care providers, and (4) the ceremonies and rituals surrounding death.[11,35,63]

The national association Share: Pregnancy & Infant Loss Support, Inc. has revised the "Rights of Parents When a Baby Dies" and "Rights of the Infant" (Box 30-3). These documents serve as guidelines for creation of protocols, checklists, and bereavement programs; affirmation and empowering tools for bereaved parents; and communication points for parents and care providers initiating the grief process.[85]

BOX 30-3 RIGHTS OF PARENTS AND INFANT WHEN AN INFANT DIES

Rights of Parents

1. To be given the opportunity to see, hold, and touch their baby at any time before or after death, within reason
2. To have photographs of their baby taken and made available to the parents or held in security until the parents want to see them
3. To be given as many mementos as possible (i.e., crib card, baby beads or bracelet, ultrasound or other photographs, lock of hair, feet and hand prints, and record of weight and length)
4. To name their child and bond with him or her
5. To observe cultural and religious practices
6. To be cared for by an empathetic staff who will respect their feelings, thoughts, beliefs, and individual requests
7. To be with each other throughout hospitalization as much as possible
8. To be given time alone with their baby, allowing for individual needs
9. To be informed about the grieving process
10. To request an autopsy; in the case of a miscarriage, to request to have or not have an autopsy or pathology examination as determined by applicable law
11. To plan a farewell ritual, burial, or cremation in compliance with local and state regulations and according to their personal beliefs, religion, or cultural tradition
12. To be provided information on support resources that assist in the healing process (i.e., support groups, counseling, reading material, and perinatal loss newsletter)

Rights of the Infant

1. To be recognized as someone who was born and died
2. To be named
3. To be seen, touched, and held by the family
4. To have life-ending acknowledged
5. To be put to rest with dignity

Modified from *SHARE pregnancy and infant loss support,* Available at www.nationalshareoffice.org.

ENVIRONMENT

The first step in facilitating grief work is to create an environment that is supportive, permissive, and conducive to the expression of feelings.[16,21,83,93] This type of environment does not depend on physical surroundings but, rather, is created and maintained by a warm, receptive, accepting, and caring staff. Such an environment centers its concern more on the people giving and receiving care than on the tasks of care.[58] This type of environment is nonjudgmental and is characterized by an attitude of openness and freedom.[19,99] People feel safe enough to ventilate a full range of feelings—sadness, anger, despair, and even humor—without the fear of condemnation or rejection. The staff become role models of open communication, facing grief, and feeling comfortable in an uncomfortable situation. The safety of such an environment generates feelings of acceptance and understanding so that grieving and healing may proceed.

Professional presence and support are essential to families in crisis because of the increased dependency needs that accompany grief and loss. Yet certain aspects of a conducive environment such as privacy, quiet, and comfort may be difficult to obtain in a noisy and busy perinatal setting. The recommendation to never leave the family alone must be balanced with their need for privacy and personal time alone with their infant (stillborn, ill, or dying). Simply saying "I will stay with you unless you ask me to leave so that you can have some private time alone with your child" or "Would you like me to leave for a while so that you can be alone with your baby?" offers both support and privacy. Many parents later regret not having time alone and not thinking to ask to be alone with their infant.

A quiet place away from the hustle and bustle of the routine may facilitate both attachment and detachment. The mother of a stillborn child who is quickly shown her infant in the delivery room as her episiotomy is being repaired is not in an optimal physical (or psychologic) environment. Attaching to and saying good-bye to her infant are better accomplished in a quieter and more private setting with significant others present.[64,82,110] Active participation of parents at the death of their newborn may not optimally occur in a busy intensive care unit. Rather, adaptation of hospice concepts to neonatal care provides a private, homelike room, with focus on palliative (comfort) care, rather than cure, to the dying newborn and the family (see Chapter 32).[21,96,107,108] When the family is too emotionally drained, they may elect to "say good-bye" and leave the hospital before life support is removed; the nurse then disconnects, holds, and rocks the baby so the infant does not die alone.[15,83] In some situations (e.g., chromosomal anomalies), parents and professionals may opt to provide end-of-life care ideally with hospice care at home.[74]

Supportive, Trusting Relationships. A relationship with a caring individual who offers consistency and support is the foundation of a therapeutic environment. During periods of crisis, when there is a temporary increase in dependency needs and feelings of loneliness, it is an adaptive behavior to seek emotional support from family, friends, and professionals.[16,68,83] Even the crisis of normal childbearing prompts many cultures to provide a doula[90] to teach the new mother and give her emotional support. For a mourning family, the relationships established with helpful professionals are more important than the physical care given.

Support, "sharing one's ego strength with another in a time of need,"[46] is particularly helpful in perinatal loss because of the threat to self-concept and self-esteem suffered by parents. Support may be as simple as remaining with the parents. "Being there" indicates not only physical presence but also an emotional availability and willingness to share their experience of loss. Often professionals, family, and friends are hampered by not knowing what to say. Usually words are initially unnecessary or do not adequately describe the moment and silent presence may better convey the message. Often it is not what is said but the mere presence of loving others that conveys empathy and support to parents and colleagues. Yet presence is not enough; meaningful interaction between parents and professionals is also necessary for a trusting relationship to develop.

The initial meeting with the professionals, including verbal and nonverbal cues, leaves a lasting impression on the family. Addressing family members by name personalizes the encounter, and a brief touch or handshake represents an extension of self, a gesture of warmth, concern, and acceptance from professional to parents. An introduction that includes a brief explanation of the professional's role in relation to them and their infant helps orient them: "Good morning, Mr. and Mrs. Black. I'm Sue, your baby's primary nurse. That means that I will be caring for Jason while he is here and working with you." Orientation to the physical surroundings and technical equipment eases the transition to an unfamiliar and often intimidating hospital environment. Providing physical comfort such as rocking chairs, privacy for interaction, and sleeping facilities for parents demonstrates the philosophy of the parents' worth and importance to their infant.

Empathy, an emotional understanding and identification with the plight of another, characterizes a helping relationship. In such a relationship, "How are you?" is asked with the emphasis on you and a genuine interest in the answer—unlike a social inquiry in which an automatic "Fine" is expected. Recognition of verbal and nonverbal cues of parental feelings (e.g., "You look tired" or "I hear that you are frustrated") communicates that these emotions are legitimate, understood, and accepted. A willingness to help, listen, console, and give encouragement and positive feedback establishes the professional as a sensitive, responsive person whom parents will trust. Supporting any and all parental involvement, supporting damaged parental egos, and helping parents succeed in the tasks of attachment and detachment are goals of effective intervention.

A qualitative study examining maternal perceptions and experiences showed that mothers had feelings of both empowerment and powerlessness with professional care after the death of their newborn.[64] Feelings of powerlessness occurred when (1) mothers felt disrespected as a person and a mother, (2) good communication between mother and professionals did not exist, and (3) the mother did not feel treated as an individual.[64] Mothers felt empowered (e.g., more confident, able to ask questions, understood and supported) when they felt that (1) professionals were "near," both psychologically and emotionally, (2) professionals supported the mother's self-esteem and confidence, and (3) professionals provided empathetic, comforting support.[64]

The tone of in-hospital perinatal settings is often determined by the nursing staff. Generally, residents, interns, and specialists remain for short periods and the private physician or permanent medical staff are not available on a minute-to-minute basis. Development of a safe, trusting environment depends on viewing parents as essential partners in care of their baby and not as visitors or "disruptors" of the ward routine.[22] Pleasant and relaxed surroundings convey the message of hospitality and "You are welcome here."

Both professional and nonprofessional support systems are available in the crisis of perinatal loss. Yet relating to many people during crisis is difficult for parents. Primary care (both medical and nursing) uses the same care provider for both the physiologic and psychologic care of the infant and the family. Thus the family is able to relate to as few professionals as possible. This special caring reassures parents that a few special people love, know, and are invested in their infant. Primary care providers share with the parents the joys of even small gains and the sorrows and tears of complications or death. Professionals and parents benefit from primary care systems in the emotional and psychologic satisfaction of such involvement. Yet this involvement is not without a price of vulnerability to an individual's feelings of loss and grief. Peer support on an individual basis or in a group setting is essential in dealing with the stress of continual attachment and loss.[32]

Normal grief reactions may be facilitated by nursing and medical professionals using others (social workers or counselors) when necessary.[7,21,69,83] Collaboration and consultation with these professionals help the staff gain insight into parental and personal behaviors and appropriate intervention strategies. The staff also may benefit from the expertise of a trained counselor in dealing with their own feelings of loss and grief.

PATHOLOGIC GRIEF

Maladaptive responses to perinatal loss are indications for referral for specialized care (see the Critical Findings box on p. 917).[127] Involvement of clergy and religious organizations is often comforting and supportive to the family.[73,82,112,125] Religious rituals (i.e., baptism, prayer service, or anointing) may be advocated by certain denominations and provide a measure of comfort and hope. Often parents in crisis do not think to request infant baptism or to call their priest, minister, or rabbi. Offering to call a clergy member of their choice or the hospital chaplain may be helpful. A national survey of pastoral care providers noted barriers to providing spiritual care: (1) inadequate numbers of pastoral care staff, (2) inability of health care providers to assess spiritual needs, and (3) being called "too late" to provide all the care that could have been provided.[41] Primary care providers who have shared intimately with the parents the experience of their child's life and death may be invited to attend the funeral or memorial service. For both care providers and parents, this may represent the final act of caring for the infant.[32]

Critical Findings

INDICATORS OF PATHOLOGIC GRIEF[61]

1. Overactivity without a sense of loss
2. Acquisition of symptoms belonging to the last illness of the deceased
3. Psychosomatic conditions
4. Altered relationships to friends and relatives
5. Furious hostility against specific others
6. Formal manner resembling schizophrenia
7. Lasting loss of social interaction patterns
8. Assuming activities detrimental to social and economic existence
9. Agitated depression

Nonprofessional support systems such as the couple, family, friends, and parent groups are often forgotten as sources of potential help to grieving parents. In our society of isolated, mobile, nuclear families, it may be erroneous to assume that a support system exists. On the other hand, it may be unrecognized because it does not fall into a traditional definition, such as the next-door neighbor or other friend who may be more supportive (and available) than the grandparents. Biologic kinship is not the only valid criterion for a support system; an emotional kinship is the most important factor.

Because professional availability and involvement with the parents is not lasting, the professional has a responsibility to identify, foster, and facilitate a nonprofessional (social) support system. Simply identifying supportive others and expecting them to automatically help in a perinatal loss situation may not be realistic. Unless those who constitute the support system are as well informed and instructed as the parents about the situation, they will not be able to offer emotional comfort. For example, if the parents wish to talk about their loss but the members of the support system empathically wish to spare them by not discussing it, no help will be given or received.

The quality and quantity of ties one has with a social network are associated with improved health status and life satisfaction.[31,110,125] For parents experiencing a perinatal loss, the quality and quantity of ties with their social network (i.e., extended family, friends, and colleagues) may be profoundly affected. In one study, most families suffered permanent loss of relationships because others were unsure of how to react, avoided talking about the baby, or made comments that diminished the intensity of the loss.[30] Fathers especially receive little personal attention as friends and colleagues focus their attention on the mother's grief.[30,31] Because grandparents grieve for their grandchild and may feel guilt and grief for their own child, they may be emotionally unavailable to support the grieving parents. To prevent social network disruption for grieving families, health care providers can (1) share information with families about reactions to expect and reasons for these reactions, (2) support families and enable them to rebuild their networks, and (3) emphasize and support the family's belief in their strengths and capacities.[30,31,83]

Open communication between the parents is essential in preserving and fostering a close relationship by the giving and receiving of mutual support. Sharing the experience presents the couple with the opportunity for personal growth and growth as a couple. Yet the individual experience of grief within the context of a couple is too often fertile ground for misunderstanding and resentment.[93] One study showed that disruption of a couple's sexual relationship occurred after the death of a child.[102]

Parental support groups offer their members an opportunity to discuss their feelings with others who have been through similar traumas.[93,121] Knowing how others who have experienced perinatal loss have felt and dealt with similar situations is emotionally comforting and stabilizing to parents experiencing their own loss. Parents provide each other with validation for their feelings and a sense that they are not alone in their pain. Each individual has different needs, different ways of adapting to crisis, and different ways of giving and receiving support. It is essential that professionals use techniques that are real and spontaneous and not adopt words or actions that are foreign to one's own self. Interventions must also be gauged to the parents' needs and pace.

In one study[119] and from clinical experience, fathers state that they receive most of their support from their spouse. They report that little attention is paid to fathers by hospital staff, causing more denial and difficulty expressing their grief. So that the father's grief is not ignored,[71] it is critical for hospital staff to address the father's feelings when addressing parental grief.[97] Suggestions to assist fathers in their grief include implementation of all-male support groups, validation of their feelings, and asking direct open-ended questions. These may include "What are you feeling right now?" "Tell me how your day is going," and "Tell me about your coping strategies." Health care providers can help a father by reflecting his statements, using his name, and assisting him with expressing his feelings. Fathers should be included and acknowledged in all discussions with staff[120] so that they are not "forgotten mourners."[57] A recent study documented that family adjustment after the NICU experience improved over time for mothers but deteriorated for fathers, especially if the infant had ongoing health problems.[31] Assessing the family as a unit rather than using the mother as a representative of the entire family, being cognizant of and responsive to gender differences in coping, and being supportive of family strengths and resources are recommendations for clinicians.[31]

Information. Information aids in intellectually understanding the crisis, thus facilitating a sense of control over it. Actively seeking and using information enable confrontation and mastery of the crisis. Knowledge about a situation strengthens the ego, because it enables "worry work" and psychologic preparation for expected events. Because "the void of the unknown is more frightening than the known; facts are more reassuring than awesome speculations,"[17] a major role of the professional is to provide and clarify facts and information relevant to the perinatal loss situation (see the Parent Teaching box at right).[16,69] In the search for meaning that always accompanies loss, medical facts may help alleviate some parental guilt about causing the tragedy. Repeating to the parents that nothing they did or did not do could have caused this problem is reassuring. Sketchy or no information only serves to contribute to parental denial of the reality or to their fantasies of causation.[99] Confronting the crisis and realizing its real element of danger and trouble starts the process of grief by giving permission for the expression of feelings of fear, sadness, and loss.

Because the family as a unit, composed of the individual members, must deal with perinatal loss, professionals should encourage and support open, interfamily communications. Keeping secrets, especially between the parents, should be discouraged because this eventually undermines trust and promotes asynchronous grief work. When parents are given the same information and talk with each other about their loss and their feelings, more synchronous grief reactions develop.[58] Telling parents together with the infant present prevents misunderstanding, misinterpretations, and "shading" of information to one parent.[82] Informed parents are better able to share their experience with each other and to participate in joint decision making with the professional.[6,14]

The questions "When to tell" and "How much to tell" the parents often arise. Parents should be told as soon as possible about perinatal complications or problems.[16,58] Receiving this information at the earliest possible time helps parents establish trust in the care provider, appreciate the reality of the situation, begin the grief process, and mobilize both internal and external support. Information must be given in its entirety, because attempts to "spare" parents by staging the truth serve only to undermine their trust in professional credibility. The couple's relation-

Parent Teaching

GRIEF

1. Grief is a normal reaction and is expected in perinatal situations: pregnancy, abortion, stillbirth, premature birth, when the baby is sick or has an anomaly, death, relinquishment, when the birth process does not meet parental expectations, and when there is postpartal depression.
2. Grief is a staged process that occurs over time and is characterized by stages: shock and disbelief, anger, bargaining, depression and withdrawal, and eventually acceptance.
3. Grief is an individualized process and may be experienced differently by the mother and father.
4. To facilitate grief reactions, the neonatal intensive care unit (NICU) will provide a safe environment for the expression of feelings, information about the infant and the infant's condition, and supportive, trusting relationships with health care providers.
5. Seeing, touching, and holding the baby are as important to the parents of a sick or dying infant or an infant with an anomaly as they are to the parents of a healthy infant.
6. When an infant dies or is dying, parents and infant(s) have the right to interact with each other, to create memories, to involve extended family and friends, and to engage in specific religious and cultural practices.
7. Parents and families are informed about the grief process, encouraged to support and care for each other, and encouraged to identify and rely on social support systems (e.g., extended family, friends, professional support services).

ship also may suffer if one parent colludes with the professional in a conspiracy of silence. This is best illustrated by the following incident:

To spare a diabetic mother from the truth about her infant's congenitally absent limbs, the physician and the father decided to tell her about his missing legs but not the missing arm. On arriving to transport the baby, the nurse asked if the mother had been told. "Yes" was the response, so she took the infant to the mother's room before transport. As she uncovered the infant, the mother gasped and looked at the physician and the father and said, "You lied to me. You didn't tell me about his arm, too."

When given the unedited truth, parents can face reality and begin the grief process without fear that something else is the matter that they are not being told. The individual's stage of grief influences not when or what will be said but how the information will be given and received. During the initial stage of shock, information, if processed, is processed slowly.[58] Often events take on a foggy, dreamlike quality so that sensory information remembered is not believed. Yet to give no information only perpetuates this frightening feeling. Communication to those in shock and denial must proceed simply, slowly, and with much repetition and reinforcement. Giving information once does not ensure that it will be retained or understood. Repetition by the professionals is necessary for gradual acceptance of the reality of the situation.[6,14] This may be a nuisance for the professional who has already given the information and wonders why the parents cannot remember it. Parents are so shocked they do not hear what is said, and information must be patiently repeated. Even though an early contact with parents almost ensures they will be in a state of shock, the tone and content of the first meeting are not forgotten.[16,58] Initial information about the infant and his or her condition may have long-term effects on the parents' ability to attach or detach. In the past, parents were given a pessimistic outlook with the belief that "It will be easier for them. They won't get so involved." Negative descriptions and initial pessimism only increase the amount of grief and detachment while effectively blocking attachment behaviors. If the sick or defective infant survives, the parents may have detached to the point of, at least emotionally, burying him or her. Knowledge of better survival rates and the quality of survival enables a truthfully optimistic outcome for many sick neonates. Therefore information must be given clearly (not medical jargon) with a minimal focus on possible complications and medical odds.[58,128]

Volunteering information to parents is essential, but encouraging their questions is equally important. As the normal mechanism for adapting to crisis and gaining mastery over a situation, questions help the professional "start where the parents are" and begin communication with their concerns. Questions and comments unrelated to the discussion may indicate either failure to comprehend or failure to send the information clearly.[128]

Direct questions deserve direct answers, because they indicate a readiness and desire for information. Indirect questions or comments by the parents may indicate concern about their own infant that cannot be directly expressed. "Baby Stevie (who died yesterday) had severe respiratory distress syndrome, didn't he?" The parents want to be reassured that their infant will not die, too.

During the crisis of perinatal loss, interpersonal communication is difficult. Therefore as few professionals as possible should relay information to the parents. Primary care providers (nurse and physician) should coordinate and provide continuity in giving information to parents because individual care providers will supply information about the same topic in different ways.[22,83] The use of varied terms, inflections, and attitudes by a multitude of professionals becomes a monumental source of confusion and anxiety for parents. A trusted relationship[14,16,19] with a primary nurse and physician through whom all communication flows minimizes unnecessary anxiety and concern for parents. It is essential that the nurse (or primary nurse) be present and assist the physician in communication with the parents. Any anxiety-producing information (poor prognosis, complication, or impending death) may not be heard or understood initially by the parents. The nurse must know exactly what information was given and how the parents were given this information. After the physician departs, the nurse must be able to offer clarification, explanation, and support to the distraught parents. Nothing is more distressing than finding a crying, upset mother who is unable to relate what the physician said, why she is upset, or even if she understood what was said.

No family or parent should have to wonder and worry about a dreaded or feared outcome without being given the proper information. If the primary care physician is unavailable to speak with the family, then someone from the health care team must assume this responsibility. No mother whose infant is ill, deformed, or dead should awaken from an anesthetized birth to find her physician absent and the nurses unable to answer "How's my baby?" A plan of action for telling individual parents must be decided and agreed on by all care providers.

Parents are interested in the daily (or hourly) progress of their infant, including both positive and negative developments. A crisis or negative development in an infant's condition is important for parents to know about as soon as possible. They are then able to participate and care for their infant through the difficulty and to trust professional communication. Parents should have unlimited access to phone or personal contact with the staff in the perinatal care setting. Phone calls to the hospital from concerned parents should be possible any time of the day or night. The knowledge that information about their infant and access to a caring professional are available at any hour often is enough to comfort parents of a critically ill infant.

Lactation suppression for the mother of a dying newborn often has been a forgotten aspect of care.[76] Engorgement creates a feedback mechanism to the maternal brain that leads to cessation of milk production; however, painful engorgement should be avoided. Using a breast pump to remove enough milk to relieve pressure and discomfort but not enough to empty the breasts will gradually result in a decrease in milk production. If the mother pumps till she is comfortable, gradually prolongs the intervals between pumping, and pumps for shorter periods, lactation gradually is suppressed. Use of a well-fitting and supportive bra relieves the discomfort/pain of heavy breasts. A recent study comparing the use of breast binding to a supportive bra found that the breast-binding group had greater breast pain/tenderness, leakage, and use of other pain-relief measures; the study recommendation was to discontinue breast binding for the more comfortable and efficacious supportive bra.[111] Mothers who have pumped and stored breast milk may wish to donate it to a mother's milk bank. A mother also may wish to continue pumping to be a human milk donor. These options should be sensitively discussed with the mother of the dying infant.

ENCOURAGING EXPRESSION OF EMOTIONS

Because grief is an emotional reaction to loss, expression of these emotions is necessary for grief work to begin and proceed. Verbalizing thoughts and feelings provides an outlet for the intense emotions accompanying grief and signifies to others that emotional support is needed.[16] For some, the open expression of emotions may be difficult because of influence from their culture, gender-specific roles, and social status. Yet the containment of intense feelings uses a great deal of emotional and physical energy that could be more productively used in moving on with the grief work. Those who are stoic and noncommunicative have symptoms of grief for a longer period than those who freely express their feelings and emotions.[9]

Experiencing the loss of an infant initiates an "ambivalent transition" into motherhood in a short period.[65] These women often feel totally confused, with broken expectations and elusive grief: "Have I or have I not become a mother?" Supporting families provides them with an opportunity to talk about their infant, confirming the baby's life as important, although short. This process assists parents to attach and subsequently begin the grieving process.[126]

Talking about the loss helps parents validate and assimilate the experience. Timing and events are clarified, including forgotten details, by discussion with each other and with their care providers. Confronting the reality enables them to work through the shock and disbelief, verbalize their fears and disappointments, and begin to cry and grieve. Expression of feelings gradually permits a clarification of the meaning of the loss to the parents. Talking lightens the burden of loss, because every time the experience is shared with another, half of the experience and the accompanying emotions are given away. Telling, retelling, reviewing, and reliving the experience are all necessary ways to understand and gain mastery over a frightening and most often unexpected situation.[16]

Verbal and nonverbal cues tell professionals where the parents are in their grief process. To elicit feelings, the professional may verbalize his or her own perceptions and observations:

- "Mrs. Green, you sound tense (upset, tired) today."
- "Mr. Brown, you look worried today."
- "I'm sorry that your baby died."

These statements indicate the listening ear and observing eye of one who cares. They set the stage for communication: "It's okay to talk with me about how you are feeling, because I acknowledge your pain."

Feeling scared, alone, and out of control, parents often deny their feelings under direct questioning. Thus "Do you think you did or didn't do something to cause your baby's problem?" may be answered negatively, even though parents are consumed with guilt. Direct questioning places parents in an awkward and vulnerable position of revealing their most personal doubts and fears. Direct questions may be reworded with safer and more indirect statements:

- "Most parents feel overwhelmed and sad when their baby is sick."
- "Many parents wonder if the cause of their baby's death is something they did or didn't do."
- "It is helpful to many parents to talk about their doubts and fears. These feelings are common and normal in such a difficult situation."

The professional gives parents information about the feelings and emotions commonly felt in similar situations. Because there is safety in numbers, if "most" or "many" parents feel this way and it is expected, then it might be safe to share their feelings. Validating parents' reactions as appropriate reassures them that they are not crazy. With this type of invitation, the feelings may be free to come spilling forth or the parents may need time to establish a relationship with this professional before they are ready to talk about such personal emotions.

Empathetic actions and comments may open communication pathways with parents.[16] A professional presence that is warm and caring may facilitate more communication than any words. Touching or holding grieving parents may help feelings be expressed. Nonverbal cues such as nodding, direct eye contact, uninterrupted attention, and the physical closeness of pulling up a chair and sitting down give positive feedback to verbal communication and indicate active listening by the professional.

Crying is the expression of feelings of sadness, sorrow, and intense longing that accompany the pain of loss.[61,128] A healthy catharsis, crying should be expected and encouraged in any loss situation. Yet the cultural, gender-specific, and professional taboos against crying have defined it as an unacceptable and inappropriate response and one that should be suppressed. Because tears are healing and therapeutic, professionals must learn to be comfortable with the crying of others. "Don't cry" is often heard from those attempting to comfort grieving parents (or colleagues). This is an admonition against the behavior rather than an empathetic comment. "It's okay to cry" or "Go ahead and cry; let it out" gives permission and acceptance to the behavior and the need for it.

By expecting tears, providing a safe environment for their expression, and encouraging the behavior by words and actions, the professional may facilitate crying in both mothers and fathers. Too often, tears are blocked in a relationship in which one partner (usually the man) is expected to be stoic and in control, whereas the other's (usually the woman's) tears are defined as too upsetting or difficult. Because the ability to cry is a healthy response, the couple must be encouraged to use this outlet together.

In the past, crying in the presence of patients and their families was defined as "unprofessional." Yet the cool, controlled exterior defined as "professional" was seen by others as noncaring and nonfeeling. When the professional cries with the parents, it is an acceptable expression of genuine emotion, a demonstration of empathy, and a role model of the appropriateness of tears given the situation. Parents do not define the tears of care providers as weak or unprofessional. Rather, they feel a special bond of love and care with professionals who have been free enough to share their grief.[16,83,93] Instead of relearning that crying is acceptable, many parents and care providers must learn for the first time.

Talking and crying about the loss are easier to facilitate than is the expression of anger.[47] Because of the social expectations of dependency of the patient role and real or imagined consequences of retaliation (against the infant or against job status), perinatal care settings are not safe environments for the expression of anger. Parents (and colleagues) will be able to vent anger only in an environment free of punishment or retaliation for their behaviors. It is the responsibility of the professionals to create an environment that allows open expression of negative criticism and anger.

SEEING AND TOUCHING

Seeing and touching are as important to the parents of a sick, deformed, or dead infant as they are to the parents of a normal, healthy one. In the past, fear that seeing a deformed or dead infant would intensify grief and be overly upsetting resulted in no contact between parents and their newborn. Despite the fact that many mothers wished to see their infants, the prevailing practice was to discourage and prevent it. Often no information, including sex or physical characteristics, was given to grieving parents, who were left to fantasize about their newborn's problems or cause of death. More recently, research and practice indicate that parental contact with the infant does not cause "unduly upsetting immediate reactions or appear to result in pathologic mourning."[56]

Recently, researchers in the United Kingdom have evaluated mothers and fathers who have seen and held their infants after stillbirth. In several of their studies, they have correlated posttraumatic stress symptoms in both mothers and fathers[114,115] and disorganized maternal-infant attachment[51] in subsequent pregnancies to seeing/holding their stillborn infant. While remarking that seeing/holding the dead infant is culturally entrenched and highly valued by parents, these researchers warn that this practice is associated, in their studies, with psychologic sequelae and that these practices were based only on clinical impression without empirical evidence of benefit.[6] However, other research cited in Table 30-1 shows how this small sample of well-adjusted and low-grieving parents valued holding their infant, being present at the time of death with family/friends, and keeping mementoes and the memory of their child alive.[14] The sequelae of seeing/holding a stillborn and the sequelae of seeing/holding a live infant who has died may not be similar; clearly more research is necessary.

The British researchers,[6] who found psychologic sequelae of parental contact with their stillborn infant, state that many parents experience great meaning and treasure the memory of time with their dead infant. They concede that some parents would choose to have contact with their dead infants, regardless of potentially harmful outcomes. They also state that parental decision to see/hold the dead infant may be heavily influenced by attending staff who may expose reluctant parents to their dead baby. Clearly, the decision to see and touch their infant is ultimately a parental one.[6,128] Making decisions *for* parents is not the professional's role; making decisions *with* parents is the professional's role. Each parent must make the decision for himself or herself; neither may decide for the other. Altruistic others, such as professionals, the spouse, or other family members, must not usurp the right to individual decision making. Often, in an attempt to protect the mother, the father or the professional decides that she should not have contact with her infant. They either actually discourage it or do nothing to facilitate it. Mothers who have not seen their infants always know who prohibited it. The couple's relationship may suffer irreparable damage if one decides for the other, even if the motive is altruistic. The professional's role is to facilitate a healthy decision by each parent so that their individual needs to see or to not see the infant are met.

Parents may not realize that seeing and touching their infant is an option, or they may just be too overwhelmed or afraid to ask if it is possible. Instead of waiting for parents to ask, the professional care provider takes a more active role by offering the possibility to the parents: "Would you like to hold your baby?"

Time is often necessary to make the decision, because initially parents are ambivalent about seeing and holding a deformed or dead infant. Most mothers and fathers want to see their child but fear what they might see and how they may feel. The care provider may alleviate the parents' ambivalence by acknowledging that being with the infant will be difficult but that the professional will remain with them unless asked to leave. The emotional support of the physical presence of an empathetic professional may allay the fear of becoming out of control. The professional can reassure the family by explaining what they will see before they hold their infant. Making such a crucial decision in the initial stages of loss is difficult. Giving parents information about the positive aspects of seeing and holding the infant in facilitating their grief process helps make their decision an informed one.[96,128]

Seeing the infant brings the dreaded impossibility of perinatal loss into stark reality.[128] Parents confirm with their own eyes that the infant is alive or dead or normal or abnormal. Contact enables claiming behaviors and identification of the infant as their own. While holding their infant, parents examine it and begin to recognize familiar family characteristics: "She has my long fingers and her father's red hair." Even small, severely deformed, or macerated infants can be recognized and claimed by the parents as part of their family. The normal, endearing characteristics that identify the child as "mine" are remembered.

Parental contact confirms the infant's own reality and eliminates the prenatal fantasy of the expected child. For the parents of an infant with an anomaly, grief work about the fantasized perfect child may begin so that the actual child may become the object of love. Early and frequent contact between the parents and the infant encourages a realistic perspective of the infant's problems. A stillborn or aborted fetus may be physically normal rather than the deformed infant imagined by the parents. Seeing the infant allays doubts and fears about the infant's normal state and about the parents' ability to subsequently have a normal child.[99] Seeing and touching enable parents to grieve the infant's reality rather than a feared and dreaded, and thus more frightening, fantasy. It is easier to grieve a real infant than a mystical, dreamlike fantasy of the infant.[58]

Whether the ultimate decision is to see or to not see the infant, the professional must honor and respect that choice.[128] Cultural taboos against viewing dead bodies may preclude some parents from seeing and touching their infant. Yet many such cultures support their members by formalizing the grief process in sanctioned ritual and ceremony. For those parents who decide to not see and touch, the professional should reassure them of their infant's normal condition (e.g., "He had 10 fingers and toes."). Describe the infant in as much detail as necessary to give parents a mental picture. Include gender, size, hair color, skin, weight, and distinguishing characteristics. A simple, realistic description of any anomaly is also helpful, because the fantasy of the defect is worse than its reality.

Adequate preparation for the first encounter with their infant includes a description of everything parents will see, hear, and feel.[128] Verbal preparation for viewing an infant with a congenital anomaly includes not only a simple description of the abnormality but also the infant's normal characteristics. Seeing a picture of the abnormality first may help parents prepare for seeing their infant. Remaining with the parents at the initial visit, the professional describes the anomaly and points out normal findings. Focusing by parents on the normal familial characteristics helps in attaching to the less-than-perfect baby. Although parents of a dead, deformed infant view the abnormality, they often focus on the normal traits and remember him or her not as "monstrous" but as beautiful.

For those who have never seen a dead body, the mind may invent frightening images and sensations. Certainly, "dead" is associated with the temperature sensation of cold. However, a newborn who has been placed under a radiant warmer or in an incubator may feel warm rather than cold shortly after death, hence the statement by a mother, "You couldn't be dead. You feel so warm." The professional must touch the infant and prepare the parents for the tactile sensation of warm or cold: "The baby will feel warm to you because she (or he) has been under the radiant warmer."

To prepare parents for seeing their infant, the professional must observe the baby. Color, skin condition, and size must all be described and are not shocking with adequate preparation: maceration—"peeling of the skin"; peripheral shutdown—"the blue-white discoloration"; and the small size—"as long as the length of my hand." Any equipment that must remain on the body should be described and explained before viewing. Even an umbilical cord clamp may cause concern in a parent who has never seen one. The reason for not removing equipment also must be explained. Respectful care of the infant's body after death shows respect for the person of the infant and for the grieving parents. Attention to details such as wrapping the infant in a blanket rather than a surgical drape or towel, cleaning the infant, and holding the infant in a cuddling position indicates care and concern.

Parents whose infant has died, is deformed, or is ill proceed with attachment behaviors of seeing and touching in the same manner as parents of normal, healthy infants.[58] Touching is important, but the distinction must be made between touching and holding. Cradling one's infant is quite different from merely touching with a hand. Holding the infant, whether healthy, sick, or dead, for the first time is a momentous event. Touching the infant who has died is not sufficient; parents must be given the opportunity to hold and cuddle the child before, during, and after death. Other parenting behaviors, such as bathing and dressing their infant, also should be offered to parents.[52,55,108]

Parents of a dead infant may need more than one chance to see and touch the infant. The first time, they attach to the reality of their infant. Subsequent encounters allow a final chance to see and hold their child. Parents have described the initial encounter as saying "Hello" and the subsequent one as saying "Good-bye." Some parents may be able to accomplish closure with one visit, whereas others who might benefit from a final visit may not ask or think to ask. Offering another contact with their infant leaves the decision with the parents.

The emotional effect of seeing the infant requires support, time, and permission to cry. Attaching is a process that occurs over time. Providing parents sufficient time with their infant takes precedence over paperwork, ward routine, or taking the infant to the morgue. Parents have indicated a need to hold their infant for a longer time and not feel pushed by care providers.[52,65] Even infants who have been removed to the morgue may be returned if parents need more time and contact for detachment.[64]

When an infant dies, opportunities for memories are limited. Professionals have the responsibility of helping parents make memories so that they will have a tangible person to mourn. Encouraging parents to name their infant gives the infant a separate identity, which helps facilitate the grieving process. Tangible mementos may include photographs, handprints and footprints, a lock of hair, hand/foot castings,[54,83,116] measurements of the infant, identification bands, the blanket the infant was wrapped in, a blessing or baptismal certificate, and birth and death certificates. Parents find most beneficial the interventions that acknowledged the infant (e.g., photographs, holding the infant, and receiving personal mementos).[14,52,55,64,86] Even when parents say they do not want mementos, the mementos should be kept in hospital files and the parents made aware that they will be available to them in the future if they want them.[64] Taking pictures of the infant, obtaining other mementos, and telling the parents that such mementos will be available to them on request not only respect their immediate decision to not see or have information on the infant but also provide a mechanism for them to "know" their infant at a later date if they wish to do so.

Before an infant is transported to a newborn special care unit, photographs should be taken and given to the parents to promote bonding. If the infant remains hospitalized for a long time or requires surgery, pictures taken at weekly intervals or before and after surgery can help confirm the reality of the child's condition and progress and assist with bonding, as well as the grief process. Despite the outcome, parents will appreciate some lasting record of their child's life.

The staff who provide emotional support for parents must also receive support from each other. Expecting the staff to immediately return to work is unrealistic. Such an emotional experience takes time and space for decompression, which is facilitated by the use of exercise, crying, and being alone for quiet time.[32] A recent study of staff and family perceptions of palliative care showed that interdisciplinary staff felt inexperienced in communicating with families about sensitive end-of-life issues and inexperienced in pain management and received inadequate education and support to deal with these families and their own personal pain.[21]

OPEN VISITING AND CAREGIVING POLICIES

Perinatal care settings with open visiting and caregiving policies foster a shared family experience and support from others. Regardless of the type of perinatal loss, no mother should experience it alone—a spouse, friend, family member, or identified supportive other should remain with her.[52,120] Members of the mother's support system will also need an outlet for the expression of their grief.

Women suffering the grief of perinatal loss should be given a choice about their room assignment. Arbitrary removal from the obstetric unit may deny the mother's maternity: "Am I a mother or not?" It also may escalate her feelings of failure, guilt, and worthlessness as a woman and a mother. Because she did not produce a normal, healthy infant, she may feel punished and banished from the maternity area by isolation on another floor. Her care may be entrusted to those without expertise in the physiologic and psychologic care of the normal postpartum period, much less a postpartum complicated by loss. Placement at the end of the hall far from the nurses' station, with the door closed and no company from staff and family, only increases her feelings of loneliness and isolation. Yet being on a happy maternity floor with normal, healthy infants and their mothers may be an exceedingly difficult and constant reminder of her loss and even complicate her recovery.[56] Information about the advantages and disadvantages of staying or leaving the maternity ward should be given by the professional. The mother, knowing what will be helpful, makes the decision.[128]

The alternative to maternal hospitalization is early discharge as soon as medically possible so the mother may join her infant when the infant has been transported to another hospital. Early discharge also facilitates an easier mobilization of supportive others in the familiar surroundings of home. Removal from the constant reminder of one's failure (i.e., other healthy infants) may let the grief work begin.[128] Early discharge is not therapeutic when the professional assumes there is a support system to provide care and no one is available. Without a plan for follow-up care and contact, early discharge merely relocates the problem.

Caregiving is as important for the parents of a sick, deformed, or dead infant as it is for the parents of a normal infant. Open visiting and caregiving policies increase interaction between the parents and their infant by actively involving them in the reality of their child's illness, deformity, or impending death. Even if the child lives only a short time, parental access and taking care of the infant complete the attachment process and enable them to begin the detachment of grief work. Even minimal caregiving helps parents overcome their sense of helplessness and be comforted by "We did all that we could have done. We cared; we made a difference to our baby." Active parental involvement decreases poor outcomes such as aberrant parenting styles, attachment problems, and unresolved grief.[14,58]

The loneliness and isolation of death are decreased for both parents and infant when they are together at the time of death. Parents are often comforted and relieved that their fantasy of the agony of the death scene is not borne out in the quiet, peaceful reality of death.[58] Having experienced the beginning of life together, parents who are present at the ending of life can feel a sense of closure and completion. Parents who can share even a brief life with their baby and the moment of death can face death's finality knowing they did not abandon their infant but provided him or her love and care.[64] Parents who are not present at death may take care of the infant afterward by seeing and holding him or her.

Parents should be given the opportunity to make final plans for their deceased infant.[83] The planning will help them face the death and facilitate the grief process. For many parents, this is their first experience with death and making final arrangements and they are not aware of the options. It is helpful to provide the family with detailed, specific verbal and written information about cremation, burial, funeral, or hospital disposal.[18,52,83]

A funeral may be chosen for religious reasons or as a declaration of the fetus or newborn as a person befitting burial rather than disposal. Burial leaves a specific place of remembrance and recognition that this infant lived. Care for the infant after death may include funeral arrangements, such as choosing the clothes or bathing and even dressing the infant. If parents choose not to have a funeral, they may wish to have a memorial service or do something special, such as plant a rosebush or tree, in memory of their infant. Regardless of their decision, the birth and death of their baby constitute a life event for the family, and one must recognize it.

AUTOPSY[87]

For parents who experience a stillbirth, spontaneous abortion, or neonatal death, knowing why the infant was deformed or died eases their recovery from grief.[58] In the search for a cause, many parents blame themselves for doing too much or too little to favorably influence the outcome. A recent study showed that neonatal autopsies reveal important new information in 26% of the cases.[12] Knowing why the infant died or the converse, that not even the "experts" know why the infant died, may help assuage their personal feelings of guilt and failure.

Approaching the family for permission for an autopsy must be done by the primary care providers (physician and nurse) with the utmost tact and respect for the family's feelings. Too often the permission for autopsy is denied because of the way the subject is broached by professionals. Telling the family about their infant's death in one breath and asking for an autopsy with the next breath is not appropriate. Parents need time to deal with the reality of the death, including seeing and holding their infant and being with each other and supportive others before they are even ready to think about an autopsy. Consideration of the family's feelings and stage of grief greatly enhances communication with the professional. Reasons for the autopsy, including a possible answer to the question of why their infant died or was deformed, are important to discuss in a relaxed and unhurried manner.[3] Parents may feel rushed to make a decision without clearly understanding the advantages and disadvantages and resist the emotional topic of a postmortem examination. Time for discussion with an empathetic professional, as well as between themselves, facilitates an informed parental decision; sometimes consultation with a religious leader is necessary.

The professional who receives permission for an autopsy is then obliged to discuss with the parents all findings.[3,56] This may entail more than one meeting with the parents, because they should be informed of the findings as soon as they are available.[82] Therefore the professional may meet with them within 24 hours of completing the autopsy to discuss gross and preliminary findings and again 2 to 8 weeks later to discuss microscopic results.[58,72] Autopsy data may indicate either a condition that has implications for subsequent pregnancies or one that has little chance of recurrence.[3] The need for genetic counseling for future pregnancies may be evident from autopsy results.[87] Discussing the results with the report in hand and offering parents a copy for future reference are also important.

ANTICIPATORY GUIDANCE

Encounters with parents after the death of their infant give professionals the opportunity for anticipatory guidance/information about what to expect from themselves and from others.[52,55] Reactions to perinatal loss differ markedly, so family, friends, and acquaintances may not act as parents might expect. Some will be supportive and emotionally empathetic, especially if they have suffered a perinatal loss. Others will be uncomfortable and, not knowing what to say or do, may choose to avoid the couple and never mention the loss, even in future conversations. Those who are unaware of the loss may question the newly nonpregnant parents about the new infant. These inquiries are both awkward and painful.

Knowledge of the universal feelings and behaviors associated with grief gives comfort and relief to parents. Knowing what to expect from grief (i.e., how it progresses and how long it takes) is valuable to those who are or will be experiencing it.[43,55,58,83,128] Knowing the stages of grief and that the accompanying behaviors and emotions are normal decreases the feeling of "going crazy." Recovery from the loss takes time and cannot be hurried or ignored. The most difficult time is immediately after birth and the first few months after the loss (2 to 4 months).[48] The emotions of grief begin to lessen toward the end of the first year.

Parents should be encouraged to support and care for each other in their time of loss. Professionals should advocate mutual support by a free expression of feelings and emotions between the parents. Although parents need each other during grief, they also need an identified support system with whom to talk and cry. Reaching outside of the nuclear family to friends, extended family, and professionals should be encouraged.[14,31,83] Professionals have a responsibility to ask to whom parents turn for help and support in a crisis. If there are no identified supportive others, parents must know whom to call for help in the initial bereavement period.

Anticipatory guidance is also essential at the discharge of an infant with an anomaly, a preterm, or a previously ill newborn. Knowing what to expect when going home with an infant with a defect or an infant who has been hospitalized for months makes the transition from hospital to society easier for parents. Evaluation of the grief process, the attachment level of the parents to a less-than-perfect infant, and the presence or potential for postpartum depression (see Chapter 29) is vital.

LONG-TERM FOLLOW-UP CARE

Follow-up care and contact with professionals are needed by grieving parents.[14,31,52,82,83] A recent study of bereaved parents highlights their needs for follow-up: (1) appointments should be scheduled with the neonatologist soon after the baby's death and certainly within 2 months, even if autopsy results are unavailable and (2) in a setting away from the hospital; (3) families value the professionals' efforts to determine how they are coping; (4) families value full, frank, sensitively delivered information and reassurance that enable them to understand what happened and assess their future risks; and (5) families do not want false reassurances, half truths, and broken promises.[72] Follow-up meetings function as a catharsis for parents, as well as an opportunity for assessment, counseling (psychologic and genetic), and possibly referral. Primary care providers (physicians, nurses, and social workers) from the perinatal care setting may provide follow-up. One study documented a significant decrease in the intensity of a mother's grief after stillbirth when she received one telephone call from the physician.[81] For the family, relating to providers with whom a relationship has been established may be easier than establishing a new relationship with a stranger.[14,19,83] However, being with those who are associated with the loss event may be uncomfortable for the parents at the height of their grief. For the professional, the ability to continue to be a source of help and comfort to families with whom one has established a relationship may help complete their grief reactions. Maintaining contact with the family may be painful as the professional relives the feelings of grief and loss associated with sharing their tragedy. Although painful, this re-experience of intense feelings gives both parents and professionals another opportunity to work toward grief resolution.

When and where to provide continuing care for families are crucial questions. Contact in the perinatal care setting both at the time of death and daily until discharge provides immediate care. However, when discharged, too often the family returns home alone to face weeks and months of unsupported and lonely grief. Without feedback about their normal reaction and society's expectation that they will shortly be "back to normal," they are abandoned to their emotions. They suffer in silence and often drift apart in their misery. With their support system withdrawn but still feeling overwhelmed with grief, parents describe the period between 2 and 4 months after the loss as the most difficult time.[56] At 2 months after perinatal loss, parents show increased symptoms of anxiety and depression that are reduced by 8 months but still higher than in parents not experiencing perinatal loss.[118] Follow-up care from professionals is most meaningful and needed by parents during this period when they feel deserted by previously supportive others.[52] Parents experience a need for spiritual support weeks and months after the loss. Meeting with families sooner (within weeks of their loss) may alleviate the effect of decreasing support as the months go by. The professional who acknowledges the withdrawal of others but can be relied on to be available provides the parents with the emotional anchor of long-term care and support.

Breaking appointments or continually not being available may be resistance to follow-up contact with the professionals but also represents a reluctance to return to the perinatal care setting with its painful memories. A visit from the professional in the home provides a nonthreatening, familiar environment for follow-up care. The more comfortable home environment enables assessment of family interactions and facilitates communication at the "feeling" level.

Each family member and the family as a unit must be assessed for their place in the grief process as follows:

- In what stage of grief is each family member?
- Is anyone "stuck" in a stage of grief?
- Are behaviors appropriate for normal grief reactions, or do altered behaviors represent pathologic grief reactions?
- Do altered behaviors warrant referral for further treatment and evaluation?
- Do the caregiving and attachment behaviors of the parents reflect resolution of grief over loss of the perfect child and adoption of the less-than-perfect child as the love object?

Just because everything was progressing normally at previous encounters does not mean that it should be assumed to still be so. As the flood of initial grief subsides, problems and questions that were not considered suddenly become of great concern. For the first time in months, the regressive behavior of siblings not only may be noticed but also may be extremely annoying to parents. The beginning of grief resolution may allow future projections such as "When can I have another baby?" or the dread of the painful anniversary of the loss.

Referral to public health nurses or visiting nursing services in the community for follow-up care is appropriate. However, a written referral alone is not enough. Involving them in the hospital care and discharge planning is essential for a smooth transition to home care. Having the new professional meet the family in the hospital with the primary care providers facilitates trust transference from the familiar to the unfamiliar. Traditionally, home care providers have been involved in care of normal mothers and infants in the community. Involvement in perinatal loss situations requires knowledge about the process of grief and willingness to share the grief of the parents. Because these may be new skills for many, continuing education programs that teach the theory and skills of effective intervention help the professional be more comfortable with a perinatal loss situation.

Additional expertise may be warranted when the professional recognizes signs and symptoms of pathologic grief, delayed or absent grief, or concurrent multiple stresses or losses. Parents may not be ready for genetic counseling, infant stimulation programs, or financial programs until months later. Between 3 and 6 months after their loss, parents may be ready to reach outside of the nuclear and extended family for help and support for the first time.[93] Suggesting a local hospital support group or the local chapter of a national support organization may at first be met with resistance. Leaving the names and phone numbers of such organizations ensures that the parents have the information at their disposal when they are ready to use it. Until their own support system has withdrawn, parents may not be ready for a support group of other parents.[93]

Throughout this section, examples of what to say and how to say it have been used to illustrate helpful interventions for grieving families. It is essential to state that there are no "scripts." Parents do not say one thing and the professionals answer with a parroted response. Each encounter is a unique situation consisting of distinct parental and professional personalities. Each situation must be evaluated separately and individual interventions instituted.[52,83] It is recommended that the professional learn by observing an experienced colleague with grieving families and that the professional "practice" with role playing and situation solving before actually attempting to intervene with the parents. Use of formalized education about grief, loss, and bereavement is also recommended for health care providers.[43,69]

Innovative bereavement programs have been developed to provide families and staff with support and follow-up care.[35,52,93] Such programs[35,52] provide education and assistance to the health care providers who care for the family at the time of their infant's death. There is follow-up care to the family for up to 1 year after the death of their infant.[52] These programs provide the needed support, education, and help to families, as well as to staff. Use of a couples-oriented program enables the following[93]:

- Participation in the group at 3 to 5 months after the loss when most other support systems have ceased
- Ability of partners to share with the group and each other gender-related differences in grief experiences
- Opportunity for men to share and hear about other men's feelings and coping skills
- Couples to learn to tolerate their differences in grief processing and to process their grief together
- Enhancement and preservation of the couple's relationship

Having an evaluation tool to assess and continually change and improve the program is essential.[52,93]

CHILDREN AND GRIEF

Explaining and helping a surviving child to understand the loss of an infant is an enormous task for parents.[108] Facilitating the child's normal feelings of sadness, worry, and anger after a loss may be difficult for parents who fear being flooded with their own emotions. Unresolved grief from the parents' own childhood may prevent the expression of grief by their children.

To maintain the myth of childhood (innocent happiness), children are often shielded from any knowledge about death, even when it is an inevitable event in their lives. Thus children are prevented from full realization, validation, and expression of their feelings and emotions. They cannot formalize and express their grief over the loss of a significant person.

Even though adults are encouraged to cry, talk, and gradually understand and integrate their feelings of grief, no one helps the child deal with the same frightening feelings. No one discusses the loss with the child, because "He might cry" and because of the adult's inadequacy and lack of understanding of how to respond and what to say. No amount of secrecy or denial of the situation will hide the fact that the child is being excluded from an important family event.

Attempts to protect children from feelings of grief and mourning because of death or other important losses isolate the child. Age and developmentally appropriate explanations include the child in the family's experience, rather than separating and excluding him from what is happening. Shielding children from the knowledge of death denies them the reality of life and the opportunity for personal growth and mastery of the experience. Like the subject of sex, death is taboo for children.

A child's grief and mourning in response to perinatal loss depend on his cognitive and developmental level, the extent of prenatal attachment and expectation about the infant, the degree of ambivalent feelings, and the response of his or her parents to the death. Because the child's understanding of death differs from that of adults, knowledge of the stages of growing awareness is essential for both parents and professionals working with children experiencing grief (see the Critical Findings box on p. 929).[1] Regardless of age or developmental stage, the universal fear of childhood is the fear of separation and abandonment. For a young child (younger than 5 years), the loss of the infant is experienced indirectly through parental grief. A young child reacts to the emotional withdrawal of grieving parents and fears loss of them (and their love).

Although children at different developmental stages have their own conceptions of death, adults must provide them with the facts about the situation in language that they can understand. They may benefit from guidance by the nurse, social worker, or other health professional about beneficial approaches to facilitate the child's grief work. The professional serves as a resource, role model, and support system to parents caring for their surviving children. Printed materials are also available to assist parents in helping their other children understand death (see "Resource Materials for Parents" at the end of this chapter). Age-appropriate storybooks concerning death can facilitate grief discussion and elicit questions and feelings from children.

Just as grieving adults need repetition, children need repeated explanations and discussions about the loss. Constantly in a state of developmental flux,

Critical Findings

A CHILD'S DEVELOPING CONCEPT OF DEATH

AGE	COGNITIVE UNDERSTANDING	HOW EXPERIENCED
Infant (to 12 mo)	None	Indirectly through parental grief expressed in: Emotional withdrawal Inability to provide concern and continuity in caregiving behaviors Overconcern for fear of recurrent loss
Toddler (1-3 yr)	Little understanding of cause and effect Death may be confused with sleeping or being away	React to changes in behavior of grieving parents and reflect their feelings and anxiety
Preschooler (3-6 yr)	View death as a temporary state and not an inevitable occurrence Believe that they are the center of the universe and can do anything, and that thinking is doing (thoughts have the power of actions)	Expect the dead to return—ask questions about "when?"
School age (6-12 yr)	Understand that death is inevitable and irreversible; 6- to 9-yr-olds personify death as a separate person (skeleton; bogeyman) About 8 yrs old: "death phobia," a normal developmental stage characterized by preoccupation with thoughts of own death and that of loved one Reasons concretely with ability to see cause-and-effect relationships	Realize death occurs in adults like parents and even in children; realize death is permanent, not temporary state May show interest in biologic aspects of death and details of funeral
Adolescent (12 yr)	Able to think abstractly about death like the adult; philosophic reasoning	Similar to that in adult

Modified from American Academy of Pediatrics, Committee on Psychosocial Aspects of Child and Family Health: The pediatrician and childhood bereavement, *Pediatrics* 105:445, 2000; Gardner SL, Merenstein GB: Helping families deal with perinatal loss, *Neonatal Netw* 5:17, 1986.

the child attempts to view the loss in new ways as a result of increasing maturation. Asking questions (usually at inopportune times) and making comments about the infant are ways the child continues to process the experience, often long after the parents have completed it. These questions and comments may seem endless and resurrect the parent's own grief. The child's inquiries must be encouraged and supported so that he or she knows that talking about the loss or death is acceptable. Exploring the child's feelings for fears of causation, guilt, or the wonder if "death is catching" enables them to be dealt with appropriately. Truthful discussion with the child dispels the worst fears and fantasies and replaces them with reality that is "not too horrible to discuss" with parents. If the cause of the infant's death is known, it is explained to the child in simple, direct terms: "Baby Bobby couldn't breathe by himself because his lungs were sick. His sick lungs only happen to little babies."

In one study, bereaved children had more frequent health care contacts for symptoms (e.g., abdominal pain, enuresis, headaches, insomnia) with no organic cause in the year after their loss.[62] Subsequent illness may precipitate worry by the child that he or she, too, will die. Often this fear is not verbalized but acted out by significant behavioral changes such as withdrawal, clinging, whining, or overactivity that is uncharacteristic for the child. Verbal reassurance that the child will not die and a reminder that "the baby died of a sickness that only little babies get; big boys and girls can't get it" are helpful.

The normal feelings that accompany grief should be acknowledged and explained to the child. "Mommy and Daddy feel sad that Baby Jean died. Sometimes we will cry because we feel sad. It's okay to cry when you feel sad." Permission for the expression of the child's feelings should also be given verbally: "You might feel sad, too. It's okay for you to cry when you're sad. Then we will talk about how you are feeling." Encouraging children to draw or write their feelings is another way of giving them permission to express their grief.

Using words such as "went away," "expired," "lost," or "went to sleep" is dangerous in describing death to children. Because young children are concrete and literal, they think they might die if they "go to sleep" or that anyone who leaves them is in danger of dying. Children also relate current experiences to past ones and interpret "lost" quite literally. In the mind of the child, if the parent only searched well enough, the misplaced (i.e., "lost") child would be found.

Including children at funeral or memorial services facilitates their grief and prevents exclusion from a significant family event. Consideration of the family value system, age of the child, and religious custom must enter into the decision to include the child. Adequate preparation includes a discussion of everything the child will see, hear, and feel, including the normal adult emotions of crying and sadness. An adult besides the grieving parents should accompany the child to reiterate what is happening and to meet the child's physical and psychologic needs. Adult support is necessary so that the child can express and deal with his or her feelings.

Helping children with their grief is also therapeutic for parents. Assisting children to master the crisis of loss ultimately augments the parents' self-esteem and restores confidence in their parenting skills.[58] Parents can deal in a healthy way with their own grief when they can facilitate the grief of their other children. Qualitative studies reveal parental spiritual needs and support of siblings after a perinatal loss[73]:

- Recognition and acknowledgment of the child's grief, which included listening and answering questions honestly; interpreting and acknowledging the meaning of the child's behaviors; shielding from the insensitivity of others; and knowing when support of the child would be more effectively handled by someone outside the immediate household
- Inclusion of the child in family events, rituals, and practices such as visiting, holding, and touching the baby in the hospital; attending the funeral/memorial service; and visiting the gravesite
- Keeping the baby alive in the family's memory by encouraging questions and comments about the baby; expressing feelings about the loss; including in viewing photos and personal items of the baby; and recognizing the deceased infant in birthday/holiday celebrations

PATHOLOGIC GRIEF

The absence of grief when it would be expected is not a healthy sign but, rather, a cause for concern.[56] The emotions of grief and their expression are healing. Early and full expression of grief is associated with an optimal outcome.[58] However, many people in grief-producing situations attempt to avoid the pain of grief and the expression of emotions, the result of which prolongs mourning, delays a return to the previous lifestyle, prevents the creation of new attachments and relationships, and ultimately results in pathologic grief (see the list on p. 917).[58]

Not grieving precludes opportunities for growth and change. No new coping styles will be attempted. No novel alternatives to problem solving and adapting to a crisis will be added to the repertoire of behavior for future use. In other words, those who choose not to do grief work say "no" to their own potential and remain frozen in development.[77] Under the stress of not resolving their grief, some may even regress in their development.

Reproductive loss is a blow to self-concept and self-esteem, as well as loss of the infant. Blocking appropriate feelings of loss, grief, and anger results in a significant decrease in one's sense of self-esteem.[28] After death of their neonates, 33% of mothers suffered severe and tragic outcomes (including psychoses, phobias, anxiety attacks, and deep depression) (see Chapter 29).[58,128] Those who cannot effectively resolve their grief may suffer lifelong emotional damage[68]; however, some empirical research shows that those who suppress feelings of grief may recover with relatively few difficulties.[6]

Not working through grief associated with repetitive contact with perinatal loss also affects the staff.[37] To cope with feelings, they may hide behind a "professional" demeanor characterized by decreased spontaneity and withdrawal. Such a provider defends against the repeated pain of loss by emotional dissociation from the situation. The real self does not respond; instead, the professional stays in the role of the omnipotent, unemotional physician or nurse. The result, self-alienation, eventually desensitizes the professional to the experience and ultimately prevents any empathy with the experience of others.[53] Emotions that cannot be acknowledged or expressed healthily are vented in ways that may be destructive to relationships in personal and professional life.

Unresolved grief does not disappear and is not dissipated. The emotions accompanying grief may never be expressed but are not forgotten by the unconscious mind. Containment of these emotions through repression or suppression takes psychic energy. A conscious, intentional decision to postpone or dismiss grief to meet others' needs or to meet immediate demands of the loss situation (e.g., funeral arrangements/care of a surviving multiple) is called ***delayed grief.***[61,68,83] For a period of time (days, weeks, or longer), there is little or no grief response when such a reaction would be expected and appropriate. Delayed grief also may be the result of repression—the unconscious content seems to have a life and energy of its own that become the sources of later emotional conflict.

Grief that is inhibited and never resolved is called ***abortive.***[68] Those who have aborted their grief work often live bereft of *joie de vivre* with no interest, concern, or enthusiasm for life. Chronic grief is characterized by an indefinite prolonging of the acute stage of depression.[68] Indeed, chronic depression may be traceable to unresolved grief from the past.

Grief that is not resolved remains buried in the psyche, waiting for an opportunity to "rear its ugly head." A current loss may remind the psyche of the unmourned grief from a previous loss or losses.[36] As the two (or more) losses become intertwined and are experienced as one and the same, repressed emotions of unresolved grief pour forth. Grieving more than one loss or a lifetime of losses is more difficult and emotionally draining than grieving one event at a time.[36] Cumulative grief work also may be occurring when a current loss of seemingly little importance overwhelms the person with intense emotions.[36,68] This flood of emotions seems disproportionate to the current loss and is only peripherally related to it. The unconscious, unresolved grief is finally uncovered when the individual is flooded with emotions. Thus the emotional components of any grief reaction may be influenced by aspects of unresolved grief from the past.[121]

Grief and loss events of the perinatal period have been equated only for a relatively short time (≈30 years). Because loss during the perinatal period is a common experience, many childbearing and older women (and men) have never grieved over their spontaneous abortion, stillbirth, or neonatal death, even 10 to 20 years after its occurrence. Parents in a current perinatal loss situation also may be dealing with unresolved grief from a previous perinatal loss. Unresolved grief (whether from perinatal or other loss events of life) may become available for resolution in subsequent crisis events. A mother who delivers a normal healthy newborn, yet is depressed postpartally, may not have postpartum depression. Instead, she may be grieving the unresolved loss of a spontaneous abortion, therapeutic abortion, or other perinatal loss. The normal grief reaction accompanying relinquishment may persist and often leads to chronic unresolved grief that may present itself during and after a subsequent pregnancy.[5] Her depressed mood could also be resulting from unresolved grief from the loss of a parent, spouse, or child. Depressed menopausal women may be experiencing the cumulative effects of a lifetime of unresolved grief (see the Critical Findings box below).

Recognizing unresolved grief has implications for facilitating grief work in a current loss, episodic care, and health maintenance. The energy to keep unresolved emotions restrained could better be used in personal growth and development, grieving, and maintaining and establishing relationships. The lifelong stress of unresolved grief contributes to both

Critical Findings

SYMPTOMS OF UNRESOLVED GRIEF

1. Vivid memory for the details of the perinatal loss event
2. Flashback to the event
3. Anniversary grief (date of birth or expected date of delivery)
4. Emotions of grief (sadness, anger, or crying) when talking about loss
5. Intense emotions with subsequent loss or crisis

psychologic and physical illness, including increased death rates and an earlier death.[88]

Not grieving a perinatal loss affects the individual involved and the relationships with significant others, including present and future children. Asynchronous grief and the absence of grief in one or more family members weaken and strain family relationships.[31,58] The irritability and preoccupation of normal grief may overly disrupt the family. Differences may be magnified to the extent that major rifts and disruptions in the relationship occur, resulting in increased incidence of separation and divorce.[58]

Exclusive dedication to the care of a deformed or ill infant to the detriment of other family relationships is symptomatic of a pathologic grief reaction.[58,106,127] The parent who neglects other children, the couple's relationship, and social outlets is so overwhelmed with guilt about having caused the baby's defect that nothing else in life matters. This guilty attachment and exclusive dedication are ways of avoiding grief work.[106] Other forms of pathologic reactions include parental rejection and intolerance of the deformed or ill infant.[58]

The parent who is emotionally withdrawn and unavailable to the family because of chronic grief and depression cannot attach to and care for present or subsequent children. Aberrant parenting styles (resulting in a vulnerable, battered, or failure-to-thrive child) may be the result of prolonged separation, unresolved grief, or grief that has progressed beyond the anticipatory phase, so that emotional ties with the infant have been severed.[58] These difficulties with caring and parenting may affect the deformed or ill child and all the children in the family. In turn, these children may grow up unable to parent subsequent generations because of the type of ineffectual parenting they received. Parents who grieve inappropriately may leave their children a legacy of psychosocial problems such as difficulty with separation, independence, and control (e.g., school phobia and toilet training); failure to thrive; and sleep disturbances.

Planning for a new pregnancy and another baby should begin after the grief process for the lost infant is complete (about 6 months to 1 year), so that parents are emotionally ready to invest in a relationship with another fetus/newborn.[58] However, because the decision to become pregnant is highly personal and individual, many women are pregnant within 6 months to 1 year after a perinatal loss.[50,95] Some women see a subsequent pregnancy as a "cure" for their overwhelming feelings of emptiness and failure,[122] whereas others are averse to a subsequent pregnancy. Pregnancy after a perinatal loss is characterized by (1) increased pregnancy anxiety, a heightened fear, concern, and vigilance about the pregnancy and baby; (2) comparisons of current and previous pregnancies; (3) less attachment to the current versus the previous pregnancy; (4) a desire to see and phone the health care provider more often; (5) a desire for more prenatal testing; and (6) the subsequent pregnancy possibly being the precipitating event for posttraumatic stress disorder (PTSD) in both mothers and fathers.* Mothers appreciate being educated by their health care providers about the benefits and risks of subsequent pregnancies so that they can make an informed choice.[33] Benefits of postponing pregnancy include (1) enabling physiologic recovery from pregnancy before another is attempted; (2) enabling psychologic recovery, progression of grief work, and an optimal state to emotionally invest in a new pregnancy and newborn; (3) avoiding anniversary dates with the second pregnancy/child; and (4) improving the maternal-infant relationship—less anxiety, overprotectiveness, overindulgence, and hypervigilance.[80,121] The time necessary for physical and emotional recovery varies widely, and parents may benefit from interconceptual counseling after a perinatal loss.[121]

REFERENCES

1. American Academy of Pediatrics: The pediatrician and childhood bereavement, *Pediatrics* 114:1126, 2004.
2. American Academy of Pediatrics, Committee on Pediatric Workforce: Ensuring culturally effective pediatric care: implications for education and health policy, *Pediatrics* 114:1677, 2004.
3. American Academy of Pediatrics and The American College of Obstetricians and Gynecologists: *Guidelines for perinatal care,* ed 6, Elk Grove, Ill, 2007, The Academy.
4. Armstrong DS: Perinatal loss and parental distress after the birth of a healthy infant, *Adv Neonatal Care* 7:200, 2007.
5. Askren H, Bloom K: Post adoptive reactions of the relinquishing mother: a review, *J Obstet Gynecol Neonatal Nurs* 28:395, 1999.

*References 4,23,25,26,33,80,114,115,121.

6. Badenhorst W, Hughes P: Psychological aspects of perinatal loss, *Best Pract Res Clin Obstet Gynaecol* 21:249, 2007.
7. Benfield D, Leib S, Reuter J, et al: Grief response of parents after referral of the critically ill newborn to a regional center, *N Engl J Med* 294:975, 1976.
8. Berezin N: *After a loss in pregnancy, help for families affected by a miscarriage, a stillbirth, or the loss of a newborn,* New York, 1982, Fireside Books.
9. Bibring GL: The death of an infant: a psychological study, *N Engl J Med* 283:370, 1970.
10. Borg S, Lasker J: *When pregnancy fails: families coping with miscarriage, stillbirth, and infant death,* Boston, 1981, Beacon Press.
11. Bracht M, Kandankery A, Nodwell S, et al: Cultural differences and parental responses to the preterm infant at risk: strategies for supporting families, *Neonatal Netw* 21:31, 2002.
12. Brodlie M, Laing I, Keeling J, et al: Ten years of neonatal autopsies in tertiary referral centre: retrospective study, *BMJ* 324:761, 2002.
13. Broen A, Moum T, Bodtker A, et al: Psychological impact on women of miscarriage versus induced abortion: a 2 year follow up study, *Psychosom Med* 66:265, 2004.
14. Brosig CL, Pierucci RL, Kupst MJ, et al: Infant end-of-life care: the parent's perspective, *J Perinatol* 27:510, 2007.
15. Burkes N: Saying good-bye, *Neonatal Netw* 23:75, 2004.
16. Byrnes A, Berk N, Cooper M, et al: Parental evaluation of informing interviews for cleft lip or palate, *Pediatrics* 112:308, 2003.
17. Cadden V: Crisis in the family. In Caplan G, editor: *Principles of preventive psychiatry*, New York, 1964, Basic Books.
18. Caplan G: *Principles of preventive psychiatry*, New York, 1964, Basic Books.
19. Carter BS: Neonatal and infant death: what bereaved parents can teach us, *J Perinatol* 27:467, 2007.
20. Clements P, Vigil G, Manno M, et al: Cultural perspectives of death, grief and bereavement, *J Psychosoc Nurs* 41:18, 2003.
21. Contro N, Larson J, Scofield S, et al: Hospital staff and family perspectives regarding quality of pediatric palliative care, *Pediatrics* 114:1248, 2004.
22. Costello AC, Gardner SL, Merenstein GB: Perinatal grief and loss, *J Perinatol* 8:41, 1988.
23. Cote-Arsenault D: The influence of perinatal loss on anxiety in multigravidas, *J Obstet Gynecol Neonatal Nurs* 32:623, 2003.
24. Cote-Arsenault D, Donato KL, Earl SS: Watching and worrying: early pregnancy after loss experiences, *MCN: Am J Matern Child Nurs* 31:356, 2006.
25. Cote-Arsenault D, Marshall R: One foot in and one foot out: weathering the storm of pregnancy after perinatal loss, *Res Nurs Health* 23:473, 2000.
26. Cote-Arsenault D, Morrison-Beedy D: Women's voices: reflecting back on pregnancy after perinatal loss, *J Nurs Scholar* 33:239, 2001.
27. Cummings ST: The impact of the child's defect on the father, *Am J Orthop* 46:246, 1976.
28. Cummings ST, Bayley HC, Rie HE: Effects of the child's deficiency on the mother: a study of mothers of mentally retarded, chronically ill, and neurotic children, *Am J Orthopsychiatry* 36:595, 1966.
29. Davies R: New understanding of parental grief: literature review, *J Adv Nurs* 46:506, 2004.
30. de Montigny F, Beaudet L, Dumas L: A baby has died: the impact of perinatal loss on family social networks, *J Obstet Gynecol Neonatal Nurs* 28:151, 1999.
31. Doucette J, Pinelli J: The effects of family resources, coping, and strains on family adjustment 18 to 24 months after the NICU experience, *Adv Neonatal Care* 4:92, 2004.
32. Downey V, Bengiamin M, Heuer L, et al: Dying babies and associated stress in NICU nurses, *Neonatal Netw* 14:41, 1995.
33. Downie J, Letendre A: Parent's experiences of midwife managed care following the loss of a baby in a previous pregnancy, *J Adv Nurs* 39:127, 2002.
34. Dyer KA: Identifying, understanding, and working with grieving parents in the NICU. I. Identifying and understanding loss and the grief response, *Neonatal Netw* 24:35, 2005.
35. Dyer KA: Identifying, understanding, and working with grieving parents in the NICU. II. Strategies, *Neonatal Netw* 24:27, 2005.
36. Eason WM: *The dying child,* Springfield, Ill, 1970, Charles C Thomas.
37. Egan K, Arnold R: Grief and bereavement, *Am J Nurs* 103:42, 2003.
38. Engel GL: Grief and grieving, *Am J Nurs* 64:93, 1964.
39. Ewing A, Carter BS: Once again, Vanderbilt NICU in Nashville leads the way in nurse's emotional support, *Pediatr Nurs* 30:471, 2004.
40. Feudtner C: Grief-love: contradictions in the lives of fathers of children with disabilities, *Arch Pediatr Adolesc Med* 156:643, 2002.
41. Feudtner C, Haney J, Dimmers M: Spiritual care needs of hospitalized children and their families: a national survey of pastoral care providers' perceptions, *Pediatrics* 111:e67, 2003.
42. Gardner SL, Merenstein GB: Helping families deal with perinatal loss, *Neonatal Netw* 5:17, 1986.
43. Gold KJ: Navigating care after a baby dies: a systematic review of parent experiences with health providers, *J Perinatol* 27:230, 2007.

44. Goldbach KR, Dunn DS, Toedter LJ, et al: The effects of gestational age and gender on grief after pregnancy loss, *Am J Orthop* 61:461, 1991.
45. Goldberg H: *The hazards of being male,* New York, 1976, Sanford J. Greenberger.
46. Gonzalez MT: Nursing support of the family with an abnormal infant, *Hosp Top* 15:68, 1971.
47. Griffin T: Facing challenges to family-centered care. II. Anger in the clinical setting, *Pediatr Nurs* 29:212, 2003.
48. Harmon R, Glicken A, Siegel R: Neonatal loss in the intensive care nursery: effects of maternal grieving and a program for intervention, *J Am Acad Child Psychiatry* 23:68, 1984.
49. Hobdell E: Chronic sorrow and depression in parents of children with neural tube defects, *J Neurosci Nurs* 36:82, 2004.
50. Hughes P, Turton P, Evans C: Stillbirth as a risk factor for anxiety and depression in the next pregnancy: does time since loss make a difference? *BMJ* 318:1721, 1999.
51. Hughes P, Turton P, Hopper RN, et al: Disorganized attachment behaviour in infants born subsequent to stillbirth, *J Child Psychol Psychiatry* 42:791, 2001.
52. Jansen J: A bereavement model for the intensive care nursery, *Neonatal Netw* 22:17, 2003.
53. Jourard S: *The transparent self* (revised edition), New York, 1971, Van Nostrand Reinhold.
54. Jung A, Milne P, Wilcox J, et al: Neonatal hand casting method, *J Perinatol* 23:519, 2003.
55. Kavanaugh K, Hershberger P: Perinatal loss in low-income African American parents, *J Obstet Gynecol Neonatal Nurs* 34:595, 2005.
56. Kennell JH, Slyter H, Klaus MH: The mourning response of parents to death of a newborn infant, *N Engl J Med* 283:344, 1970.
57. Kitson C: Commentary on: Fathers experienced in stillbirth as a waste of life and needed to protect their partners and express grief in their own way, *Evid Based Nurs* 5:61, 2002.
58. Klaus M, Kennell J: *Parent-infant bonding,* ed 2, St Louis, 1982, Mosby.
59. Kübler-Ross E: *On death and dying,* New York, 1969, Macmillan.
60. Leonard L: Prenatal behavior of multiples: implications for families and nurses, *J Obstet Gynecol Neonatal Nurs* 31:248, 2002.
61. Lindemann E: Symptomatology and management of acute grief, *Am J Psychiatry* 101:141, 1944.
62. Lloyd-Williams M, Wilkinson C, Lloyd-Williams F: Do bereaved children consult the primary health care team more frequently? *Eur J Cancer Care* 7:120, 1998.
63. Lobar S, Youngblut J, Brooten D: Cross-cultural beliefs, ceremonies and rituals surrounding death of a loved one, *Pediatr Nurs* 32:44, 2006.
64. Lundqvist A, Nilstun T, Dykes A: Both empowered and powerless: mother's experience of professional care when their newborn dies, *Birth* 29:3, 2002.
65. Lundqvist A, Nilstun T, Dykes A: Experiencing neonatal death: an ambivalent transition into motherhood, *Pediatr Nurs* 28:621, 2003.
66. Maifield M, Hahn S, Titler M, et al: Decision making regarding multifetal reduction, *J Obstet Gynecol Neonatal Nurs* 32:357, 2003.
67. Mallow G, Bechtel G: Chronic sorrow: the experience of parents with children who are developmentally disabled, *J Psychosoc Nurs* 27:31, 1999.
68. Marris P: *Loss and change,* New York, 1974, Pantheon Books.
69. Matzo M, Sherman D, Lo K, et al: Strategies for teaching loss, grief and bereavement, *Nurse Educ* 28:71, 2003.
70. McCarthy M: *Gender differences in reactions to perinatal loss: a qualitative study of couples* doctoral dissertation, San Diego, Calif, 2002, California School of Professional Psychology.
71. McCreight B: A grief ignored: narratives of pregnancy loss from a male perspective, *Sociol Health Illn* 26:326, 2004.
72. McHaffie H, Laing I, Lloyd D: Follow up care of bereaved parents after treatment withdrawal from newborns, *Arch Dis Child Fetal Neonatal Ed* 84:F125, 2001.
73. Meert K, Thurston C: Spiritual needs of bereaved parents: a qualitative study, *Pediatr Res* 55:378, 2004.
74. Milstein J: Detoxifying death in the neonate: in search of meaningfulness at the end of life, *J Perinatol* 23:333, 2003.
75. Mitchell L: Women's experiences of unexpected ultrasound findings, *J Midwifery Womens Health* 49:228, 2004.
76. Moore D, Catlin A: Lactation suppression: forgotten aspect of care for the mother of a dying child, *Pediatr Nurs* 29:383, 2003.
77. Moore M, Moos M: *Cultural competence in the care of childbearing families,* New York, 2003, March of Dimes Birth Defects Foundation.
78. Nystrom K, Axelsson K: Mother's experience of being separated from their newborns, *J Obstet Gynecol Neonatal Nurs* 31:275, 2002.
79. Ohlshansky S: Chronic sorrow: a response to having a mentally defective child, *Soc Case* 43:190, 1962.
80. O'Leary J: Grief and its impact on prenatal attachment in the subsequent pregnancy, *Arch Womens Ment Health* 7:7, 2004.
81. Parkes CM: *Bereavement: studies of grief in adult life,* New York, 1972, International Universities Press.
82. Pector E: Views of bereaved multiple-birth parents on life support decisions, the dying process, and discussions surrounding death, *J Perinatol* 24:4, 2004.

83. Pector E: How bereaved multiple-birth parents cope with hospitalization, homecoming, disposition for deceased, and attachment to survivors, *J Perinatol* 24:714, 2004.
84. Pector E, Smith-Levitin M: Bereavement in multiple birth. I. General considerations, *Female Patient* 26:31, 2001.
85. Primeau M, Lamb J: When a baby dies: rights of the baby and parents, *J Obstet Gynecol Neonatal Nurs* 24:206, 1995.
86. Primeau M, Recht C: Professional bereavement photos: one aspect of a perinatal bereavement program, *J Obstet Gynecol Neonatal Nurs* 23:22, 1994.
87. Putman, M: Perinatal perimortem and postmortem examination: obligations and considerations for perinatal, neonatal and pediatric clinicians, *Adv Neonatal Care* 7:281, 2007.
88. Rahe R, Meyer M, Smith M, et al: Social stress and illness onset, *J Psychosom Res* 8:35, 1964.
89. Rapaport L: The state of crisis: some theoretical considerations. In Parad H, editor: *Crisis intervention*, New York, 1965, Family Service Association of America.
90. Raphael D: *The tender gift: breastfeeding*, New York, 1973, Schocken Books.
91. Ray L: Parenting and childhood chronicity: making visible the invisible work, *J Pediatr Nurs* 17:424, 2002.
92. Reddick B, Catlin E, Jellinek M: Crisis within crisis recommendations for defining, preventing, and coping with stressors in the NICU, *J Clin Ethic* 12:254, 2001.
93. Reilly-Smorawski B, Armstrong A, Catlin E: Bereavement support for couples following death of a baby: program development and 14-year exit analysis, *Death Stud* 26:21, 2002.
94. Roberts K: Providing culturally sensitive care to the childbearing Islamic family: Part II, *Adv Neonatal Care* 3:250, 2003.
95. Robertson P, Kavanaugh K: Supporting parents during and after a pregnancy subsequent to a perinatal loss, *J Perinat Neonatal Nurs* 12:63, 1998.
96. Romesberg T: Understanding grief: a component of neonatal palliative care, *J Hosp Palliat Care Nurs* 6:161, 2004.
97. Samuelsson M, Radestad I, Segesten K: A waste of life: fathers' experience of losing a child before birth, *Birth* 28:124, 2001.
98. Sandelowski M, Barroso J: The travesty of choosing after positive prenatal diagnosis, *J Obstet Gynecol Neonatal Nurs* 34:307, 2005.
99. Saylor D: Nursing response to mothers of stillborn infants, *J Obstet Gynecol Neonatal Nurs* 8:39, 1977.
100. Schoenberg BA: *Anticipatory grief*, New York, 1974, Columbia University Press.
101. Schoenberg BA, Carr A, Perety D, et al: *Loss and grief: psychological management in medical practice*, New York, 1970, Columbia University Press.
102. Schwab R: Effects of a child's death on the marital relationship: a preliminary study, *Death Stud* 16:141, 1992.
103. Seidman R, Kleine P: A theory of transformed parenting: parenting a child with developmental delay/mental retardation, *Nurs Res* 44:38, 1995.
104. Shah M: *Transcultural aspects of perinatal health care: a resource guide,* Washington, DC, 2004, National Perinatal Association.
105. Simons C, Ritchie S, Mullett M: Parents' perceptions of medical diagnoses and related issues for their high-risk infants, *J Pediatric Health Care* 12:118, 1998.
106. Solnit A, Stark M: Mourning and the birth of a defective child, *Psychoanal Study Child* 16:523, 1961.
107. Stringer M, Shaw V, Savani R: Comfort care of neonates at the end of life, *Neonatal Netw* 23:41, 2004.
108. Sudia-Robinson T: Palliative care. In Kenner C, McGrath J, editors: *Developmental care of newborns and infants: a guide for health professionals,* St Louis, 2004, Mosby.
109. Swanson K, Karmali Z, Powell S, et al: Miscarriage effects on couples' interpersonal and sexual relationships during the first year after loss: women's perspectives, *Psychosom Med* 65:902, 2003.
110. Swanson P, Pearsall-Jones J, Hay D: How mothers cope with the death of a twin or higher multiple, *Twin Res* 5:156, 2002.
111. Swift K, Janke J: Breast binding…is it all that it's wrapped up to be? *J Obstet Gynecol Neonatal Nurs* 32:332, 2003.
112. Taylor L, Scott S, Leuthner S: Experience of prenatal palliative care consultation, *Pediatr Res* 31:72, 2004.
113. Traxler P: *Poem for my son, blood calendar*, New York, 1975, William Morrow.
114. Turton P, Badenhorst W, Hughes P, et al: The psychological impact of stillbirth on fathers in subsequent pregnancy and puerperium, *Br J Psychiatry* 188:165, 2006.
115. Turton P, Hughes P, Evans C, et al: Incidence, correlates and predictors of post-traumatic stress disorder in the pregnancy after stillbirth, *Br J Psychiatr* 178:556, 2001.
116. Ufema J: A need for gentleness, *Nursing* 34:66, 2004.
117. Van P, Meleis A: Coping with grief after involuntary pregnancy loss: perspectives of African American women, *J Obstet Gynecol Neonatal Nurs* 32:28, 2003.
118. Vance J, Boyle F, Najman J, et al: Couple distress after sudden infant or perinatal death: a 30-month follow up, *J Paediatr Child Health* 38:368, 2002.
119. Wagner T, Higgins P, Wallerstedt C: Perinatal death: how fathers grieve, *J Perinatal Educ* 6:4, 1997.

120. Wallerstedt C, Higgins P: Facilitating perinatal grieving between the mother and the father, *J Obstet Gynecol Neonatal Nurs* 25:389, 1996.
121. Wallerstedt C, Lilley M, Baldwin K: Interconceptional counseling after perinatal and infant loss, *J Obstet Gynecol Neonatal Nurs* 32:533, 2003.
122. Wheeler S: A loss of innocence and a gain in vulnerability: subsequent pregnancy after a loss, *Illness Crisis Loss* 8:310, 2000.
123. Whitfield M: Psychosocial effects of intensive care on infants and families after discharge, *Semin Neonatol* 8:185, 2003.
124. Wilson AL, Fenton LJ, Stevens DC, et al: The death of a newborn twin: an analysis of parental bereavement, *Pediatrics* 70:587, 1982.
125. Wilson S, Miles M: Spirituality in African-American mothers coping with a seriously ill infant, *J Soc Pediatr Nurses* 6:116, 2001.
126. Workman E: Guiding parents through the death of their infant, *J Obstet Gynecol Neonatal Nurs* 30:569, 2001.
127. Young RK: Chronic sorrow: parent's response to the birth of a child with a defect, *MCN Am J Matern Child Nurs J* 2:38, 1977.
128. Zahourek R, Jensen J: Grieving and the loss of the newborn, *Am J Nurs* 73:836, 1973.

RESOURCE MATERIALS FOR PARENTS

Balter L: *A funeral for Whiskers*, New York, 1991, Barron's Educational Services.

Berezin N: *After a loss in pregnancy*, New York, 1982, Fireside Books.

Borg S, Lasker J: *When pregnancy fails*, Boston, 1981, Beacon Press.

Boyle F: *Mothers bereaved by stillbirth, neonatal death, or sudden infant death syndrome*, Ashgate, United Kingdom, 1997, Aldershot.

Brown L, Brown M: *When dinosaurs die: a guide to understanding death*, Boston, 1996, Little, Brown.

Burns L, Ilse S: *Miscarriage: a shattered dream*, Maple Plain, Minn, 2000, Wintergreen Press.

Buscaglia L: *The fall of Freddie the leaf*, Thorofare, NJ, 1982, Slack.

Cardin N: *Tears of sorrow, seeds of hope. A Jewish spiritual companion for infertility and pregnancy loss*, Woodstock, Vt, 2001, Jewish Light Publishing.

Case B: *Living without your twin*, Portland, Ore, 2001, Tibbutt.

Cirulli C: *Pregnancy after loss: a guide to pregnancy after a miscarriage, stillbirth, or infant death*, New York, 1999, Berkeley Books.

Davis D: *Empty cradle, broken heart*, Golden, Colo, 2000, Fulcrum Publishing.

Davis D, Stein M: *Parenting your premature baby and child: the emotional journey*, Golden, Colo, 2004, Fulcrum Books.

Dyer KA: *Journey of hearts*, Website: www.journeyofhearts.org.

Eddy ML, Raydo L: *Making loving memories: a gentle guide to what you can do when your baby dies*, Omaha, Neb, 1990, Centering Corp.

Eldon K, Eldon A: *Angel catcher: a journal of loss and remembrance*, San Francisco, 1998, Chronicle Books.

Emswiler M, Emswiler J: *Guiding your child through grief*, New York, 2000, Bantam Trade.

Grollman E: *Talking about death: a dialogue between parent and child*, Boston, 1990, Beacon Press.

Grollman E: *Straight talk about death to teenagers*, Boston, 1993, Beacon Press.

Harrison H: *The premature baby book*, New York, 1983, St Martin's Press.

Isle S: *Empty arms*, Maple Plain, Minn, 1996, Wintergreen Press.

Leon IC: *When a baby dies: psychotherapy for pregnancy and newborn loss*, New Haven, Conn, 1990, Yale University Press.

Limbo R, Wheeler S: *When a baby dies: a handbook for healing and helping*, La Crosse, Wis, 1998, Lutheran Hospital—La Crosse.

Linden D, Paroli E, Doron M: *The essential guide for parents of premature babies*, New York, 2000, Pocket Books.

March of Dimes: *The bereavement kit*, New York, 2002, March of Dimes Birth Defects Foundation.

Miller S: *Finding hope when a child dies*, New York, 1999, Simon & Schuster.

Mundy M: *Sad isn't bad: a good-grief guidebook for kids dealing with loss*, (Elf-Help Books for kids) St. Meinrad, Ind, 1999, Abbey Press.

Pector, E: *Multiplicity: resources for loss, prematurity and special needs*, Website: www.synspectrum.com/multiplicity.html.

Read B, Bryan E, Hallett F: *When a twin or triplet dies*, London, 1997, The Multiple Births Foundation.

Shriver M: *What's heaven?* New York, 1999, Golden Books.

Standucher C: *Men and grief*, Oakland, Calif, 1991, New Harbinger Publications.

Thomas P: *I miss you: a first look at death*, Hauppauge, NY, 2001, Barron's Educational Series.

Tracy A, Maroney D: *Your premature baby and child*, New York, 1999, Berkley Books.

Woodward J: *The lone twin: understanding twin bereavement and loss*, London, 1998, Free Association Books.

Zaichkin J: *Newborn intensive care: what every parent needs to know*, ed 3, Petaluma, Calif, 2009, NICU Inc.

VIDEOS, DVDS, AND PROFESSIONAL MODULES

Gemma P, Arnold J: *Loss and grieving in pregnancy and the first year of life: a caring resource for nurses*, White Plains, NY, 2003, March of Dimes.

Grieving in the NICU: *Supporting families and the health team when a baby dies and Grieving in the NICU: mending broken hearts when a baby dies*, Website: www.grievingforbabies.org.

What do I tell my children? Newton, Mass, 1990, Life-cycle Productions.

When a baby dies, La Crosse, Wis, 1991, Resolve Through Sharing, La Crosse Lutheran Hospital.

NATIONAL ORGANIZATIONS

American Academy of Pediatrics: The pediatrician and childhood bereavement, *Pediatrics* 105:445, 2000.

Angel babies forever loved, Website: www.angels4ever.com/multiples.

A place to remember de-Ruyter-Nelson Publications, Inc., 1885 University Ave., Suite 110, St Paul, MN 55104; Phone: (800) 631-0973 Website: www.aplacetoremember.com.

Association for Death Education and Counseling: Website: www.adec.org.

Bereavement Services/RTS, 1910 South Ave, La Crosse, WI 54601; Phone: (608) 791-4747, Website: www.gundluth.org/bereave.

Center for Loss in Multiple Birth: Inc: Website: www.climb-support.org.

Centering Corp. and Grief Digest: Box 3367, Omaha, NE 68103-0367; Phone: (402) 553-1200; Website: www.centering.org.

Climb, Inc., Center for Loss in Multiple Birth, Inc: PO Box 91377, Anchorage, AK 99509; Phone: (907) 222-5321, Website: www.climb-support.org.

Hygeia Foundation, Inc: Website: www.hygeia.org.

March of Dimes Birth Defects Foundation: 1275 Mamaroneck Ave., White Plains, NY; Phone: 1-888-663-4637, Website: www.marchofdimes.com/loss.

Memories Unlimited, Inc: 9511 Johnson Point Loop NE, Olympia, WA 98516-9529; Phone: (360) 491-9819.

Mothers in Support and Sympathy (MISS) Foundation: Website: www.missfoundation.org.

Parents of Stillborn, 5570 South Langston Road, Seattle, WA, 98718; Phone: (206) 772-5338.

Perinatal Hospice: Website: www.perinatalhospice.org.

Pregnancy Loss and Infant Death Alliance: Website: www.plida.org.

Remember When (Video and DVD tributes), Phone (720) 859-1122, Website: www.rememberwhenvideo.com.

RTS Bereavement Program: Website: www.bereavement-programs.com.

SHARE Pregnancy and Infant Loss Support, Inc: St Joseph's Health Center, 300 First Capitol Drive, St Charles, MO 63301; Phone: (800) 821-6819, Website: www.nationalshareoffice.com.

The Compassionate Friends, Inc: PO Box 3696, Oak Brook, IL 60522-3696; Phone: (630) 990-0010, Website: www.compassionatefriends.org.

31 DISCHARGE PLANNING AND FOLLOW-UP OF THE NEONATAL INTENSIVE CARE UNIT INFANT

DONNA K. DAILY, ANGEL CARTER, AND BRIAN S. CARTER

Parents with infants in the neonatal intensive care unit (NICU) have immediate worries about whether their newborn infant will survive but soon thereafter start having concerns about how their child will do through infancy and into adulthood. As the infant's convalescence begins, so does discharge planning; this brings to the forefront questions about outcomes. Unfortunately, it is almost impossible to know the outcome of any individual infant at the time of discharge from the NICU. **Caregivers within the NICU must be knowledgeable of the latest outcomes literature to respond to these questions and to guide parents in the importance of follow-up care.**

Of the many reasons that newborns require neonatal intensive care, the most common one is preterm birth. Numerous publications report the outcomes of very-low-birth-weight (VLBW, birth weights <1500 g) and extremely-low-birth-weight (ELBW, birth weights <1000 g).[3,23,28,33,65] Recent studies have focused on the survival and outcome of even more immature infants with birth weights below 750 g, or on infants born at the limits of viability, 22 to 25 weeks' gestation.[45,64,68,84] Late preterm infants have been a topic of renewed interest because they are at risk for a unique set of problems with adverse outcomes.[2,52] Infants with intrauterine growth restriction (IUGR) are also vulnerable to a wide range of complications requiring neonatal intensive care, especially if they are also preterm and experience extrauterine growth failure.[32,80] Full-term infants with meconium aspiration syndrome (MAS), persistent pulmonary hypertension of the newborn (PPHN), infection, congenital diaphragmatic hernia (CDH), or neonatal encephalopathy also require intensive care and are at risk for health and developmental sequelae.[121] Finally, a number of infants with multiple congenital anomalies require surgery or neonatal intensive care.

PLANNING FOR DISCHARGE

An organized, well-implemented discharge plan is the beginning of successful follow-up of a NICU graduate. A family-centered multidisciplinary team approach uses the expertise of many disciplines, along with the family, to formulate and implement the discharge and follow-up plan. The team can comprise parents, grandparents, other caregivers, physicians, nurses, case managers, dietitians, therapists, developmental specialists, and social workers.

Integrating family-centered principles into the discharge process as a continuation of family-centered care practiced throughout the NICU stay facilitates better parental adaptation to the transition to home.[62] For many infants, the NICU stay has been lengthy and complex, and families may experience varying degrees of anxiety and stress as they prepare for the infant to come home. In some cases, attachment and bonding may have been affected by a long, complicated medical course.[41] A survey of preterm mothers found that symptoms of psychologic distress (fatigue, depressive mood, anxiety, physical symptoms) persisted up to a year after the birth of their premature baby.[57] Families may need

Please note that the **PURPLE** type in each chapter is intended to make it easier to identify clinically applicable material.

extra attention paid to these issues before they can successfully attend to the discharge process. A thorough assessment of caregiver needs, environmental issues, and knowledge of their infant's care before discharge is an important part of the planning process. Implementation of a parent educational-behavioral intervention program during the NICU stay may be one mechanism to reduce stress, depression, and anxiety and effect more positive interactions of parents with their infant, a shorter NICU stay, and shorter total hospital stay.[86] In addition, an assessment tool may be considered in efforts to quantify the discharge readiness of the family.[111]

Considerations Before Discharge

INSURANCE

Many parents may need assistance to enroll their infant in their existing insurance policy or to identify the procedures necessary to apply for medical assistance. This process can take many weeks and must be accomplished before discharge in order to select a pediatrician for follow-up care. Social workers, case managers, and financial counselors are valuable resources to assist families in this process.

IDENTIFICATION OF A FOLLOW-UP PROVIDER

A pediatric health care professional to follow the infant after discharge, trained in the care of NICU graduates, should be identified before discharge. Ideally, this provider has been identified early in the admission to facilitate regular communications regarding the infant's medical course. Immediately before discharge, a written summary should be provided, with follow-up recommendations regarding nutrition and growth, developmental surveillance, and subspecialty referrals, along with verbal notification of the discharge date. Parents should be advised to keep this summary with the infant at all times because this written documentation of the NICU stay is invaluable if the infant needs to be seen on an emergency basis shortly after hospital discharge. Providing families with a "care notebook" containing specialized forms and organizing tools can be a valuable addition to the discharge process, particularly for those with anticipated complex follow-up needs. The American Academy of Pediatrics (AAP) also provides a form for summarizing the history and current needs of children with special health care needs.

CAREGIVER EDUCATION

In a family-centered environment, families have been partners in caring for their infant throughout the hospital stay. Discharge teaching then becomes a process of reinforcing and attending to final details. In some instances, however, this teaching may be limited by the inability of the family to be present because of transportation and family or job constraints. In these cases, readiness of the caregivers and home environment should be thoroughly evaluated (Box 31-1).

HOME EQUIPMENT

When a home apnea monitor is used, a clear plan outlining the reasons for initiating home monitoring and the indications for discontinuing it should be discussed with the family and the primary care provider before discharge.[5] Any necessary durable medical equipment or supplies, such as an apnea monitor, feeding pump, ventilator, suction equipment, or oxygen for home use, should be delivered to the hospital before discharge to give parents practice using the equipment. The company supplying the equipment should provide training in its use. NICU nurses or respiratory therapists should verify the parents' understanding of the purpose of the equipment and its operation and also ensure that home caregivers for the baby have been trained in cardiopulmonary resuscitation (CPR).

ROOMING IN

Whether or not an infant is going home with equipment, giving family caregivers the opportunity to provide "independent" care of their infant with professional caregivers nearby for assistance has been shown to increase parental competence and provide confirmation of readiness for independent care at home.[39] One intensive care nursery's experience in establishing a step-down unit where mothers provided all basic care for their infant under supervision resulted in earlier discharge to home with no increases in short-term complications or readmissions.[29]

DISCHARGE CRITERIA

Clearly defined discharge criteria provide both the family and the staff a point of reference from which to judge the infant's progress. Discharge criteria should be reviewed in a multidisciplinary team meeting with the family. Setting goals that

BOX 31-1 CAREGIVER EDUCATION

- Every encounter with the parents is a teaching opportunity. Assess each individual family's readiness for discharge.
- Inform parents verbally and in writing about the tests included in the newborn genetic screening and how they will receive the results.
- Teach parents the special nutritional needs of preterm infants after discharge, including nutritional supplementation, lactation support and intervention to promote breast feeding, and use of alternative feeding methods, if necessary.
- Teach parents the importance of maintaining their infant on home oxygen therapy (e.g., for growth and development, sleep, and feeding) at designated pulse oximetry targets until pulse oximetry studies (e.g., awake, feeding, asleep) document that the infant can tolerate weaning and discontinuing the supplemental oxygen.
- Teach parents to dress their infant appropriately to maintain adequate axillary temperature.
- Teach parents appropriate safety precautions:
  - Proper positioning (supine) for sleep: "Back to Sleep"
  - Proper use of car seats
  - Importance of a smoke-free environment
  - Never shake the baby! Dangers of shaking infants include blindness, brain damage, developmental delays, seizures, paralysis, and death
  - Information, in writing, about all medications for their infant including name, action, dose, route, side effects, schedule
  - Provide parents opportunity to participate in infant CPR class
- Teach parents the importance of follow-up care and appointments:
  - Timely follow-up for infants with retinopathy of prematurity (ROP) provided verbally and in writing
  - Timely follow-up for hearing screen and referral for re-screening
  - Need for monthly RSV immunizations throughout the RSV season
- Give parents the newborn immunization record.
- Teach parents the importance of their own self-care, and assist in identifying resources for support.

the infant, parents, and staff must accomplish before discharge helps keep everyone focused and prevents important components of the discharge process from being overlooked.

For preterm infants, the attainment of a weight of 5 pounds is no longer the criterion for discharge. Rather, the ability of a preterm or recovering neonate to maintain physiologic stability and the ability of the family to care for the infant's physiologic and developmental needs are the criteria for discharge (Box 31-2). There are significant variations across NICUs for specific discharge criteria, with assessment of apnea and feeding behavior significantly influencing the duration of hospitalization in a healthy preterm infant.[49] The recently published AAP policy statement "Hospital Discharge of the High-Risk Neonate" provides guidance that should minimize such variations.[6]

TRANSFER

Some infants are not discharged home from the regional or tertiary NICU but, instead, are transferred from a regional referral center to a community unit or facility for the duration of their hospital stay. **Transfer to a community hospital may be beneficial to families because they are often closer to the parents' home (especially if the NICU is part of a regional referral center). Possible locations for transfer, as well as the criteria for transfer, should be discussed with the parents early in the hospitalization if this is an expected possibility. Communication of a comprehensive discharge plan should take place with the receiving hospital before transfer.**[66,79] As the capacity for back-transporting convalescing neonates to community hospitals has increased in the United States over the past 20 years, persistent issues of communication, trust, and psychosocial support remain for parents.[44]

EARLY DISCHARGE

Preterm infants are often discharged between 35 and 37 weeks chronologic age.[89] **Parental concerns at the time of discharge may include their ability to have adequate rest, their readiness to learn and assume self-care and newborn care, their readiness to parent, and availability of support systems.** Concerns about the newborn may include transition from the intensive care nursery to the home care environment, ability to feed and hydrate adequately, and the early development and recognition of complications.[117] In addition, late-preterm infants (34 to 36 weeks gestational age) are sometimes discharged early (<48 hours) using criteria developed for term infants. Tomashek et al demonstrated that late-preterm, early discharged, breast-fed infants were 1.5 times more likely to require hospital-related care and 2.2 times more likely to be readmitted than term infants who were breast fed, with jaundice and infection accounting for the majority of readmissions.[132] Early discharge requires appropriate post-discharge follow-up and monitoring to prevent morbidity. Numerous studies document the positive effects of home visitation programs to assist with post-discharge education and support.[95,102,146]

BOX 31-2 SELECTED CRITERIA FOR DISCHARGE OF THE PREMATURE INFANT OR NEONATE WITH SPECIAL NEEDS

Infant

- Sustained weight gain of sufficient duration
- Maintain normal body temperature, clothed in an open bed, at normal room temperature (20° to 25° C)
- Establish and maintain competent breast or bottle feeding without cardiopulmonary problems
- Nutrition assessment and dietary management provided as indicated
- Hematologic assessment and management provided as indicated
- Documented physiologically mature and stable cardiopulmonary function of sufficient duration
- Parents have been given a report of neurodevelopmental and neurobehavioral status
- Completed metabolic, hearing, and indicated funduscopic screenings
- Appropriately immunized, including (respiratory syncytial virus [RSV] prophylaxis) and plan for subsequent injections
- A completed car seat evaluation
- A completed review of the hospital course, pending medical problems noted, and follow-up plans identified
- A home-care plan, individualized to the patient's needs, has been provided by all disciplines

Parents, Family, and Home Environment

- Identify and assess at least two caregivers for home.
- Assess psychosocial and parenting strengths and risks.
- Consider the home environment and on-site visit as indicated.
- Review resource availability (including financial, utilities, and transportation).
- Determine caregiver availability, ability, and commitment to the following:
  - Provide basic infant care: diapering, bathing, dressing, cord and circumcision care.
  - Maintain infant's thermal state: able to take temperature and dress appropriately.
  - Feed infant (breast, bottle, or alternative method—nasogastric tube, gastrostomy, parenteral nutrition), and demonstrate formula preparation if required.
  - Manage home feeding tube, infusion pump, intestinal stoma care, and other devices as indicated.
  - Manage home monitoring, oxygen, and other equipment as indicated; address initial problem solving; demonstrate CPR and initial emergency interventions.
  - Maintain safe environment, car seat, heat, electricity, telephone, transportation, smoke-free, emergency resuscitation.
  - Recognize signs of illness, and identify when to call primary care provider or emergency services.
  - Have support system identified to assist in infant's care.
  - Demonstrate medication administration and recognize signs of medication adverse effects (e.g., toxicity); understand importance of follow-up care, and know whom to call for questions or concerns.

Modified from American Academy of Pediatrics, Committee on Fetus and Newborn: Hospital discharge of the high-risk neonate, *Pediatrics* 122:1119, 2008.

Screening

GENETIC SCREENING

Initial screening of sick or premature infants is performed as soon as possible after birth, before the administration of blood or antibiotics. Although it is common for these infants to have some relatively abnormal results—especially for thyroid function or amino acid profiles while on parenteral nutrition—early screening is recommended to identify in a timely manner those infants who may have an inborn metabolic disorder, congenital endocrinopathies, hemoglobinopathies, or infectious processes so that early treatment can be initiated.[12,109] **Subsequent screenings should take place according to an established routine, depending on state requirements.** Recommendations for continued screenings after discharge should be clearly outlined in the discharge summary.

HEARING

All infants, especially those who need NICU admission for more than 5 days, should be screened for hearing loss using otoacoustic

emissions or auditory brainstem response testing. This initial screening should be performed once the infant is medically stable, and if there are any concerns that warrant a secondary screen, re-screening should occur before 1 month of age. Infants who do not pass (are "referred" after secondary screening) should have a full-scale auditory diagnostic evaluation by 3 months of age. Infants with confirmed hearing loss should receive intervention by 6 months of age from an infant hearing specialist.[11,134] Those infants with an increased risk for hearing impairment should be assessed by a pediatric audiologist with a follow-up schedule outlined for the parents (Box 31-3). The goal of early detection and intervention is to maximize language, cognitive, literacy, and social development of the hearing impaired.[126]

BOX 31-3 CONDITIONS ASSOCIATED WITH INCREASED RISK FOR HEARING LOSS

- Neonatal intensive care unit (NICU) admission for more than 5 days or any of the following regardless of length of stay: extracorporeal membrane oxygenation (ECMO), assisted ventilation, exposure to ototoxic medications (gentamicin and tobramycin) or loop diuretics (furosemide/Lasix), hyperbilirubinemia requiring exchange transfusion
- Syndromes associated with hearing loss such as neurofibromatosis, osteopetrosis, and Usher syndrome
- Family history of hereditary childhood hearing loss
- Craniofacial abnormalities
- Congenital infections such as cytomegalovirus, toxoplasmosis, bacterial meningitis, syphilis, herpes, and rubella
- Physical findings (white forelock) associated with syndromes known to include hearing loss
- Neurodegenerative disorders (e.g., Hunter syndrome) or sensory motor neuropathies (e.g., Friedreich ataxia and Charcot-Marie-Tooth syndrome)
- Culture-positive postnatal infections such as bacterial and viral (especially herpes and varicella) meningitis
- Chemotherapy
- Caregiver concerns regarding hearing, speech, language, or developmental delay

Modified from American Academy of Pediatrics and Joint Committee on Infant Hearing, Year 2007 Position Statement: Principles and guidelines for early hearing detection and intervention programs, *Pediatrics* 120(4):898, 2007.

VISION

Development of severe retinopathy of prematurity (ROP) may still be a concern at the time of NICU discharge for infants born prematurely. Infants born at less than 32 weeks' gestation or less than 1500 g birth weight, as well as infants with a birth weight between 1500 and 2000 g or born at more than 32 weeks with an unstable clinical course, should have a retinal screening examination with pupillary dilation.[13] Follow-up of infants should be according to the ophthalmologist's recommendations based on retinal findings. Arrangements for follow-up examinations should be made before discharge. Current research indicates that the risk to visual development in preterm infants does not end when the risk for ROP has passed. Any infant born prematurely, whether or not they develop ROP, are at increased risk for amblyopia/strabismus and refractive errors.[97]

IMAGING

Premature infants are at increased risk for injuries to the brain, potentially causing permanent damage. The most common form of damage and the leading cause of chronic neurologic morbidity is periventricular white matter injury.[25] Identification of infants at high risk for poorer outcomes related to brain injury allows for timely referrals to early intervention therapies. A recent Cochrane review indicates that early intervention can improve cognitive outcomes up to preschool age.[127] Imaging techniques for routine screening for white matter injury have traditionally been the cranial ultrasound, although the ability of ultrasound to predict developmental outcome is inferior to magnetic resonance imaging (MRI).[90] A recent review of MRI screening to identify risks of suboptimal neurologic outcomes suggests the following be considered as indications for screening by MRI at approximately 36 weeks postmenstrual age[67]:

- Grade III to IV intraventricular hemorrhage
- Periventricular hemorrhagic infarction
- Cystic periventricular white matter damage
- Cerebellar hemorrhage or other abnormalities on ultrasound
- Suspected white matter abnormalities on ultrasound (echodensities/echolucencies)
- Post–hemorrhagic hydrocephalus
- Abnormal neurologic examination
- Other conditions warranting detailed neuroimaging (metabolic disorders or suspected congenital structural abnormality)

Preventive Care

IMMUNIZATIONS

Infant immunizations are recommended for all NICU infants, according to the guidelines issued by the Centers for Disease Control and Prevention (CDC) and approved by the AAP.[37] Immunizations administered in the NICU should appear in the discharge summary. When immunizations have been declined by parents, this should be clearly indicated in the discharge summary, along with follow-up recommendations.

RESPIRATORY SYNCYTIAL VIRUS INFECTION PROPHYLAXIS

Respiratory syncytial virus (RSV) infection poses a risk for serious morbidity or even death for infants who were born prematurely, especially those with chronic heart or lung disease. **For qualifying infants, RSV prophylaxis should be initiated with intramuscular palivizumab before discharge into the community setting during RSV season.** RSV infection prophylaxis should be coordinated with the follow-up pediatrician for subsequent monthly injections.

Assessments

CAR SAFETY

All 50 states require infants to be restrained in a safety seat while riding in a motor vehicle, although laws vary from state to state. The AAP's recent clinical report on transporting infants home states that "Infants with documented oxygen desaturation, apnea, or bradycardia in a semiupright position should travel in a supine or prone position in an Federal Motor Vehicle Safety Standard (FMVSS) 213–approved car bed after an observation period that is free of such events as described in point 1 above [e.g., 'increased frequency of oxygen desaturation and episodes of apnea or bradycardia while sitting in car safety seats…preferably their own…for a minimum of 90 to 120 minutes or the duration of travel, whichever is longer…']." This may need to be revised as new evidence becomes available from future research.[4,7,9]

Discharge of smaller infants results in the use of car seat restraint devices that were designed for 7- to 8-pound term infants. **In these devices, preterm infants may experience oxygen desaturations and apnea and bradycardia caused by head slouching and airway obstruction.**[105] Use of rolled diapers/blankets may be necessary to support upright posture, prevent slouching, and enable the preterm to maintain stability while in the car seat. A recent study of a foam insert that enabled the preterm's head to be maintained in a neutral position showed a significant reduction in the rate of apneas.[133] In addition, infants with certain conditions (e.g., Down syndrome, osteogenesis imperfecta, myelomeningocele, Pierre Robin syndrome, cerebral palsy) may benefit from special-needs car restraints.[82]

A car seat challenge before discharge is recommended for all infants born less than 37 weeks' gestation; this includes "late preterm" infants (i.e., 34 to 36$^{6}/_{7}$ weeks) who are cared for and discharged from level I/normal newborn nurseries.[7,9] Although the car seat challenge has not been standardized, certain components are common: (1) using the car seat purchased by the parents, (2) positioning the infant in the car seat immediately before discharge while on cardiorespiratory and pulse oximetry monitoring, (3) for a prescribed period of time (e.g., 30 to 90 minutes), and (4) recording respiratory/heart rates, oxygen saturations, apnea/bradycardia events. Although this is a recommended practice, limitations have been identified. First, little objective evidence supports the ability of this challenge to absolutely confirm safe travel for an infant.[60] A recent Cochrane review of the literature found no randomized controlled trials that fulfilled eligibility criteria for their review and were unable to recommend or refute a car seat challenge before discharge.[106] Further, common clinical practice has been to recommend the use of a car bed as a safe alternative to infants failing the car seat challenge, although recent studies have failed to prove any difference in apneic events.[77,119] A recommendation has been put forth regarding changing the notion of a "test" or "challenge" to a car seat "orientation" in which the emphasis would be on education on proper positioning, limiting duration of automobile travel, and close observation during travel.[60]

NUTRITION AND GROWTH

Before discharge, (1) current growth trends should be reviewed; (2) either breast feeding, if desired, should be established or guidelines given for increasing and monitoring; and (3) special feeding considerations such as the use of increased calorie formula, vitamin and mineral supplementation, and use of "special" formulas, tube feedings, or home total parenteral nutrition

(TPN) should be outlined.[144] In studies of infants who experienced extrauterine growth restriction (EUGR), commonly defined as weight less than the 10th percentile for corrected gestational age (CGA) at discharge, the period from discharge to 30 months is shown to be a critical period for growth.[116] Nutritional intake at this time sets the trajectory for growth and neurodevelopment in childhood and adolescence. VLBW children who have low weight gain in early years of life have a higher probability of cognitive deficits; conversely, those with excessive weight gain had a higher likelihood of obesity, cardiovascular disease, and diabetes.[36]

NEURODEVELOPMENT

Some premature infants may have recognized risks to their later development evident at discharge. For these infants, early evaluation of their functional neurologic status may facilitate referrals to early intervention services soon after discharge.[104] Early intervention has been shown to improve neurobehavioral development with improved cognitive outcomes and parent-child interactions.[31,98]

Technology-Dependent Infants

Infants who rely on long-term technologic support are being discharged home in increasing numbers. In the past, children who were ventilator dependent, who had tracheostomies, gastrostomies, or jejunostomies, and even those who required long-term intravenous (IV) access for medications or parenteral nutrition would remain hospitalized, separated from their families and susceptible to other morbidities associated with long hospital stays (e.g., infection, delayed development, impaired mental health). With this increase of technology-dependent children discharged into the community comes a greater need for support services for the parents, providers, and the infants themselves.[142] Numerous investigators have undertaken projects to understand the impact that caring for these children has on the individual child and the family as a whole. Carnevale et al described the experiences of 12 families with technology-dependent children at home.[35] They identified key themes in this population to include (1) parental responsibility being stressful and, at times, overwhelming; (2) the devotion of significant energy in trying to "normalize" their home life; (3) living in isolation and feeling like strangers in their own communities; and (4) an overall theme of "daily living with distress and enrichment."[35]

In-home nursing care, extensive parent training, and an identified primary care provider comfortable with all aspects of the child's care are essential for successful discharge of technology-dependent children to home.[70] Developing home care plans that contain emergency and resuscitation procedures, as well as parental support and respite services, is vital.[91] Parents need training around all the details of their child's care, including early signs of illness and emergency procedures, whether or not home shift nursing will be provided. **Rooming in with their infant for one or more nights is an important safety net to evaluate their abilities and confidence in caring for their child.** Communication and care coordination among the subspecialties following these infants are crucial.

NEURODEVELOPMENTAL FOLLOW-UP OF HIGH-RISK INFANTS

Ideally, parents of all NICU infants would be offered comprehensive, coordinated, developmentally based, family-centered follow-up for their child through infancy and childhood (Figure 31-1). Each infant is unique, as is each infant's family. The following are the primary objectives of follow-up care:

- To counsel the family about their child's development so that they are empowered to optimize the child's health, growth, and development
- To recognize and diagnose (early) significant health conditions and neurodevelopmental disabilities to facilitate appropriate referrals for community services
- To anticipate future difficulties and needs so that optimal development is promoted and secondary complications are avoided or minimized

The ultimate goal is to promote the child's integration into the family, school, and community.

Follow-up resources are generally limited, however, and today health insurance plans (both public and private) determine how children will access care. Consequently, criteria for developmental follow-up of NICU infants vary widely. Some high-risk infants are routinely referred to early intervention programs for developmental care, but implementation of these programs varies among states. The dynamics of development are such that periodic assessments of the child's

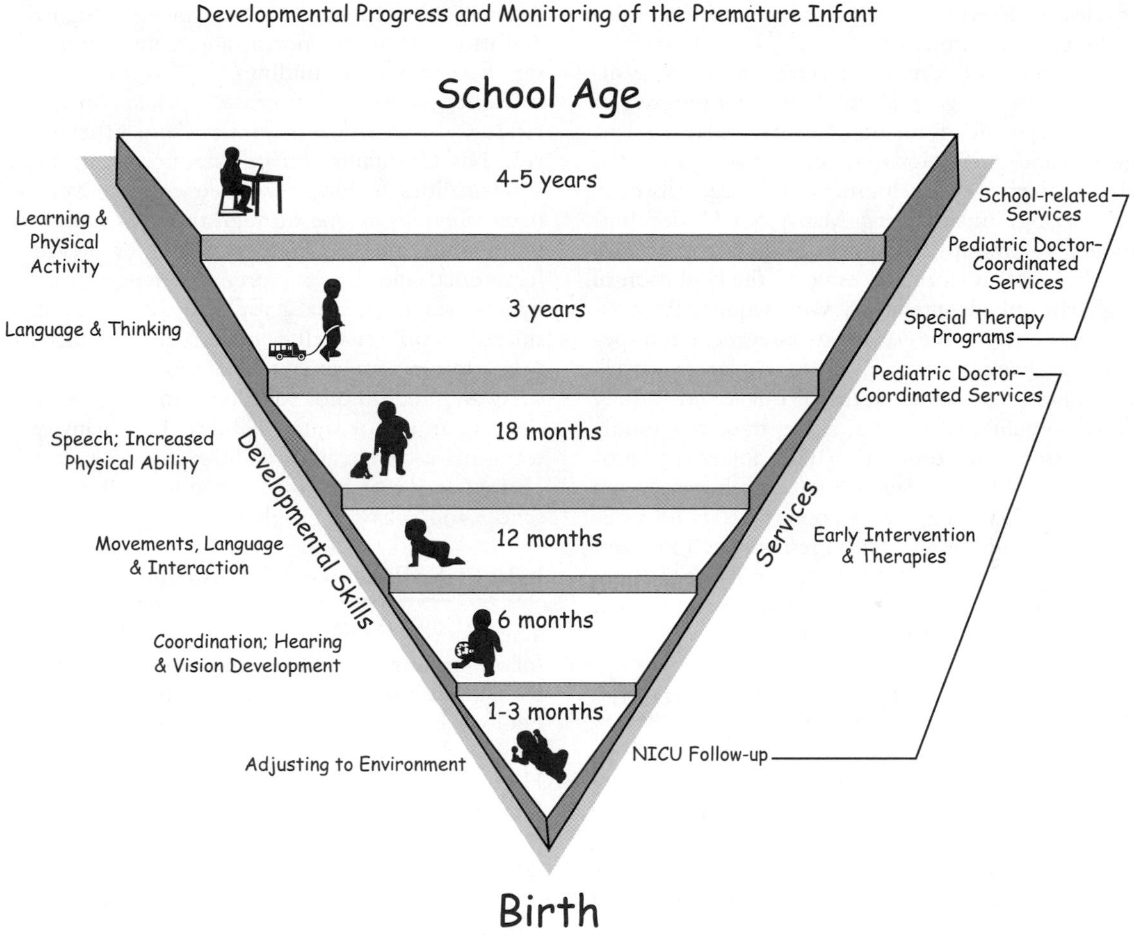

FIGURE 31-1 Developmental progress and monitoring of the premature infant. (Courtesy Angel Carter, Brian S. Carter, and Donna K. Daily, Vanderbilt University Medical Center.)

health and developmental progress are needed to determine whether current interventions are effective and sufficient. Parents often need guidance to better understand what to expect from their child, how to interpret their own observations of their child, and how health care and community services can support their child's development. The AAP has emphasized that each child have a "medical home," and especially the child with complex health and developmental needs. Unfortunately, the care of these children often is fragmented among numerous subspecialists and therapists.[10] Well-organized NICU follow-up clinics can facilitate developmental and health care of the NICU infant in coordination with the primary care provider and the family.

Developmental Milestone Attainment

In developmentally based follow-up, much of the information about the child's development comes from a careful interview of the parent about the child's health status and developmental milestone attainment. Noting the age of acquisition of the gross-motor, fine-motor, language, and adaptive-behavioral milestones helps determine a possible developmental delay. Parents are very good historians of their child's current functioning and recent accomplishments, which is why eliciting a history of milestone attainment during serial clinic visits is so useful in assessing a child's rate of development. Sometimes additional explanation may be needed to clearly determine the age of acquisition, especially language milestones.

A number of accurate screening tools are available to monitor general developmental progress or domain-specific evaluation.[58] Early delay in language and self-help milestones raises concerns about cognitive development, language disorder, or hearing impairment.[1] Many NICU developmental follow-up clinics rely on pediatric clinical psychologists to formally evaluate the cognition of high-risk infants, preferably with sequential assessments but sometimes with one assessment at a specific age (e.g., at 18 to 24 months corrected age). For infants, the Bayley Scales of Infant and Toddler Development, 3rd edition, is the most commonly used assessment tool in NICU follow-up programs in the United States.[27] For preschool-age and school-age children, several cognitive tests are available, including the Wechsler Preschool and Primary Scale of Intelligence (WPPSI), the Stanford-Binet Intelligence Scales, and the Kaufman Assessment Battery for Children (K-ABC II).[75,112,145]

Correction for Degree of Prematurity

One controversy that arises in monitoring developmental scores of preterm infants is whether to correct for degree of prematurity (i.e., whether to use the child's chronologic age, calculated from birth, or to use corrected age for degree of prematurity). The best evidence supports correcting for degree of prematurity, but whether it is best to correct throughout infancy is controversial, and there is no agreement as to when one should stop correcting for degree of prematurity.[138] **By convention, most practitioners correct through 2 years of age.** It is necessary to be very cautious when interpreting corrected age scores at 12 months or less for ELBW infants. Parental understanding may lead to an overly optimistic outlook that will not be supported by testing at a later date.

Neurodevelopmental Examination

For high-risk infants, the standard pediatric neurologic examination is expanded to include a detailed assessment of posture, muscle tone, reflexes, postural reactions, and functional abilities. Interpretation of the examination requires a thorough understanding of the normal pattern of development over time, the examiner's skill at assessing the infant's performance, recognizing deviations from the norm, and determining the significance of these findings.[1,15,18,51]

Abnormalities of posture, muscle tone, and reflexes are common in preterm and other high-risk NICU infants during the first year. These abnormalities include asymmetries of movement, marked extensor tone through the neck and trunk with significant shoulder retraction or elevation, hypotonia, and lower extremity hypertonia and hyperreflexia. Cerebral palsy (CP) should be considered in infants with persistent abnormalities in tone, posture, movement, and motor delay. Mild delay and neuromotor tone variation suggest transient neuromotor abnormalities. For many preterm infants, these abnormalities can no longer be elicited at 1 year but they remain at risk for later school and behavior problems.[76]

NICU Follow-up Guidelines

The issue of how to do NICU developmental follow-up and how to conduct follow-up studies for high-risk infants has been complex. The methodology can lead to inadequate interpretation of published studies. The National Institute of Child Health and Human Development (NICHD), the National Institute of Neurologic Disorders and Stroke, and the CDC convened a workshop in 2002 to address these issues. Their purpose was to provide standardized guidelines for follow-up care, especially for tertiary care centers with neonatal fellowship training programs in the United States. The results of that workshop have been published and address topics such as risk factors that affect outcome, appropriate assessments, correction for prematurity, assessment tools, and research-related subjects.[138]

Again, these criteria may not fit the need or focus of every program. The resources available across states, within communities, and in individual hospitals and the commitment within the NICU strongly drive follow-up programs in different communities. Programs that wish to have developmental follow-up for quality care surveillance and to provide families with information about their high-risk infant can be resourceful in developing partnerships with local early intervention programs and community physicians. Programs that address scientific questions generally need a focused approach or a research network to approach the study.[135]

It is now recognized that survival to the end of the NICU stay is a very short-term outcome. It is generally recommended that NICU graduates be followed until at least 8 years of age, but most programs do not have the resources to do this. Furthermore, it has become apparent that the effects of prematurity may extend throughout the life span.[64] This is important to know but clearly goes beyond the capability of most NICU follow-up programs.

NEURODEVELOPMENTAL DISABILITIES

Neurodevelopmental disabilities are a group of chronic, nonprogressive disorders of central nervous system (CNS) function that occur as result of malformation of or insult to the developing brain.[1] **There is a spectrum of neurodevelopmental disabilities, from the major disabilities (CP and mental retardation [MR]), to sensory impairments, and to the more subtle disorders of higher cortical functioning (Box 31-4).** Preterm infants are at an increased risk for major disabilities and also for more subtle disabilities. Both may have a long-term impact on their life.[151]

The World Health Organization (WHO) has revised its definition of disability, impairment, and handicap to an International Classification of Functioning, Disability and Health (ICF) and places emphasis on the interaction of functioning and disability, health condition of the individual, and factors of the environment. The ICF is structured around the following components: (1) body functions and structure, (2) activities and participation, and (3) additional information on severity and environmental factors.[150] This view has aided our thinking not only of the specific disability but also how it affects a child's ability to function physically and socially within his or her home and community.

BOX 31-4 NEURODEVELOPMENTAL DISABILITIES

1. Major disability
    - Cerebral palsy
    - Global developmental delay or mental retardation
2. Sensory impairment
    - Hearing impairment
    - Visual impairment
3. Subtle disorders of higher cortical function
    - Language delay or disorder
        - Expressive language delay
        - Receptive and expressive language delay
    - Developmental coordination disorder
        - Fine-motor incoordination
        - Sensorimotor integration problems
    - Learning disability
        - Variable cognitive abilities
        - Visual-perceptual problems
    - Behavior problems
        - Attention deficit hyperactivity disorder
        - Social emotional adaptation

Modified from Accardo PJ, editor: *Capute and Accardo's neurodevelopmental disabilities in infancy and childhood*, ed 3, Baltimore, Md, 2008, Paul H Brookes; Wolraich ML, editor: *Disorders of development and learning*, ed 3, Hamilton, Ontario, Canada, 2003, BC Decker.

Cerebral Palsy

Cerebral palsy "describes a group of permanent disorders of the development of movement and posture, causing activity limitation, that are attributed to non-progressive disturbances that occurred in the developing fetal or infant brain."[114] Important to this current definition is the recognition of the accompanying disturbances of sensation, perception, cognition, communication, and behavior and by epilepsy and secondary musculoskeletal problems. CP is the most disabling motor impairment found in preterm infants and is difficult to diagnose with any degree of certainty before 6 to 12 months of age. It sometimes takes until the child is 2 years or older before the diagnosis becomes clear. Cerebral palsy occurs in 7% to 18% of preterm infants and is more common in the most immature infants.[33,92]

CP has traditionally been classified by physiologic type (tone abnormality), topography (i.e., muscle groups involved), and severity.[1] Again, the most recent recommendation for definition and classification has been expanded and relates to the WHO ICF.[114,150] Components of the currently recommended classification stress motor abnormalities, accompanying impairments, anatomic and neuroimaging findings, and causation and timing. Because consensus has not been clear on the definition of level of severity, the Gross Motor Classification Scale is now commonly used to address motor function, and scales are being developed to more reliably measure other important areas of functioning, such as hand control, speech, and swallowing.[101,114] Persistently increased muscle tone and increased deep tendon reflexes with persistence of pathologic reflexes (e.g., Babinski) are early signs of spasticity. Variable tone with persistent primitive reflexes, often with involuntary movements, is a sign of extrapyramidal CP. The child may be 2 to 3 years old before involuntary movements are seen. Children who manifest signs of both spasticity and extrapyramidal CP have mixed CP. Extrapyramidal CP is generalized, but spasticity should be further typed according to which limbs are most significantly involved.

Spastic diplegia, the most common form of CP in preterm infants, is characterized by spasticity in both lower extremities, with mild or minimal involvement of the upper extremities.[1,92] ***Spastic hemiplegia*** is characterized by involvement of one side of the body, with the upper extremity more involved than the lower. Because intrauterine and perinatal strokes are usually unilateral, children who had strokes often demonstrate spastic hemiplegia. ***Quadriplegia*** is the most severe form of spastic CP, with involvement of both upper and lower extremities and the lower more severely affected than the upper. Children with neonatal encephalopathy (whether caused by hypoxia/ischemia, metabolic disorders, or other causes) who develop CP are most likely to have spastic quadriplegia or severe mixed CP.

Global Developmental Delay and Mental Retardation

Developmental delay is used to describe a deficit in any of the five developmental domains (cognition, motor, language, adaptive, social-emotional skills). *Global developmental delay* is used to define deficits in two or more areas of development with scores more than two deviations below norm referenced standards.[123] Currently in the United States, a child may receive services through his or her local school district special education program with a diagnosis of developmental delays until almost 8 years of age before the definition may be switched to mental retardation, again based on standardized testing. Standardized tests, such as the Bayley, 3rd edition, have score groupings and definitions to match, such as low average and borderline, for each domain.[27] It is during this early period of detection that early intervention services become important for the high-risk infant.[31,98,104]

Mental retardation is a global impairment of cognitive functioning resulting from injury to or malformation of the developing brain that impairs the child's ability to adapt and function in society.[1,150] MR frequently manifests with an early delay in language and problem-solving abilities. A diagnosis of MR requires a comprehensive evaluation of the child, with neuropsychologic testing of intelligence and assessment of adaptive (functional) abilities, which can be reliably done only at school age.

Neuropsychologic testing includes an assessment of a child's intelligence quotient (IQ). Intelligence is not one entity but, rather, many different abilities, including auditory and visual memory, visual-perceptual abilities, and understanding complex language concepts. The older the child is, the greater the number of functions that can be tested and therefore the more accurate the tests are in assessing intelligence. Intelligence and functional ability tests for school-age children and adults consist of a variety of subtests. Most children with MR have lower abilities for age across all domains of development, so severity of MR is easily classified. Many preterm children have a significant variability in cognitive functions, with high scores on some subtests and low scores on others, which makes them more difficult to classify and appropriate educational services more difficult to determine.

MR is classified in terms of severity, from profound (IQ below 20), severe (IQ 20 to 34), moderate (IQ 35 to 49), to mild (IQ 50 to 70).[1,150] Children with an IQ of 70 to 80 or 85 have borderline intelligence, not MR. They are capable of academic learning but may have trouble keeping up with their class. The most important characteristics of children with cognitive impairments that enhance adult functioning are interpersonal skills and ability to communicate and relate to other people.

Sensory Impairments

Hearing impairment occurs in 1% to 10% of NICU infants.[136] Most states require hearing screening for all newborns using a 2-step process: initial screening with otoacoustic emissions, followed by auditory evoked responses if the first test is failed.[11,134] Because of the risk

for progressive hearing impairment, infants with congenital cytomegalovirus (CMV) infection, primary pulmonary hypertension, and congenital diaphragmatic hernia and infants treated with extracorporeal membrane oxygenation (ECMO) should have serial hearing evaluations during infancy and early childhood, as should infants with recurrent ear infections.[11,14,56,110,131]

Neonates demonstrate hearing thresholds similar to those of older children and adults. Even preterm infants as early as 24 to 25 weeks' gestation demonstrate an immature brainstem waveform in response to sound stimuli, although the pattern of the waveform matures to a normal waveform as the infant reaches near-term equivalence. Infants hear and process language throughout their first year, beginning at birth.

Retinopathy of prematurity (ROP) results from injury to the very immature developing retina, which causes abnormal proliferation of blood vessels. Severe ROP, which tends to occur in the most immature and sickest preterm infants, is treated with laser to try to prevent retinal detachment and blindness. Preterm infants may develop medically related eye complications (retinal detachment, cataract, glaucoma) and are at increased risk for refractive errors, strabismus, and amblyopia.[96] There are no well-delineated guidelines for eye care follow-up of the preterm infant once ROP has resolved. Infants who have structurally normal eyes, no refractive error, and a history of no or low-level regressed ROP may be dismissed by the ophthalmologist after 12 to 18 months of age but should continue to receive routine child-care eye screening based on the AAP recommendations for routine preventive care.[97] Late preterm and term infants with other neonatal complications and neurodevelopmental sequelae will often have visual impairments and need ongoing ophthalmologic follow-up.

Infants with congenital CMV infection or toxoplasmosis should be examined by ophthalmologists for chorioretinitis. Neonates symptomatic with congenital infection (e.g., CMV infection, rubella, toxoplasmosis) have a high risk (20% to 30%) of visual and/or hearing impairment.[141] Preterm infants in the NICU with varying types of postnatal sepsis syndromes have also been identified as having an increased risk for neurodevelopmental impairment.[129] If infants with neonatal encephalopathy develop disability, they tend to have severe multiple disabilities, including cortical visual impairment or processing and hearing impairment.[108]

Subtle Disorders of Higher Cortical Function

Even if the NICU graduate does not develop major disability or sensory impairment, he or she remains at increased risk for the more subtle disorders of higher cortical function (see Box 31-4). These disorders, because they are milder than the major disabilities, may not manifest in infancy or may be associated with only nonspecific symptoms in infancy (e.g., irritability, posturing, feeding problems). Diagnostic criteria, and even nomenclature, for these disorders vary widely, and few reports of preschool and school-age outcome studies have a comparison group evaluated in the identical manner.

Language delay may manifest as early as 6 to 12 months as delay or deviance (i.e., nonsequential) in language milestone acquisition.[1,147] Expressive language delay, either alone or in combination with receptive language delay, is common in preterm and other NICU infants. Every child who manifests with delayed language should have a hearing test and neuropsychologic testing to distinguish between language disorder, hearing impairment, and cognitive impairment.

Developmental coordination disorder (DCD), also referred to as ***minor neuromotor dysfunction,*** presents as mild delay or deviant motor milestone acquisition in conjunction with mild or transient neuromotor abnormalities.[33,42,76] These are children who sit by 1 year of age and walk by 2 years, although they may have an atypical pattern to their motor progress (e.g., transient low or high tone, toe-walking, persistent wide-base gait). These children generally look normal by 3 to 5 years of age, although they may continue to have some balance or motor planning problems. Fine-motor incoordination, visual-perceptual deficits, and sensorimotor inefficiencies may accompany DCD, but they may not be recognized until preschool or school age.[21,33,41] Visual-perceptual deficits, often in combination with fine-motor incoordination, are manifest by an inability to recognize and copy figures, letters, and numbers; complete puzzles and mazes; or copy block designs; or by some level of difficulty with these tasks. Fine-motor incoordination makes it difficult to button, zip, cut with scissors, draw, and write. Sensorimotor inefficiencies are characterized by difficulty following directions that include demonstrating an action (e.g., tying shoelaces) and tolerating motion through space (e.g., swinging on a swing) or different tactile sensations (e.g., clothing or food textures).

For children with DCD, fine-motor incoordination or sensorimotor inefficiencies and failures in school and on the playground erode self-esteem and peer relationships.

Language disorder, visual-perceptual problems, DCD, transient neuromotor dysfunction, and variable cognitive disabilities are associated with learning disability (LD) and other school problems.[1,21,33,41,147] LD means difficulty learning one or more academic subjects (reading, writing, arithmetic) in children with normal intelligence who have had adequate exposure to school. Some children have more of a learning inefficiency, in that they do well in the early grades of school but have a relative inefficiency in reading or writing that causes them trouble as the work becomes more complex. Their intelligence and resiliency help them make adaptations in learning, but they become overwhelmed in situations in which speed and accuracy are viewed as important.

Behavior problems are more common in preterm and other NICU children.[19,23,28,73,93] Some children have attention deficit hyperactivity disorder (ADHD), characterized by marked distractibility, short attention span, and impulsivity. ADHD can occur with or without hyperactivity: the child may be restless, always on the move, or constantly busy or may just demonstrate difficulty paying attention and impulsiveness. One must recognize these more subtle problems as soon as possible. Counseling parents and teachers can prevent the devastating effect these "mild" disabilities have on self-esteem, peer relationships, and performance in school and at home.

Diagnosis of Disability

The major disabilities may be recognized and diagnosed in the first 2 years after birth. The more severe the disability, the sooner it may be recognized and diagnosed. Occasionally a child may have significant motor delay initially but seems to "catch up" by 1 to 2 years, with concomitant improvement in neuromotor abnormalities. These are often children with ongoing health problems (e.g., chronic lung disease [CLD]/bronchopulmonary dysplasia [BPD]) and are diagnosed with developmental coordination disorder but have a high risk for learning disability at school age. Language disorders, visual-perceptual difficulties, and fine-motor incoordination are generally recognized and diagnosed during the preschool years (ages 3 to 5 years). Specific learning disabilities and attentional difficulties cannot be diagnosed until school age, usually around 7 to 8 years of age. Mild LD or learning inefficiencies may not be recognized until middle school or high school.

Because there is so much overlap among the neurodevelopmental disabilities, whenever abnormality in one area is detected, the child should have a comprehensive, multidisciplinary evaluation of all his or her abilities. Services are now available to all children through the Individuals with Disabilities Education Act (IDEA 2004).[71] Children from birth to 3 years of age receive services through their early intervention program and after the age of 36 months, receive services through their local public school's special education program.

PERINATAL RISK FACTORS FOR NEURODEVELOPMENTAL DISABILITY

Many conditions that require neonatal intensive care also increase risk for neurodevelopmental disability, including prematurity, PPHN, hypoxic-ischemic encephalopathy, necrotizing enterocolitis (NEC), maternal chorioamnionitis, neonatal sepsis, and IUGR. Perinatal risk factors can be used to identify NICU infants with a high risk for neurodevelopmental disability so that they can be followed closely and referred for comprehensive evaluations and early intervention programs when appropriate (Box 31-5).

Risk does not imply causation; it is merely a marker of brain injury. As markers of brain injury, intraventricular hemorrhage (IVH), intraparenchymal hemorrhage, and white matter injury are all important neonatal risk factors.[87] Evidence of brain injury on neuroimaging studies, specifically MRI, has been strongly predictive of adverse neurodevelopmental outcomes.[22,147] There is a great deal of variability in how predictive other individual risk factors are of neurodevelopmental outcome. Very low Apgar scores, especially at 5 to 10 minutes or more after birth, are associated with later CP. These low Apgar scores are signs of severe perinatal depression. However, the signs and symptoms of neonatal encephalopathy predict CP far better than do low Apgar scores.[88] Even within a risk factor category, the degree of risk can vary. Infants who are symptomatic with congenital CMV infection at birth are far more likely to develop

BOX 31-5

PERINATAL RISK FACTORS FOR NEURODEVELOPMENTAL DISABILITIES

- Maternal characteristics
  - Socioeconomic status
  - Education
  - Race/ethnicity
- Obstetric/prenatal complications
  - Maternal illness
  - Chorioamnionitis
  - Maternal ingestions (alcohol, drugs, medications)
  - Congenital infection
  - Multiple gestation
  - Labor or delivery complications
  - Placental abnormalities
- Physical characteristics
  - Prematurity
  - Postmaturity
  - Intrauterine growth restriction
  - Small for gestational age
  - Macrosomia
  - Gender
  - Microcephaly
  - Congenital anomalies
  - Dysmorphic features
- Condition at birth
  - Apgar scores
  - Cord pH
  - Meconium staining
  - Need for and response to resuscitation
- Neonatal complications
  - Hypoxia
  - Acidosis
  - Hypotension/shock
  - Apnea and bradycardia
  - Chronic lung disease
  - Sepsis
  - Meningitis
  - Seizures
  - Hypoxic-ischemic encephalopathy
- CNS structure and function
  - Intraventricular hemorrhage
  - Intraparenchymal hemorrhage or infarction
  - Ventricular dilation
  - Cortical atrophy
  - Periventricular leukomalacia
  - Burst-suppression pattern on EEG
  - Abnormal neurologic examination

Modified from Taeusch W, Ballard R, Gleason C, editors: *Avery's diseases of the newborn*, ed 8, Philadelphia, 2005, Saunders.
CNS, Central nervous system; *EEG*, electroencephalogram.

CP, MR, and sensory impairment than infants who are asymptomatic at birth with congenital CMV infection.[40,110] **Multiple risk factors increase an infant's risk for neurodevelopmental disability, and the effects may be more than additive.** As a group, preterm infants or full-term infants with IUGR tend to have lower mean IQ than full-term appropriate for gestational age (AGA) infants.[115,140] Infants with both prematurity and IUGR are vulnerable to the complications of each condition.

SPECIFIC NEURODEVELOPMENTAL OUTCOMES

This section summarizes reported neurodevelopmental outcomes for some of the most frequently encountered conditions in the NICU. A systematic approach (see Box 31-5) allows the clinician to assess the risk factors that may affect developmental outcome. Preterm infants and their medical sequelae are most commonly encountered in neonatal intensive care. However, term infants with pulmonary disease, encephalopathy, or congenital defects also may require intensive care and have significant sequelae. Finally, while we have focused our attention in recent years on smaller and smaller babies in tertiary care centers, it has become apparent that we have often neglected issues for larger "late-preterm" infants (see Chapter 5). These infants are more typically followed in level II or transitional nurseries but are not without risk. It is beyond the scope of this chapter to cover congenital malformations or genetic conditions (see Chapter 27), but it is well known that these infants often require complex multidisciplinary care and the principles of follow-up outlined previously apply to them as well.

Prematurity

For more than 50 years, the medical literature has described the neurodevelopmental outcome of preterm VLBW infants (birth weight <1500 g). With the beginning of modern neonatal intensive care in the mid-1960s, tertiary care NICUs began reporting the incidence or prevalence of major disability (i.e., CP and MR) in survivors.[3] Initially, there was a great deal of variability in reported incidences because of differences in populations studied, neonatal intensive care practices, definitions of disability (e.g., whether they include children with mild CP or children with borderline intelligence), and age at follow-up. Because of these issues of study methodology, outcomes are now more frequently reported from large regional studies or research consortiums.

Among a number of studies published between 1988 and 2001, 5% to 19% of ELBW infants with birth weights below 1000 g had CP, with a mean of 10.2%.[33,81,99,118] A number of studies reporting CP by gestational age note a prevalence of CP at 8% to 21% for infants born at less than 26 weeks' gestation. Studies of populations of VLBW and ELBW children find that their mean intelligence quotients are 0.3 to 0.6 standard deviation below that of full-term controls, or a 4-point to 9-point difference (at times up to a 17-point difference).[23] This is most meaningful when one considers how many more preterm children there are with MR or borderline intelligence. As many as 37% of ELBW children have IQs below 70.[118,136,137,139,148]

A recent study of 6-year-old children who were born at less than 26 weeks gestational age found that 12% had disabling CP and 21% had moderate to severe cognitive impairment (IQ <70).[84] When compared with full-term controls, 41% of these extremely preterm children had moderate to severe cognitive impairments; one quarter had borderline intelligence; 10% had hearing loss (profound in 3%), and 7% had visual impairments (2% were blind). The lower border of viability is currently 23 to 24 weeks' gestation and approximately 500 g birth weight. There have been rare survivors reported to have been born at 22 weeks' gestation or at 300 to 500 g birth weight.[68] Few, if any, of the survivors at these extremes have been reported as demonstrating normal development. **The largest study of infants born at less than 26 weeks' gestation and followed to age 6 years found that 22% had severe disability, 24% had moderate disability, 34% had mild disability, and only 20% were normal.**[83,84]

As many as 50% of VLBW children and 60% to 70% of ELBW children have school problems, including LD, failed grades, and special education requirements.[23,93] Studies that have compared the outcomes of normally intelligent VLBW children with full-term control subjects have found that VLBW children have more language delay, more visual-perceptual problems, lower reading quotients, greater difficulty with arithmetic, and more problems with attention and behavior. Compared with full-term controls, ELBW children are three to five times more likely to require special resources in school, and this increases to 8 to 10 times more likely by adolescence.[64]

Recent reviews and meta-analyses of outcomes of children who were born prematurely do not show improvement over time in rates of CP or presence of cognitive impairment.[30,92,99,113] While rates of CP are higher in the ELBW infant, there is also an independent increase in cognitive impairment with a correlation between cognitive impairment and birth weight or gestational age.[20,28] Advances in neuroimaging techniques are starting to correlate newborn brain injury with developmental outcome, but as yet, they are not of sufficient sensitivity and specificity to give predictive information to families.[67,149]

Late Preterm Infants

In the past decade, there has been renewed interest and concern in the health and development of the larger preterm infant. While these infants make up the greater proportion of all preterm infants, their neonatal course is generally less complicated and they may actually receive their care in a level I or II nursery. Moderately-low-birth-weight infants (between 1500 and 2500 g) have been reported to have increased risk for neurodevelopmental sequelae and account for between 18% and 37% of all children with CP and 7% and 12% of children with mental retardation.[15] Even larger preterm infants, now called *late preterm infants,* make up 75% of all preterm births and are defined as infants born between 34 and 36 completed weeks. These infants are physiologically and metabolically immature, which predisposes them to special transitional care needs.[53] If these needs are not met or recognized, such as post-discharge hyperbilirubinemia, these infants may be placed at risk for neurodevelopmental sequelae.[2,52] Recent outcome information about this group of infants suggests that they are likely to have more problems with school readiness and that even CP and developmental delay (DD)/MR rates are increased when compared with term gestation.[2,85,103]

Intrauterine Growth Restriction and Extrauterine Growth Restriction

Prenatal and postnatal growth can seriously affect neurodevelopmental outcomes of high-risk infants. The neurodevelopmental outcome of IUGR infants is strongly associated with the cause of IUGR; with the timing, severity, and duration of the insult; and with perinatal complications the IUGR infant encounters (see Box 31-4). Early severe IUGR often reflects a chromosomal anomaly, other severe genetic disorder, or congenital infection that occurred early to cause organ malformation or significant injury. Some causes of IUGR result in death (e.g., trisomy 18) or severe disability. Some carry a high risk for neurodevelopmental disability (e.g., fetal alcohol syndrome). Others are associated with only mild disability (e.g., an increased incidence of attention and behavior problems in infants born to mothers who took narcotics or cocaine during pregnancy).

One of the most common causes of IUGR is uteroplacental insufficiency, generally a diagnosis of exclusion. The fetus responds in many adaptive ways when the supply of nutrients or oxygen is limited.[16,17] There is first a decrease in subcutaneous tissue, resulting in lower birth weight, and then a decrease in length, before head and brain growth are affected (symmetric growth restriction). Nevertheless, the problem may be severe enough to overwhelm these adaptations and lead to brain injury. In addition, a chronically compromised fetus, with decreased glycogen and nutrient stores, has more difficulty with the stresses of labor and delivery, leading to perinatal depression, cold stress, hypoglycemia, and hypocalcemia. Polycythemia may result from chronic intrauterine hypoxia but may result in the complications of hyperviscosity.[115]

Prospective studies of full-term infants with IUGR do not show an increased risk for major disability, but retrospective studies of CP and MR have demonstrated that more disabled children had IUGR than was expected.[3] Prospective studies of full-term IUGR school-age children compared with full-term AGA children showed that more IUGR children had language problems, learning disability, minor neuromotor dysfunction, hyperactivity, and attention and behavior problems. Postnatal growth may also be affected, but this will largely depend on whether the infant has symmetric or asymmetric IUGR. **Preterm IUGR children demonstrate the disadvantages of both prematurity and IUGR, but which is more important in determining outcomes is not clear.** The degree of IUGR may influence early delivery, either spontaneous or induced, because of concerns of fetal well-being. The most striking findings in studies of preterm IUGR children and preterm AGA controls are the high rates of major disability (7% to 23%) and LDs (36% to 50%).[80]

Extrauterine growth restriction, that is delayed growth after birth, also occurs commonly in ill preterm newborns.[36,116] The long-term effects of this early delayed growth have been unclear.[74] However, infants in the lower quartiles of growth in the NICU have higher incidences of neurodevelopmental impairment at 18 to 22 months follow-up in the NICHD-Neonatal Research Network. Although markers of illness severity such as NEC or BPD had a significant effect on outcome, poor postnatal growth itself may exert an independent effect.[47] **Post-discharge growth failure for preterm infants is also a common problem, especially in those with associated CLD. Transitional formulas, occasionally with caloric concentration, may be needed to optimize growth and subsequent development.**[46,61]

Neonatal Encephalopathy

The extent and nature of an initial hypoxic-ischemic event cannot be easily determined for individual infants, leading clinicians to rely on recognizable signs and symptoms of neonatal encephalopathy to predict outcome. These signs and symptoms include the following:

- Poor feeding
- Hypotonia or extensor hypertonia
- Lethargy or hyperexcitability
- Apnea
- Seizures
- Abnormalities on neuroimaging studies, which are far more predictive than low Apgar scores
- The need for positive pressure ventilation or CPR at birth
- Initial response to resuscitation

Many infants with congenital brain malformations or prenatal brain injury may present with perinatal cardiorespiratory depression. They do not breathe normally at birth and may require positive-pressure ventilation or further resuscitation. It is very difficult to distinguish these infants from those with encephalopathy caused by hypoxia or ischemia. Metabolic problems or neonatal sepsis may also present with these signs. Therefore the term ***neonatal encephalopathy*** **is preferred over the term** ***hypoxic-ischemic encephalopathy (HIE),*** **because etiology cannot always be determined with certainty.** However, the clinician must evaluate the history and relevant factors in each infant to address the etiology of their encephalopathy. The etiology may be important in decisions about treatment, prognosis, and follow-up, as well as for family planning.

In the absence of a confirmed specific etiology, the stages of encephalopathy described in 1976 by Sarnat and Sarnat remain highly predictive of outcome.[120] Infants with stage 3 (severe) encephalopathy and coma, severe hypotonia or increased extensor tone, intermittent decerebration, decreased or absent reflexes, variable pupil reactivity, and abnormal electroencephalogram (EEG) generally will die or have multiple severe disabilities. Only 20% to 30% of infants with stage 2 (moderate) encephalopathy with lethargy or coma, mild hypotonia, overactive reflexes, seizures, abnormal EEG, and generalized parasympathetic function (constricted pupils, bradycardia, profuse secretions, and diarrhea) have multiple severe disabilities. The remainder of newborns with stage 2 encephalopathy have lower scores on tests of cognition, vocabulary, reading, spelling, and arithmetic than children with stage 1 (mild) encephalopathy (hyperalert state, jitteriness, overactivity and easily elicited reflexes, increased sympathetic function, dilated pupils, and decreased gastrointestinal motility) or healthy control children. Infants with neonatal encephalopathy should be evaluated with both EEGs and neuroimaging studies. Very-low-voltage EEG patterns (signifying little brain activity) and burst-suppression EEG patterns carry an extremely poor prognosis, as does diffuse encephalomalacia detected by MRI.[108,128] Infants with moderate encephalopathy may benefit from the newer technique of hypothermic treatment, commonly called "cooling," (see Chapter 26) leading to increased survival without disability. The results from all published trials in North America and Europe are most promising for encephalopathies of less than a severe nature.[24,63,122] Mild encephalopathy with only a subarachnoid hemorrhage carries a good prognosis, although these children should be monitored for later subtle learning difficulties.

Infants with ischemic perinatal stroke are another group of infants with brain injury who are at risk for long-term developmental sequelae. This entity is generally distinctly different from diffuse ischemia seen in the so-called "watershed" injury of perinatal HIE. Timing of the event may also be less easily determined, but the infant may present with focal or generalized seizures or less-defined clinical signs such as poor perfusion ("dusky" or "gray" spells), respiratory distress or apnea, poor feeding, or low neuromotor tone in the first few days of life. MRI is the most reliable method of diagnostic detection in the newborn period if timed appropriately. Neurologic deficits have been reported in 50% to 75% of survivors, and hemiplegic CP is most commonly found. Later difficulties with sensory impairment or learning difficulties are also present, thus requiring long-term follow-up.[107]

Persistent Pulmonary Hypertension of the Newborn/Meconium Aspiration Syndrome

PPHN and MAS often overlap clinically, and many of these infants require neonatal intensive care technologies, including inhaled nitric oxide, high-frequency ventilation, and ECMO. Full-term survivors of this care have an increased risk for major disability (2% to 26%) and milder impairments (8% to 49%), including minor neuromotor dysfunction, borderline intelligence, language delay, and attention problems.[43,59] Both CLD (seen in 7% to 40%) and hearing impairment (seen in 20% to 50%) are common sequelae of PPHN or ECMO. Most recent studies of ECMO that include venovenous as opposed to venoarterial flow report a lower incidence (≈15%) of developmental disabilities. In the past decade, inhaled nitric oxide has become a more common treatment of pulmonary hypertension in the newborn, and follow-up studies indicate that these infants have a developmental disability rate of 14% to 19%.[38,50] Because the hearing impairment associated with either PPHN or ECMO may be progressive, serial hearing evaluations during infancy and early childhood are required.[56]

Bronchopulmonary Dysplasia/ Chronic Lung Disease

BPD or chronic lung disease (CLD) is the most common morbidity in surviving preterm infants.[55] The etiology of neonatal lung injury appears to have changed over time as methods of treatment of respiratory failure have changed and as an increasing number of extremely immature preterm infants survive.[26,72] **Regardless of specific cause, the risk for pulmonary hypertension, post-discharge growth failure, recurrent hospitalizations, and adverse neurodevelopmental outcomes persists in children with BPD.**[19,78,100,124,125] Many of these infants exhibit low tone and early motor delays, often consistent with developmental coordination disorder.[69] Cerebral palsy is highly associated with infants of extremely low birth weight, as is BPD, but varies in infants with BPD from 11% to 27% based on severity of BPD. Likewise, lower cognitive scores are related to severity of BPD and may be present in 50% of infants with severe BPD.[48,124]

TRACKING HEALTH OUTCOMES: THE PRIMARY CARE PROVIDER

Primary Care Follow-up

At the time of discharge, the NICU staff must provide the primary care pediatrician and the parents with a complete and accurate history of the child's NICU course including recommendations for ongoing care. Special health concerns, specific to the premature infant, should be closely monitored and surveillance of these should supplement the AAP guidelines for preventive, "well-child" care. These additional areas of special concern for the premature infant would include such things as the following:

- Neurodevelopmental follow-up
- Visual and hearing outcomes
- Growth, nutrition, and feeding issues
- Osteopenia of prematurity
- Dental enamel defects
- Sequelae related to issues during hospitalization including pulmonary, gastrointestinal, hematologic, and surgical conditions

Along with the subspecialty medical follow-up, **the primary care provider will also need to coordinate other supportive services such as early intervention programs and developmental follow-up through an NICU follow-up program, if available.**[34] **Recommendations for specialized follow-up of the late preterm infant have also been proposed with the focus on feeding, sleeping, temperature regulation, jaundice, and infection in an effort to reduce post-hospital morbidities and rehospitalization of these infants.**[52,143]

Growth, Nutrition, and Feeding

Premature infants are at increased risk for growth deficits after discharge—many are discharged below the body weight of their healthy term counterparts. **The failure to achieve adequate growth is known as *extrauterine growth restriction (EUGR)* and is defined by weight less than the 10th percentile for CGA at the time of discharge.**[116] These infants remain at risk for long-term adverse health and neurodevelopmental outcomes. As such, early nutrition and feeding support are essential.

Recommendations from the European Society for Paediatric Gastroenterology, Hepatology and Nutrition (ESPGHAN) Committee on Nutrition support breast feeding of AGA infants or formula with long-chain polyunsaturated fatty acids for formula-fed, appropriately grown infants.[54] **For those infants with evidence of growth deficits present at discharge (EUGR), breast milk should be supplemented with a human milk fortifier. Formula-fed infants should receive a special post-discharge formula, with increased protein, minerals, and long-chain polyunsaturated fatty acids, for at least the first 9 months.**[8] Serial measurements of head circumference, weight, length, and weight/length ratio should be closely monitored.[130]

Some infants do not achieve full breast feeding before discharge. It is essential, therefore, to provide **clear verbal and written instruction to the breast-feeding mother about how to assess her infant's hydration status if the transition from partial to full breast feeding is to occur at home, along with ensuring that the mother has access to medically sound breast-feeding support from the child's pediatrician or a qualified lactation consultant.**

Although premature infants are at an increased risk for childhood obesity and the metabolic syndrome associated with excess weight gain, this risk is thought to be small when compared with the risk for growth failure and should be considered with other risk factors such as parental size, adolescent weight, and lifestyle factors.[61] Nutritional status should be monitored closely to intervene for either deficient or excessive weight variations.

Medically Fragile and Chronically Ill Infants

Increasing survival of infants with post-NICU morbidities, including those associated with congenital diaphragmatic hernia (CDH), short bowel syndrome, and others, has increased the need for detailed parent training, home health care arrangements, and comprehensive, coordinated, multidisciplinary follow-up. The AAP has recently issued extensive follow-up guidelines for infants with CDH including monitoring neurodevelopment, managing pulmonary morbidities such as pulmonary hypertension and chronic lung disease, assessing hearing function at regular intervals, providing early therapies for feeding difficulties such as oral aversion and gastroesophageal reflux, and monitoring for hernia recurrence, which have been reported in 8% to 50% of CDH infants.[14] Brodsky and Ouellette recommend close monitoring of infants with a history of NEC and/or short bowel syndrome to include neurodevelopmental delays; growth, nutrition, and feeding concerns; dehydration and electrolyte imbalances; and signs of associated complications such as infection, late strictures, and cholestatic liver disease.[34]

LONG-TERM NEURODEVELOPMENTAL FOLLOW-UP

During hospitalization, parents may ask questions about outcome that simply cannot be answered. **Although the infant's risk for cognitive and motor impairment should be discussed, parents must understand that the certain diagnosis of developmental delay or disability cannot be made before 12 to 24 months of age. This need to "wait and see" creates an additional burden for families that the NICU staff should help the family anticipate.** Referral to a multidisciplinary developmental follow-up clinic should provide the family with ongoing information about their child's progress and give parents the opportunity to speak with professionals about their concerns. These clinics often provide families with concrete, focused tasks to undertake with their child that may optimize infant development and help parents feel they are contributing to their child's success.

An additional concern that has more recently surfaced is even longer-term outcome issues for high-risk children. Because many children may be seen once for a multidisciplinary evaluation (18 to 24 months corrected age) or may not be followed beyond 3 to 5 years of age in the NICU follow-up clinic, it is important that parents be informed before release from specialty follow-up care about longer-term concerns regarding health and development, especially possible challenges with academics and social-emotional issues.[64,93,94,151]

Pediatric health care professionals need to be aware also that recent reports delineate some more lifelong impacts on the former NICU patient's quality of life as a child and adolescent, daily personal and social functions, and overall experiences with health and disease. Although much of this information may be speculative and studies remain ongoing, it is nonetheless important to inform the family that their child's long-term health and quality of life issues may relate to their child with a history of prematurity, regardless of the developmental status of the child when seen in the first few years of life.

REFERENCES

1. Accardo PJ: *Capute and Accardo's neurodevelopmental disabilities in infancy and childhood,* ed 3, Baltimore, Md, 2008, Paul H Brookes.
2. Adams-Chapman I: Neurodevelopmental outcome of the late preterm infant, *Clin Perinatol* 33:947, 2006.
3. Allen MC: Preterm outcomes research: a critical component of neonatal intensive care, *Ment Retard Dev Disabil Res Rev* 8:22, 2002.
4. American Academy of Pediatrics: Transporting children with special health care needs, *Pediatrics* 104:988, 1999.
5. American Academy of Pediatrics, Committee on Fetus and Newborn: Apnea, sudden infant death syndrome, and home monitoring, *Pediatrics* 111:914, 2003.
6. American Academy of Pediatrics, Committee on Fetus and Newborn: Hospital discharge of the high-risk neonate, *Pediatrics* 122:1119, 2008.
7. American Academy of Pediatrics, Committee on Injury and Poison Prevention: Safe transportation of newborns at hospital discharge, *Pediatrics* 104:986, 1999.
8. American Academy of Pediatrics, Committee on Nutrition: Nutritional needs of the preterm infant.

In Kleinman RE, editor: *Pediatric nutrition handbook*, ed 5, Elk Grove Village, Ill, 2004, The Academy.

9. American Academy of Pediatrics, Committee on Injury and Poison Prevention and Committee on Fetus and Newborn: Safe transportation of preterm and low birth weight infants at hospital discharge, *Pediatrics* 123:1424, 2009.
10. American Academy of Pediatrics, Council on Children with Disabilities: Care coordination in the medical home: integrating health and related systems of care for children with special health care needs, *Pediatrics* 116:1238, 2005.
11. American Academy of Pediatrics, Joint Committee on Infant Hearing, Year 2007 Position Statement: Principles and guidelines for early hearing detection and intervention programs, *Pediatrics* 120:898, 2007.
12. American Academy of Pediatrics, Newborn Screening Authoring Committee: Newborn screening expands: recommendations for pediatricians and medical homes—implications for the system, *Pediatrics* 121:192, 2008.
13. American Academy of Pediatrics, Section on Ophthalmology: Screening examination of premature infants for retinopathy of prematurity, *Pediatrics* 117:572, 2006.
14. American Academy of Pediatrics, Section on Surgery and the Committee on Fetus and Newborn: Postdischarge follow-up of infants with congenital diaphragmatic hernia, *Pediatrics* 121:627, 2008.
15. Amiel-Tison C, Allen MC, Lebrun F, et al: Macropremies: underprivileged newborns, *Ment Retard Dev Disabil Res* 8:281, 2002.
16. Amiel-Tison C, Cabrol D, Denver R, et al: Fetal adaptation to stress. I. Acceleration of fetal maturation and earlier birth triggered by placental insufficiency in humans, *Early Hum Dev* 78:15, 2004.
17. Amiel-Tison C, Cabrol D, Denver R, et al: Fetal adaptation to stress. II. Evolutionary aspects; stress-induced hippocampal damage; long-term effects on behavior; consequences on adult health, *Early Hum Dev* 78:81, 2004.
18. Amiel-Tison C, Gosselin J: *Neurological development from birth to six years,* Baltimore, Md, 2001, Johns Hopkins University Press.
19. Anderson PJ, Doyle LW: Neurodevelopmental outcome of bronchopulmonary dysplasia, *Semin Perinatol* 30:227, 2006.
20. Anderson PJ, Doyle LW: Cognitive and educational deficits in children born extremely preterm, *Semin Perinatol* 32:51, 2008.
21. Arnaud C, Daubisse-Marliac L, White-Koning M, et al: Prevalence and associated factors of minor neuromotor dysfunctions at age 5 years in prematurely born children, *Arch Pediatr Adolesc Med* 161:1053, 2007.
22. Arzoumanian Y, Mirmiran M, Barnes PD, et al: Diffusion tensor brain imaging findings at term-equivalent age may predict neurologic abnormalities in low birth weight preterm infants, *AJNR Am J Neuroradiol* 24:1646, 2003.
23. Aylward, GP: Cognitive and neuropsychological outcomes: more than IQ scores, *Ment Retard Dev Disabil Res Rev* 8:234, 2002.
24. Azzopardi D, Edwards AD: Hypothermia, *Semin Fetal Neonatal Med* 12:303, 2007.
25. Back SA, Riddle A, McClure MM: Maturation-dependent vulnerability of perinatal white matter in premature birth, *Stroke* 38(Suppl 2):724, 2007.
26. Bancalari E, Claure N: Definitions and diagnostic criteria for bronchopulmonary dysplasia, *Semin Perinatol* 30:164, 2006.
27. Bayley N: *Bayley scales of infant and toddler development*, ed 3, San Antonio, Tex, 2006, The Psychological Corporation.
28. Bhutta AT, Cleves MA, Casey PH, et al: Cognitive and behavioral outcomes of school-aged children who were born preterm: a meta-analysis, *JAMA* 288:728, 2002.
29. Bhutta ZA, Khan I, Salat S, et al: Reducing length of stay in hospital for very low birthweight infants by involving mothers in a stepdown unit: an experience from Karachi (Pakistan), *BMJ* 329:1151, 2004.
30. Blair E, Watson L: Epidemiology of cerebral palsy, *Semin Fetal Neonatal Med* 11:117, 2006.
31. Bonnier C: Evaluation of early stimulation programs for enhancing brain development, *Acta Paediatr* 97:853, 2008.
32. Bos AF, Einspieler C, Prechtl HF: Intrauterine growth retardation, general movements, and neurodevelopmental outcome: a review, *Dev Med Child Neurol* 43:61, 2001.
33. Bracewell M, Marlow N: Patterns of motor disability in very preterm children, *Ment Retard Dev Disabil Res Rev* 8:241, 2002.
34. Brodsky D, Ouellette M, editors: *Primary care of the premature infant*, Philadelphia, 2008, Saunders.
35. Carnevale FA, Alexander E, Davis M, et al: Daily living with distress and enrichment: the moral experience of families with ventilator-assisted children at home, *Pediatrics* 117:e48, 2006.
36. Casey PH: Growth of low birth weight preterm children, *Semin Perinatol* 32:20, 2008.
37. Centers for Disease Control and Prevention: Recommended immunization schedules for persons aged 0-18 years—United States, *MMWR* 56(51&52):Q1, 2008.
38. Clark RH, Huckaby JL, Kueser TJ, et al: Low-dose nitric oxide therapy for persistent pulmonary hypertension: 1-year follow-up, *J Perinatol* 23(4):300, 2003.
39. Costello A, Chapman J: Mother's perceptions of the care-by-parent program prior to hospital discharge of their preterm infants, *Neonatal Netw* 17:37, 1998.
40. Dahle AJ, Fowler KB, Wright JD, et al: Longitudinal investigation of hearing disorders in children with

congenital cytomegalovirus, *J Am Acad Audiol* 11:283, 2000.

41. Davis L, Edwards H, Mohay H, et al: The impact of very premature birth on the psychological health of mothers, *Early Hum Dev* 73:61, 2003.
42. Davis NM, Ford GW, Anderson PJ, et al, and the Victorian Infant Collaborative Study Group: Developmental coordination disorder at 8 years of age in a regional cohort of extremely-low-birth-weight or very preterm infants, *Dev Med Child Neurol* 49:325, 2007.
43. Desai SA, Stanley C, Gringlas M, et al: Five-year follow-up of neonates with reconstructed right common carotid arteries after extracorporeal membrane oxygenation, *J Pediatr* 134:428, 1999.
44. Donohue PK, Hussey-Gardner B, Sulpar LJ, et al: Parents' perception of the back-transport of very-low-birth-weight infants to community hospitals, *J Perinatol* 29(8):575, 2009.
45. Doyle LW: Outcome at 5 years of age of children 23 to 27 weeks' gestation: refining the prognosis, *Pediatrics* 108:134, 2001.
46. Dusick AM, Pindexter BB, Ehrenkranz RA, et al: Growth failure in the preterm infant: can we catch up? *Semin Perinatol* 27:302, 2003.
47. Ehrenkranz RA, Dusick AM, Vohr BR, et al: Growth in the neonatal intensive care unit influences neurodevelopmental and growth outcomes of extremely low birth weight infants, *Pediatrics* 117:1253, 2006.
48. Ehrenkranz RA, Walsh MD, Vohr BR, et al: Validation of the National Institutes of Health consensus definition of bronchopulmonary dysplasia, *Pediatrics* 116:1353, 2005.
49. Eichenwald EC, Blackwell M, Lloyd JS: Inter-neonatal intensive care unit variation in discharge timing: influence of apnea and feeding management, *Pediatrics* 108:928, 2001.
50. Ellington M, O'Reilly D, Allred EN, et al: Child health status, neurodevelopmental outcome, and parental satisfaction in a randomized, controlled trial of nitric oxide for persistent pulmonary hypertension of the newborn, *Pediatrics* 107:1351, 2001.
51. Ellison PH, Daily DK: The neurologic examination of the preterm and full-term neonate and of the infant. In David RB, editor: *Child and adolescent neurology,* ed 2, Oxford, UK, 2005, Blackwell Publishing.
52. Engle WA, Tomashek KM, Wallman C: Late-preterm infants: a population at risk, *Pediatrics* 120:1390, 2007.
53. Escobar GJ, Clark RH, Greene JD: Short-term outcomes of infants born at 35 and 36 weeks gestation: we need to ask more questions, *Semin Perinatol* 30:28, 2006.
54. ESPGHAN Committee on Nutrition: Feeding preterm infants after hospital discharge: a commentary by the ESPGHAN Committee on Nutrition, *J Pediatr Gastroenterol Nutr* 42:596, 2006.
55. Fanaroff AA, Stoll BJ, Wright LL, et al: Trends in neonatal morbidity and mortality for very low birthweight infants, *Am J Obstet Gynecol* 196:147.e1, 2007.
56. Fligor BJ, Neault MW, Mullen CH, et al: Factors associated with sensorineural hearing loss among survivors of extracorporeal membrane oxygenation therapy, *Pediatrics* 115:1519, 2005.
57. Garel M, Dardennes M, Blondel B: Mothers' psychological distress 1 year after very preterm childbirth: results of the EPIPAGE qualitative study, *Child Care Health Dev* 33:137, 2007.
58. Glascoe FP: Screening for developmental and behavioral problems, *MRDD Res Reviews* 11:173, 2005.
59. Glass P, Bulas DI, Wagner AE, et al: Severity of brain injury following neonatal extracorporeal membrane oxygenation and outcome at age 5 years, *Dev Med Child Neurol* 39:441, 1997.
60. Greenberg JM: The challenge of car safety seats, *J Pediatr* 150:215, 2007.
61. Greer FR: Post-discharge nutrition: what does the evidence support?, *Semin Perinatol* 31:89, 2007.
62. Griffin T, Abraham M: Transition to home from the newborn intensive care unit: applying the principles of family-centered care to the discharge process, *J Perinat Neonatal Nurs* 20:243, 2006.
63. Gunn AJ, Wyatt JS, Whitelaw A, et al: Therapeutic hypothermia changes the prognostic value of clinical evaluation of neonatal encephalopathy, *J Pediatr* 152:55, 2008.
64. Hack M: Young adult outcomes of very low birth weight children, *Semin Fetal Neonatal Med* 11:127, 2006.
65. Hack M, Wilson-Costello D, Friedman H, et al: Neurodevelopment and predictors of outcomes of children with birth weights of less than 1000 g: 1992-1995, *Arch Pediatr Adolesc Med* 154:725, 2000.
66. Hanrahan K, Gates M, Attar MA, et al: Neonatal back transport: perspectives from parents of Medicaid-insured infants and providers, *Neonatal Netw* 26:301, 2007.
67. Hart AR, Whitby EW, Griffiths PD, et al: Magnetic resonance imaging and developmental outcome following preterm birth: review of current evidence, *Dev Med Child Neurol* 50:655, 2008.
68. Hoekstra RE, Ferrara TB, Couser RJ, et al: Survival and long-term neurodevelopmental outcome of extremely premature infants born at 23-26 weeks' gestation age at a tertiary center, *Pediatrics* 113:e1, 2004.
69. Holsti L, Granau R, Whitfield MF: Developmental coordination disorder in extremely low birth weight children at nine years, *J Dev Behav Pediatr* 23:9, 2002.
70. Hummel P, Cronin J: Home care of the high-risk infant, *Adv Neonatal Care* 4:354, 2004.

71. Individuals with Disabilities Education Act (IDEA): 2004, website: http://idea.ed.gov/.
72. Jobe AH: The new BPD, *NeoReviews* 7:e531, 2006.
73. Johnson S: Cognitive and behavioural outcomes following very preterm birth, *Semin Fetal Neonatal Med* 12:363, 2007.
74. Kan E, Roberts G, Anderson PJ, and the Victorian Infant Collaborative Study Group: The association of growth impairment with neurodevelopmental outcome at eight years of age in very preterm children, *Early Hum Dev* 84:409, 2008.
75. Kaufman AS, Kaufman NL: *Kaufman assessment battery for children*, ed 2, Circle Pines, Minn, 2004, AGS Publishing.
76. Khadilkar V, Tudehope D, Burns Y, et al: The long-term neurodevelopmental outcome for very low birthweight (VLBW) infants with "dystonic" signs at 4 months of age, *J Paediatr Child Health* 29(6):415, 1993.
77. Kinane TB, Murphy J, Bass JL, et al: Comparison of respiratory physiologic features when infants are placed in car safety seats or car beds, *Pediatrics* 118:522, 2006.
78. Kobaly K, Schluchter M, Minich N, et al: Outcomes of extremely low birth weight (<1 kg) and extremely low gestational age (<28 weeks) infants with bronchopulmonary dysplasia: effects of practice changes in 2000 to 2003, *Pediatrics* 121:73, 2008.
79. Lainwala S, Perritt R, Poole K, et al: Neurodevelopmental and growth outcomes of extremely low birth weight infants who are transferred from neonatal intensive care units to level I or level II nurseries, *Pediatrics* 119:e1079, 2007.
80. Leonard H, Nassar N, Bourke J, et al: Relation between intrauterine growth and subsequent intellectual disability in a ten-year population cohort of children in Western Australia, *Am J Epidemiol* 167:103, 2007.
81. Lorenz JM: The outcome of extreme prematurity, *Semin Perinatol* 25:348, 2001.
82. Lovette B: Safe transportation for children with special needs, *J Pediatr Health Care* 22:323, 2008.
83. Marlow N: Neurocognitive outcome after very preterm birth, *Arch Dis Child Fetal Neonatal Ed* 89:F224, 2004.
84. Marlow N: Outcome following extremely preterm birth, *Curr Obstet Gynaecol* 16:141, 2006.
85. McCormick MC, Brooks-Gunn J, Buka SL, et al: Early intervention in low birth weight premature infants: results at 18 years of age for the Infant Health and Development Program, *Pediatrics* 117:771, 2006.
86. Melnyk BM, Feinstein NF, Alpert-Gillis L, et al: Reducing premature infants' length of stay and improving parents' mental health outcomes with the Creating Opportunities for Parent Empowerment (COPE) neonatal intensive care unit program: a randomized, controlled trial, *Pediatrics* 118:e1414, 2006.
87. Ment LR, Vohr BR: Preterm birth and the developing brain, *Lancet Neurol* 7:378, 2008.
88. Mercuri E, Rutherford M, Barnett A, et al: MRI lesions and infants with neonatal encephalopathy: is the Apgar score predictive? *Neuropediatrics* 33:150, 2002.
89. Merritt TA, Pillers D, Prows SL: Early NICU discharge of very low birth weight infants: a critical review and analysis, *Semin Neonatol* 8:95, 2003.
90. Mirmiran M, Barnes PD, Keller K, et al: Neonatal brain magnetic resonance imaging before discharge is better than serial cranial ultrasound in predicting cerebral palsy in very low birth weight preterm infants, *Pediatrics* 114:992, 2004.
91. Montagnino BA, Mauricio RV: The child with a tracheostomy and gastrostomy: parental stress and coping in the home—a pilot study, *Pediatr Nurs* 30:373, 2004.
92. Msall ME: The panorama of cerebral palsy after very and extremely preterm birth: evidence and challenges, *Clin Perinatol* 33:269, 2006.
93. Msall ME, Park JJ: The spectrum of behavioral outcomes after extreme prematurity: regulatory, attention, social, and adaptive dimensions, *Semin Perinatol* 32:42, 2008.
94. Msall ME, Tremont MR: Measuring functional outcomes after prematurity: developmental impact of very low birth weight and extremely low birth weight status on childhood disability, *Ment Retard Dev Disabil Res Rev* 8:258, 2004.
95. Norr KF, Crittenden KS, Lehrer EL, et al: Maternal and infant outcomes at one year for a nurse-health advocate home visiting program serving African Americans and Mexican Americans, *Public Health Nurs* 20:190, 2003.
96. O'Connor AR, Fielder AR: Visual outcomes and perinatal adversity, *Semin Fetal Neonatal Med* 12:408, 2007.
97. O'Connor AR, Fielder AR: Long term ophthalmic sequelae of prematurity, *Early Hum Dev* 84:101, 2008.
98. Ohgi S, Fukuda M, Akiyama T, et al: Effect of an early intervention programme on low birthweight infants with cerebral injuries, *J Paediatr Child Health* 40:689, 2004.
99. O'Shea M: Cerebral palsy, *Semin Perinatol* 32:35, 2008.
100. O'Shea TM, Goldstein DJ, deRegnier RA, et al: Outcome at 4 to 5 years of age in children recovered from neonatal chronic lung disease, *Dev Med Child Neurol* 38:830, 1996.
101. Palisano R, Rosenbaum P, Walter S, et al: Development and reliability of a system to classify gross motor function in children with cerebral palsy, *Dev Med Child Neurol* 39:214, 1997.
102. Paul IM, Phillips TA, Widome MD, et al: Cost-effectiveness of postnatal home nursing visits for prevention of hospital care for jaundice and dehydration, *Pediatrics* 114:1015, 2004.

103. Petrini JR, Dias T, McCormick MC, et al: Increased risk of adverse neurological development for late preterm infants, *J Pediatr* 154:169, 2009.
104. Picciolini O, Gianni ML, Vegni C, et al: Usefulness of an early neurofunctional assessment in predicting neurodevelopmental outcome in very low birthweight infants, *Arch Dis Child Fetal Neonatal Ed* 91:F111, 2006.
105. Pilley E, McGuire W: The car seat: a challenge too far for preterm infants? *Arch Dis Child Fetal Neonatal Ed* 90:F452, 2005.
106. Pilley E, McGuire W: Pre-discharge "car seat challenge" for preventing morbidity and mortality in preterm infants, *Cochrane Database Syst Rev* 1: CD005386, 2008.
107. Raju TN, Nelson KG, Ferriero D, et al, and the NICH-NINDS Perinatal Stroke Workshop Participants: Ischemic perinatal stroke: summary of a workshop sponsored by the National Institute of Child Health and Human Development and the National Institute of Neurological Disorders and Stroke, *Pediatrics* 120:609, 2007.
108. Rennie JM, Hagmann CF, Robertson NJ: Outcome after intrapartum hypoxic ischemia at term, *Semin Fetal Neonat Med* 12:398, 2007.
109. Rinaldo P, Lim JS, Tortorelli S, et al: Newborn screening of metabolic disorders: recent progress and future developments, *Nestle Nutr Workshop Ser Pediatr Program* 62:81, 2008.
110. Rivera LB, Boppana SB, Fowler KB, et al: Predictors of hearing loss in children with symptomatic congenital cytomegalovirus infection, *Pediatrics* 110:762, 2002.
111. Robison M, Pirak C, Morrell C: Multidisciplinary discharge assessment of the medically and socially high-risk infant, *J Perinat Neonatal Nurs* 13:67, 2000.
112. Roid GH: *Stanford-Binet Intelligence Scales*, ed 5, Itasca, Ill, 2003, Riverside Publishing.
113. Romantseva L, Msall MM: Advances in understanding cerebral palsy syndromes after prematurity, *NeoReviews* 7:575, 2006.
114. Rosenbaum P, Paneth N, Leviton A, et al: A report: the definition and classification of cerebral palsy—April 2006, *Dev Med Child Neurol* 49(Suppl 109):8, 2006.
115. Rosenberg A: The IUGR newborn, *Semin Perinatol* 32:219, 2008.
116. Ruth VA: Extrauterine growth restriction: a review of the literature, *Neonatal Netw* 27:177, 2008.
117. Saenz P, Cerda M, Cordobes JL, et al: Psychological stress of parents of preterm infants enrolled in an early discharge program from the neonatal intensive care unit: a prospective randomized trial, *Arch Dis Child Fetal Neonatal Ed* 94:F98, 2008.
118. Saigal S, Szatmari P, Rosenbaum P, et al: Cognitive abilities and school performance of extremely low birth weight children and matched term control children at age 8 years: a regional study, *J Pediatr* 118:751, 1991.
119. Salhab WA, Khattak A, Tyson JE, et al: Car seat or car bed for very low birth weight infants at discharge home, *J Pediatr* 150:224, 2007.
120. Sarnat HB, Sarnat MS: Neonatal encephalopathy following fetal distress: a clinical and electroencephalographic study, *Arch Neurol* 3:696, 1976.
121. Schiariti V, Klassen AF, Hoube JS, et al: Perinatal characteristics and parents' perspective of health status of NICU graduates born at term, *J Perinatol* 28:368, 2008.
122. Shankaran S: Neonatal encephalopathy: treatment with hypothermia, *Neurotrauma* 26:437, 2009.
123. Shevell M, Ashwal S, Donley D, et al: Practice parameter: evaluation of the child with global developmental delay—report of the Quality Standards Subcommittee of the American Academy of Neurology and The Practice Committee of the Child Neurology Society, *Neurology* 60:367, 2003.
124. Short EJ, Kirchner HL, Asaad GR, et al: Developmental sequelae in preterm infants having a diagnosis of bronchopulmonary dysplasia: analysis using a severity-based classification system, *Arch Pediatr Adolesc Med* 161:1082, 2007.
125. Singer L, Yamashita T, Lilien L, et al: A longitudinal study of developmental outcome of infants with bronchopulmonary dysplasia and very low birth weight, *Pediatrics* 100:987, 1997.
126. Sleifer P, da Costa SS, Coser PL, et al: Auditory brainstem response in premature and full-term children, *Int J Pediatr Otorhinolaryngol* 71:1449, 2007.
127. Spittle AJ, Orton J, Doyle LW, et al: Early developmental intervention programs post hospital discharge to prevent motor and cognitive impairments in preterm infants, *Cochrane Database Syst Rev* 2: CD005495, 2007.
128. Spitzmiller RE, Phillips T, Meinzen-Derr J, et al: Amplitude-integrated EEG is useful in predicting neurodevelopmental outcome in full-term infants with hypoxic-ischemic encephalopathy: a meta-analysis, *J Child Neurol* 22:1069, 2007.
129. Stoll BJ, Hansen NI, Adams-Chapman I, et al: Neurodevelopmental and growth impairment among extremely low-birth-weight infants with neonatal infection, *JAMA* 292:2357, 2004.
130. Sullivan MC, McGrath MM, Hawes K, et al: Growth trajectories of preterm infants: birth to 12 years, *J Pediatr Health Care* 22:83, 2008.
131. Temple RO, Pass RF, Boll TJ: Neuropsychological functioning in patients with asymptomatic congenital cytomegalovirus infection, *J Dev Behav Pediatr* 21:417, 2000.
132. Tomashek KM, Shapiro-Mendoza CK, Weiss J, et al: Early discharge among late preterm and term newborns and risk of neonatal morbidity, *Semin Perinatol* 30:61, 2006.
133. Tonkin SL, McIntosh CG, Nixon GM, et al: Can we reduce episodes of haemoglobin desaturation in

full-term babies restrained in car seats? *Acta Paediatr* 97:105, 2008.
134. U.S. Preventive Services Task Force: Universal screening for hearing loss in newborns: U.S. Preventive Services Task Force recommendation statement, *Pediatrics* 122:143, 2008.
135. Vohr BR: How should we report early childhood outcomes of very low birth weight infants? *Semin Fetal Neonatal Med* 12:355, 2007.
136. Vohr BR, Msall ME: Neuropsychological and functional outcomes of very low birth weight infants, *Semin Perinatol* 21:202, 1997.
137. Vohr BR, Wright LL, Dusick AM, et al: Neurodevelopmental and functional outcomes of extremely low birth weight infants in the National Institute of Child Health and Human Development Neonatal Research Network, 1993-1994, *Pediatrics* 105(6):1216, 2002.
138. Vohr BR, Wright LL, Hack M, et al: Follow-up care of high-risk infants, *Pediatrics* 114:1377, 2004.
139. Vohr BR, Wright LL, Poole WK, et al: Neurodevelopmental outcomes of extremely low birth weight infants <32 weeks' gestation between 1993 and 1998, *Pediatrics* 116:635, 2005.
140. Walker DM, Marlow N: Neurocognitive outcome following fetal growth restriction, *Arch Dis Child Fetal Neonatal Ed* 93:F322, 2008.
141. Wallon M, Kodjikian L, Binquet C, et al: Long-term ocular prognosis in 327 children with congenital toxoplasmosis, *Pediatrics* 113:1567, 2004.
142. Wang KK, Barnard A: Technology-dependent children and their families: a review, *J Adv Nurs* 45:36, 2004.
143. Wang ML, Dorer DJ, Fleming MP, et al: Clinical outcomes of near-term infants, *Pediatrics* 114:372, 2004.
144. Washington State Department of Health: *Low birth weight neonatal intensive care unit graduate: critical elements of care*, 2005, website: www.medicalhome.org.
145. Wechsler D: *The Wechsler Preschool and Primary Scale of Intelligence-III*, San Antonio, Tex, 2002, The Psychological Corporation.
146. Willis V: Parenting preemies, *Adv Neonatal Care* 8:221, 2008.
147. Wolraich ML: *Disorders of development and learning,* ed 3, Hamilton, Ontario, Canada, 2003, BC Decker.
148. Wood NS, Marlow N, Costeloe K, et al: Neurologic and developmental disability after extremely preterm birth. EPICure Study Group, *N Engl J Med* 343:378, 2000.
149. Woodward LJ, Anderson PJ, Austin NC, et al: Neonatal MRI to predict neurodevelopmental outcomes in preterm infants, *N Engl J Med* 355:685, 2006.
150. World Health Organization: *International Classification of Functioning, Disability and Health (ICF),* Geneva, 2001, The Organization.
151. Zwicker JG, Harris SR: Quality of life of formerly preterm and very low birth weight infants from preschool age to adulthood: a systematic review, *Pediatrics* 121:366, 2008.

RECOMMENDED RESOURCES

American Academy of Pediatrics (AAP): *Policies/recommendations,* Website: http://aappolicy.aappublications.org/.
Brodsky D, Ouellette MA, editors: *Primary care of the premature infant,* Philadelphia, 2008, Saunders.
Critical elements of care for the low birth weight neonatal intensive care graduate: guidelines for care and follow-up of NICU graduates, Website: www.medicalhome.org.
Davis D, Stein MT: *Parenting your premature baby and child: the emotional journey,* Golden, Colo, 2004, Fulcrum.
Developmental and Behavioral Pediatrics: *Information on pediatrics and developmental screening,* Website: www.dbpeds.org/
Individuals with Disabilities Education Act (IDEA): Website: http://idea.ed.gov/
Kenner C, McGrath J, editors: *Developmental care of newborns and infants,* St Louis, 2004, Mosby.

32 ETHICS, VALUES, AND PALLIATIVE CARE IN NEONATAL INTENSIVE CARE

JULIE R. SWANEY, NANCY ENGLISH, AND BRIAN S. CARTER

Clinical decision making is influenced by the values of the individuals involved. In the neonatal intensive care unit (NICU), these values include preserving life, decreasing morbidity, and relieving pain and suffering. Sound clinical skills and judgment, combined with societal and personal values, result in the art of clinical practice.

Technologic advances in medicine have benefited many patients. We are better able to prolong life; at the same time, we are more often in a position to make deliberate decisions about when and how death will occur. Concomitantly, it has become necessary for society to reassess whether the value of prolonging life conflicts with other values, such as relieving pain and suffering and reducing morbidity. In such cases, values of society, the family, and the health care professional necessarily enter into and influence the decision-making process.

Ethical reasoning insists that we understand the role of values, as well as medical data, in making decisions.

HISTORICAL OVERVIEW

Historically, ethical concerns in neonatal care focused on the risks and benefits of available technology (Table 32-1). An example is oxygen therapy with the offsetting dilemma that treatment could cause degrees of blindness or residual lung damage, whereas nontreatment might result in death or brain damage (1960s). Treatment of premature infants and those with birth defects became technically possible in the 1950s with development of infant ventilators and refined surgical techniques. Because these new technologies not only failed to eliminate all bad outcomes but also added new problems, controversies developed over when and how much to use them. Care of newborns with spinal cord defects is illustrative.

Zachary[80] and Shurtleff[65] advocated aggressive management, which increased survival rates but offered questionable quality of life for those more severely affected. Lorber[49,50] was less optimistic about the effects of aggressive management of infants with meningomyelocele and is recognized for his selective nontreatment of some of these infants. Today, open neural tube defects are routinely closed in the immediate neonatal period, and research is ongoing to assess the potential for fetal surgery to close these defects to mitigate long-term morbidity in what is clearly acknowledged as a nonlethal condition.[17]

Discussion of treatment of seriously ill newborns was stimulated by the 1973 publication of Duff and Campbell.[28] Their seminal article described the selective nontreatment or withdrawal of treatment for 43 seriously ill newborns at Yale–New Haven Hospital (between 1970 and 1972) whose "prognosis for meaningful life was extremely poor or hopeless." According to Duff and Campbell[28]:

> Both treatment and nontreatment constitute unsatisfactory dilemmas for everyone. When maximum treatment was viewed as unacceptable by families and physicians in our unit, there was a growing tendency to seek early death as a management option,[18] to avoid that cruel choice of gradual, often slow, but progressive deterioration of the child.

They recognized that most survivors of NICUs are healthy; however, they also recognized that some infants remain severely disabled by congenital

Please note that the **PURPLE** type in each chapter is intended to make it easier to identify clinically applicable material.

TABLE 32-1 SELECTED ISSUES IN PERINATAL/NEONATAL HISTORY OF ETHICAL IMPORT

TIME	FETAL DIAGNOSIS	FETAL THERAPY	NEONATAL THERAPY
1900s (early)			Temperature regulation, nutrition; limited survival in low-birth-weight and anomalous infants Recognition of congenital rubella syndrome Cardiovascular surgery in the newborn period Modern incubator developed Oxygen therapy for respiratory distress
1950s		Tocolysis (ETOH)	Erythroblastosis fetalis (EBF) (Rh) incompatibility recognized Oxygen toxicity recognized: retrolental fibroplasia/blindness in treated infants; cerebral palsy and mortality in those untreated Other iatrogenic diseases Antibiotic usage broadens
1960s	Placentocentesis Early ultrasonography Fetal heart rate monitoring Fetal scalp pH assessment Amniocentesis Chromosomal analysis	Intraperitoneal blood transfusion for EBF	Birth of "modern" neonatal intensive care units Field of teratology develops after thalidomide disaster Improved outcome for infants <2500 g Surgical management of meningomyelocele becomes an issue
1970s	Fetoscopy Real-time ultrasonography Improved structural, chromosomal, and metabolic diagnostics	Intravascular blood transfusion for EBF Beta-adrenergic agonists for tocolysis Corticosteroids for lung maturation Legalization of abortion	Continuous positive airway pressure, modern neonatal ventilator Improved outcome for infants <1500 g Bronchopulmonary dysplasia (BPD) recognized Problems of the very-low-birth-weight infant: intraventricular hemorrhage, bronchopulmonary dysplasia, necrotizing enterocolitis Total parenteral nutrition/hyperalimentation (TPN/HAL) becomes available Improved pediatric surgery Newborn metabolic screening
1980s	Chorionic villus sampling Cordocentesis Doppler flow studies of placenta and umbilical vessels New reproductive technology Alpha fetoprotein monitoring	Fetal surgery Prophylactic penicillin for group B streptococcus infection Treatment of fetal dysrhythmias via maternal medications	High-frequency ventilation Surfactant replacement therapy Improved survival in infants <1000 g Extracorporeal membrane oxygenation Intravenous immunoglobulin
1990s	Fetal cell isolation in maternal blood Polymerase chain reaction and genetic amplification		Liquid ventilation Recombinant erythropoietin Nitric oxide therapy
2000	First-trimester high-resolution ultrasonography	Further advances in fetal surgery (including that for nonlethal anomalies)	
2000-2010	Genetic testing Expanded perinatal, genetic, and metabolic screening	Potential genetic treatments	Sildenafil for pulmonary hypertension

ETOH, Alcohol.

malformations that, until recently, would have resulted in premature death. They were legitimately concerned about the quality of life for these infants and their families.

The majority of newborns treated in NICUs do grow up to lead active, productive lives, but not all fare well with even the most aggressive treatments.[40,41] Consequently, there is increasing concern over what is "appropriate" treatment of newborns, particularly seriously ill or disabled ones. Recognizing the risks and benefits of technology over 30 years ago, Eisenberg[30] stated, "At long last, we are beginning to ask, not *can* it be done, but *should* it be done."

Baby Doe (1982) and Baby Jane Doe (1983) became the focus of controversy over the issue of withholding treatment and nutrition from handicapped infants.[11,20,52,71] Today, new issues require our attention. Recent advances in fetal surgery raise the question of whether interventions for nonlethal conditions warrant the attendant risks of preterm birth and treatment postnatally in the NICU.[17] Assisted reproduction technologies (ARTs) contribute to increasingly greater numbers of very-low-birth-weight (VLBW) infants born as multiples (twins, triplets, and higher-order multifetal gestations) in NICUs. At what point these well-intended services should be restrained or curtailed to prevent prematurity and its associated morbidities poses new ethical questions.

Throughout this short but focused "history" of ethical issues in neonatal care, it has become increasingly apparent that there are significant issues about appropriate treatment and the limits of treatment.[37,53] Not only numerous issues but also many individuals are involved in the decision-making process about treatment and nontreatment options. More people become involved as technologic advances increase treatment options. Parents have always been presumed to be the best decision makers on their child's behalf. Health care providers also have been committed to providing what is in the best interests of their patients. Historically, decisions were made privately between parents and their physician. In the modern NICU, treatment goals and decisions are made in the context of a health care team composed of professionals from various moral communities who offer specialized input into the care of the neonate and the family. Parents must be included in the team, because their values are of paramount importance in establishing goals and making decisions about their infant's care. Societal concerns generally have focused on protecting infants against decisions that are detrimental to their best interests by statutes on child abuse and neglect. Professional groups such as the American Academy of Pediatrics (AAP),[7,8] the American College of Obstetricians and Gynecologists (ACOG),[9] and the Canadian Pediatric Society (CPS)[19] have now addressed these concerns in published guidelines for care of critically ill infants. Community groups[27,29,76] are addressing limitations of care for high-risk newborns as well. Clinical decision making is affected by parents, the health care team, professional groups, and society. Respect for clinical decision making, preferably made by parents and clinicians together, the appropriateness of care, and the protection of children against harm are constantly being balanced.

DEFINITION OF BIOETHICS

Ethics is the study of rational processes for determining the most morally desirable course of action in view of conflicting value choices. Ethics is a branch of philosophy that considers competing values to obtain the best possible outcome to a given situation. When values conflict and each value is morally justifiable, an ethical dilemma exists. For an ethical dilemma to exist, a real choice between possible courses of action must exist.

Bioethics seeks to determine the most morally desirable course of action in health care given the conflicting values inherent in varying treatment options.[10] Most often, when a conflict of values does not exist, moral conflict does not exist. That is, when the health care providers and parents all agree that it is most beneficial to an infant to not treat the infant aggressively and to allow the infant to die, no dilemma or conflict between them exists. Of course, that they agree does not mean that conflict does not exist with moral views of outside parties or principles. Regardless, the goal is to determine the most morally desirable course of action under a given set of circumstances.

THEORIES OF ETHICS

An ethical theory provides a basis for making morally appropriate decisions. There are many theories or approaches to ethics to consider. ***Principle-based ethics*** identifies fundamental principles that form the foundation of ethical deliberation. This approach emphasizes the centrality of principles and rules to determine moral duty. Principles commonly recognized are autonomy, beneficence, nonmaleficence, and justice.[14] ***Virtue ethics*** is character-based and, as such, identifies the virtues of the moral agents involved, rather than the applied principles, as essential to ethical outcome. Various views of the moral life emphasize different virtues as more primary than others. In modern bioethics, primary virtues include respect, fidelity, honesty, and benevolence. ***Casuistry is case-based ethics*** in which the claims, grounds, and warrants of a particular case are compared with similar cases. The basic question for moral casuistry is how a general moral precept is to be understood in similar sets of circumstances. ***Narrative ethics*** is story-based in which the narrative itself is a method of ethical reasoning. Every case has different "narratives" to consider, such as medical knowledge, personal identity, patient experience, and the doctor-patient relationship. Although the medical model may focus on disease, psychopathology, objectivity, and diagnosis, the narrative model may focus correspondingly on illness, "the person," subjective experience, and caring. ***Feminist ethics*** is relationship-based and considers primarily the ethics of care. All of these approaches are important to consider. Deciding which moral theory is operative is important to proceeding.

CLINICAL DILEMMAS IN THE NEONATAL INTENSIVE CARE UNIT

Personhood

Decision making in the NICU often revolves around the concept of personhood. When is one a person? Determining what this means depends on which moral community is consulted. Designation of personhood is morally significant because it determines whether and what duties and obligations are owed to a particular newborn.

Some communities believe personhood is present at the moment of conception; they equate "human" with "person." Shelp[64] refers to this as the "genetic theory of personhood." Others believe personhood depends on the presence or absence of certain basic human qualities. Shelp calls this moral theory "property based." Although with the latter theory there is agreement that the concept of personhood is nongenetic, there are differences about which qualities qualify for "person" status.

Fletcher[36] and Engelhardt[31] support the "property-based" stance. They believe that there are human lives that are "subpersonal." Fletcher said, "It is not what is natural but what is personal which has the first-order value in ethics."[36] Both researchers believe that neocortical function is necessary for personhood. Engelhardt[31] related qualities such as self-consciousness, rationality, and self-determination to personhood. He distinguished between persons in a moral sense and persons in a social sense. Infants are deemed persons only in a social sense, not a strict sense by which societal rights are obligatory. The rights of the infant, according to Engelhardt, are held in trust by his or her parents; therefore "decision(s) about treatment belong properly to the parents because the child belongs to them in a sense that it does not belong to anyone else, even to itself."[31]

Tooley[70] suggested that "The ability to see oneself as existing over time is a necessary condition for the possession of a right to life."[45] If Tooley's reasoning is correct, then no infant has a right to life, at least not for some time. Although the "pro-life" moral community assigns person status to all with potential life, Tooley denied that potential has anything to do with a right to life. He advocated a quality-of-life standard. When a life is full of intractable pain and suffering, death is seen as a morally acceptable option. In fact, it is sometimes considered a relatively better outcome than continuing life.

Ramsey[60] and Robertson[62] held a contrasting view. For them, death is never better than life; quality-of-life assessments are not part of their moral reasoning. Life is considered sacred, an absolute good. Both the fetus and newborn are considered persons with a right to live. Therefore "death must always be imposed nonhumanly by God or nature or some other cosmic arbiter."[36] This "pro-life" position supports the moral right of deformed fetuses and deformed newborns to whatever care would be given a normal infant, implying that abortion and infanticide are morally reprehensible. If antibiotics would be given to a normal infant, then they also must be administered to a newborn infant with trisomy 18.

If one is deemed a "person," then society owes one certain obligations and expects certain duties. If one is not deemed a "person," then it is morally reasonable for societal benefits to be withheld or withdrawn. Whatever justification is needed for a particular moral dilemma in the NICU extends from this beginning. Clearly, there is no final definition of personhood, and differing definitions must be considered.

Patienthood

A primary problem confronting a perinatal clinician is this fundamental question: Who is the patient? The adult patient is generally competent and worthy of respect as a moral agent. However, in the case of a newborn, the newborn, the family, and in some circumstances, society have been variously considered the "patient." The accordance of rights to the newborn as an independent agent is a relatively recent occurrence. Neonatal cases are inextricably bound in the context of varying definitions of personhood and of complicated family and societal situations. This fundamental question remains: To whom is the moral duty owed? To the infant? To the family as "patient"? To society? If there are competing moral obligations, then it is essential to determine to whom the primary moral duty is owed.

Professional-Patient Relationship

The importance of the professional-patient relationship cannot be overestimated, because this is the human context in which decision making occurs. With neonates, this includes a relationship between parents as surrogates and the health care team.

When the four major principles—autonomy, beneficence, nonmaleficence, and justice—are applied to health care relationships, several moral rules can be derived. These moral rules include fidelity, truth telling, and confidentiality. The professional-patient relationship is considerably affected by the meaning and extent of these rules.

Fidelity, or promise keeping, may be derived from the principle of autonomy. The duty to keep promises may promote the greatest good (utilitarian) or be seen as an obligation (formalist). Many relationships between professionals and patients (or surrogates) involve promises or contracts, whether implicitly or explicitly made. For example, once professionals have established a relationship with a patient, their duty of fidelity includes not abandoning or neglecting that patient. An obvious problem in dealing with surrogates may be conflicting duties to the surrogates and the patient. Promises made by professionals are binding except when they are superseded by stronger obligations.

Truth telling, like fidelity, can be derived from the principle of autonomy or respect for persons. It assumes an implicit contract between parties that the truth will be told. At the heart of truth telling is trust, which gives professional-patient relationships their integrity. Lying violates implicit contracts, respect for persons, and trust. It also impedes informed consent.

Utilitarians and formalists may agree on the duty to tell the truth, although they may disagree on the duty not to deceive. Cases have been made for "benevolent deception," when intentional deception is morally justifiable if its primary intent is for the benefit of the patient. In such cases, telling the truth may be a violation of ***beneficence and nonmaleficence.*** Others argue that deception, benevolent or not, is morally wrong, because it violates respect for persons and trust. Ultimately, the professional-patient relationship erodes. Respect for persons involves acknowledging patient autonomy to know or not to know the truth of his or her particular situation.

It is generally agreed that ***confidentiality*** should prevail in professional-patient relationships. With minors, confidentiality extends to the parents or legal guardians. Part of the implied contract is that information gained by both parties will be kept confidential. From the earliest days of medicine, protecting the patient's privacy has been a fundamental tenet of clinical practice. There are, of course, instances in which confidentiality is justifiably breached. It is at this point that many ethical dilemmas arise.

Breach of confidentiality may be morally and legally justified to protect the life of a patient or the lives of others who may be endangered. The value of human life overrides the relationship, but the professional should be able to demonstrate clear danger before violating a patient's privacy. This also may be seen as a violation of autonomy. "The health care professional's breach of confidentiality thus cannot be justified unless it is necessary to meet a strong conflicting duty."[14]

Obviously, health care professionals can be torn between conflicting moral obligations, such as between the patient and society. Such instances in which a breach may be justified include child abuse and neglect and certain communicable diseases. However, there is strong justification among both utilitarians and formalists for maintaining the privacy and confidentiality of patient information. Most important, the genuine integrity of the professional-patient relationship will be enhanced and preserved when confidentiality, like fidelity and truth telling, is respected and upheld. This integrity of relationship then becomes the basis of the decision-making process.

Informed Consent

The issue of valid informed consent is repeatedly raised in the environment of the NICU. All relevant information for a decision must be given. Voluntary consent, free of coercion, by competent persons must be obtained. Information given to parents may be poorly understood for many reasons, including the complex nature of the information; the emotional or physical state of the parents after the birth of a sick, premature, or anomalous infant; physical separation of the parents from their newborn; and feelings of bewilderment and intimidation leading to uncontested paternalism. Indeed, there are indications that valid informed consent is an ideal toward which we work but one that, within the realities of practice, may rarely be obtained. Consent should be sought, however, and open lines of communication and parental education established to facilitate some level of understanding and enable more than token participation in decision making by the parents.[2,42,68]

One standard that has been put forth in an effort to accomplish informed consent is the "reasonable person standard." It asks, "What would a reasonable person want in this circumstance?"

There are several ways in which the ***reasonable person standard*** might be enacted in the NICU, thus ensuring that more valid informed consent is obtained. First, early contact should be made with the parents or family about the expected course of problems and special management needs of the newborn. This consultation may be initiated even before delivery. Second, information should be provided by the clinical staff in a factual, compassionate manner. Parents may need continued orientation or reorientation to the NICU environment. This may be necessary especially for parents who are geographically separated from their infant. Third, phone calls and photographs are important means for parents to maintain emotional involvement with their baby. Fourth, social workers, chaplains, or other support resources should be contacted and utilized early to manage emotional distress and facilitate communication. Fifth, regular patient care conferences with the parents should be scheduled. This will keep parents apprised of the newborn's status and will keep the staff informed about the parents' level of understanding, perspectives, and values. Additional efforts to communicate must be made at the time of special procedures, tests, or therapies to enhance everybody's understanding and the informed consent process.

An integral part of the informed consent process and one that directly affects decision making is the principle of fidelity, commonly called *truth telling,* as discussed. **Issues of what to tell, how and when to tell, and whom to tell become a daily part of the staff's interaction with each other and the families of affected newborns.**

In practice, the issue of truth telling is considered an essential component of the professional-patient relationship. Information should be shared among staff members and presented to the family truthfully, compassionately, and without bias. However, it is often best for a single voice (e.g., the attending neonatologist or primary care clinician) consistently to relate information and interpret facts for families to minimize confusion or misinformation.

Double Effect

The principle of "double effect" asserts that an action may be considered good if the intent of the action is a positive value, even if the secondary effects of the action might be considered harmful if undertaken as the primary goal; further, the good effect should be commensurate with the harm. Double effect is used frequently in the NICU. An example is the use of opioids (morphine or fentanyl) in a newborn for whom there has been a compassionate life-support withdrawal from assisted ventilation: the positive goal is reduction of air hunger and suffering, even at an acknowledged low risk for causing some degree of respiratory depression.

Problems of Uncertainty

A major difficulty in ethical decision making is the medical uncertainty that exists around such decisions. It is difficult to determine what may be in the best interest of the child when the prognosis remains unclear. Even when the prognosis seems clear, there are always those children who confound science, whose outcomes are far from expected.

Some of the most frequent problems in working with perinatal cases arise as a result of this uncertainty. Parents always ask, "Will my baby be okay when he (or she) grows up?" Answers are often unsatisfying or incomprehensible. In most cases with premature infants, truth telling may compel an answer that, when reduced to its simplest form, says, "I don't know." A statistical approach to answering the question may be "Most babies like yours grow up to be normal" or "Some babies like yours have serious problems." These answers are often followed by a litany of statistical probabilities of each morbidity. Neither approach answers the mother's question of what her particular baby will be like. Such approaches serve to complicate the clinician's relationship with parents over issues such as expertise, veracity, and disclosure. The statistical approach may answer the NICU staff's question of quality of care, but few parents understand such statistics or are willing to apply them to a loved one. Nonetheless, uncertainty is a way of life in many perinatal cases, and this observation significantly compromises the resolution of ethical problems in the NICU.

In considering medical uncertainty, it may be helpful to recognize two general classes of perinatal cases. NICU patients can be generally classified as either premature infants without known anomalies or near-term infants with major anomalies, either syndromic or nonsyndromic. For infants with known syndromes or major anomalies, prognoses from the literature are describable with reasonable accuracy. Thus the prognosis for an infant with trisomy 18 can be given with a fairly high degree of accuracy, permitting reasonable application of these processes.

A detailed review of neonatal outcome is beyond the scope of this chapter, but several conclusions appear justified. First, infant mortality has declined rapidly since the establishment of NICUs and the major mortality groups are in lower weight and younger gestational age groups.[1,25,44] Second, coincident with the decline in mortality have come major improvements in neonatal morbidity (both neurodevelopmental and pulmonary) from nearly 50% in the pre-NICU era to current figures in the range of 15% from many institutions.[25] Third, the absolute number of normal premature survivors has increased dramatically and the absolute number of moderately and severely affected survivors appears to have increased as well.[25]

"Extreme prematurity, on the other hand, is characterized by an enormous uncertainty. In these cases predictions of outcome at birth are probabilistic at best."[61] Accordingly, attempts have been made to establish guidelines for treatment of extremely-low-birth-weight (ELBW) infants.[9,19,27,29,76] The morbidities in premature survivors are variable in nature, but central nervous system morbidities generally include visual impairment and blindness, speech and hearing impairment, neuromuscular impairment, and serious cognitive impairment.[57] Few premature survivors require long-term institutional care.[25] The combined risk for one or more of these disabilities is in the range of 15% to 20%.[26,40,41,78] Most people agree that these are indeed serious disabilities, with major effect on the patient and family. However, do they justify withholding or withdrawing treatment? If so, under what circumstances?

For perinatal clinicians for whom quality of life is a major consideration, it remains an exceedingly difficult practical problem to predict which particular child will be significantly impaired and in what manner. The predictive value of nursery evaluations in estimating long-term disability is low.

The intent of raising these questions is to underscore the complexity of ethical discussions as particularly applied to problems in the modern NICU. This in no way reduces the enormity of such problems for the patient, family, health care providers, or society. Technologic advances may resolve old uncertainties but often seem to carry new uncertainties that are equally perplexing.

Setting Goals

Treatment goals should be established so that incremental decisions can be made. Preferably, parents should establish goals based on their values for their child. **Parents should be involved, not just informed, in determining the overall goals of treatment.** Decisions toward that end then can be made. Goals expressed by parents may be living a "normal" life, living with a debilitating outcome but without persistent pain or suffering, existence without any notable "quality of life," and so on. Accordingly, treatment goals may be to improve an infant's health, help the infant to maintain the current state of health, or help the infant die with supportive palliative care. Too frequently, decisions are made before the treatment goal is established. The parents and health care team members may be working toward different goals. **The physician, health care team, and parents all should be guided by established goals so that beneficial treatment can be offered.** The AAP Committee on Fetus and Newborn has stated that although the role of parents in goal setting and decision making must be respected[7]:

> [t]he physician is not obligated to provide inappropriate treatment or to withhold beneficial treatment at the request of the parents. Treatment that is harmful, of no benefit, or futile and merely prolonging dying should be considered inappropriate. The physician must ensure that the chosen treatment, in his or her best medical judgment, is consistent with the best interest of the infant.

Treatment and Nontreatment

For parents to be involved in determining overall treatment goals and the decision-making process, they must be fully informed to consent to or refuse treatment for their child. Infants should be treated humanely and with respect in an environment that is conducive to maximum comfort and healing. Humane judgments should be made in determining how infants can most benefit from treatment in any given situation. Palliative care should be provided to all infants at all times.[15] As noted in Chapter 12, sufficient analgesic should be administered to infants having surgery because they can indeed experience physical and psychologic pain. Staff and parents should maximize the development of premature infants and offer every possible benefit to them. The nursery environment should be as free from excessive overstimulation as possible.

Other perplexing ethical questions arise when the benefit of treatment is unclear. Even the most perfunctory of decisions should be based on the patient's best interests, yet "best interests" are often difficult to determine. Should a baby born with anencephaly be resuscitated or receive life-sustaining interventions solely for the purpose of organ transplantation? Should an ELBW infant receive aggressive ventilatory therapy? Medical and ethical decisions involve considering not only what kind of treatment serves the patient's best interest but also whether the treatment is appropriate at all. Limited or nontreatment decisions are agonizing and regularly result in ethical discussions. **A nontreatment decision is sometimes incorrectly called withholding or withdrawing *care*. Only *treatment* may be withheld or withdrawn. *Care* always should be provided, whether curative or palliative.**

"Nonbeneficial" Treatment

The concept of "nonbeneficial" [or futile] medical treatment may be as perplexing as the concept of benefit. It does, however, deserve attention, because there are increasing circumstances in which treatment may be considered to be nonbeneficial and thus withheld or withdrawn. There is no ethical obligation to offer nonbeneficial treatment, yet there is no one definition of "nonbeneficial."

Most often, judgments about benefit are based on medical or physiologic data. It may be medically nonbeneficial to resuscitate an infant under certain conditions, because the treatment cannot alter the course of the illness or problem, yet there are psychologic, social, and religious reasons that such treatment might be offered. If, because of the treatment, the family has time to hold the infant and say good-bye, the resuscitation may not be considered by them to have been nonbeneficial. Of course, the opposite is also true; that is, what may not be physiologically nonbeneficial may be considered to be nonbeneficial by the family or surrogates based on religious or other reasons. Again, there is no ethical obligation to offer nonbeneficial treatment. It is possible to get a medical effect but not a medical benefit.[63] The distinction can be significant. Determination of the appropriateness of treatment should be based on medical benefit as determined by family goals for the patient, which include physiologic, psychologic, social, and religious data.[46] By attending to all of these aspects of care, which include staff and family input alike, a determination of what is nonbeneficial therapy and thus what is beneficial therapy can be made.

Research Ethics

A persistent and controversial issue in neonatal care has been the introduction of new therapies or procedural interventions into the NICU without appropriate research into their safety, efficacy, net benefit, and long-term outcomes for those critically ill infants who receive them. Appropriate studies in animal models ideally are followed by randomized, controlled clinical trials in human newborns (see Chapter 1). Extracorporeal membrane oxygenation (ECMO), high-frequency ventilation, and recombinant erythropoietin all have been examples of interventions that crept into neonatal care before controlled trials were conducted. In recent years, the use of glucocorticoids either to enhance fetal lung maturity antenatally or to prevent or treat bronchopulmonary dysplasia (BPD) postnatally is an example worth evaluating.

Although the benefits of a two-dose regimen of antenatal steroids was demonstrated in 1972,[48] the development of recent practice patterns in which multiple doses of steroids were used over successive weeks of pregnancy was unsubstantiated by randomized clinical trials designed to address the efficacy or safety of such practices. Subsequently the National Institutes of Health held a Consensus Development Conference and published a statement advising that repeat courses of steroids not be used routinely.[53] Research conducted after these practice patterns were established demonstrated increased maternal infection and suppression of the normal hypothalamic-pituitary-adrenal axis and both fetal and neonatal decreased somatic and brain growth, adrenal suppression, neonatal sepsis, chronic lung disease, and increased mortality. In addition, neurodevelopmental outcome studies suggested an increase in psychomotor delay and behavioral problems.

The acute, seemingly beneficial effects of administering systemic steroids to newborns with lung disease, however, were not met with significantly improved mortality or long-term outcome. It is also associated with a number of acute side effects (e.g., gastrointestinal perforation, hypertension, hyperglycemia) and possible long-term harmful consequences on lung and central nervous system function.[13,55,67] Recent studies that caution about the poor postnatal brain growth among some ELBW NICU survivors raise additional concerns about the wisdom of adding risks associated with steroid treatment to an already at-risk newborn.[55,67] Research into the future use of steroids in premature infants should be well designed and adequately powered to provide answers and should include an evaluation of long-term neurodevelopmental outcome.[34]

DECISION MAKING IN THE NEONATAL INTENSIVE CARE UNIT

In the NICU, decisions of serious proportion are encountered regularly, based on medical facts and nonmedical values. From the moment of birth, and in some cases even earlier, a foremost issue is that of determining the appropriate level of treatment (or nontreatment) of sick or anomalous newborns. Entire texts have been devoted to this issue.[45,74] Primary concerns are when to treat, when to limit treatment or not offer curative treatment at all, and who should be involved in the decision-making process.

A frequently encountered treatment problem requiring attention, other than the much-publicized anomalous infant, is the extremely premature or VLBW infant whose course is marked by slow or absent progress despite appropriate and seemingly heroic intervention. The development of complications from disease is of further concern. In concert, these may portend a guarded or very poor prognosis. Recognizing this, the CPS and the Society of Obstetricians and Gynecologists of Canada have published guidelines for the care of women at 22 to 25 weeks' gestation.[19]

These cases may prompt "quality of life" and "ordinary versus extraordinary treatment" discussions. The President's Commission[59] noted that "there is no basis for holding that whether a treatment is common or unusual, or whether it is simple or complex, is in itself significant to a moral analysis of whether treatment is warranted or obligatory"—a view that had been voiced previously by moral philosophers. The AAP has published a strategy for the initiation and withdrawal of treatment for high-risk newborns.[5] General recommendations include the importance of ongoing evaluation, parental participation, establishing the goals of humane care, and upholding the best interests standard seeking to benefit the infant: "It is inappropriate for life-prolonging treatment to be continued when the condition is incompatible with life or when the treatment is judged to be futile."[5] The AAP Committee on Bioethics further "supports individualized decision making about life-sustaining medical treatment for all children, regardless of age. These decisions should be jointly made by physicians and parents."[5] If we are honest about our professions, we must realize that "quality of life" is what we are all about. Health care professionals are entrusted by society to advance the health and well-being of the mind and body of all persons so that they can lead their lives and function as part of the human family, individually or collectively. No individual is capable of establishing what is an acceptable "quality of life" for all persons in all circumstances. Each case requires our collective efforts to facilitate the best decision for that particular patient.

Steps in Ethical Decision Making

The approach should follow a method that clearly demonstrates the practice of applied clinical ethics. As stated by Pellegrino,[56] the goal of applied ethics is making right and good moral decisions for and with a particular patient. Such a decision requires first that a decision maker be determined. The decision maker, whether a parent, health care provider, or other, must understand his or her own (1) philosophy of relationship to the patient (or family), (2) interpretation of ethical principles and values, (3) theoretic basis of ethics used (e.g., utilitarian, deontologic), and (4) source from which morality is derived.

An ethical "workup" is then undertaken in which substantive issues are identified and worked through, resulting in a decision.[69] Implementing decisions requires determining who shall decide, by what criteria they shall be allowed to do so, and subsequently how the decisions or actions are to be implemented.

Box 32-1 presents the essential steps to decision making in neonatal cases in which a dilemma exists. Consider all involved values and possible solutions to the problem, realizing that alternative solutions may uphold different principles and result in different (positive or negative) consequences. Options that may appear acceptable to the family may be unacceptable to the health care team, or vice versa. There may be societal (legal) constraints on certain actions. In some instances, only one option will be consistent with the rules and principles to which the decision maker subscribes. Other options may present apparent conflicts between competing values or result in unacceptable consequences. In a decision, there will probably be some give and take. Some priority must be assigned to a certain set of values, rules, principles, or resultant effects of any action or inaction. A decision should be made in light of these issues. This process need not always be invoked in full. Often, when the case is carefully dissected and medical facts, values, treatment alternatives, and expected prognoses are revealed, issues that at first seemed in question are clarified and it becomes apparent that no real dilemma exists.

BOX 32-1 APPROACH TO ETHICAL DILEMMAS IN NEONATAL CARE

1. Consider who is involved in making and implementing the decision (family, guardians, clinicians, society).
2. Decide who will make the final decision. Is referral to an ethics committee indicated?
3. Clarify all of the medical facts within the case; consider indications, alternatives, and consequences of each action or inaction.
4. Understand significant human factors and values (for patient, family, and health care team).
5. Identify the ethical dilemma or conflict.
6. Make a decision:
   a. List options as solutions to the problem.
   b. Weigh and prioritize values.
   c. Make a decision.
7. Check for moral and rational defensibility.

Data from Brody H: *Ethical decisions in medicine,* Boston, 1981, Little, Brown; and Francoeur RT: From then to now. In Harris CC, Snowden F, editors: *Bioethical frontiers in perinatal intensive care,* Natchitoches, La, 1985, Northwestern State University Press.

Good ethics, then, starts with good facts and effective communication. All parties involved should be aware of all relevant facts, be they medical, social, human value, or legal in nature. Decisions should not be based on personal opinion or insufficient data. The value placed on one's medical well-being may differ between the health care team and the patient or family, and discrepancy may lead to a perceived problem. This serves to remind us of the need for a formal approach to problem solving in hard cases.

A viable patient-professional relationship that clarifies facts (taking into account uncertainties and the difficulties of prognosticating), human values and feelings, and the interests of all relevant parties is essential to ethical decision making. **Decisions made should reflect a moral choice that is beneficial to the patient as determined by the established, informed decision makers.** We should all work toward achieving a position that is both morally congruent with the values deemed of greatest worth in an individual case and applicable within the moral community as a whole.

Although it may be arguable whether the patient is the neonate, family, or another societal group, it is prudent to develop a consensus wherever possible and thus minimize conflict among the interested parties. **Efforts should be made to involve the parents early in the care of their child and listen carefully to their values, goals, and dreams. Clinical information should be presented sensitively and thoroughly.** These efforts may help minimize the stresses on the parents and prepare them to participate in decision making about the care of their child. These efforts will also assist staff as they participate with the parents in the decision-making process. With careful attention to the needs of patients, families, and staff, many conflicts can be resolved at an early stage before positions are hardened and emotional investment is high.

In most cases, consensus is reached. In a minority of cases, conflict is unavoidable. In some cases, medical care raises issues that are highly controversial either within the group of clinicians providing care or in the broader context of societal problems. In many cases, the family is far from homogeneous in its expression of wishes. Many parents are young and in the process of achieving independent adulthood with well-developed values. Single-parent families are not uncommon. The birth of a critically ill infant may serve as a focus to crystallize disagreements between spouses or may aggravate conflicts between the parent (or parents) and the extended family. In such cases, a more formal process, such as a formal conference between clinicians and the family, appeal to an ethics committee, or even involvement of the legal system, may help resolve or minimize conflicts of values. It is preferable, however, that decisions be made by involved parties as close to the bedside as possible.

Proxy Decision Makers

In dealing with newborns who are, by their very nature, incompetent and cannot make decisions for themselves, value conflicts must be resolved with the input of a proxy or surrogate decision maker acting on the infant's behalf. This may be the parents, a family member, friend, guardian ad litem, or the physician. To be considered a valid surrogate, the person should be competent, knowledgeable of integral values of the patient or family, free from conflicting interests, and without serious emotional conflicts in dealing with the case.

Society has for many reasons allocated to the parents the primary authority role in collaboration with health care providers in making decisions about their newborn's care. In most instances, the parents are best suited for deciding such matters and have the infant's best interests in mind. They are usually present when possible, are concerned for their infant's well-being, and are willing to hear the facts of their infant's condition, as well as learn of needed therapies. Of all people, they also know best the values of the family culture or environment in which the infant will be raised.

Yet parents may be less than dispassionate decision makers. They are understandably overwhelmed at times, both physically and emotionally exhausted, and baffled or intimidated by the high-technology environment of the NICU and the complexities of their infant's care. Amid feelings of grief, fear, anxiety, and wonderment over their premature or anomalous infant, they may be uncertain of their proper role and responsibilities as parents. Health care providers should give daily updates on the infant's condition and anticipated course. Parents' needs for emotional support and avenues to both vent their frustrations and explore their concerns over economic, marital, family or sibling, and career effects of their predicament make resources such as nurses, social workers, and chaplains essential in providing assistance to allow them to participate in goal setting and difficult decision making. Occasionally it will be necessary to assess the level of parental competency in assuming the role of surrogate, recognizing when additional help or support for them is needed to fulfill this role.

Reliance on physicians as decision makers, an often-cited traditional paternalistic role, is yet another option. They know and understand the complexities of the medical condition and treatment more than parents do and should promote the patient's best interests in advocating treatment. They may be more objective about individual cases and are not emotionally overwhelmed, as the parents might be. Also, based on experience, they offer a perspective of effectiveness of treatments and can be consistent in treating similar cases.

However, physicians also may encounter problems when they act as the principal decision makers. Although their knowledge of medical facts is the most complete of all persons, it is at the same time, unfortunately, incomplete. Accurate diagnoses and certainty in prognoses are elusive at times. Medical knowledge does have limits. Statistics are helpful for groups of similarly affected patients, but individual outcomes are difficult to predict. Further, while having an advanced degree of specialized information and knowledge, physicians do not necessarily possess any more moral expertise than that of parents or others.

Treatment versus nontreatment decisions are ultimately moral, not simply medical, decisions. These decisions are weightier than most clinical decisions that physicians make. More is involved than a rote, rational process employed in isolation from the family or health care team. The physician must contend with his or her own values and emotions, as well as the medical facts, in each individual case. He or she must facilitate parental and health care team communication and interaction and ultimately order the provision or withdrawal of treatment.

Fortunately, physicians do not work in isolation from the health care team when making decisions about patients. Nurses, child life workers, social workers, and chaplains are vital members of the decision-making team. A potential problem with each of these clinicians as surrogates is that a conflict of interest may exist between them and the patients for whom they are deciding. Members of the health care team may be biased toward the prolongation of life, have preconceived and strong biases about euthanasia, or be influenced by issues unrelated to the patient, including advancement of care, financial issues, or societal issues. Hence they may not fully consider the best interests of the patient or the values of the involved family. In contrast to parents, they do not live with the results of their decisions and actions. Also, consistency in their application of principles to similar cases may be lacking, and they may give in to strong pressures (real or perceived) exerted by the law or very assertive parents.

Various factors should contribute to minimizing the potential problems in parents and health care professionals reaching morally defensible decisions in the best interest of the premature or anomalous infant. The professionalism of health care team members who are committed to serving the health and interests of their patients is a foremost consideration that serves this purpose. A sense of duty leads these professionals to assist families in achieving their life goals through facilitating open communication and discussion of their varied concerns. A great sense of personal and professional satisfaction may be derived by helping families accept and deal with their emotions, questions, and concerns for their infant and their own circumstances. Professionals may benefit from the support afforded by each other, and they certainly will avoid problems if they try to communicate well with each other.

In recent years, hospital ethics committees have been given an increasing role in facilitating ethical decision making for sick neonates and have, in rare instances, actually functioned as proxy decision makers. As more institutions are establishing committees, their roles are more focused on education, policy interpretation, and advisory functions than on decision making. Decision making by committees might be problematic in that it may threaten the traditional physician-patient or family relationship and usurp both the physician's authority and the parents' autonomy. Siegler[66] noted a number of ways in which a committee "can constrain and modify physician-patient decisions," including the imposition of administrative and regulatory burdens. The mechanics of the committee process, time, and distant relationship to the family and case also have been raised as problems in using committees.

Weir[74] noted that a committee, especially an infant bioethics committee, may have the potential of meeting all of the criteria for a proxy decision maker. Ethics committees are multidisciplinary in composition and have the goals of emotional stability, objectivity, impartiality, and consistency. Ideally, they may facilitate the resolution of conflicts between parents and physicians in matters of treatment and be more capable of both addressing and working through the ethical or moral aspects of cases than parents, health care professionals, or other individuals. In reality, their most useful role seems to be one of improving effective communication between staff and families. Finally, they may prove to be a safeguard for infants for whom parents and professionals are working toward an end that may be perceived as contrary to the infant's best interests.

Surely, much reflective thinking should be invested in our decisions, as individuals, parents, or members of a committee. However, a small number of cases will proceed beyond institutional review to a court. Courts may employ many of the criteria for being good proxies—they are disinterested parties, free of emotional involvement, and mostly consistent in reasoning from case to case. They can ensure that all relevant facts are presented and considered, and judges are capable of exercising unmatched control of data collection, investigation, questioning of experts, and seeking of alternative solutions. A judge also can appoint a guardian ad litem to be the patient's advocate when necessary.

Yet there are at least a few weaknesses in courts as proxies. They are removed from the NICU and have no contact with the case, patient, staff, or family whose problem they are deciding; hence they are more remote than other possible proxy decision makers. Working through cases may be time-consuming, which may result in additional problems, changes in pertinent facts, or prolongation of suffering. Decisions rendered by judges also may reflect some bias based on personal considerations of the judge, rather than consistent judicial decisions across lines of legal jurisdiction. Also, some would argue that courts are by design adversarial, using force to resolve conflict rather than promoting cooperation.

Standard of Best Interest

The best-interest standard has been advocated by the President's Commission and others seeking to accomplish valid moral decision making in difficult neonatal cases.[59,73,74] We are obliged "to try to evaluate benefits and burdens from the infant's own perspective."[59] This standard is accepted in the case of newborns over the autonomy—promoting "substituted judgment," because substituted judgment can only be applied hypothetically to a never-competent newborn. This standard is accepted as the best method available to "reasonable" adults who have to make decisions for neonates.

The potential for self-seeking by the decision maker is easy to understand and has been recognized. The interests of parents, siblings, physicians, hospital staff or administration, and society may all seem to compete with those of the newborn. But the interests of others—be they emotional, economic, or otherwise problematic—cannot justifiably override those of the patient[12,43] based on the actual or potential personhood of the critically ill neonate. Individual or societal problems or perceived burdens generally are not viewed on the same moral plane as a person's claim to life.

Certainly some cases stretch the best-interest standard to its limits. Cases of protracted treatment with uncertain prognoses beg the question of quality of existence (in which nonmaleficence is the principle of concern) and require consideration of more than mere suffering and pain.[43] Indeed, in the words of Arras,[12] "Sometimes circumstances may be so extreme and the consequences so dreadful that the priority of justice can no longer be maintained." In this sense, we have to find the best balance of beneficence, nonmaleficence, and justice.

We also must consider other morally relevant concerns of neonates who may be doomed to brief lives with less-than-recognizably-"human" existence. Human capacities (e.g., ability to think, be aware of self, relate to other people) may be different from biologic human life. The preservation of biologic human life bereft of the benefit of distinctly human capacities is controversial and has been challenged in quality-of-life decisions.[12,28,45,49,74] Walters has written of the "proximate personhood" model.[72] Arras[12] suggested the "relational potential standard" (Does this child have the ability, or potential, to relate to physical space and time and to communicate to others?) as a means to address these concerns more aptly than the "misapplied best interest standard," calling on society itself to inquire "into the conditions of valuable human life."

Priority should be given to attempts at effecting a cure in these ill infants; when a cure cannot be achieved, patient comfort should be sought. Some maintain that life itself may not always be an absolute good; thus it may be morally justifiable to withhold or withdraw futile treatment associated with inhumane risks or harms that would prolong dying. Mitchell, while a member of the American Nurses Association Committee on Ethics, has stated[52]:

> Some infants are so premature and underweight, so profoundly impaired, so hopelessly diseased, or so severely asphyxiated that their foreshortened lives are full of misery for them and those around them. For infants who are so impaired that medical therapies are futile or would only prolong suffering, invasive medical procedures and surgery are morally, as well as medically inappropriate.

She calls on nurses to shift their focus in such cases to "seek primarily to provide comfort, relieve suffering and help a grieving family."

Creating an Ethical Environment

Ethical decisions do not happen in a vacuum. Environments should exist that promote ethical behavior and deliberation. Such environments should be institutional (the nursery, the hospital, the community, social and political structures) and attitudinal. Attitudes include those in which families and staff are empowered to express their opinions and engage in the decision-making process, all voices are valued, information is openly and honestly shared (including uncertainties), respect for all individuals is upheld, and the predominant concern is to benefit the patient, whether that be minimizing overstimulation of patients, administering the appropriate analgesic, or providing appropriate palliative care.[77] **Routine ethics rounds or ethics committee and palliative care consults, along with family care conferences and generally good**

family communication, are recognized means of enhancing such an environment in the NICU. Yet none of these replace the responsibility of all staff members consistently to promote an overall ethical milieu in the nursery in which ethical practice is the standard of care.

Recent literature has focused on the concept of moral distress, particularly among nursing staff. Moral distress occurs when conflict exists between personal values and treatment being given. **The most commonly reported cause of distress is following orders to support patients at end of life with advanced technology when palliative or comfort care would be, from the perspective of the caregivers, more humane.**[32]

Some institutions hold weekly staff conferences for education, clarification, and open and informed communication among staff members. Information can be clarified, and family care conferences can be arranged. When the NICU staff enter into these dialogs with parents or when an ethics consultant joins in, the ability to clarify the goals of care and understand the present condition of the patient and potential future concerns of all parties as they view the patient is enhanced.

ETHICS COMMITTEE OR PALLIATIVE CARE CONSULTATION?

Generally in practice, it is preferable to keep the decision-making responsibility within the professional-patient relationship. In the vast majority of cases, members of the health care team and the parents do have the infant's best interests in mind. Yet in view of the vast dimension and difficulties of some of the required decisions, many clinicians will consult with a hospital ethics committee (HEC), infant bioethics committee (IBC), or palliative care team (PCT). Some institutions have all three of these committees—the IBC falling under the HEC—but many do not have an IBC, PCT, or palliative care consultant. For those who have both ethics and palliative care consultation available, it is reasonable to question whom to call, and when, for consultation. **When there is agreement about a treatment plan, both the ethics committee and palliative care might be consulted for confirmation of that plan.** When there is a dispute about a proposed course of treatment, the HEC (and/or IBC) might be consulted for clarification of ethical principles, values, and various treatment options that would be consistent with ethical and legal standards. The PCT or consultant might also be used for consultation on goals clarification and the development of a comprehensive palliative treatment plan to include comfort measures, specific symptom management, and support to the infant, family, and caregivers.

The stimulus to the establishment of IBCs in the United States was the controversy over and death of Baby Doe in Bloomington, Indiana, when society (and government) became acutely aware of the moral issues surrounding what many perceived to be wrongful nontreatment of a handicapped newborn.[58] Resulting government regulations, along with AAP policies, have focused on the importance of ethics consultation to promote quality decisions about treatment of ill newborns. HECs, composed of members from different disciplines, are a resource for consultation and advice. They are not a decision-making body, although some groups are moving toward a consensus model. Different committees have different procedures.[35,47] Committee functions and responsibilities may include (1) offering counsel and ethical review, (2) educating hospital personnel, (3) retrospectively and prospectively reviewing pertinent government guidelines, and (4) developing appropriate institutional policies. **In most institutions, *anyone* involved in a particular case may request a consultation from the HEC.**

Palliative care as a discipline has, in more recent years, focused on comprehensive, compassionate comfort and support. Many domains of palliative care are appropriate for all patients. Palliative care may, however, be especially important—and become the predominant paradigm of care—when an infant is on the threshold of viability, is gravely ill or has an uncertain outcome, or is dying despite appropriately applied intensive care measures.[15] **Palliative care consultation should be sought (1) any time there is a question about comfort or support, (2) any time there is a question about pain and symptom management specific to the realm of comfort and end-of-life, and (3) when an infant has a life-threatening condition or is dying despite life-sustaining interventions.** Palliative care services generally work collaboratively with HEC members and the clinical team to ensure maximum comfort and minimal suffering for babies whether their conditions are improving or worsening. Such consults, along with good family communication, enhance patient care and the ethical environment of the NICU.

COMMUNICATING WITH FAMILIES

The most important element in communicating with families is listening to them. Indeed, consistent, sensitive, and thorough communication of clinicians with families is essential to good patient care. **The more complex the medical situation, the more crucial it is that parents receive consistent information, perhaps from a single designated person on the health care team.** Parents often are confused by the various prognostications offered by multiple subspecialists and cannot synthesize the data into a "larger picture" of what is happening to their baby. **Yet in the urgency to communicate information, clinicians sometimes forget to listen to the grief, fears, and concerns of parents for their child.**[39] These feelings can profoundly influence decisions that are made and how they are made. Ethics as a rational process must also consider the range of human emotions involved in life-and-death issues, not just clinical information. What parents would not be distraught over the premature birth of their infant? Overwhelmed by their severely disabled infant? The prospect of lifetime rehabilitation? The reality or prospect of suffering? The prospect of death of their newborn?

Good communication with parents is essential, because parents play a vital role in the decision-making process. They, along with the infant, are the most affected.[16] No matter what their religious or sociocultural background, almost all parents experience shock and grief over their infant's need for intensive care.[39] They deal with this in better and worse ways. For many parents, the ability to participate in ethical decision making is impaired while they are in such an acute stage of shock. Usually, prenatal diagnosis of anomalies gives parents time to adjust to their baby's condition before birth or before decisions have to be made. This adjustment time can be most valuable. To participate in ethical decision making, particularly decisions about withholding or withdrawing treatment, parents must have achieved some degree of emotional reorganization and acceptance. Staff assistance in helping them move from emotional disorganization to reorganization is crucial to further decisions that should be made. At this point, parents may be better able to absorb medical data, ethical values, and principles. **Although a theoretic difference may not exist between withholding and withdrawing treatment, there is a large emotional difference. The sound clinician, as well as the ethicist, must be sensitive to this distinction.**

Choices about treatment and nontreatment do affect the grieving process. Questions such as "Am I just prolonging suffering by keeping her alive?" are countered by "Am I not giving her a chance and playing God by allowing her to die?" Duff and Campbell[28] report families experiencing "a normal mourning for their losses" after allowing their seriously ill infants to die. What remains for many parents are doubts that their choice was correct. For some, decisions based on certain religious principles or other value criteria offer moral justification of behavior that assists in the mourning process. For others, the justification may be logically but not emotionally clear. In these instances, grieving can become more complex and difficult.

A valuable role of an ethics committee and/or ethics consultant may be to offer input into, if not confirmation of, the parents' decision in a way that helps allay guilt that can interrupt normal grieving. Ethics, although at once highly theoretic and intellectual, must consider that the situations with which it most intimately deals are highly emotional. For parents, the psychologic trauma will affect their ethical considerations and ethical decisions will have further psychologic effect.

A real value of an interdisciplinary health care team is the particular attention paid to the many complex aspects of a patient's living and dying. **When parents are facing the death of their baby, the entire team may be involved in assisting them. Nurses and physicians, social workers, chaplains, and psychologists may all be intimately involved with monitoring the patient's comfort level and deteriorating course and with comforting grieving parents.** Baptisms (when appropriate) and especially funerals are important ritualistic ways of organizing the meaning of the traumatic event. **The entire staff should encourage parents to offer all that they can to their dying infant.** They should provide active palliative care—maximum comfort for the patient and maximum support to the family. Helping patients and families cope with death is a privilege. It can be personally and professionally satisfying, and ultimately immeasurably helpful to everyone involved, to enter emotionally into this process. Often care of the living means care of the dying.

Good communication among staff members is also important. The effect on the health care team members of helping an infant die also should be recognized because their concern and involvement with the infant usually are significant. **Helping someone through the dying process can be a difficult, though rewarding, experience.** In such instances, professionals may agree with the decision (preferably the parents') to withhold or withdraw treatment. Professionals may also disagree with the decision but may place a higher value on the parents' autonomy to decide than on the decision itself. Respecting this, they may abide by the parents' wishes for their baby. **No one should be forced to compromise personal or professional integrity, however, and in cases in which one's ethics or integrity is being violated, the case may be transferred. Catlin et al suggest "conscientious objection" as a potential response to the moral distress experienced by neonatal nurses.**[23] Preferably, professionals can learn about the range of ethically defensible options and can support the parents in choices different from their own.

How does the clinician discuss such sensitive issues, especially dying, with parents? In many ways. First and foremost, listen to their thoughts, feelings, and concerns as they express them. Clinicians should consider the vulnerability of parents who are frequently overwhelmed by the delivery, their baby's condition, and other related stressors. **Clinicians should be compassionate not only in their listening but also in their communication to parents.** What are they feeling, perceiving, wondering about, fearing, hoping for? Box 32-2 suggests some questions to engage in empathic conversation. Such questions are relevant to the parents of the infant whose condition is improving, the infant whose future is uncertain, the infant for whom parents must make agonizing decisions, and the infant who is clearly dying. **Empathic communication with families is a critical component of the ethical environment of the NICU.**

BOX 32-2 SUGGESTED QUESTIONS TO ENGAGE EMPATHIC CONVERSATION

- What do you understand is going on with your baby?
- Who is your main doctor? What has he or she told you?
- Do you have the medical information you need, or do you want more?
- What kind of information would help you the most right now?
- What are you expecting for your baby?
- What do you think your baby feels?
- What do you see your baby doing?
- Who is your very best support person right now?
- Is he or she available?
- What is your greatest concern about your baby?
- What would give you a sense of peace or comfort in the midst of this, if that is possible?
- What is happening at home?
- Faith and beliefs can be very important in the grief and healing process. Is there anything about your faith or beliefs that we should know to be able to take care of you and your baby?
- Who or what is helping you get through this?
- This may be or is the best condition your baby will ever be in. When this is the case, we usually focus on keeping him or her warm and comfortable until he or she dies rather than on curing. How do you feel about this for your baby?
- Our goals in health care are to (1) improve health, (2) maintain health, and (3) help someone die.
- How can we ease this experience for you?

INTEGRATING PALLIATIVE CARE IN THE INTENSIVE CARE SETTING

Neonatal palliative care offers families comprehensive, compassionate, and supportive care when their baby's diagnosis has an uncertain outcome or a condition that may end in death. Palliative care is not synonymous with comfort care but can include comfort care at a certain point when life-prolonging interventions are no longer of benefit to the infant. Two thirds of all infant deaths will occur during the neonatal period, and the majority of these deaths will occur in the intensive care setting.[33]

The AAP suggests that a palliative care model can be integrated into a variety of pediatric settings.[6] **Palliative care for infants and children has emerged from the adult palliative/hospice care philosophy and can be defined as an interdisciplinary approach to care for families when their infant has a condition that is life-threatening or life-limiting (will lead to premature death in childhood).** It further recognizes that families experience unmitigated stress when there is even a remote possibility that their infant could die or have severe disabilities. These families require intensified support from palliative care professionals to address their psychosocial stress and conflicts within a spiritually and culturally sensitive context as they evolve under circumstances essentially out of their control.

The term *life-threatening* evades a common definition among health care professionals. It is suggested that life-threatening conditions are the following[33]:

- Those that carry a substantial probability of death in childhood even though the treatment may prolong life (e.g., short gut syndrome in which nutritional supplementation is a palliative procedure for an indefinite time; extreme prematurity <500 g)
- Those that are perceived as potentially having a fatal outcome (e.g., palliative surgical repair of certain heart defects)

The words *"We need to take your baby to the intensive care unit now"* can remain etched in the mind of a parent forever. In the intensive care setting, families face uncertainty, fear, and anxiety as they make decisions concerning the life or death of their baby. Decisions concerning continuing or discontinuing life support, initiating enteral feedings, and even the need for prolonged ventilator support can affect a family's life and financial resources for years.

These decisions often involve considerations and circumstances surrounding the quality of the life and the developmental needs of the infant as he or she matures. Often these discussions are approached with caution by the NICU staff. Yet, addressing and ensuring "quality of life" are central to palliative care philosophy. **Palliative care recognizes that quality of life is an individual value that families must decide for themselves after being fully informed of the intended outcome that decisions will have on the infant's development and, in turn, their family.**[33]

An interdisciplinary palliative care team can help families navigate the unfamiliar world of the NICU. The palliative care team can facilitate decisions, clarify diagnoses, and offer education regarding the potential outcomes of all the treatment options offered by the NICU staff. A palliative care nurse or social worker may act as a resource professional who offers support to the family from the time of admission through and after discharge. The nurse or social worker forms a trusting relationship with the family and may serve as a care navigator in the foreign and complex world of the NICU and children's hospital.

Integrating palliative care in a NICU may present challenges in an environment that emphasizes technical advances directed to saving lives of newborns.[38] Yet certain conditions of the newborn could benefit from, but are not limited to, the palliative care team's involvement when the newborn is admitted to the NICU[21,22,33]:

- Neonates on the threshold of viability—typically <23 weeks' gestation or <500 g birth weight
- Neonates with congenital malformations considered incompatible with life—certain complex cardiac conditions or congenital diaphragmatic hernias
- Neonates with conditions in which life-sustaining interventions no longer benefit their life:
  - Overwhelming sepsis
  - Severe neurologic injury
  - Insurmountable loss of bowel function or length

A palliative care model, as proposed by the authors, includes the palliative care team and the ethics consultant in supporting families' understanding of the infant's condition and care (Figure 32-1):

Phase I: Admission to NICU. A plan of care is initiated that includes support for the family, as well as information about the nature of the infant's condition. Family support is offered by the palliative care interdisciplinary team including pastoral care. A care navigator (palliative care nurse or social worker) is assigned. The plan of care includes an assessment of family dynamics, cultural and spiritual preferences, and the family's own religious and community support.

Phase II: Ongoing Assessment. If the infant's condition is judged to be either declining or not improving, a family conference is initiated. This should include all involved medical, nursing, social work, and pastoral care staff. At times, an ethics committee member may be asked to facilitate or reflect upon a discussion about the risks and benefits of continuing life-prolonging interventions. Nurses and child life specialists can help family members enhance communication with their infant through touch and recordings of heartbeats and siblings' and grandparents' voices. Families are allowed time to process information and work toward their decisions. The palliative care nurse may well need to follow up with the family and clarify discussions from the conference. Future meetings are often necessary.

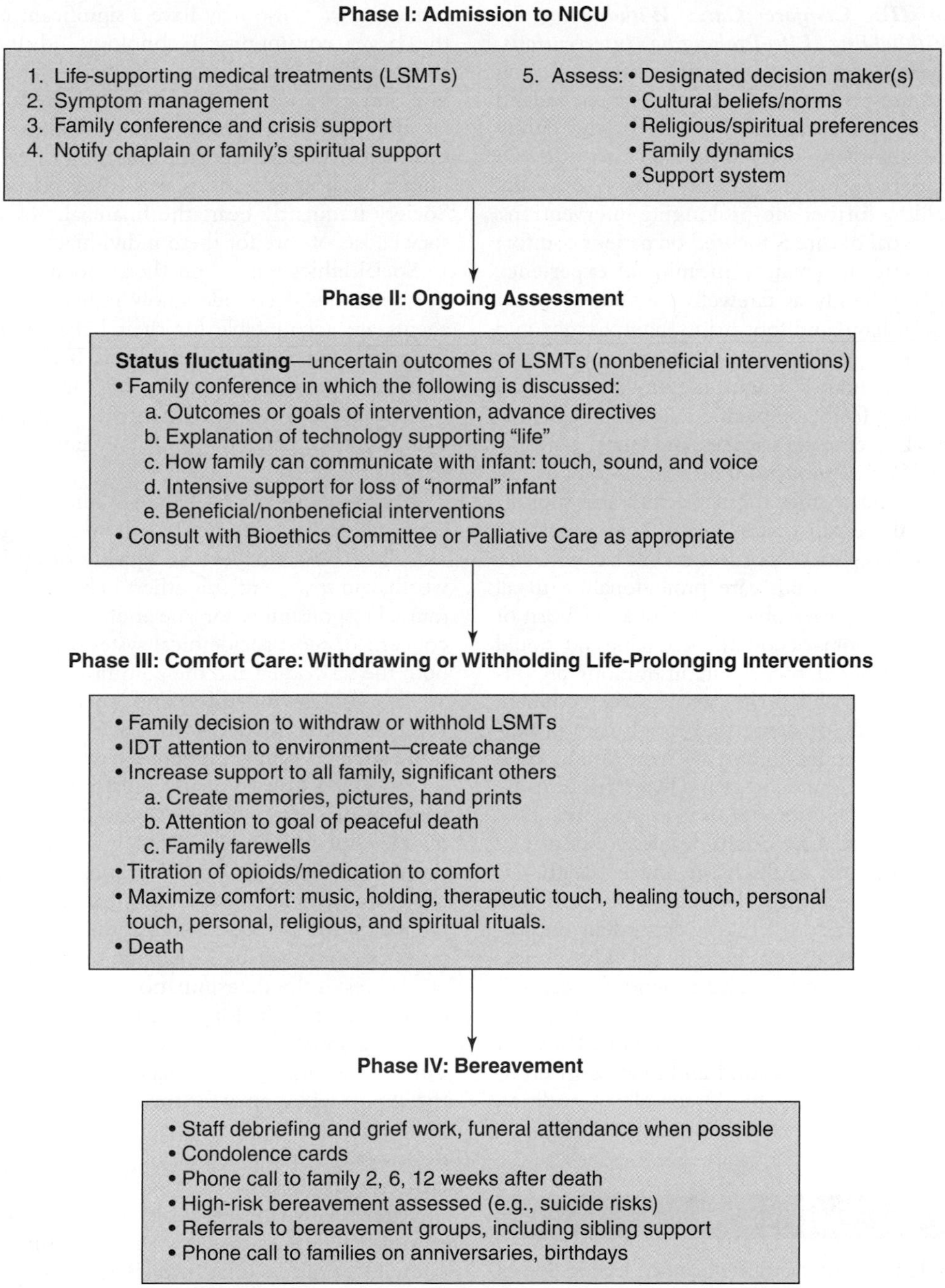

Phase I: Admission to NICU
1. Life-supporting medical treatments (LSMTs)
2. Symptom management
3. Family conference and crisis support
4. Notify chaplain or family's spiritual support
5. Assess: • Designated decision maker(s)
• Cultural beliefs/norms
• Religious/spiritual preferences
• Family dynamics
• Support system
Phase II: Ongoing Assessment
Status fluctuating—uncertain outcomes of LSMTs (nonbeneficial interventions)
• Family conference in which the following is discussed:
a. Outcomes or goals of intervention, advance directives
b. Explanation of technology supporting "life"
c. How family can communicate with infant: touch, sound, and voice
d. Intensive support for loss of "normal" infant
e. Beneficial/nonbeneficial interventions
• Consult with Bioethics Committee or Palliative Care as appropriate
Phase III: Comfort Care: Withdrawing or Withholding Life-Prolonging Interventions
• Family decision to withdraw or withhold LSMTs
• IDT attention to environment—create change
• Increase support to all family, significant others
a. Create memories, pictures, hand prints
b. Attention to goal of peaceful death
c. Family farewells
• Titration of opioids/medication to comfort
• Maximize comfort: music, holding, therapeutic touch, healing touch, personal touch, personal, religious, and spiritual rituals.
• Death
Phase IV: Bereavement
• Staff debriefing and grief work, funeral attendance when possible
• Condolence cards
• Phone call to family 2, 6, 12 weeks after death
• High-risk bereavement assessed (e.g., suicide risks)
• Referrals to bereavement groups, including sibling support
• Phone call to families on anniversaries, birthdays

FIGURE 32-1 Integrating palliative care and bioethics in neonatal intensive care: an interdisciplinary approach. *IDT,* Interdisciplinary team.

Phase III: Comfort Care: Withdrawing or Withholding Life-Prolonging Interventions. The status of the infant's condition is declining and life-prolonging interventions are judged to be nonbeneficial. Once again, the family and interdisciplinary team come together to support each other in withdrawing or withholding further life-prolonging interventions. The goal of care is focused on patient comfort and ways to create a meaningful experience for the family as farewells are said. Memory books, hand and foot prints, photographs, and a lock of hair can provide tangible memories of their infant's unique identity. Pastoral staff can help facilitate specific religious or spiritual rituals, memorial services, and burial plans.

Phase IV: Bereavement. The staff, as well as the family, need time for debriefing and support after the death of the infant. Support groups for parents who have lost a child are valuable. Contact by health care professionals with all families experiencing the loss of a newborn or young infant is of documented value and should be considered broadly in institutions providing neonatal intensive care.[51,75] A bereavement coordinator or designated health care professional continues contact with the family for at least 1 year. Condolence and memorial cards are valued by families after the loss of an infant.

This model of palliative care promotes continuity of care from diagnosis to discharge and/or death.[54] It acknowledges the family's decisions about care even when it means that the child is dependent on life-prolonging interventions indefinitely. This model promotes communication and support for the difficult decisions that are necessary for families to make in a time of crisis and uncertainty. Palliative care recognizes the profound and long-term emotional impact that a child's complex condition and/or death has on a family and a community.

SOCIAL ETHICS

Moral judgments made in the hospital setting do not occur in isolation from the larger social context of which institutions and individuals are a part. Such judgments can be considerably affected by prevailing social values and perspectives. Further, although decisions in the NICU generally are interpersonal in nature, they also may have a significant effect on the larger community. Technologic advancements have enabled some severely disabled infants to survive and grow, albeit with varying degrees of mental and physical disabilities. Indeed, these are not the majority of newborns, but they often require numerous hospitalizations and costly rehabilitation. Society frequently bears the financial, physical, and social costs of care for these individuals.

Social ethics reflects on the sociocultural aspects of human life. It considers how individuals as moral agents are accountable for their behavior in social structures and public policy issues. It also can refer to shared patterns of moral judgment. Moreover, it focuses on how social contexts influence individual moral behavior and the range of moral responsibility.

In a pluralistic society like the United States, there is no one social ethic. Some believe in rugged individualism; others believe in equality of opportunity, worth, and treatment; still others believe that we bear mutual responsibility for one another. An underlying concern of most socioethical systems is concern for both the individual and the common good.

In NICUs, bioethics and social ethics converge. Treatment decisions have social implications; societal values influence treatment decisions. As described, government regulations highlight the paradox of societal values about the treatment of disabled infants. These federal guidelines advocate the use of "reasonable medical judgment" in treating disabled infants, yet their effect may be seen as increasing the perceived obligation to treat—to the point of "unreasonable." Through government, society expresses the determination to treat, yet societal commitment to the long-term care of special-needs NICU graduates and families is wholly insufficient. Public funds for such care have been reduced while the expressed urgency for treatment of all babies has increased. The values inherent in our public policy decisions about initial and long-term treatment are curiously disparate.

After comparing the health care and social policies of the United States with the seemingly more equitable policies of Great Britain and Sweden, Young[79] concluded, "We need to strive for a better balance between aggressive treatment in the neonatal intensive care units initially, and the resources currently allocated for the long-term care of the disabled." Such a balance might include being more selective about aggressive treatment, as well as learning more about prematurity and trying to prevent it. Young continued, "To the extent that society fails to ensure that seriously ill newborns have the opportunity for an adequate level of continuing care, its moral authority, to intervene on behalf of a newborn whose life is in jeopardy, is compromised."[79]

Recognizing this disparity, various community groups have attempted to establish guidelines for standards of care that are fiscally, morally, and medically responsible to guide parents and clinicians in goal setting and decision making. They have recognized the high cost, in every respect, of neonatal and pediatric intensive care. Their impetus has been to determine community "agreed-upon" values for treatment and nontreatment of disabled infants to effect a standard of care for the extreme premature, severely disabled, and critically ill infant. Managed care organizations are also assessing the ethics of reasonable care and the limits of treatment to be offered. Although not wholly able to determine "agreed upon" values for treatment and nontreatment standards of care, these community and professional groups have offered important social voices to the complexity of neonatal care.

GLOSSARY

- ***Best Interest:*** A standard used to determine the validity of proxy consent in decision making. Treatment decisions are based on what most "reasonable persons" would assess as the burdens and benefits that would likely accompany the child's life. This standard leads clinicians to seek treatment resulting in a "net benefit" to the child.
- ***Casuistry:*** Case-based ethics in which the claims, grounds, and warrants of a particular case are compared with similar cases. The basic question for moral casuistry is how a general moral precept is to be understood in similar sets of circumstances.
- ***Deontology (Formalism):*** A theory of ethics that holds that the moral rightness of an act must be decided totally independent of the consequences of that act. Duty is independent of consequential good, and certain moral commands (rules) operative under fundamental principles must be obeyed under all circumstances.
- ***Dilemma:*** A situation in which more than one possible course of action exists and differing values are held for each possible course of action by the parties involved. Moral dilemmas arise when an appeal to moral considerations can be made for opposing courses of action—when it is apparent that an act can be considered both morally right and morally wrong, and that on moral grounds there is a sense of "ought" and "ought not" to perform the act.
- ***Double Effect:*** A principle, often viewed within the larger context of nonmaleficence, that claims that an act having a harmful effect is not always morally prohibited. Any harmful effect of an act is viewed as indirect, unintended, or simply a foreseen effect but not as the direct and intended effect (e.g., if an act, as in treatment, brings about death, it is not always to be prohibited). Four conditions are often given to clarify this principle for specific acts:
    - The action itself must be "good" or at least morally indifferent.
    - The agent must intend only the good effect and not the harmful effect.
    - The harmful effect cannot be a means to the good effect.
    - There should be a favorable balance between the good and harmful effects of the action.
- ***Ethics:*** The study of moral conduct, systems, and ideas.
- ***Morals:*** The conduct and codes of conduct of individuals and groups. Three popular uses of the term exist: (1) in contrast to immoral (right vs. wrong); (2) in contrast to nonmoral (actions that have no bearing or question of right and wrong); and (3) "morals" (the behavior pattern of an individual or group).
- ***Nonbeneficial Treatment:*** The notion that the efficacy of treatment is very low. There is no ethical obligation to offer nonbeneficial treatment. Nonbenefit may best be judged by the overall medical benefit, not just effect, that a given treatment has on a patient. Treatment is nonbeneficial if it is useless. Physiologic, psychologic, religious, and social data should be considered in making a determination of nonbenefit. Determination of nonbeneficial treatment should be based on medical benefit in consort with family goals for the patient.

- ***Palliative Care:*** An approach that improves the quality of life of patients and their families facing problems associated with life-threatening illness, through the prevention and relief of suffering by means of early identification and impeccable assessment and treatment of pain and other problems: physical, psychosocial, and spiritual. Palliative care for children is the active total care of the child's body, mind, and spirit and involves giving support to the family.
- ***Personhood:*** A characteristic that may be used in decision making that is based on the idea (1) that possession of certain capabilities (typically higher brain functions such as consciousness, rationality, perception of space and time, and the ability to communicate) constitutes personhood and (2) that only "persons" have any moral claim to life, treatment, and so on.
- ***"Proxy" (Surrogate) Decision Maker:*** A designated person who will act on behalf of an individual who is incapable of making decisions.
- ***Reasonable Person Standard:*** A standard by which the validity of informed consent is measured. Information to be disclosed is determined by referring to a hypothetical "reasonable person" and determining whether such a person would see any significance in the information in assessing risk and deciding whether to submit to a treatment or procedure.
- ***Rights:*** Those things to which people have a just claim; a claim to a condition to which the individual is entitled.
- ***Utilitarianism (Consequentialism):*** A theory in ethics that holds that an act is right when it brings about a good outcome for the greatest number of people, upholds the greatest balance of "good" over "evil," and seeks to effect "utility" or the most useful outcome. "The end justifies the means." This may be developed into rules that are adhered to to maximize benefits and minimize harms (rule utilitarian) or simply appealed to in individual actions (act utilitarian).
- ***Values:*** Those things that have worth or are desirable to an individual or group.
- ***Virtues:*** A habit, disposition, or trait that a person may possess or aspire to possess; specifically, a moral virtue upholds what is morally right or praiseworthy.

REFERENCES

1. Ajayi-Obe M, Saeed N, Cowan FM, et al: Reduced development of cerebral cortex in extremely preterm infants, *Lancet* 356:1162, 2000.
2. Allmark P, Mason S, Gill AB, et al: Obtaining consent for neonatal research, *Arch Dis Child Fetal Neonatal Ed* 88:F166, 2003.
3. Reference deleted in proofs.
4. Reference deleted in proofs.
5. American Academy of Pediatrics, Committee on Bioethics: Ethics and the care of critically ill infants and children, *Pediatrics* 98:149, 1995.
6. American Academy of Pediatrics, Committee on Bioethics and Committee on Hospital Care: Palliative care for children, *Pediatrics* 106:2, 2000.
7. American Academy of Pediatrics, Committee on Fetus and Newborn: Noninitiation or withdrawal of intensive care for high-risk newborns, *Pediatrics* 119:401, 2007.
8. American Academy of Pediatrics, Committee on Fetus and Newborn: Perinatal care at the threshold of viability, *Pediatrics* 96:974, 1995.
9. American College of Obstetricians and Gynecologists, Committee on Ethics: *Patient choice: maternal-fetal conflict*, (ACOG committee opinion 55), Washington, DC, 1987, ACOG.
10. American Hospital Association, Report of the Special Committee on Biomedical Ethics: *Values in conflict: resolving ethical issues in hospital care,* Chicago, 1985, American Hospital Publishing.
11. Angell M: The Baby Doe rules, *N Engl J Med* 314:642, 1986.
12. Arras JD: Toward an ethic of ambiguity, *Hastings Cent Rep* 14:25, 1984.
13. Bancalari E: Corticosteroids and neonatal chronic lung disease, *Eur J Pediatr* 157:S31, 1998.
14. Beauchamp T, Childress J: *Principles of biomedical ethics,* ed 6, New York, 2008, Oxford University Press.
15. Bhatia J: Palliative care in the fetus and newborn, *J Perinatol* 26(Suppl 1):524, 2006.
16. Board R, Ryan-Wenger N: State of the science on parental stress and family functioning in pediatric intensive care units, *Am J Crit Care* 9:2, 2000.
17. Bruner J: Intrauterine surgery in myelomeningocele, *Semin Fetal Neonatal Med* 12:471, 2007.
18. Buus-Frank ME: Sometimes a time to be born is also a time to die, *Adv Neonatal Care* 6:1, 2006.
19. Canadian Pediatric Society and Society of Obstetricians and Gynecologists of Canada: Management of the woman with threatened birth of an infant with extremely low gestational age, *Can Med Assoc J* 155:547, 1994.
20. Caplan AL, Murray TH, editors: *Which babies shall live? Humanistic dimensions of the care of imperiled newborns,* Clifton, NJ, 1985, Humana Press.

21. Carter BS, Bhatia J: Comfort/palliative care guidelines for neonatal practice: development and implementation in an academic medical center, *J Perinatol* 21:279, 2001.
22. Carter BS, Hubble C, Weise KL: Palliative medicine in neonatal and pediatric intensive care, *Child Adolesc Psychiatr Clin North Am* 15:759, 2006.
23. Catlin A, Armigo C, Volat D, et al: Conscientious objection: a potential neonatal nursing response to care orders that cause suffering at the end of life?, *Neonatal Netw* 27:101, 2008.
24. Reference deleted in proofs.
25. Congress of the United States, Office of Technology Assessment: *Neonatal intensive care for low birth weight infants: costs and effectiveness,* Washington, DC, 1987, U.S. Government Printing Office.
26. Costeloe K, Hennessy E, Gobson AT, et al: The EPICURE study: outcomes to discharge from hospital for infants born at the threshold of viability, *Pediatrics* 106:659, 2000.
27. Doroshow RW, Hodgman JE, Pomerance JJ, et al: Treatment decisions for newborns at the threshold of viability: an ethical dilemma, *J Perinatol* 20:379, 2000.
28. Duff R, Campbell AGM: Moral and ethical dilemmas in the special care nursery, *N Engl J Med* 289:890, 1973.
29. ECHO: Extreme Care, Human Options: *Community recommendations for appropriate, humane medical care for dying or irreversibly ill patients,* Carmichael, Calif, 1997, Sacramento Health Care Decisions.
30. Eisenberg L: The human nature of human nature, *Science* 176:123, 1972.
31. Engelhardt HT Jr: Viability and use of the fetus. In Bondeson WB, editor: *Abortion and the status of the fetus,* Dordrecht, Netherlands, 1983, D Reidel Publishing.
32. Ferrell B: Understanding the moral distress of nurses witnessing medically futile care, *Oncol Nurs Forum* 33:922, 2006.
33. Field MJ, Behrman RE: *When children die: improving palliative and end-of-life care for children and their families*, (Report of the Institute of Medicine Task Force), Washington, DC, 2003, National Academy Press.
34. Finer NN, Craft A, Vaucher YE, et al: Postnatal steroids: short-term gain, long-term pain? *J Pediatr* 137:9, 2000.
35. Fleischman A, Murray T: Ethics committees for Infants Doe? *Hastings Cent Rep* 13:5, 1983.
36. Fletcher J: *Humanhood: essays in biomedical ethics,* Buffalo, NY, 1979, Prometheus Books.
37. Francoeur RT: From then to now. In Harris CC, Snowden F, editors: *Bioethical frontiers in perinatal intensive care,* Natchitoches, La, 1985, Northwestern State University Press.
38. Gale G, Brooks A: Implementing a palliative care program in a newborn intensive care unit, *Adv Neonatal Care* 6:37, 2006.
39. Gardner S, Hauser P, Merenstein G: Grief and perinatal loss. In Merenstein G, Gardner S, editors: *Handbook of neonatal intensive care,* ed 6, St Louis, 2006, Mosby.
40. Hack M, Taylor G, Klein N, et al: Functional limitations and special health care needs of 10- to 14-year-old children weighing less than 750 grams at birth, *Pediatrics* 106:554, 2000.
41. Hack M, Wilson-Costello D, Friedman H, et al: Neurodevelopment and predictors of outcomes of children with birth weights of less than 1000 g, *Arch Pediatr Adolesc Med* 154:725, 2000.
42. Kodish E: Informed consent for pediatric research: is it really possible? *J Pediatr* 142:89, 2003.
43. Koogler TK, Wilfond BS, Ross LF: Lethal language, lethal decisions, *Hastings Cent Rep* 3:37, 2003.
44. Koops BL, Morgan LJ, Battaglia FC: Neonatal mortality risk in relation to birth weight and gestational age: update, *J Pediatr* 101:969, 1982.
45. Kuhse H, Singer P: *Should the baby live?* New York, 1985, Oxford University Press.
46. Lantos JD, Singer PA, Walker RM, et al: The illusion of futility in clinical practice, *Am J Med* 87:81, 1989.
47. Leiken S: Children's hospital ethics committees, *Am J Dis Child* 141:954, 1987.
48. Liggins GC, Howie RN: A controlled trial of antepartum glucocorticoid treatment for prevention of the respiratory distress syndrome in premature infants, *Pediatrics* 50:515, 1972.
49. Lorber J: Results of treatment of myelomeningocele, *Dev Med Child Neurol* 13:279, 1971.
50. Lorber J: Early results of selective treatment of spina bifida cystica, *BMJ* 4:201, 1973.
51. Meert KL, Eggly S, Pollack M, et al, and the National Institute of Child Health and Human Development Collaborative Pediatric Critical Care Research Network: Parents' perspectives regarding a physician-parent conference after their child's death in the pediatric intensive care unit, *J Pediatr* 151:50, 2007.
52. Mitchell C: Care of severely impaired infant raises ethical issues, *Am Nurse* 16:9, 1984.
53. National Institute of Health: *NIH Consensus Statement: Antenatal corticosteroids revisited—repeat courses,* Bethesda, Md, 2000, The Institute.
54. Nelson-Marten P, Braatan J, English NK: Critical caring: dying in the intensive care unit, *Crit Care Nurs Clin North Am* 13:577, 2001.
55. O'Shea TM, Kothadia JM, Klinepeter KL, et al: Randomized placebo-controlled trial of a 42-day tapering course of dexamethasone to reduce the duration of ventilator dependency in very-low-birth-weight infants: outcome of study participants at 1-year adjusted age, *Pediatrics* 104:15, 1999.
56. Pellegrino ED: The anatomy of clinical ethical judgments in perinatology, *Semin Perinatol* 11:202, 1987.

57. Peterson BS, Vohr B, Staib LH, et al: Regional brain volume abnormalities and long-term cognitive outcome in preterm infants, *JAMA* 284:1939, 2000.
58. Pless JE: The story of Baby Doe, *N Engl J Med* 309:663, 1983.
59. President's Commission for the Study of Ethical Problems in Medicine and Biomedical and Behavioral Research: *Deciding to forego life-sustaining treatment*, Washington, DC, 1983, U.S. Public Health Service, Health and Human Services.
60. Ramsey P: *Ethics at the edges of life,* New Haven, Conn, 1978, Yale University Press.
61. Rhoden NK: Treating Baby Doe: the ethics of uncertainty, *Hastings Cent Rep* 16:34, 1986.
62. Robertson JA: Involuntary euthanasia of defective newborns. In Mappes TA, Zembaty JS, editors: *Biomedical ethics,* ed 2, New York, 1986, McGraw-Hill.
63. Schneiderman LJ, Jecker NS, Jonsen AR: Medical futility: its meaning and ethical implications, *Ann Intern Med* 112:949, 1990.
64. Shelp EE: *Born to die? Deciding the fate of critically ill newborns*, New York, 1986, The Free Press.
65. Shurtleff D: Care of the myelodysplastic patient. In Green M, Haggerty R, editors: *Ambulatory pediatrics,* Philadelphia, 1986, Saunders.
66. Siegler M: Ethics committees: decisions by bureaucracy, *Hastings Cent Rep* 16:22, 1986.
67. Stark AR, Waldemar AC, Tyson JE, et al: Adverse effects of early dexamethasone treatment in extremely-low-birth-weight infants, *N Engl J Med* 344:95, 2001.
68. Stenson BJ, Becher J-C, McIntosh N: Neonatal research: the parental perspective, *Arch Dis Child Fetal Neonatal Ed* 89:F321, 2004.
69. Thomasma DC: Training in medical ethics: an ethical workup, *Forum Med* 1:33, 1978.
70. Tooley M: *Abortion and infanticide,* New York, 1983, Oxford University Press.
71. Victoroff M: The ballad of Baby Doe: parental discretion or medical neglect? *Prim Care* 13:271, 1986.
72. Walters JW: Approaches to ethical decision making in the neonatal intensive care unit, *Am J Dis Child* 142:825, 1988.
73. Weil WB: Issues associated with treatment and nontreatment decisions, *Am J Dis Child* 138:519, 1984.
74. Weir RF: *Selective nontreatment of handicapped newborns,* New York, 1984, Oxford University Press.
75. Williams C, Cairnie J, Fines V, et al, for the With Care Team: Construction of a parent-derived questionnaire to measure end-of-life care after withdrawal of life-sustaining treatment in the neonatal intensive care unit, *Pediatrics* 123:e87, 2009.
76. Wisconsin Association for Perinatal Care: *Position statement: guidelines for the responsible utilization of neonatal intensive care,* Madison, Wis, 1997, Lawrence University.
77. Wolfe, J: Suffering in children at the end of life: recognizing an ethical duty to palliate, *J Clin Ethics* 11:157, 2000.
78. Wood NS, Marlow N, Costeloe K, et al: Neurologic and developmental disability after extremely preterm birth, *N Engl J Med* 343:378, 2000.
79. Young EWD: Caring for disabled infants, *Hastings Cent Rep* 13:15, 1983.
80. Zachary R: Ethical and social aspects of treatment of spina bifida, *Lancet* 2:274, 1968.

RESOURCE MATERIALS

Books and Journals

Carter B, Hubble C, Weise K: Palliative medicine in neonatal and pediatric intensive care, *Child Adolesc Psychiatr Clin N Am* 15:759-777, 2006. A complete outline of the issues involved in implementing palliative care for infants and children in an intensive care setting. It also describes select programs that have a palliative care service in intensive care.

Carter B, Levetown M: *Palliative care for infants, children, and adolescents: a practical handbook*, Baltimore, Md, 2004, Johns Hopkins University Press. Excellent chapter on decision making in the pediatric setting.

Gale G, Brooks A: A parent's guide to palliative care, *Adv Neonatal Care* 6(1):54, 2006. Directed to parents, this article describes what palliative care is, who it may benefit, where and how long it may be provided for babies.

Johnson A, Siegler M, Winslade WJ: *Clinical ethics: a practical approach to ethical decisions in clinical medicine,* ed 5, New York, 2002, McGraw-Hill.

Leuthner S, Jones EL: Fetal concerns program: a model for perinatal palliative care, *MCN Am J Matern Child Nurs* 32(5):272, 2007.

Neonatal Netw 27(6):2008. This entire issue addresses the needs of infants on the margin of viability, 23 to 27 weeks' gestation.

WEBSITES

The Initiative for Pediatric Palliative Care: *A comprehensive resource on educational resources including videotapes and other resources,* Website: www.ippcweb.org.

When children die: improving palliative and end-of-life care for children and their families, Washington, DC, 2003, The National Academies Press. Website: www.nap.edu/catalog/10390.html.

End of Life Physicians Education Resource Center. Educational resources for physicians (includes pediatrics): Website: www.eperc.mcw.edu.

Website: www.grievingforbabies.org. A website that provides access to materials addressing both the needs of grieving family members and perinatal professional staff. Includes available DVDs addressing topics such as initial shock, grief, effects on siblings and grandparents, and the role of health care professionals, including chaplains, throughout the hospital and bereavement process.

Ian Anderson Continuing Education Program in End of Life Care with a pediatric module on decision making and more in development. Website: www.cme.utoronto.ca/endoflife.edu.

National Association of Neonatal Nurses: *1999 Position statement for NICU nurse involvement in ethical decisions* (treatment of critically ill newborns), 2003. Website: www.nann.org.

End-of-Life Nursing Education Consortium pediatric palliative care training program, from the American Association of Colleges of Nursing: Website: www.aacn.nche.edu/ELNEC/Pediatric.htm.

VIDEOS

Family and Neonatal Staff Education: *You are not alone*, Denver, Colo, 1998, The Colorado Collective for Medical Decisions, Neonatal Care subcommittee, Nickel's Worth Productions.

INDEX

b indicates boxed material, *f* indicates illustrations, and *t* indicates tables.

E

M